Clinical
Geriatrics

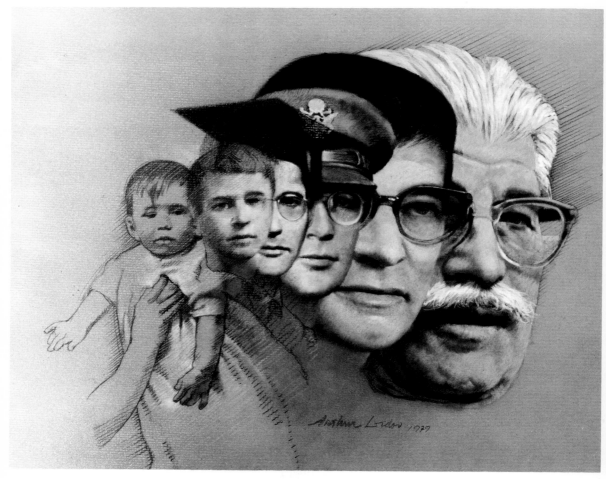

Acrylic and pastel painting by Arthur Lidov, 1979

Clinical
Geriatrics

Edited by

Isadore Rossman, M.D., Ph.D.

Medical Director, Home Health Agency
Montefiore Hospital and Medical Center
Professor Emeritus, Epidemiology and Social
Medicine
Associate Clinical Professor Emeritus, Dept. of
Medicine,
Albert Einstein College of Medicine
Bronx, New York

With 54 Contributors

Third Edition

J. B. Lippincott Company   Philadelphia
London   Mexico City   New York
St. Louis   São Paulo   Sydney

Acquisitions Editor: Lisa A. Biello
Sponsoring Editor: Sanford J. Robinson
Copy Editor: Jeanne M. Carper
Manuscript Editor: Don Shenkle
Indexer: Barbara Farabaugh
Art Director: Tracy Baldwin
Designer: Kate Nichols
Production Supervisor: Kathleen P. Dunn
Production Coordinator: George V. Gordon
Compositor: Ruttle, Shaw & Wetherill, Inc.
Printer/Binder: Halliday Lithograph

3rd Edition

Library of Congress Cataloging in Publication Data

Main entry under title:

Clinical geriatrics.

Includes bibliographies and index.
   1. Geriatrics.   2. Aging.   I. Rossman, Isadore,
1913–   . [DNLM: 1. Aging.   2. Geriatrics.   WT 100
C645]
RC952.C537   1986   618.97   85-10098
ISBN 0-397-50672-4

The authors and publisher have exerted every effort to ensure that drug selection and dosage set forth in this text are in accord with current recommendations and practice at the time of publication. However, in view of ongoing
research, changes in government regulations, and the constant flow of information relating to drug therapy and drug reactions, the reader is urged to
check the package insert for each drug for any change in indications and
dosage and for added warnings and precautions. This is particularly important when the recommended agent is a new or infrequently employed drug.

Clinical Geriatrics III is
for Jonathan Rossman, also 3.

Contributors

John Agate, C.B.E., M.O., F.R.C.P.
Consulting Physician in Geriatrics
Ipswich & East Suffolk Hospital,
Ipswich, England

Joan Albin, M.D.
Assistant Professor of Medicine,
Albert Einstein College of Medicine;
Attending in Medicine,
Director of Diabetes Clinic,
Montefiore Hospital and Medical Center,
Bronx, New York

William M. Anderson, M.D.
Assistant Professor of Medicine,
Louisiana State University School of
    Medicine—Shreveport,
Shreveport, Louisiana

Reubin Andres, M.D.
Clinical Director,
National Institute on Aging,
Gerontology Research Center,
Francis Scott Key Medical Center,
Baltimore, Maryland

Hugh R. K. Barber, M.D.
Professor and Chairman, Department of
    OB/GYN,
New York Medical College;
Director, Department of OB/GYN,
Lenox Hill Hospital,
New York, New York

David W. Bentley, M.D.
Associate Professor of Medicine,
University of Rochester School of
    Medicine;

Head, Infectious Diseases,
Monroe Community Hospital,
Rochester, New York

Frank G. Berson, M.D.
Assistant Professor of Ophthalmology,
Harvard University Medical School;
Assistant Chief of Ophthalmology,
Massachusetts Eye and Ear Infirmary;
Director, Glaucoma Service,
Beth Israel Hospital,
Boston, Massachusetts

Henry Black, M.D.
Associate Clinical Professor of Medicine,
Yale University School of Medicine,
New Haven, Connecticut

Dan Blazer, M.D., Ph.D.
Associate Professor of Psychiatry,
Director, Affective Disorders Program,
Duke University Medical Center,
Durham, North Carolina

Lawrence J. Brandt, M.D.
Director, Division of Gastroenterology,
Montefiore Hospital and Medical Center;
Professor of Medicine,
Albert Einstein College of Medicine,
Bronx, New York

**Ronald D. T. Cape, B.Sc., M.D.,
    F.R.C.P.(E), F.R.C.P.(C), F.A.C.P.**
Professor, Department of Medicine,
Chairman, Division of
    Geriatric Medicine,
The University of Western Ontario,
London, Ontario

**S. George Carruthers, M.D.,
M.R.C.P.(UK), F.R.C.P.(C), F.A.C.P.**
Associate Professor of Medicine and
  Pharmacology and Toxicology,
University of Western Ontario;
Clinical Pharmacologist,
University Hospital,
London, Ontario

**Alan Barham Carter, M.A., M.D. (Cantab),
F.R.C.P., D.P.M. (Lond.)**
Honorary Consulting Physician,
  St. George's Hospital;
Advisor in Neurology, Ministry of
  Defense, London;
Consulting Physician Emeritus, Ashford
  Hospital,
Middlesex, England

Paul T. Costa, Jr., Ph.D.
Chief, Section on Stress and Coping,
Gerontology Research Center,
National Institute on Aging,
National Institutes of Health,
Baltimore, Maryland

Faith B. Davis, M.D.
Associate Professor of Medicine,
State University of New York at Buffalo
  School of Medicine;
Endocrinologist, Erie County Medical
  Center,
Buffalo, New York

Paul J. Davis, M.D.
Professor and Vice-Chairman, Head,
  Endocrinology Division,
Department of Medicine,
State University of New York at Buffalo
  School of Medicine;
Chief, Medical Service, Veterans
  Administration Medical Center,
Buffalo, New York

Deryck Duncalf, M.B., Ch.B., F.F.A.R.C.S.
Chairman, Department of
  Anesthesiology,
Montefiore Hospital and Medical Center,
Professor of Anesthesiology, Albert
  Einstein College of Medicine,
Bronx, New York

Eben I. Feinstein, M.D.
Associate Professor of Clinical Medicine,

University of Southern California School
  of Medicine,
Los Angeles, California

Jerome L. Fleg, M.D.
Cardiologist, Gerontology Research
  Center,
National Institute on Aging,
National Institutes of Health;
Assistant Professor of Medicine,
Johns Hopkins University School of
  Medicine,
Baltimore, Maryland

Selwyn Z. Freed, M.D.
Chief of Urology,
Montefiore Hospital and Medical Center,
Professor and Chairman, Department of
  Urology,
Albert Einstein College of Medicine,
Bronx, New York

Barbara A. Gilchrest, M.D.
Chief, Cutaneous Gerontology
  Laboratory,
U.S.D.A. Human Nutrition Research
  Center on Aging at Tufts University;
Professor and Chairman, Department of
  Dermatology,
Boston University School of Medicine,
Boston, Massachusetts

Mervyn L. Goldstein, M.D., F.A.C.P.
Director of Education in Hematology,
Montefiore Hospital and Medical Center;
Associate Clinical Professor of Medicine,
Albert Einstein College of Medicine,
Bronx, New York

Victor Goodhill, M.D.
Adjunct Professor,
Department of Head and Neck Surgery
  (Otology),
U.C.L.A. Medical Center,
Los Angeles, California

Edward T. Habermann, M.D.
Professor and Chairman, Department of
  Orthopaedic Surgery,
Albert Einstein Medical Center;
Orthopaedic Surgeon in Charge,
Montefiore Medical Center and Albert
  Einstein Medical Center

Henry Haimovici, M.D.
Clinical Professor Emeritus of Surgery,
Albert Einstein College of Medicine;
Chief Emeritus, Vascular Surgery, and
  Senior Consultant,
Montefiore Medical Center

David Hamerman, M.D.
Division of Geriatrics,
Montefiore Hospital,
Professor of Medicine,
Albert Einstein College of Medicine;
Head of Unified Division of Geriatric
  Medicine,
Bronx, New York

Melvin H. Jahss, M.D.
Chief Foot Surgeon,
Hospital for Joint Diseases,
Orthopaedic Institute;
Professor of Orthopaedic Surgery,
Mount Sinai Medical Center,
New York, New York

Lissy F. Jarvik, M.D., Ph.D.
Professor and Chief, U.C.L.A. Section on
  Neuropsychiatrics,
The Neuropsychiatric Institute,
University of California, Los Angeles;
Chief, Psychogeriatric Unit,
West Los Angeles Veterans
  Administration Medical Center,
  Brentwood Division,
Los Angeles, California

Lorin K. Johnson, Ph.D.
Senior Scientist,
California Biotechnology, Inc.,
Mountain View, California

Beatrice Kastenbaum, M.S.N.
Instructor, College of Nursing,
Arizona State University,
Tempe, Arizona

Robert Kastenbaum, M.D., Ph.D.
Professor of Gerontology,
Director of Adult Developmental and
  Aging Program,
Arizona State University,
Tempe, Arizona

Edith R. Kepes, M.D.
Clinical Professor Emeritus of
  Anesthesiology,
Albert Einstein College of Medicine,
Clinical Professor of Anesthesiology;
Director, Pain Treatment Center,
Montefiore Hospital and Medical Center,
Bronx, New York

Lois Kramer, R.D.
Merion Health Center,
Peoria, Illinois;
Metabolic Section,
Veterans Administration Hospital,
Hines, Illinois

Edward G. Lakatta, M.D.
Chief, Cardiovascular Section,
Gerontology Research Center,
National Institute on Aging,
National Institutes of Health,
Baltimore City Hospital,
Baltimore, Maryland;
Associate Professor of Medicine,
Johns Hopkins School of Medicine;
Associate Professor of Physiology,
University of Maryland School of
  Medicine

Keith R. Latham, Ph.D.
Research Professor of Medicine,
Department of Medicine,
Uniformed Services University of the
  Health Sciences,
Bethesda, Maryland

Steven S. Matsuyama, Ph.D.
Associate Research Geneticist,
Department of Psychiatry and
  Biobehavioral Sciences,
University of California, Los Angeles;
Research Geneticist,
West Los Angeles Veterans
  Administration Medical Center,
  Brentwood Division,
Los Angeles, California

Kevin P. Morrissey, M.D.
Associate Professor of Clinical Surgery,
Cornell University Medical College;
Associate Attending Surgeon,
The New York Hospital,
New York, New York

Marvin Moser, M.D.
Clinical Professor of Medicine,
Yale University School of Medicine,
New Haven, Connecticut;
Senior Medical Consultant,
National High Blood Pressure Education
  Program,
National Heart, Lung, and Blood
  Institute,
Bethesda, Maryland

Charles P. Pollak, M.D.
Head, Sleep-Wake Disorders Center;
Acting Director, Institute of
  Chronobiology,
New York Hospital–Cornell Medical
  Center, White Plains, New York

Harold Rifkin, M.D.
Clinical Professor of Medicine,
Albert Einstein College of Medicine;
Principal Consultant, Diabetes Research
  and Training Center,
Albert Einstein College of Medicine—
  Montefiore Medical Center, Bronx,
  New York

Herbert Ross, M.D.
Associate Clinical Professor of Medicine,
Albert Einstein College of Medicine;
Attending in Medicine,
Montefiore Hospital and Medical Center,
Bronx, New York;
Associate Attending in Medicine,
White Plains Hospital Medical Center,
White Plains, New York

Isadore Rossman, M.D.
Medical Director, Home Health Agency,
Montefiore Hospital and Medical Center;
Professor Emeritus, Epidemiology and
  Social Medicine, Associate Clinical
  Professor Emeritus, Department of
  Medicine, Albert Einstein College of
  Medicine,
Bronx, New York

Gene G. Ryerson, M.D.
Associate Professor of Medicine,
University of Florida College of
  Medicine,
Gainesville, Florida

Clarence J. Schein, M.D.
Chief of Surgery, Professor in
  Department of Surgery,
Albert Einstein College of Medicine
  Hospital,
Bronx, New York (Deceased)

Stephen J. Sontag, M.D.
Metabolic Section,
Veterans Administration Hospital,
Hines, Illinois;
Department of Medicine, Loyola
  University Stritch School of Medicine,
Maywood, Illinois

Herta Spencer, M.D.
Professor of Medicine,
Loyola University Stritch School of
  Medicine,
Maywood, Illinois;
Chief, Metabolic Section,
Veterans Administration Hospital,
Hines, Illinois

Martha Storandt, Ph.D.
Professor, Department of Psychology
  and Neurology,
Director of Aging and Developing
  Program,
Washington University,
St. Louis, Missouri

Kakarla Subbarao, M.D.
Professor of Radiology,
Department of Radiology,
Albert Einstein College of Radiology and
  Montefiore Hospital Medical Center,
Bronx, New York

Jerome Tobis, M.D.
Professor and Chairman,
Department of Physical Medicine and
  Rehabilitation;
Director of Program in Geriatric Medicine
  and Gerontology,
Attending in Physical Medicine,
University of California Medical Center,
Irvine, California

Norman Trieger, D.M.D., M.D.
Chairman and Professor,
Department of Dentistry, Oral and
  Maxillofacial Surgery,

Albert Einstein College of Medicine and
  Montefiore Hospital and Medical
  Center,
Bronx, New York

Marc E. Weksler, M.D.
Director, Division of Geriatrics and
  Gerontology;
Irving Sherwood Wright Professor of
  Medicine,
Department of Medicine,
Cornell University Medical College,
New York, New York

Mark Williams, M.D.
University of North Carolina at Chapel
  Hill,
Division of General Medicine,
Chapel Hill, North Carolina

Fred Winsberg, M.D.
Professor of Radiology,

New York Medical College,
Valhalla, New York;
Ultrasonix, Inc.,
5 Odell Plaza,
North Yonkers, New York

James W. Wynne, M.D.
Clinical Associate Professor of
  Medicine,
University of Florida College of
  Medicine,
Gainesville, Florida

Leo Zach, D.D.S.
Associate Attending, Departments of
  Dentistry and Pathology,
Montefiore Hospital and Medical Center
  and North Central Bronx Hospital,
Bronx, New York (Deceased)

Preface

Over recent years interest in geriatric medicine has been growing laudably in contrast to the comparative neglect in 1970, when the first edition was written. An unforeseen geriatric population explosion (Ch. 6), the emergence of the National Institute on Aging, and a rapidly expanding knowledge base have all quelled the carping concerning the viability of this area of internal medicine. The necessarily enlarged third edition of *Clinical Geriatrics* contains much new material reflecting this increased growth. Some of the new chapters deal with age-related immunologic alterations with longitudinal aging changes, infections, sleep, falls, incontinence, and the endocrines. It has been estimated that almost half the complaints of elderly ambulatory patients relate to the digestive tract. The major clinical importance of this area is recognized in the three new chapters by Dr. Lawrence Brandt. Other chapters have been extensively rewritten and, in some instances, done over by new authors with fresh points of view.

As with its predecessors, this edition has been conceptualized as a readable text to help the primary care physician, both generalist and internist, in the daily struggles with geriatric morbidity. The emphasis continues to be on useful material that too often receives short shrift, if not inattention, in the usual texts of medicine. In keeping with this conception has been the need to place usefulness above formal considerations, and thus *Clinical Geriatrics* continues to be multidisciplinary and rather wide in range. It is lamentable that textbooks traditionally have been detached and dry to a degree that withers interest and makes them difficult reading. I have spent many hours trying to modify this tradition and also to make it clear that this book deals not only with diseases, but also with human beings.

Isadore Rossman, M.D., Ph.D.

From the Preface to the First Edition (1971)

Suddenly the geriatric group in our population has assumed a burgeoning importance in medical practice. Many of the strides forward in the care of the young and the middle aged have inevitably led to a marked increase in the absolute number of the elderly, and Medicare legislation has further emphasized the impact of the geriatric group in office and hospital practice. More medical practitioners are discovering that this is one of the most challenging and difficult areas of clinical practice, calling for unusual skills and a knowledgeability not readily derived from standard textbooks of medicine.

When our Department at Montefiore Hospital and Medical Center agreed to give medical care to more than 500 patients in nursing homes and extended care facilities, we found that even our relatively seasoned clinicians were hampered by the absence of textual material that would serve as a guide to their geriatric practice. This text was, therefore, conceived as an everyday aid to the clinician in understanding and treating his elderly patients. To overcome the gaps that sometimes exist between theory, practice and necessity, the many contributors to this book were selected for their special interest in and clinical experience with elderly patients. Because of the importance attached to clinical experience, some of the contributors sought out were clinicians attached to hospitals or to care facilities concerned with the elderly, rather than traditional academicians. It has been equally rewarding from this point of view to seek out chapters from some of our esteemed British colleagues, contributors to the clinical science of geriatrics in a tradition that had its beginnings somewhat earlier than that in the United States. To all these contributors, busy with their practices and other duties, the editor expresses his special thanks.

Those who are familiar with the neat edifices constructed in standard medical texts may encounter new emphases and some seeming asymmetries in *Clinical Geriatrics*. This derives from two editorial concerns: the contributors were charged not to repeat the details of familiar material available in standard texts, but rather to accent that which was characteristic or unique in dealing with the elderly. The apparent asymmetry evolves from the nature of clinical practice with the elderly. Many of the major medical problems and some of the everyday threats to this fragile group give new dimensions to diseases and events that may be uncommon or inconsequential in younger persons. Osteoporosis and fractures; loss of ambulation and decubiti; diminished hearing and vision; loss of proprioception; the threat of vertigo; the rising incidence of postural hypotension; the impairment of homeostasis even in heat-regulating capacity, as represented by hypothermia and hyperthermia; these and many other problems acquire new importance and carry different therapeutic implications. Out of this everyday stuff of geriatric practice emerged the substance of the chapters in this book. The editor and the contributors are certain that those quite familiar with standard texts will find rewarding further reading in *Clinical Geriatrics*.

Isadore Rossman, M.D., Ph.D.

Contents

I

Aging Changes

1   The Anatomy of Aging

Isadore Rossman

By the time the eighth or ninth decade is achieved, most persons have undergone a number of progressive aging changes that if not recognized as normal can raise troublesome diagnostic problems. Sometimes, because of loss of sweat glands and hair, with slowed cerebration, hypothyroidism may be suggested. The bloodless aspect of the face may seem to confirm an accompanying anemia. The extensive loss of pubic and axillary hair may suggest other forms of endocrinopathy. Shrinkage of muscles, weakness, and ptosis of the lids, all very common in the elderly, can suggest a primary muscle disorder or myasthenia. Loss of subcutaneous fat and atrophic epidermal changes make the usual tests for tissue turgor useless. Elongation of the aorta can produce buckling of the innominate or carotid artery and can present a pulsating mass in the neck (which has been mistaken for aneurysm) or can simulate a tumor on the chest roentgenogram. Thus it is necessary to know geriatric anatomy not only because of its intrinsic interest but also because it serves as a basis for rational differential diagnosis. Some overviews of gross and microscopic anatomical changes and body composition alterations with aging have appeared in recent years.[28,73]

When we judge the age of persons, we do so on the basis of various criteria for senescence. However, it is advisable to remain skeptical of some criteria. Aging changes that are purely local may indicate only an unusual individual exposure (*e.g.*, wrinkling owing to much solar exposure) or that a genetic event has been operative (*e.g.*, early familial graying). Accompanying senescent changes are a number of what might be termed time-related pathologic events.[58] The importance of this distinction is indicated by the fruitfulness of research in atherosclerosis and osteoporosis when these disorders came to be considered time-related pathologic events, not inevitable consequences of aging. But for descriptive purposes in dealing with the aged, the complexities of pathogenesis can be bypassed. Perhaps many of the changes should not imply inescapable, universal sequences, and it is important to call attention to the existence of variability. The geriatrician is in no sense looking at an unbroken chain of events in the decline and fall of humanity, and perhaps in those who fall outside the limits of the standard deviations one may seek important clues to constructive therapy.

CHANGES IN STATURE AND POSTURE

The geriatric population, with its disproportionately large number of women, is a short group, but other factors besides a preponderance of females contribute to this. Many elderly persons, in addition to kyphosis, undergo postural changes, among which slight flexion at the knees and at the hips tends to contribute further to diminished stature (Fig. 1-1). A progressive statural decline also seems apparent in the two generations found in a geriatric facility. Women in their 90s are shorter than those in their 70s. Shrinkage in height with aging is well recognized, and its extent has been quantitated by longitudinal studies of a large number of persons. The problem is somewhat complicated by the increase in stature occurring during the 20th century. Records of incoming freshmen in American colleges indicate they are 1 to 2 inches taller than were their parents and grandparents at the same age.[15] Because many persons seen in a

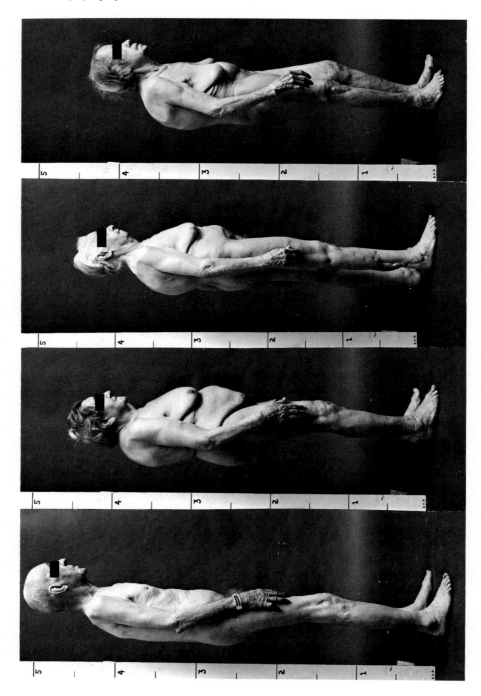

FIG. 1-1. Four randomly selected patients from the ambulatory section of a nursing home, illustrating short stature, osteoporotic kyphosis, and relatively long extremities. From left to right: T.H., age 82, L.B., age 78, A.I., age 79, A.S., age 94. (Photo by DeWayne Dalrymple)

geriatric institution were born at the turn of the century, we are probably looking at a moiety of humans who were originally of shorter stature.

Trotter and Gleser[85] have reported an unmistakable upward trend in the stature of American whites and blacks born between 1840 and 1924. The increase in stature occurring in the 20th century amounted to an average of 3.6 cm in white males. It has been well established by anthropometric studies that a constant relation exists between height at maturity and the length of such long bones as the tibia and femur. Thus, in *Homo sapiens* and any immediate forerunners, one can accurately calculate original stature from measurements of selected long bones. By using such measurements Trotter and Gleser[84] obviated the pitfall caused by shortening owing to spinal osteoporosis. Although humans are getting taller, aging does reverse this. Trotter and Gleser noted a statistically significant decline in stature for each age-group past maturity. This rate of decrement was uniform in all groups, in whites and blacks of both sexes. It was estimated to be 1.2 cm per 20 years.

Thus, if one assembles a number of persons of different ages, the older ones will typically be shorter than their juniors (Fig. 1-2). It has sometimes been held that being short favors survival and that a selective process may tend to weed out taller members of the population. However, there is no evidence that height is related to survival.[59]

Clear-cut evidence of statural decline with aging comes from studies in which persons of varying ages were measured and then remeasured after a suitable interval. The changes are more complex than had been thought. Thus Büchi[11] found the lower extremities decreasing in length past maturity, the rate being maximal in the third decade in males and in the fourth in females. Sitting height increased well into the middle years. In a similar study Miall and co-workers[64] noted an increase in height of some Welshmen from ages 25 to 40, with declining stature taking over past age 50; the lifetime loss thereafter was on the order of 1.5 cm. In a less favored group of males from a mining area, the decline began somewhat earlier and exceeded 2.5 cm thereafter. In females in both groups, loss in height began earlier and was more marked (see Fig. 1-2).

Understandably, very few studies have dealt with persons much past age 80.[36] The impression

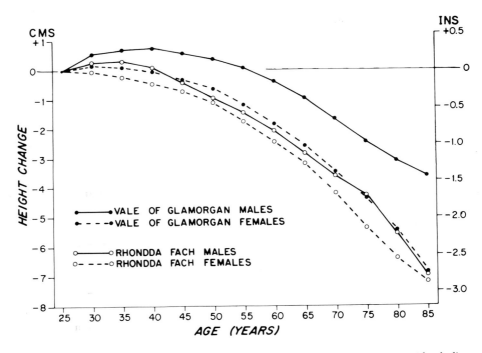

FIG. 1-2. Decrements in height for two groups in Wales, based on remeasurements. The decline appears somewhat earlier and is more marked in the Rhondda Fach (mining area) group, presumably reflecting poorer environmental circumstances. (Miall WE, Ashcroft MT, Lovell HG, Moore F: A longitudinal study of the decline of adult height with age in two Welsh communities. Hum Biol 39:445, 1967, reprinted by permission, Wayne State University Press)

is that the decline is even more accelerated in very old age. Rössle's data for reduction in height[72] are given in Table 1-1.

In the centenarians studied by Basilevich,[3] the women on average were just about 5 feet (152 cm) tall, and the men were 2 to 3 inches taller.

Because the long bones do not undergo significant shortening with age, much of the loss in stature must be ascribed to shortening in the spinal column. Shortening of the vertebral column results from narrowing of the disks plus loss in height of individual vertebrae. Thinning of the disks appears to be the major reason for shrinking stature in the middle years, and diminution in height of the vertebrae is the major reason for the progressive loss in height thereafter. Moderate to marked degrees of osteoporotic vertebral narrowing are nearly universal in elderly women and less so in men. The elderly are thus characterized by shortened trunks and comparatively long extremities, proportions that are the reverse of those seen in infancy and early childhood (Fig. 1-3).

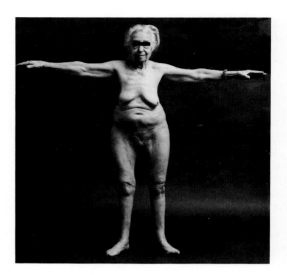

FIG. 1-3. A 79-year-old woman illustrating the maintenance of span in spite of decreasing height (span is 145 cm; height 136 cm).

SPAN

For both sexes a 2% reduction in span in the 65- to 73-year age-group, progressing to a 3% reduction thereafter was recorded by Büchi.[11] Decline in stature exceeds this by a considerable amount particularly in aging women. Hence span measurements, even uncorrected, can lead to a rough estimate of height at maturity in the presence of much kyphosis or bowing of the lower extremities. Brown and Wigzell[10] measured a group of elderly patients in hospital and, on the assumption that span and height were roughly equal at maturity, constructed Table 1-2.

Similar findings are reported by Dequeker and associates.[19] They noted in one group of women

that length exceeded span by 1 cm in the fourth and fifth decades; from the sixth decade on, span exceeded length, and this progressed in successively older groups. By the ninth decade, the mean span was 8 cm greater than the mean body length.

It is thus apparent that the loss of height becomes progressively more severe in the eighth and ninth decades, largely owing to an increasing progression in osteoporotic collapse of the spine. On average one can expect an approximate 2-inch loss in height in both men and women in the 50-year span from the second to the seventh decade. Stoudt and co-workers[79] reviewed a variety of studies and constructed height–weight tables for white Americans from birth on (Table 1-3).

TABLE 1-1   Heights of Subjects of Different Ages

Age	Height (cm)
20	169.2
40	167.0
60	165.8
80	164.2
90	160.8

(Rössle R, Roulet F: Zahl und Mass in Pathologie Berlin, Springer-Verlag, 1932)

TABLE 1-2   Relationship Between Age, Length, and Span in 125 Hospital Subjects

Age in years	65–74	75–84	85–94
Number of subjects	45	53	28
Mean length/span ratio (× 100)	97.34	96.70	95.15
Equivalent loss in inches	1½	2	3

(Brown OT, Wigzell FW: The significance of span as a clinical measurement. *In* Anderson WF, Isaacs B (eds): Current Achievement in Geriatrics. London, Cassell, 1964)

TABLE 1-3 Average Heights and Weights by Age and Sex: U.S. Health Examination Study 1960-1962*

	Males		Females	
Age	*Height (in)*	*Weight (lb)*	*Height (in)*	*Weight (lb)*
18–24	68.7	160	63.8	129
25–34	69.1	171	63.7	136
35–44	68.5	172	63.5	144
45–54	68.2	172	62.9	147
55–64	67.4	166	62.4	152
65–74	66.9	160	61.5	146
75–79	65.9	150	61.1	138

*Based on a nationwide probability sample of 7710 persons. Averages and 50th percentiles were quite equal. Both secular trends and aging changes are mirrored by such measures as the 3-inch difference in height of younger and older males.

(Stoudt HW, Damon A, McFarland RH, Robert J: Weight, height, and selected body measurements of adults—US, 1960–62. Public Health Service publication 1000, series 11, No. 8. Washington, DC, US Government Printing Office, 1965)

BONE AND JOINT CHANGES

Throughout the middle and later years, the bony skeleton undergoes a complex of changes in which growth, regression, and proliferation are interwoven. Although osteoporosis may be severe, and arthritic changes may dominate the picture from the clinician's viewpoint, concurrent bone growth is also to be recognized.

Postmaturational Bone Growth

The skull is unique in being free from the weight bearing and other stresses that occur in the axial skeleton and extremities. With aging, the skull exhibits anabolic changes. Todd[82] noted thickening of the cranial vault into the 60s, and in Büchi's longitudinal study,[11] head circumference increased continuously in both sexes into old age, with persons over 65 exhibiting a more than 2% increment over persons 20 years old. Israel has presented longitudinal data and roentgenograms that show a continued growth of the craniofacial complex from early adulthood into later life.[47–49] All skull diameters increased in thickness as did the endocranial dimensions, with a disproportionately greater increase in the size of the sella turcica and frontal sinuses. Todd and Lyons[83] found endocranial suture closure to occur in bursts through-

out a person's life. For example, the masto-occipital suture begins to close only at around age 30, with a final episode of suture closure at around age 80; and the parietomastoid suture does not attain complete closure until age 80 or later. Appositional bone growth through the seventh and eighth decades has been demonstrated at many sites: rib,[22] metacarpal,[28] and femur.[63] Femoral changes are of particular importance. The femoral diameter at midshaft progressively increases in aging women. This gain in width is 3.5 to 5.0 mm between ages 45 and 49 and ages 75 and 90.[63] Because this is accompanied by osteoporosis, the net result is a wider and weaker bone. The pelvis also widens with age in both males and females. This amounted to a 3.5% increase in the bi-iliac diameter in the group of male white veterans reported by Damon and co-workers.[17]

The complexity of other osseous change is illustrated in the scapula.[32] Over the life span the scapula exhibits gross deterioration in its vascular patterns and musculotendinous indentations. The originally well-delineated vascular patterns show increasing disarray after age 50. Ossification of the glenoid cartilage progresses while, simultaneously, atrophic spots, initially minute, become merging areas of bone atrophy. A distortion owing to progressive folding or wrinkling of the initially relatively smooth surface is first noted in the early 30s. In old age, areas of atrophy become so common that the bone appears spotty or moth-eaten.

Osteoarthritic Changes

The universality of arthritic change in such joints as the knee and spine makes it a matter of definition as to whether it should be considered as an inevitable aging change or a pathologic change (see also Chapters 6 and 29). In the spine, changes progress in an irregular but predictable fashion involving narrowing of the disks and joint spaces with proliferation of osteophytes at the margins. It is possible to grade such changes and give reasonable estimates of the age of the person. Nathan,[67] in a study of 400 vertebral columns, found osteophyte formation to be age related; minor grades were found in many persons in their 20s, but 100% of the vertebral columns of persons in their 40s exhibited them. With advancing age, the severity of osteophytosis also increased with complete bridging of intervertebral spaces seen in the older columns. Other findings included (1) anterior osteophytes were more prevalent in the lower cervical, lower thoracic, and lumbar regions, corresponding to their greater mobility; (2) posterior osteophytes were less frequent and had a marked peak in the cervical spine, with relatively few in the thoracic and upper lumbar areas; and (3) osteophytes were less marked on the left side of the thoracic spine than on the right. This asymmetry was ascribed to the presence of the aorta on the left. Howells[44] found the best correlation between vertebral lipping and age in the C5–7 and L2–4 regions. The knee joint, as described by Bennett and associates,[4] undergoes progressive changes with aging. The earliest changes, seen in the second decade, involve fibrillar degeneration of the cartilage. Progressive degeneration in the cartilage is followed in succeeding decades by osteophytes, loss of cartilage, and eburnation (Fig. 1-4).

Osteoporosis

As indicated previously, loss of bone matrix outpaces appositional growth in most bones. The net effect leads to osteoporosis, an age-related process, which appears to be greater for females than for males and greater for whites than for blacks. Thus bowing of the spine with loss of height typically appears earliest in white females of light build, who are also most subject to the common fractures of the femur and to Colles' fracture. The subject is discussed in detail in Chapter 30.

OTHER ASSOCIATED CHANGES

The loss in height of the vertebral column also affects the neck. To compensate for kyphosis of the upper thoracic spine, there may be a backward tilting of the head, producing an even further reduction of the occiput-to-shoulder distance. Thus viewed from the left side, the head-on-trunk configuration, particularly in women, resembles a figure three. In association with neck shortening, the thyroid gland may descend in relation to the clavicles, to be remembered in palpating the lower poles for possible adenoma. Lengthening of the aorta with elevation of the aortic arch may bring the right innominate artery up into the neck and may result in kinking of the artery and of the right common carotid artery, producing a pulsating swelling palpable and occasionally visible behind the clavicular portion of the right sternocleidomastoid muscle. Buckling of the innominate artery is more common in women than in men, and in association with hypertension. In the 104 angiograms of patients with hypertensive or arteriosclerotic heart disease studied by Honig and co-workers,[42] there were 12 such instances of significant buckling; of these, 8 were in women and 6 were normotensive. A related change affecting the left innominate vein has been described by Smith.[77] Compression of the vein by the enlarged rigid

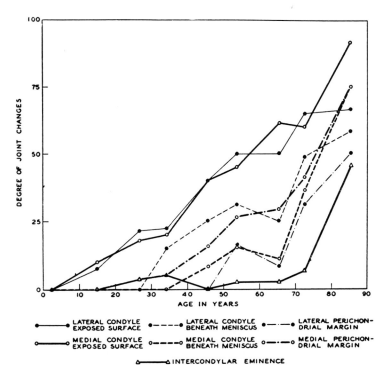

FIG. 1-4. Average degenerative and proliferative changes in the articular surfaces and perichondrial margins of the tibia at each age decade. Changes are apparent in the second decade. A marked increment occurs after the sixth decade. (Bennett GA, Waine H, Bauer W: Changes in the Knee Joint at Various Ages—With Particular Reference to the Nature and Development of Degenerative Joint Disease, p 97. New York, The Commonwealth Fund, 1942)

aorta leads to a dilation of the left external jugular vein. This unilateral vein fullness is best observed with the subject sitting up in bed at a 45° angle.

A number of anthropometric studies have quantitated the other changes associated with aging.[11,16,17,43,69] Some derived from cross-sectional measurements of male veterans in the Boston normative aging study are shown in Figure 1-5. The nose and the ears lengthen and become broader. The width of the shoulders decreases, the chest depth increases, and the pelvis widens. Abdominal depth increases, while body weight decreases.

Most studies agree in finding the chest width apparently increasing through the middle years, with decreases noted in the oldest subjects, particularly the females. Thus, in the group of women reported by Parot,[69] transverse chest diameter, recorded as averaging 24.4 cm at 25 years of age, was 20.7 cm at 85, while the anteroposterior diameter increased from 17.3 cm to 20.8 cm. Longitudinal studies indicate that the left ventricle thickens with aging in normotensive persons, an incremental change to be contrasted with the de-

cline in skeletal muscle (Fig. 1-6) (see Chap. 11), and this may well be a normal aging change. Thus, the point of maximum cardiac impulse may present in the anterior axillary line in elderly women without necessarily indicating pathologic hypertrophy. Edge and co-workers[20] ascribed the increase in the cardiothoracic ratio of elderly women to contraction of the thoracic cage.

CHANGES IN WEIGHT AND SUBCUTANEOUS FAT

The widespread belief that being overweight militates against survival is only partially true.[1] Most reports have dealt with urban Europeans and Americans and thus have recorded the effects of an abundant food supply and often an increasingly sedentary pattern of life. When calories are abundant, a significant number of older persons can maintain an obese status. Hollifield and Parson[41] studied 700 persons over the age of 65 and found 11% of the males and 16% of the females to be

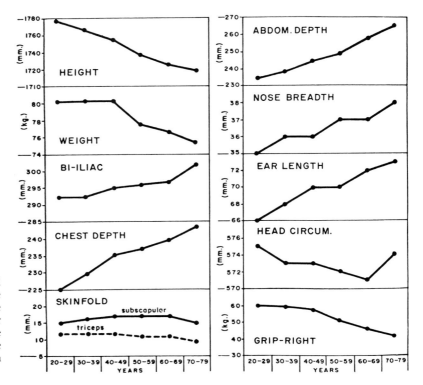

FIG. 1-5. Cross-sectional age-associated changes in the Boston group of male white veterans. (Damon A, Seltzer CC, Stoudt HW, Bell B: Age and physique in healthy white veterans at Boston. Aging Hum Dev 3:202, 1972)

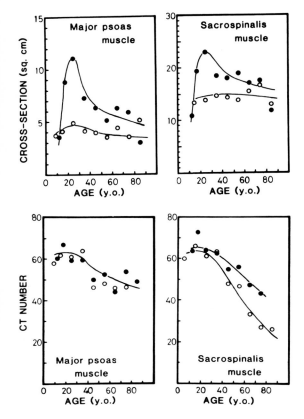

FIG. 1-6. Computed tomographic scans of muscle cross-section and density in relation to age. (Solid circles, males; open circles, females. Upper two figures cross section in sq cm; lower two figures CT number in Hounsfield units) (Imamura K, Ashida H, Ishikawa T, Fujii M: Human major psoas muscle and sacrospinalis muscle in relation to age: A study by computed tomography. Gerontol 38:678, 1983)

20% or more above average weight for their height and age. They noted a tendency for weight to plateau between ages 65 and 74 and to fall thereafter. Their data suggest that the incidence of overweight in this older group was at least as great as it is in younger adults. Hejda[37] studied persons 82 to 100 years of age selected from the normal population and found moderate or severe obesity in 15% of the older men and 21% of the older women. However, most persons in the group studied had reached their maximum weight at around age 42. In Table 1-3 an average weight of around 172 pounds for males in all the age-groups from 25 to 54 is recorded. This drops steadily thereafter with an apparent weight decline of more than 20 pounds. In females, in contrast, weight is approximately the same in age-groups 25 to 34 and 75 to 79. The male-female difference here may reflect the greater shrinkage of muscle in the aging male. Also to be considered is a factor of differential mortality that may favor the survival of a leaner person, particularly the males. Master and co-workers[59] found that for the 65- to 97-year age-group the percentage of overweight males steadily decreased over the 30-year span to only 10% of

the total group; during the same time span, the number of underweight men increased from 20% to 50%. For the same age-groups, the percentage of overweight females decreased from 40% to 10%, with underweight females increasing from 20% to 55%.

The manner in which subcutaneous fat is distributed over the body undergoes significant changes during a lifetime. These differences reflect changes in body weight and sex differences in youth and maturity. Some of the age-related changes may reflect socioeconomic and nutritional status. In the study of Lee and Lasker,[55] only slight changes in the thickness of subcutaneous fat at different sites were seen in elderly compared with middle-aged indigent men. There was no significant age trend in their group; those in their 40s weighed about the same as those in their 80s. Typically, men and women tend to gain weight in their 40s and 50s but need not exhibit the same body contours they did earlier in life at the same weight. Thus, there may be a loss of fat from the face along with a simultaneous deposition on the abdomen and hips. In the women studied by Wessel and colleagues,[87] there was a marked gain in the skin-fold thickness of the pubis (+ 10.8 mm) and umbilicus (+ 16.5 mm) between 59 and 69 years. But as an illustration of the vagaries of fat deposition, skin-fold thicknesses are maintained throughout the sixth and seventh decades at the pubis, umbilicus, and waist, though the scapular measurements decrease markedly.

Skin-fold measurements of various age-groups were reported by Hejda.[37] The thickness of skin folds at 12 different sites was reported and averaged. For males aged 25 to 39, the average skin fold was 1.2 cm. This decreased to 1.0 cm at ages 65 to 79 and to 0.9 cm in those over 80. In women there was but little tendency for a change in the averages throughout their lifetime, with a 1.5-cm thickness at ages 25 to 39 and a 1.4-cm measurement in those over 80. In men the most reliable measurement in relation to weight was that taken from the right of the umbilicus, with the next most reliable that over the hip; in women the most useful predictive measurements were from the umbilicus and upper arm.

Although, in general, increases in weight up until the 60s are due to thickening of preexisting fat depots, this is not true of the anterior leg.[29] Here the skin-fold measurement decreases despite weight gains and increases in skin-fold elsewhere. In persons in their 80s and 90s, gross inspection reveals that the fatty depots tend to disappear from the periphery, although fat deposition is still apparent over the hips and abdomen. Most striking is the loss of subcutaneous fat from the forearms observed in elderly persons in good nutrition, who may in fact be somewhat overweight. In some of them, the forearm skin fold is extremely reduced to an extent that illustrates the selective atrophy of a fat depot. Ryckewaert and co-workers[75] have drawn attention to aging changes in the skin fold of the dorsum of the hand. This decreases rapidly after age 45 in the female, though body weight continues to rise. This decrement occurs later in males.

In aging women the breasts undergo changes that partially mirror changes in the fat elsewhere. As described by Herrmann,[39] there is atrophy not only of the glandular elements but, in most instances, also of the fat envelope. This may make tumors, such as fibroadenomas, that have been present for years more prominent. Cases in which such tumors have calcified may be mistaken clinically for carcinoma. Shrinkage and fibrotic changes may cause retraction of the nipple, which may mimic the retraction produced by cancer. However, the nipple can usually be everted, and no associated tumor mass is palpable, so that the

differential diagnosis can usually be established without surgery. In some elderly women, the terminal ducts become more readily palpable and are easily outlined because of fibrosis and calcification. These firm linear strands may appear at first in one breast and then in the other and have occasionally created a suspicion of malignancy. In many women, the breasts may hang at a lower level, a feature accentuated by kyphosis (see Fig. 1-1).

Contour Changes

Because subcutaneous fat is the padding that fills out and rounds the body's contours, its loss in old age leads to an increasing sharpness of contour and a deepening of previous hollows. This occurs in the hollows of the orbits and axillas, in the supraclavicular and the intercostal spaces, in the pelvic contour, and elsewhere. Bony landmarks become increasingly prominent, and formerly hidden landmarks become easily visible. Typically, the tips of the vertebrae, the angles of the scapula, the ribs, the xiphisternum, the crests and spines of the ilium, the patella, the arch of the foot, and the metatarsal heads become more prominent. This contributes to the well-known bony appearance of the aged. When advanced, the net change is similar to that seen in cachexia. Because this bony appearance is largely due to atrophy of fat, it is not significantly reversible by increasing the caloric intake.

Muscle contours also become more prominent. Muscle bundles and their tendinous points of attachment may become startlingly distinct. The accentuation of muscle contours occurs despite the absolute loss of muscle substance. Thus Korenchevsky,[52] using figures from Rössle and Roulet,[72] gives a weight of 536 g to 538 g for the triceps muscle in each decade between ages 20 and 50; this decreases to 478 g between ages 50 and 60 and to 457 g after 70. The total weight of all the skeletal muscles averages 452 g/kg of body weight in the third decade and decreases to 339 g in the seventh decade and to 270 g after age 70. Because some replacement of muscle substance by fat occurs in the older age-groups, the absolute weight of muscle is doubtless less than these figures suggest. Thus in the morphologic study of Ingelmark and Gustafsson,[46] aging is shown to result in a variable atrophy of the muscle fibers so that their formerly uniform diameter becomes quite variable and the amount of intramuscular fat increases.

Computed tomographic scanning has made possible measurement of muscle *in vivo*[7] and clearly indicates progressive declines with aging in cross-sectional studies (see Fig. 1-6), which are most striking in the male.[45]

BODY HAIR

Many elderly subjects present with states of hairlessness that would be considered diagnostic of an endocrinopathy were they younger. In a few, the loss of hair over the body may be comparable to that in alopecia totalis.

Multiple factors—racial, genetic, and sex-linked—determine the maximum amount of hair a person possesses and the subsequent changes with age. Many white Europeans are obviously a great deal hairier than are persons of Asian or black ancestry. Males of American Indian origin have strikingly little body and face hair. Hamilton[35] has delineated some of the differences between white and Japanese subjects. White males were found to have far heavier beards, with peak values attained earlier in life, and with an earlier onset of graying. These differences were also found to hold true for axillary hair. In female subjects, no case of facial hirsutism was observed in Japanese women ranging up to 88 years, in contrast to the considerable incidence of facial hirsutism in aging white women. In comparing the two groups of women 60 or more years of age, Hamilton found complete loss of axillary hair in 196 of the 200 Japanese women examined. In all groups, aging generally produces a considerable decrease in hair everywhere, with the single exception of the face. In this location, especially in whites, some men past 40 develop hairiness of the ears, and women past 40 often sprout hairs above their lips and on their chins.

The hair of the head is subject to the greatest variations because of sex-linked factors. Patterns of baldness that affect men alone are inherited from the mother, with the genetic decree effectuated only in the presence of testosterone. A number of patterns for hair loss from the scalp have been described. The onset is variable but not uncommonly in the 20s, with what has been termed the M-shaped pattern, in which hair loss occurs to either side of the midline. Another commonly involved area consists of a patch over the vertex. Extension of these areas occurs with the passage of the years, often resulting in their coalescence. However, a small but cosmetically important patch of hair isolated to the midline may survive. In advanced baldness, more than half the scalp is affected, though here and there fine scattered hairs may survive. In the severer degrees of

sex-linked baldness, hair may be limited to the area above the ear, where if it is followed posteriorly it swings down below the vertex toward the nape of the neck and then generally symmetrically curves upward to the opposite ear. In men not subject to this form of baldness and in women, the hair loss is not patterned. There is, rather, a slow thinning out; the hairs become less numerous, and many become thinner with the passage of the years, especially after age 60. Graying tends to precede hair loss. Because it too is progressive, with more and more hairs becoming depigmented, the net effect of aging on the scalp is the transformation of darker, thicker, and more numerous hairs to lighter, thinner, and less numerous ones. In some elderly persons, unusual shades of yellow to yellow-green may appear.

Axillary hair is sensitive both to the passing of time and to changes in hormonal status. As Hamilton[35] pointed out, coarse axillary hairs are secondary sex characteristics. They appear only at sexual maturation and fail to grow in men castrated before puberty. They tend to regress in the castrated male adult. Axillary hairs appear centrally first and then peripherally, with the central hairs distinctly longer and thicker. Aging reverses the sequence seen with puberty. There occurs a gradual loss of axillary hair that proceeds from the periphery to the center. With the passage of time, the remaining central hairs tend to become thinner, less kinky, and grayer. Melick and Taft[61] surveyed the hair in 167 males and 189 females past the age of 60. In one sixth of the males and one half of the females, most or all of the axillary hair was lost. The loss progressed with age. Obvious loss of pubic hair was seen in one-fifth of the males and one third of the females. Complete loss of pubic hair occurred in one man and five women. Melick and Taft observed a loss of hair in the outer third of the eyebrows in one sixth of the group; these subjects otherwise appeared euthyroid. Coarse facial hairs were seen in three fourths of the women. These did not progress with age. Leg hair was absent or scanty in both sexes; in contrast, arm hair was often plentiful in males, though scanty in females.

The appearance, as well as disappearance, of some body hair in women, can perhaps be correlated with such endocrine transitions as menopause. Thomas and Ferriman[81] found that abdominal hair in women—specifically the hair extending from pubis to umbilicus—though present in 7% to 11% of women between 15 and 45, abruptly disappeared postmenopausally. Such abdominal hairs were found in only 1 of 108 women in the 45- to 54-year age-group and none of 186 women in the 55- to 84-year age-group. However, there was a gradual increase in the number of women with significant amounts of chin hairs. The incidence rose from 6% in the 45- to 54-year age-group to 41% in the 75- to 84-year age-group. The extensiveness of the beard in elderly women in such institutions as nursing homes is often not recognized. Compassionate nurses may go to some lengths to keep these patients shaven.

FACIAL CHANGES

The muscles of expression give the human face a play of emotion unknown in any other species but are responsible also for the characteristic wrinkling produced by time. The creasing of the skin resulting from the repeated use of these muscles tends to occur at right angles to the axis of their contraction. In this way, habitual patterns of expression, such as frowning, pursing the mouth, and smiling, produce characteristic wrinkles in some persons earlier in life than in others. But these and other changes have a variable onset. They are determined by factors such as the toughness and elasticity of the skin, solar radiation, the extent to which subcutaneous fat is maintained during aging, and individual states of nutrition. Dieting with loss of the subcutaneous fat in persons of middle age or beyond accentuates wrinkling, a fact that often deters reducing.

Among the first wrinkles to form are those on the forehead related to the activity of the occipitofrontalis muscle. This bilaterally symmetrical muscle sweeps upward from above each eyebrow and inserts at around the level of the hairline. A variable area in the midline is free of muscle fibers. Thus when the muscle contracts, the skin of the forehead is raised, producing curvilinear wrinkles more or less parallel to each orbital region and dipping toward the midline. Wrinkling of the forehead starts in the 20s and increases in the 30s and 40s; the initially thin tracings become deeper and thicker with the passage of the years. Roughly paralleling this development temporally are the wrinkles that radiate fanwise from the lateral canthus. Known for centuries as crow's-feet, the more prominent middle one has sometimes been referred to as the "over-40 line."

Other facial wrinkles near the eyes include the two vertical or comma-shaped frown lines on either side of the root of the nose and the various wrinkles involving the upper and lower lids. The play of expression around the mouth, especially as a result of smiling, tends to accentuate the nasolabial groove, which may become a deep furrow. It can also produce an equally deep groove extending downward from the area adjacent to the mouth toward the chin. This develops in the 50s and deepens thereafter. Attributable to the action of the orbicularis oris muscle and arising usually past the 60s are multiple fine wrinkles of the upper and lower lips, which radiate away from the vermilion border. This wrinkling has been compared to the folding produced by tightening a purse string.

In addition to the progressive wrinkling produced by the play of facial muscles, wrinkling results from the loss of fat and elastic fibers characteristic of aging skin. This leads to a laxness of skin, which then drapes itself chiefly in accordance with gravitational pull and produces a ptosis of lids, ears, jowls, and submental wrinkling. In a few persons, sagging of the tissues of the neck combined with fat deposition produces a double chin. More often, the neck undergoes shrinking and wrinkling that may become more marked than the facial changes. A characteristic development that may appear in the 50s is the appearance of two prominent lines coursing up the neck on either side of the midline, ascribed in large measure to the action of the platysma muscle. The lines come closest together at the midneck and diverge as they approach the medial ends of the clavicles. A course reticulation of the neck skin may proceed to an elaborate patterning, and a number of accentuated circular lines may appear both anteriorly and posteriorly.

Other Facial Changes

The edentulous state progressively leads to resorption of bone from the mandible and maxilla. When advanced, this produces marked shrinkage in the lower portion of the face, an increased infolding of the mouth, and a slow closing of the distance between chin and nose. A slight elongation of the nose has also been recorded by several investigators. Somewhat more marked is elongation of the ears, which according to Fleischer[24] averages 12 mm by age 80. The elongation has been attributed by him to loss of elasticity, causing the lobe to become more pendulous. Because cartilage not exposed to weight bearing shows little aging changes, ear elongation is due largely to sagging of the lobe, which also becomes wrinkled.

In many elderly persons, the skin of the face appears pale and strikingly uniform in coloration. It has an opaque, dull white, or putty-colored appearance, with little or no evidence of a hemal component over such areas as the cheek, and indeed the bloodless tone might at first glance suggest anemia. Various factors contribute to this graying of the skin, with loss of capillaries perhaps predominant.[74] In addition, aging is accompanied by a marked loss of functioning melanocytes,[23] and doubtless a continuous life indoors, the frequent fate of the very old, also contributes to their pallor.

Other aging changes alter the appearance of the face, particularly in relation to the eyes, jaws, and ears. Puffiness, particularly below the lower lids, may develop in the 40s and 50s, largely owing to herniation of fat into this area, which is often associated with some fluid retention. When associated with venous hyperemia or pigmentation, this produces the dark bags sometimes unjustly attributed to keeping late hours or having irregular pursuits, but later in life these seem to recede and disappear. The sunken appearance of elderly eyes is due to loss of fat from the orbit, leading to an enophthalmos that can be severe by the time the 80s are reached and progressing thereafter. In a group of centenarians, Gall recorded exophthalmometer readings varying from 5 mm to 16 mm, with a mean for 45 eyes of 11.3 mm. A further change in ocular appearance is introduced by ptosis, as the upper lid droops backward and then anteriorly over the superior surface of the eyeball. In unusual instances, geriatric ptosis may interfere with vision.

Arcus Senilis

Because of its striking appearance and its name, arcus senilis has been given undue importance as evidence of aging. When fully developed, it appears grossly as a white line encircling the cornea. When it first appears, it is thin, does not quite reach the outermost border of the limbus, and may be limited to the upper portion of the eye. As it progresses, it becomes thicker and denser, and it completely encircles the cornea. In some old persons, it forms a moundlike elevation. Arcus senilis is a misnomer, much like senile telangiectasia, in that both not infrequently occur early in life. Nascher,[66] who is said to have coined the term *geriatrics* and wrote one of the early American texts in the field, stated: "The arcus senilis which is always found in the aged does not interfere with sight nor does it denote fatty degeneration of the heart as was formerly thought. (The author has a well-marked arcus senilis which was shown to the class during his school days.)" Although it is true

that virtually all older persons have some degree of arcus, the association is variable and dominated by individual, familial, and racial factors.[40,57] Macaraeg and co-workers[57] called attention to its early onset in blacks, in whom significant degrees of arcus are found in the third and fourth decades in nearly half the cases studied. A complete absence of arcus was occasionally found in both black and white persons, even in their 70s and 80s. Despite various claims in the past that linked arcus senilis to atherosclerosis, myocardial infarction, cerebrovascular accident, and hypertension, Macaraeg and co-workers were unable to establish such significant correlations. However, there is little doubt that the arcus does appear earlier in life in familial hypercholesterolemia. That some degree of arcus is found in almost everyone past age 65 does give it a highly positive correlation with chronologic age, whatever else its biological significance may be. Whether very old persons who fail to develop significant arcus have any other concomitant slowing of aging processes has not been established.

CHANGES IN BODY COMPOSITION

The body tissue that undergoes the widest fluctuations throughout growth, maturity, and old age is fat (Fig. 1-7). The overt differences between the slender adolescent, the overweight middle-aged person, and the withered old person constituting the backbone of the nursing home population underline the importance of subcutaneous fat in the appearance and weight of a person. Even though obesity does not preclude achievement of senescence,[1] the great majority of patients encountered by the geriatrician appear to have lost much of their fat. Because fat is the only tissue lighter than water, one might anticipate that the specific gravity of the body would increase in old age. In fact, the reverse occurs. Although it may come as no surprise to find the specific gravity dropping from well-muscled youth to flabbier middle age, there can be no doubt that the specific gravity of the human body continues to diminish progressively well into advanced old age. Because the muscle compartment is shrinking, and bone is becoming more porous, it is clear that the diminishing specific gravity is the net result of alterations in all major body compartments. Specific gravity can be readily determined by underwater weighing, using Archimedes' principle, after a suitable correction for volume of residual lung air. Figure 1-8 illustrates some aspects of the changes in body com-

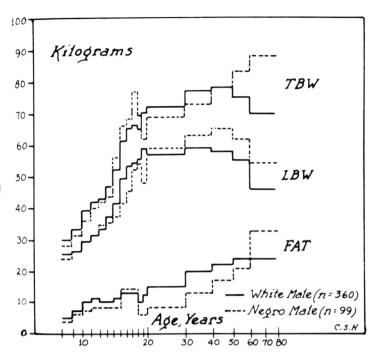

FIG. 1-7. The decrease in lean body weight (LBW) progresses at an increasing rate past middle age. The relative percentage of fat in the body continues to increase in old age, in spite of a decrease in total body weight (TBW). (Meneely GR, Heyssel RM, Ball COT, Weiland RL, Lorimer AR, Constantinides C, Meneely EU: Analysis of factors affecting body composition determined from potassium content in 915 normal subjects. Ann NY Acad Sci 110:271, 1963)

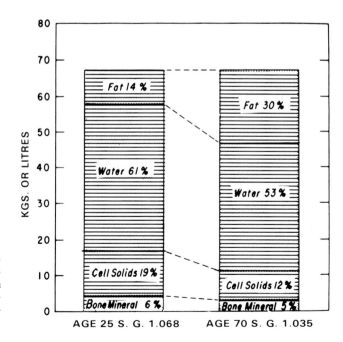

FIG. 1-8. A comparison of major body compartments and their changes with the aging process. (Fryer JH: Studies of body composition in men aged 60 and over. In Shock NW (ed): Biological Aspects of Aging, p 75. New York, Columbia University Press, 1962)

partments with aging and emphasizes the fat increment. Since skin-fold measurements attest to the decrease in the fatty subcutaneous tissue, the fat increment apparently occurs elsewhere—in and about the viscera and the muscles.

Potassium is present in high concentration (150 mEq/liter of cell water) in cells and is virtually absent from neutral fat and other noncellular components of the body. Quantitatively, more than half the body potassium is in skeletal muscle, with the rest chiefly in organ parenchyma and the nervous system. These tissues, which collectively define the lean body mass, have been characterized by Moore[65] as "the engine of the body." Although it is possible to alter the lean body mass by exercise and sports that increase muscle mass, it tends to remain stable year in and year out, whatever the fluctuations in fat and body weight may be. An inexorable manifestation of the aging process is the slowly progressive diminution of the lean bodymass. Moore has summed this up by stating: "the engine shrinks within the chassis."

Good approximation of lean body mass has been achieved with specific gravity measurement such as underwater weighing and by an independent method, after the introduction of potassium chloride [42]K. Extensive studies using the isotope dilution technique were reported by Moore and his co-workers.[65] They were able to demonstrate

that the total exchangeable potassium decreases linearly with advancing age. They concluded that the decrease was primarily due to a change in the relation between intracellular and extracellular components of the body and could be ascribed to a progressive relative predominance of extracellular components such as the dermis, collagen, tendon, fascia, and cortical bone. Measurements of body water showed a decrease with age, also reflecting, at least in part, some of the loss of lean body mass. Although there is no good indirect way of estimating the weight of bone in a living subject, several acceptable ways of estimating this are available. It is thus possible to estimate the changes in proportions of major body compartments at various ages by these methods (see Fig. 1-8).

A further advance in technique was made possible by whole body counting of the naturally occurring radioactive [40]K in the body, which enables estimation of lean body mass without administration of an isotope. The most important factors affecting lean body mass are age and sex.[68] The normal age- and sex-specific curves are seen in Figure 1-9. Race is an additional significant factor: Asians show a markedly lower lean body mass and lower fat values than either white or black American subjects. Because "fat" Asians do not differ from average Americans, it is likely that the lower lean body mass of most Asians relates en-

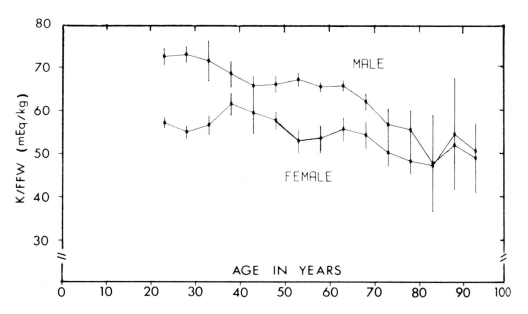

FIG. 1-9. Potassium/fat-free weight vs. age over 20. Fat measured by anthropometry. The decline in potassium with age is calculated from total body counting. (Pierson RN Jr, Lin DHY, Phillips RA: Total body potassium in health: Effects of age, sex, height, and fat. Am J Physiol 226:206, 1974)

tirely to fat and the skeletal and muscle increase it obligates. A study of 915 normal subjects, reported by Meneely and co-workers,[62] showed slight differences in the lean body mass between white and black subjects early in life. The total body weight of white males reached a peak in the fifth decade; that of black males rose steadily from a mean of 70 kg in the third decade to 88 kg in the seventh and eighth decades. Possibly these weight changes reflect differences in work patterns and energy expenditures, as well as other socio-economic differences. In both races, beginning at about age 40, the estimated lean body weight as a fraction of total body weight progressively diminished.

All cross-sectional and longitudinal studies of the body's ^{40}K content corroborate a marked loss with aging indicative of a decline in the lean body mass. Burmeister and Bingert[12] found this shrinkage to be on the order of 25% in males and 15% in females. In the study of over 3000 subjects of all ages reported by Pierson and co-workers,[70] males showed a peak of 53.8 mEq/kg at age 20. This decreased at an average of 0.25 mEq/kg/year thereafter. In females, the ratio of potassium to weight decreased continuously from puberty onward because of added fat. In females, the total potassium value was constant from age 20 to age 45 and then declined (see Fig. 1-9). The sex difference may be due to earlier shrinkage in the muscle component of the male. Forbes and Reina[25,26] have demonstrated the validity of the larger cross-sectional studies by re-measurements of persons years to decades later; aging invariably led to loss of lean body mass even when considerable weight gain had occurred.

THE AGING BRAIN

The foremost organ in *Homo sapiens,* the brain, has been intensively studied with regard to aging changes and function. It, too, undergoes decremental changes, which are far more complex but perhaps comparable with those in striated muscle, another irreplaceable tissue composed of postmitotic cells. It has generally been accepted that the size and weight of the brain diminish with aging.[5,72] Older autopsy figures indicated a loss of 100 g to 150 g of tissue over the life span; these figures doubtless included an unknown number of patients with both early and late senile dementia of the Alzheimer type in whom a considerable abnormal degree of brain shrinkage generally oc-

curs. Simple weighing of the organ or naked eye inspection for shrinkage of gyri and widening of sulci were markedly improved by the methodology of Davis and Wright.[18] These researchers developed a technique for accurate assessment of brain volume and cranial cavity volume. After showing that the latter did not change significantly over the life span, they found that the ratio of brain to cranial cavity volume of around 0.92 up to age 60 progressively fell to around 0.80 in the succeeding 3 decades.

Shrinkage of the brain within its cavity would be expected to lead to an increase in the size of ventricles and cisterns, changes that are quantifiable on computed tomographic scans. In one study of 1000 Japanese who had no neurologic findings but were not free of other disease (*e.g.,* hypertension, diabetes, ischemic heart disease), a brain atrophy index was constructed by calculating the ratio for cerebrospinal fluid volume and brain cavity volume.[80] By this measure, atrophy was found to increase logarithmically past age 30 in both sexes. Again in the study, cranial cavity volume was remarkably constant in the different age-groups. The cerebrospinal fluid space volume increased progressively past age 40, as shown in Table 1-4. Cranial cavity volume in all the age brackets was approximately 1050 ml for males and 950 ml for females. Other computed tomographic studies have also shown that dilatation of ventricles up to a certain point appears to be part of normal aging. Because of considerable overlap, it is impossible to draw a distinction between the decrement in brain of the normal elderly individual and that observed in the scans of patients with early and even moderate degrees of dementia.

TABLE 1-4   Brain Cerebrospinal Fluid Space Volume by Age and Sex*

Age	Males	Females
10–19	20.7 ± 10	19.1 ± 8.5
20–29	23.1 ± 10.9	15.4 ± 7.2
30–39	21.0 ± 8.7	15.4 ± 8.7
40–49	32.0 ± 20.4	20.3 ± 10.2
50–59	39.9 ± 25.1	29.3 ± 16.0
60–69	59.6 ± 28.6	43.6 ± 21.7
70–79	84.0 ± 34.1	66.0 ± 28.4
80–89	124.3 ± 63.0	98.1 ± 29.0

* Based on computed tomographic scans of 980 Japanese (Data from Takeda S, Matsuzawa T: Brain atrophy during aging: A quantitative study using computerized tomography. J Am Geriatr Soc 32:520, 1984)

The counting of neurons in microscopic preparations indicates that cellular loss begins even earlier than is suggested by some functional studies. In a classic study, Brody[9] showed that cerebral neuronal loss occurred from the 20s onward, with a total loss of about 30% by age 90. Of considerable importance are the regional variations. There was much loss in the superior temporal gyrus, the precentral gyrus, and the inferior temporal gyrus. Using a computerized scanning analyzer, Henderson and associates[38] estimated a cell loss on the order of 40% to 50% over the life span in pooled counts from 11 cortical areas. Large declines in Purkinje cells[34] and anterior horn neurons also take place with aging. In contrast, the brain stem nuclei, such as the abducens nucleus, with its approximately 6500 cells, show no decrement over the life span.[86]

The loss of cells from the substantia nigra that results in Parkinson's disease is an example of a pathologic regional neuronal loss. What produces the striking regional variations seen with aging is unknown.

It would appear that widespread cell loss associated with aging occurs in all manners of tissues from brain to fat, including such diverse elements as nephrons, hepatocytes, muscle, and even skin structures such as hairs. However, cell loss *per se* may play only a minor part in some age-related declines in organ function; declines in cellular capabilities and reactivities are more important.[51]

AGING AS INVOLUTION

It has long been known that most organs of the healthy aged are smaller than those of youth[8,13,72] (Fig. 1-10). Exceptions are the prostate, lungs, and heart (see Chapter 11). That this decline in organ size is a true one is validated by the parallel findings in laboratory animals followed through their life. Striated muscle, an example of specialized postmitotic cells, is particularly subject to a senescent involution (see Fig. 1-6). This is regarded by Gutmann[33] as a genetic program of cellular death. Although disuse atrophy often plays a role in the shrinking muscle mass of the elderly, the fact that the continually used eye and vocal cord muscles shrink with aging emphasizes the intrinsic nature of the process.[76] Cellular loss and concomitant shrinkage in such widely different tissues as brain, muscle, kidney, even some subcutaneous fat depots, point to a widespread involutionary or degenerative process for which there is at present no unitary explanation.

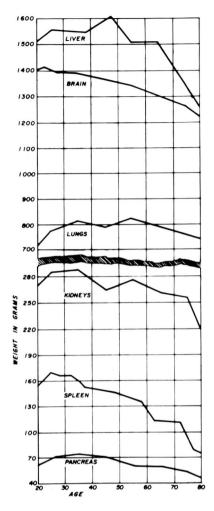

FIG. 1-10. The decrease in weight of body organs with aging. With the exception of the prostate and the heart, all organs shrink with age. This is an anatomical corroboration of the more precise studies based on the counting of intracellular radioactive potassium. (Redrawn from Rössle R, Roulet F: Zahl und Mass in Pathologie. Berlin, Springer-Verlag, 1932)

SIMPLE PARAMETERS FOR AGING

Our most reliable measures of rate of aging include decline in lean body mass as measured by ^{40}K counting, increased cross-linking of the body's collagen molecules, and the dwindling of cell populations in many sites from brain to skin. None of these nor a number of other age-related changes (see Fig. 1-4) answer the clinician's need for some simple parameter to serve as an index to biologic rather than chronologic age. Some that have been suggested are also, interestingly enough, said to be related to coronary artery disease. Thus the arcus senilis, a lipid infiltration of the corneal limbus, tends to progress with aging, though, as noted, it may be found in young blacks. Hickey and associates[40] related the progress of coronary artery disease in 534 males to both age and alcohol intake. There were no positive correlates to total serum lipids, cigarette smoking, or obesity. Rosenman and co-workers[71] in their multivariate analysis found the arcus in younger subjects (ages 39 to 49) to be positively related to increased heart attacks, though this did not hold for their older subjects.

The diagonal ear crease, unilateral and bilateral, is fairly common in whites past 50 and has also been related to an increased rate of myocardial infarction[27,56,] and to increased cardiac complications following anesthesia.[78] In a survey of 1000 admissions to an urban hospital, Elliott concluded that a high degree of correlation did exist between the ear crease and coronary artery disease.[21] Almost simultaneously the opposite conclusion was drawn by Gral and Thornburg.[31] Graying of the hair is one of the classic signs of aging, though quantitative attempts to relate rate of graying to biologic aging or age-related disease are few. Damon[16] in the longitudinal normative aging study found graying to be the most reliable index to biologic age. Keogh and Walsh studied 8720 subjects and found more complete graying appeared earlier in fair than in dark-haired subjects and concluded that for their sample, "it seems a fair approximation to say that at 50 years of age, 50 percent of people are at least 50 percent gray, irrespective of sex or hair color."[50] However, ethnic differences are important and have not been reported in detail. Lasker and Kaplan noted that hair graying occurred later in Mexicans than has been reported for Irish subjects.[54]

CONCLUSION

Visible evidences of the aging process appear with a lamentable inevitability, but fortunately their rate of progress can be quite variable. Thus, it is seldom that graying, diminishing body hair, loss of dermal fat, or the formation of arcus senilis progress in lockstep. Also, some pathologic events mimic aging. Thus, the early onset of idiopathic osteoporosis may lead to the shortening of stature and bowed appearance common in the aged. Atrophy of muscle is often correctly attributable to disuse but also simulates the irreversible shrinking associated with aging. Even that everyday criterion,

wrinkling of the skin of the face, is so accelerated by solar exposure that it is an erratic measuring rod. Clearly, none of these changes, singly or even in small groupings, confirms the existence of significant aging, and the expert may detect them as isolated phenomena not in harmony with the absence of other aging changes.

The existence of localized or regional aging changes implies that to gauge true aging we must look for evidence of a systemic involutionary process, apparently operative at both anatomical and physiologic levels, the somatic mirror of "the force of mortality."[60] An analogy that can be drawn is with the effect of x-rays. Applied to the face, as in the now obsolete treatment of acne, it produced premature aging of the skin accompanied by atrophy and wrinkling. This can be compared with the effects of whole-body irradiation, which leads to aging of the body as a whole.[14]

It becomes apparent that the diagnosis of aging, like the diagnosis of rheumatic fever, has both major and minor criteria, and the existence of one or more findings does not necessarily ensure the presence of others., Even one of our best criteria— the steady decline in the body's potassium content after age 40—is modifiable by exercise and is otherwise quite variable. Some of our long-accepted minor criteria, like the arcus senilis, seem almost too variable to be used as criteria.[57] However, that the arcus is seen in some persons in their 20s may be comparable to an early onset of graying. The occurrence of early onset need not completely invalidate the worth of such criteria. Thus, diminution of elasticity in the crystalline lens and diminution of auditory acuity appear to be aging changes established by the third or fourth decades of life. The conception of aging changes existing in young manhood may be a verbal paradox but not a biologic one.

Pediatricians have long been aware of the variations in growth and maturation in their patient population. One measure of this has been the concept of bone age. Far greater discrepancies between biologic and chronologic age occur at the geriatric end of the scale, discrepancies that are of prime clinical importance. Even though the criteria for aging are singly not hard and fast, collectively they are important not only in assessing the rate of aging but also in having some prognostic value.[6] One would far rather operate on a "young" patient of 80 than an "old" patient of 70. It is a commonly held clinical impression that in long-lived families the onset and progression of aging changes occurs at an identifiably slower pace. Because most of the changes the clinician observes are chiefly ectodermal—regression and degenerative changes in skin, hair, and eyes—and inferentially of the underlying mesenchymal tissue, it is conceivable that they mirror the hypothetical force of aging. Perhaps, as Medawar[60] has pointed out, the gears are in mesh even though the major one that drives the others has not as yet been identified.

The examination of the elderly gives the clinician the opportunity to observe at first hand the entropy produced by the force of mortality, as distinct from acute and chronic pathologic events. It leads to the tentative conclusion that if we project the curve of our slow geriatric therapeutics, we can still foresee the area in which, even if disease does not progress, aging will. Thus, if the human's unfortunate tendency to sclerose is prevented, the bone is protected against demineralization by fluorides or other agents, and the skin is sheltered against all exogenous aging factors, a recognizably old human will still emerge.

REFERENCES

1. Andres R: Effect of obesity on total mortality. Int J Obesity 4:381, 1980
2. Andrew W: The Anatomy of Aging in Man and Animals, p 259. New York, Grune & Stratton, 1971
3. Basilevich I: The Medical Aspects of Natural Old Age: An Introduction to Clinical Gerontology, p 317. Munich, 1958. Also privately printed, Howard, Rhode Island, 1959. Rhode Island State Hospital, 1959
4. Bennett GA, Waine H, Bauer W: Changes in the Knee Joint at Various Ages—with Particular Reference to the Nature and Development of Degenerative Joint Disease, p 97. New York, The Commonwealth Fund, 1942
5. Blinkov SM, Glezer II: The Human Brain in Figures and Tables. New York, Basic Books, 1968
6. Borkan GA, Norris AH: Assessment of biological age using a profile of physical parameters. Gerontol 35:177, 1980
7. Borkan GA, Hults DE, Gerzof SG, Robbins AH, Silbert CK: Age changes in body composition revealed by computed tomography. Gerontol 38:673, 1983
8. Bourlière F: The Assessment of Biological Age in Man. Public Health Papers, No. 37. Geneva, World Health Organization, 1970
9. Brody H; Organization of cerebral cortex: III. A study of aging in human cerebral cortex. J Comp Neurol 102:511, 1955
10. Brown OT, Wigzell FW: The significance of span as a clinical measurement. In Anderson WF, Isaacs B (eds): Current Achievements in Geriatrics, pp 246–251. London, Cassell & Co, 1964
11. Büchi EC: Änderung der Körperform beim erwachsenen Menschen, eine Untersuchung nach der Individual-Methode. Anthrop Forsch, Heft 1. Anthrop Gesel, Wien, 1950
12. Burmeister W, Bingért A: Die quantitativen Veränderungen der menschlichen Zellmasse zwischen dem 8 und 90 Lebensjahr. Klin Wochenschr 45:409, 1967
13. Calloway NO, Foley CF, Lagerbloom P: Uncertainties in geriatric data: II. Organ size. J Am Geriatr Soc 13:20, 1965
14. Curtis HJ: Biological Mechanisms of Aging, p 113. Springfield, IL, Charles C Thomas, 1966
15. Damon A: Secular trend in height and weight within old American families at Harvard 1870–1965: I. Within twelve four-generation families. Am J Phys Anthropol 29:45, 1968
16. Damon A: Predicting age from body measurements and observations. Aging Human Dev 3:169, 1972
17. Damon A, Seltzer CC, Stoudt HW, Bell B: Age and physique in healthy white veterans at Boston. Aging Human Dev 3:202, 1972
18. Davis PJM, Wright EA: A new method for measuring cranial cavity volume and its application to the assessment of cerebral atrophy at autopsy. Neuropathol Appl Neurobiol 3:341, 1977
19. Dequeker JV, Baeyens JP, Claessens J.: The significance of stature as a clinical measurement of aging. J Am Geriatr Soc 17:169, 1969
20. Edge JR, Millard FJC, Reid L, Simon G: The radiographic appearance of the chest in persons of advanced age. Br J Radiol 37:769, 1964
21. Elliott WJ: Earlobe crease and coronary artery disease: 1000 patients and review of the literature. Am J Med 75:1024, 1983
22. Epker BN, Frost HM: Periosteal appositional bone growth from age two to age seventy in man: A tetracycline evaluation. Anat Rec 154, 573, 1966
23. Fitzpatrick TB, Szabo G, Mitchell RE: Age changes in the human melanocyte system. In Montagna W (ed): Advances in Biology of Skin Aging, 6th ed, pp 35–50. New York, Pergamon Press, 1965
24. Fleischer K: Das Alternde Ohr. Aesthet Med 16:95, 1967
25. Forbes GB: The adult decline in lean body mass. Hum Biol 48:161, 1976
26. Forbes GB, Reina JC: Adult lean body mass declines with age: Some longitudinal observations. Metabolism 19:653, 1970
27. Frank ST: Aural sign of cornary artery disease. N Engl J Med 289:327, 1973
28. Garn SM, Robmann CG, Wagner B, Ascoli W: Continuing bone growth throughout life: A general phenomenon. Am J Phys Anthropol 26:313, 1967
29. Garn SM, Young RW: Concurrent fat loss and fat gain. Am J Phys Anthropol 14:497, 1956
30. Gerstenblith G, Frederiksen J, Yin FCP, Fortuin NJ, Lakatta EG, Weisfeldt ML: Echocardiographic assessment of a normal adult aging population. Circulation 56:273, 1977
31. Gral T, Thornburg M: Earlobe creases in a cohort of elderly veterans. J Am Geriatr Soc 31:134, 1983

32. Graves WW: Observations on age changes in the scapula. Am J Phys Anthropol 5:21, 1922

33. Gutmann E: Muscle. In Finch C, Hayflick L (eds): Handbook of Biology of Aging, pp 445–469. New York, Van Nostrand Reinhold, 1977

34. Hall TG, Miller AKH, Corsellis JAN: Variations in the human Purkinje cell population according to age and sex. Neuropathol Appl Neurobiol 1:267, 1975

35. Hamilton JB: Age, sex, and genetic factors in the regulation of hair growth in man: A comparison of Caucasian and Japanese populations. In Montagna W, Ellis RA (eds): Biology of Hair Growth, pp 399–433. New York, Academic Press, 1958

36. Haranghy L (ed): Gerontological Studies on Hungarian Centenarians, p 166. Budapest, Akademiai Kiado, 1965

37. Hejda S: Skinfold in old and longlived individuals. Gerontologia 8:201, 1963

38. Henderson G, Tomlinson BE, Gibson PH: Cell counts in human cerebral cortex in normal adults throughout life using an image analyzing computer. J Neurol Sci 46:113, 1980

39. Herrmann JB: Personal communication, 1970

40. Hickey N, Maurer B, Mulcahy R: Arcus senilis: Its relation to certain attributes and risk factors in patients with coronary heart disease. Br Heart J 32:449, 1970

41. Hollifield G, Parson W: Overweight in the aged. Am J Clin Nutr 7:127, 1959

42. Honig EI, Dubilier W, Steinberg I: Significance of the buckled innominate artery. Ann Intern Med 39:74, 1953

43. Hooton EA, Dupertuis CW: Age changes and selective survival in Irish males. In Studies in Physical Anthropology, vol 2. American Association of Physical Anthropologists and Wenner-Gren Foundation, 1951

44. Howells WW: Age and Individuality in Vertebral Lipping: Notes on Stewart's data. Homenaje a Juan Comas, vol 2. Mexico City, Instituto Indigenista Interamericano, 1965

45. Imamura K, Ashida H, Ishikawa T, Fujii M: Human major psoas muscle and sacrospinalis muscle in relation to age: A study by computed tomography. J Gerontol 38:678, 1983

46. Ingelmark BE, Gustafsson L: The aging of calf muscles in women, a morphological and roentgenological study. Acta Morphol Neerl Scand 1:173, 1957

47. Israel H: Continuing growth in the human cranial skeleton. Arch Oral Biol 13:133, 1968

48. Israel H: Continuing growth in sella turcica with aging. Am J Roentgenol Radium Ther Nucl Med 108:516, 1970

49. Israel H: Age factor and the pattern of change in craniofacial structures. Am J Phys Anthropol 39:111, 1973

50. Keogh EV, Walsh RS: Rate of greying of human hair. Nature 207:877, 1965

51. Knook DL: Organ ageing in relation to cellular aging, p 213. In Viidik A (ed): Lectures on Gerontology, vol. 1, On Biology of Aging. London, Academic Press 1982

52. Korenchevsky V: Physiological and Pathological Aging, p 514. New York, Hafner, 1961

53. Lakatta EG: Alterations in the cardiovascular system that occur in advanced age. Fed Proc 38:163, 1979

54. Lasker GW, Kaplan B: Graying of the hair and mortality. Soc Biol 21:290, 1974

55. Lee MMC, Lasker GW: The thickness of subcutaneous fat in elderly men. Am J Phys Anthropol 16:125, 1958

56. Lichtstein E, Chadda KD, Naik P, Gupta PK: Diagonal ear-lobe crease: Prevalence and implications as a coronary risk factor. N Engl J Med 290:615, 1974

57. Macaraeg PVJ Jr, Lasagna L, Snyder B: Arcus not so senilis. Ann Intern Med 68:2, 345, 1968

58. McKeown F: Pathology of the Aged. London, Butterworth & Co, 1965

59. Master AN, Lasser RP, Beckman G: Tables of average weight and height of Americans, aged 65 to 94 years etc. JAMA 172:658, 1960

60. Medawar PB: The Definition and Measurement of Senescence—Ciba Foundation Colloquia on Aging, vol 1, p 4. Boston, Little, Brown & Co, 1955

61. Melick R, Taft P: Observations on body hair in old people. J Clin Endocrinol Metab 19:1575, 1959

62. Meneely GR, Heyssel RM, Ball COT, Weiland RL, Lorimer AR, Constantinides C, Meneely EU: Analysis of factors affecting body composition determined from potassium content in 915 normal subjects. Ann NY Acad Sci 110:271, 1963

63. Merz AL, Trotter M, Peterson RR: Estimation of skeleton weight in the living. Am J Phys Anthropol 14:589, 1956

64. Miall WE, Ashcroft MT, Lovell HG, Moore F: A longitudinal study of the decline of adult height with age in two Welsh communities. Hum Biol 39:445, 1967

65. Moore FD: The Body Cell Mass and Its Supporting Environment, p 535. Philadelphia, WB Saunders, 1963

66. Nascher IL: The Diseases of Old Age and Their Treatment, Geriatrics, pp 36, 517. Philadelphia, P Blakiston & Son, 1914

67. Nathan H: Osteophytes of the vertebral column. J Bone Joint Surg 44:243, 1962

68. Oberhausen E, Onstead CO: Relationship of potassium content of man with age and sex. In Radioactivity in Man, pp 179–185. Springfield, IL, Charles C Thomas, 1965

69. Parot S: Recherches sur la biométrie du vieillissement humain. Bull Mém Soc Anthropol 299, 1961

70. Pierson RN Jr, Lin DHY, Phillips RA: Total body potassium in health: Effects of age, sex, height and fat. Am J Physiol 226:206, 1974

71. Rosenman RH, Brand RJ, Sholtz RI, Friedman M: Multivariate prediction of coronary heart disease

during 8.5-year follow-up in the western collaborative group study. Am J Cardiol 37:903, 1976

72. Rössle R, Roulet F: Zahl und Mass in Pathologie. Berlin, Springer-Verlag, 1932
73. Rossman I: Anatomic and body composition changes with aging. In Finch C, Hayflick L (eds): Handbook of Biology of Aging, pp 189–221. New York, Van Nostrand Reinhold, 1977
74. Ryan TJ: The microcirculation of the skin in old age. Gerontol Clin 8:327, 1966
75. Ryckewaert A, Parot S, Tamisier S, Bourlière F: Variations, selon l'âge et le sexe, de l'epaisseur du pli cutané mesuré au dos de la main. Rev Fr Etudes Clin Biol 12:803, 1967
76. Sato T, Tauchi H: Age changes in human vocal muscle. Mech Ageing Dev 18:67, 1982
77. Smith KS: The kinked innominate vein. Br. Heart J 22:110, 1960
78. Sprague DH: Diagonal ear-lobe crease as an indicator of operative risk. Anesthesiology 45:363, 1976
79. Stoudt HW, Damon A, McFarland RA, Roberts J: Weight, height, and selected body measurements of adults—US 1960–62. Public Health Service, publication 1000, series 11, No. 8. Washington, DC, US Government Printing Office, 1965
80. Takeda S, Matsuzawa T: Brain atrophy during aging: A quantitative study using computerized tomography. J Am Geriatr Soc 32:520, 1984
81. Thomas PK, Ferriman DG: Variation in facial and pubic hair growth in white women. Am J Phys Anthropol 15:171, 1957
82. Todd TW: Thickness of the male white cranium. Anat Rec 27:245, 1924
83. Todd TW, Lyons DW Jr: Endocranial suture closure: Its progress and age relationship: I. Adult males of white stock. Am J Phys Anthropol 7:325, 1924
84. Trotter M, Gleser G: The effect of aging on stature. Am J Phys Anthropol 9:311, 1951
85. Trotter M, Gleser G: Trends in stature of American whites and Negroes born between 1840 and 1924. Am J Phys Anthropol 9:427, 1951
86. Vijayashankar N, Brody H: A study of aging in the human abducens nucleus. J Comp Neurol 173:433, 1977
87. Wessel JA, Ufer A, VanHuss WD, Cederquist D: Age trends of various components of body composition and functional characteristics in women aged 20–69 years. Ann NY Acad Sci 110:608, 1963

2

Patterns of Age Changes

Paul T. Costa, Jr., and Reubin Andres

The dominant model of aging is one of universal decline in all functions, physiologic and psychological. We will show that such a model is a serious distortion and, at best, a major oversimplification. The facts are that all functions and organ systems do not show decline. Some functions show great stability, while others show improvements. Moreover, it is incorrect to attribute lower levels of functioning to biologic aging when they are in fact caused by disease. Finally, even when functions do show decline, averages or group means obscure and even mask the noteworthy variability among different individuals of the same age.

In this brief chapter we summarize some of the major themes and findings that have emerged from the Baltimore Longitudinal Study of Aging (BLSA). The first section acknowledges the importance of the specificity of aging processes, and the second identifies five patterns of change important for an adequate understanding of aging processes. For an extended discussion of the many cross-sectional and longitudinal studies and findings the reader is referred to *Normal Human Aging* by Shock and colleagues.[13] A number of questions about physiologic, psychological, and psychosocial variables in the processes of aging are considered in that text, which can be viewed as a progress report on the first quarter-century of the Baltimore Longitudinal Study.

SPECIFICITY AND INDIVIDUALITY OF AGING

Aging cannot be equated with a disease or disorder, nor should there be hope for a "magic bullet" that will cure it or stop it. In the past 20 years most gerontologists have recognized the distinctly limited use of a simple and sovereign notion of aging. Instead of hypothesizing a unitary or unicausal process of aging, researchers have emphasized the need to consider the interacting influences of biologic processes, personality and behavioral factors, social and environmental forces, and idiosyncratic health behaviors and stresses of the individual. The BLSA experience has revealed the complexity of aging processes. Instead of a single underlying mechanism, aging is now regarded as reflecting the expression of a host of processes that independently and in concert bring about the changes we recognize as aging.

The BLSA experience indicates that aging is a highly individual process. Although cross-sectional observations show a significant decline in many physiologic variables over the total age span, individual differences are very large. For some variables, individual 80-year-old subjects may perform as well as the average 50-year-old. A recent longitudinal study on creatinine clearance illustrates this principle.[10] Although, on the average, longitudinal decline in renal function is striking (Fig. 2-1, *top panel*), there are marked individual variations. There is a small percentage of individuals who show no decline in creatinine clearance over a period of many years and indeed show statistically significant, albeit small, increases in function with time (Fig. 2-1, *bottom panel*). Aging is highly specific not only for each individual but also for each organ system within the individual.

Because of the high degree of specificity of aging among different subjects and among different organ systems, chronologic age itself is not a very reliable predictor of performance in individual adults. Recognition of this great diversity may prove of value in devising interventions to improve

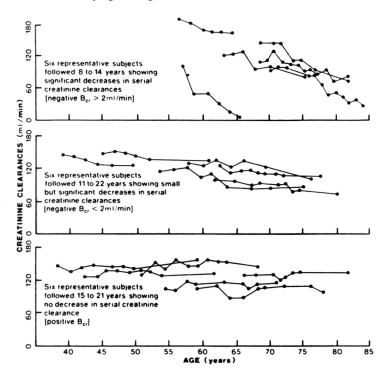

FIG. 2-1. Individual plots of serial creatinine clearance versus age in years for representative subjects.

performance in normal aging subjects. Although no single treatment is likely to be discovered that will improve various kinds of performance in all or most persons, a variety of different interventions or treatments tailored to critical personal characteristics might be developed.

The discrete character of various physiologic and behavioral functions has been confirmed by several analyses that have found no general aging factor.[1,2] The conclusions—that there is no single process of aging and that so-called physiological indices of aging provide no better predictors of individual performance than chronological age[3]— justify the BLSA's choice of a multidisciplinary and multivariate approach.

PATTERNS OF CHANGE WITH AGE

From the research results of the BLSA, we can readily conclude that there is no one uniform age course for all variables. The evidence is conclusive that there is a variety of changes with age. The changes that have been documented fall into five main categories:

1. Stability, or absence of change
2. Change that results from disease
3. Compensatory change
4. Secular change
5. Change intrinsic to aging

The Absence of Change

An obvious example of a physiologic function that remains stable across the age-span is resting heart rate, although most functions that show little or no change with aging (or change only very late in life) are predominantly psychosocial. In the personality arena, a substantial number of investigators unanimously agree that individuals change very little in self-reported personality traits over periods of up to 30 years and over the age range from 30 to 90. The degree of individual consistency in personality traits over time is shown by re-test correlations, or stability coefficients, that assess the magnitude of personality consistency or change in the relative ordering of individuals in a group (regardless of absolute level). Only repeated testing of the same individuals can speak to the degree of stability of individual differences. The consistency of personality in men from the BLSA over 12 years as tested by the Guilford-Zimmerman Temperament Survey (GZTS) is shown in Table 2-1.[4]

These results are typical of a body of studies that obtain similar results using a variety of different measures and a variety of different samples

TABLE 2-1   Twelve-year Re-test Coefficients for Guilford-Zimmerman Temperament Survey Scales in Different Age-groups

		AGE		
SCALE	**TOTAL (20-76)**	*Young (20-44)*	*Middle (45-59)*	*Old (60-76)*
General activity	.77 (192)	.77 (60)	.82 (93)	.78 (39)
Restraint	.72 (193)	.61 (62)	.74 (94)	.76 (37)
Ascendance	.83 (194)	.85 (62)	.85 (95)	.77 (37)
Sociability	.74 (182)	.64 (62)*	.81 (88)	.66 (32)
Emotional stability	.70 (203)	.63 (68)	.76 (96)	.71 (39)
Objectivity	.69 (191)	.66 (64)	.76 (87)	.59 (40)
Friendliness	.74 (193)	.74 (64)†	.68 (88)‡	.87 (41)
Thoughtfulness	.73 (199)	.78 (64)	.71 (94)	.71 (41)
Personal relations	.68 (188)	.70 (62)	.64 (89)	.73 (37)
Masculinity	.72 (200)	.73 (66)	.71 (94)	.70 (40)
M stability	.73	.72	.75	.73

Note: *n*s are given in parentheses; numbers in parentheses in column headings are age at first time. All correlations significant at $p < .001$.
 * Difference between young and middle significant at $p < .05$.
 † Difference between young and old significant at $p < .05$.
 ‡ Difference between middle and old significant at $p < .01$.

(for women as well as men, in other countries besides the United States, and for adolescents as well as older adults). McCrae and Costa[11] offer a detailed and extensive review of the evidence from large-scale longitudinal studies conducted over the past 40 years that documents the consistency or stability of personality through adulthood and older ages. The findings that personality is relatively unchanging and that cognitive functions decline only late in life point to the need to identify the underlying mechanisms by which stability is maintained and change occurs.

Change That Results From Disease

The second pattern of change is characterized by declines with age that are not due to aging *per se* but to illnesses associated with age. Thus, although earlier studies reported a significant decline in plasma-testosterone levels with age, analyses performed on subjects who were carefully screened for disease revealed no such age differences among healthy men.[6] Similarly, cardiac output, both at rest and at maximal exercise, does not decline with age, provided subjects are screened for coronary artery disease by treadmill stress testing with thallium scanning. The percentage of BLSA subjects aged 51 to 90 years with clinically detectable coronary disease is only 13% to 20% but jumps to 24% to 50% when results of stress testing with

thallium scanning are added to the results of the history and physical examination. The pervasive occurrence of such occult disease mandates that comprehensive screening is essential if true age changes are to be disentangled from effects of disease on performance and functioning (secondary aging).

Changes that occur precipitously in old age represent a variant of this pattern; such changes are often expressions of acute disease processes. Sudden decrements in function, whether physiologic, psychological, or—as in dementia—a combination of the two, should serve as a warning sign for practitioners, alerting them to the need for therapeutic intervention. For researchers in all fields of gerontology and geriatrics, the task is to identify the patterns of pathology that are likely to be manifest and to weigh the comparative merits of various interventions.

Compensatory Change

In its study of both physiologic and psychological functions the BLSA has found evidence of changes that in part compensate for declines that accompany aging. Two examples of compensatory change can be considered: the first involves only one system, and the second illustrates how decline in one system can be offset by compensatory change in another system. The example of a compensatory mechanism at work within a single organ system occurs with physical exercise. Despite the decrease in maximal heart rate with age, cardiac output is maintained by a compensatory change—dilation of the heart with consequent increase in stroke volume, a recruitment of the Frank-Starling mechanism.[9] The example of a compensatory multisystem change involves the hypothalamic–posterior pituitary–renal axis for the conservation of water. Intravenous infusion of hypertonic saline (3%) in BLSA participants created a condition of hyperosmolality, a challenge to the hypothalamic-pituitary system. The increase in serum osmolality, from 290 mOsm to 306 mOsm/kg, was the same in older as in younger subjects, despite the fact that overall renal function decreases with age. Under this infusion condition, the need to conserve water loss is met by posterior pituitary secretion of the antidiuretic hormone, arginine vasopressin.[7] The responses of arginine vasopressin in older subjects significantly exceeded that of younger adults (4.5- vs. 2.5-fold increase over basal). Thus, the age decline in one system—renal function—is compensated for by an age increase in another system—the hypothalamic-pituitary system.

Other compensatory changes may result either from voluntary action (*e.g.*, a person stops smoking) or from adjustments of which he is unaware (*e.g.*, a deficit in learning and memory is in part offset by an increase in knowledge). Identification of the mechanisms by which such change occurs and an understanding of how they work suggest possible interventions to enhance the quality of life of the elderly, a development that becomes more urgent as our elderly population continues to increase.

Secular Change

Secular change occurs with the passage of time and has little or nothing to do with age, or with health and disease, but reflects changes that are of importance in interpreting research data on aging. A clear example of change that affects a whole population irrespective of age (and thus of birth cohort) is the wholesale decline of serum cholesterol levels found in subjects in the BLSA.[8]

Studies of many populations have shown that the age curve of serum cholesterol is that of an inverted U, rising from early adult to middle age and then falling in the late years of life. Since elevated cholesterol levels are associated with increased mortality rates, it is possible that the late life fall in average cholesterol levels represents an

example of the influence of selective mortality: individuals with high values die first, leaving survivors in old age with low levels. Longitudinal analysis of the changes in cholesterol during the years 1963 through 1971 (Fig. 2-2, *upper panel*) showed, however, that the fall in the later years was not due to selective mortality. In fact, the mean slopes for the individual age decades followed the cross-sectional pattern very accurately. In the years 1969 through 1977, however, a remarkable difference in pattern occurred (Fig. 2-2, *lower panel*). Here every age-group showed a marked decline in cholesterol. The overall pattern differed sharply from the cross-sectional picture.

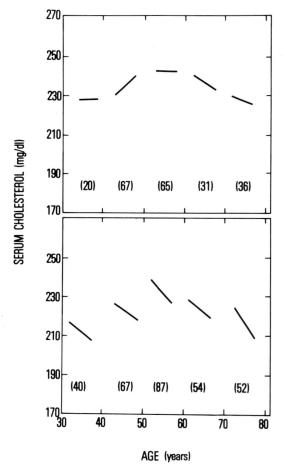

FIG. 2-2. Longitudinal changes in serum cholesterol concentration. Upper panel shows mean slopes for individual age-groups during the years 1963 through 1971; the slopes closely follow the cross-sectional pattern. Lower panel shows slopes derived during the years 1969 through 1977; the slope for each age-group declines, forming a dissimilar pattern from the cross-sectional age trend.

Clearly, the changes in those years had to be caused by a secular factor or an exogenous effect on the cholesterol level. Unfortunately, efforts to identify more precisely the nature of those effects (the "epidemiologic search for an etiology" as the authors put it) did not succeed.

Longitudinal study of dietary patterns has shown some additional changes with time that affect the whole cohort. Using the technique of the 7-day dietary diary, Elahi and colleagues[5] presented a detailed analysis of several dietary constituents using a schema that efficiently presents the actual values obtained in numerous age-groups over several time periods, permitting cross-sectional, longitudinal, and time-series analyses of the data. The schema for one of the dietary variables, the polyunsaturated/saturated fatty acid ratio, is shown in Figure 2-3 as an illustration of the analytical complexities involved in attempts to unravel changes that occur with time. The results are characteristic of secular changes. When these data are plotted (Fig. 2-4) by connecting data points for each of the eight birth cohorts, the pattern is one of uniformly sharply rising values with time. The discontinuity of the resulting slopes is similar to the discontinuity reflected in the serum cholesterol

values of the 1970s; this is in contrast to the continuity pattern described by values for creatinine clearance.

The primary nutrients, protein, carbohydrate, and fat, expressed as percentages of the total caloric intake, show differing patterns with age (Fig. 2-5). The protein fraction is remarkably constant at 15% to 16%. Intake of carbohydrate and fat is identical in the youngest age-group (42% each), but with increasing age there is a tendency to increase the carbohydrate fraction with a compensatory decrease in the fat fraction.

Change Intrinsic to Aging

The last pattern of change describes steady decline in functioning despite good health or the absence of disease; creatinine clearance is a classic illustration of intrinsic change. Studies of renal function also illustrate the difficulty in differentiating true age changes from those secondary to disease. Cross-sectional studies of the 24-hour creatinine clearance (an index of the kidney's glomerular filtration rate) in humans show a progressive decline from early to late adult life. Primary diseases of the urinary system, as well as many diseases of

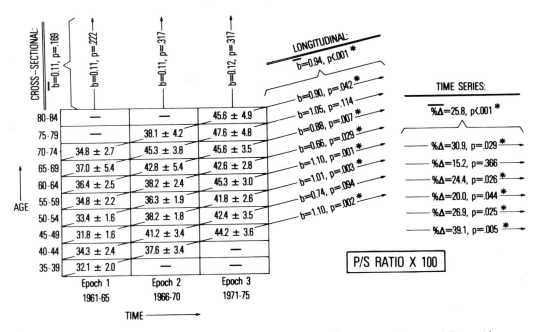

FIG. 2-3. Schema for presentation of longitudinal data: dietary polyunsaturated/saturated fatty acid ratio X 100. Data are presented for each of eight age cohorts over three epochs of time. The mean P/S ratios are presented in each box. Analyses are presented for (1) cross-sectional age differences (vertical dimension), (2) longitudinal age changes (upward slanting dimension), and (3) time-series changes (horizontal dimension).

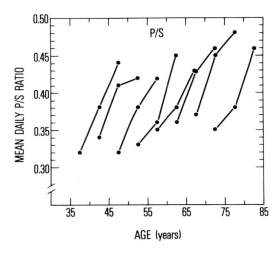

FIG. 2-4. Longitudinal changes in dietary polyunsaturated/saturated (P/S) fatty acid ratio. An increase in the ratio occurred in each of the eight age cohorts.

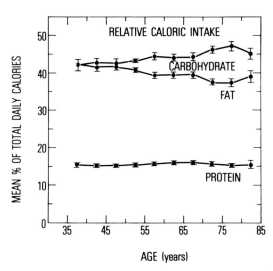

FIG. 2-5. Mean percent of total daily calories from specified nutrient, by age and epochs combined.

other organ systems that could secondarily cause a decline in clearance, occur with increasing frequency with age. Thus, the age differences shown by these cross-sectional studies could reflect simply the declining health status of individuals rather than true biologic aging effects on the kidney. To test this possibility, Rowe and his colleagues[12] meticulously performed a ''clinical clean-up'' of the population in order to eliminate all individuals with evidence of any disorder or medication that could influence this physiologic function. The results showed that there was a sharp decline in creatinine clearance not only cross-sectionally but also longitudinally (Fig. 2-6).

Finally, it is necessary to examine causal mechanisms to understand the true nature of aging changes. An additional complexity in the interpretation of physiologic data is that of the appropriate reference base. Numerous cross-sectional studies have shown marked decline in total body oxygen consumption under basal conditions. This is true whether the oxygen consumption was expressed per whole body, per kilogram of body weight or per square meter body surface area. The use of body size as a reference, however, assumes that all tissues contribute equally to body metabolism. In reality, adipose, bone, and connective tissues have very low oxygen demands in comparison with other tissues' greater oxygen consumption. Since the major oxygen-consuming tissue of the body, even under basal conditions, is muscle, this decline in the basal metabolic rate could be due to a change in body composition. Tzankoff and Nor-

ris,[14] therefore, made estimates of muscle mass from the 24-hour urinary creatinine excretion rate. They showed a progressive loss of muscle mass with increasing age (Fig. 2-7). Thus the basal metabolic rate drop could simply reflect a relative loss of active metabolizing tissue with a gain in relatively poorly metabolizing tissues, especially adipose tissue.

CONCLUSION

One of the fundamental endeavors of the BLSA has been to study the effects of aging as distinct from those of disease. Routine medical examinations have been supplemented by diagnostic procedures, such as stress testing, that make it possible to identify deseases that would otherwise remain occult. Screening for these illnesses allows investigators to study aging in large samples in the absence of clinically detectable illness. At the same time, longitudinal data from individuals who develop specific conditions can be used to follow the course of those diseases.

Analysis of BLSA longitudinal data indicates that a precipitous drop in any physiologic or behavioral function is likely to be a manifestation of a pathologic condition. A corollary is the hypothesis that, in variables that remain essentially stable over the adult life span, any significant change may be a manifestation of pathology. Further study of this hypothesis will be an important part of future BLSA analyses.

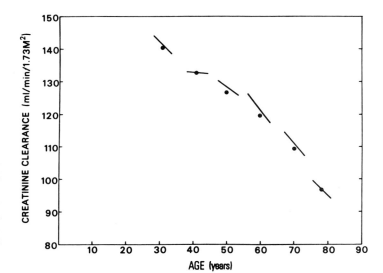

FIG. 2-6. Comparison of cross-sectional age differences and longitudinal age changes in creatinine clearance. The longitudinal changes (the six individual slopes) follow the cross-sectional results (the black dots) quite closely. Declines in renal function occurred in subjects with no evidence of renal disease.

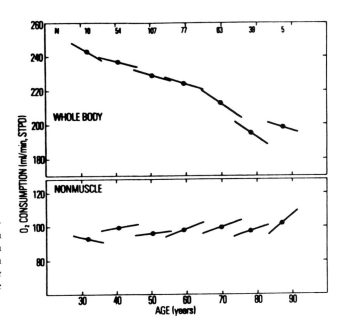

FIG. 2-7. Mean changes with age in whole-body and nonmuscle oxygen consumption in basal state. The decline in whole-body oxygen consumption contrasts to the stability of oxygen consumption of nonmuscle tissues. The decline in basal metabolic rate with age is attributable to a change in body composition with age (*i.e.,* a loss of muscle mass).

BLSA researchers are generating a large data base with numerous serial measurements that invite sophisticated investigations of questions about aging. The findings of the BLSA contained in *Normal Human Aging* now constitute a kind of gerontologic agenda for the future. The work of the BLSA is just beginning.

REFERENCES

1. Borkan GA: The Assessment of Biological Age During Adulthood, dissertation. Ann Arbor, University of Michigan, 1978
2. Costa PT Jr, McCrae RR: Functional age: A conceptual and empirical critique. In Haynes SG, Feinleib M (eds): Proceedings of the Second Conference on Epidemiology of Aging, pp 23–47. Bethesda, MD, National Institute on Aging, 1980
3. Costa PT Jr, McCrae RR: Concepts of functional or biological age: A critical view. In Andres R, Bierman EL, Hazzard WR (eds): Principles of Geriatric Medicine, pp 30–37. New York, McGraw-Hill, 1985
4. Costa PT Jr, McCrae RR, Arenberg D: Enduring dispositions in adult males. J Pers Soc Psychol 38:793–800, 1980
5. Elahi VK, Elahi D, Andres R, Tobin JD, Butler NG, Norris AH: A longitudinal study of nutritional intake in men. J Gerontol 38:162–180, 1983
6. Harman SM, Tsitouras PD: Reproductive hormones in aging men: I. Measurement of sex steroids, basal luteinizing hormone, and Leydig response to human chorionic gonadotropin. J Clin Endocrinol Metab 51:35–40, 1980
7. Helderman JH, Vestal RE, Rowe JW, Tobin JD, Andres R, Robertson G: The response of arginine vasopressin to intravenous ethanol and hypertonic saline in man: The impact of aging. J Gerontol 33:39–47, 1978
8. Hershcopf RJ, Elahi D, Andres R, Baldwin HL, Raizes GS, Schoken DD, Tobin JD: Longitudinal changes in serum cholesterol in man: An epidemiologic search for an etiology. J Chronic Dis 35:101-114, 1982
9. Lakatta, EG: Length of modulation of muscle performance: The Frank-Starling law of the heart. In Fozzard HM, Haber E, Jennings RB, Katz AM, Morgan HE (eds): Handbook of Experimental Cardiology. New York, Raven Press, in press
10. Lindeman RS, Tobin JD, Shock NW: Rates of decline in renal function with age. J Am Geriatr Soc 33:278, 1985
11. McCrae RR, Costa PT Jr: Emerging Lives, Enduring Dispositions: Personality in Adulthood, p 142. Boston, Little, Brown & Co, 1984
12. Rowe, JW, Andres R, Tobin, JD, Norris AH, Shock NW: The effect of age on creatinine clearance in men: A cross-sectional and longitudinal study. J Gerontol 31:155–163, 1976
13. Shock NW, Greulich RC, Andres RA, Arenberg D, Costa PT Jr, Lakatta EW, Tobin JD: Normal Human Aging: The Baltimore Longitudinal Study of Aging, publication No. 84-2450. Bethesda, MD, National Institute of Health, 1984
14. Tzankoff SP, Norris AH: Longitudinal changes in basal metabolism in man. J Appl Physiol 45:536–539, 1978

3

Aging at the Cellular Level

Keith R. Latham and Lorin K. Johnson

Most gerontologists are optimistic that during the next 10 years we will see a rapid increase in our understanding of the basic aging processes and that these insights will find increasing therapeutic expression in geriatric medicine with more emphasis on preventive measures. Owing to the integration of body functions by the endocrine, immune, and nervous systems, many age-related changes are the result of a sequence of causal events that leads to a final, often complex pattern of pathologic and eugeric expression. It is probable that primary aging events occur quite early in life and that even developmental processes set the stage for the decline and, ultimately, the death of the organism. It is therefore appropriate to discuss the causes and the effects of aging in the context of the processes of differentiation and development.

A fundamental tenet in gerontology is that age-dependent processes (including pathologic ones) have some set of cellular processes that form an etiologic rubric; the cellular sequence that can ultimately lead to cell death (differentiation → mitostasis → biochemical decline → cell death) is causal to the organism's life-cycle program (development → maturity → physiologic decline → organism death).

COMPARATIVE GERONTOLOGY AND AGING POPULATIONS

One of the universal principles of aging is that various animal and plant species have different life spans. The fact that humans live longer than mice seems commonplace, but from a biologist's view, it is astounding that the life span of different mammalian species can vary by 86-fold (between mice and humans).[28] This fact supports the conclusion that the mechanism that modulates the life span is intrinsic to the organism rather than to a set of external factors that would be nearly the same for all species.

In the total diversity of life on earth, plants and animals have developed highly divergent patterns of aging in response to very different selection pressures. The aphagous insects that die because they cannot eat (they lack a functional digestive system) should not be considered in the same context with human aging or aging in certain plant species that maintain a structural identity for thousands of years.[29] The major mammalian species diverged only 30 to 40 million years ago. Yet, even different mammals have developed significant physiologic diversity. For instance, bats and other animals that hibernate probably live longer by spending a considerable part of their lives in minimal metabolic states.[11] Thus, aging in each species should be considered within the framework of its reproductive cycle and its environmental constraints. In this chapter we will emphasize aging in mammals or mammalian cells in culture.

The various life spans of mammals seem to have evolved as an evolutionary compromise between the stress of the environment and reproductive capacity (fecundity). For example, there is a correlation between fecundity and maximum life span of various mammalian species (Fig. 3-1).[19,112,127] However, the average life span of monotocous mammals (averaging close to one offspring per birth), including monkeys, horses, whales, elephants, and humans, appears to form a component that is separate from animals that have litters (polytocous). It is probable that certain animals have evolved extremely adaptive structures, such as advanced brains, or have discovered

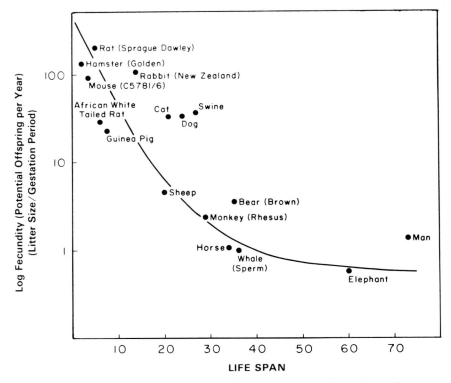

FIG. 3-1. Relationship between the maximal reproductive rate (fecundity) and average life span for various mammalian species. Monotocous and polytocous animals appear to form separate correlation components. (Data from Comfort A: The Biology of Senescence. New York, Holt, Rinehart & Winston, 1956; Rockstein, M, Chesky JA, Sussman MJ: Comparative biology and evolution of aging. In Finch C, Hayflick L [eds]: Handbook of the Biology of Aging. New York, Van Nostrand Reinhold, 1977; and Sigmund OH [ed]: The Merck Veterinary Manual, 3rd ed. Rahway, NJ, Merck & Co, 1967)

an especially forgiving environmental niche and thereby escaped high predation. Improved parental care, for instance, could supplant high fecundity; an extended life span would then be selected to permit an optimal period of offspring rearing as well as a sufficient number of reproductive cycles. Thus, the process of aging appears to be tightly coupled to reproduction.

Additional support for tight coupling of reproduction and life span comes from experiments originally performed by McCay[86] in which the life span of rats was doubled by starvation. He found that only the prepubertal developmental program could be extended by the starvation regimen.[9]

If the number of surviving organisms from a large population of a single species is measured as a function of time (age), several different parameters relating to species-specific life span and environmental stress can be deduced. Figure 3-2 shows these data plotted as a survivorship curve. The maximum life span is the projection of the

curve to the abscissa (about 120 years in humans) and is remarkably constant for a given species, excluding certain genetic diseases in highly inbred subpopulations. The average life span (the average age of death) can vary and is dependent on the degree of environmental stress and, in the limit, on the maximum life span. In addition, the shape of the survivorship curve gives a good measure of the degree of environmental stress. In India in 1925 many persons died of disease early in life (see Fig. 3-2). By contrast, the relatively "squared off" curve representing the United States in 1940 indicates a higher rate of survival into late life. Throughout recorded history, the average life span of humans has increased from about 20 years (500 BC in Greece[125]) to about 73 (69 in men, 77 in women) years in the United States today. This has been due mostly to decreased infant mortality. During this same period, with infectious diseases largely eliminated in some populations, the estimated maximum life span has lengthened by less

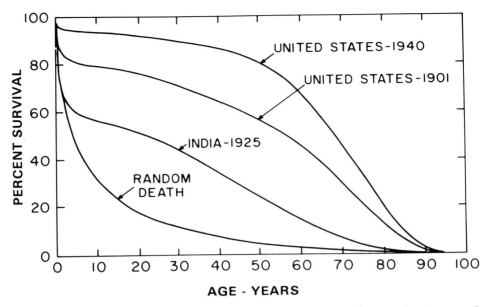

FIG. 3-2. Survivorship curves for human populations with various degrees of environmental stress. Decreased infant mortality was the major change between 1901 and 1940 in the United States; very little change in adult life span has occurred in this century. All eukaryotic organisms that reproduce sexually show a survivorship profile that is somewhere between an exponential decline (random death) and a hypothetical "squared off" curve in which all animals would die at the same instant. (Modified from Curtis H: Biological Mechanisms of Aging, p 4. Springfield, IL, Charles C Thomas, 1966)

than 5 years.[141] Animals in the wild often have survival curves that show a nearly exponential decay from birth, indicating that death is a random process (see Fig. 3-2). For field mice, high predation results in very few old individuals. However, survival curves of wild animals provided with an optimal environment are qualitatively similar to those for humans in the United States in 1940, but with a characteristic maximal life span that seems to be intrinsic to a given species.

After about age 30 in humans, there is an exponential increase in the probability of death in a given population. This relationship is very predictable and was formalized in the following equation over 150 years ago by Gompertz:[42]

$$R/R_o = e^{-\alpha t}$$

where R/R_o is the percent of individuals remaining at time t (age), e is the natural logarithm base, and α is a constant that is proportional to the mortality rate (in humans, α is about equal to 0.01 when t is measured in years). Other authors have derived more complex formulations that also take into account environmental stress and viability factors.[115,133]

It is interesting that a detailed analysis of the "tail" of the human survivorship curve shows that at the highest ages, the probability of death deviates from predicted values.[20] Apparently, the very old represent a particularly robust subgroup that has been winnowed by life's insults.

The rate of decline of a large number of physiologic and performance measures has been shown to be gradual and linear after age 30.[126,130] Performance decrements occur during a period of exponential rise in specific pathologies and death rates.[74] To explain this difference, several authors have argued that small linear declines in a number of integrative physiologic functions can result in disproportionate (exponential) changes in the death rate.[115,133] This hypothesis is in part supported by the data obtained when a physiologic parameter that relies heavily on a number of integrated body functions is examined. As shown in Figure 3-3, the age records for both male and female marathon runners show an exponential, *not* linear, decline with age after the mid 20s. Regardless of the precise relationship between loss of physiologic function and death rate, it is clear that such changes do not occur until after the organism has attained reproductive maturity. Reproductive

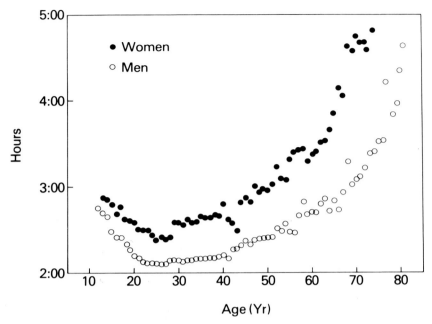

FIG. 3-3. Marathon running times for men and women of various ages. (Data from tables published in Runners World, annual edition, p 29, 1982)

maturity and senescent decline occur at characteristic times for each species. Thus, insights into post-reproductive decrements in function may come from an examination of events occurring during development and differentiation.

DEVELOPMENT, DIFFERENTIATION, AND AGING

The evolution of multicellular organisms was of considerable adaptive significance because it allowed certain cell types to become highly specialized or differentiated. Because not all cells had to perform all functions, a greater variety of different cell tasks could be more efficiently undertaken. The specialized cells of the germ line evolved mechanisms to ensure that the information in the genetic program is passed accurately from generation to generation. Thus, germ lines that incorporated information directing the differentiation of support cells had a selective advantage. This resulted in sequestered multipotent germ-line cells that are dependent on somatic cells to maintain a suitable internal environment. It was probably the advent of such programs for differentiation and development that set the stage for the aging process in metazoans.

Programs that result in specialized somatic cells and tissues have a number of elements that are common to all mammals. For example, among land animals, selection has defined optimal body size in each species. In these animals, skeletal and most tissue development slows and finally stops shortly fter reproductive matuty is ttained. Interestingly, in marine mammals that live in an environment where large size is not prohibitive owing to the buoyant force of the water, growth does not cease and the ultimate life span appears to be substantially lengthened compared with their terrestrial counterparts. Such selected developmental events must have their roots in the molecular mechanisms that regulate cell division and turnover, and they suggest that continued replacement of molecular structures through cell division may allow escape, at the cellular level, from a finite life span.

In light of these observations, it is not surprising that in rodents and fowl, the life span can be extended by slowing the developmental program, including skeletal maturity, by underfeeding.[115.] Such experiments are quite conclusive and consistently show that the reproductive phase is delayed by underfeeding. In more recent studies, rats were maintained on a tryptophan-deficient diet from birth; starting a normal diet at 22 months of age initiated the normal developmental sequence, including successful reproduction.[123,124] Their age-matched controls were clearly senescent and incapable of reproduction. This result demonstrates that the molecular mechanisms that maintain the homeostasis of the organism and its constituent cells are not influenced as much by chronologic time as they are by their position with respect to their reproductive program. Reproductive programming was probably selected for as an adaptive function; temporary fluctuations in food supply would delay development and thereby avoid waste of reproductive effort in a low-survival environment. It is apparent that the extension of the developmental period by starvation also results in a delay of the aging program. This coupling of development and aging would occur if cellular commitments are made during the developmental program that permit an optimal reproductive period but then become limiting later in life.

Most of the differentiated cell types complete their programs by the time of reproduction. For example, the number of ova present during the life of the human female is determined at a very early developmental stage. Thus, the ova in an adult woman are as old as the woman herself. As ova accumulate defects with time,[59] it is not surprising that the incidence of maternal birth defects (*e.g.,* mongolism) rises sharply toward the end of the reproductive years.[10,95] Menopause may be a selective safeguard against adding such age-dependent birth defects to the gene pool.

A sharp decline in reproductive capacity does not occur in the male in whom spermatogenesis and paternity can continue into the eighth or ninth decade of life. The continued generation of viable sperm from stem cells seems to preclude in sperm the senescent changes that occur in postmitotic ova. Another *in vivo* example of this apparent escape from aging by cell division is the intestinal lining. Continued replenishment of this cell population occurs by division of progenitor cells in the base of the crypts; daughter cells migrate along the villi to be finally sloughed into the lumen of the gut. These cells continue to divide throughout the life of the organism and, like spermatogonia, show no major change with age after maturity in their ability to divide (Fig. 3-4).[138] It was observed that the G_1 phase of the cell cycle may be somewhat lengthened in intestinal epithelial cells derived from older animals.[138] However, this age change is minor in contrast to the normal developmental shift in the position of dividing cells along the villi due to cell cycle modification.

It is clear that the developmental programs optimized by higher metazoans to provide maximal reproductive capacity may result in restricted genetic expression in differentiated cell types. In this process, ova and neuronal, skeletal, and heart-muscle cells all lose their mitotic capabilities and may be "hot spots" for age-related defects. It is also apparent from the underfeeding studies that the capacity for vigorous and efficient growth is not necessarily a function of absolute time but is the result of a developmental program that has evolved solely for the maintenance of homeostasis

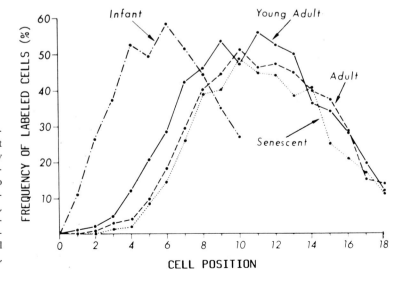

FIG. 3-4. Effect of age on the division potential of intestinal crypt cells. Cell division was measured by the incorporation of labeled nucleotides for each age-group of mice. No significant age difference after maturity is apparent. (Thrasher JD, Greulich RC: The duodenal progenitor population: I. Age-related increase in the duration of the cryptal progenitor cycle. J Exp Zool 159:39, 1965)

throughout the reproductive period. Thus it is not surprising that the major decrements in physiologic function begin after the reproductive phase begins. It appears that the processes in the organism's life span that occur before reproductive capacity is attained are under the direct control of the genetic sequence information that was selected through the enhanced survival of its own progenitors. However, once the germ line has been replicated, the finite life span of the somatic cells is determined by the quality of the structure built by the developmental program and by its interactions through time with its environment.

AGING "HOT SPOTS"

Physiologic function begins to decline in many tissues shortly after the reproductive part of the life cycle. This decrease proceeds at different rates for different tissues. Although some declines in function may be tolerated for a majority of the postpubertal years, certain cell types are more critical to continued survival. Intact immune and cardiovascular systems are essential to survival. The nervous system, especially the brain and its integration of total body function through the pituitary and its hormones, is also critical to survival. Thus, such organ systems are ideal for the study of intrinsic cellular age changes that may affect the entire functioning of the organism.

Included in this group are the cells of the nervous system, certain endocrine cells, cells of immune and cardiovascular systems, skeletal muscle cells, and certain kidney cells. One characteristic feature of all of these systems is that their constituent cells are mitostatic (nondividing or postmitotic). For example, neurons and cardiac and skeletal muscle cells do not divide after early developmental events while cells of the immune system continue on a program that fixes their mitotic rate later in development. This implies that such cells must repair or replace most of their intracellular structural components and enzymatic machinery on a regular basis to obviate the accumulation of damaged molecular components with time. In the absence of cell division there would be no selection against the accumulation of altered cells resulting from inadequate component repair and replacement. Researchers in gerontology have termed such critical organ systems and the mitostatic cells that make them up as aging *hot spots* because they are nondividing and play a critical

role in maintaining the homeostasis of the entire organism[91]. Many investigators have turned their attention to these hot-spot tissues because they may represent the pacemakers of aging.[31,32] These tissues are the most probable sites for the accumulation of defects with age that could cause decrements in function and eventually become life limiting. One important example of hot-spot aging is in the immune system.

AGING OF THE IMMUNE SYSTEM

There is little doubt that, in the natural state, all complex organisms are a constant repository of bacterial, viral, and fungal infections, as well as aberrant, potentially cancerous cells. The role of the immune system is to maintain an equilibrium against these onslaughts to ensure host viability through the reproductive phase of life. That the human immune system loses competence with age is evidenced by the nearly exponential increase in incidence of infectious and autoimmune diseases and certain cancers after age 25.[144] Because an intact immune system is essential to survival in complex animals and the deficits observed with age can be traced to specific cell types, the immune system has been a model *in vivo* cell culture system for the study of aging.

All peripheral immunologic cells appear to be derived from bone marrow, but certain cells are processed through the thymus (T lymphocytes) and are thereby conferred competency in cell-mediated responses (immunity against tumors, transplanted tissue rejection, and delayed hypersensitivity). Other bone-marrow–derived cells develop into macrophages (as well as other formed blood elements) and B lymphocytes, which are responsible for the humoral antibody response. The primary antibody responses of B lymphocytes may also require T-lymphocyte interactions. Macrophages not only scavenge foreign materials but also appear to mediate some T- and B-lymphocyte function by presenting scavenged materials for antigenic recognition. Further descriptions of the complexities and subtleties of immune response should be pursued in more detailed treatises.[17,89]

In mice as well as humans the number of circulating white blood cells has been shown to remain almost constant throughout life.[90] However, B-lymphocyte function increases during adolescence and then declines with post-reproductive age in humans and mice (Fig. 3-5).[90] In light of

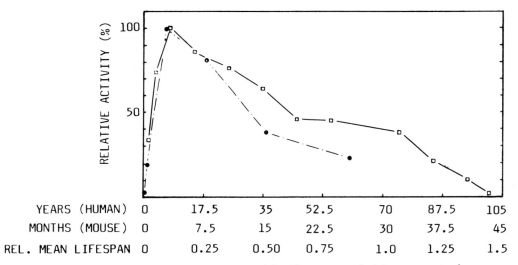

FIG. 3-5. Effect of age on B-lymphocyte immune activity. The serum agglutinin response to sheep red blood cells in mice is compared with naturally occurring serum anti-A isoagglutinin titers in humans. With the life spans normalized, the profile of this B-lymphocyte index is remarkably similar between mice and humans. (Makinodan T, Adler WH: Effects of aging on the differentiation and proliferation potentials of cells of the immune system. Fed Proc 34:154, 1975)

the B- and T-lymphocyte synergism mentioned previously, it is possible that this decline in function is not a primary B-lymphocyte defect.

Alterations of T-lymphocyte immune functions with age have been demonstrated in several systems. The most striking decline has been measured in T lymphocytes derived from BC3F mice (a long-lived strain) in which a 97% decline with age in mitogenic response to phytohemagglutinin (PHA) stimulation was demonstrated (Fig. 3-6).[64] These experiments were performed *in vitro* on isolated, spleen-derived T lymphocytes; the measured deficit is, therefore, intrinsic to the cells. It is possible, however, that their limited PHA response was a result of their long-term exposure to an aging environment *in vivo*. Declining T-lymphocyte function could, therefore, cause the observed increased incidence of infection and tumors and may also affect the specificity of antibody production through B-lymphocyte synergism.

The biochemical basis for the loss in proliferative capacity in aged T lymphocytes has not been pursued in as much detail as other *in vitro* aging systems. However, of note is correlated decline in the levels of cyclic guanosine monophosphate (GMP)[58] and a decrease in histone acetylation after PHA stimulation,[101] indicating the possibility of age-related defects at a number of loci in the sequence of events between PHA binding to cell surface receptors and the mitogenic response.

In mammals, it appears that the immune system has also been selected for optimal function in relation to the reproductive period. The pubertal involution of the thymus (a key organ in the development of cell-mediated immune competence) seems to result in a primary dose of T lymphocytes early in life. As a result, the adult must rely on an early developmental endowment of T lymphocytes for the remainder of his life. These cells remain virtually nondividing until antigenically stimulated, and over time they show a decline in proliferative capacity. By contrast, the continuously dividing bone marrow cells, the stem-cell population from which the T lymphocytes arose, do not appear to lose their proliferative capacity with age.[53] Thus, continued division of the relatively undifferentiated stem-cell population appears to ensure continued division potential, whereas highly differentiated postmitotic cells apparently have lost the ability to escape a finite life span.

Biochemical measurements at the cellular level are confounded by the question of whether the cells are responding to an aging environment or if the changes observed are intrinsic to the cells being studied. For instance, cells *in vivo* may respond to changing concentrations of components in the blood (*e.g.*, hormones). Changes with time in the extracellular microenvironment (*e.g.*, owing to collagen cross-linking) could restrict the access of nutrients and hormones from the blood.[48] One

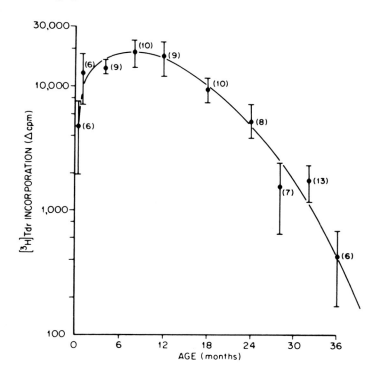

FIG. 3-6. Effect of age on T-lymphocyte proliferation. The mitogenic response to phytohemagglutinin (PHA) of spleen-derived T lymphocytes in BC3F mice (a long-lived strain) declines after about 7 months of age. (Hori Y, Perkins EH, Halsall MK: Decline in phytohemagglutinin responsiveness of spleen from aging mice. Proc Soc Exp Biol Med 144:48, 1973)

approach to this dilemma has been the study of aging in isolated, cultured cells where the environment can be controlled.

AGING IN CELL CULTURE

Studies on the life span of cloned tissue cells *in vitro* have addressed two main parameters: (1) the effect of time in culture and (2) the effect of cumulative doublings. The latter has been by far the more studied of the two. An additional question that has received little attention is the effect of time on the cells once replication has ceased. Although it is not yet clear whether attenuation of capacity for cell division in culture actually represents an expression of aging *in vitro*, it is now well documented that normal diploid cell clones propagated in culture under certain conditions do not have an infinite life span. The classic work of Hayflick is illustrative of this general phenomenon (Fig. 3-7).[56] In these experiments embryonic human lung fibroblasts were shown to proceed through an average of 50 population doublings before a sharp decline in proliferative capacity ensued. Such observations have been substantiated by many different workers using various normal diploid cell lines,[82,107,139] and the effect appears to be quite general. Detailed genetic analyses of cell

lines that do not show this limited division potential have usually demonstrated that the cells were not diploid.[26,92] Thus normal diploid cells do have a finite doubling capacity in culture under the conditions employed, while cell lines derived from cancerous tissues or transformed cultures do not. This demonstration of limited division potential under controlled culture conditions implicates a causal molecular mechanism that is intrinsic to normal cells in culture.

If normal cells *in vivo* are in fact also limited in their growth potential, then one would expect cells from donors of different ages to display growth potentials inversely related to the age of the donor. Studies by Hayflick[56] and later by Martin and co-workers[93] have shown this to be the case. In the latter work, tissue specimens from 100 subjects showed a regression coefficient of −0.20 population doublings per year between the first and ninth decades. Confirmation of this has also been made by Schneider and Mitsui[120] and by LeGuilly and associates[80] using liver biopsies. Thus cells from older human donors do have a decreased potential for cell division *in vitro*.

Organisms age at different rates and have distinct species-specific life spans. This implies that cells from long-lived species should proceed through more population doublings than those of short-lived donors if such phenomena reflect ac-

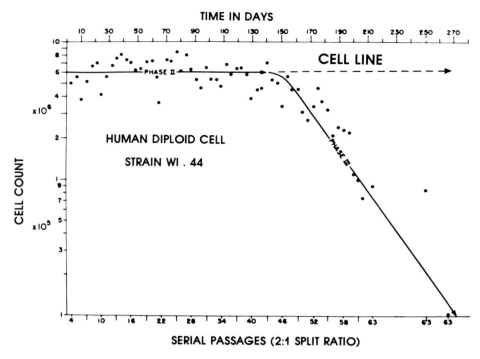

FIG. 3-7. Loss of cell-division potential in normal human fibroblasts. After about 45 doublings, WI-44 cells lose their ability to continue division. A cell line will continue to divide indefinitely in culture. (Hayflick L: The limited *in vitro* lifetime of human diploid cell strains. Exp Cell Res 37:614, 1965)

tual aging *in vivo*. Although no complete study has been performed to date, reports of various workers using a variety of different species for primary explants indicate that this is the case (Table 3-1). Embryonic cells from the long-lived Galapagos tortoise (life span, 175 years) displayed 90 to 125 population doublings,[40] while human (110 years) cells underwent 40 to 60 doublings,[57] chicken cells (25 years) showed 15 to 35 doublings,[81] and mouse cells (3.5 years) doubled 19 to 28 times.[139] Also, fibroblasts from a 9-year-old donor with the rare genetic disease progeria doubled only twice.[41]

No evidence exists to indicate that the life span is limited by a lack of replenishment of the cell types that normally continue to divide throughout life, but there is general agreement that the nondividing (postmitotic or potentially mitotic) cells in certain key systems are most limiting to general physiologic functions and, therefore, represent the major age-defective loci (hot spots). Cells from vascular tissue have been focused on because aging of the vascular system is a key component of age-associated atherosclerosis. For example, age changes in the ability of the vascular endothelia to repopulate wounds could play a significant role

in the initiation of microthrombi, local platelet degranulation, and resulting stimulation of intimal smooth muscle proliferation due to platelet-derived growth factor (PDGF). Normally, vascular endothelial cells are potentially mitotic, dividing only in response to wounding. Thus, these cells may divide only rarely at some relatively quiescent vascular sites, but turnover may be rather constant at sites such as vessel bifurcations where turbulent shear force in the blood may be high. They therefore represent a cell population that in their differentiated state must remain postmitotic but must also maintain the capacity to proliferate rapidly on wounding.

When examined in culture, the proliferative life span of bovine aortic endothelial cells is certainly not less than and probably greater than that observed for diploid human or bovine fibroblasts.[70,97] As these cells senesce, large, multinucleate cells accumulate, a process that is concomitant with an exponential decline in their ability to proliferate. Thus, this differentiated cell type is similar to fibroblasts in having a finite life span in culture. Few studies have been performed on the effects of calendar time on nondividing cultured cells. How-

TABLE 3-1   The Finite Lifetime of Cultured Embryonic Fibroblasts

Species	Range of Population Doubling for Cultured, Normal Embryo Fibroblasts	Mean Maximum Life Span (years)
Galapagos tortoise	90–125	175
Human	40–60	110
Mink	30–34	10
Chicken	15–35	30
Mouse	14–28	3.5

(Hayflick L: The cell biology of human aging. N Engl J Med 295:1302, 1976)

ever, two early studies are noteworthy. Hay and Strehler kept chick fibroblasts in a mitostatic phase using an agar overlay technique.[55] At various times thereafter the cells were removed and allowed to divide. Surprisingly, all cultures stopped dividing, not after the same number of divisions but after similar total times in culture. Other studies by McHale and co-workers[88] used low serum concentration to keep embryonic human fibroblasts from dividing for various times and also observed the cultures to be limited by calendar time and not by the number of cumulative population doublings. Although both studies have been objected to on technical grounds,[23] the results stand in direct contrast to the Hayflick studies.

An important topic is the analysis of cultured cells at various times after cell division has ceased. With the right experimental model, one could address the hypothesis that cell division allows an escape from a finite life span, as is observed with transformed cell lines. Cultures of bovine aortic endothelial cells were propagated up to 80% of their known maximum life span (about 125 doublings). The cultures were then either maintained as confluent mitostatic monolayers or continued to be passaged weekly (Fig. 3-8A). At various times (T_1,T_2,T_3) the cultures were assayed for their colony size distribution, an index of their ability to proliferate. The surprising finding was that the cultures that were maintained confluent actually increased over time in their capacity to proliferate (Fig. 3-8B) while the cultures that continued to divide decreased in their capacity to proliferate. When confluent cultures of these cells were examined it was apparent that the continuously proliferating cells continued to accumulate large, seemingly senescent cells (Fig. 3-8, panel b) while

the cultures that were maintained postconfluent actually lost these senescent cells from the culture (compare panels T_1, T_2, T_3, Fig. 3-8). This suggests that the large senescent cells may be either less viable or less adherent with time but not with cumulative population doublings in culture. Of additional interest is the observation that the loss of cell confluency in the stationary monolayers produced by the death of the large senescent cells does not appear to stimulate repopulation by the surrounding small cells even after extended periods of time. Normally such "wounds" would be rapidly repopulated within 24 hours.[121] Such observations may be related to the findings of Chandrasekher and co-workers,[16] who showed that the fibronectin isolated from old fibroblast cultures was defective in its ability to promote attachment of old as well as young cells to the extracellular matrix.

The relationship between differentiation and growth potential has also been studied in normal diploid cells. Rheinwald and co-workers found that the limiting event in the culture life span of human foreskin keratinocytes is terminal differentiation and not the number of cumulative population doublings.[110] After about 60 doublings, these cells produce a cornified envelope and cease replicating under normal conditions. However, the addition of epidermal growth factor (EGF) prolongs their life span to greater than 100 doublings, possibly by delaying terminal differentiation. Analogous to these studies are those of Gospodarowicz and co-workers,[43] who observed that fibroblast growth factor (FGF) maintains the proliferation of bovine granulosa cells in culture and delays terminal differentiation. Once FGF was removed from the culture medium, however, the

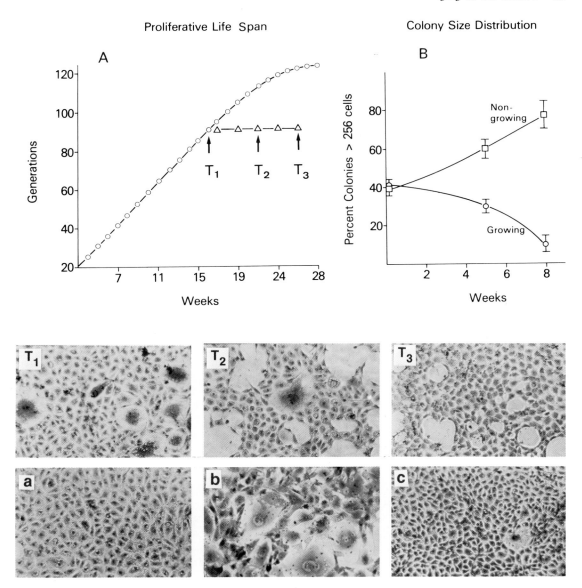

FIG. 3-8. Influence of mitostasis on the division potential and phenotype heterogeneity of bovine aortic endothelial cells. Primary cultures of aortic endothelial cells were propagated to 80% of their maximum proliferative life span. At that point some cultures were maintained as confluent, mitostatic monolayers (Δ), while others were propagated to their finite life span (o). At various times (*arrows*) cells from the mitostatic and proliferative cultures were reseeded at clonal densities, and after a 2-week period the percentage of colonies containing greater than 256 cells (eight doublings) was quantitated. The phenotypic heterogeneity of these clones was also examined by light microscopy (bottom six panels) for comparison with the phenotypes displayed at times T_1, T_2, and T_3 by the parent mitostatic cultures (top three panels). The clones propagated at times T_1 and T_3 are shown in panels *a* and *c*, respectively. For comparison, panel *b* shows the phenotype of the proliferative cells (o) at 28 weeks when they are no longer able to divide. It is apparent that the mitostatic cultures selectively lose the large senescent cells while the proliferative cultures continue to accumulate them (compare panel T_3 with panel *b*).

granulosa cells quickly ceased dividing and differentiated, producing large amounts of lipid and progesterone. In these cases the decline in proliferation capacity *in vitro* is triggered by differentiation events similar to those that occur *in vivo*. It is also clear that if they are maintained in a proper hormonal environment, permitting a high division rate, even normal diploid cells will continue to proliferate, possibly indefinitely.

The effect of EGF on the proliferation of WI-38 embryonic fibroblasts was tested by Ladda and coworkers,[77] who found that treated cultures did not decline in proliferative capacity after 50 doublings as was originally observed. Similar results with WI-38 are also reported by Cristofalo[22] using hydrocortisone, a glucocorticoid known to enhance the growth stimulation by FGF on mouse 3T3 cells.[45] In addition to specific growth factors, the extracellular matrix on which the cells rest has also been shown to influence the mitotic rate and subsequent proliferative life span. This has been observed for bovine corneal[38] and vascular endothelial[44] cells maintained continuously on preformed extracellular matrix produced by vascular smooth muscle cells.[84] Of potential significance is the possiblity that such culture conditions more closely reflect the type of extracellular substrate with which these cells interact *in vivo*. Thus, even when using cells known to be involved in a major age-associated pathology *in vivo*, the consensus is that a finite life span in terms of proliferative potential does exist *in vitro* at least when examined using the most optimal conditions known. These results provide strong support for the idea that normal diploid cells cultured under the conditions originally used by Hayflick and coworkers may be mitotically limited primarily by their program of differentiation rather than a finite number of cell divisions. However, once the rate of cell division slows, either as a function of the developmental program or by manipulation of their hormonal environment in culture, an intrinsic biologic clock may set an upper limit on their continued viability. It follows that cells in such a stationary culture could accumulate damaged molecular components in many of their more long-lived intracellular as well as extracellular structural elements unless adequate repair and replacement mechanisms are operative. Furthermore, in the absence of cell division there exists no mechanism to select against cells that cannot efficiently repair structures altered with time. This implies that, in stationary cultured cells and in mitostatic cells *in vivo*, the limitations on cell viability after replication has ceased should have a detectable biochemical basis.

INFORMATION-TRANSDUCING MECHANISMS

The cells of the body are constantly bathed by a dynamic set of hormones in the blood that include corticosteroids, thyroid hormones, catecholamines, pituitary hormones, insulin, glucagon, and many others. In addition, certain cells receive input through direct innervation by the nervous system. Because hormonal and nervous signals to target cells are essential to the integration of body function, an age-dependent loss of this information flow could cause systemic disturbances that would contribute to the decline of the system. A given target cell (target for any subset of hormonal and neural signals) could become less functional with time if its environment is aging, that is, if the hormonal/neural information presented to the cell changes with time. For instance, changes in the hormone regulatory feedback loops involving the brain, pituitary, and target tissues could result in a declining level in total body integration with time because the hormones involved in these regulatory loops interact with virtually every cell in the body.[30,32] Specific systemic aging factors have also been proposed.[13,27,46]

On the other hand, a given target-cell type could change with time in its ability to sense the hormonal/neural environment, owing to changes intrinsic to the cell. This could result in an altered cellular phenotype that may be inappropriate to its own survival or the survival of other cells that depend on its gene products. Because neurons and muscles are postmitotic from early developmental stages, the hot-spot theory would predict that the interaction of these two cell types would show age changes. In fact, age changes in muscle, which in many respects resemble denervation and disuse atrophies, have been recognized for years and may be an indication of decreasing sensitivity to acetylcholine at the neuromuscular junction. This possibility is supported by the measured decrease in postsynaptic cholinesterase activity in senile muscle end-plates.[50] However, it is known that testosterone, and possbily other androgens, play a permissive role in muscle function, suggesting that extrinsic hormonal factors may also be involved in establishing the senile neuromuscular unit.[49]

The molecular mechanisms of hormone action are quite varied, depending on the target cell and hormone type. Corticosteroid and thyroid hormones interact with cytoplasmic or intrinsic chromatin proteins, respectively, to form complexes that modulate the transcription of specific genes. On the other hand, polypeptide hormones and catecholamines bind to membrane receptors to initiate steps that are mediated by cyclic adenosine monophosphate (AMP). In spite of the complexity of the molecular details, it is safe to conclude that all hormone action is mediated by target cell receptors. It is, therefore, reasonable to measure possible changes with age in these critical cellular sites that mediate hormone action. The continued search for this type of age defect is encouraged by accumulating evidence that demonstrates changes in tissue responsiveness to hormone stimulation with age.[2]

Decreases in levels of glucocorticoid-binding proteins have been reported for some tissues derived from senescent animals.[78,113] However, cytosols derived from various brain regions of senescent mice did not show a significant decline in corticosterone binding.[98] It is important to emphasize again that the interpretation of receptor studies using tissues derived from senescent animals is complicated by the possibility that the cells were responding to a changing (aging) hormonal environment. In addition, the levels of receptors in several systems have been shown to be autoregulated by the level of the corresponding hormone.[35, 96]

The striking correspondence between the gross aspects of aging and hypothyroidism[67] led to the early proposal that aging was due to a progressive loss of thyroid function.[8,87] However, this hypothesis was largely rejected when blood levels of thyroxine and 3,5,3'-triiodo-L-thyronine were not found to change significantly with age in healthy individuals.[14, 47, 66, 147] However, a study measuring nuclear thyroid hormone receptor levels showed a significant decrease in receptor number per cell in specific tissues.[79] Although liver and kidney remained the same with age, the levels of heart receptors decreased by 60% and cerebellar receptor levels decreased by 56% in male rats. Female rats showed a similar pattern. Interestingly, the affinity of hormone binding remained constant in the age range studied (3 to 17 months). These findings suggest that certain tissues containing mitostatic cells (heart and cerebellum) may become functionally hypothyroid due to their progressive loss of nuclear thyroid hormone receptors.

Changes in responsiveness to cyclic AMP-mediated hormones have also been reported. Greger-

man and Bierman[46] have summarized the evidence that there is an age-related decline in catecholamine activation of adenyl cyclase, although the interpretation of *in vivo* data is again subject to aging environment objections.

The indications are that the ability of tissues to transduce hormonal information declines with age. Because a similar decline in response can be demonstrated in aging cells in culture, it can be argued that at least some of the changes in tissue response are attributable to the cells as opposed to a changing hormonal environment.

INFORMATION STORAGE

Genetic information stored within the nucleus of a eukaryotic cell is sequestered into a highly compact but ordered structure called chromatin. It is now accepted that two each of the four basic nuclear proteins called core histones (H_{2a}, H_{2b}, H_3, H_4) interact to form a globular structure or nucleosome around which the double helix of DNA is wrapped.[75] A fifth histone (H_1) functions as an internucleosome bridge along which the DNA follows from nucleosome to nucleosome. In the electron microscope, this yields the classic "beads on a string" structure, a 100-nm fiber described by Olins and Olins.[102] It has been suggested that the interbead histone H_1 also functions to affect the higher order coiling of nucleosomes into a superstructure called a solenoid of 300-nm diameter.[33] Other as yet unidentified molecules then cause a further condensation of the solenoid into a hollow tube, termed the *super solenoid,* observed by Bak and co-workers.[6] The final packing ratio of the DNA in this structure is calculated to be 10,000:1.[6] Thus, the majority of base sequences are probably sequestered from most enzymatic and other chemical interactions. For transcription of genetic information to occur, regions of the chromatin structure must unfold sufficiently for RNA polymerase to read specific DNA sequences. This requires the assistance of other enzymatic modification reactions, such as phosphorylation,[85] acetylation,[68] methylation,[102] and adenosine diphosphate (ADP) ribosylation,[99] that probably serve to loosen the interactions of the histones and other proteins with the DNA, allowing the structure to relax and permit transcription. In calf thymus, only about 10% of the DNA is maintained in this active or heterochromatin conformation.[15] In mitostatic cells, the remaining 90% of the DNA remains folded and compacted throughout the entire life span of the individual. Because DNA and histones are only synthesized during the S phase of the cell cycle, the chromatin of the G_o phase in fixed mitostatic cells is a repository of long-lived proteins and nucleic acids, while in dividing cells such molecular components would be resynthesized and replaced at each division (every 24 to 48 hours in most cultured cells). Thus, mitostatic, differentiated cells are locked, during development, into an irreversible sequestering of most of their genetic information.

All cells in adult mammals are at some stage of relative differentiation in that their phenotype is the result of an expression of a subset of the total potential gene products that are encoded in the DNA. In addition, a given differentiated pattern of genomic expression is inherited with a high level of accuracy by daughter cells. Although there may be a cytoplasmic component to this inheritance, the pattern of genetic expression in a given cell type represents a level of inheritance that is possibly more labile over time than are processes (*e.g.,* point mutations) that would involve changes in actual DNA base sequences. Thus, in a given cell type, quantitative and qualitative changes could occur with time in the information encoded within the DNA and in the pattern of expressed information. This raises two central questions: (1) Are there irreversible changes that would accumulate in the long-lived components of compacted chromatin that would affect the normal functioning of nondividing cells? and (2) Do the relatively exposed (transcribed) regions of DNA have an increased probability of random hits (*e.g.,* from radiation or chemical damage) owing to higher exposure to the nuclear environment?

With respect to the first question, it has been known for some time that the chromatin from thymus cells of old animals displays a higher melting temperature than the chromatin of young cells.[142] The difference could be obliterated on removal of the histones and thus is probably a result of a histone–histone cross-linkage and not DNA strand cross-linkage. Obviously such a process would have profound influences on those nondividing cells, such as the T lymphocytes, that are episodically required to divide throughout life. Histone cross-linkages could result in insufficient unfolding during DNA replication or transcription; thus, certain T-lymphocyte clones would be unable to participate in the antigenic response. It should be reiterated that the division capabilities of mouse T lymphocytes decline with time in mitostasis (see Fig. 3-6). Because the physiologic integrity of eukaryotic systems depends on the main-

tenance of differentiated cellular expression, a drift in genome expression over time could result in a direct loss in cellular viability or contribute to a loss in homeostasis in the organism.[117] This type of drift could be responsible for the apparent activation of some genes with age (*e.g.,* hairy pinna in men[128]), although it would be difficult to distinguish these changes from those with an endocrine basis.

The second question is related to the probability of random hits within the genome of the cell. Such events might arise through exposure to radiation,[3] highly reactive free radicals, chemical carcinogens, or aberrant enzymatic activities in the nucleus, some of which would be more likely to affect the template-active portion of chromatin because of its greater accessibility. Much research has been performed on the effects of radiation on the life span of a variety of species, and it is apparent that even large doses of radiation do not mimic the effects of age. In one species of the wasp, *Habrobracon,* both haploid and diploid individuals were shown to have identical survivorship curves,[18] while a 5000-rad dose of ionizing radiation actually increased the survivorship of *Drosophila.*[131] Using mice, Curtis and co-workers[24] measured the number of chromosomal aberrations in hepatocytes as a function of age and found that doubling the rate of mutation accumulation with low levels of radiation did not significantly alter the life span. Similarly, Alexander and co-workers[4] reported that chemical mutagens were not effective inducers of premature senescence. Thus, mutations in the DNA of the type produced by radiation are not sufficient to account for the major functional declines characteristic of aged cells and tissues. This could be because radiation-induced and some chemically induced mutations would probably occur in a random manner, with the majority accumulating in nonfunctional chromatin regions that are not expressed in the cell. However, other types of modifications of the DNA, for instance those produced by free radicals such as superoxide, might be preferentially localized in those regions of greater template accessibility. These could accumulate to a life-limiting level within relatively short periods of time, if the cell did not have an efficient repair and replacement system for its DNA. In this regard, it is noteworthy that an increased number of strand breaks have been observed in senescent as compared with young neurons in fixed sections of mouse brain.[108] Because these assays were performed with an exogenous DNA polymerase derived from calf thymus (the enzyme initiates DNA synthesis at strand breaks), it is likely that enzyme binding was localized to those regions of chromatin that are in the extended conformation. Thus, template active regions may be more susceptible to DNA strand scission simply on a statistical basis.

To counteract the greater potential for time-dependent DNA damage in these regions, higher organisms have developed efficient repair systems. In fact, as is shown in Figure 3-9,[54] there is a striking correlation between the repair capacity of fibroblast cells from a number of different species and the maximum longevity of that species.[60] Although it is not clear whether enhanced DNA repair actually allows for a longer life span or is simply required for the extended developmental periods of longer lived animals, it appears to permit the long life spans of mitostatic cells, which are not replicating their DNA on a regular basis. It is of additional interest to note the qualitative similarity between Figures 3-1 and 3-9, suggesting a relationship between fecundity and DNA repair.

Another form of damage that could occur in template-active regions of chromatin, in spite of an efficient repair system, is deletion of genes duplicated in tandem. In fact, a more efficient repair enzyme could even accelerate such deletions. As proposed by Strehler,[132] the two DNA strands in regions of tandemly duplicated cistrons, such as those coding for rRNA and tRNA, might reassociate out of register after RNA polymerase is read through. This could occur because adjacent genes

would still be stabilized by base pairing with genes downstream from one another. The unpaired single-stranded loops on each strand of the DNA would then be excised by the repair system and gaps would be filled in by an appropriate DNA polymerase. The dosage of genes for rRNA and tRNA is known to be amplified during the development of certain tissues[12]; if the dosage declines later in life, serious limitations may occur, especially during periods of increased protein synthetic demand (*e.g.*, in cardiac hypertrophy). Such events would also be expected to accumulate at a greater rate in mitostatic cell populations because there would be no mechanism for selection against cells with decreased viability.

Johnson and co-workers tested this possibility directly in aged mitostatic tissues of beagles.[71,72] DNA from brain, heart, skeletal muscle, and kidney all showed significant decreases in the hybridization to labeled rRNA while liver (a dividing tissue) did not. This was not confirmed in initial studies by Gaubatz and co-workers[34] using C57BL/6J mice. However, in later studies using human myocardial tissue, Johnson and co-workers[69] and Strehler and co-workers[134] found a significant decline in rRNA hybridizability using DNA from 30 individuals. These results are shown in Figure 3-10. Such a decrement (30% to 40%) could account for some of the loss of vigor characteristic of aged postmitotic tissues, especially in neurons and myocardium in which high levels of protein

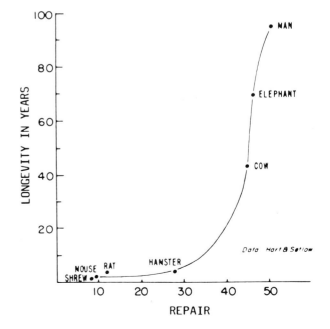

FIG. 3-9. Relationship between DNA repair and life span for various mammalian species. DNA repair was measured in ultraviolet-irradiated fibroblasts by incorporation of radiolabeled nucleotides. (Hart R, Setlow R: Correlation between deoxyribonucleic acid excision repair and life span in a number of mammalian species. Proc Natl Acad Sci USA 71:2169, 1974)

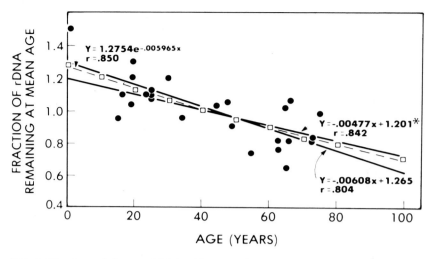

FIG. 3-10. Loss of ribosomal DNA with age. Values represent the relative degree of hybridization between labeled ribosomal RNA and DNA isolated from human myocardial tissue at the various ages. (Data from Johnson L, Johnson R, Strehler B: Cardiac hypertrophy, aging and changes in cardiac ribosomal RNA genes dosage in man. J Mol Cell Cardiol 7:125, 1975; Strehler B, Chang MP, Johnson L: Substantial loss of ribosomal DNA in DNA obtained from human myocardium. Mech Age Dev, 11:371, 1979)

synthesis are required. Thus, changes in DNA could account for some of the age-related changes in cellular function, although such changes may only occur in certain closely related gene classes because of their tandem arrangement in the genome.

In many cases, the level of specific protein production is directly dependent on the steady-state levels of translatable mRNA coding for that protein. This has been well established for certain hormonally activated genes such as ovalbumin,[106] tyrosine aminotransferase,[7] α_{2u}globulin,[76] and cells infected with mouse mammary tumor virus.[111] Thus, any age-dependent effects on the flow of genetic information from DNA to RNA could profoundly influence the functioning of cells by limiting their adaptive response to hormonal stimulation.

TRANSCRIPTION AND TRANSLATION

In all nucleated cells (certain anuclear cells such as mammalian erythrocytes being excluded), RNA is continually being transcribed from specific DNA regions. After considerable processing, during which most of the RNA is degraded, an RNA fraction results (mRNA), which is translated by the cytoplasmic protein synthetic machinery (including ribosomes, various initiation and termination factors, amino acylsynthetases and tRNAs) into

new protein. Post-translational events, including modification and degradation, are also important to protein expression and economy in the cell. Although the transcription of DNA to RNA could be subject to modulation or error with age (post-developmental), no conclusive studies have been reported on the fidelity of transcription or HnRNA processing with age.

The protein synthetic sequence is a potential source of nongenetic error that could result in faulty protein synthesis by the insertion of the wrong amino acids. It is reasonable that cells can live with a low level of such mistakes, because the nonfunctional products would represent a minor population. However, certain proteins are themselves functional parts of the protein synthetic machinery (*e.g.,* RNA polymerases, initiation and termination factors, and tRNA aminoacyl synthetases) and are therefore responsible for their own synthesis. For these proteins, an error feedback loop could occur in which an increasing error rate would finally result in an unacceptably high level of defective proteins, and the cell would die of error catastrophe.[103–105]

In certain fungi (*Neurospora* and *Podospora*), the degenerative changes that occur during prolonged vegetative growth can be shown to have a cytoplasmic basis and seem to involve an increase in error in protein synthesis.[62] For example, the leu-5 mutant of *Neurospora* has a defective leucyl tRNA synthetase (an enzyme that normally couples leucine to its specific acceptor tRNA) that can change leucyl tRNA with other amino acids that would subsequently substitute for leucine to produce defective proteins. In addition, this error rate is temperature dependent; if cultures growing at 23°C are shifted to 37°C, the rate of substitution for leucine increases and senescent decline rapidly ensues.[62]

The evidence for this type of process is not as clear in mammalian cells. Loftfield[83] has estimated the rate of substitution for leucine into ovalbumin (a protein that does not normally contain leucine) in 2-year-old chicken oviduct to be 1/3000. However, this error is not too different from the value predicted by the rate of DNA point mutations measured in cell culture (4×10^{-4} per gene per generation[146]). For example, the cells in 2-year-old chicken oviduct would have accumulated about 146 generations (assuming 5 days per generation). The accumulated errors per gene (by multiplication) are therefore about 0.6×10^{-3}, a value that is not far from the estimation of leucine substitution for ovalbumin.

The specific activity of certain enzymes should be a sensitive indicator of faulty protein synthesis caused by the insertion of inappropriate amino acids because small resulting changes in protein conformation could affect the subtle interactions between the enzyme and substrate in the active site. In this regard, studies by Holliday and Tarrant[63] on protein denaturation and studies by Gershon and Gershon[37] on inactive enzymes supported the error catastrophe hypothesis. However, in some systems, data have accumulated that do not show decreased fidelity of protein synthesis. For example, protein production from viral message is as accurate in aged human fibroblasts as in young ones.[61,140]

Strehler and co-workers have prepared an alternative and encompassing theory for aging and development involving protein synthesis, which depends on the degeneracy of the trinucleotide genetic code.[135] Because some amino acids can be represented by more than one codon (61 code words are used to specify only 20 amino acids), the same primary amino acid sequence can be specified by different codon languages. Therefore, the successful translation of a given mRNA would require language-matched translational machinery. The theory proposes that a sequence of languages, each preparing for the next, could permit a program of differentiation and development. Cellular aging could then result from a lack of critical cellular proteins due to an inability to translate the message for those proteins. New support for parts of this theory has come from DNA sequencing of specific genes in which the code words for certain amino acids are selectively used.[122]

ORGANELLES AND MEMBRANES

The effect of time on organelles and other subcellular macrostructures, such as mitochondria, lysosomes, ribosomes, and membrane components, is apparent only where the rate of turnover is exceeded by the rate of accumulation of altered molecules. Such accumulation will, in general, occur at a greater rate in the long-lived, fixed mitostatic cells. In dividing cell populations, there is a continual requirement for the synthesis of new membranes and organelles. However, even in mitostatic cells, it is likely that an ongoing program of degradation and resynthesis of these structures is operative. This turnover is most apparent in ribosomes in which the half-life of ribosomal RNA is estimated to be 4.8 days for a variety of tissues.[119] Such a turnover rate implies that these structures are not merely repaired on a regular basis but are in fact degraded and resynthesized *de novo*. It is not surprising that age-related effects on ribosomal efficiency in translation have not been reported, attesting to the continued fidelity of ribosome synthesis during the normal program of replacement.[140] Thus, it is probable that the ribosomes of senescent, postreplicative cells are no older than those of rapidly dividing cells in the body, such as bone marrow or intestinal mucosa, and would, therefore, not display diminished functions with age. However, due to the rapid degradation rate of these structures, it is possible that the steady-state level of functional ribosomes is grossly influenced by the rates of synthesis of ribosomal RNA precursors and ribosomal proteins. This implies that age-related reductions in the availability of rDNA cistrons for transcription (either by direct gene loss as previously described or by other means such as protein cross-linking[143]) could prove to be a limiting factor in the rate of induction of proteins in the cells in older animals.[1]

Mitochondria, the semi-autonomous energy-providing organelles of eukaryotic cells, are also turned over at a regular rate; in liver they have a half-life of 10 to 12 days, which is not different in young and old tissue.[94] Sulkin and Sulkin[137] found that, in nondividing cardiac muscle, the morphology of mitochondria from young (10 day) and old (100 day) rats was observed at the electron microscope level to be quite similar. However, exposure of the rats to low oxygen tension (5.5% O_2) caused the mitochondria from the older tissue to become swollen and fragmented, while those of young tissue remained unchanged. Similarly, the mitochondria of old autonomic ganglion cells also showed an increased volume and loss of cristae at low oxygen tension. Such observations suggest that although the basal functioning of mitochondria may not be altered with age, their response to environmental changes may be severely affected in older tissues. These alterations appear to be more localized in the insoluble membranous components of these organelles because oxidative phosphorylation mediated by the soluble enzymes of mitochondria does not change with age in rat liver, heart, and kidney.[39] Although mitochondria are turned over regularly like ribosomes, their increased complexity may be a basis for time-dependent alterations to occur in response to a changing intracellular environment. This could then result in decreased adaptive responses to increased functional demands.

Membrane components of nondividing cells, especially those in brain tissue, are relatively long-lived molecules. This is most apparent in the isotope retention studies of Gee and co-workers.[36] Radioactive carbon from radiolabeled acetate was retained in various lipid fractions of tissue homogenates in much higher levels than radioactive carbon retained in various protein fractions that were labeled with ^{14}C-leucine.[100] In general, nondividing tissues were also much more effective in retaining acetate-derived carbon than were tissues such as skin, liver, spleen, and lung. Thus, the replacement of membrane components is much less active in quiescent cells and could result in the accumulation of altered membrane or cell surface structures. Results documenting the accumulation of massive disulfide cross-linked glycoprotein networks (fibronectin), secreted by some cells at confluency in cell culture but less so during proliferation,[65] may explain the observations that the membranes of contact-inhibited cells are much more rigid than those of growing or neoplastic cells.[114] Thus, membrane components of highly differentiated mitostatic cells may be long-lived, static structures, susceptible to a variety of age-dependent alterations, such as cross-linkage or oxidative polymerization. Such alterations, within the membrane itself or at the cell surface, could significantly alter the permeability of the cell to a variety of small ions, amino acids, or lipids, thereby producing major alterations in the intracellular environment of senescent cells.

Although little evidence is available regarding the extent of membrane alteration with age, the accumulation of lipofuscin (age pigment) in a variety of postmitotic tissues may reflect an abortive attempt by the cell to deal with such time-worn membrane components.[109] Isolated age pigments consist of phospholipids, corticosteroids, and protein components, leading most researchers to believe that lipofuscin is derived from oxidative degradation of unsaturated lipids and cross-linked membrane structures.[60] Lipofuscin accumulation is most apparent in myocardial cells and neurons[109] but has also been reported in interstitial cells of the adrenal cortex.[118] In the case of human myocardial tissue (Fig. 3-11), the amount of pigment increases linearly with age and averages about 6% of the intracellular volume by the ninth decade, while in rat neurons this value can approach 25% of the cell volume.[136] It is also interesting to note that the rate of age pigment accumulation in the myocardium of dogs is about five times that of humans, while dogs generally attain no greater than one fifth of the natural life span of humans.[148] Occlusion of major portions of the cytoplasm by relatively inert, nondegradable components could significantly reduce the functional capacity of post-replicative cells.

In most cells, the degradation of cellular components is effected by hydrolytic enzymes contained within organelles, known as lysosomes. Because the membranes surrounding such structures are probably similar in composition to the plasma membrane, it is likely that membrane alterations might also occur in these structures. This would be particularly harmful if the lysosomes became more permeable to the hydrolytic enzymes contained within. The instability of lysosomes with age has been central to the "death bag" theories of aging.[21] However, this process does not appear to occur in aged cells or tissues, possibly because the primary function of the organelle (fusing with a phagosome to become a digestive vacuole) results in the dissolution of the entire structure. Thus, lysosomes are relatively short-lived organelles within the cell. However, even those that are newly synthesized would be subject to any changes occurring in the intracellular environment with age.

It appears that some subcellular components such as ribosomes, mitochondria, and lysosomes are turned over on a regular basis and display few age-related decrements in function, although mitochondria are much less adaptable to a changing environment as the cells age. In contrast, the

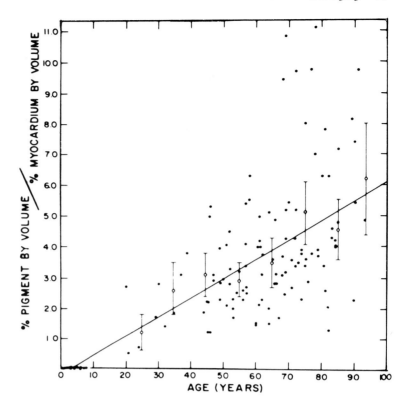

FIG. 3-11. Effect of age on cellular age pigment accumulation in human myocardium. (Strehler BL, Mark D, Mildvan A, Gee M: Rate and magnitude of age pigment accumulation in the human myocardium. J Gerontol 14:430, 1959)

membrane components of post-replicative cells are much longer-lived structures. This results in the accumulation of altered membranes, possibly by cross-linkage and oxidation, and may be reflected in the accumulation of age pigment in nondividing, terminally differentiated cells.

EVOLUTION AND AGING

It is interesting to speculate about the origin of aging in an evolutionary sense.[73,129,149] In this speculation it is essential to remember that evolution plays a game with simple rules. It asks only how well one generation of individuals can ensure the survival and reproductive competency of the next generation. It is a game played against the rigors of the environment. To survive, the earliest cells, which contained the minimal machinery for information storage and retrieval, had to reach a compromise between elaborate mechanisms to compensate for thermodynamic and chemical deterioration of the individual and cell division in which the entire structure of the cell is duplicated and the identity of the individual is lost in the daughter cells.

A significant event in the evolution of life on earth was the appearance of oxygen-producing cyanophytes or blue-green algae. These organisms initiated a rapid transition, starting about 2 billion years ago, from a reducing atmosphere, estimated to contain hydrogen, carbon dioxide, ammonia, and methane, to the present oxidative atmosphere, containing about 79% nitrogen, 20% oxygen, low levels of carbon dioxide, and trace gases. Although this high level of oxygen permitted the evolution of animals that use oxygen metabolically, it also represents a source of toxicity to living cells. Since many biomolecules can spontaneously oxidize under these conditions, elaborate physiologic and biochemical strategies evolved in both plants and animals to protect delicate cellular structures from damage by oxygen directly and also from free radicals (highly reactive species that are natural sequelae of high oxygen levels and leaky electron transport systems in an aqueous milieu). For example, plants synthesized tocopherols (vitamin E) as antioxidants that were subsequently adopted by co-evolving animals by ingestion of plants. In animals, various strategies evolved, such as mucous protection of air passages, careful molecular sequestering of oxygen by hemoglobin transport, and tight coupling to myoglobin and enzymes involved in adenosine triphosphate (ATP) generation.

The intrinsic cellular toxicity of oxygen and free radicals and their potential abundance in biologic systems led to the proposal that reactive free radicals may form an etiologic basis for some aspects of the aging process.[51,52] This "free radical" theory of aging is in many respects the most comprehensive of the theories in integrating and explaining the various aspects of the aging process.[5] The free radical theory would argue that the ultimate life span of postmitotic cells, or animals that depend on tissues containing postmitotic cells, may be determined by the effectiveness of the biochemical strategies they have evolved to block the accumulation of oxidative, free-radical damage.

On one hand, extensive cellular free radical scavenging and repair mechanisms had a low probability of arising spontaneously and were metabolically costly.[73] On the other hand, cell replication has an intrinsic chance for error and also requires energy. However, rapid cell division, coupled with an intrinsic error rate in information duplication, permitted the stepwise formation and trial of new, more adaptive organisms; these are the basic (and necessary) ingredients for evolutionary adaptation and survival. A certain level of repair was needed to attenuate the relative number of lethal experiments and to ensure an effective period of nutrient accumulation in preparation for the next cell division. Thus, early cells probably learned to escape thermodynamic aging and death by rapid cell division coupled with an intrinsic error rate (mutation) and a minimal, but sufficient, level of repair capacity.

Metazoans evolved because there was a great advantage in having specialized (differentiated) cells and tissues. Cell differentiation also provided an efficient receptacle to protect and propagate the highly specialized cells of the germ line; information could be stored in the germ line in a relatively inert state. This division between somatic cells and cells of the germ line was probably the origin of aging as we think of it because after reproduction the individual became expendable.[145] Improvements such as increased viability of mitostatic cells were made in germ-line support tissues (somatic cells) only to improve reproductive efficiency. Elaborate food-gathering mechanisms (including teeth, claws, mobility) and behavior patterns were selected for their enhancement of reproductive function. As pointed out by Sacher[116] and more recently by Cutler,[25] there appears to be a strong positive correlation between the evolution of the

hominid cephalization index (intelligence) and the maximum life-span potential. During this same evolutionary period the length of the growth (maturation) period has also been greatly extended in absolute time but remains as a rather fixed percentage of the maximum life span (about 20%).

One explanation for these curious correlations may be that in long-lived species evolution has selected first for an intelligence development period during which a maximum amount of information can be acquired, processed, and imprinted. Since the rate of information acquisition and imprinting is fixed by the frequency of significant environmental events and the speed with which the mammalian brain can convert them to long-term memory, it is not surprising that reproductive age in humans is not reached until the middle of the second decade. Such timing would promote the survival of the next generation by benefiting from parental experiences spanning the previous decade. The parents need only to survive until their offspring attain reproductive age, when there is no longer an immediate adaptive consequence of parental death on the survival of the germ line. This may be the reason why in humans most physiologic functions remain optimum until about age 30 (roughly twice the maturation period). Thus, the ability of the brain to promote survival of the organism by choosing adaptive behaviors based on experience was highly selected for because it increased the probability of offspring survival. The key cellular and molecular events that ultimately limit the length of life are therefore probably the same events that were selected through evolution to extend the developmental period. Obviously, repair and turnover of cellular components, as well as cellular differentiation, play key roles in maintaining the human organism through the first 30 years.

However, the process of differentiation in certain cell types essential to the organism's survival resulted in regulatory choices that precluded further cell division. These cells became hot spots for aging. They became life limiting because they could not escape thermodynamic and biochemical decline through cell division and were limited in their repair capacity. In addition, the life spans of the critical hot-spot cells were selected, in each species, only if they became limiting to reproductive efficiency. Thus, a rodent in the field, which may have an average life span of only several months owing to high predation, would not have been selected to have long-lived (*e.g.*, 50 years) mitostatic cells in critical organs.

Selection for or against a population of aged

individuals can also occur at other levels. There may be certain specific instances, for example in environments with restricted food or space, in which a large, non-reproductive-aged population would be selected against on the basis of competition for resources. However, most animals in the wild never reach reproductive senescence, owing to high predation (including disease). On the other hand, in human populations, elderly persons may contribute experience and information to the younger. In this case, one could postulate selection for a longer post-reproductive life.

CONCLUSION

Our ultimate understanding of life-cycle processes, including aging, will require an integration of changes at the molecular, cellular, and whole organism levels; molecular events affect cell function to become expressed ultimately as a decreased ability of the organisms to survive (Fig. 3-12). Some critical tissues contain populations of mitostatic cells that are terminally differentiated; their loss of division capacity precludes an escape from aging by new synthesis and replacement of defective cellular components during cell growth. Since populations of highly differentiated cells are requisite for the efficient functioning of complex organisms and since differentiation is tantamount to loss of division potential, it is probable that our next major advance in blocking senescent decline will be to minimize the chemical and thermodynamic processes that cause mitostatic cells to lose function. It is possible that the accumulation of cellular defects resulting from thermal denaturation and reaction with chemical species like free radicals form the molecular basis for cellular aging and may be modulated pharmacologically. In cell culture, nondividing or slowly dividing cells also senesce by a number of critieria. Normal diploid cells appear to have an upper limit on their divi-

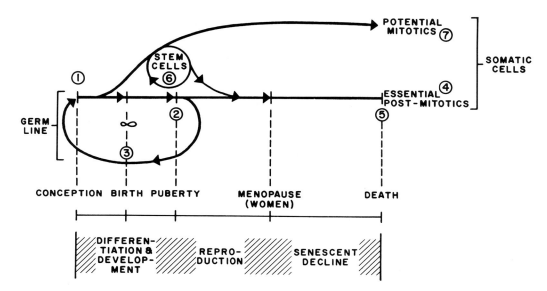

FIG. 3-12. This model of development and aging in mammals is an attempt to summarize what we know about cellular aging from cell culture and *in vivo* systems. The process of development, which requires cellular differentiation and proliferation, is initiated by the event of conception (1). In an evolutionary sense, the culmination and goal of the developmental sequence is to prepare the organism for reproduction, beginning at puberty (2). Reproduction can replenish the potentially immortal germ-cell line (3). In association with optimum reproductive capacity, certain cells become terminally differentiated and thereby lose their ability to divide. In cell culture, it has been shown that rapidly dividing cells can escape senescent changes, but when their division rate is slowed or stopped, they differentiate and begin to lose viability. Certain nondividing cells in the organism may, therefore, become less functional with time. The molecular mechanisms creating these changes in cell function are unknown. If these cells are critical to continued body function [essential postmitotic cells (4)] like the cells of the immune, nervous, and cardiovascular systems, their curtailed function may become life limiting (5). Other cells may continue to divide (6) throughout life (*e.g.,* intestinal mucosa cells) or become nondividing potential mitotics (4) that are not life limiting.

sion potential in culture, but tumor derived or transformed cells appear to be unlimited in their proliferative life span. It is interesting that certain cells, such as vascular endothelia (see Fig. 3-8), are potentially mitotic and may be encouraged to repopulate defective vascular surfaces to counter senescent decline of the blood vessels.

In geologic time, life, and finally human life, came only recently. As the hominid brain became increasingly self-aware, aging became, in a sense, a uniquely human dilemma. Only humans anticipate their own death and can regret physical and mental decline relative to a more vigorous youth. We are beginning a new phase of human evolution in which we are learning how to increase the probability of our own survival, both by elimination of disease and by intervention into the fundamental processes of human aging. These new capabilities may short circuit the evolutionary scheme by preserving maladapted genes that would otherwise be eliminated from the gene pool. On the other hand, they will allow us to establish our own set of criteria, not for who shall survive but for the ultimate goals of prolonged survival.

REFERENCES

1. Adelman RC: Age-dependent effect in enzyme induction—a biochemical expression of aging. Exp Gerontol 6:75, 1971
2. Adelman RC: Macromolecular metabolism during aging. In Finch CE, Hayflick L (eds): Handbook of the Biology of Aging. New York, Van Nostrand Reinhold, 1977
3. Albertini RJ, and DeMars R: Detection and quantification of x-ray induced mutation in cultured diploid fibroblasts. Mutat Res 18:199, 1973
4. Alexander P, and Cornell D: Shortening of the life-span of mice by irradiation with x-rays and treatment with radiomimetic chemicals. Radiant Res 12:38, 1960
5. Armstrong D: Free radical involvement in the formation of lipopigments. In Armstrong D, Sohal RS, Cutler RG, Slater TF (eds): Free Radicals in Molecular Biology, Aging and Disease. New York, Raven Press, 1984
6. Bak A, Zenthen J, Crick F: Higher-order structure of human mitotic chromosomes. Proc Natl Acad Sci USA 74:1595, 1977
7. Beck J, Beck G, Wong K, Tompkins G: Synthesis of inducible tyrosine aminotransferase in cell-free extract from cultured hepatoma cells. Proc Natl Acad Sci USA 69:3615, 1972
8. Bellamy D: Hormonal effects in relation to aging in mammals. In Bellamy D (ed): Aspects of the Biology of Aging, p 428. New York, Academic Press, 1967
9. Berg B, Simms H: Nutrition and longevity in the rat: III. Food restriction beyond 800 days. Nutr 74:23, 1961
10. Bodner W: Effects of maternal age on the incidence of congenital abnormalities in mouse and man. Nature 190:1134, 1961
11. Bourliere F: The comparative biology of aging: A physiological approach. In Welstenholme GEW, O'Connor M (eds): Ciba Foundation Colloquia on Aging, vol 3. Boston, Little, Brown, & Co, 1964
12. Brown D, Blacker A: Specific gene amplification in oocytes. Science 160:272, 1973
13. Bullough WS: Aging of mammals. Nature 229:608, 1971
14. Caplan RH, Glasser JE, Davis K, Foster L, Wickus G: Thyroid function tests in elderly hyperthyroid patients. J Am Geriatr Soc 26:116, 1978
15. Cedar H, Felsenfeld G: Transcription of chromatin *in vitro*. J Mol Biol 77:237, 1973
16. Chandrasekher S, Sorrentino JA, Millis AJT: Interaction of fibronectin with collagen: Age-specific defect in the biological activity of human fibroblast fibronectin. Proc Natl Acad Sci USA 80:4747, 1983
17. Claman HN, Chaperon EA: Immunologic complementation between thymus and marrow cells. Transplant Rev 1:92, 1969
18. Clark A, Rubin M: The modification by x-rays of the life span of haploids and diploids of the wasp, *Habrobracon* species. Radiat Res, 15:244, 1961
19. Comfort A: The Biology of Senescence. New York, Holt, Rinehart and Winston, 1956
20. Comfort A: The Process of Aging. New York, New American Library, 1964
21. Comfort A: The prevention of aging in cells. Lancet 2:1325, 1966
22. Cristofalo V: Metabolic aspects of aging in diploid human cells. In Holeckova E, Cristofalo V (eds): Aging in Cell and Tissue Culture. New York, Plenum Publishing, 1970
23. Cristofalo V: Animal cell cultures as a model system for the study of aging. In Strehler BL (ed): Advances in Gerontological Research, vol IV, pp 55–56. New York, Academic Press, 1972
24. Curtis H: Biological Mechanisms of Aging. Springfield, IL, Charles C Thomas, 1966
25. Cutler RG: Evolution of human longevity and the genetic complexity governing aging rate. Proc Natl Acad Sci 72:4664, 1975
26. Deaven L, Petersen D: The chromosomes of CHO, an aneuploid chinese hamster cell line: G-band, C-band, and autorodiographic analysis. Chromosoma 41:129, 1973
27. Denckla WD: Role of the pituitary and thyroid glands in the decline of minimal O_2 consumption with age. J Clin Invest 53:572, 1974
28. Denckla WD: A time to die. Life Sci 16:31, 1976
29. deRopp RS: Man Against Aging. New York, St. Martin's Press, 1960
30. Dillman VM: Age-associated elevation of hypothalamic threshold to feedback control, and its role

in development, ageing, and disease. Lancet 2:1211, 1971

31. Finch CE: Comparative biology of senescence: Some evolutionary and developmental considerations. In Animal Models for Biomedical Research, vol 4. Washington, DC, National Academy of Sciences, 1971

32. Finch CE: The regulation of physiological changes during mammalian aging. Q Rev Biol 51:49, 1976

33. Finch J, Klug A: Solenoidal model for superstructure in chromatin. Proc Natl Acad Sci USA 73:1897, 1976

34. Gaubatz J, Prashad N, Cutler R: Ribosomal RNA gene dosage as a function of tissue and age for mouse and human. Biochim Biophys Acta 418:358, 1976

35. Gavin JR III, Roth J, Neville DM Jr, Demeyts P, Buell DN: Insulin-dependent regulation of insulin receptor concentrations: A direct demonstration in cell culture. Proc Natl Acad Sci USA 71:84, 1974

36. Gee M, Nordgren R, Menzies R, Hirsch G, Kutsky R, Strehler B: Evidence for long-lived lipid components in developing mouse tissues. Exp Gerontol 4:27, 1969

37. Gershon H, Gershon D: Inactive enzyme molecules in aging mice: Liver aldolase. Proc Natl Acad Sci USA 70:909, 1973

38. Giguere L, Cheng J, Gospodarowicz D: Factors involved in the control of proliferation of bovine corneal endothelial cells maintained in serum-free medium. J Cell Physiol 110:72, 1982

39. Gold P, Gee M, Strehler B: Effect of age on oxidative phosphorylation in the rat. J Gerontol 23:509, 1968

40. Goldstein S: Aging *in vitro:* Growth of cultured cells from the Galapagos tortoise. Exp Cell Res 83:297, 1974

41. Goldstein S, Littlefield J, Soeldner J: Diabetes mellitus and aging: Diminished plating efficiency of cultured human fibroblasts. Proc Natl Acad Sci USA 64:155, 1969

42. Gompertz B: On the nature of the function expressive of the law of human mortality and a new mode of determining the value of life contingencies. Phil Trans R Soc Lond 115:513, 1825

43. Gospodarowicz D, Bialecki H: The effects of the epidermal and fibroblast growth factors or the replicative lifespan of cultured bovine granulosa cells. Endocrinology 103:854, 1978

44. Gospodarowicz D, Ill CR: The extracellular matrix and the control of proliferation of vascular endothelial cells. J Clin Invest 65:1351, 1980

45. Gospodarowicz D, Moran J: Stimulation of division of sparse and confluent 3T3 cell populations by a fibroblast growth factor, dexamethasone and insulin. Proc Natl Acad Sci USA 71:4584, 1974

46. Gregerman RI, Bierman EL: Aging and hormones. In Williams RH (ed): Textbook of Endocrinology. Philadelphia, WB Saunders, 1974

47. Gregerman RI, Davis PJ: Effects of intrinsic and extrinsic variables on thyroid hormone economy: Intrinsic physiologic variables and non-thyroidal illness. In Werner SC, Ingbar SH (eds): The Thyroid, pp 223–246. New York, Harper & Row, 1978

48. Gross J: Aging of connective tissue: The extracellular components. In Bourne GH (ed): Structural Aspects of Aging. New York, Hafner, 1961

49. Gutmann E, Hanzlikova V: Age Changes in the Neuromuscular System. Bristol, Scientechnica, 1972

50. Gutmann E, Hanzlikova V: Changes in neuromuscular relationships in aging. In Ordy JM, Brizzee KR (eds): Neurobiology of Aging. New York, Plenum Publishing, 1975

51. Harman D: Aging: A theory based on free-radical and radiation chemistry. J Gerontol 11:298, 1956

52. Harman D: Free radical theory of aging: Dietary implications. Am J Clin Nutr 25:839, 1972

53. Harrison DE: Normal production of erythrocytes by mouse marrow continuous for 73 months. Proc Natl Acad Sci USA 70:3184, 1973

54. Hart R, Setlow R: Correlation between deoxyribonucleic acid excision repair and life span in a number of mammalian species. Proc Natl Acad Sci USA 71:2169, 1974

55. Hay R, Menzies R, Morgan H, Strehler B: The division potential of cells in continuous growth as compared to cells subcultivated after maintenance in stationary phase. Exp Gerontol 3:35, 1965

56. Hayflick L: The limited *in vitro* lifetime of human diploid cell strains. Exp Cell Res 37:614, 1965

57. Hayflick L, Moorhead P: The serial cultivation of human diploid cell strains. Exp Cell Res 25:585, 1961

58. Heidrick ML: Imbalanced cyclic-AMP and cyclic-GMP levels in concanavalin-A stimulated spleen cells from aged mice. J Cell Biol 57:139a, 1973

59. Henderson S, Edwards R: Chiasma frequency and maternal age in mammals. Nature 218:22, 1968

60. Hendley D, Mildvan A, Reporter M, Strehler B: The properties of isolated human cardiac age pigment: II. Chemical and enzymatic properties. J Gerontol 18:250, 1963

61. Holland JJ, Kohne D, Doyle MV: Analysis of viral replication in ageing human fibroblasts. Nature New Biol 245:316, 1973

62. Holliday R: Errors in protein synthesis and clonal senescence in fungi. Nature 221:1224, 1969

63. Holliday R, Tarrant GM: Altered enzymes in aging human fibroblasts. Nature New Biol 238:26, 1972

64. Hori Y, Perkins EH, Halsall MK: Decline in phytohemagglutinin responsiveness of spleen cells from aging mice. Proc Soc Exp Biol Med 144:48, 1973

65. Hynes RO, Destree A: Extensive disulfide bonding at the mammalian cell surface. Proc Natl Acad Sci USA, 74:2855, 1977

66. Ingbar SH: The influence of aging on human thyroid hormone economy. In Greenblatt R (ed): Geriatric Endocrinology. New York, Raven Press, 1978

67. Ingbar, SH, Woeber KA: The thyroid gland. In Williams RH (ed): Textbook of Endocrinology, pp 208–214. Philadelphia, WB Saunders, 1981

68. Jackson V, Shires A, Chalkley R, Granner D: Studies on highly metabolically active acetylation and phosphorylation of histones. J Biol Chem 250:4856, 1975

69. Johnson L, Johnson R, Strehler B: Cardiac hypertrophy, aging and changes in cardiac ribosomal RNA gene dosage in man. J Mol Cell Cardiol 7:125, 1975

70. Johnson LK, Longenecker JP: Senescence of aortic endothelial cells *in vitro:* Influence of culture conditions and preliminary characterization of the senescent phenotype. Mech Aging Dev 19:1, 1984

71. Johnson R, Chrisp C, Strehler B: Selective loss of ribosomal RNA genes during the aging of postmitotic tissues. Mech Ageing Dev 1:183, 1972

72. Johnson R, Strehler B: Loss of genes coding for ribosomal RNA in aging brain cells. Nature New Biol 240:412, 1972

73. Kirkwood TBL: Evolution of aging. Nature 270:301, 1977

74. Kohn RR: Human aging and disease. J Chronic Dis 16:6, 1963

75. Kornberg R: Chromatin structure: A repeating unit of histones and DNA. Science 184:868, 1974

76. Kurtz D, Sippel A, Feigelson P: Effect of thyroid hormones on the level of the hepatic mRNA for α_{2u} globin. Biochemistry 15:1031, 1976

77. Ladda R, Gianopoulos T, McCormick L: Increased proliferative response of human skin fibroblasts exposed to EGF. Ped Res 12:395, 1978

78. Latham KR, Finch CE: Hepatic glucocorticoid binders in mature and senescent C57BL/6J male mice. Endocrinology 98:1480, 1976

79. Latham KR, Tseng YL: Nuclear thyroid hormone binding activities and serum iodothyronine levels in aging rats. J Am Aging Assoc 2:48, 1985

80. LeGuilly Y, Simon M, Lenoir P, Bourel M: Long-term culture of human adult liver cells: Morphological changes related to *in vitro* senescence and effect of donors age on growth potential. Gerontologia 19:303, 1973

81. Lima L, Macieira-Coelho A: Parameters of aging in chicken embryo fibroblasts cultivated *in vitro.* Exp Cell Res 70:279, 1972

82. Lithner F, Ponten J: Bovine fibroblasts in long-term tissue culture: Chromosome studies. Int J Cancer 1:579, 1966

83. Loftfield RB, Vanderjagt D: The frequency of errors in protein biosynthesis. Biochem J 128:1353, 1972

84. Longenecker JP, Kilty LA, Ridge JA, Miller LD, Johnson LD: Proliferative variability of endothelial clones derived from adult bovine aorta: Influence of smooth muscle extracellular matrix and fibroblast growth factor. J Cell Physiol 114:7, 1983

85. Louie A, Candido E, Dixon G: Enzymatic modifications and their possible roles in regulating the binding of basic proteins to DNA and in controlling chromosomal structure. Cold Spring Harbor Symp Quant Biol 38:803, 1973

86. McCay CM: Chemical aspects and the effect of diet upon aging. In Cowdry EV (ed): Problems of Ageing, 2nd ed. Baltimore, Williams & Wilkins, 1942

87. McGavack TH: Aging as seen by the endocrinologist. Geriatrics 18:181, 1963

88. McHale J, Mouton M, McHale J: Limited culture life-span of human diploid cells as a function of metabolic time instead of division potential. Exp Gerontol 6:89, 1971

89. Makinodan T: Immunity and Aging. In Finch CE, Hayflick L (eds): Handbook of the Biology of Aging. New York, Von Nostrand Reinhold, 1977

90. Makinodan T, Adler WH: Effects of aging on the differentiation and proliferation potentials of cells of the immune system. Fed Proc 34:153, 1975

91. Martin G: Cellular aging: I. Clonal senescence; II. Post replicative cells. Am J Pathol 89:484, 1977

92. Martin G, Ogburn C: Cell, tissue and organoid cultures of blood vessels. In Rothblatt G, Cristofalo V (eds): Growth, Nutrition and Metabolism of Cells in Culture, vol 3.

93. Martin G, Sprague C, Epstein C: Replicative life-span of cultivated human cells: Effect of donor's age, tissue and genotype. Lab Invest 23:86, 1970

94. Menzies R, Gold P: The turnover of mitochondria in a variety of tissues of young adult and aged rates. J Biol Chem 246:2425, 1971

95. Meredith R, Taylor AI, Ansi FM: High risk of Down's syndrome at advanced maternal age. Lancet 1:564, 1978

96. Mickey J, Tate R, Lefkowitz RJ: Subsensitivity of adenylate cyclase and decreased β-adrenergic receptor binding after chronic exposure to isoproterenol *in vitro.* J Biol Chem 250:5727, 1975

97. Mueller SN, Rosen EM, Levine EM: Cellular senescence in a cloned strain of bovine fetal aortic endothelial cells. Science 207:889, 1980

98. Nelson JF, Holinka CF, Latham KR, Allen JK, Finch CE: Corticosterone binding in cytosols from brain regions of mature and senescent male C57BL/6J mice. Brain Res 115:345, 1978

99. Nishizuka Y, Ueda K, Yoshihara K, Yamamura H, Takeda M, Hayaishi O: Enzymic adenosine diphosphoribosylation of nuclear proteins. Cold Spring Harbor Symp Quant Biol 34:781, 1969

100. Nordgren R, Hirsch G, Menzies R, Hendley D, Kutsky R, Strehler B: Evidence for long-lived components in developing mouse tissues labeled with leucine. Exp Gerontol 4:7, 1969

101. Oh YH, Conrad RA: Effect of aging on acetate incorporation in nuclei of lymphocytes stimulated with phytohemagglutinin. Life Sci 11:677, 1972

102. Olins A, Olins D: Spheroid chromatin units (v bodies). Science 183:330, 1974

103. Orgel LE: The maintenance of accuracy of protein synthesis and its relevance to aging. Proc Natl Acad Sci USA 49:517, 1963

104. Orgel LE: The maintenance of accuracy of protein synthesis and its relevance to aging: A correction. Proc Natl Acad Sci USA 67:1476, 1970

105. Orgel LE: Ageing of clones of mammalian cells. Nature 244:441, 1973

106. Palmiter R, Smith L: Synergistic effects of oestrogen and progesterone on ovomucoid and conalbumin mRNA synthesis in chick oviduct. Nature New Biol 246:74, 1973

107. Ponten J: The growth capacity of normal and *Rous*-virus transformed chicken fibroblasts *in vitro*. Int J Cancer 6:323, 1970

108. Price G, Modak S, Makinodan T: Age-associated changes in the DNA of mouse tissue. Science 171:917, 1971

109. Reichel W, Hallander J, Clark J, Strehler B: Lipofuscin accumulation as a function of age and distribution in rodent brain. J Gerontol 23:71, 1968

110. Rheinwald J, Green H: Epidermal growth factor and the multiplication of cultured human epidermal keratinocytes. Nature 265:421, 1977

111. Ringold G, Yamamoto K, Bishop J, Varmus H: Dexamethasone mediated induction of mouse mammary tumor virus RNA: A system for studying glucocorticoid action. Cell 6:299, 1975

112. Rockstein M, Chesky JA, Sussman MJ: Comparative biology and evolution of aging. In Finch C, Hayflick L (eds): Handbook of the Biology of Aging. New York, Van Nostrand Reinhold, 1977

113. Roth GS: Age-related changes in glucocorticoid binding by rat splenic leukocytes: Possible cause of altered adaptive responsiveness. Fed Proc 34:183, 1975

114. Rutishauser U, Sacks L: Receptor mobility and the binding of cells to lectin-coated fibers. J Cell Biol 66:76, 1975

115. Sacher GA: Life table modification and life prolongation. In Finch C, Hayflick L (eds): Handbook of the Biology of Aging. New York, Van Nostrand Reinhold, 1977

116. Sacher GA: Longevity and aging in vertebrate evolution. Bioscience 28:497, 1978

117. Salser JS, Balis ME: Alterations in deoxyribonucleic acid bound amino acids with age and sex. J Gerontol 27:1, 1972

118. Samorajski T, Ordy M: The histochemistry and ultra structure of lipid pigment in the adrenal glands of aging mice. J Gerontol 22:253, 1967

119. Schimke RT, Ganschow R, Doyle D, Arias IM: Regulation of protein turnover in mammalian tissues. Fed Proc 27:1223, 1968

120. Schneider E, Mitsui Y: The relationship between *in vitro* cellular aging and *in vivo* human age. Proc Natl Acad Sci USA 73:3584, 1976

121. Schwartz SM, Haudenschild CC, Eddy EM: Endothelial regeneration: I. Quantitative analysis of intimal stages of endothelial regeneration in rat aortic intima. Lab Invest 381:578, 1978

122. Seeburg P, Shine J, Martial J, Baxter J, Goodman H: Nucleotide sequence and amplification in bacteria of the structural gene for rat growth hormone. Nature 270:486, 1977

123. Segall P, Timiras P: Pathophysiologic findings after chronic tryptophan deficiency in rats: A model for delayed growth and aging. Mech Ageing Dev 5:109, 1976

124. Segall P, Timiras P: Neural and endocrine development after chronic tryptophan deficiency in rats. Mech Ageing Dev 7:1, 1978

125. Shock NW: Trends in Gerontology, 2nd ed. Stanford, CA, Stanford University Press, 1957

126. Shock NW: Energy metabolism, caloric intake and physical activity of the aging. In Carlson LA (ed): Nutrition in Old Age: Tenth Symposium of the Swedish Nutrition Foundation. Stockholm, Almqvist and Wiksell, 1972

127. Sigmund OH (ed): The Merck Veterinary Manual, 3rd ed. Rahway, NJ, Merck & Co, 1967

128. Slatis HM, Apelbaum A: Hairy pinna of the ear in Israeli populations. Am J Hum Genet 15:74, 1963

129. Sokal RR: Senescence and genetic load: Evidence from tribolium. Science 167:1733, 1970

130. Strehler BL: Origin and comparison of the effects of time and high-energy radiation on living systems. Q Rev Biol 34:117, 1959

131. Strehler BL: Studies on the comparative physiology of aging: III. Effects of x-radiation dosage on age-specific mortality rates of *Drosophila melanogaster* and *Campanularia flexuosa*. J Gerontol 19:83, 1964

132. Strehler BL: Aging at the cellular level. In Rossman I (ed): Clinical Geriatrics. Philadelphia, JB Lippincott, 1971

133. Strehler BL: Time, Cells and Aging, 2nd ed. New York, Academic Press, 1977

134. Strehler B, Chang MP, Johnson L: Loss of hybridizable ribosomal DNA from human post-mitotic tissues during aging: I. Age-dependent loss of human myocardium. Mech Ageing Dev 11:371, 1979

135. Strehler B, Hirsch G, Gusseck D, Johnson R, Bick M: Codon restriction theory of aging and development. J Theor Biol 33:429, 1971

136. Strehler B, Mark D, Mildvan A, Gee M: Rate and magnitude of age pigment accumulation in the human myocardium. J Gerontol 14:430, 1959

137. Sulkin N, Sulkin D: Age differences in response to chronic hypoxia on the fine structure of cardiac muscle and autonomic ganglion cells. J Gerontol 22:485, 1967

138. Thrasher J, Greulich R: The duodenal progenitor population: II. Age-related changes in size and distribution. J Exp Zool 159:385, 1965

139. Todarao G, Green H: Quantitative studies of the growth of mouse embryo cells in culture and their development into established lines. J Cell Biol 17:229, 1963

140. Tomkins GA, Stanbridge, EJ, Hayflick L: Viral probes of aging in the human diploid cell strain WI-38. Proc Soc Exp Biol Med 146:385, 1974

141. Vital Statistics of the United States, vol 2, section 5. Life Table 5-5, 1963

142. vonHahn HP: Age-related alterations in the structure of DNA: II. The role of histones. Gerontologia 10:174, 1964

143. vonHahn HP: A model of "regulatory" aging of the cell of the gene level. J Gerontol 21:291, 1966

144. Walford RL: The immunologic theory of aging: Current status. Fed Proc 33:2020, 1974

145. Weismann A: Essays upon Heredity and Kindred Biological Problems. London, Oxford University Press (Clarendon), 1891

146. Welch JP: Somatic mutations and the aging process. Adv Gerontol Res 2:1, 1967

147. Westgren U, Burger A, Ingemansson S, Melander A, Tibblin S, Wahlin E: Blood levels of 3,5,3'-triiodothyronine and thyroxine: Differences between children, adults, and elderly subjects. Acta Med Scand 200:493, 1976

148. Whiteford R, Getty R: Distribution of lipofuscin in canine and porcine brain as related to aging. J Gerontol 21:31, 1966

149. Williams GC: Pleiotropy, natural selection, and the evolution of senescence. Evolution 11:398, 1957

4

Biologic Basis and Clinical Significance of Immune Senescence

Marc E. Weksler

Although a primary role of immune senescence in the process of aging has been suggested,[77] it is doubtful that the aging of any single physiologic system directly causes the age-associated changes in all organ systems. More likely the effect of age on physiologic function reflects changes in vital cellular processes such as cell replication, energy metabolism, and detoxification, which occur in all tissues and organ systems. As these functions decline, the capacity of the organism to adapt, as is required to maintain homeostasis, is compromised. This loss of homeostatic reserve with age, I have termed *homeostenosis*.

Changes in immune function with age have been known for more than 50 years. However, the systematic study of immune senescence began in the early 1960s when Makinodan and Walford and their colleagues established the field of immunogerontology. In the past 2 decades considerable understanding of the age-associated changes in immune function and their biologic mechanisms have been achieved. The relative importance of immune senescence to the diseases of aging has been difficult to establish. Even with infectious diseases, in which immunity plays such a clear role in resistance and recovery to infection, the precise contribution of immune deficiency to infection in the elderly patient is not clear. For example, many changes in the respiratory system that occur with age lead to infection. Alterations in bacterial adherence, mucus production, and ciliary action at the mucosal surface; changes in the inflammatory response including chemotaxis, phagocytosis, complement activation, as well as

This research was supported in part by grants AG 00239 and AG 00541 from the National Institutes of Health.

the generation of fever; and immune senescence all contribute to the predisposition of the elderly to respiratory infections. This chapter is an update of my review of immune senescence published in 1983.[80]

BIOLOGIC BASIS OF IMMUNE SENESCENCE

Thymic Involution

The involution of the thymus gland is a universal accompaniment of aging in both man and experimental animals. The loss of the cellular mass of the thymus begins at sexual maturity and is complete by 45 to 50 years of age in humans.[11] At this time the thymus retains only 5% to 10% of its maximal mass. The striking involution of the thymus gland during the first half of life can, to a considerable extent, be related to the altered form and function of the immune system observed during the second half of life.

Two functions of the thymus gland have been recognized: (1) the production of a family of polypeptide hormones and (2) the maturation of T-lymphocyte precursors from the bone marrow. Thymic hormones are important in the differentiation of pre- and post-thymic lymphocytes. In humans, thymic hormone activity in serum is maintained from birth until the age of 20 to 30 and then declines.[48] Thymic hormone can no longer be detected in healthy normal humans over 60 years of age. It has been suggested that the low level of serum thymic hormone activity is due to the presence of inhibitors.[24]

Immature lymphocytes from the bone marrow enter the cortex of the thymus gland. With age,

57

fewer immature lymphocytes enter the thymus and the gland loses its capacity to facilitate the differentiation of these cells.[56,69] Perhaps as a consequence of these events, immature T lymphocytes are found in increased numbers in the blood of elderly humans.[53] Thus, with age, serum thymic hormone activity declines and the percentage of immature lymphocytes within the thymus gland and in the peripheral blood increases.

Age-Associated Changes in Lymphocytes

Most investigators·have found that the total number of lymphocytes and the number of T or B lymphocytes in peripheral human blood do not change with age. Most studies, however, have quantitated lymphocytes in a single or limited number of lymphoid compartments. It remains possible that the total number or distribution of lymphocytes within the organism changes with age. A decrease in germinal centers in lymph nodes and an increase in plasma cells and lymphocytes in the bone marrow occur with age.[7] The maintenance of cell number does not imply functional competence. It is likely that although the number of T lymphocytes does not change with age, these long-lived cells may circulate in a postmature state, viable but lacking the replicative capacity required for immune competence.

Although the total number of T lymphocytes in blood does not change, the representation of T-lymphocyte subpopulations in peripheral blood does change with age: immature autorosetting T lymphocytes increase[53]; T-gamma lymphocytes increase[35]; helper/inducer T lymphocytes identified by the OKT4 monoclonal antibody increase[53]; and suppressor/cytotoxic T lymphocytes identified by the monoclonal OKT8 antibody decrease[53]. Although the changes in the proportion of T-lymphocyte subsets are modest, they may be important in the regulation of immune function.

The cell surface characteristics of lymphocytes change with age. New antigenic determinants are expressed on lymphocytes from old mice that are recognized by young syngeneic animals.[14] The density of some surface determinants such as theta on T lymphocytes and surface immunoglobulin on B lymphocytes decreases with age, and the capping of these surface receptors decrease with age.[29] It is likely that these changes in the number, affinity, and mobility of surface determinants contribute to the altered function of lymphocytes with age.

The metabolic functions of lymphocytes depend on enzymes. Lymphocyte adenylate cyclase has been reported to increase and guanylate cyclase to decrease with age.[72] Other enzymes, deficient in certain immunodeficiency states, are also reported to be decreased in lymphocytes with age. The activity of purine nucleoside phosphorylase has been reported to be decreased in spleen cells from old mice.[68] The activity of ecto-5'-nucleotidase has also been found to be reduced in lymphocytes from immunologically deficient and elderly humans.[10]

Lymphocytes from both elderly experimental animals and humans are more susceptible to damage induced by ionizing radiation, ultraviolet light, and mutagenic drugs.[71,78] The instability of chromosomes in lymphocytes from old subjects may contribute not only to the impaired capacity of these cells to divide but also to the increased susceptibility of elderly humans to neoplastic disease. Finally, chromosomal instability and increased susceptibility to cell cycle arrest may explain the increased toxicity of certain drugs in elderly patients.

ALTERATIONS IN IMMUNE FUNCTION WITH AGE

Humoral Immunity

The total concentration of immunoglobulins in serum changes little with age, although minor shifts in the distribution of immunoglobulin class have been reported: the concentration of IgA and IgG in serum is increased in older humans while the concentration of IgM is decreased.[37] In this study, humans in whom the serum concentration of IgG fell had a reduced life expectancy.[12] The concentration of IgA and IgG in cerebrospinal fluid is also reported to increase with age.[54]

The first evidence that the function of the immune system changes with aging came from the measurement of natural antibodies in serum from humans of different ages. It was found that the concentration of isoagglutinins, of antibody to sheep erythrocytes and to *Salmonella* flagellin, was lower in elderly humans.[59,65,74] Subsequently, it became clear that autoantibodies and monoclonal immunoglobulins increase with age.[4,66] Autoantibodies to nucleic acids, immunoglobulin, and thyroglobulin have all been found with increased frequency in serum from old humans, and two thirds of elderly subjects in one study had one or more of these autoantibodies.[37] My experience suggests that a smaller fraction of healthy elderly humans living in the community have autoantibodies. Although old experimental animals and humans express autoantibodies, autoimmune disease is not increased in frequency. In fact, old animals are no more susceptible to autoimmune disease induced by cross-reacting antigens (a common method to induce autoantibodies) than young animals, although there is an increased number of lymphocytes that secrete autoantibodies in old animals.[32]

One class of autoantibodies, auto-anti-idiotypic antibodies, plays an important role in the "down" regulation of the immune response. Anti-idiotypic antibodies in old animals inhibit the secretion of idiotype-bearing antibodies. Old mice have been shown to produce excessive auto-anti-idiotypic antibody during the immune response, and this response contributes significantly to the difference in the apparent antibody response between old and young mice.[33]

The frequency of monoclonal immunoglobulin, like autoantibodies, increases with age in humans and experimental animals. Less than 0.1% of humans under age 50 have benign monoclonal gammopathies, while almost 2% of humans over age 70 have these immunoglobulins.[4] In one study, 19% of humans over age 95 had monoclonal immunoglobulins.[63] These homogeneous proteins reflect disordered immune regulation of normal B lymphocytes and not the neoplastic transformation of plasma cells seen in multiple myeloma. Until recently the relationship between monoclonal gammopathy and thymic involution was only conjecture. Old CBA mice show an increased prevalence of monoclonal immunoglobulins by 30 months of age. It has been found that neonatal thymectomy increased the age at onset of monoclonal gammopathies to 6 to 9 months of age.[62] By 30 months of age, 65% to 75% of neonatally thymectomized mice had monoclonal immunoglobulins instead of the usual prevalence of monoclonal immunoglobulins of 5% to 10% at this age in these mice. In addition to the increased incidence of autoantibodies and monoclonal immunoglobulins and the decreased levels of natural antibodies, the response of elderly humans and of experimental animals to foreign antigens decreases with age. The antibody response to Japanese B encephalitis, influenza, and parainfluenza virus vaccine is lower in old as compared with young humans.[19,67] Similarly, the antibody response to pneumococcal polysaccharide, *Salmonella* flagellin, and tetanus toxoid is lower in old humans.[2,47,65]

The class of immunoglobulin generated in the immune response also changes with age.[31] The more thymic-dependent IgG antibody response is more impaired than the more thymic-independent IgM response. The antibody response is also maintained for a shorter time in old as compared with young individuals. These findings and the findings in experimental animals that thymectomy accelerates the onset of these age-associated changes and that young thymocytes or thymic hormones can augment the IgG and high affinity antibody response of old mice[79] clearly point to the contribution of thymic involution to immune senescence.

The age-associated changes in the immune system discussed so far do not indicate whether these changes are intrinsic to the immune system or the result of the environment within an elderly host. Evidence that the age-associated changes in immune function are intrinsic to the immune system is derived from *in vivo* transfer studies in experimental animals and from *in vitro* studies of the function of lymphocytes from young and old experimental animals and humans.

The transfer of lymphocytes from old mice to young, syngeneic recipients revealed an intrinsic functional defect. Thus, young thymectomized recipients of old lymphocytes displayed the characteristic immune response expressed by intact old animals: a reduced immune response to foreign antigens with a preferential loss of high affinity and IgG antibodies.[31] Mixed transfer studies in which B lymphocytes and T lymphocytes from old and young mice were combined in various combinations revealed that the predominant defect in lymphocytes from old animals resided in the T lymphocyte preparation. Helper T-lymphocyte activity in old spleen cells was only one-third to one-tenth that found in spleen cell preparations from young mice.[52] Furthermore, the immune response of recipients of old lymphocytes could, to a considerable extent, be corrected if thymocytes from young animals were mixed with old spleen cells or if lymphocytes from old animals were transferred to irradiated young recipients with intact thymus glands.[79] This suggested that the thymus of the young recipient was able to facilitate the maturation of immature lymphocytes transferred from old animals.

It has been found that self-reconstitution of old mice also reestablishes immune function of young mice. In these studies the increased auto-anti-idiotypic antibody response was reversed in old mice following total nodal irradiation and reconstitution from the shielded bone marrow.[44a] Finally, it has been found that old mice treated with thymic hormone or recipients reconstituted with lymphocytes from old animals incubated *in vitro* with thymic hormones had improved immunologic competence.[79]

The humoral immune response can also be studied *in vitro*. Specific antibody, total antibody, and the number of antibody-forming cells can be determined after incubation of human lymphocytes with polyclonal B-lymphocyte activators. Lymphocytes from old humans produced significantly less specific antibody following *in vivo* immunization or *in vitro* activation with polyclonal B-lymphocyte activators.[2,47,57] However, there was no decrease in the total amount of immunoglobulin produced or in the total number of antibody-forming cells.

The major defect in specific antibody secretion *in vitro* by lymphocyte preparations from old humans was due to impaired T lymphocyte function. As was observed in cell transfer studies, a deficiency of helper T lymphocytes and/or an increase in suppressor T lymphocyte activity was found. B lymphocyte function appeared to be less affected by age. Specific antibody produced by human B lymphocytes from young and old subjects after polyclonal B lymphocyte activation showed no significant changes with age.[45] Studies with murine lymphocytes, in which it is possible to generate hapten-specific immune responses to both thymic-independent and thymic-dependent antigens *in vitro*, have revealed decreased response to both classes of antigens with age.[21] Spleen cells from mice more than 20 to 24 months of age express significant suppressor T lymphocyte activity. Suppressor activity contributes to, but cannot account totally for, the immune deficiency of aging as the impairment in antibody response develops before suppressor cells can be demonstrated and because removal of suppressor T lymphocytes does not reverse the impaired response of B lymphocytes to thymic-independent antigens.

It has been found that the decrease in T-lymphocyte function in elderly humans and old animals can be in part related to their decreased capacity to produce and to bind Il-2.[28] Although the *in vitro* proliferative response of T lymphocytes from old humans stimulated by mitogen was not augmented by exogenous T-lymphocyte growth factor, the plaque-forming cell response and the proliferation of splenic T lymphocytes from old mice cultured with antigen were augmented by the addition of T-lymphocyte growth factor.[73]

The proliferation of B lymphocytes from humans and experimental animals can also be studied *in vitro*. The proliferative response induced by anti-immunoglobulin antibody does not decline with age.[13,73] Most investigators report that the proliferative response of murine lymphocytes to lipopolysaccharide is modestly if at all impaired with age. Even when the proliferative response of T and B lymphocytes has been found to be impaired with age, the T-lymphocyte response is more greatly impaired than the B-lymphocyte response.

Macrophages are required for antigen processing, lymphocyte proliferation, and antibody synthesis.They also phagocytize and destroy microbial agents. Several studies have reported that both the number of macrophages and their antigen-processing capabilities are not altered with age.[26] The *in vitro* phagocyte activity of peritoneal macrophages from old mice is equal to or better than that of young mice. The ability of old and young antigen-pulsed peritoneal macrophages to stimulate both primary and secondary immune responses was comparable. In addition, the capability of macrophages to support lymphocyte proliferation was unaltered with age. Finally, the ability of human macrophages to secrete T-lymphocyte replacing factor when exposed to lipopolysaccharide or to phagocytize and kill *Candida albicans* was not different in old and young individuals.[26,45] Thus, it appears that macrophage function is not significantly altered with age.

In summary, the humoral immune response is impaired in old subjects. This is predominately due to a decrease in helper T-lymphocyte activity, although increased suppressor activity and defects in B-lymphocyte function may also play a role. It is important to note that although specific antibody responses are greatly impaired with age, the number of lymphocytes, the concentration of serum immunoglobulin, the total number of antibody-producing cells, and the total amount of antibody formed following antigenic stimulation are little, if at all, altered. These observations suggest that the production of other antibodies (*e.g.*, autoantibodies and homogeneous antibodies by the aged subject) makes up for the loss of specific antibody production.

Cell-mediated Immunity

Cell-mediated immunity depends on the functional integrity of thymic-dependent lymphocytes. As thymic involution is a universal accompaniment of aging, studies of immune senescence have examined the *in vivo* functions of T lymphocytes, delayed hypersensitivity, and graft rejection. Elderly humans have less vigorous delayed hypersensitivity reactions to common skin testing antigens such as *Candida,* purified protein derivative of tuberculin (PPD), and mumps, than do young individuals.[65] The impaired response of the elderly to these antigens might reflect an altered response to antigenic challenge, the loss of immunologic memory, or both. Differences in the interval between sensitization and challenge can be eliminated by sensitizing individuals of different ages to a new antigen (*e.g.,* dinitrochlorobenzene) and then challenging all subjects after the same interval of time. Using this protocol, 30% of humans over age 70 failed to respond to dinitrochlorobenzene while only 5% of subjects under age 70 failed to respond.[76]

Ethical constraints prevent the direct assessment of other cell-mediated reactions such as the graft-versus-host reaction or tissue and tumor graft rejection in humans. However, the lymphocyte transfer test, a cutaneous model of the graft-versus-host reaction, has been studied in individuals of different ages. Lymphocytes from old donors were less able to induce a positive transfer reaction than lymphocytes from young donors.[3]

Graft-versus-host reactivity as well as tumor and skin graft rejection have been studied in animals of different ages. Lymphocytes from old mice were less capable of eliciting a graft-versus-host reaction or of rejecting tumor or skin grafts than were lymphocytes from young mice.[25,46,50] Lymphocytes from old mice were impaired in generating a graft-versus-host reaction *in vivo* and *in vitro.* However, incubation of lymphocytes from old animals with thymic hormone reconstituted their capacity to manifest a vigorous *in vitro* graft-versus-host reaction.[25]

Graft rejection depends on an integrated series of immune reactions including alloantigen recognition, helper T lymphocyte proliferation, and the generation of cytotoxic T lymphocytes. Cytotoxic T lymphocytes are effector cells in graft rejection. The impaired rejection of tissue and tumor grafts in old mice is associated with the impaired generation of cytotoxic T lymphocytes *in vitro.*[5]

Immunity to viral infection also depends on the generation of cytotoxic T lymphocytes. Older mice are impaired in their capacity to generate T-lymphocyte mediated immunity to influenza[23] and lymphochoriomeningitis virus[22] and to *Listeria monocytogenes.*[58] Old animals infected with *Listeria* develop only one-thousandth the level of T-lymphocyte immunity found in young mice.

A syngeneic graft-versus-host reaction follows the transfer of lymphocytes from old animals to syngeneic young recipients.[34] This reaction does not occur when lymphocytes from young animals are transferred to syngeneic recipients of the same age. This suggests the presence of "autoimmune" T lymphocytes in old animals. Thus, the increase in autoimmune reactivity seen with age is expressed by both humoral and cell-mediated immunity.

The function of T lymphocytes has also been studied *in vitro.* The proliferative response of lymphocytes from old humans is impaired in their response to T-lymphocyte mitogens.[37,43] Lymphocytes from elderly persons sensitized to *Mycobacterium tuberculosis* or *varicella zoster* virus did not proliferate to the same degree observed with lymphocytes from young donors when cultured with these antigens.[51,55] The defect in the proliferative response to mitogens in cultures from old humans could not be explained by a deficiency in the number of T lymphocytes, since the impaired proliferative response was also expressed when purified T lymphocytes from old subjects were cultured with mitogen.

My colleagues and I have studied the cellular basis of the impaired proliferative response of T lymphocytes from old humans in considerable detail. A number of independent techniques have revealed that the T-lymphocyte preparations from old humans contain only one fifth to one half as many mitogen-responsive cells as do similar preparations from young humans.[43] Not only are there fewer mitogen-responsive T lymphocytes in the blood of old humans, but their capacity to divide sequentially in culture is impaired.[39] After 96 hours in culture with phytohemagglutinin, the number of lymphocytes from old subjects dividing for the third time was only one fourth that found in cultures containing lymphocytes from young subjects. The number of cells dividing for the second time in cultures from old subjects was only one half that found in cultures from young subjects, although the number of cells dividing for the first time was the same in cultures of lymphocytes from old or young donors.

We have begun studies that attempt to pinpoint the intracellular site of the proliferative defect. The number and affinity of receptors for phytohemagglutin are the same in lymphocytes from old and young donors. The generation of a cytoplasmic factor that stimulates ^{3}H-Tdr incorporation by isolated nuclei is comparable in lymphocytes from young or old humans incubated with phytohemagglutinin.[36] On the other hand, we have found in preliminary studies that nuclei isolated from lymphocytes of old humans are impaired in their response to the cytoplasmic factor that stimulates DNA replication when compared with nuclei from young donors. Thus, it appears that lymphocytes produce cytoplasmic factors that stimulate DNA replication in nuclei from other cells but the nuclei in old lymphocytes fail to respond to these cytoplasmic signals.

Calcium ions (Ca^{2+}) have been shown to play an important role in cell activation. Using divalent cation chelators, lymphocytes from old subjects were found to be more sensitive to increased amounts of chelating agents such as EDTA and EGTA. Furthermore, lymphocytes from old persons required greater amounts of CA^{2+} supplements to restore their proliferative response after inhibition.[44] Verapamil, a calcium channel blocker, inhibits activation of lymphocytes from old humans to a greater degree than it does that of lymphocytes from young.[9]

In summary, cell-mediated immunity is impaired in old animals and humans. The cellular basis of the impaired response of lymphocytes from old humans reflects a decreased number of responsive T lymphocytes as well as an impaired proliferative capacity of these cells. The proliferative defect appears to be due to the failure of the nucleus to carry out DNA replication despite the fact that many of the cell surface and cytoplasmic changes that follow activation appear to occur normally.

CLINICAL CONSEQUENCES OF IMMUNE SENESCENCE

Clinically, immune senescence leads to a moderate T-lymphocyte–immunodeficient state. Since the degree of immune deficiency associated with aging is relatively modest, opportunistic infections with *Pneumocystis* or *Aspergillus,* seen in severe immunodeficient states, do not occur in normal elderly subjects. However, there can be no doubt that immune senescence increases the susceptibility to and severity of certain viral and bacterial diseases in elderly persons. The strongest case for a causal relationship between immune senescence and infectious disease can be made for the reactivation of latent varicella-zoster and mycobacterial disease. Reactivation of these diseases is almost always associated with defects in cell-mediated immunity that occur with aging, the acquired immune deficiency syndrome, neoplastic disease, and immunosuppressive or cytotoxic drug therapy.

Zoster or shingles is the reexpression of latent varicella-zoster infection. Virtually all adults have been infected with the varicella-zoster virus during a childhood symptomatic (chickenpox) or asymptomatic infection with this virus. Convalescence from this disease and resistance to its reexpression depends on cell-mediated immunity. Patients with humoral immune defects (*e.g.,* X-linked agammaglobulinemia) handle the varicella-zoster infection normally. Antibody does play a role in resisting initial infection, and passive antibody can prevent infection of susceptible individuals with varicella-zoster.

A latent viral infection remains after recovery from varicella-zoster. The virus is believed to enter the dorsal root ganglia and remain latent for the life span of the individual. In a small number of healthy individuals the varicella-zoster virus is expressed between the ages of 15 and 45. However, beginning at the age of 45 the incidence of reexpression of varicella-zoster increases. In the 40 years between 45 and 85 the incidence of varicella-zoster disease increases fivefold.[41] This is related to the loss of specific cell-mediated immunity to the varicella-zoster virus, although humoral immunity to the virus remains intact.[8]

The reactivation of tuberculosis in the elderly also appears to be related to the declining vigor of cell-mediated immunity. Cell-mediated immunity plays a crucial role in host resistance to tuberculosis. The same clinical circumstances that lead to the exacerbation of varicella-zoster infection lead to reactivation of tuberculosis. Usually tuberculosis in the elderly results from the reexpression of latent mycobacterial disease. The nature of the latent state in tuberculosis is less clear, but it is likely that local inflammatory processes contain viable bacteria. Breakdown of local barriers release infectious microorganisms that can disseminate if specific cell-mediated immunity is impaired. The defects in cell-mediated immunity to mycobacterial antigens in elderly subjects has been demonstrated by testing cutaneous delayed-type hypersensitivity. Patients of various ages with culture-proven tuberculosis have been tested. With the use of the optimal technique, 10% of tubercular patients under age 55 were found to be unresponsive to PPD while 30% of patients with tuberculosis over 55 were unresponsive.[40] Epidemiologic evidence over the past 40 years indicates that tuberculosis in the United States is a disease of the elderly. The absolute morbidity and mortality from tuberculosis has decreased, although the relative morbidity and mortality has increased moderately in patients over 45 years of age and dramatically in patients over 65 years of age.[15]

Many factors contribute to the increased susceptibility of the elderly to other infectious diseases, although the precise role of immune senescence is difficult to quantitate. Nonspecific resistance factors that are part of the inflammatory response, such as fever, are impaired in the elderly. Hippocrates in his "Aphorisms," states "Old men have little innate heat, and for this reason they need but little fuel; too much fuel puts it out. For this reason too, the fevers of old men are less acute than others, for the body is cold." In one study, 90% of afebrile patients with culture-proven bacteremia were elderly.[39] As the febrile response augments immune reactions,[70] a blunted febrile response also compromises the defenses to infection. Leukocytosis has been reported to be less marked in the elderly with pneumonia.[18] Clearance of bacteria from the blood may be decreased if opsonization necessary for complement activation is impaired or phagocytosis is depressed. Phagocytosis and intracellular killing by leukocytes from aged humans have been reported to be impaired.[17]

Structural changes that accompany age in the urinary tract, including prostatic hypertrophy and relaxation of the pelvic floor, lead to the accumulation of residual urine. The loss of elastic recoil of the lungs, decreased mucus production, and impaired ciliary action, as well as the dampened cough reflex, lead to aspiration and contamination of the lungs, which contribute to respiratory infection.[61]

Gram-negative bacterial colonization of the respiratory and urinary system increases with age, immobility, debility, chronic disease, and level of care required for the patient.[75] One factor that leads to bacterial colonization is increased adherence of bacteria to mucosal cells of the upper respiratory or urogenital tract.[81] This appears to be due to increased protease activity in secretions and decreased amounts of fibronectin and possibly other bactericidal factors such as IgA antibody. The role of protein in preventing bacterial adherence is supported by the fact that exposure of mucosal cells to trypsin increases adherence of gram-negative bacteria. Compromise of these natural barriers in the elderly probably contributes to their increased susceptibility to bacterial colonization, infection, and sepsis. Bacteremia is more common in old as compared with young patients with urinary and respiratory infection.

Pneumonia was identified as a special risk for the elderly in 1836, less than 20 years after Laennec's classic description of the disease.[42] This fact derives no doubt from the many factors including increased bacterial colonization, decreased pulmonary clearance, and blunting of the cough reflex. In addition, it is likely that deficient alveolar macrophage and T-lymphocyte production of lymphokines, which draw accessory cells into the lungs that contribute to the normal inflammatory response as well as decreased local IgA production, compromise local defense mechanisms. Mucosal IgA production has not been adequately studied in humans of various ages, but in one report it was suggested that nasal secretion of IgA decreases with age.[1] The increased severity of pneumonia in the elderly is obvious from the increased incidence of bacteremia, morbidity, and mortality from this disease in older patients.

The availability of a polyvalent pneumococcal vaccine, proved to be clinically useful in young miners, has been recommended for elderly persons, although clinical effectiveness of the vaccine in the elderly has not been proven. The antibody response to the vaccine in the elderly is lower than that in young subjects, although it is believed to be "adequate".[2] It is important to realize that humoral immunity, which is a satisfactory index of immunity in the young, may not correlate with immune protection in the elderly. This caution is based on the fact that virtually all elderly persons have antibodies to the varicella-zoster virus, although one third of these subjects lack T-lymphocyte immunity to the varicella-zoster virus.[8] It is the defective T-lymphocyte immunity despite humoral immunity that explains the reactivation of the virus in the elderly. Studies in mice support the importance of defense mechanisms beyond antibody production. Immunization of mice with pneumococcal polysaccharide stimulates old and young mice to produce comparable amounts of antibody to this thymus-independent antigen, although old mice suffer very much greater morbidity and mortality when old and young immunized mice are challenged with the pneumococcus.*

The elderly are also more susceptible to influenza and its complications. For this reason the use of influenza vaccine has been recommended for the elderly. Although the antibody response to the vaccine is lower in the elderly than the young,[60] the vaccine when used in relatively healthy, free living elderly subjects has been effective in preventing influenza and its consequences.[6] On the other hand in studies of institutionalized elderly in whom the antibody response is probably more compromised than in noninstitutionalized elderly, no protection by vaccination was demonstrated.[20] As discussed before, the generation of cell-mediated immunity or local IgA antibody production may be more important for immunity than the level of circulating antibody.

---

* Erschler W: Personal communication, 1985.

The complexity of assigning a role for immune senescence in bacterial disease is also illustrated when the increased susceptibility and severity of the elderly to bacterial infection of the intestinal tract is considered. In part, the increasing prevalence of achlorhydria leads to an increased number of coliform bacteria in the stomach and upper intestine.[27] Such bacterial overgrowth can cause malabsorption in the elderly in the absence of "blind loops."[64] The particular susceptibility of the elderly to *Salmonella* infection is well recognized.[16] Whether the increased frequency of *Salmonella* bacteremia and mortality is due to achlorhydria or to defects such as the local production of IgA antibody, mucus, and other bacteriocidal substances requires more attention.

CONCLUSION

The immune system changes with age. Cell-mediated and humoral immune responses to foreign antigens are decreased, while the response to autologous antigens is increased. These defects can be related to the involution of the thymus and the alteration in the balance among regulatory T lymphocytes and the altered balance between idiotypic and anti-idiotypic activity. The increased susceptibility of the elderly to infections, neoplastic disease, and perhaps vascular injury may be a consequence of immune senescence. The contribution of autoantibodies to the pathobiology of aging is less certain. It has been suggested that autoantibodies and circulating immune complexes, which can damage tissues and organs, contribute to the pathologic changes of the vasculature that occur with age.

If the pathobiology of aging were related to the loss of immune competence with age, the survival of individuals with an impaired immune response would be expected to be shorter than of individuals in whom immune competence was well maintained. Three studies have examined this thesis. In one study, more humans with severely impaired delayed hypersensitivity reactions died within a 2-year period than did age-matched controls who had well-maintained delayed hypersensitivity responses.[65] In another study, humans with autoantibodies had a shorter survival than did age-matched individuals without autoantibodies.[49] A third study showed that the elderly humans with reduced suppressor cell activity had a shorter survival than did age-matched subjects with normal suppressor activity.[38] These studies could not distinguish between an alteration in the immune re-

sponse causing the shortened survival or an alteration in the immune response resulting from the factors that lead to reduced survival.

In the past decade, many of the changes in the immune system that accompany aging have been defined and related to the involution of the thymus gland. The potential contribution of immune senescence to the diseases of aging has been studied. Whether immune senescence is a primary or secondary contributor to the pathology of aging, it is likely that increased knowledge of immune senescence and the increasing ability to correct immune defects that occur in elderly subjects will offer insight into the diseases and pathology of aging.

REFERENCES

1. Alford RH: Effects of chronic bronchopulmonary disease and aging on human nasal secretion IgA concentrations. J Immunol 101:984, 1968
2. Ammann AJ, Schiffman G, Austrian R: The antibody responses to pneumococcal capsular polysaccharides in aged individuals. Proc Soc Exp Biol Med 164:312, 1980
3. Andersen E: The influence of age on transplantation immunity: Reactivity to normal lymphocyte transfer at different ages. Scand J Haematol 9:621, 1972
4. Axelsson U, Bachmann R, Hallen J: Frequency of pathological proteins (M-components) in 6,995 sera from an adult population. Acta Med Scand 179:235, 1966
5. Bach M: Influence of aging on T cell subpopulations involved in the *in vitro* generation of allogeneic cytotoxicity. Clin Immunol Immunopathol 13:220, 1979
6. Barker WH, Mullooly JP: Influenza vaccination of elderly persons: Reduction in pneumonia and influenza hospitalizations and deaths. JAMA 244:2547, 1980
7. Benner R, Haaijman JJ: Aging of the lymphoid system at the organ level. Exp Comp Immunol 4:591, 1980
8. Berger R, Florent G, Just M: Decrease of the lymphoproliferative response to varicella-zoster virus antigen in the aged. Infect Immun 32:34, 1981
9. Blitstein-Willinger E, Diamanstein T: Inhibition by isoptin (a calcium antagonist) of mitogenic stimulation of lymphocytes prior to the S-phase. Immunology 34:303, 1978
10. Boss GR, Thompson RF, Speigelberg HL, Pichler WJ, Seegmiller JE: Age-dependency of lymphocyte ecto-5'-nucleotidase activity. J Immunol 125:679, 1980
11. Boyd E: The weight of the thymus gland in health and in disease. Am J Dis Child 43:1162, 1932
12. Buckley CS III, Buckley EG, Dorsey FC: Longitu-

dinal changes in serum immunoglobulin levels in older humans. Fed Proc 33:2036, 1974

13. Callard RE: Immune function in aged mice: III. Eur J Immunol 8:697, 1978

14. Callard RE, Basten A, Blanden RV: Loss of immune competence with age may be due to a qualitative abnormality in lymphocyte membranes. Nature 281:218, 1979

15. Centers for Disease Control: Tuberculosis in the United States. Atlanta, CDC bulletin No. 00-329, 1977

16. Centers for Disease Control: *Salmonella* bacteremia: Reports to the Centers for Disease Control, 1968–1969. J Infect Dis 143:743, 1981

17. Charpentier B, Fournier C, Fries D, Mathew D, Noury J, Bach JF: Immunological studies in human aging: I. *In vitro* function of T-cells and polymorphs. J Clin Lab Immunol 5:87, 1981

18. Chatard JA: The leukocytes in acute lobar pneumonia. Johns Hopkins Hosp Rev 15:89, 1910

19. Czlonkowska A, Korlak J: The immune response during aging. J Gerontol 34:9, 1979

20. D'Alessio DJ, Cox PM Jr, Dick EC: Failure of inactivated influenza vaccine to protect an aged population. JAMA 210:485, 1969

21. DeKruyff RH, Kim YT, Siskind GW, Weksler ME: Age-related changes in the *in vitro* immune response: Increased suppressor activity in immature and aged mice. J Immunol 125:142, 1980

22. Doherty PC: Diminished T cell surveillance function in old mice infected with lymphocyte choriomeningitis virus. Immunology 32:751, 1977

23. Effros RB, Walford RL: Diminished T-cell response to influenza virus in aged mice. Immunology 4:387, 1983

24. Fabris N, Amadio L, Licastro F, Mocchegiani E, Zannotti M, Franceschi C: Thymic hormone deficiency in normal aging and Down's syndrome: Is there a primary failure of the thymus? Lancet 1:983, 1984

25. Friedman D, Keiser V, and Globerson A: Reactivation of immunocompetence in spleen cells of aged mice. Nature 251:545, 1974

26. Gardner ND, Lim STK, Lawton JWM: Monocyte function in ageing humans. Mech Ageing Dev 16:233, 1981

27. Giannella RA, Broitman SA, Zamcheck N: Gastric acid barrier to ingested microorganisms in man: Studies *in vivo* and *in vitro*. Gut 13:251, 1972

28. Gillis S, Kozak R, Durante M, Weksler ME: Immunological studies of aging: Decreased production of response to T cell growth factor by lymphocytes from aged humans. J Clin Invest 67:937, 1981

29. Gilman S, Woda BA, Feldman JD: T-lymphocytes of young and aged rats: I. Distribution, density and capping of T antigens. J Immunol 127:149, 1981

30. Gleckman R, Hibert D: Afebrile bacteremia. JAMA 248:1478, 1982

31. Goidl EA, Innes JB, Weksler ME: Immunological

studies of aging: II. Loss of IgG and high avidity plaque-forming cells and increased suppressor cell activity in aging mice. J Exp Med 144:1037, 1976

32. Goidl, EA, Michelis M, Siskind GW, Weksler ME: Effect of age on the induction of autoantibodies. Clin Exp Immunol 44:24, 1981

33. Goidl EA, Thorbecke GJ, Weksler ME, Siskind GW: Production of auto-anti-idiotypic antibody during the normal immune response: Changes in the auto-anti-idiotypic antibody response and the idiotype repertoire associated with aging. Proc Natl Acad Sci USA 77:6788, 1980

34. Gozes Y, Umiel T, Asher M, Trainin M: Syngeneic GvH induced in popliteal lymph nodes by spleen cells of old C57BL/6 mice. J Immunol 121:2199, 1978

35. Gupta S, Good RA: Subpopulation of human T lymphocytes: X. Alterations in T, B, third population cells, and T cells with receptors for immunoglobulin M or G in aging humans. J Immunol 122:1214, 1979

36. Gutowski JK, Innes, J, Weksler ME, Cohen S: Induction of DNA synthesis in isolated nuclei by cytoplasmic factors: II. Normal generation of cytoplasmic stimulatory factors by lymphocytes from aged humans with depressed proliferative responses. J Immunol 132:559, 1984

37. Hallgren HM, Buckley GC, Gilbertsen VA, Yunis EJ: Lymphocyte phytohemagglutinin responsiveness, immunoglobulins and autoantibodies in aging humans. J Immunol 111:1101, 1973

38. Hallgren HM, Yunis EJ: In Segre D, Smith L (eds): Immunological Aspects of Aging. New York, M Dekker, 1980

39. Hefton JM, Darlington GJ, Casazza BA, Weksler ME: Immunologic studies of aging: V. Impaired proliferation of PHA responsive. J Immunol 125:1007, 1980

40. Holden M, Dubin MR, Diamond PH: Frequency of negative intermediate-strength tuberculin sensitivity in patients with active tuberculosis. N Engl J Med 285:1506, 1971

41. Hope-Simpson RE: The nature of herpes zoster: A long term study and a new hypothesis. Proc Roy Soc Med 58:9, 1965

42. Hourman, DeChambre: Pneumonia chez les vieillards. Arch Gen Med *(Paris)*. 10:269, 1836

43. Inkeles B, Innes JB, Kuntz MM, Kadish AS, Weksler ME: Immunological studies of aging: III. Cytokinetic basis for the impaired response of lymphocytes from aged humans to plant lectins. J Exp Med 145:1176, 1977

44. Kennes B, Hubert C, Brohee D, Neve P: Early biochemical events associated with lymphocyte activation in ageing: I. Evidence that Ca^{2+} dependent processes induced by PHA are impaired. Immunology 42:119, 1981

44a. Kim YT, Goidl EA, Samarut C, Weksler ME, Thorbecke GJ, Siskind GW: Bone marrow function I: Peripheral T cells are responsible for the increased auto-antiidiotype response of older mice. J Exp Med 161:1237, 1985

45. Kim YT, Siskind GW, Weksler ME: Cellular basis of the impaired immune response in elderly people. In Fauci AS (ed): Human B-Lymphocyte Function Activation and Immunoregulation, pp 129–139. New York Raven Press 1982

46. Kishimoto S, Shigemoto S, Yamamura Y: Immune response in aged mice. Transplant 15:455, 1973

47. Kishimoto S, Tomino S, Mitsuya H, Fujiwara H, Tsuda H: Age-related decline in the *in vitro* and *in vivo* synthesis of anti-tetanus toxoid antibody in human. J Immunol 125:2347, 1980

48. Lewis VM, Twomey JJ, Bealmear P, Goldstein G, Good RA: Age, thymic involution and circulating thymic hormone activity. J Clin Endocrinol Metab. 47:145, 1978

49. Mackay I: Aging and immunological function in man. Gerontologia 18:285, 1972

50. Menon M, Jaroslow BN, Koesterer R: The decline of cell-mediated immunity in aging mice. J Gerontol 29:499, 1974

51. Miller AE: Selective decline in cellular immune response to varicella-zoster in the elderly. Neurology 30:582, 1980

52. Miller RA: Age-associated decline in precursor frequency for different T-cell–mediated reactions, with preservation of helper or cytotoxic effect per precursor cell. J Immunol 132:63, 1984

53. Moody CE, Innes JB, Staiano-Coico L, Incefy GS, Thaler HT, Weksler ME: Lymphocyte transformation induced by autologous cells: XI. The effect of age on the autologous mixed lymphocyte reaction. Immunology 44:431, 1981

54. Nerenberg ST, Prasod R: Radioimmunoassays for Ig classes G, A, M, D and E in spinal fluids: Normal values of different age groups. J Lab Clin Med 86:887, 1975

55. Nilsson BS: *In vitro* lymphocyte reactivity to PPD and phytohaemagglutinin in relation to PPD reactivity with age. Scand J Resp Dis 52:39, 1971

56. Pahwa RN, Moodak MJ, McMorrow T, Pahwa S, Fernandes G, Good RA: Terminal deoxynucleotidyl transference (TdT) enzyme in thymus and bone marrow. Cell Immunol 58:39, 1981

57. Pahwa SG, Pahwa R, Good RA: Decreased *in vitro* humoral immune responses in aged humans. J Clin Invest 67:1094, 1981

58. Patel PJ: Aging and antimicrobial immunity. J Exp Med 154:821, 1981

59. Paul JR, Bunnell WW: Anti-SRBC agglutinin with age. Am J Med Sci 183:90, 1932

60. Phair J, Kauffman CA, Bjornson A, Adams L, Linneman C Jr: Failure to respond to influenza vaccine in the aged: Correlation with B-cell number and function. J Lab Clin Med 92:822, 1978

61. Puchelle E, Zahm J-M, Bertrand A: Influence of age on bronchial mucociliary transport. Scand J Resp Dis 60:307, 1979

62. Radl J, DeGlopper E, Vandenberg P, VanZwieten MJ: Idiopathic paraproteinemia: III. Increased frequency of rare proteinemia in thymectomized aging C57BL/KaLwRij and CBA/BrARij mice. J Immunol 125:31, 1980

63. Radl J, Sepers JM, Skuaril F, Morell A, Hijmans W: Immunoglobulin patterns in humans over 95 years of age. Clin exp Immunol 22:84, 1975

64. Roberts SH, Jarvis EH, James O: Bacterial overgrowth syndrome without "blind loop": A cause for malnutrition in the elderly. Lancet 2:1193, 1977

65. Roberts-Thomson IC, Whittingham S, Youngchaiyud U, Mackay IR: Ageing, immune response, and mortality. Lancet 2:368, 1974

66. Rowley MJ, Buchanan H, Mackay IR: Reciprocal change with age in antibody to extrinsic and intrinsic antigens. Lancet 2:24, 1968

67. Sabin AB, Ginder DR, Matumoto M, Schlesinger RW: Serological response of Japanese children to Japanese B encephalitis mouse brain vaccine. Proc Soc Exp Biol Med 67:135, 1947

68. Scholar EM, Rashidian M, Heidrick ML: A denosine deaminanse and purine nucleoside phosphorylase activity in spleen cells of aged mice. Mech Ageing Dev 12:323, 1980

69. Singh J, Singh AK: Age-related changes in human thymus. Clin Exp Immunol 37:507, 1979

70. Smith JB, Knowlton RP, Agarwal SS: Human lymphocyte responses are enhanced by culture at 40°C. J Immunol 121:691, 1978

71. Staiano-Coico L, Darzynkiewicz Z, Hefton JM, Dutkowski R, Darlington GJ, Weksler ME: Increased sensitivity of lymphocytes from people over 65 to cell cycle arrest and chromosomal damage. Science 219:1335, 1983

72. Tam CF, Walford RL: Alterations in cyclic nucleotides and cyclase activities in T lymphocytes of aging humans and Down's syndrome subjects. J Immunol 125:1665, 1980

73. Thoman ML, Weigle WO: Lymphokines and aging: Interleuken-2 production and activity in aged animals. J Immunol 127:2102, 1981

74. Thomsen O, Kettel K: Die Starke der menschlichen Isoagglutinine und entsperchenden Blutkorperchenrezeptoren in verschiedenen Lebensaltern. Z Immunitatsforsch 63:67, 1929

75. Valenti WM, Trudell RG, Bentley DW: Factors predisposing to oropharyngeal colonization with gram-negative bacilli in the aged. N Engl J Med 298:1108, 1978

76. Waldorf DS, Wilkens RF, Decker JL: Impaired delayed hypersensitivity in an aging population: Association with antinuclear reactivity and rheumatoid factor. JAMA 203:831, 1968

77. Walford R: The Immunologic Theory of Aging. Copenhagen, Munksgaard, 1969

78. Walford RL, Bergmann K: Influence of genes associated with the main histocompatibility complex on deoxyribonucleic acid excision repair capacity

and bleomycin sensitivity in mouse lymphocytes. Tissue Antigens 14:336, 1979

79. Weksler ME, Innes JB, Goldstein G: Immunological studies of aging: IV. The contribution of thymic involution to the immune deficiencies of ageing mice and reversal with thymopoietin$_{32-36}$. J Exp Med 148:996, 1978

80. Weksler ME: Senescence of the immune system. Med Clin North Am 67:263, 1983

81. Woods DE, Straus DC, Johanson WG Jr, Bass JA: Role of salivary protease activity in adherence of gram-negative bacilli to mammalian buccal epithelial cells *in vivo.* J Clin Invest 68:1435, 1981

5 Genetic Aspects of Aging

Lissy F. Jarvik and Steven S. Matsuyama

"You are old, Father William," the young man cried,
"The few locks which are left you are gray;
You are hale, Father William, a hearty old man—
Now tell me the reason, I pray."

Southey (1799)

Despite the dramatic advances made in medical science during the past century, we are as incapable today of explaining Father William's's relative resistance to senile decline as were the physicians of his time. Of the many reasons for our persisting ignorance, lack of interest in individual differences is being recognized as most important.

As a consequence of the spectacular control achieved over known infectious diseases, disorders of idiopathic etiologies have assumed major epidemiologic importance and spurred a renewed interest in the host-specific factors of individual variability. Among them are the chief causes of mortality and morbidity among the aged of today—cardiovascular diseases, malignant neoplasia, and mental disorders—all of which have significant genetic components.

At a time when genetic determinants of illness are assuming greater importance, the geriatrician is in the unenviable position of lacking sufficient information for distinguishing between hereditary diseases and their phenocopies, or between independent diseases and diverse manifestations of a single basic abnormality. The prodigious strides

This research was supported in part by National Institute of Mental Health grant MH36205 and by the Veterans Administration. The opinions expressed herein are those of the authors and not necessarily those of the Veterans Administration.

made in deciphering the genetic code and elucidating a variety of genetic mechanisms have been concerned chiefly with hereditary disorders attributable to single major gene mutations manifested early in life by severe dysfunction. The genetic aspects of aging, however, remain, but for a modest beginning, virtually unexplored.

GENETIC ANALYSIS AND LIFE SPAN

Pedigrees

One of the oldest methods of genetic investigation in humans is the study of individual family histories (pedigrees). Successful utilization of the pedigree method, however, requires an understanding of its limitations, some of the key ones consisting of the small size of human families, the difficulty in gathering accurate information for ancestral generations (particularly when many generations are involved, as in genealogies extending back some 300 years), and the tendency to report pedigrees that are characterized by an accumulation of affected people.

The pedigree method does not lend itself readily to the exploration of the hereditary basis for normal, or common, conditions such as height (except for the extremes of dwarfism and gigantism), intelligence, graying of hair, loss of teeth, and the gradual decline in sensory, perceptual, and psychomotor processes characteristic of advancing age. There are at least two reasons for this. First, common conditions frequently escape notice, and, therefore, reporting tends to be inaccurate for preceding generations. Second, the traits often are the result of graded characters and represent the effects of many genes, any of which, alone, produces only minor effects (polygenic inheritance).,

Further, as pointed out by Cohen[23] in a careful critique regarding the pedigree and other methods of investigating human life span, the combination of several genealogies fails to take into account the possible influence of social factors and different mortality patterns among different social strata. Clearly then, the pedigree method is not suited to an exploration of the hereditary factors in longevity. And yet, it was on the basis of family histories that the first hypotheses of the inheritance of longevity were formulated. Early in this century, Bell[11] reported on the genealogy of the Hyde family and determined that among offspring who survived until age 80, almost half had fathers who had reached the age of 80. In the United States, Pearl[146] devised the concept of total immediate ancestral longevity (TIAL) as an indicator of the hereditary contribution toward longevity, when a centenarian examined by Pearl had six direct ancestors whose average age at death was also close to 100 years. An example of a longevous family from our own study of senescent twins illustrates this concept (Fig. 5-1). Another of our families exemplifies the many instances in which grandparental ages cannot be determined and relatives' life spans are short despite the longevity of the index case, emphasizing the need for other approaches toward understanding extended life span (Fig. 5-2).

Population Samples

Another approach to understanding longevity is demography. The demographic approach is useful for determining relationships that can be elicited with relatively uncomplicated enumerative procedures, such as hospital admissions, vital statistics, and differential mortality rates. Studies of this kind have provided information on the association of blood groups with disease (*e.g.*, the increased frequency of duodenal ulcer among persons with type O blood), as well as on differential mortality trends, particularly the longer life expectancy of women in all human populations in which the risk of childbirth has been reduced to a minimal level.

This difference in life span has been attributed to the more protected life of the woman. It has been said, for example, that unlike the man, who has to work under stress in highly competitive civilizations, the modern woman has been released from the burden of housekeeping duties by an increasing variety of mechanical devices. In an attempt to assess the validity of this hypothesis, Madigan and Vance[115] found a 10% difference in

life expectancy of 9,813 brothers and 32,041 sisters in American Catholic teaching orders, approximating the life-span differential in the general population, despite negligible sex differences in occupational hazards and relatively sheltered lives for both men and women.

In nearly every species in which sex-specific longevity variations have been studied in detail, the female outlives the male.[170] The average differences range from about 10% in the fruit fly (33 versus 31 days) to more than two and one-half times in the spider (271 versus 100 days).

Is the presence of a second X chromosome in humans responsible for the lower mortality of women and, throughout most of life, their lower morbidity as well? To some extent, although a very small one, the answer already is positive. In sex-linked recessive conditions with random mating, the effects of deleterious genes located on one X chromosome are neutralized by the action of normal genes on the second X chromosome, so that in hemophilia and other sex-linked conditions, it is only the male who manifests the abnormal condition.

Further answers may eventually come from the study of more persons with abnormalites of the sex chromosomes. Thus, males with an extra X chromosome (XXY, Klinefelter's syndrome) characteristically have seminiferous tubular dysgenesis with consequent gynecomastia and sterility; yet they have survived into their 80s and have been found among patients suffering from senile mental disorders.[113] Their female counterparts (XXX) are often entirely normal in appearance and fertility, and their investigation should shed further light on the role of the X chromosome in longevity.

The presence of an extra Y chromosome, like that of extra X chromosomes, is often associated with mental deficiency. In addition, however, XYY men tend to be unusually tall and to display aggressive, antisocial behavior, which militates against a prolonged life span.[30,65,83] Among possible mechanisms through which differences in sex chromosome constitution may be mediated are hormones. Thus, a study of more than 1000 institutionalized mentally retarded males suggests that prepubertal castration may extend the life span, on the average, by more than 13 years.*

Fluorescent techniques help to identify the Y chromosome[162] and extra or missing X chromosomes. A scraping from the buccal mucosal epithelium of a woman shows a dark staining mass (chromatin or Barr body) in approximately 30%

---

* Hamilton JB: Personal communication.

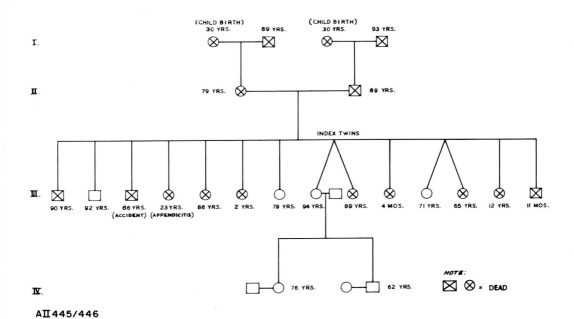

AII 445/446

FIG. 5-1.   Pedigree of longevous twin family.

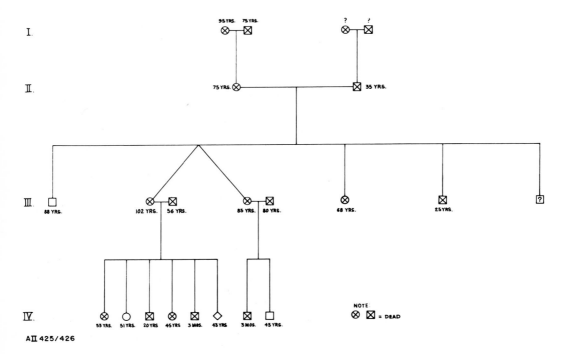

AII 425/426

FIG. 5-2.   Pedigree of longevous twin index pair.

of her cells, whereas a man's buccal mucosal smear contains no, or very few, such chromatin-positive cells. The chromatin body, characteristic of female cells, is believed to consist of one partly inactive X chromosome. According to the Lyon hypothesis, only one functioning X chromosome is required postembryonically; all others condense to form chromatin bodies. The number of chromatin bodies, therefore, is one less than the number of X chromosomes. Persons have been reported with as many as four X chromosomes, and they have had three Barr bodies.[106]

Twin and Twin-Family Samples

Twin studies are based on the regular occurrence of two types of twins, monozygotic (one-egg) and dizygotic (two-egg). Monozygotic twins (Fig. 5-3), derived from a single fertilized ovum, are of the same sex and have the same complement of genes, barring mutation or mosaicism, so that differences between them are attributable to developmental and environmental variations. By contrast, dizygotic twins (Fig. 5-4) are the product of two separate ova, fertilized by two different spermotazoa, and they are genetically no more alike than two ordinary siblings born at different times, who on the average have 50% of their genes in common (see Fig. 5-4). Of course, there may be wide divergence from this average, as illustrated by the physical features of siblings. Some resemble one another closely, others hardly at all.

Dizygotic pairs are expected to show considerably smaller rates of concordance (*i.e.,* both affected) for pathologic conditions controlled by major genes than is true for monozygotic pairs.[72] With respect to the distribution of genetically determined variations in graded characters (*e.g.,* height), the intrapair differences observed in dizygotic pairs are apt to be decidedly larger than those in the monozygotic group. To establish accurately the zygosity of each pair, the methods usually employed are the General Similarity Method (based on comparison of characteristics known to be largely genetically determined like eye color, hair color, and shape of ears), dermatoglyphics, and blood groups.

Most limitations of the original twin-study method can be remedied by a refinement that increases the number of genotypes available for comparison. This twin-family method is based on the study of a random sample of twin pairs (monozygotic and dizygotic) and their full siblings, half siblings, and stepsiblings.[87] The usefulness of the

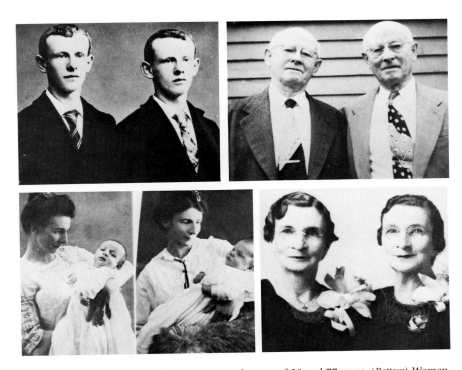

FIG. 5-3. Monozygotic twins. (*Top*) Men, at the ages of 20 and 77 years. (*Bottom*) Women, at the ages of 25 and 60 years.

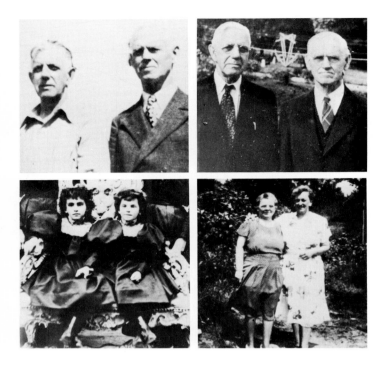

FIG. 5-4. Dizygotic twins. (*Top*) Men, at the ages of 59 and 70 years. (*Bottom*) Women, at the ages of 10 and 61 years.

twin-family method has clearly been shown in studies of the genetic aspects of chronic reinfection tuberculosis, with the demonstration of marked individual differences in susceptibility to the tubercle bacillus.[88]

The twin-study method has also been used for the evaluation of genetic influences on longevity. It has been found that mean intrapair differences in same-sex dizygotic pairs exceeded those in monozygotic pairs (Fig. 5-5).[80] This held true even for the oldest pairs, despite the fact that any group of aging persons is expected to show increasing homogeneity as the upper limits of life expectancy are approached, owing to the restricted years of remaining life, as well as their having been selected for superior health and survival values. This effect is manifested earlier in men than in women because of their shorter life span. Gradually, both male and female two-egg twins approach the low levels of intrapair differences in length of life characteristic of one-egg twins at any age.

Even though, on the average, monozygotic twins die within 5 years of each other, pairs have been observed in which differences in age at death exceeded a decade. The "E" twins, for example, were among the most similar twins in our series in physical appearance, health, interests, occupational choice, and general living conditions (Fig. 5-6). Nonetheless, "A. E." died 16 years earlier than "E. E." In both cases, the cause of death was

myocardial failure and general arteriosclerosis (according to physicians' reports, no autopsies having been performed). When "A. E." was seen at the age of 72, he prided himself on the excellent care he always took of himself by wrestling, boxing, and gymnasium work. Nonetheless, he died a year later. "E. E." also prided himself on his active life, and at the age of 73 he continued to work around the house and walked a great deal each day at a rapid pace. "E. E." died at the age of 89, having been bedridden for just 7 days before his death.

A detailed analysis of cases such as this may one day furnish the clues to the pertinent environmental variables that either shorten or prolong the life of a given genotype.

GENETICS AND COMMON DISORDERS OF THE AGED

For many of the ills most commonly afflicting the aging person, such as senile cataracts, there is little or no information concerning hereditary factors. Despite the well-known differences in incidence between the sexes and among different population groups,[3,7] osteoporosis, for example, appears to be characterized genetically only when it is associated with other diseases (*e.g.,* homocystinuria, diabetes mellitus), chromosomal disorders (*e.g.,* XO), or syndromes such as osteogenesis imperfecta or pseudogliomatous blindness and osteoporosis.[138]

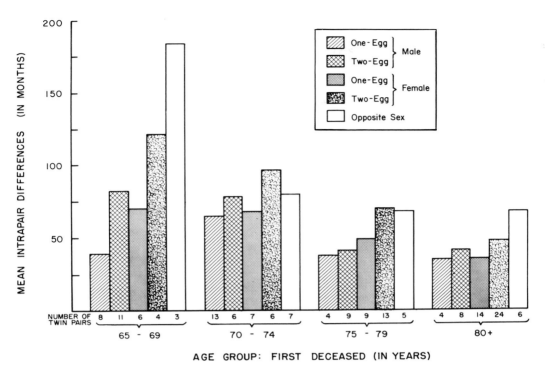

FIG. 5-5. Life-span differences for 167 twin pairs. (Both partners died of natural causes.) (Jarvik LF, Falek A, Kallman FJ, Lorge I: Survival trends in a senescent twin population. Am J Hum Genet 12:170, 1960)

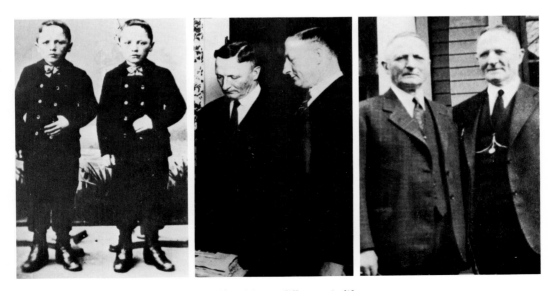

FIG. 5-6. The monozygotic "E" twins, with a 16-year difference in life span.

For benign prostatic hypertrophy, there appears to be no information on genetic determinants except for statements that affirm the importance of genetic factors (*e.g.,* in producing individual differences in metabolism, in androgen secretions, and in density of prostatic androgen-binding receptor sites). In the less common disorder of Dupuytren's contracture, an autosomal dominant mode of inheritance has been proposed,[112] but patterns of genetic transmission have not always followed this model. Chromosome mosaicism has been reported in cells cultured from the palmar fascia of one patient,[19] but the significance of this finding has not as yet been established.

An elevated frequency of certain human lymphocyte antigens (HLA) has been associated with a number of diseases. Thus, ankylosing spondylitis and juvenile rheumatoid arthritis have both been associated with HLA-B27,[153,160] and so has clinical expression of rheumatic disease.[6] HLA-Dw4 was also reported to be significantly more frequent in patients with rheumatoid arthritis than in controls.[114] In these diseases, however, onset is usually long before the age of 60, and the rest of this chapter is primarily concerned with conditions that most commonly occur in the seventh decade of life and beyond.

Cardiovascular Diseases

Familial aggregations of hypertension, hyperlipidemia, and coronary artery disease have long been known, but the genetic mechanisms have remained largely unknown, as have the modes of operation of environmental influences that clearly help determine the occurrence of cardiovascular diseases. The following summarizes the information accumulated to date on hereditary influences in these disorders.

Hypertension

In men, as in mice, inheritance of normal variations in blood pressure seems to follow a polygenic model,[68] whereas certain specific forms of hypertension, like those due to pheochromocytoma and polycystic kidneys, are attributable to single autosomal dominant defects. There is no unanimity of opinion about the most common form—essential hypertension. However, clinicians have long recognized that hypertension is common among relatives of hypertensives, and recent observations suggest that familial aggregation of blood pressure levels is primarily the result of heredity.[16,163]

Animal studies indicate that psychic stress has selective effects in producing hypertension, depending on genetic predisposition of the animal. Thus, genetically susceptible rats showed persistent elevations in systolic blood pressure when they were chronically exposed to an approach–avoidance conflict, while rats genetically resistant to hypertension showed no such elevation. In humans, results of twin studies point to the importance of genetic determinants,[8,54,110,120] without specifying either the mode of hereditary transmission or the distinction between essential hypertension as a specific disorder and blood pressures that represent the upper end of the normal distribution curve.

Excess salt ingestion has been related to the development of primary hypertension in laboratory animals; in humans, the evidence is indirect[168] and includes the observation that population groups that consume small quantities of salt tend to be relatively free of hypertension.[34,177,178] The suggestion has been made that the decreased taste threshold for salt found among persons with hypertension, as well as their relatives, may be related to the development of essential hypertension.[175] Indeed, the correlations of salt-taste threshold and sodium excretion in female siblings of hypertensives have been reported as high as those for height and other anthropometric data.[103] Even though no relationship between either salt-taste threshold or salt preference and blood pressure was detected in schoolchildren,[105] study of older subjects may be required to determine whether there is a relationship that is clearly age dependent. Another study concluded that "an abnormality of NaCl taste acuity, *per se,* is not a constituent factor of hypertension in man," because salt-taste thresholds in patients with hypertension fell into the normal range for all but four of the 49 patients with essential hypertension.[58] Since most of the patients showed thresholds in the upper rather than the lower ranges of normal, the issue remains unsettled.

Coronary Artery Disease

Genetic factors have been assigned great weight in the etiology of coronary artery disease, the risk having been shown to increase markedly in relatives of afflicted persons.[33,109,166] A strong genetic component has also been reported in the electrocardiograms of twins[120] and in the anatomical pattern of gross arborization and intercoronary anastomoses.[111] Moreover, selective coronary arteriography has demonstrated close similarities in location and extent of arteriosclerotic lesions in identical twins with premature coronary artery disease, findings that the authors believe are best explained by genetic influences.[100]

In early reports, however, concordance rates for coronary occlusion were only slightly higher for monozygotic than for dizygotic pairs,[55] so that we must await further studies to shed light on this area. There is also the now well-known association between coronary heart disease and Type A behavior (intensely competitive, driving, and time-pressured), as described by Friedman and Rosenman.[40] The extent to which Type A behavior is influenced by genetic factors is under investigation.[39]

Last, and perhaps most important, is the association of increased frequency of atherosclerosis with elevated serum lipid levels. A single autosomal gene defect appears to be the cause, as it is in rare syndromes, such as essential familial hypercholesterolemia,[48,49] in which a deficiency in cell-surface receptors for low-density lipoproteins has been proposed as the primary genetic defect.[20,50] More complex is the question of variations in serum lipid levels in normal populations. Thus, in a study covering the entire community of Tecumseh, Michigan, positive correlations for serum cholesterol were obtained for first-degree blood relatives but not for spouses, pointing toward genetic influences.[34] Yet, comparison of the serum lipid levels of monozygotic and dizygotic twin partners indicate that both genetic and environmental factors could produce measurable variations.[142,150] In our own study of aging twins, data obtained on 17 same-sex pairs, ranging from 78 to 89 years, were not conclusive.[73]

As early as the 1940s, an increasing number of lipoprotein markers had been recognized and a beginning made in studying their inheritance.[1] Despite suggestive evidence linking lipoproteins to arteriosclerosis, the exact relationship remains to be determined. A step in that direction has been taken by researchers at the University of Washington who used hyperlipidemic survivors of myocardial infarction as a source of probands for family studies. Their results indicate that hypertriglyceridemia may be as important a risk factor for coronary disease as hypercholesterolemia, since one of five survivors under 60 years of age had some form of simply inherited hyperlipidemia. So far, five distinct lipid disorders have been identified, three of them apparently representing dominant expression of three different autosomal genes. The relationship between elevated serum lipid levels and coronary disease awaits further identification. Either can exist without the other,

and even within populations with relatively homogeneous dietary customs, there is still much unexplained variation.[57,95,131]

Finally, mention must be made of findings that suggest the operation of immunogenetic mechanisms in the etiology of vascular disease by way of linkage to certain histocompatibility antigens.[121,122,158]

Neoplastic Diseases

That genetic factors play a role in the etiology of cancer (used in its broadest sense) has been inferred from the following six observations:

1. Family studies indicate single-factor inheritance for a few rare forms of cancer (*e.g.*, retinoblastoma) and familial aggregations for several other, more common forms (*e.g.*, breast and stomach cancer). It has been reported by numerous investigators, with great consistency, that the frequency of cancer that affects a specific organ is considerably higher in the relatives of patients who also suffer from cancer at that particular site than in other poulation groups.[63]

2. The incidence of various types of neoplastic disease differs for diverse populations, as exemplified by the high frequency of carcinoma of the stomach in Japan and its relative rarity in the United States.

3. Substances that are mutagenic, such as ionizing radiations and specific chemical agents, are also carcinogenic. Somatic mutations with consequent genic imbalance have, for many years, been considered significant in the etiology of cancer.[18]

4. Down's syndrome, with its extra chromosome, and a few rare genetic syndromes, such as Bloom's syndrome and Fanconi's aplastic anemia, are associated with an increased frequency of leukemia.[45,161] The frequency of both cancer and Down's syndrome is greater than expected in siblings of leukemic children.[130] The importance of chromosomal, single-gene, and polygenic factors in clinical oncology and cancer prevention has become increasingly apparent.[99,132]

5. Nonrandom chromosomal changes are common in certain forms of neoplasia.[184] In chronic myelogenous leukemia, for example, there is a reciprocal exchange between the long arms of chromosomes 9 and 22. Further advances will ensue as cytogenetic studies are

complemented with recombinant DNA technologies.

6. Animal studies have shown a higher incidence of a variety of neoplastic growths among some strains than among others, and it has been possible selectively to breed cancer-susceptible and cancer-resistant strains.[62]

Of particular interest to geriatricians is the position that normal age changes and carcinogenic changes may be diametrically opposed. Carcinogenic change may represent mutations that interfere with growth regulation and therefore lead to rapid uncontrolled growth. By contrast, normal cells from aged persons show less growth than those of younger persons, and the mammalian life span may be limited by the number of divisions that cells are programmed to undergo. In aging, then, growth is reduced; in malignant neoplasia it is accelerated and uncontrolled.

More recently, defects in repair mechanisms have come to the fore as major determinants of cancer development, following the model of xeroderma pigmentosum. In this autosomal recessive disorder, the skin is extremely sensitive to sunlight so that affected persons readily develop skin cancer. It is believed that their decreased ability to excise ultraviolet photoproducts and perform DNA repair replication (in contrast to their ability to repair, with normal efficiency, DNA breaks caused by other mechanisms) may be due to a specific enzymatic defect, although more than one variant has already been described.[118] Despite the convincing evidence of genetic determinants of xeroderma pigmentosum, the manifestation of this hereditary predisposition to skin cancer clearly depends on environmental exposure (amount of ultraviolet radiation).

For cancer, broadly diagnosed, twin studies have generally confirmed a higher concordance for monozygotic than for dizygotic twin partners, especially regarding the site of lesions, even though most of the studies suffer from the handicap of limited follow-up after diagnosis or death of one twin. When the observation period extended over 15 years, prolonged temporary discordance was noted, one dizygotic pair becoming concordant only after 15 years and one monozygotic pair after 10 years.[79]

Clearly, exogenous agents must play an important role in the etiology of these kinds of neoplasia to account for so marked a difference in time of onset in identical twins. Yet evidence is mounting that endogenous host defense mechanisms against viral, toxic, or other noxious agents are at least partly under genetic control. The identification of high-risk patients (relatives of cancer patients, especially discordant monozygotic twins) assists in uncovering factors that tend either to precipitate or to suppress neoplasia, and early detection as a result of frequent follow-ups may reduce fatalities. Thus, Lynch and colleagues, as a result of their survey of familial cancer syndromes, pointed out the importance of communicating genetic and diagnostic information to primary care physicians, especially for precancerous states characterized by simple Mendelian inheritance and clinically apparent phenotypes (*e.g.,* polyposis coli) or biochemical markers (*e.g.,* Sipple's syndrome with its multiple endocrine neoplasia).[107] The physician must also be aware that multiple primary malignant neoplasms are the rule, and not the exception, in nearly all hereditary forms of cancer[108] and that heritable as well as nonheritable forms of cancer occur at virtually all sites. Indeed, they are histologically indistinguishable from one another in cancer of the breast, colon, skin, and uterus (all being subgroups with autosomal dominant inheritance), so that an accurate family history is a crucial element in the diagnosis. Even in those forms of cancer in which etiology remains unknown, hereditary transmission has been observed in certain families, for example in intraocular malignant melanoma.

According to a popular model, carcinogenesis is a two-stage event, the first being mutational and heritable; the second, somatic and not hereditary but attributable to environmental carcinogens such as viruses, radiation, and chemicals.[98] An intriguing attempt has been made to link genetic predisposition to bronchogenic carcinoma with levels of the microsomal oxidase aryl hydrocarbon hydroxylase,[94] but this remains to be confirmed.[145,174] Similarly, attempts have failed to link serum levels of carcinoembryonic antigen with malignant transformations of hereditary adenomatosis of the colon and rectum.[5] Although tissue levels may still be useful, this antigen is unlikely to detect genetic predispositions to cancer reliably and is not recommended for the screening of elderly populations.[173]

Another approach to the prediction of likelihood of cancer is the association of different rates of breast cancer in different population groups, with their rates of production of wet-type cerumen.[147] Asians exhibit low, Western Europeans high, and Middle Easterners intermediate rates of both. The association is plausible since ceruminous, mammary, and certain axillary sweat glands are histologically of the apocrine type with biochemically similar secretions. Nonetheless, a subsequent large-scale case-control study failed to confirm the hypothesis,[69] although more complex relationships have not been ruled out.[148]

The role of genetic factors has been clearly established for certain immunodeficiency diseases,[116,179] and decline in efficiency of immunologic surveillance has been suggested as one reason for the increasing frequency of malignant neoplasia with advancing age.[93,141]

Increasing length of exposure to exogenous carcinogens is clearly a major factor, as well.[151] There is also the possibility that the increasing DNA repair required with increasing age leads to the manifestation of genetically determined deficiencies in repair mechanisms (see Chapter 3). Pursuit of the various leads that relate genetics, cancer, and aging may provide clues to the basic processes that determine age-associated and neoplastic changes.

Mental Diseases

Genetic elements tend to be ignored in the psychiatric aspects of aging, owing to general lack of knowledge of the role played by genetic factors in the dementias, the most prominent mental disorders of old age. More than 30 years ago, Kallmann commented:[87]

In mental conditions peculiar to the senium and presenium, clearer genetic evidence is avilable for those specific and relatively rare disorders distinguished by prematurity and the presence of gross but circumscribed lesions than it is for the more common types of senile dementia.

And it is true that the most cogent information about hereditary transmission has been provided for the presenile brain atrophies (onset generally between the ages of 45 and 64) by the accumulation of pedigrees with Alzheimer's, Pick's, and Creutzfeldt-Jakob disease. There are presently no data on genetic factors in neuroses or personality disorders in the aged.

Presenile Dementias

Creutzfeldt-Jakob disease is a rare, rapidly progressive neurologic disease that occurs throughout the world, affects both sexes equally, and shows a highly variable age at onset.[126] In a review of the world literature, May[127] found patients as young as 21 years and as old as 79 years. Symptoms, too, are variable, and Slater and Roth discussed two clinically different types, one being characterized by a rapidly developing dementia with death ensuing within 3 to 6 months, and the second typically showing a longer course terminated by death within 1 to 2 years.[167]

Cutler and co-workers[31] reported that a patient with neuropathologically confirmed Creutzfeldt-Jakob disease survived for 16 years. There is also one report of a patient who apparently had a spontaneous remission from this usually fatal disease.[117]

At initial presentation, there may be fatigue, dizziness, apathy, irritability or confusion, memory impairment, and speech disturbances. Dementia is accompanied by the development of a variety of neurologic disturbances, including cerebellar ataxia, myoclonus, seizures, and pyramidal and extrapyramidal signs.

There is reasonable certainty that Creutzfeldt-Jakob disease is a transmissible spongiform encephalopathy. The disease has been transmitted successfully by intracerebral inoculation first to primates[47] and then to cats, guinea pigs, and other species. There are also reports of suspected accidental transmission in humans via neurosurgery and corneal transplantation.[13,35,43] The transmissible agent is believed to be a slow virus[42] similar to the scrapie agent in goats and sheep. Merz and colleagues[129] have observed abnormal fibrils, possibly representing the infectious agent, in synaptosomal preparations of scapie-infected brains, in brain fractions of patients with Creutzfeldt-Jakob disease, as well as in spleen extracts of experimentally infected animals. Prusiner[152] coined the term *prion* (proteinaceous infectious agent) for the slow infectious agent causing scrapie. Prions represent ''unconventional viruses'' since no nucleic acid genome has been identified; yet they replicate. Whether the scrapie-associated abnormal fibrils are the same as prions is not known, but ongoing research should provide an answer.

Even though an infectious agent has been identified, approximately 15% of the cases show a familial pattern.[119] In the hereditary form, published pedigrees are consistent with an autosomal dominant mode of inheritance,[125] so that a slow virus infection may be superimposed on a preexisting, genetically determined dysfunction, which allows for invasion or activation of the agent. In familial Creutzfeldt-Jakob disease, the agent might be incorporated in the genome of the family members and transmitted in this manner until it is activated.[176]

Pick's disease, another form of presenile dementia, is also a rare disorder (less than 0.1%), and, clinically, it is probably indistinguishable from Alzheimer's disease, the prominent features being an insidous onset of confusion, deteriorating memory, and defects in judgment, terminating eventually in severe dementia and death. Differences in regional cerebral blood flow have been reported to distinguish Pick's disease from other dementias,[53] but the techniques are experimental rather than clinical, and without specific treatments there has not been much interest in the antemortem distinction of presenile dementias. Postmortem, however, they are readily distinguishable. In Pick's disease, cerebral atrophy affects primarily the frontal and temporal lobes, and microscopic findings include neuronal loss, gliosis, and the distinctive Pick cell, a neuronal cell with a large argyrophilic cytoplasmic inclusion body.[29]

Ongoing studies of Pick's disease in the United States suggest geographical variability in incidence, with Minnesota having higher rates than New York.* Information on the heritable aspect of this disorder is based on very few studies.[125] The largest is the systematic investigation by Sjögren and colleagues in Sweden, identifying 44 patients with Pick's disease (18 histopathologically confirmed) and reporting an increased morbidity risk for presenile dementia for their parents (19%) and siblings (6.8%).[165] They concluded that an autosomal dominant major gene with modifiers was the most likely mode of inheritance.

An autosomal dominant mode also fits the data accumulated by Schenk in a longitudinal study of a single pedigree extending over five generations.[159] This family was reexamined after 20 years, and the pedigree now covers six generations and includes 25 patients with the clinical diagnosis of Pick's disease (14 autopsy-proven) and 7 patients in whom the diagnosis was considered likely.[51] These authors systematically reviewed the literature but found no additional families with the autosomal dominant pattern of inheritance exhibited by the Schenk family. Thus, at the moment, the genetics of Pick's disease must await further reports of large families who have been systematically studied.

Huntington's disease is not considered presenile dementia because of its earlier onset (age range, 5–70 years; highest frequency, ages 35–40 years), but it is included here because it must be considered in the differential diagnosis. It, too, is characterized by an insidious onset, and early symptoms include changes in personality, with a variety of nonspecific cognitive, affective, behavioral, or

psychotic symptoms, followed by the appearance of involuntary movements, which usually, but not always, progress to choreic movements, and eventually profound dementia. Clinical features vary, with early onset patients characterized by a more rapid progression and a more profound dementia than patients with late onset. This pattern suggests genetic heterogeneity. The mean duration of life after onset is approximately 16 years.[154] Overall prevalence rates range from 4 to 7 per 100,000 population.[134] Accurate diagnosis is essential for a number of reasons, including the institution of appropriate therapy should the disease be other than Huntington disease (*e.g.*, neurologic disorder with hyperkinetic symptoms or schizophrenia) or, in the case of a positive diagnosis, for purposes of genetic counseling.

Huntington's disease exhibits an autosomal dominant mode of inheritance with complete penetrance.[75,181] On the average, half the offspring are affected, with equal probability of transmission from either parent. Some studies, however, reported that the younger the age at onset, the greater the probability that the disease was inherited from the father, even though boys and girls were affected in equal proportion, among juvenile patients (under age 19). The later onset, the greater the chance that inheritance was from an affected mother, leading Myers and colleagues[133] to suggest that this pattern may be due to heritable extrachromosomal factors.

To our knowledge, there are no systematic studies of twins in the literature on Huntington's disease. Hayden[56] found reports of 13 monozygotic pairs (all concordant for the disease) and five dizygotic pairs (only one concordant).

The principal neuropathologic feature is neuronal fallout, particularly in the striatum and cerebral cortex, although cell loss is also seen in other regions of the brain. In areas of neuronal loss, there is extensive astrocytic gliosis. Positron emission tomography (PET) scans have shown decreased glucose metabolism in the caudate with normal cortical metabolism.[101]

Despite clear genetic determinants known for over a century (since Huntington's original description in 1872), little is known of the etiology and pathogenesis.[10,22] Changes have been reported in neurotransmitter receptors.[38] The possibility that Huntington's disease is due to a membrane defect has been an area of intense research investigation.[15,27] A number of different peripheral tissues (*e.g.*, fibroblasts, lymphocytes, red blood cells) have been examined by various techniques

---

* Heston LL: Personal communication, 1984.

(*e.g.,* electron spin resonance, cell culture, immunologic assessments). Unfortunately, due to research design problems as well as methodologic issues, conflicting results have been obtained and, at the moment, there is no consensus.

Recombinant DNA technologies have begun to provide a plethora of new genetic markers. Restriction fragment length polymorphisms (RFLPs) are available for use in attempts to map disorders with a genetic basis for which neither the biochemical nature of the trait nor the molecular basis of the DNA change responsible are known (*e.g.,* Huntington's disease). Using this technique, Gusella and associates[52] located the Huntington disease gene in two families on chromosome 4. Since there is the possibility of genetic heterogeneity, the general applicability of this finding for carrier identification awaits confirmation from additional informative families.

Dementia of the Alzheimer Type

Dementia of the Alzheimer type (DAT) includes both the presenile and senile forms of the disease, a differentiation based solely on age at onset (prior to or after age 65). This is not satisfactory, since overlapping ages of onset among probands are included in a number of studies. Furthermore, age at onset is difficult to determine accurately. The neuropathologic findings and clinical symptomatology are identical in both the presenile- and senile-onset forms, and the tendency is to include both under the category of DAT. Other investigators have reported neuropathologic and neurochemical differences in patients dying before age 80, compared with those over 80 years of age.[17,156,157] The available literature, however, differentiates between Alzheimer's disease and senile dementia, and this distinction will be maintained here.

DAT is a dementia of insidious onset with early clinical symptoms of loss of memory, in particular for recent events, and inefficiency in social or occupational functioning. There is progressive deterioration with impairment of judgment and abstract thinking, and there may be changes in personality. Finally, the individual is reduced to a vegetative state and eventually dies.

Neuropathologically, DAT is characterized by diffuse cerebral atrophy and senile (neuritic) plaques, neurofibrillary tangles in the hippocampus and neocortex, and neuronal degeneration in several regions of the brain. The individual variability detected on neuropathologic examination

suggests the possibility of genetic heterogeneity. However, at the moment, confirmation of the clinical diagnosis of DAT is based on the quantitative assessment of plaques and tangles.

Presenile Onset. Several pedigree studies, published as early as the 1930s, indicated a high familial incidence of Alzheimer's disease and suggested an autosomal dominant mode of inheritance for this disorder. The first systematic study, in 1952, is still the classic study. Using the detailed records maintained in Sweden, Sjögren and colleagues collected a series of 36 index cases of Alzheimer's disease, 18 with histopathologically verified diganosis.[165] Genealogical data were then collected from parish records and personal visits made to the families of index and secondary cases. In addition, all those suspected of having the disorder were psychiatrically evaluated (or hospital records were reviewed for those who had died prior to the investigation) for clinical symptoms of dementia. From these data, morbidity risks for Alzheimer's disease were calculated at 10% for parents and 3.8% for siblings. The general population rate in Sweden being 0.1% first-degree relatives thus exhibited a 38- to 100-fold increase in risk.

Sjögren and colleagues suggested a polygenic mode of inheritance, while data from a major Swiss study were interpreted as supporting an autosomal dominant mode of inheritance with reduced penetrance.[28] There, the risk figures for siblings were 3.3% and for parents 1.4%. Although the risk for siblings was similar in both the Swiss and Swedish studies, the risk for parents was much lower in the former, possibly due, at least in part, to the fact that Constantinides and associates[28] relied on hospital records, and Sjögren and colleagues[165] carried out personal psychiatric interviews. In the United States, data from a study of 30 well-documented index cases with Alzheimer's disease were compatible with both an autosomal dominant (low penetrance) and a polygenic model.[60] They yielded much higher recurrence risks than those in the previous literature (23% for parents and 10% for siblings), perhaps because Heston and Mastri[60] regarded Alzheimer's disease and senile dementia (Alzheimer type) as a single entity (the only difference being the age at onset) and, therefore, included both when they calculated their risk figures. These investigators also reported a marked increase in the frequency of Down's syndrome and myeloproliferative diseases among the families of patients with Alzheimer's disease, the first such observation, although it had been known before that patients with Down's syndrome, if they survived, developed dementia at relatively early ages (*i.e.*, in their 30s and 40s) with characteristic Alzheimer-type brain changes and also had an increased risk of leukemia. On the basis of these associations, Heston and Mastri[60] hypothesized a defect in the spatial organization of microtubules as a common pathologic mechanism.

Whalley and associates[180] reported on 74 probands with neuropathologically confirmed Alzheimer's disease identified through the neuropathology departmental records in Edinburgh, Scotland, who had died between 1959 and 1978. Scottish public records were used to identify family members, and attempts were made to trace all first-degree relatives. The frequency of secondary cases of presenile dementia was considerably higher than that expected in the general poulation (0.3). Unfortunately, no information was provided regarding the relationship of affected individuals (*i.e.*, parent, sibling, or child). These investigators considered their results compatible with a polygenic model of inheritance. Contrary to Heston and Mastri's report,[60] they found no increase in either the familial incidence of Down's syndrome or immunoproliferative disorders. However, the small sample size precluded a definitive refutation of Heston and Mastri's hypothesis. In contrast, Heyman and colleagues[64] noted a significantly increased frequency of Down's syndrome among the relatives of their probands. However, unlike Heston and Mastri, they did not find an increased frequency of hematologic cancers. Whalley and associates[180] did find significantly increased maternal and paternal ages at birth of the probands compared with controls; Heyman and associates[64] did not.

The preliminary data of Heyman and colleagues[64] on their study of 68 probands with a clinical diagnosis of Alzheimer's disease and age at onset of 70 years or less included information on 1278 relatives. The exclusion of secondary cases of possible dementia with onset after age 75 results in a minimum estimate. The cumulative incidence of dementia among the parents and siblings at age 75 was 14.4% and 13.9%, respectively. A new association to emerge from their investigation was the increased frequency of a history of documented thyroid disease among the women probands.[64] In a review of our own records of patients with DAT and controls, the frequency of prior thyroid disease was similar in both groups. Genetic markers to identify persons at increased risk have not as yet been detected, with attempts

to use blood groups, dermatoglyphics, and chromosomes all unsuccessful. A brief review of the various markers investigated is presented later in this chapter.

The available data provide evidence for a genetic factor in the etiology of Alzheimer's disease. The mode of inheritance may vary between families; autosomal dominant with reduced penetrance, autosomal recessive, and polygenic models have been proposed.

Senile Onset.   Evidence for genetic factors comes from family and twin studies that date to the 1920s and is compatible with both an autosomal dominant and a polygenic mode of inheritance. The hereditary factors are specific for senile dementia rather than generally increasing the risk for psychoses.

In the monumental study by Larsson and associates,[104] 2675 relatives and index cases yielded morbidity risks for senile dementia among first-degree relatives 4.3 times higher than for the general population. Not a single case of the presenile Alzheimer or Pick diseases was said to have been discovered among the relatives. No evidence for sex linkage was found, and sociomedical factors have not yet appeared to influence the morbidity risk for senile dementia in this or any other study. Since accurate diagnosis is of primary importance in quantitative genetic analysis, further analyses were carried out only for those 217 probands who displayed typical insidious onset and progression. The ages at onset were unknown for 8 individuals, and for the remaining 209 probands they ranged from 56 to 90 years (17 under 65 years). Field investigations identified 29 secondary cases in 22 families. Only in 9 cases was there direct transmission through two generations. We calculated the morbidity risk for siblings at 11.9 ± 3.0% and for parents at 20.8 ± 13.4%.

In another Swedish study, an entire population was surveyed, and a markedly elevated risk for parents and siblings was noted.[2] The rate for siblings 60 to 70 years of age was 7.1% and rose to 30.8% for those over 80 years of age, while for parents the rates were 60 to 70 years, 5.6%; 70 to 80 years, 8.7%; and over 80 years, 23.1%.

Heston and associates[61] reported their findings on the relatives of 125 probands with histopathologically confirmed DAT (the presenile and senile onset cases were combined). This report expands on their initial 30 probands with Alzheimer's disease, presenile onset, by adding new information on an additional 95 senile-onset cases. From these 95 families, 69 secondary cases were identified in

37 families. There were 19 families with two or more affected generations. Overall, 59.2% (74/125) of the probands represented sporadic cases of DAT. The morbidity risk for siblings was 19.5%, and for parents, 22.7%. The association between DAT and Down's syndrome was confirmed, while the initial association between DAT and hematologic malignancies was limited to solid lymphoproliferative cancers.

In addition to these family studies, there is one twin study in the literature.[87] In that study, concordance rates were 8% for dizygotic twins and 42.8% for monozygotic twins, with frequencies of 6.5% for siblings and 3% for parents.

Together, the family and twin studies provide strong evidence that genetic factors play a role in senile dementia, although the mode of inheritance remains unknown.

The consensus in the medical and scientific community is that Alzheimer's disease, presenile and senile onset, is a single entity, differing only in age at onset. In an attempt to gain a more comprehensive understanding of the genetics of Alzheimer's disease, we reviewed all family study reports in the literature, including those discussed previously as well as the numerous studies with small sample sizes, combining investigations when possible for quantitative genetic analysis.[125] Adequate information was available to allow analysis on a total of 515 probands. One hundred and thirteen (21.9%) of them had at least one other affected family member. However, only 58 (11.3%) of these exhibited transmission through two or more generations.

Unfortunately, the critical estimate that is of primary importance in genetic counseling (*i.e.*, the risk for the children of parents with DAT) is limited to the report by Constantinides and associates.[28] Briefly, children of patients with Alzheimer's disease, presenile onset, had a risk of 2.4% (1.6% and 0.8%, respectively, for presenile and senile onset). For children of senile-onset patients, the risk was 6% (3.2% for senile onset and 2.8% for presenile onset). Further data are required and will become available once longitudinal follow-up investigations of families have been completed.

Additional evidence for the potential role of genetic factors in DAT is provided by other lines of research. Chromosome studies have been carried out on patients with DAT, and in the initial studies women with senile dementia but not with cerebrovascular (multi-infarct) dementia showed a significant increase in chromosome loss in comparison to normal women of comparable age.[76,140] Later studies examining abnormalities in chromosome number[123,125] have reported conflicting reports that remain unexplained. Aberrations in chromosome structure have also been investigated in DAT patients and, once again, the results differ. However, the importance of chromosomal abnormalities has received further support from Heston's report of an increased frequency of Down's syndrome and hematologic malignancy in the families of patients with Alzheimer's disease, including senile dementia.[59] Heston[59] hypothesized a defect in the spatial organization of microtubles as a common underlying pathologic mechanism.

The association between DAT and Down's syndrome has directed an examination of the relationship of DAT and maternal age in light of the well-known increased frequency of Down's syndrome with increased maternal age. Maternal age is known to be an etiologic factor in Down's syndrome, but, aside from the initial report,[25] subsequent efforts[64,97] have failed to confirm an elevated maternal age at the birth of DAT patients. Other evidence is provided by the work of Stam and Op den Velde, who reported an increased Hp[1] gene frequency among patients with DAT.[71] However, another investigation, also carried out in the Netherlands,[36] failed to detect an association of DAT with Hp[1]. By contrast, we found an increased Hp[2] gene frequency in patients with clinically diagnosed DAT. In light of these conflicting results, the association between haptoglobin and DAT remains an open question. The HLA histocompatibility complex has also been investigated in DAT. Although some studies suggest an association between DAT and HLA, especially the B7 and Cw3 antigens, other studies have failed to demonstrate HLA disequilibria. In two multigenerational families, HLA haplotypes did not segregate with the disease. To accommodate exogenous influences, Albert suggested that what is inherited is a " special cerebral sensitivity," which may involve immunologic factors.[4] This is supported by a number of different observations.

Yugoslavian investigators, using the delayed skin hypersensitivity reaction to human brain protein, found a higher proportion of positive responders (69%) among their patients with cerebral atrophy than among schizophrenics (35%) or controls (2.5%).[71] Nandy[136] has identified brain-reactive antibodies in the γ-globulin fraction of serum from old but not from young mice, while Ingram and colleagues[70] described an age-associated increase in a neuron-binding globulin fraction in human serum, suggesting the existence of a similar brain-reactive antibody in aged humans; in line with this suggestion are Nandy's preliminary data that show an increase with age in brain-reactive antibodies in humans as well as higher levels in persons with Alzheimer's disease (both presenile and senile forms) than in control subjects of similar ages.[137]

Immune changes are also consistent with the involvement of an infectious agent in the etiology of senile dementia, suggested on the basis of the increased frequency of Down's syndrome and myeloproliferative disorders among the relatives of patients with Alzheimer's disease,[59,60] and the report that cultured neurons from fetal human cerebral cortex, exposed to an extract of Alzheimer's diseased brain, developed the paired helical filaments characteristic of neurofibrillary tangles.[32] These results must be interpreted cautiously because of difficulties with reproducibility and also because brains damaged by some other underlying pathology may be attacked by a transmissible viral agent not directly involved in the pathogenesis of the final disorder.

The primary problem in genetic research on senile dementia is diagnostic accuracy. Most information comes from clinical data, and, without autopsy findings, diagnostic distinctions are exceedingly difficult, especially since multiple syndromes that present as senile dementia suggest genetic heterogeneity.[12]

Multi-Infarct Dementia

Vascular dementia, the other major type of organic mental disorder common in old age, is clinically similar to senile dementia, except that there are more frequent focal neurologic signs, patchy deterioration, and a stepwise, rather than continuously progressive, decline in intellectual function. Diagnosis is often unclear, even on pathologic examination, because both kinds of dementia frequently coexist. The current theory is that vascular dementia is not the result of atheromatous changes within the cerebral vessels but that repeated infarcts, many of them small, are responsible for the dementia, hence the change in name from "arteriosclerotic" or "cerebrovascular" to "multi-infarct" dementia.

A sex difference has been reported for multi-infarct dementia, the disorder being more common in men than in women.[91,139] Constantinides and associates,[28] however, did not find a sex difference in their family investigation of 423 patients with the diagnosis of cerebral arteriosclerosis, which yielded morbidity risks of 7.3% for siblings and 3.9% for parents. They believed their data were consistent with an autosomal dominant mode of

inheritance with reduced penetrance. Furthermore, among these same relatives, the morbidity risk for senile dementia of the Alzheimer type was lower than expected.

Akesson's study also provided data that support the role of genetic factors in the vascular type of dementia.[2] Among the families of patients with the diagnosis of arteriosclerotic psychosis, he calculated a morbidity risk of 5.6% for siblings 60 years of age or older, and 9.6% for parents who lived to be 60 years of age or over, compared with the population incidence figures of 0.52%.

Sourander and Walinder[169] reported on a single family with five cases of similar vascular disease that began acutely in individuals whose general health was good and who were not hypertensive. The neuropsychiatric syndrome, including degree of dementia, was interpreted in terms of multiple focal lesions within the central nervous system, together with observed central and cortical atrophy. Histopathologic examinations of these cases ruled out nonvascular presenile dementia. The age at onset was between 29 and 38 years, and survival varied from 12 to 15 years in all but one of the deceased patients (5 months). The pattern of inheritance in this family was consistent with an autosomal dominant mode.

The above studies support the view that patients with multi-infarct dementia have a hereditary predisposition to develop this disease. It must be borne in mind that the dementia is secondary to vascular disease, and that vascular disease is believed to be related to environmental factors as well as to other conditions with genetic components (*e.g.*, hyperlipidemia[131] and hypertension[144]).

Ostfeld[143] reported that heart disease, hypertension (particularly systolic when diastolic is normal), and diabetes are risk factors for stroke. Surprisingly, there was no evidence for an association with blood lipid levels or cigarette smoking. Not all stroke patients are demented; yet the clinical features that increase an individual's risk for multi-infarct dementia have not been delineated. Ladurner and associates[102] examined this issue by comparing stroke patients with dementia to those without dementia. Demented stroke patients had higher incidences of cardiac problems, hypertension, and diabetes, but only hypertension was significantly higher. It may be difficult, therefore, to separate the genetic factor specific to multi-infarct dementia. In a follow-up of the twins who participated in the New York State Psychiatric Institute longitudinal study,[89] we reported an increased frequency of multi-infarct dementia among the children of parents who had a stroke.[84] In this small sample, we found that among the six parents of three twin pairs concordant for multi-infarct dementia, four (67%) had suffered a stroke as compared with only four of the 34 parents (12%) of twin pairs concordant for the absence of dementia. This finding suggests that stroke in a parent may constitute a risk factor for the development of vascular dementia among individuals prone to cerebrovascular accident. Despite the low correlation between cardiovascular and cerebrovascular disease, the understanding of multi-infarct dementia clearly depends on the progress that is made in the investigation of the other arteriosclerotic diseases.

It is possible that separate genetic mechanisms, as well as exogenous factors, are responsible for the various forms of this disorder. That identical genotypes can lead to markedly different histories of arteriosclerosis is exemplified by the monozygotic "O" twins. These brothers were first separated at the age of 25, when one of them left Europe to come to the western hemisphere (Fig. 5-7). His twin followed a year later. Marriage and the incompatibility of their mates markedly diminished their contact. Both continued in good health until the age of 59, when one developed symptoms of cardiovascular disease. Because of his Christian Scientist wife, no physician was consulted until his death at 61. According to the death certificate, he died of an acute coronary thrombosis. His twin received regular medical attention before and after he developed arteriosclerotic heart disease at 81. At 87 he was still active.

The "M" twins were also distinguished by intimate and constant contact until well into adult life (Fig. 5-8). Their health histories did not begin to diverge until they were in their 70s, when "A" developed hypertension. At the age of 82, "A" suffered a stroke, the following year a severe gastrointestinal hemorrhage, and a year later a probable coronary thrombosis. At age 85, "A" had a right hemiparesis, retinal hemorrhages in the right eye, left ventricular hypertrophy, and atrial premature beats with coupling. He was mentally confused and unable to care for himself and died within a year. His twin brother, W, was still rated in good physical and mental health without signs or symptoms of arteriosclerotic disease and was active socially and vocationally apparently until the age of 88 when he developed carcinoma of the stomach, which was fatal within 6 months.

Although differences in the health histories of the "M" twins did not become obvious until the second decade of our 20-year study of them, differential patterns of intellectual decline emerged during the first decade of follow-up. Whereas "W" showed the classic pattern associated with aging (a decrement on speeded motor tasks), 'A," in addition, evidenced the specific decline on tests of cognitive function defined as "critical loss," which has been found useful in predicting 5-year mortality (Table 5-1).[77] Because the terminal illness in the twins with "critical loss" was cardiovascular or cerebrovascular, this specific cognitive decline may be a sensitive indicator of cerebral ischemia. It is likely, therefore, that further twin studies will yield valuable information on the interaction of genetic and environmental factors in the production of mental changes associated with aging.

Affective Disorders

Unlike the dementias, affective disorders are not predominantly disorders of old age; yet depression is very common among the aged. Nonetheless, little is known about it and its relation to depressive illnesses of younger years[74] or about the role played by genetic factors in the depressions of later life. Genetic variability is an important determinant of reactions to psychotherapeutic agents, both in clinical efficacy and side reactions. Gene-controlled individual differences are not restricted to psychotropic drugs but also have been estab-

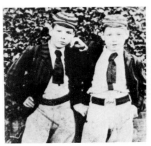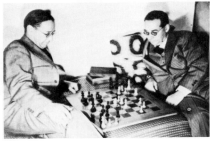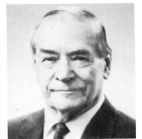

FIG. 5-7. The "O" twins at ages 13 and 60; (*right*) the survivor at age 80.

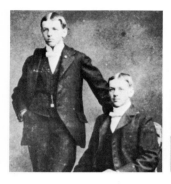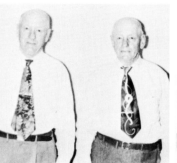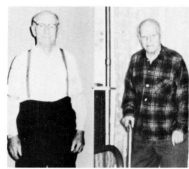

FIG. 5-8. The "M" twins at ages 16, 74, and 84 years.

lished for other drugs, including isoniazid, phenylbutazone, and antipyrine. Pharmacogenetics is expected to provide valuable guidelines to the clinician in the selection of dosages for individual patients. A major advance already attributable to this new discipline is the identification of persons who would react unfavorably to the administration of muscle relaxants, such as succinylcholine, important in the use of electroconvulsive therapies.

A confounding factor in studies of depressive disorders is the ongoing change in diagnostic concepts. Involutional melancholia, once a distinct diagnostic category, is now considered part of the major affective disorders, either unipolar or bipolar, and it is believed that previous studies included patients with depressions of heterogeneous etiology. Thus, Stenstedt, who excluded subjects with known manic-depressive disease from his genetic investigation of involutional melancholia in Sweden, did not find an increase in the incidence of involutional melancholia in primary relatives, compared with general population expectancy rates.[172] However, he did find the rate of "endogenous" affective disorder (including both involutional melancholia and manic depressive illness) in primary relatives to be approximately twice that expected for the Swedish general population (6.1% versus 3%) and believed that his data suggested that the diagnosis of "involutional melancholia" included patients with exogenous depression as well as late-onset manic-depressive illness.

Kallmann's twin-family study of "involutional psychosis" in the United States (patients in whom compulsive-delusional symptoms, nonperiodical forms of depression, or agitated anxiety states were observed after age 50 and before age 70) disclosed morbidity rates for siblings of 6 ± 1.61%; for dizygotic twins, 6 ± 3.36%; and for monozygotic twins, 60.9 ± 10.8%. By contrast, Kallmann found a low rate of manic-depressive psychosis

and a high rate of schizophrenia in the primary relatives of these patients and suggested that, according to his data, involutional psychosis was related to schizophrenia rather than to manic-depressive psychosis.[86] In contrast to Kallmann, Kay and Roth[92] found the morbidity risk for schizophrenia to be only slightly increased in relatives of their Swedish patients with late-onset affective disorders. They also compared patients with early- and late-onset affective disorders and noted that those with early onset had a significantly higher incidence of first-degree relatives with affective disorders. They concluded that patients with late-onset affective disorder are a heterogeneous group with frequent exogenous or symptom factors playing an etiologic role. Hopkinson[66] also reported that the morbidity risk for primary relatives was significantly greater for younger patients. If symptoms appeared before age 50, the risk was 20.1 ± 3.6%, compared with 8.3 ± 1.9% after age 50. For patients specifically diagnosed with "involutional melancholia" (diagnostic criteria not specified), the risk of affective illness in primary relatives was 10.2 ± 3.4%. The incidence of schizophrenia in first-degree relatives did not exceed the general population expectation for patients diagnosed with involutional melancholia. In a subsequent study, Hopkinson and Ley confirmed that the age at onset of affective illness was a significant variable in predicting morbidity risk for affective illness in first-degree relatives, with age 40 being the most significant differentiating age, and suggested that many of the depressions after age 40 might be secondary to other exogenous factors.[67] However, an American study did not disclose any relationship between medical illness or bereavement and the presence or lack of family history of affective disorders in depressed aged patients, although with onset after age 50 a positive family history of similar disease was less frequent than with earlier onset.[183]

TABLE 5-1   Critical Loss and Survival

Critical Loss*	Both 5 Years		Survival One 5 Years		Neither 5 Years	
	Monozygotic	*Dizygotic*	*Monozygotic*	*Dizygotic*	*Monozygotic*	*Dizygotic*
Neither partner	10	2		3		
One partner†	2	2	5	1	1	
Total	12	4	5	4	1	

* Critical loss is defined as a combination of at least two of the following: an annual decrement in score of at least 20% on Digit Symbol Substitution or 10% on Similarities subtests of the Wechsler Bellevue, or any decline on Vocabulary.

† In no pair did both partners show a critical loss. Where only one twin had a critical loss, it was always that twin who showed the earlier mortality.

(Data from Jarvik LF, Blum JE: Cognitive declines as predictors of mortality in twin pairs: A twenty-year longitudinal study of aging. In Palmore E, Jeffers FC (eds): Prediction of Life Span. Toronto, DC Heath, 1971)

In the major affective disorders (unipolar and bipolar), with onset at younger ages but often persisting into old age, significant genetic components have been uncovered by twin, family, and adoption studies, especially in bipolar disease (formerly termed *manic-depressive illness*), in which in some families a sex-linked dominant mode of inheritance has been described.[21,46,128,182] Nonetheless, there are still many questions about the genetics of affective disorders.[96, 149]

A potential marker for affective disorders in some familial cases has been reported.[135] Specifically, these investigators, using cultured skin fibroblasts and the family study methodology, detected a higher mean density of cholinergic receptors in patients and their affected relatives than in normal controls. Nonaffected relatives had mean values similar to controls. There is need to replicate these intriguing preliminary data on larger sample sizes. The cholinergic mechanism, however, is an unlikely candidate for explaining the underlying defect in all affective disorders, since it does not encompass the popular biogenic amine hypothesis.

Paranoid Disorders

Paranoid symptoms often accompany the organic mental syndromes of later life (including both senile and multi-infarct dementias). In addition, paranoid symptoms in elderly patients may occur in the course of preexisting schizophrenia or appear for the first time in old age (late paraphrenia), when they have also been related to schizophrenia. However, in one of the few genetic studies carried out with late-life paranoid disorders, the morbidity risk for schizophrenia for first-degree relatives was found to be much lower (ranging between 3.6% and 5.6%) than that for relatives of

schizophrenics with onset at younger ages.[90] It was concluded that there was a genetically determined predisposition to late paraphrenia but that it was of less importance than were genetic factors in schizophrenic illness that occurred in earlier life.[92] Other investigators also reported increased frequencies of nonspecific mental illness among relatives of aged paranoid patients, but further data are clearly needed.[41,164] At present, there is essentially no information about the mode of transmission of genetic factors in late-life paraphrenia.

MENTAL FUNCTIONING IN NORMAL AGING

Even though a decline in intellectual performance is frequently found with advancing age, data on the influence of genetic factors on mental functioning in old age are limited. The most extensive study has been the twin study carried out by Kallmann and colleagues.[9,78,80,89] In this long-term investigation, a set of 134 twin pairs, both alive, of 1603 twin "index cases," 60 years of age and over, were used for psychological assessments and followed for approximately 30 years. The initial psychometric results demonstrated that the mean intrapair differences in test scores were smaller for monozygotic twins than for dizygotic twins, but, at later testings, the differences were no longer statistically significant, perhaps owing to the smaller sample sizes and increasing homogeneity of those dizygotic pairs in which both partners survived.

Longevity and psychological test scores were also found to be positively correlated, suggesting a possible relationship between genetic factors in survival and intellectual performance.[78,81] A common underlying biologic mechanism responsible for these interrelated associations might be chromosomal. It is now well established that the proportion of hypodiploid cells (cells with 45 or fewer chromosomes instead of the normal 46) increases with advancing age, particularly in older women who show a greater loss of C-group chromosomes (including the X chromosome) than might be expected by chance.[44,85] For men, most investigations failed to detect an increase in hypodiploidy but nonetheless found an increased loss of G-group chromosomes (including the Y chromosome) with age. These cross-sectional findings have been confirmed in the only longitudinal study on aged subjects, a six-year follow-up of aged twins.[85]

Chromosome loss has been reported to correlate significantly with mental functioning, specifically with loss of certain cognitive functions, such as memory.[14,82] As mentioned earlier, chromosome loss has also been associated with dementia of the Alzheimer type and, again, the associations have been found primarily in women. Since women live longer than men, the possibility exists that the mental impairment associated with X-chromosome loss in women is an undesirable accompaniment of an otherwise successful mechanism for survival.

Evidence has begun to accumulate suggesting that the immune system may mediate the relationship between chromosome loss and intellectual impairment.[24,26,155] Both a direct and an indirect relationship have been reported between serum immunoglobulin levels and vocabulary score, leading Eisdorfer and colleagues[37] to suggest that a curvilinear function may best describe the relation between immune response and cognition. This association, as well as that between chromosome changes and levels of serum immunoglobulins observed in a small pilot study of aging twins,[124] require further investigation. In summary, genetic factors are implicated in the preservation of mental functioning into old age and chromosomal changes may represent the mechanism that underlies individual differences in both intellectual performance and survival in old age.

CONCLUSIONS

The potential for reducing the effects of many of the current life-shortening influences is inherent in our understanding of genetically determined variability, whether as individual differences in

susceptibility to specific diseases, in comparative resistance to senile decline, or in total longevity. Despite the paucity of studies dealing directly with genetic factors in aging, such factors have been demonstrated whenever an adequate search for etiologic components has been undertaken. Knowledge of genetic mechanisms is assuming enhanced importance as a substrate from which rationally directed therapies can evolve.

The longitudinal twin study from which much of our information on aging and longevity has been derived was initiated and guided, until his death in 1965, by Franz J. Kallmann.

REFERENCES

1. Adlersberg D, Parets AD, Boas EP: Genetics of atherosclerosis: Studies of families with xanthoma and unselected patients with coronary artery disease under the age of 50 years. JAMA, 141:246, 1949
2. Akesson HO: A population study of senile and arteriosclerotic psychoses. Hum Hered 19:546, 1969
3. Albanese AA: Bone Loss, Causes, Detection and Therapy. In Current Topics in Nutrition and Disease, vol 1. New York, Alan R. Liss, 1977
4. Albert E: Discussion contribution to "epidemiology and genetics of senile dementia." In Muller C, Ciompi L (eds): Senile Dementia, pp 65–68. Bern, Switzerland, Hans Huber Verlag, 1968
5. Alm T, Wahren B: Carcinoembryonic antigen in hereditary adenomatosis of the colon and rectum. Scand J Gastroenterol 10:875, 1975
6. Arnett FC Jr, Schacter BZ, Hochberg MC, Hsu SH, Bias WB: Homozygosity for HLA-B27: Impact on rheumatic disease expression in two families. Arthritis Rheum 20:797, 1977
7. Avioli LV: Senile and postmenopausal osteoporosis. Adv Intern Med 21:391, 1976
8. Awano I, Takahashi S: The twin studies in essential hypertension: Heredity and environment in essential hypertension. Jpn J Hum Genet 11:208, 1966
9. Bank LI, Jarvik LF: A longitudinal study of aging twins. In Schneider EL (ed): Genetics of Aging. New York, Plenum Publishing, 1978
10. Barbeau A, Chase TN, Paulson GW (eds): Huntington's chorea. In Advances in Neurology, vol 1, pp 1872–1972. New York, Raven Press, 1973
11. Bell AG: The Duration of Life and Conditions Associated with Longevity: A Study of the Hyde Genealogy. Washington, Judd and Detweiler, 1918
12. Bergmann K: The epidemiology of senile dementia. Br J Psychiatry 9:100, 1975

13. Bernouilli C, Siegfried J, Baumgartner G, Regli F, Rabinowitz T, Gajdusek DC, Gibbs CJ: Danger of accidental person-to-person transmission of Creutzfeldt-Jakob disease by surgery. Lancet 1:478, 1977

14. Bettner LG, Jarvik LF, Blum JE: Stroop color-word test, non-psychotic organic brain syndrome, and chromosome loss in aged twins. J Gerontol 26:458, 1971

15. Beverstock GC: The current state of research with peripheral tissues in Huntington disease. Hum Genet 66:115, 1984

16. Biron P, Mongeau JG, Bertrand D: Familial aggregation of blood pressure in 558 adopted children. Can Med Assoc J 115:773, 1976

17. Bondareff W: Age and Alzheimer disease. Lancet 1:1447, 1983

18. Boveri I: The Origin of Malignant Tumors. Baltimore, Williams & Wilkins, 1929

19. Bowser-Riley S, Bain AD, Noble J, and Lamb DW: Chromosome abnormalities in Dupuytren's disease. Lancet 2: 1282, 1975

20. Brown MS, Goldstein JL: Receptor mediated control of cholesterol metabolism. Science 191:150, 1976

21. Cadoret RJ: Evidence for genetic inheritance of primary affective disorder in adoptees. Am J Psychiatry 135:463, 1978

22. Caine ED, Hunt RD, Weingartner H, Ebert MH: Huntington's dementia: Clinical and neuropsychological features. Arch Gen Psychiatry 35:377, 1978

23. Cohen BH: Family patterns of mortality and life span. Q Rev Biol: 39:130, 1964

24. Cohen D, Eisdorfer C: Behavioral-immunologic relationships in older men and women. Exp Aging Res 3:225, 1977

25. Cohen D, Eisdorfer C, Leverenz J: Alzheimer's disease and maternal age. J Geriatr Soc 30:656, 1982

26. Cohen D, Matsuyama SS, Jarvik LF: Immunoglobulin levels and intellectual functioning in the aged. Exp Aging Res 2:345, 1976

27. Conneally PM: Huntington disease: Genetics and epidemiology. Am J Hum Genet 36:506, 1984

28. Constantinides J, Garrone G, de Ajuriaguerra J: L'heredité des demences de l'age avance. Encephale 51:301, 1962

29. Corsellis JAN: Ageing and the dementias. In Blackwood W, Corsellis JAN (eds): Greenfield's Neuropathology, pp 796–848. London, Edward Arnold, 1976

30. Court Brown WM, Price WH, Jacobs PA: Further information on the identity of 47 XYY males. Br Med J 2:325, 1968

31. Cutler NR, Brown PW, Narrayan T, Parisi JE, Janotta F, Baron H: Creutzfeldt-Jakob disease: A case of sixteen years' duration. Ann Neurol 15:107, 1984

32. de Boni U, Crapper DR: Paired helical filaments of the Alzheimer type in cultured neurones. Nature 271:566, 1978

33. deFaire U: Ischaemic heart disease in death discordant twins. Acta Med Scand 568 (suppl):1, 1974

34. Deutscher S, Epstein FH, Kjelsberg MO: Familial aggregation of factors associated with coronary heart disease. Circulation 33:911, 1966

35. Duffy P, Wolf J, Collins G, De Voe AG, Steeten B, Cowen D: Possible person-to-person transmission of Creutzfeldt-Jakob disease. N Eng J Med 290:692, 1974

36. Eikelenboom P, Vink-Starreveld ML, Jansen W, Pronk JC: C3 and haptoglobin polymorphism in dementia of the Alzheimer type. Acta Psychiatr Scand 69:140, 1984

37. Eisdorfer C, Cohen D, Buckley CE: Serum immunoglobulins and cognition in the impaired elderly. In Katzman R, Terry RD, Bick KL (eds): Alzheimer's Disease: Senile Dementia and Related Disorders, pp 401–407. New York, Raven Press, 1978

38. Enna SJ et al: Huntington's chorea: Changes in neurotransmitter receptors in the brain. N Engl J Med 294:1305, 1976

39. Feinleib M et al: The National Heart and Lung Institute twin study of cardiovascular disease risk factors: Organization and methodology. Acta Genet Med Gemollol 25:125, 1976

40. Friedman M, Rosenman RH: Association of specific overt behavior pattern with blood and cardiovascular findings. JAMA 169:1286, 1959

41. Funding T: Genetics of paranoid psychoses in later life. Acta Psychiatr Scand 37:267, 1961

42. Gajdusek DC: Unconventional viruses and the origin and disappearance of kuru. Science 197:943, 1977

43. Gajdusek DC, Gibbs CJ, Earle K, Dammin CJ, Schoene W, Tyler HR: Transmission of subacute spongiform encephalopathy to the chimpanzee and squirrel monkey from a patient with papulosis maligan of Kohlmeier Degos. In Subriana A, Espadaler JM, Burrows EH (eds): Proceedings of the Tenth International Congress of Neurology, Barcelona, pp 390–392. Amsterdam, Excerpta Medica, 1974

44. Galloway SM, Buckton KE: Aneuploidy and aging: Chromosome studies on a random sample of the population using G-banding. Cytogenet Cell Genet 20:78, 1978

45. German J: Bloom's syndrome: I. Genetical and clinical observations in the first twenty-seven patients. Am J Hum Genet 21:196, 1969

46. Gershon ES, Bunney WE Jr, Leckman JF, Van Eerdewegh M, DeBauche BA: The inheritance of affective disorders: A review of data and of hypotheses. Behav Genet 6:227, 1976

47. Gibbs CJ, Gajdusek DC, Asher DM, Alpers MP,

Beck E, Daniel PM, Matthews WB: Creutzfeldt-Jakob disease (spongiform encephalopathy) transmission to the chimpanzee. Science 161:388, 1968

48. Goldstein JL, Brown MS: The low-density lipoprotein pathway and its relation to atherosclerosis. Annu Rev Biochem 46:897, 1977

49. Goldstein JL, Schrott HG, Hazzard WR, Bierman EJ, Motulsky AG: Hyperlipidemia in coronary heart disease: II. Genetic analysis of lipid levels in 176 families and delineation of a new inherited disorder, combined hyperlipidemia. J Clin Invest 52:1544, 1973

50. Goldstein JL, Sobhani MK, Faust JR, Brown MR: Heterozygous familial hypercholesterolemia: Failure of normal allele to compensate for mutant allele at a regulated genetic locus. Cell 9:195, 1976

51. Groen JJ, Endtz LJ: Hereditary Pick's disease—second reexamination of a large family and discussion of other hereditary cases, with particular reference to electroencephalography and computerized tomography. Brain 105:443, 1982

52. Gusella JF, Wexler NS, Conneally PM, Naylor SL, Anderson MA, Tanzi RE, Watkins PC, Ottina K, Wallace MR, Sakaguchi AY, Young AB, Shoulson I, Bonilla E, Martin JB: A polymorphic DNA marker genetically linked to Huntington's disease. Nature 306:234, 1983

53. Gustafson L, Brun A, Hagberg B, Ingvar, DH, Risberg J: Presenile dementia: A prospective, clinical neurophysiological and neuropathological investigation. Abstracts from the meeting of the VI World Congress of Psychiatry, p 79. Honolulu, 1977

54. Harvald B, Hauge M: Hereditary factors elucidated by twin studies. In Neel JV, Shaw M, Schull WJ (eds): Genetics and the Epidemiology of Chronic Diseases, publication 1163, pp 61–76. Washington, DC, US Department of Health, Education and Welfare, Public Health Service, 1965

55. Hauge M et al: The Danish twin register. Acta Genet Med Gemellol 17:315, 1968

56. Hayden MR: Huntington's Chorea. New York, Springer-Verlag, 1981

57. Hazzard WR, Goldstein JL, Schrott HG, Motulsky AG, Bierman EL: Hyperlipidemia in coronary heart disease: III. Evaluation of lipoprotein phenotypes of 156 genetically defined survivors of myocardial infarction. J Clin Invest 52:1569, 1973

58. Henkin RI: Salt taste in patients with essential hypertension and with hypertension due to primary hyperaldosteronism J. Chronic Dis 27:235, 1974

59. Heston LL: Alzheimer's disease, trisomy 21, and myeloproliferative disorders: Associations suggesting a genetic diathesis. Science 196:322, 1976

60. Heston LL, Mastri AR: The genetics of Alzheimer's disease: Associations with hematologic malignancy and Down's syndrome. Arch Gen Psychiatry 34:976, 1977.

61. Heston LL, Mastri AR, Anderson VE, White J: Dementia of the Alzheimer type: Clinical genetics, natural history, and associated conditions. Arch Gen Psychiatry 38:1085, 1981

62. Heston WE: Genetics of cancer. J Hered 65:262, 1974

63. Heston WE: The genetic aspects of human cancer. Adv Cancer Res 23:1, 1976

64. Heyman A, Wilkinson WE, Hurwitz BJ, Schmechel D, Sigmon AH, Weinberg T, Helms MJ, Swift M: Alzheimer's disease: Genetic aspects and associated clinical disorders. Ann Neurol 14:507, 1983

65. Hook EB: Behavioral implications of the human XYY genotype. Science 179:139, 1973

66. Hopkinson G: A genetic study of affective illness in patients over 50. Br J Psychiatry 110:244, 1964

67. Hopkinson G, Ley P: A genetic study of affective disorder. Br J Psyciatry 115:917, 1969

68. Humerfelt S: Distribution of blood pressure in a population group begun in 1963–1964: Epidemiological aspects. Tidssk Nor Laegeforen 88:1406, 1968

69. Ing R, Ho HC: Evidence against association between wet cerumen and breast cancer. Lancet 41:7793, 1973

70. Ingram CR, Phegan KJ, Blumenthal HT: Significance of an aging-linked neuron binding gammaglobulin fraction of human sera. J Gerontol 29:29, 1974

71. Jankovic BD, Jakulic S, Horvat J: Cerebral atrophy: An immunological disorder. Lancet 2:219, 1977

72. Jarvik LF: Genetic variations in disease resistance and survival potential. In Kallmann FJ (ed): Expanding Goals of Genetics in Psychiatry. New York, Grune & Stratton, 1962

73. Jarvik LF: Genetic aspects of aging. In Rossman I (ed): Clinical Geriatrics, pp 85–105. Philadelphia, JB Lippincott, 1971

74. Jarvik LF: Aging and depression: Some unanswered questions. J Gerontol 31:324, 1976

75. Jarvik LF: Genetic modes of transmission relevant to psychopathology. In Sperber MA, Jarvik LF (eds): Psychiatry and Genetics. New York, Basic Books, 1976

76. Jarvik LF, Altshuler KZ, Kato T, Blumner B: Organic brain syndrome and chromosome loss in aged twins. Dis Nerv Syst 32:159, 1971

77. Jarvik LF, Blum JE: Cognitive declines as predictors of mortality in twin pairs: A twenty-year longitudinal study of aging. In Palmore E, Jeffers FC (eds): Prediction of Life Span. Toronto, DC Heath, 1971

78. Jarvik LF, Blum JE, Varma O: Genetic components and intellectual functioning during senes-

cence: A 20-year study of aging twins. Behavioral Genetics, 2:159, 1972

79. Jarvik LF, Falek A: Comparative data on cancer in aging twins. Cancer 15:1009, 1962

80. Jarvik LF, Falek A, Kallmann FJ, Lorge I: Survival trends in a senescent twin population. Am J Hum Genet 12:170, 1960

81. Jarvik LF, Kallmann FJ, Falek A: Intellectual changes in aged twins. J Gerontol 17:289, 1962

82. Jarvik LF, Kato T: Chromosomes and mental changes in octogenarians. Br J Psychiatry 115:1193, 1969

83. Jarvik LF, Klodin V, Matsuyama SS: Human aggression and the extra Y chromosome—fact or fantasy? Am Psychol 28:674, 1973

84. Jarvik LF, Matsuyama SS: Parental stroke: Risk-factor for multi-infarct dementia? Lancet 2:1025, 1983

85. Jarvik LF, Yen FS, Fu TK, Matsuyama SS: Chromosomes in old age: A six year longitudinal study. Hum Genet 33:17, 1976

86. Kallmann FJ: The genetics of psychoses: An analysis of 1,232 twin index families. In Congres International de Psychiatrie, Rapports, vol. 6, pp. 1–27. Paris, Hermann, 1950

87. Kallmann FJ: Heredity in Health and Mental Disorder. New York, WW Norton, 1953

88. Kallmann FJ, Jarvik LF: Twin data on genetic variations in resistance to tuberculosis. Collana di Monographie Analecta. Genetica 6:15, 1958

89. Kallmann FJ, Sander G: Twin studies on senescence. Am J Psychiatry 106:29, 1949

90. Kay D: Observations on the natural history and genetics of old age psychoses: A. Stockholm material 1931–1937. Proc R Soc Med 52:791, 1959

91. Kay DWK, Beamish P, Roth M: Old age mental disorders in Newcastle-upon-Tyne: Part I. A study of prevalence. Br J Psychiatry 110:146, 1964

92. Kay D, Roth M: Environmental and hereditary factors in the schizophrenias of old age (late paraphrenia) and their bearing on the general problem of causation in schizophrenia. Br J Psychiatry 107:649, 1961

93. Kay MMB, Makinodan T: Immunobiology of aging: Evaluation of current status. Clin Immunol Immunopathol 6:394, 1976

94. Kellermann G, Luyten-Kellermann M, Shaw CR: Genetic variation of aryl hydrocarbon hydroxylase in human lymphocytes. Am J Hum Genet 25:327, 1973

95. Keys A, Brues AM, Sacher GA (eds): Aging and Levels of Biological Organization. Chicago, University of Chicago Press, 1965

96. Kidd K, Weissman MM: Why we do not yet understand the genetics of affective disorders. In Cole J, Schatzberg A, Frazier SH (eds): Depression: Biology, Dynamics, and Treatment. New York, Plenum Publishing, 1977

97. Knesevich JW, LaBarge E, Martin RL, Danziger WL, Berg L: Birth order and maternal age effect in dementia of the Alzheimer type. Psychiatr Res 7:345, 1982

98. Knudson AG Jr: Genetics of human cancer. Genetics, 79 (suppl):305, 1975

99. Knudson AG, Strong LC, Anderson DE: Heredity and cancer in man. Prog Med Genet 9:113, 1973

100. Kreulen TH, Cohn PF, Gorlin R: Premature coronary artery disease in identical male twins studied by selective coronary arteriography. Cathet Cardiovasc Diagn, 1:91, 1975

101. Kuhl DE, Phelps ME, Markham CH, Metter J, Riege WH, Winter J: Cerebral metabolism and atrophy in Huntington's disease determined by 18FDG and computed tomographic scan. Ann Neurol 12:425, 1982

102. Ladurner G, Iliff LD, Lechner H: Clinical factors associated with dementia in ischaemic stroke. J Neurol Neurosurg Psychiatry 45:97, 1982

103. Langford HG, Watson RL: A study of the urinary sodium, salt-taste threshold and blood pressure resemblance of siblings. Johns Hopkins Med J 131:143, 1972

104. Larsson T, Sjögren T, Jacobson G: Senile dementia: A clinical sociomedical and genetic study. Acta Psychiatr Scand 39 (suppl):1, 1967

105. Lauer RM, Filer LJ Jr, Reiter MA, Clarke WR: Blood pressure, salt preference, salt threshold, and relative weight. Am J Dis Child 130:493, 1976

106. Levine H: Clinical Cytogenetics. Boston, Little, Brown & Co, 1971

107. Lynch HT, Guirgis HA, Lynch PM, Lynch JF, Harris RE: Familial cancer syndromes: A survey. Cancer 39:1867, 1977

108. Lynch HT et al: Role of heredity in multiple primary cancer. Cancer 40:1849, 1977

109. McGill HC, Mott GE: Genetic mechanisms in atherosclerosis: Comparative pathology of the heart. Adv Cardiol 13:108, 1974

110. McIlhany ML, Shaffer JW, Hines EA: The heritability of blood pressure: An investigation of 200 pairs of twins using the cold pressor test. Johns Hopkins Med J 136:57, 1975

111. McKusick VA: Coronary artery disease. In Neel JV, Shaw M, Schull WJ (eds): Genetics and the Epidemiology of Chronic Diseases, publication 1163, pp 133–143. Washington, DC, US Department of Health, Education and Welfare, Public Health Service, 1965

112. McKusick VA: Mendelian Inheritance in Man: Catalogs of Autosomal Dominant, Autosomal Recessive and X-Linked Phenotypes, 6th ed. Baltimore, Johns Hopkins University Press, 1983.

113. Maclean N, Court-Brown WM, Jacobs PA, Menth DJ, Strong JA: A survey of sex chromatin abnormalities in mental hospitals. J. Med Genet 5:165, 1968

114. McMichael AJ, Sasazuki T, McDevitt HO, Payne RO: Increased frequency of HLA-Cw3 and HLA-

Dw4 in rheumatoid arthritis. Arthritis Rheum 20:1037, 1977

115. Madigan FC, Vance RB: Differential sex mortality: A research design. Social Forces 35:193, 1957

116. Makinodan T, Yunis E (eds): Immunology and aging, 1. In Good RA, Day SB (eds): Comprehensive Immunology. New York, Plenum Publishing, 1977

117. Manuelidis EE, Manuelidis L, Pincus JH, Collins WF: Transmission from man to hamster of Creutzfeldt-Jakob disease with clinical recovery. Lancet 2:40, 1978

118. Marx JL: DNA repair: New clues to carcinogenesis. Res News Sci 100:518, 1978

119. Masters CL, Gajdusek DC, Gibbs CJ Jr: The familial occurrence of Creutzfeldt-Jakob disease and Alzheimer disease. Brain 104:535, 1981

120. Mathers JAL, Osborne RH, DeGeorge FV: Studies of blood pressure, heart rate, and the electrocardiogram in adult twins. Am Heart J 62:634, 1961

121. Mathews JD: Ischaemic heart disease: Possible genetic markers. Lancet 2:681, 1975

122. Mathews JD et al: Antigen and haplotype frequencies in essential hypertension and ischaemic heart disease. In Dausset J, Svejgaard A (chairmen): International Symposium on HLA and Diseases. Paris, Editions INSERM, 1976

123. Matsuyama SS: Genetic factors in dementia of the Alzheimer type. In Reisberg B (ed): Alzheimer's Disease—The Standard Reference, pp 155–160. New York, The Free Press, 1983

124. Matsuyama SS, Cohen D, Jarvik LF: Hypodiploidy and serum immunoglobulin concentrations in the elderly. Mech Ageing Dev 8:407, 1978

125. Matsuyama SS, Jarvik LF, Kumar V: Dementia: Genetics. In Arie T (ed): Recent Advances in Psychogeriatrics, in press

126. Matthews WB: Epidemiology of Creutzfeldt-Jakob disease in England and Wales. J Neurol Neurosurg Psychiatry 38:210, 1975

127. May WW: Creutzfeldt-Jakob disease: I. Survey of the literature and clinical diagnosis. Acta Neurol Scand 44:1, 1968

128. Mendlewicz J, Rainer JD: Adoption study supporting genetic transmission in manic-depressive illness. Nature 268:327, 1977

129. Merz PA, Somerville RA, Wisniewski HM, Manuelidis L, Manuelidis EE: Scrapie-associated fibrils in Creutzfelt-Jakob disease. Nature 306:474, 1983

130. Miller RW: Congenital malformations and cancer in the sibships of leukemic children—further considerations. In Neel JF, Shaw, MW, Schull WJ (eds): Genetics and the Epidemiology of Chronic Diseases, publication 1163, pp 373–381. Washington, DC, US Department of Health, Education and Welfare, Public Health Service, 1965

131. Motulsky AG: Current concepts in genetics: The genetic hyperlipidemias. N Engl J Med 294:823, 1976

132. Mulvihill JJ: Congenital and genetic diseases. In Fraumeni JF Jr (ed): Persons at High Risk of Cancer: An Approach to Cancer Etiology and Control. New York, Academic Press, 1975

133. Myers RH, Goldman D, Bird ED, Sax DS, Merril CR, Schoenfeld M, Wolf PA: Maternal transmission in Huntington's disease. Lancet 1:208, 1983

134. Myrianthopoulos NC: Huntington's chorea: Review article. J Med Genet 3:298, 1966

135. Nadi NS, Nurnberger JI, Gershon ES: Muscarinic cholinergic receptors on skin fibroblasts in familial affective disorder. N Eng J Med 311:225, 1984

136. Nandy K: Immune reactions in aging brain and senile dementia. In Nandy K, Sherwin I (eds): The Aging Brain and Senile Dementia, pp 181–196. New York, Plenum Publishing, 1977

137. Nandy K: Neuroanatomical changes in the aging brain. Presented at the South Central RMEC symposium on Biomedical Aspects of Senile Dementia and Related Disorders. St. Louis, 1978

138. Neuhauser G, Kaveggia EG, Opitz JM: Autosomal recessive syndrome of pseudogliomatous blindness, osteoporosis and mild mental retardation. Clin Genet 9:324, 1976

139. Nielsen J: Geronto-psychiatric period—prevalence investigation in a geographically delineated population. Acta Psychiatr Scand 38:307, 1962

140. Nielsen J: Chromosomes in senile, presenile, and arteriosclerotic dementia. J Gerontol 25:312, 1970

141. Oleinick SR: Mechanisms of tumor immunology. In Fromlich ED (ed): Pathophysiology: Altered Regulatory Mechanisms in Disease, 2nd ed. Philadelphia, JB Lippincott, 1976

142. Osborne RH, DeGeorge FV: Genetic Basis of Morphological Variation. Cambridge, MA, Harvard University Press, 1959

143. Ostfeld AM: A review of stroke epidemiology. Epidemiol Rev 2:136, 1980

144. Page LB: Epidemiologic evidence on the etiology of human hypertension and its possible prevention. Am Heart J 91:527, 1976

145. Paigen B et al: Questionable relation of aryl hydrocarbon hydroxylase to lung-cancer risk. N Engl J Med 297:346, 1977

146. Pearl R: Studies on human longevity: IV. The inheritance of longevity: Preliminary report. Hum Biol 3:245, 1931

147. Petrakis NL: Cerumen genetics and human breast cancer. Science 173:347, 1971

148. Petrakis NL, King MC: Genetic markers and cancer epidemiology. Cancer 39:1861, 1977

149. Petterson U: Manic-depressive illness: A clinical, social and genetic study. Acta Psychiatr Scand 269 *(Suppl)*: 1, 1977

150. Pikkarainen J, Takkunen J, Kulonen E: Serum cholesterol in Finnish twins. Am J. Hum Genet 18:115, 1966

151. Pitot HC: Carcinogenesis and aging—two related phenomena? A review. Am J Pathol 87:444, 1977

152. Prusiner SB: Novel proteinaceous infectious particles cause scrapie. Science 216:136, 1982

153. Rachelefsky G, Terasaki PI, Katz R, Stiehm ER: Increased prevalence of W27 in juvenile rheumatoid arthritis. N Engl J Med 290:892, 1974

154. Reed TE, Chandler JH: Huntington's chorea in Michigan: Demography and genetics. Am J Hum Genet 10:201, 1958

155. Roseman JM, Buckley CE: Inverse relationship between serum IgG concentrations and measures of intelligence in elderly persons. Nature 254:55, 1975

156. Rossor MN, Iverson LL, Reynolds GP, Mountjoy CQ, Roth M: Neurochemical characteristics of early and late onset types of Alzhemier's disease. Br Med J 288:961, 1984

157. Roth M: Senile dementia and related disorders. In Wertheimer J, Marois M (eds): Senile Dementia: Outlook for the Future, pp 493–515. New York, Alan R Liss, 1984

158. Ryder LP, Svejgaard A: Report from the HLA and Disease Registry of Copenhagen. Copenhagen, LP Ryder and A Svejgaard, 1976

159. Schenk VWD: Reexamination of a family with Pick's disease. Ann Hum Genet 23:325, 1959

160. Schlosstein L, Terasaki PI, Bluestone R, Pearson CM: High association of an HLA antigen, w27, with ankylosing spondylitis. N. Engl J Med 228,704, 1973

161. Schroeder TM, Anschutz F, Knopp A: Spontane Chromosomenaber-rationen bei familiarer Panmyelopathie. Humangenetik 1:194, 1964

162. Schwarzacher HG: Analysis of interphase nuclei. In Schwarzacher HG, Wolf U, Passarge E (eds): Methods in Human Cytogenetics pp 207–234. New York, Springer-Verlag, 1974

163. Schweitzer MD, Gearing FR, Perera GA: Family studies of primary hypertension: Their contribution to the understanding of genetic factors. *In* Stamler J, Stamler R, Pullman TN (eds): The Epidemiology of Hypertension (Proceedings of an International Symposium). New York, Grune & Stratton, 1967

164. Sjögren H: Paraphrenic, melancholic and psychoneurotic states in the presenile-senile period of life. Acta Psychiatr Scand 176 (*suppl*):1, 1964

165. Sjögren T, Sjögren H, Lindgren AGH: Morbus Alzheimer and Morbus Pick. Acta Psychiatr Neurol Scand 82 (*suppl*):1, 1952

166. Slack J, Evans KA: The increased risk of death from ischaemic heart disease in first degree relatives in 121 men and 96 women with ischaemic heart disease. J Med Genet 3:239, 1966

167. Slater E, Roth M: Clinical Psychiatry, 3rd ed. Baltimore, Williams & Wilkins, 1969

168. Smith W: Epidemiology of hypertension. Med Clin North Am 61:468, 1977

169. Sourander P, Walinder J: Hereditary multi-infarct dementia: Morphological and clinical studies of a new disease. Acta Neuropathol 39:247, 1977

170. Spector WS (ed): Handbook of Biological Data. Philadelphia, WB Saunders, 1956

171. Stam FC, Op den Velde W: Haptoglobin types in Alzheimer's disease and senile dementia. In Katzman R, Terry RD, Bick KL (eds): Alzheimer's Disease: Senile Dementia and Related Disorders, pp 279–285. New York, Raven Press, 1978

172. Stenstedt A: Involutional melancholia: An etiologic, clinical and social study of endogenous depression in later life, with special reference to genetic factors. Acta Psychiatr Neurol Scand 127(*suppl*):1, 1959

173. Stevens DP Mackay IR, Cullen KJ: Carcinoembryonic antigen in an unselected elderly population: A four year follow up. Br J. Cancer 32:147, 1975

174. Strong LC: Genetic and environmental interactions. Cancer 40:1861, 1977

175. Topinka I, and Sova, J: The taste threshold of NaCl, its genetic bondage and possible importance for the etiology of hypertension. Cas Lek Cesk 106:689, 1967

176. Traub R, Gajdusek DC, Gibbs CJ: Transmissible virus dementia: The relation of transmissible spongiform encephalopathy to Creutzfeldt-Jakob disease. In Smith WL, Kinsbourne M (eds): Aging and Dementia. New York, Spectrum Publication, 1977

177. Trowell HC: Hypertension and salt. Lancet 2:204, 1978

178. Von Behren PA, Lauer RM: The significance of blood pressure measurements in childhood. Med Clin North Am 61:487, 1977

179. Waldmann TA et al: Role of suppressor T cells in pathogenesis of common variable hypogammaglobulinemia. Lancet 2:609, 1974

180. Whalley LJ, Carothers AD, Collyer S, De Mey R, Frackiewicz A: A study of familial factors in Alzheimer's disease. Br J Psychiatry 140:249, 1982

181. Whittier JE: Research on Huntington's chorea: Problems of privilege and confidentiality. J Forensic Sci 8:568, 1963

182. Winokur G, Cadoret R, Dorzab J, Baker M: Depressive disease: A genetic study. Arch Gen Psychiatry 24:135, 1971

183. Woodruff R, Pitts FN, Winokur G: Affective disorder: II. A comparison of patients with endogenous depressions with and without family history of affective disorder. J Nerv Ment Dis 139:49, 1964

184. Yunis JJ: The chromosomal basis of human neoplasia. Science 221:227, 1983

II

The Aged Patient— General Principles

6

Mortality and Morbidity Overview

Isadore Rossman

As will be noted repeatedly in this volume, old age is characterized by many physiologic declines and an accretion of pathologic disorders. Many of them are inevitable, irreversible, and additive; hence, aging is often regarded with varying degrees of negativism by both professionals and the public. There is little doubt that much of the negativism is related to symbolic rather than factual thought processes. This is evidenced by the over-reaction to landmark birthdays—40, 65—to graying of hair, and even to the first pair of bifocals. These are commonly perceived as threats or onslaughts, perhaps heralding an oncoming decrepitude. Irreversibility is the essence of virtually all the age-related diseases noted as challenges for research by a National Institute on Aging task force more than a decade ago: atherosclerosis, cancer, diabetes mellitus, obesity, osteoporosis, osteoarthritis, benign prostatic hypertrophy, emphysema, cataracts, depressive illness and senile dementia, and parkinsonism.[41]

Functional declines in many organ systems are generally distinguishable from disease as such, are age-related (see Chapter 2), and are universal. Despite these bleak prospects for our future selves, functional ability often persists at excellent levels, so that individuality and variability are equally valid key concepts. A 75-year-old man may have significant atherosclerosis, harbor a nidus of carcinoma in his prostate, have indisputable glucose intolerance, need intermittent treatment for osteoarthritis, and still perform outstandingly as head of state. It is mandatory for the physician to avoid the *idée fixe* and all the other variants of symbolistic thinking with patients of any age. Unconscious categorization can dampen therapeutic effort, produce defects in differential diagnosis, and

lead to lapses in reevaluation and to unwarranted poor prognoses. Clinical practice is replete with evidence that radiculopathies improve despite impressively stable osteophytes, that organic mental syndromes get better on discontinuing medications, and that dyspepsia may not be due to a previously identified hiatal hernia, cholelithiasis, or diverticulosis but to a new treatable peptic ulcer.

To be both objective and informed, the geriatrician should be well grounded in the data that relates to morbidity and mortality in his unique patient population. Some of this material will in fact illustrate how well older patients cope with the inevitable disorders of somatic decline. It will also become clear that the data base of vital statistics sometimes has only a shaky correlation with the facts of clinical practice. Finally, some actuarial formulations such as those dealing with the force of mortality should be regarded as of importance to the informed geriatrician.

The widespread belief that old age is synonymous with major impairments and chronic illness is of course a marked exaggeration. In the 1972 Health Interview Survey 82.4% of the over-65 age-group had no limitation of mobility. Slightly over 5% were confined to their homes, another 6.7% needed help in getting about, and 5.8% had trouble getting around alone. Some of the major disorders contributing to limitation of activity are listed in Table 6-1.

Although many of the disorders can be helped, there are few that are curable. There are also many that may not limit activity but can impair the quality of life. Thus in the 65- to 74-year age-group, 16.4% are obese and more than 45% are edentulous. The impaired elderly often have a number of significant conditions simultaneously. Lake,[30] in a

TABLE 6-1   Some Conditions Contributing to Limitation of Activity in US Population Over 65

Condition	%
Heart conditions	23.5
Arthritis and rheumatism	23.2
Visual impairments	9.8
Diabetes	6.8
Cerebrovascular disease	4.9
Emphysema	4.4
Paralysis, complete or partial	3.6
Mental and nervous conditions	3.4
Hearing impairments	2.3
Malignant neoplasms	2.2

(US Department of Health, Education and Welfare publication No. HRA 77-1537. Limitation of Activity Due to Chronic Conditions, United States, 1974. National Center for Health Statistics, 1977)

postmortem analysis of 713 men in a hospital and home for the aged, found 80% to have between three and nine significant lesions.

Osteoarthritis is an outstanding example of a disease virtually universal in the elderly, which may contribute to mild or major disability. Lawrence and co-workers[31] found five or more joint groups involved in 37% of the males and 49% of the females over age 65. Changes in the knee[4] and in the lumbar and cervical spine[25,40] have been shown to increase with age in a predictable manner. In the spine the most marked changes occur in the regions of greatest mobility, the lower cervical and lumbar areas, and it seems reasonable to relate the progressive changes to use, a function, therefore, of time and aging. There is a variability with respect to the hip that points to other possible factors, although again the age relationship is clear (Fig. 6-1). Intermittent or recurrent pain related to osteoarthrosis is more common than is indicated in Table 6-1. In the majority of old persons it does not attain a level that makes for significant disability. The entirely distinct entities of rheumatoid arthritis and polymyalgia rheumatica are also strongly age related. These topics are discussed further in Section IV, Musculoskeletal Problems.

MORTALITY FORMULATIONS

In addition to the more or less inevitable appearance of impairments, intimations of mortality hover rather closely over this patient population.

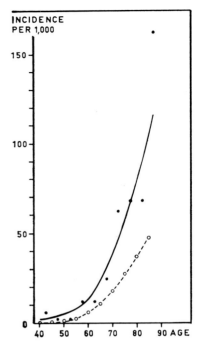

○ — — ○ Patients who have sought medical advice
● ———— ● Coxarthrosis found at examination of 3,903 colon roentgenographies

FIG. 6-1.   Incidence of primary coxarthrosis per 1,000 inhabitants in Malmö. (Danielsson LG: Incidence of osteoarthritis of the hip. Clin Orthop 45:67, 1966)

The syllogistic fact that all humans are mortal has been a propulsive force in theology, philosophy, and medicine and has even been made into a psychodynamic fundamental by Becker.[3] It is the sine qua non of actuaries and insurance companies who have compiled extensive life tables and dealt with the effects of medical impairments in detail.[57] The basic formulation for human mortality is that of Gompertz:[18]

$$q_x = q_o e^{ax}$$

expressed logarithmically as

$$\log q_x \text{ (mortality for age } x) = {}^a\log x$$

in which *a* is known as the Gompertz coefficient. For practical purposes the equation describes the common observation that mortality in a population rises exponentially with the passage of time: past age 30, mortality rates double approximately every 8.5 years.

The Gompertz equation has been subjected to

a great deal of discussion and modification. It has been pointed out that a fairly constant number of persons in a population die off at any age from the onslaught of accidents, intercurrent epidemics, and other causes not related to the aging process. This dropout led to the revision proposed by Makeham:[36]

$$q_x = q_o e^{ax} + A$$

in which *A* is known as Makeham's correction. Makeham's law defines the form of the mathematical function dealing with mortality and yields numerical measurements when appropriate values for the parameters are chosen. In its present form,

$$\mu x = A + Bc^x$$

the parameters are usually confined to the following:

$$.001 < A < .003$$
$$10^{-6} < B < 10^{-3}$$
$$1.08 < c < 1.12$$

Various other formulas have dealt with correction for neonatal and infant mortality, accidents in youth, and so on. Because these are not relevant to mortality in the aged, the original equations can be regarded as reasonable approximations.

Life Expectancy

The expectation of life has progressed steadily during the 20th century and in the United States in 1980 was 70.7 years for white males (up from 48.2 in 1900) and 78.1 (up from 51.0 in 1900) years for white females. This is the expectation at birth. The life span experienced rises as one gets older and thereby demonstrates successful coping with the force of mortality. For healthy older people life expectancy is often greater than some physicians believe; it can certainly be greater than is indicated in Table 6-2, which is a statistical compilation that covers the ill and feeble together with the well. The life expectations contained in the table are thus subject to questions of applicability in actual practice, in which the physician is likely to find patients with one, two, or more significant impairments. The life-span impact of most such impairments, singly or collectively, is still far from comprehensively understood. There is an absence of detailed studies, and the vast pooled experience of life insurance companies deals mostly with those under 65 and is thus barely relevant to our problem. For example, our present body of knowledge indicates that a severe dementia is far more

TABLE 6-2 Expected Remaining Years of Life at Beginning of Age Interval

Age	Males		Females	
	White	*Black*	*White*	*Black*
65	14.2	12.9	18.5	16.5
70	11.3	10.5	14.8	13.4
75	8.8	8.3	11.5	10.7
80	6.7	6.3	8.6	8.2
85 +	5.0	4.5	6.3	6.1

Vital Statistics of the US: 1980 Life Tables, vol 11, sec. 6, DHHS Publication No. (PHS) 84-1104. Washington, DC, US Government Printing Office, 1984)

likely to shorten the life span of an elderly man than most other infirmities.[17] This may be more likely in an institution than in the home so that environment as well as disorder have to be considered. The geriatrician generally has to rely on a scattered body of literature, some of which will be noted here, plus his own accumulation of clinical experience. In Table 6-3 the leading causes of death in the current decade are listed for the United States. To be noted is the preponderance of a few diseases. Atherosclerotic disease and malignancies, for example, are responsible for three fourths of the total mortality.

Changing Aspects of Morbidity

There have been rapid changes in morbidity and mortality over recent years, to an extent that were not foreseen even by demographers. An example discussed by Manton concerns the US Census Bureau forecast in 1972 that there would be 24 million Americans over age 65 by 1980.[35] When the census figures came in, the total turned out to be 25.6 million, a 1.6 million underestimate, thus a 6.6% error in the forecast. The decline in death rate far exceeded expectations. For example, the mortality from stroke declined by 6% per year over this period. In fact, the largest single favorable event over the past 30 years has been the 60% decline in stroke mortality. Over the same period, mortality from coronary artery disease declined 30%.[32] Marked changes are to be noted over relatively short periods. Thus in Table 6-4, the changes in mortality in males in the 65- to 74-year age-group for the decade 1968–1977 showed steep declines in pneumonia–influenza, ischemic heart disease, and stroke. In contrast, mortality from cancer has increased, as would be expected

TABLE 6-3   Deaths and Death Rates for 15 Leading Causes of Death in Age-Groups 65 and Over in Both Sexes in the United States in 1981

Rank Order	Cause of Death	Number	Rate (per 100,000)
	All causes	1,341,796	5,109.5
1	Diseases of heart	590,896	2,250.1
2	Cancer	264,464	1,007.1
3	Cerebrovascular diseases	140,205	533.9
4	Chronic obstructive pulmonary diseases	46,085	175.5
5	Pneumonia and influenza	45,035	171.5
6	Atherosclerosis	26,720	101.7
7	Diabetes mellitus	25,182	95.9
8	Accidents	23,743	90.4
	Motor vehicle accidents	5,879	22.4
	All other accidents	17,864	68.0
9	Nephritis and nephrosis	13,585	51.7
10	Cirrhosis of liver	9,709	37.0
11	Septicemia	7,542	28.7
12	Hypertension	6,089	23.2
13	Stomach ulcer	4,996	19.0
14	Suicide	4,478	17.1
15	Hernia	4,354	16.6
	All other causes	128,713	490.1

from a logarithmically age-related disorder for which current treatment often fails.

ATHEROSCLEROTIC DISEASE

The dominating disease the geriatrician must deal with, in the Western world at least, is atherosclerosis. In its three major categories of coronary, cerebral, and peripheral arterial disease it becomes virtually ubiquitous in an aged population. Thus, the sudden or unexpected cardiovascular catastrophe of the early and middle years becomes the almost commonplace event of the later years (Table 6-5). Although some recent clinical evidence and animal models indicate that the process may be interrupted or even partially reversed, the classic teaching still describes a pathologic process that starts early in life and becomes more widespread with the decades. Thus in Finland, a country with the highest incidence of myocardial infarction in Europe, studies of accident victims indicate that raised lesions both in the aorta and in the coronary arteries of males begin at ages 15 to 24. Onset of these lesions in the coronary arteries of females occurs about 10 years later. The deposition progresses steadily in ensuing decades (Fig. 6-2).[46]

Innumerable studies, monographs, and books have dealt with the problem of atherosclerosis. There has been a great deal of study of the influence of cigarette smoking and serum and dietary lipids. For some manifestations of the disease process, a specific factor seems to have greater weight. Thus, hypertension is of singular importance for the stroke problem, and cigarette smoking appears to be more important in the genesis of peripheral vascular and coronary artery disease than of brain infarction. Epidemiologic evidence delineates a multifactorial disease process of arteries with variable manifestations in different organ systems.[19]

Age and Risk Factors

The long-term study of the population of Framingham, Massachusetts, has been one of the important studies dealing with the variables involved

TABLE 6-4   Changing Mortality of Males Aged 65 to 74: 1968–1977

Cause of Death	1968	1977
Pneumonia–influenza	248.3	152.5
Cancer	1162.5	1289.3
Diabetes	126.1	101.4
Ischemic heart disease	2044.8	1510.1
Stroke	869.4	513.6
Chronic respiratory disease	131.2	137.6

(Data from Manton KM: Changing concepts of morbidity and mortality in the elderly population. Milbank Mem Fund Q 60:183, 1982)

TABLE 6-5 Percentage Probabilities of Having Cardiovascular Disease* within 8 Years According to Age and Risk Factors—Framingham Study: 18-Year Follow-Up

Age (yr)	Men			Women		
	Average Risk	Low Risk†	High Risk†	Average Risk	Low Risk†	High Risk†
35	1.8	0.6	60.2	0.5	0.4	19.5
40	4.1	1.2	70.8	1.2	0.7	28.4
45	7.5	2.2	77.8	2.5	1.3	38.0
50	11.5	3.7	81.9	4.8	2.2	47.0
55	15.9	5.5	84.1	8.0	3.4	54.7
60	19.3	7.4	84.8	11.9	5.1	60.6
65	21.2	9.0	84.0	16.0	7.0	64.9
70	22.9	10.0	81.7	19.9	9.0	67.5

* Cardiovascular disease = coronary heart disease, brain infarction, intermittent claudication or congestive heart failure.

† Low risk = systolic blood pressure of 105 mm Hg,, serum cholesterol of 185 mg/dl, nonsmoking, no glucose intolerance, no left ventricular hypertrophy by electrocardiogram; high risk = systolic blood pressure of 195 mm Hg, serum cholesterol of 335 mg/dl, cigarette smoking, glucose intolerance, left ventricular hypertrophy by electrocardiogram.

(Kannel WB: Some lessons in cardiovascular epidemiology from Framingham. Am J Cardiol 37:269, 1976)

in cardiovascular disease. As the study unfolded, developing concepts related to personality factors[14] and to high density lipids[7,37] served to reemphasize the multifactorial hypothesis. For the most part the Framingham variables have firmed with time. For example, highly positive correlations between coronary angiograms and these risk factors have been described by Sallel and co-workers.[53] Table 6-5 illustrates the predictive value of grouping various risk factors and how they yield clinical expectations of considerable validity. Aging in itself is an important, if not the most important, single risk factor, although it is of interest to note that a low-risk male of 70 has perhaps one-sixth the probability of cardiovascular disease over the ensuing 8 years as a high-risk male half his age. The potency of the age factor is clear as between the 35- to 40-year age-group and the 70-year olds. As Kannel summarizes it, "Age is still a potent factor, especially in low-risk persons, although having multiple risk attributes is equivalent to being considerably older than one's chronologic age."[26] This then becomes the epidemiologic confirmation of Osler's clinical observation early in the century that a man was as old as his arteries.

Of special clinical interest is not only the prevalence of these disorders but also the interrelationships between the broad categories of atherosclerotic disease. It is clear that elderly patients presenting with one of these clinical disorders are at high risk for the others. The combinations are not always clinically obvious, as in the patient with hemiplegia and aphasia of sudden onset, thereby unable to reveal that his stroke was brought on by a myocardial infarction with temporary hypotension. Although coronary artery disease tends to appear earliest, it is well to regard any patient with evidence of atherosclerosis at any site as carrying the clinical potential for episodes elsewhere (Fig. 6-3). For example, in the Framingham study, the relative risk of developing intermittent claudication in persons with coronary heart disease was four times the standard risk. Victims of angina proved to have three times the standard risk for intermittent claudication.

Coronary Artery Disease

Of the atherosclerotic diseases, that of coronary arteries is certainly the most important because it alone produces 35% of all deaths. In 1982 in the United States there were 555,000 deaths attributable to coronary artery disease, with approximately 52% due to acute myocardial infarction and 47% to chronic ischemic heart disease. The disease presents in a variety of acute and chronic manifestations. It is the chief cause of sudden unexpected death, but as an almost entirely different clinical disorder it produces decreasing cardiac output and failure in the older age group. As shown in Table 6-6, coronary artery mortality is strongly age-related, with the rates rising by at least 50% for each 5-year period past age 50 in both males and females. However, there has been a 30% decline over the past 30 years,[32] although the excess mortality of males continues to be marked. In the 35- to 64-year age-group, the male-to-female ratio is approximately 4:1. There are also striking worldwide variations in mortality. These are not ascribable to differences in reporting. Thus, in the 45- to 74-year age-group, the annual death rate per 100 thousand in 1972 was 886 for Finland, 830 for the United States, 707 for the United Kingdom, 552 for Sweden, 208 for France, and 180 for Spain.

Cerebrovascular Disease

Winter and co-workers[64] scored multiple sites of cerebral vessels by degree of luminal narrowing in females of different ages. Narrowing was greatest

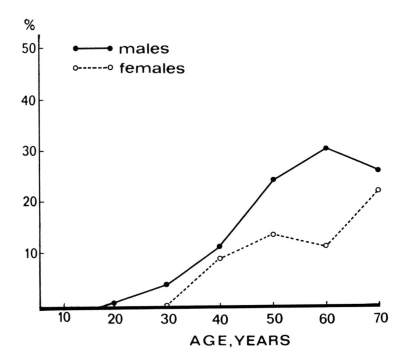

FIG. 6-2. Mean values for the percentage areas of raised lesions in all coronary arteries in accident victims (Finland). The age-related rise occurs earlier and is more marked in males until onset of the seventh decade. (Rissanen V, Pyörälä K: Aortic and coronary atherosclerosis in the Finnish population. Atherosclerosis 19:221, 1974)

in the middle cerebral and somewhat less marked in the anterior cerebral and internal carotid. In all the vessels a steep rise with age was noted after the fourth decade. Klassen and co-workers[29] have reported extensively on cerebral atherosclerosis and its relation to other atherosclerotic diseases in 3942 adult subjects at autopsy. The study was based on assigning numerical grades of 0 through 4 to the degree of luminal encroachment by lesions at each of 22 sites in the circle of Willis and its major branches. The scores were computed separately for hypertensive and nonhypertensive subjects. Age-related aspects are shown in Figure 6-3 and Figure 6-4. Thus, in Figure 6-3 it is clear that lesions of atherosclerotic heart disease rise with age and parallel those of cerebrovascular disease. The sex distinction is manifest in the early decades in which the figures are higher for males than for females. In the presence of atherosclerotic heart disease there was generally more marked cerebral atherosclerosis in both sexes (Figure 6-4). With or without hypertension, scores were somewhat lower when malignant neoplasm or peptic ulcer disease was present. But no matter what the cause of death listed clinically or pathologically, the strong age correlation existed. Diabetes mellitus was a notable aggravating factor, without, as well as with, hypertension (Fig. 6-5). The increased incidence of cerebral infarction in diabetics in this and other studies indicates that death owing to

cerebrovascular disease occurs in 5% to 7% of diabetic subjects. An increase in cerebral atherosclerosis presumably owing to the frequent occurrence of hypertension was found in patients with chronic renal disease.

In the Framingham study, risk of cerebral infarction was almost five times as great in persons with coronary heart disease; stroke within 6 months of a myocardial infarction was excluded, thereby omitting possible cases of embolus from a mural thrombus. Intermittent claudication was also associated with an increased incidence of strokes. It has also been shown that coronary attacks are more frequent in stroke victims than controls.[26] Still a further example of the interrelationships among cardiovascular events is the finding that transient ischemic attacks (TIAs) may be important harbingers for acute myocardial infarction. In two clinical outcome studies there were two and one-half to three times more deaths from myocardial infarction than brain infarction in patients who had experienced TIAs.[39,61]

Peripheral Vascular Disease

In the study of Singer and Rob,[56] 24% of patients with intermittent claudication had evidence of previous ischemic heart disease and over a 3-year follow-up period a further 24% of episodes of myocardial ischemia, half fatal, occurred. Of the

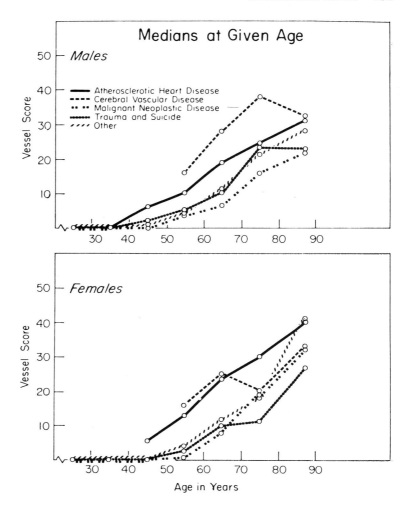

FIG. 6-3. Quantitative scoring of cerebral blood vessels for atherosclerosis as related to age and diagnosis. Higher scores noted with clinical or pathologic diagnosis of cerebrovascular and atherosclerotic heart disease, lower scores with neoplasms, trauma, and suicide. (Klassen AC, Loewenson RB, Resch JA: Cerebral atherosclerosis in selected chronic disease states. Atherosclerosis 18:321, 1973)

major cardiovascular events followed in the Framingham study, intermittent claudication ranked lowest, well behind coronary heart disease, brain infarction, and congestive heart failure. The course of intermittent claudication was quite benign.[28] Of

TABLE 6-6   Death Rates from Ischemic Heart Disease in the United States in 1981

Age	Rate
45–54	128.5
55–64	359.9
65–74	892.1
75–84	2,124.7
85 +	5,359.8

(National Center for Health Statistics, vol. 33, No. 3, supplement, June 1984)

1062 persons with intermittent claudication, essentially untreated until rest pain and tissue loss began, only four progressed to major amputations and three to toe loss. In Framingham, signs of coronary heart disease very often preceded intermittent claudication. Men with preceding uncomplicated angina had three times and women five times the risk of claudication compared with the risk in the congestive heart disease–free cohorts. In Tillgren's study,[59] 5 years after hospital observation only 36 of 294 patients with intermittent claudication attributed to atherosclerosis required amputations. The amputation rate of nondiabetics was quite low. In the Silbert and Zazeela study,[55] the risk of amputation in the diabetic appeared to be four times that of the nondiabetic. In Tillgren's study, myocardial infarction also was a common fate of those afflicted with intermittent claudication, with one in four developing an infarction

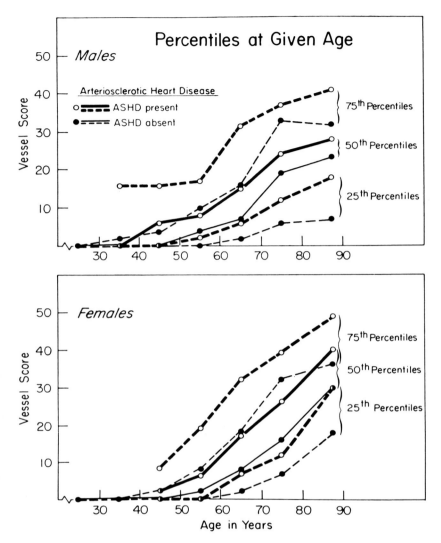

FIG. 6-4. The severity of cerebral atherosclerosis is greater in the presence of atherosclerotic heart disease at all decades. Note earlier onset in males and the steeper rate of rise in females past 50. (Klassen AC, Loewenson RB, Resch JA: Cerebral atherosclerosis in selected chronic disease states. Atherosclerosis 18:321, 1973)

during an average 5-year period of observation. The Framingham study found the risk for other cardiovascular disease significantly higher in those who developed intermittent claudication. Within 4 years, 25% had developed coronary heart disease, and 13% had developed brain infarctions. The overall death rate was 20% for the ensuing 5 years. Hence Peabody and co-workers[42] stated, "The conclusion seems inescapable that the major problem of a patient with intermittent claudication is his high risk for the other cardiovascular events, and attention to the ischemic limb is not enough."

CANCER

Cancer accounts for a fourth of all deaths and ranks second to cardiovascular-renal disease in the mortality of the aged. The age relationship has led some to relate the rising cancer incidence to a decreasing immunologic competence in the elderly. Clinical examples of its steep rise with age would include cancer of the colon, lung, stomach, skin, and others (Fig. 6-6). Of interest also are those cancers that deviate from the expected age-related rise. Thus Wilms' tumor, osteogenic sar-

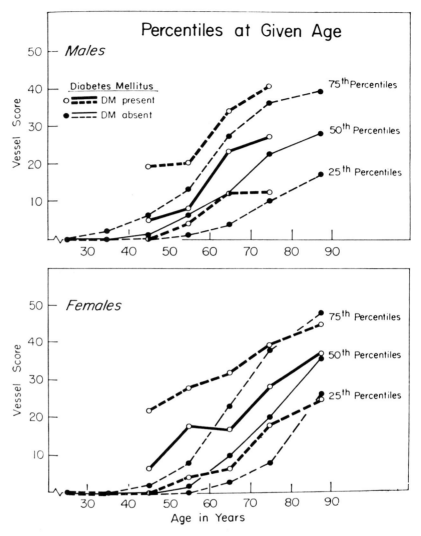

FIG. 6-5. The degree of severity of cerebral atherosclerosis is generally higher in diabetics in the different age-groups, but the difference is no longer apparent in the oldest females. (Klassen AC, Loewenson RB, Resch JA: Cerebral atherosclerosis in selected chronic disease states. Atherosclerosis 18:321, 1973)

coma, and neuroblastoma are characteristic of childhood. Carcinoma of the testis peaks sharply at around age 30 and declines rapidly thereafter. Other departures from an exponential relationship with aging are seen in such cancers as those of the cervix, which begin their rise in the third decade but do not increase in incidence after about 45 years of age.

Doll[12] ascribes peak incidences in childhood, adolescence, or early adult life to periods of heightened mitotic activity in the tissue or to a brief exposure to a carcinogenic agent. For the much

larger group in which progressive and often rapid increase occurs with age he suggests that the tissue may have to be regularly exposed to a carcinogenic agent over a long period of time. For those, Doll[12] and Cook and colleagues[9] proposed the equation

$$I = b(t - w)^K.$$

In this, I is the incidence of the cancer; t, the age of the subjects at risk; and w, the sum of the preexposure period; the length of time needed for the pathologic development of the tumor before clinical recognition, b, is proportional to the mean

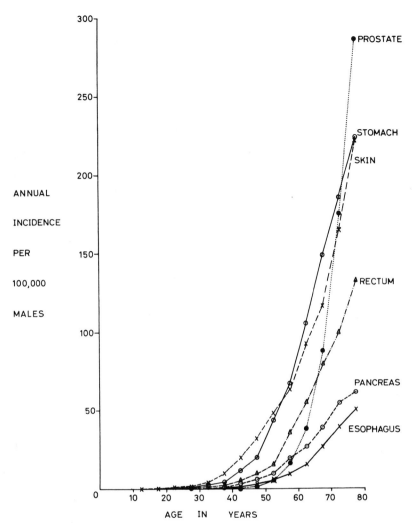

FIG. 6-6. Age-related incidence of various carcinomas illustrating the steep rise characteristic of the digestive tract and prostate. (Doll R: The Age Distribution of Cancer in Man, pp 15–36. Thule International Symposia—Cancer and Aging Symposium. Stockholm, Nordiska Bokhandelns Förlag, 1968)

daily dose of the agents; and *K* for many epithelial tumors is approximately 5. Doll explains unusually rapid increase in incidence with age, as is the case with cancer of the prostate, as being due to either a long pre-exposure period, a prolonged development time, or a reduction in the exposure of successive cohorts to environmental carcinogens. Similarly a break in the progressive increase with age followed by a slower rate of increase or a steady incidence, as in cancer of the breast and cervix, is ascribed to reduction in or complete cessation of exposure to carcinogenic agents. Table 6-7 indicates some common cancers in the US population and their age incidence.

Cancers in the aged may be both overt and unsuspected. In McKeown's series of 1500 autopsies of patients over age 70,[34] 302 deaths were due to cancer and a further 10% exhibited tumors that, although they did not contribute to death, were also often unsuspected clinically. In order of incidence the tumors were of the large bowel, stomach, lung, prostate, and bladder Table 6-8. Suen and co-workers[58] reported an autopsy study of 3535 cancer patients over 65, performed over the 10-year period 1960 to 1970. In this series by rank, lung was 18.1%; prostate, 16.5%; colon, 11.3%; stomach, 6.3%; rectum, 4.2%; breast, 4.2%; and uterus, 4.1%. Twenty-nine percent of the total

TABLE 6-7 Death Rates for Selected Cancers by 5-Year Age-Groups in the United States in 1981

Site of Disease	Age Group				
	65–69	*70–74*	*75–79*	*80–84*	*85+*
Lung	223.3	252.2	251.7	224.9	177.3
Prostate Total, male	76.2	146.4	252.5	406.8	605.1
Breast Total, female	100.6	109.0	119.4	137.7	171.9
Stomach	22.8	33.2	43.8	59.3	75.6
Colon	71.0	103.6	145.7	195.8	249.0
Rectum, sigmoid	13.7	19.6	25.9	36.0	53.9

(Vital Statistics, National Center for Health Statistics 44(3) [Suppl], June 1984)

number of cancers were not suspected in life and did not contribute to the death. Of these, 66% were in the prostate; of the remainder, 31.5% were found in the colon, 20.5% in the lung, and 16.6% in the breast. Their data suggest that there were fewer metastases in the very old and a slight falloff in incidence in the over 84-year age-group. That cancer may diminish in aggressiveness in the very old was also indicated in the study by Bussey,[6] who concluded, "Cancer of the large intestine is a disease the incidence of which rises throughout life and the malignancy of which diminishes with increasing age." Because colonic cancer has a better prognosis than cancer of the lung, mortality rates do not truly reflect incidence. Berge and coworkers[5] concluded the incidence of colorectal cancer was 56.8 per 100,000 in a defined population for which both surgical and postmortem figures were available. During life 18.7% were undiagnosed. The incidence rose sharply after the sixth decade (Fig. 6-7) and is to be contrasted to the 8.9% incidence for Japan, the 3.5% incidence for Uganda calculated by Burkitt, and the 51.8% incidence reported from Connecticut.

Some of the difficulty in diagnosing cancer in the older age-group is indicated in the series from Boston City Hospital.[2] One fourth of all their autopsies exhibited cancer, and 40% of the 2,734 patients had serious clinical errors in the diagnosis. Cancer was undiagnosed in 26% of all patients, in 45% of whom the neoplasms were fatal. In the Suen study, the number of unsuspected neoplasms rose with age-groups: 20.7% in the 66- to 75-year age-group, 29.4% in the 76- to 85-year age-group, and 36.2% in the 86 and over age-group. In this study, a fall-off in the percentage of cancer displaying metastases was also noted with rising age. Suen and co-workers suggested that this may reflect a lesser aggressiveness of neoplasia in old age but that a number of other explanations were

possible, for example, that elderly patients are frequently affected by intercurrent disease that becomes fatal before there is time for the development of metastatic cancer. Many of these clinical aspects of cancer in the elderly were considered in depth at a conference sponsored by the National Institutes of Health in 1982.[65]

PNEUMONIA AND INFLUENZA

The pneumonias occupied a special place in geriatric pathology, even before Osler dubbed them "Captain of the Men of Death." They have long been recognized as the most frequent terminal event in a variety of clinical sequences seen on all the services of the modern hospital. In many of these patients, it is difficult to determine whether pneumonia *per se* was the cause of death or whether it was a terminal event that was incidental rather than causal. In McKeown's series bronchopneumonia was found in 11% of all autopsies. It was adjudged the direct cause of death in 3.6% and a terminal or contributory factor in 7.4%. McKeown records it as occurring as a more frequent complication in heart failure, cerebrovascular disease, and urinary tract disorders. The incidence may well vary with different patient groupings and geriatric settings as different as the home, the general hospital, and the chronic care facility. In Lake's[30] study, 59.5% of 713 men over 70 years of age in a hospital and home for the aged had bronchopneumonia at autopsy.

In a study of consecutive autopsies at a chronic care facility, bronchopneumonia was believed to be the primary cause of death in 22.8% of all deaths.[50] The major associated disease in deaths from bronchopneumonia was chronic organic mental syndrome. This was accounted for by the fact that many of these patients have to be fed and

TABLE 6-8   Incidence of Malignant Disease (In 1500 Consecutive Autopsies, Age 70 and Over)

Site	Fatal Cases	Total Number
Large intestine	73	82
Stomach	37	54
Lung	37	41
Prostate	27	93 (including carcinoma *in situ*)
Bladder	19	24
Esophagus	18	18
Pancreas	14	14
Breast	10	12
Miscellaneous	67	112
Totals	302	450

(McKeown F: Pathology of the Aged, p 361. London, Butterworth & Co, 1965)

may aspirate. In others, the dementia may make it impossible for them to report early symptoms. The high correlation between organic mental syndromes and death by bronchopneumonia has been commented on by others.[63,43]

Pneumococcal pneumonia both in its classic lobar form and as patchy infiltrates has its greatest impact on mortality rates at the extremes of the life span, in infancy and in old age. The rising incidence in old age has been attributed to attenuation of defense mechanisms including declines in antibody levels. The precise attack rate in the elderly is not known because much pneumonia is treated without culture. It has been estimated that, in persons 50 years of age and older and in those with chronic underlying systemic illness, bacteremic pneumococcal pneumonia has a mortality of approximately 30% (R. Austrian). One reason for a high mortality in an era of antibiotics is the atypical course pneumonia may pursue in the elderly, as was emphasized by Zeman and Wallach.[66] In some elderly patients, the illness may develop almost without fever and with few symptomatic complaints. By the time the diagnosis is made in a previously weakened or bedridden patient, antibiotic administration may come too late. Also, as Zeman and Wallach pointed out, the course may be atypical as, for example, the cases of pneumonia that simulate a cerebrovascular accident. Immunization with a polyvalent antipneumococcal vaccine does reduce illness owing to pneumococcal infection in old age.[45] The geriatrician must therefore consider the possibility that more lives may be saved by antipneumococcal vaccines than by the currently accepted routine influenza vaccination.

For obvious reasons, mortality reports generally combine influenza with pneumonia. New influenza mutants have produced great pandemics with characteristicslly high mortality in the elderly, as was observed in the 1958–1959 pandemic due to Hong Kong A strain. The analysis of the excess mortality indicates the importance of certain background factors such as heart disease.[24] This has led to advocacy of routine influenza immunization on an annual basis for those over age 65. In recent years the dictum has been somewhat obscured by confusion over which clinical illnesses are in fact influenza and to troublesome forecasting and vaccine problems. Thus the 1976–1977 immunization debacle in the United States was due to failure of the anticipated swine flu (A New Jersey '76) to materialize plus a slight increase in Guillain-Barré syndrome post vaccination. Sabin[52] in reviewing this subject, indicated that many influenzalike illnesses were not influenza by serum typing. Sabin was of the opinion that the routine annual administration of influenza vaccine to the elderly would at best save few lives and was not indicated except in special pandemic years. In direct contrast, influenza surveillance facilities, such as the one in Houston, Texas, relying on actual viral isolates, found influenza to be epidemic in each respiratory season studied over the years 1974 to 1981.[16] Mortality from pneumonia–influenza peaked about 2 weeks following the peak in influenza; this did not occur in the absence of increased influenza. By far the highest mortality occurred in the age-group of 65 years and over. These epidemiologic studies amply justify the recommendation of the Centers for Disease Control: "The availability of a safe, inexpensive, and effective vaccine justifies the long-standing recommendation for annual vaccination of persons at high risk of dying from influenza and mandates the continuation of this policy."[22]

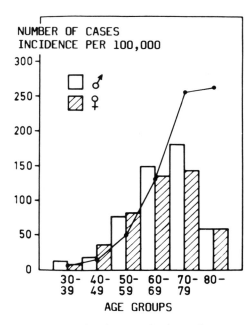

NUMBER OF CASES
INCIDENCE PER 100,000

FIG. 6-7. Age distribution of colorectal cancer cases from combined surgical and postmortem reports. The plotted curve shows that the incidence at least doubles for each of the decades from 40 up to 80. (Berge T, Ekelund G, Mellner C, Pihl B, Wenchert A: Carcinoma of the colon and rectum in a defined population. Acta Chir Scand [Suppl] 438, 1973)

PULMONARY EMBOLISM

In their review, Dalen and Alpert[10] estimated the total number of symptomatic episodes of pulmonary embolism per year in the US population to be 630,000, making it about half as common as acute myocardial infarction and three times as common as cerebrovascular accident. When one considers the large number of institutionalized or homebound elderly, many confined to wheelchair or bed, one would anticipate an increased incidence of thromboembolism. The figures reported in the vital statistics fail to reveal the anticipated high rate of such embolic phenomena. This is due to coding procedures for death certificates in which the antecedent cause (the condition that initiated a chain of consequences) is alone reported as cause of death. Thus, if an elderly patient dies of a pulmonary embolus following a fractured hip, a myocardial infarct, a stroke, or associated with congestive failure, the death will be coded under hip fracture or whatever disease process preceded the fatal thromboembolism. This leads to severe underreporting of pulmonary embolism as a cause of death.[49] In one instutitionalized elderly population the incidence of death owing to pulmonary em-

bolism was 6.4%.[50] This corresponds to the 6.8% noted by Moran in a custodial institution.[38] A figure of 14.2% was found by Towbin[62] in a custodial and psychiatric population in a state hospital. Towbin emphasized the age relatedness with the rate rising from 20% in the fifth decade to over 40% in the ninth.

Many such deaths are clinically indistinguishable from myocardial infarction, with many of them occurring within a few minutes or within an hour of the clinical event. In Gorham's study,[20] only 19% had evidence of venous thrombosis, and most of the cases were diagnosed as myocardial infarction. Similarly, Horowitz and Tatter[23], in reviewing 316 cases of fatal pulmonary embolism, found 22% diagnosed as myocardial infarct, 15 percent as cerebrovascular accident, and 14% as pneumonia. In McKeown's study,[34] 3.5% died directly of pulmonary embolism. The overall incidence was 14%, which she thought was an underestimate because small emboli are readily overlooked.

One must conclude that the age-related incidence of pulmonary embolism, the many known predisposing factors including congestive failure, immobility, known or unsuspected malignancy, and frequency of falls, all put the geriatric population at high risk for thromboembolism. Obviously, prophylactic measures are the solution of choice. This has been documented in studies using low dosage of heparin in various surgical procedures.[44] It seems not unreasonable to consider other procedures, perhaps prophylactic aspirin or other platelet inhibitors, as measures that may be applicable to a considerable number of older patients. For the present, the geriatrician must adopt the view that pulmonary embolism is the Damocles' sword that hangs over many of his patients. It should be thought of first with any nonambulatory or otherwise limited elderly person who exhibits increased dyspnea, cough, and tachycardia and in the differential diagnosis of pneumonia and myocardial infarctions.

ACCIDENTS

Mortality owing to accidents ranks eighth in the list presented in Table 6-3. As Rodstein[47] points out, 72% of all fatal falls, 30% of pedestrian fatalities, and 29% of deaths owing to burns and fires occurred in the population aged 65 and over. Neurologic deficits such as impairments of sight, hearing, smell, balancing reflexes, and reaction time contribute to the toll. The ability to perceive an oncoming automobile and to rapidly get out of harm's way is diminished. Comfort[8] regarded such abilities as parameters for an organism's coping behavior and points out that the curve for pedestrian fatalities rises steadily with age in the same manner as the Gompertz curve. Cardiovascular problems alone make an important contribution. Rodstein and Camus[48] analyzed 140 falls in aged persons and found 37 to be associated with acute changes in cardiac status, chiefly arrhythmias. Other contributory causes were diseases such as parkinsonism, hemiplegia, cancer, and acute events such as respiratory infection, gastrointestinal bleeding, and hypoglycemia. It would appear wise, therefore, to run through a differential diagnosis with the patient who has sustained a fall and not regard it as an inevitability owing to central nervous system changes as is postulated for drop attacks. The effect of drugs and of postural hypotension are often overlooked. Because of frailty and the latent threat owing to disorders such as osteoporosis, preventive measures are especially applicable. Such measures are evaluated in the paper of Rodstein[47] and include non-skid carpets, grab bars, hand rails, painted steps, hi-low beds, bed rails, safety lights, and anti-slip devices in bathtubs. The subject is discussed in further detail by Cape (see Chapter 41).

DIABETES MELLITUS

The incidence of diabetes in the general population is said to be 1% to 2%, but in the over 65 age-group the incidence is much higher but difficult to define (see Chapter 37). Mortality ascribable to diabetes other than coma and Kimmelstiel-Wilson syndrome is doubtless heavily underreported. It may appear instead as mortality owing to various cardiovascular disorders such as stroke (Fig. 6-5), myocardial infarction, and amputations, all of which are multiplied several times by the presence of diabetes. By still other pathways, such as blindness owing to retinopathy and locomotor incapacity due to neuropathy and myopathy, it makes its contribution to the accident mortality. Mild diabetes and chemical diabetes may not present any clinical problem in control and, hence, often go unmentioned in death certificates. Even the more severe grades of diabetes may not be entered as an antecedent or contributing cause of mortality. Tokuhata and coworkers[60] showed that the incidence of diabetes in Pennsylvania was eight times higher than one would gather from death certificates. They concluded, "Diabetes has a very poor visibility as a public health problem."

In the Framingham study, diabetes was estimated to produce a two- to threefold increase in clinical atherosclerotic disease. The relative impact was greatest for intermittent claudication and congestive heart failure.[27] Chemical diabetes, either undiagnosed in an aging patient or dismissed as unimportant, may still be associated with typical renal glomerular lesions or other metabolic disorders of significant impact. Hence, the full extent of cardiovascular mortality that should be attributed to diabetes, undiagnosed as well as diagnosed, remains moot.

PROSTATIC HYPERPLASIA

Benign prostatic hypertrophy was the subject of a symposium held at the National Institutes of Health in 1975.[51] The incidence and epidemiology of benign prostatic hypertrophy was there reviewed by Rotkin. Clinically significant benign prostatic hypertrophy is far from being a universal fate for the aging male. As judged by mortality figures, the risk level varies greatly in different countries. The low is the 1.2 per 100,000 mixed-sex population in the Philippines. It is 7.1 in Japan, and twice that level in the United States (14.4). Although the highest mortality appears for European nations, the geographic variability cannot be accounted for by inadequacies in reporting. The high rates reported for Iceland of 82.5 and for Germany of 75.1 are to be compared with the 31.3 for Sweden and 27.5 for England-Wales (Table 6-9). Thus the Icelandic mortality is triple that of England-Wales. There is a relative freedom from benign prostatic hypertrophy in the Orient, and, of interest, the same freedom extends to prostatic cancer.

All studies agree that age is the major risk factor for benign prostatic hypertrophy. The highest frequency occurs between 60 and 70 years of age. Blacks have an earlier onset by about 5 years. Because prostatic cancer is also strongly age-related (Fig 6-8),[33] the coincidence of both disorders in the same patient is predictable. However, the interrelationship between hyperplasia and neoplasia is still debated with exactly opposite conclusions reported in two prospective studies.[1,21] The possible influence of other factors such as diabetes, which seems to increase the incidence of benign prostatic hypertrophy, as against hypertension, cirrhosis, and coronary artery disease (all questionable) is discussed by Rotkin. Rotkin estimated that in the United States 75% of white and black males past age 70 have benign prostatic hypertrophy.

TABLE 6-9 BPH Mortality per 100,000 Mixed-Sex Population

Relative Incidence	Country	Mortality
Low	Philippines	1.2
	Taiwan	4.0
	Hong Kong	5.5
	Japan	7.1
Low-moderate	United States	14.4
	Poland	18.7
	Spain	19.6
	Canada	20.5
	N. Ireland	23.7
	Scotland	27.3
	England–Wales	27.5
	Greece	29.8
High-moderate	Sweden	31.3
	France	33.7
	Italy	42.4
	Ireland	42.9
High	Netherlands	50.5
	Denmark	53.1
	Rumania	55.9
	Germany	75.1
	Iceland	82.5

(Rotkin ID: Epidemiology of benign prostatic hypertrophy. In Grayhack JT, Wilson JD, Scherbenske MJ (eds): Benign Prostatic Hyperplasia. Department of Health, Education, and Welfare publication No. NIH 76–1113. Washington, DC, US Government Printing Office, 1976)

PREVENTIVE MEDICINE IN GERIATRICS

The two great achievements of medicine in the 20th century have been the virtual abolition of pediatric mortality and an unprecedented postponement of geriatric mortality. The latter is for the most part the result of a marked improvement in the toll of cardiovacular disease. The 60% decline in mortality from stroke from 1950 to 1980[32] was the serendipitous outcome of the introduction of orally active diuretics in 1958 and, subsequently, of other effective drugs. It serves as a striking example of the impact of preventive measures in geriatric medicine, in this instance prevention of stroke. Manton has discussed the implications of such advances for aging individuals and their society.[35] As an example, one could consider the consequences of the abolition of an otherwise fatal stroke on the life span (Table 6-10). As can be seen, a man who might have died of a cerebrovascular accident at age 75 acquires on average another 6.18 years of life. Similar calculations can

be made for ischemic heart disease, chronic obstructive pulmonary disease, and other clinically important entities. The marked decline in mortality from cardiovacular disease has had financially draining repercussions on the Social Security system and other actuarily based retirement systems. It has also fueled more active thinking about the consequences of geriatric preventive medicine.

It is apparent from the mortality figures of Table 6-4 that further significant advances can be contemplated. Thus mortality from chronic obstructive pulmonary disease, chiefly the result of bronchitis and emphysema, could be virtually abolished with cessation of cigarette smoking. A similar improvement could occur for cirrhosis of the liver with control of alchoholism. The identification of the risk factors for ischemic heart disease, not to mention coronary artery surgery and advances in medical therapy, is likely to yield further improvement, albeit at a slower rate. Other promising areas are enhanced use of pneumococcus vaccination, expansion of influenza vaccination, and continued prophylactic emphasis on antithrombotic measures for the geriatric patient in medical or surgical contexts where thromboembolism poses increased risk.

Even in the statistically unyielding area of cancer mortality, improvement should be anticipated. Lung cancer, to the extent that it is attributable to cigarette smoking, is a preventable disease. Conceivably even nonspecific measures such as the administration of carotenoids or similar substances may have some favorable influence on cancer incidence and mortality. Technical advances such as made colonoscopy possible will doubtless further improve the cancer mortality picture.

The outcome of these advances has led to two quite opposed scenarios: One, argued for by Fries and Crapo,[15] pictures an increasingly older population still in relative good health as symbolized by "the little old lady in jogging shoes." An important feature of this scenario is the possibility of practical modification of rate of progression of disease. For example, there seems to be enough clinical and epidemiologic data to suggest that although the human species is vulnerable to atherosclerosis, slowing down its rate could keep the disorder from clinical manifestations over the course of the genetically decreed life span (see Table 6-10). Old subjects would thus die from noncardiovascular causes because of only modest life-time accumulations of atherosclerosis. Another opposing viewpoint is that enunciated by Schneider and Brody:[54] even with the abolition of one or many major categories of illnesses, chronic

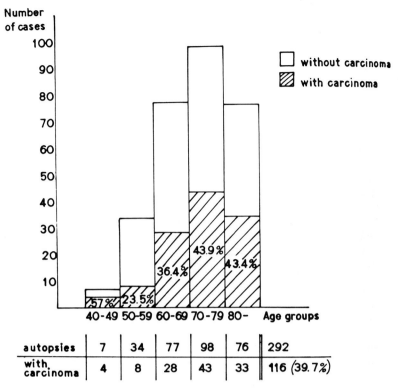

FIG. 6-8. Age-related rise in prostatic carcinoma searched for at routine autopsies. The incidence exceeds 43% in the later decades. (Lundberg S, Berge T: Prostatic carcinoma. Scand J Urol Nephrol 4:93, 1970)

disease and frailty would continue to produce an increasing toll in the elderly. As an example, avoidance of death at 75 from a cerebrovascular accident, in the hypothetical male of Table 6-10 would not enable him to escape frailty, progressive osteoarthritic impairment, or Alzheimer's disease later in life and wind up with long-term impairments sufficient to warrant admission to a nursing facility. This, of course, is in sharp contrast to the Fries and Crapo vision of a long life span quite free of serious disease, with a relatively brief terminal phase symbolized by sudden collapse. In geriatric medicine, unfortunately, abolition of one category of disease may increase the probability of acquiring an illness in another category. Thus, since the incidence of Alzheimer's disease in the 80-year age-group is on the order of 4% per year, abolition of cardiovascular and cancer mortality will predictably increase the prevalence of dementia in an aging population. This does not negate the value of our successes so much as it underlines the continuity of the challenges to preventive geriatric medicine.

TABLE 6-10 Alternate Estimates of Life-Expectancy Changes in US Males in 1969*

Years Delay	Population	Individual
1	0.08	0.54
5	0.34	2.33
10	0.57	3.94
15	0.71	4.94
Eliminated	0.89	6.18

*Effect of postponement or elimination of stroke in 75-year-old US males. Elimination of the disease leads to almost 6.2 years of additional life for the individual and to a 0.89-year extension of life expectancy for the population.

(Data from Manton KM: Changing concepts of morbidity and mortality in the elderly population. Milbank Mem Fund Q 60:183, 1982)

CONCLUSION

It is clear that morbidity is widespread in the geriatric population but is not necessarily a cause of major disability. The common diseases of old age are remarkable for the narrowness of their number and their widespread, sometimes universal, occurrence. Equally noteworthy are the stealthiness and atypism of their presentation, although again the range of presentation may be strikingly narrow. Thus a myocardial infarction, gastrointestinal bleeding, an arrhythmia, a pulmonary embolism, and a febrile infection may all present as an acute confusional state (see Chapters 11, 14, and 26). In clinical geriatrics, Sherrington's "final common path" is the cerebral cortex, rather than the neurons of the anterior horn.

Many of the impaired, as well as the healthy, elderly have a stronger love of life than the youthful who attend them would anticipate. Life-span considerations continue to play an important but even more complex role with the geriatric group. Morbidity and mortality considerations become ponderous and complicate decision making. Thus it may be sound clinical judgment to recommend against procedures that would be mandated in younger persons be they a cholecystectomy, coronary angiography, or a vascular bypass. Another example of age as a turning point in clinical decisions is illustrated in the paper of Emerson and associates.[13] These authors compared the risk of pulmonary embolism in myocardial infarction patients under and over age 70 plus other factors in a prospective study of 98 patients (see Table 6-11). Age was the gravest risk factor. The incidence of deep vein thrombosis was 12.5% under 50 and 71% over 70. Oddly, in the 50- to 70-year age-group, smokers without a history of thromboembolism or varicosities had a markedly lessened risk than nonsmokers. From this and a consideration of the probability of fatal bleeding with heparin therapy (5 per 1000 under 70; 2 per 100 over 70)

they conclude that heparin should be given routinely to those over 70 with a myocardial infarction who enter a coronary care unit.

Anomalous situations may arise in which one must ponder the rate of growth of a malignancy as one variable and the host's life-span expectations as another. Some tumors grow so slowly in the very old that one may anticipate no significant shortening of the life span and, hence, may not treat. In other instances a judicious decision may elect palliation by irradiation rather than cure by surgery. A significant immediate mortality and morbidity ascribable to anesthesia and surgery are avoided by conservatism.

Although medical judgment has historically been dominated by experience with the young and the middle-aged, there has been a growing trend to an egalitarian assessment of the elderly. While at one time the elderly were deemed too old for renal dialysis or cardiac surgery, the reevaluation is based on not denying the elderly either the quantitative or qualitative life benefits of our new technology, even if the benefits are measured in months rather than years or decades. There are many pros and cons derived from such antithetic foundations as humanistic ethics and cost-effectiveness. As in all emergent areas, nothing has been codified, and individual judgment remains dominant. Chronic brain syndrome, especially if advanced, is deemed by many to be a major contraindication in clinical assessment and treatment. However, in most other circumstances a familiarity with life-span data can be used in the patient's behalf and be tempered by the foreknowledge that actuarial data are only useful abstractions in the treatment of any individual patient.

TABLE 6-11   Probabilities of Deep-Vein Thrombosis (DVT) Complicating Myocardial Infarction

| | Age Less Than 50 Years | Age 50-70 Years | | | Age More Than 70 Years |
| | | Varicose Veins or Previous Thromboembolism | No Varicose Veins or Previous Thromboembolism | | |
			Non Smokers	Smokers	
No DVT	7	5	13	31	6
DVT	1	4	9	7	15
Incidence	12.5%	44%	41%	17.5%	71%

(Emerson PA, Teather D, Handley AJ: The application of decision theory to the prevention of deep-vein thrombosis following myocardial infarction. Q J Med, 43:389, 1974)

REFERENCES

1. Armenian HK, Lillienfeld AM, Diamond EL, Bross IDJ: Relation between benign prostatic hyperplasia and cancer of the prostate—a prospective and retrospective study. Lancet 2:115, 1974

2. Bauer FW, Robbins SL: An autopsy study of cancer patients: I: Accuracy of the clinical diagnosis (1955 to 1965, Boston City Hospital). JAMA 221:1471, 1972

3. Becker E: The Denial of Death, p. 315. New York, The Free Press, 1973

4. Bennett GA, Waine, H, Bauer W: Changes in the Knee Joint at Various Ages With Particular Reference to the Nature and Development of Degenerative Joint Disease. New York, The Commonwealth Fund, 1942

5. Berge T, Ekelund G, Mellner C, Pihl B, Wenckert A: Carcinoma of the colon and rectum in a defined population. Acta Chir Scand Suppl. 438, 1973

6. Bussey HJR: Age and Cancer of the Large Intestine. Thule International Symposia—Cancer and Aging Symposium, pp 203–214. Stockholm, Nordiska Bokhandelns Förlag, 1968

7. Castelli WP, Doyle JT, Gordon T, Hames, CG, Hjortland MC, Hulley SB, Kagan A, Zukel WJ: HDL cholesterol and other lipids in coronary heart disease. Circulation 55:767, 1977

8. Comfort A: The biological approach in the comparative study of aging. In Ciba Foundation Colloquia on Aging, vol. 3, p 202. Boston, Little, Brown & Co, 1957

9. Cook PJ, Doll R, Fellingham SA: A mathematical model for the age distribution of cancer in man. Int J Cancer 4:93, 1969

10. Dalen JE, Alpert JS: Natural history of pulmonary embolism. Prog. Cardiovasc Dis, 17:259, 1975

11. Danielsson LG: Incidence of osteoarthritis of the hip. Clin Orthop 45:67, 1966

12. Doll R: The age distribution of cancer in man. Thule International Symposia—Cancer and Aging Symposium, pp 15–36. Stockholm, Nordiska Bokhandelns Folag, 1968

13. Emerson PA, Teather D, Handley AJ: The application of decision theory to the prevention of deep-vein thrombosis following myocardial infarction. QJ Med 43:389, 1974

14. Friedman M, Rosenman RH: Type A Behavior and Your Heart, p. 276. New York, Alfred A Knopf, 1974

15. Fries JF, Crapo LM: Vitality and Aging, p 172. San Francisco, WH Freeman, 1981

16. Glezen WP: Serious morbidity and mortality associated with influenza epidemics. Epidemiol Rev 4:25, 1982

17. Goldfarb AI: Predictors of mortality in the institutionalized aged. In Palmore E, Jeffers FC (eds): Prediction of Life Span, pp 79–93. Lexington, MA, DC Heath & Co, 1971

18. Gompertz B: On the Nature of the Function Expressive of the Law of Human Mortality and on a New Mode of Determining the Value of Life Contingencies. Phil Trans R Soc 115:513, 1825

19. Gordon T, Kannel WB: Multiple risk functions for predicting coronary heart disease: The concept, accuracy and application. Am Heart J 103:1031, 1983

20. Gorham LW: A study of pulmonary embolism. Arch Intern Med 108:8, 1961

21. Greenwald P, Kirmss V, Polan AK, Dick VS: Cancer of the prostate among men with benign prostatic hyperplasia. J Natl Cancer Inst 53:335, 1974

22. Gregg MB, Bregman DJ, OBrien RJ, Millar JD: Influenza-related mortality. JAMA 239:115, 1978

23. Horowitz RE, Tatter D: Lethal pulmonary embolism. In Sherry S (ed): Thrombosis, pp 19–28. Washington, DC, National Academy of Sciences, 1969

24. Houswirth J, Langmuir AD: Excess mortality from epidemic influenza 1957–1966. Am J Epidemiol 100:40, 1974

25. Howells WW: Age and individuality in vertebral lipping: Notes on Stewarts' data. Mexico DF, Homenaje a Juan Comas 2:169, 1965

26. Kannel WB: Some lessons in cardiovascular epidemiology from Framingham. Am J Cardiol 37:269, 1976

27. Kannel WB, McGee DL: Diabetes and cardiovascular disease. JAMA 241:2035, 1979

28. Kannel WB, Shurtleff D: The natural history of arteriosclerosis obliterans. Cardiovasc Clin 3:38, 1971

29. Klassen AC, Loewenson RB, Resch JA: Cerebral atherosclerosis in selected chronic disease states. Atherosclerosis 18:321, 1973

30. Lake B: Morbid conditions at death in old men. J Chronic Dis 21:761, 1969

31. Lawrence JS, Bremner JM, Bier F: Osteoarthritis—prevalence in the population and relationship between symptoms and x-ray changes. An Rheum Dis 25:1, 1966

32. Levy RL, Moskowitz J: Cardiovascular research: Decades of progress, a decade of promise. Science 217:121, 1982

33. Lundberg S, Berge T: Prostatic carcinoma. Scand J Urol Nephrol 4:93, 1970

34. McKeown F: Pathology of the Aged, p 361. London, Butterworth & Co, 1965

35. Manton KM: Changing concepts of morbidity and mortality in the elderly population. Milbank Mem Fund Q 60:183, 1982

36. Makeham WM: On the law of mortality. J Inst Actuaries 13:325, 1867

37. Miller NE, Førde OH, Thelle DS, Mjøs OD: The Tromsø heart study: High-density lipoprotein and coronary artery disease: A prospective case-control study. Lancet 1:965, 1977

38. Moran TJ: Pulmonary embolism in nonsurgical patients with prostatic thrombosis. Am J Clin Pathol 17:205, 1947

39. Muuronen A, Kaste M: Outcome of 314 patients with transient ischemic attacks. Stroke 13:24, 1982

40. Nathan H: Osteophytes of the vertebral column. J Bone Joint Surg Am 44A:243, 1962

41. National Institute on Aging Task Force: Our Future Selves. U.S. Department of Health, Education and Welfare publication No. (NIH) 78-1445. Washington, DC, US Government Printing Office, 1978

42. Peabody CN, Kannel WB, McNamara PM: Intermittent claudication—surgical significance. Arch Surg 109:693, 1974

43. Peck A, Wolloch L, Rodstein M: Mortality of the aged with chronic brain syndrome. J Am Geriatr Soc 21:264, 1973

44. Prevention of fatal postoperative pulmonary embolism by low doses of heparin: An international multicentre trial. Lancet 2:45, 1975

45. Riley ID, Andrews M, Howard R, Tarr PI, Pfeiffer M, Challands P, Jennison G, Douglas RM: Immunization with a polyvalent pneumococcal vaccine. Lancet 1:1338, 1977

46. Rissanen V, Pyörälä K: Aortic and coronary atherosclerosis in the Finnish population. Atherosclerosis 19:221, 1974

47. Rodstein M: Accidents among the aged: Incidence, causes, and prevention. J Chronic Dis 17:515, 1964

48. Rodstein M, Camus AS: Interrelation of heart disease and accidents. Geriatrics 28:87, 1973

49. Rossman I: True incidence of pulmonary embolization and vital statistics. JAMA 230:1677, 1974

50. Rossman I, Rodstein M, Bornstein A: Undiagnosed diseases in an aging population. Arch Intern Med 33:366, 1974

51. Rotkin ID: Epidemiology of benign prostatic hypertrophy. Grayhack JT, Wilson JD, Scherbenske MJ (eds): Benign Prostatic Hyperplasia, pp 105–117. Department of Health, Education and Welfare, Publication No. NIH 76-1113. Washington, DC, US Government Printing Office, 1976

52. Sabin AB: Mortality from pneumonia and risk conditions during influenza epidemics. JAMA 237: 2823, 1977

53. Salel AE, Fong A, Zellis R, Miller RM, Borhani NO, Mason DT: Accuracy of numerical coronary profile correlation of risk factors with arteriographically documented severity of atherosclerosis. N Engl J Med 296:1447, 1977

54. Schneider EI, Brody JA: Aging, natural death and the compression of morbidity: Another view. N Engl J Med 309: 854, 1983

55. Silbert S, Zazeela H: Prognosis in arteriosclerotic peripheral vascular disease. JAMA 166:1816, 1958

56. Singer A, Rob C: The fate of the claudicator. Br Med J 2:633, 1960

57. Singer RB, Levinson L (eds): Medical Risks: Patterns of Mortality and Survival. Lexington, MA, DC Heath & Co, 1976

58. Suen KC, Lau LL, Yermakov V: Cancer and old age—an autopsy study of 3,535 patients over 65 years old. Cancer 33:1164, 1974

59. Tillgren C: Obliterative arterial disease of the lower limbs: II. A study of the cause of disease. Acta Med Scand 178:103, 1965

60. Tokuhata GK, Miller W, Digon E, Hartman T: Diabetes mellitus: An underestimated public health problem. J Chronic Dis 28:23, 1975

61. Toole JF, Yuson CP, Janeway R et al. Transient ischemic attacks: A prospective study of 225 patients. Neurology 28:746, 1978

62. Towbin A: Pulmonary embolism—incidence and significance. JAMA 156:209, 1954

63. Varsamis J, Zuchowski T, Maini KK: Survival rates and causes of death in geriatric psychiatric patients. Can Psychiatr Assoc J 17:17, 1972

64. Winter MD Jr, Sayre GP, Millkan CH, Barker NW: Relationship of degree of atherosclerosis of internal carotid system in the brain of women to age and coronary atherosclerosis. Circulation 18:7, 1958

65. Yancik R (ed): Perspectives on Prevention and Treatment of Cancer in the Elderly. New York, Raven Press, 1983

66. Zeman FD, Wallach K: Pneumonia in the aged. Arch Intern Med 77:678, 1946

7   Principles of Drug Treatment in the Aged

S. George Carruthers

SPECIAL PROBLEMS

Although the use of medications in patients of all ages requires careful consideration, drug therapy in the elderly demands special attention for the following reasons:

Social isolation, bereavement, and mental changes associated with aging increase the likelihood that older patients will receive mood-altering and other psychotropic medications.

It is common for the elderly, and especially the very aged, to suffer from at least one physical disease in which drug treatment may be beneficial.

The elderly are much more likely to have multiple concurrent disease states and receive multiple treatments, so that the risks of adverse drug reactions and drug interactions are increased.

"Normal" changes in weight, body composition, renal function, and hepatic function tend to alter the disposition of drugs in the elderly, and these changes may be further enhanced by actual disease in the organs responsible for drug elimination.

Age-related changes in receptors, tissue responsiveness, and homeostatic control mechanisms may predispose the elderly to altered effectiveness of drug treatment or altered predisposition to adverse effects.

Because they expect to experience medical problems associated with their advancing age, older patients may be reluctant to question the possibility that medications are responsible for some of their problems.

Likewise, since physicians by training and experience have an inherent expectation for older patients to suffer from medical problems associated with aging, they, too, may be unwilling to blame medications for some of the health problems of the elderly, especially if the adverse effects are subtle or differ from the usual adverse effects in younger patients.

Failure to evaluate the elderly patient adequately, to provide appropriate drug and nondrug therapy, and to continue to assess the patient's response in terms of benefit or adverse effects may cause deterioration in organ function or unmask preexisting disease[21] and may even lead to the development of an "illness-medication spiral."[9] With larger numbers of medications, the elderly patient is at increased risk of an adverse reaction to individual drugs and of interaction of two or more drugs. The resulting loss of therapeutic benefit or the development of new "disease" may not be interpreted appropriately, with the result that further medications are prescribed, often in addition to existing therapy. It is easy to see how the original disease may become obscured by the development of additional symptoms and signs (Table 7-1).

It has become fashionable in reviewing drug therapy in the elderly to focus almost exclusively on the specific aspects of pharmacokinetics and pharmacodynamics. Although many of the most important recent developments in the knowledge of drugs at both extremes of life have been made in these areas and will be discussed later, it is imperative that both topics are kept in perspective. It is crucial that the general aspects of health care delivery in the elderly should not be neglected,[8] since treatment with drugs is only one aspect of the care provided. Integration of the therapeutic activities of family physicians, internist–geriatricians, psychogeriatricians, public health nurses,

114

TABLE 7-1 Drug–drug Interactions in Which Pharmacologic Effects Are Additive

Interacting Drugs		Effects
β-blockers	+ Verapamil Quinidine Disopyramide	Atrio-ventricular dissociation and Cardiac decompensation
Diuretics	+ Corticosteroids	Hypokalemia
Potassium-sparing diuretics	+ Potassium salts	Hyperkalemia
Metoclopramide	+ Phenothiazines	Extrapyramidal movement disorders
Tricyclic antidepressants	+ Disopyramide Antihistamines	Anticholinergic effects of urine retention, constipation, and glaucoma
Levodopa	+ Tricyclic antidepressants	Hypertension

social workers, and others involved in the complex management of the elderly patient is paramount. The elderly patient or his relatives may be excused if they do not review each aspect of the patient's condition at each encounter with a health professional. One clinician must accept ultimate responsibility for the assimilation of the data base generated by the others to avoid delays in appropriate initiation or discontinuation of medication. Sometimes, when the situation becomes unclear, the responsible clinician may have little choice but to review each diagnosis in a critical manner and undertake a major revision of drug therapy.

EXTENT OF DRUG USE

Skoll and associates[49] reviewed the prescription of drugs for the elderly in Saskatchewan during 1976. One year earlier, the Saskatchewan Prescription Drug Plan had begun providing universal benefits to an eligible population of almost 1 million patients of whom 11% were 65 years of age or older at that time. These investigators found that 77.3% of this elderly populace had received at least one prescription drug from the Saskatchewan Formulary. Compared with a middle-aged group of individuals between the ages of 35 and 54 years, the elderly received a higher average number of prescriptions and medications. All subgroups of the elderly (65–74, 75–84, 85 +) received more prescriptions for anti-infective, autonomic, cardiovascular, central nervous system, diuretic, hormone, and skin and mucous membrane preparations than their "middle aged" counterparts. Greatest differences were observed for autonomic (2.2 times), cardiovascular (5.7 times), central nervous system (1.9 times), and diuretic groups of medications (6.4 times). The numbers in parentheses refer to the relative frequency of use of individual groups of medications. Despite its known risk of causing depression, reserpine was prescribed 9.6 times as often for all patients over 65 as for younger hypertensives and the very elderly (greater than 75 years of age) received an alarming 11.8 times as many prescriptions for reserpine! Patients 85 years of age and older were 14.5 times as likely to receive thioridazine and 24.1 times as likely to receive chloral hydrate prescriptions as younger individuals.

A more detailed evaluation of psychoactive drug prescribing for the chronically ill elderly was undertaken by Achong and colleagues in Hamilton, Ontario.[1] Their survey of drug therapy in 1431 ill elderly patients showed that psychoactive drugs had been prescribed for about one fourth of the patients. They express concern about the prolonged use of benzodiazepines and chloral hydrate, despite evidence that these drugs may become ineffective in improving sleep after extended use and may contribute to considerable adverse effects in the elderly.[4]

More recent experience in another Canadian province has been described by Aoki and colleagues who reviewed relatively heavy drug use (more than $50 worth of prescription drugs per year) in Manitoba in 1978.[2] Of 117,000 Manitobans over the age of 65 at that time, 6.5% received 12 or more prescription drugs, a probable underestimate since residents of hospitals or other institutions were not included in their survey.

A British study conducted by Law and Chalmers[37] found that 87% of 151 patients aged 75 years and over were on regular medications and that 44% of patients within this age-group consumed three or more medications daily while 20% consumed three or more medications on an occasional basis. The major prescription drugs in this particular study, which was conducted in a family practice setting in London, were psychotropic, cardiovascular, analgesic, genitourinary,

and metabolic agents. Over-the-counter preparations, particularly analgesics and laxatives, were
frequently used and were also hoarded by elderly
patients for intermittent use.

Segal and Bornstein[47] conducted a survey of
drug use in long-term health care facilities in metropolitan Toronto. They monitored intensively the
drug use of a 1% sample of 12,168 residents. Three
fourths of the patients studied were female and
one fourth were male. The average age was 82
years. The average number of diagnoses was 3.3,
with a range from none to 8. Almost a fourth of
the residents had five or more diagnosed ailments.
The top five diagnostic groupings were cardiovascular diseases (85%), psychiatric disturbances
(48%), musculoskeletal disorders (46%), disorders
of the eyes and ears requiring medications (23%),
and hormonal disorders (18%).

The range of drugs prescribed simultaneously
for each resident ranged from none to 19, with an
average figure of 6.6 prescribed drugs per resident
per day or two medications for each diagnosed
disease. Sixty-one percent of medications were
prescription drugs, while 39% were over-the-
counter drugs. Fifty-six percent of the medications
were prescribed on a regular basis, and 44% on
an as needed basis. The cost of the medications
involved for each resident averaged $34.20 per
month. The wasted costs from drug surplus
amounted to an average of $1.79 per patient per
month.

Segal and Bornstein[47] also examined potential
drug–drug interactions. They found that potential
interactions with digitalis preparations accounted
for over half of those documented (digitalis with
potassium-depleting diuretics, 31.4%; digitalis
with antacids, 21.4%). Other potential interactions
were relatively uncommon but included two cases
of potential interaction with alcohol (an antihistamine in one case and acetylsalicylic acid in the
other). The high use of digitalis preparations was
consistent with the 85% incidence of cardiovascular disease diagnosed in the study population.
The well-known but sometimes subtle adverse effects of digoxin, especially in the elderly, and increasing evidence that many patients on digoxin
either suffer from subtle adverse effects[26] or derive
little benefit from it[30] make the continued widespread use of digoxin in the elderly a problem that
deserves further attention.

COMPLICATIONS

As indicated previously, the consequences of such
heavy drug use cannot be ignored. A survey conducted in hospitals in Belfast disclosed an overall
incidence of drug reactions of 10.2% in the 1160
patients studied who were receiving drug therapy.[29] The incidence of reactions was 15.4% in
those over the age of 60 years compared with 6.3%
in those under this age (Fig. 7-1). Adverse reactions to drugs were responsible for admission to

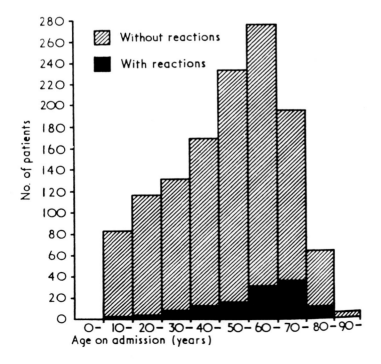

FIG. 7-1.   Incidence of adverse drug reactions in 1160 patients studied after admission to hospital. The incidence rises
with age. (Hurwitz N, Wade OL: Intensive hospital monitoring of adverse reactions to drugs. Br Med J 1:531, 1969)

hospital of 2.9% of patients, and the median age of these patients was 60 years.[28]

Another study of almost 2000 consecutive admissions to British geriatric units revealed that 248 adverse reactions were recorded in 1625 patients taking medications at the time of hospitalization, and 209 of these adverse effects were considered serious enough to be a major cause for the patient's admission to hospital. Drugs contributing to morbidity were antihypertensives, antiparkinsonian agents, digoxin, and various psychotropic drugs.[56] The authors of this report, Williamson and Chopin, agree with Hurwitz[28] that the number of prescribed drugs was an important predictor of the frequency and severity of adverse effects.

It should not be surprising that the admission of many elderly patients is precipitated by drug treatment and that complications of treatment often arise during the course of the patient's stay in hospital. Such problems arise particularly in elderly patients being treated for congestive cardiac failure, diabetes mellitus, arthritis, and mental disturbances, notably the high prevalence disorders in the studies by Skoll and colleagues,[49] Law and Chalmers,[37] Aoki and associates,[2] and Segal.[47] One must wonder if these diagnoses have been reached in a critical manner, with an adequate data base, or if the predominant symptoms in a particular patient (*e.g.*, lethargy, tiredness, weakness, dyspnea, cough, dyspepsia, aches and pains) have swayed the physician toward a more serious organic diagnosis (rather than a temporary functional disorder) simply because the patient was an older individual. There appears to be an unfortunate tendency to prescribe drug therapy in the elderly before a comprehensive data base is developed. Perhaps this is true for all age-groups, but the elderly are more likely to suffer for the reasons stated earlier.

Preexisting dementia (often unrecognized), defective hearing and vision, and parkinsonism are predisposing factors in the development of confusional states, which may be precipitated by pneumonia, cardiac failure, urinary infection, carcinomatosis, and metabolic disturbances such as hypokalemia.[25] To this list must be added the consequences of the very medications that may then be used to control the overt psychological disturbances experienced by the elderly patient! A study of drug use in the elderly in Houston concluded that potential interactions between psychotropic drugs represented a considerable hazard for older patients.[3] The World Health Organization[57] has reported the concerns of an advisory panel on the issues of polypharmacy and the apparently excessive use of psychotropic drugs.

PHARMACOKINETICS

Pharmacokinetics is the science of drug disposition in the body. In brief, pharmacokinetics is the study of what the body does to a drug. It defines in both physiologic terms and in mathematical models how drugs are absorbed, distributed, metabolized, and excreted from the body. Descriptive terms include the nature, extent, and rate of drug absorption, apparent volume of distribution, distribution compartments, intercompartmental rate constants, elimination rate constant, elimination half-life, and total body clearance.[12,23,39]

Absorption

Although there are theoretic concerns about alterations in drug absorption in older individuals because of changes in intestinal mucosa, blood flow, and motility, there is no convincing evidence that changes in absorption actually occur. Presumably, this reflects the enormous reserve of the gastrointestinal mucosa.

Following their absorption, all drugs pass in the portal circulation to the liver where some undergo substantial presystemic metabolism, a phenomenon known as the first-pass effect. A reduction in hepatic metabolic activity is likely to be reflected in a reduced first-pass effect and improved systemic bioavailability following oral administration of the drug. A list of medications that undergo substantial first-pass clearance is presented below:

Desipramine
Labetalol
Meperidine
Methadone
Methyldopa
Morphine
Nortriptyline
Oral nitrates (*e.g.*, isosorbide dinitrate)
Pentazocine
Propoxyphene
Propranolol
Terbutaline

Distribution

The age-related decline of serum albumin concentration has been shown to produce significant increases in unbound plasma concentrations of several drugs that are strongly bound to protein (*e.g.*, salicylates, sulfadiazine, and phenylbutazone).[54] The adverse effects of corticosteroids occur more frequently in patients with low serum albumin concentrations. This results from the saturation of specific and nonspecific corticosteroid binding proteins. Increased concentrations of cortisol result in higher concentrations of unbound cortisol as transcortin binding sites are saturated and binding to albumin is less avid. Exogenous corticosteroids likewise depend on albumin for their binding. There is an increase in unbound warfarin concentration in plasma in the elderly,[24] and this may predispose older patients to increased risk of bleeding.

The role of α_1-acid glycoprotein in drug binding in the elderly has not been well established. Concentrations of this binding protein increase during acute illness and alter the free or unbound plasma concentration of several basic drugs such as propranolol, lidocaine, and quinidine.[42]

Changes in body composition with increasing age alter drug disposition in the body tissues. With decreasing muscle mass and decreasing body water and replacement by adipose tissue, the apparent volume of distribution of water-soluble drugs should diminish while the apparent volume of distribution per unit of total body mass should increase for fat-soluble drugs. Caird and Kennedy[7] have shown the apparent volume of distribution of digoxin in the elderly is in the range of 250 to 350 liters compared with the value of about 500 to 600 liters in younger subjects. Castleden and colleagues[10] found higher plasma concentrations of practolol in the elderly and related this to the smaller apparent volume distribution of practolol in older patients. The volume of distribution of morphine in healthy older subjects (mean age 64) was about half of the volume of distribution in younger subjects (mean age 25).[41]

Metabolism

The microsomal enzyme system in the liver is the major site of drug metabolism. Antipyrine is commonly used as an index drug for oxidative metabolism. O'Malley and colleagues[40] have shown that the mean plasma elimination half-life of antipyrine is almost 50% longer in the elderly compared with younger controls. There is an overall tendency for the metabolic activity of older individuals to be less efficient than in younger individuals, as is shown in the compilation of data assembled by Ritschel (Fig. 7-2).

The extent to which drug metabolism in the elderly can be altered by substances that induce or inhibit oxidative metabolism has not been studied in very great detail. However, available evidence indicates that the mixed function oxidase system in the elderly is inhibited by agents such as cimetidine but, in general, mixed-function oxidase

activity does not appear to be induced as readily in the elderly by drugs such as dichloralphenazone[45] or rifampin.[51] Nevertheless, occasional elderly patients appear responsive to enzyme-inducing drugs such as phenytoin and rifampin and should be monitored carefully when receiving these drugs to ensure that the therapeutic actions of other agents such as theophylline and quinidine are not diminished. The elimination of theophylline is enhanced in smokers of all age-groups.[13]

A study of pharmacokinetic differences between younger and older individuals of the tricyclic antidepressant nortriptyline at steady state found that patients over the age of 70 years had higher plasma concentrations of nortriptyline even when their plasma concentrations were corrected for dosage and weight.[36] It was also noted that nortriptyline plasma concentrations rose during episodes of acute inflammatory disease, and this elevation was associated with an increase in the sedimentation rate. The authors of this Danish study, Kragh-Sorensen and Larsen, surmise that changes in the acute reactive protein α_1-acid glycoprotein may be responsible for the changes in plasma concentrations of the antidepressant medication, but the exact clinical relevance of this change is not certain. It seems likely that measurement of the unbound plasma concentration of the antidepressant drug would be more useful in predicting its therapeutic efficacy and its possible contribution to toxicity.

Excretion

For some drugs (*e.g.*, the aminoglycoside antibiotics and digoxin) the kidney is the major route of elimination. For many other agents, renal excretion is an important means of eliminating unchanged drug or active metabolites. Drugs that undergo extensive renal clearance and are therefore likely to accumulate in elderly patients include the following:

Amantidine
Aminoglycosides (*e.g.*, amikacin, gentamicin, streptomycin, tobramycin)
Atenolol
Cimetidine
Co-trimoxazole
Digoxin
Disopyramide
Lithium
Nadolol
Procainamide
Sulfonamides

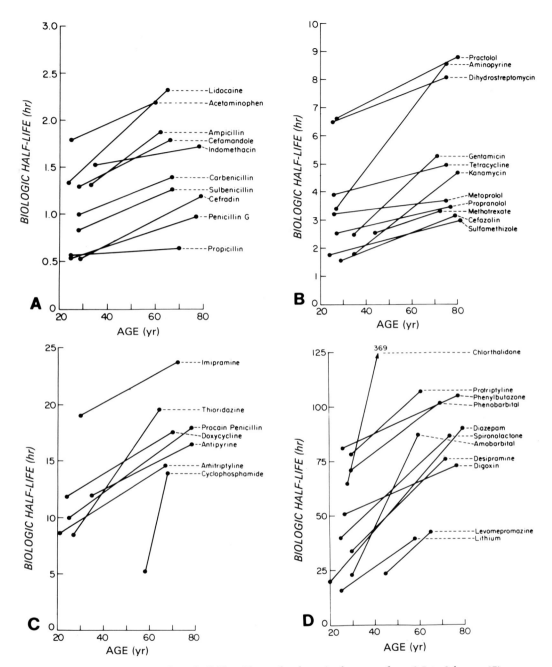

FIG. 7-2. (*A*) Increase in biologic half-life with age for drugs in the range from 0.5 to 3 hours. (*B*) Increase in biologic half-life with age for drugs in the range from 1 to 10 hours. (*C*) Increase in biologic half-life with age for drugs in the range from 5 to 25 hours. (*D*) Increase in biologic half-life with age for drugs in the range from 20 to 400 hours.

In all of the above, the straight lines between the half-lives of the young and elderly do not necessarily imply linear increase with age, nor is extrapolation permitted beyond the age range given. (Ritschel WA: Pharmacokinetics of Drugs in the Elderly Patient. Tarrytown, New York, The New York Academy of Medicine, Section on Geriatric Medicine with The New York State Council of Hospital Pharmacists, 1978)

Changes in renal function associated with aging have important pharmacokinetic implications for these agents. An age-related fall in glomerular filtration occurs such that patients 80 years of age have a fall of approximately 40% in creatinine clearance from the creatinine clearance measured in healthy 20-year-old subjects.[44] The serum creatinine level may remain within the usual range for younger patients despite the fall in creatinine clearance. However, it is possible to make a reasonable estimation of renal function if age, sex, and weight are taken into consideration.[32] Apart from this "normal" or usual decline in renal function, many elderly patients show an additional decrement in renal function due to dehydration, congestive cardiac failure, and intrinsic renal disease. The plasma elimination half-life of digoxin is increased from 36 hours to as much as 72 hours in otherwise healthy older individuals.[17]

The elderly are at risk of reduced clearance and resulting accumulation of the parent drug and the active metabolites of the benzodiazepines flurazepam[22] and diazepam.[35] The pharmacokinetics of oxazepam are not altered by age or liver disease, apparently making its use in the elderly relatively safe. However, the elimination half-life of oxazepam is extended from 10 hours to 25 hours in patients with renal insufficiency.[38]

The need to study the disposition of metabolites as well as parent drug is demonstrated in the study of desipramine and hydroxydesipramine pharmacokinetics in older and younger patients.[34] Plasma concentrations of hydroxydesipramine increased with age and were related to the decrease in glomerular filtration associated with aging. The renal clearance of the metabolite exhibited a strong negative correlation with age. Since there is evidence that the metabolite has both therapeutic and toxic effects, the accumulation of the metabolite in older patients with impaired renal function has important therapeutic considerations. The pharmacokinetics of the analgesic acetaminophen were studied by Divoll and colleagues.[16] They noted a slight decline in acetaminophen clearance with age in both sexes but considered the changes to be clinically insignificant and did not recommend any dosage adjustment in elderly patients.

PHARMACODYNAMICS

Pharmacodynamics describes the response of the body to drugs (*i.e.*, the pharmacologic, therapeutic, and toxic effects of the drugs on receptors, tissues, and organ systems). The response ultimately reflects the ability of the free or unbound concentration of the drug to react with specific cell components and to initiate an action. That action is modified by factors such as homeostatic control mechanisms, the influence of disease states, and concurrent medications.

ALTERED RESPONSIVENESS

Much of what has been stated already about the relationship between plasma concentrations of drugs and their therapeutic and toxic effects has assumed an age-independent plasma concentration-effect relationship. However, disturbances in distribution, changes in the diffusion or transportation of drugs into the cells on which they act, alterations in the metabolic and synthetic activities of the cells, and modifications in homeostatic or counterregulatory mechanisms may result in the appearance of altered tissue responsiveness. There is increasing evidence that age may alter responsiveness to drugs. Castleden and colleagues[11] have reported an increased level of responsiveness of the aging brain to the benzodiazepine nitrazepam.

Although the majority of reports indicates that the elderly are more "sensitive" to the central nervous system effects of drugs, elderly women exhibited a lack of sedation after diphenhydramine while younger individuals exhibited sedative/hypnotic effects.[5]

Isoprenaline infusion produces less increase in heart rate in older patients than in younger individuals, suggesting that there are reduced numbers or decreased affinity of β-adrenergic receptors for isoproterenol on sinoatrial nodal activity.[52] Likewise, Bertal and associates[6] demonstrated evidence of decreased responsiveness to β-adrenergic receptor blocking drugs in older patients.

The production of cyclic adenosine monophosphate (AMP) by lymphocytes was used as an index of β-adrenergic receptor–mediated responsiveness to isoproterenol to compare β-adrenergic receptor responsiveness in young and old subjects.[15] The mean response of the elderly was less than that of the younger subjects to all doses of isoproterenol used; the maximum response of cyclic AMP production was a little more than half in elderly compared with younger subjects. The authors of this study point out that much of the information about β-blocker activity is derived from studies in younger individuals; yet the drugs are commonly used in older patients whose responsiveness may be quite different.

Leukocyte β-adrenergic receptor affinity was

studied in healthy individuals aged 21 to 74 years by Feldman and colleagues.[19] They made several interesting but not fully understood observations. The leukocyte β-adrenergic receptor affinity for agonists was correlated inversely with age. With increasing age there was evidence of a reciprocal relationship between plasma norepinephrine concentration and the β-receptor affinity for agonists. However, there was no correlation between age and β-receptor density or β-receptor affinity for antagonists. In the supine position there was a lower proportion of high-affinity binding sites for agonists in older subjects than in the young. With upright posture, the high-affinity binding receptors for agonists were reduced in younger subjects but were not altered in the elderly. Reduced β-receptor affinity for agonists such as norepinephrine and isoproterenol may explain altered β-adrenergic sensitivity in older subjects.[48]

Kaiko[31] has investigated the possibility of age-related differences in analgesia following intramuscular administration of morphine. Although his study population was fairly well matched in terms of weight and initial pain intensity, he noted that the aged had superior analgesia when pain relief was expressed in magnitude and duration of action. The role of pharmacokinetic and pharmacodynamic alterations in responsiveness to narcotic analgesics remains an area of debate.[41]

The complexity of interpreting kinetic and dynamic components of central nervous system toxicity is presented by Schentag and his associates[46] in a study of cimetidine disposition in health and in disease. These workers concluded that age itself had little influence on the distribution or elimination of cimetidine. They found that patients with liver disease were more likely to experience adverse neurologic effects of cimetidine and related this to an apparent change in the blood–brain barrier to cimetidine in the presence of liver disease. For a given plasma concentration, almost twice as much cimetidine crossed the blood–brain barrier in a patient with liver disease as in a patient with normal liver function. The plasma concentrations of cimetidine were increased by as much as ten times in patients with both renal failure and liver disease. Substantial reductions in cimetidine dosage are necessary to avoid producing mental confusion in such patients.

CONTROVERSIAL ASPECTS

When a drug is administered to a patient with a specific disease, there should be a reasonable expectation for benefit in that patient. The properly designed and well-executed clinical trial has become the "gold standard" for evidence of drug efficacy. Unfortunately, there is a serious dearth of good studies and many common therapeutic maneuvers are based on tradition or anecdotal experience. The problems are compounded in the elderly because they are often excluded from even the better trials because of (arbitrary) age limitations or specific criteria that forbid entry into studies by patients with concurrent disease states.

Sound clinical practice requires that all outcomes are examined and some concept formulated of a benefit–risk ratio for treating the patient. This is a difficult concept since many of the judgments are qualitative. Cost–benefit ratios must also be considered, but judgments in this area are also difficult, again because of the qualitative decisions involved. Many of these decisions are made on the basis of what is termed "common sense." Our ignorance in many of these areas and our lack of solid evidence that costly treatments reduce morbidity or mortality in many diseases make it difficult to develop forceful arguments for interventional therapy in the elderly. Obvious examples include the level of aggressiveness in the treatment of malignant disease in the very elderly. The treatment may have a relatively low likelihood of success, there may be a high risk of adverse effects, the treatment may be costly for the patient or for society at large, the quantity of remaining life may not be particularly prolonged, and the quality of remaining life may be seriously disturbed. Given these considerations, it is tempting to accept the passive course of no interference; yet it is likely that some patients would benefit from the aggressive approach. The development of clinical paradigms based on science rather than conjecture or convenience is badly needed.

With increasing numbers of older patients and with increasing diagnosis of common disorders such as hypertension and maturity-onset diabetes mellitus, it is critical that we optimize our therapeutic strategies. There is little doubt that elevated blood pressure and blood glucose levels contribute to morbidity and mortality in all age-groups. However, the evidence is far from clear that the normalization by drugs of either blood pressure or blood glucose in entirely asymptomatic patients contributes to improved longevity, reduced morbidity, or a more desirable quality of life in the older patient. Resolution of these issues by properly conducted clinical trials that attempt to measure many of the variables necessary to make these judgments will be costly and time consuming. While adhering to the principle that age in itself should not be the determining factor in providing drug therapy, it would be naive to urge the reader to ignore age completely in therapeutic decision making. Until adequate studies are performed, it is likely that the debate will continue with extremes of opinion ranging from "appropriate active intervention" to "meddlesome interference."

PRACTICAL CONSIDERATIONS

Theoretic considerations become irrelevant unless they can be translated into practical strategies for helping the elderly patient gain optimal benefit with minimum risk of adverse effect from necessary and appropriate medications. The elderly have special difficulties. Forgetfulness may lead to poor compliance with the potential of either underdosing or overdosing. Failing vision, small print on medication labels, and ambiguity of tablet size or color[27] make it relatively easy for the elderly patient to err in taking tablets as directed. Such errors may be compounded by the common practice of mixing medications in a single container. There is evidence that the elderly may comply poorly if they perceive that the medications are either ineffective[14] or are thought to be the possible cause of adverse drug reactions.

There is little evidence that education by itself is an effective means of dealing with these problems. There is, therefore, considerable onus on the physician, pharmacist, and/or community nurse to develop strategies that reduce the likelihood of the development of problems.[55] The patient should be encouraged to obtain both prescription and non-prescription medications from the same pharmacy. The patient should be encouraged to discuss the proposed use of the medication and to consider possible interactions with other drugs. Labeling should be large and clear, and, if possible, the physician should include the indication in the instructions for labeling, such as "for blood pressure," "sleeping pill," "for arthritis," so that the patient and relatives or friends can recognize the proposed role of the medication.

Patients should be encouraged to dispose of medications that are no longer being used to avoid possible confusion with necessary medications at a later date and to reduce the risk of interaction or adverse effect if a hoarded medication is taken at a later date for what the patient believes to be a recurrence of the problem for which it was first prescribed. It may be important for the patient to have a further clinical assessment rather than use,

for example, an antibiotic that has been sitting in the drug cabinet for the past 6 months.

A simple chart of medications and the times at which they are to be taken can be helpful. It is critical, of course, that the names used are those that will appear on the medication bottles. There is much potential for confusion in the use of approved names and various trade names at different times.

Optimal dosing strategies include the supervision of medication by a friend, neighbor, or relative, and, if this cannot be achieved, the use of a Dosett or a similar container in which medications for several days can be provided conveniently.

The pharmacist should ensure that the medication is in a container that can be readily opened by an elderly individual, whose weakness, joint deformities, painful hands, or lack of coordination may make it virtually impossible to open the usual childproof containers.

RECOMMENDATIONS

All physicians have a very great responsibility to ensure that the perceived need for a drug can be justified by solid evidence of disease, that there is a reasonable expectation that the patient will be helped by drug therapy, and that the exhibition of the drug achieves the therapeutic goal at the minimum dosage and with the least toxicity possible.

The approach to treatment must ensure a proper working diagnosis based on adequate laboratory and clinical data. There is a place for both therapeutic nihilism and polypharmacy in the care of the elderly. When there is no convincing evidence that drug therapy has a place, the physician must learn to appreciate this and must develop appropriate nondrug treatments. There is a place for the judicious use of psychotherapeutic agents.[18,20,50] A physician should not avoid the issue of polypharmacy by denying drug treatments that are effective in given disease states but must be careful to choose the drug and dosage that achieves the optimal benefit–risk ratio. Given the increased numbers of elderly patients and the rapidly increasing costs of drugs for this group, the physician has an important social responsibility to ensure that therapy is achieved with minimal cost and least potential for drug wastage.

Follow-up should ensure that therapy has achieved the desired goals without the development of drug interaction or adverse effect. The duration of therapy must take into consideration the natural history of disease. Drugs that are clearly ineffective should be discontinued. Drugs that cause adverse effects should be reduced or replaced with safer alternatives. If there are doubts about the role of a medication in a patient's deterioration, the need for it should be carefully reviewed and temporary discontinuation should be considered.

One would do well to remember the admonition of Wade,[53] who has emphasized the need to observe "two simple rules of wise and proper use of drugs": (1) no drug should be administered unless there is a good reason and (2) as few drugs as possible should be given at any one time.

REFERENCES

1. Achong MR, Bayne JRD, Gerson LW, Golshani S: Prescribing of psychoactive drugs for chronically ill elderly patients. Can Med Assoc J 118:1503, 1978
2. Aoki FY, Hildahl VK, Large GW, Mitenko PA, Sitar DS: Aging and heavy drug use: A prescription survey in Manitoba. J Chronic Dis 36:75, 1983
3. Armstrong WA Jr, Driever CW, Hays RL: Analysis of drug-drug interactions in a geriatric population. Am J Hosp Pharm 37:385, 1980
4. Barton R, Hurst L: Unnecessary use of tranquillizers in elderly patients. Br J Psychiatry 112:989, 1966
5. Berlinger WG, Goldberg MJ, Spector R, Chiang C-K, Ghoneim MM: Diphenhydramine: Kinetics and psychomotor effects in elderly women. Clin Pharmocol Ther 32:387, 1982
6. Bertal O, Buhler FR, Kiowski W, Lutold BE: Decreased beta-adrenoceptor responsiveness as related to age, blood pressure and plasma catecholamines in patients with essential hypertension. Hypertension 2:130 1980
7. Caird FI, Kennedy RD: Digitalisation and digitalis detoxication in the elderly. Age Ageing 6:21, 1977
8. Cape RDT, Valberg LS: Care of the elderly: The role of the internist. Can Med Assoc J 121:990, 1979
9. Carruthers SG: Clinical pharmacology of aging. In Cape RDT, Coe RM, Rossman I (eds): Fundamentals of Geriatric Medicine. New York, Raven Press, 1983
10. Castleden CM, Kaye CM, Parsons RL: The effect of age on plasma levels of propranolol and practolol in man. Br J Clin Pharmacol 2:303, 1975
11. Castleden CM, George CF, Marcer D, Hallet C: Increased sensitivity to nitrazepam in old age. Br Med J 1:10, 1977
12. Crooks J, O'Malley K, Stevenson IH: Pharmacokinetics in the elderly. Clin Pharmacokinet 1:280, 1976
13. Cusack B, Kelly JG, Lavan J, Noel J, O'Malley K: Theophylline kinetics in relation to age: The importance of smoking. Br J Clin Pharmacol 10:109, 1980
14. D'Arcy PF: Drug reactions and interactions in the elderly patient. Drug Intell Clin Pharm 16:925, 1982
15. Dillon N, Chung S, Kelly J, O'Malley K: Age and beta adrenoceptor-mediated function. Clin Pharmacol Ther 27-769, 1980
16. Divoll M, Abernethy DR, Ameer B, Greenblatt DJ: Acetaminophen kinetics in the elderly. Clin Pharmacol Ther 31:151, 1982
17. Ewy GA, Kapadia GG, Yao L, Lullin M, Marcus FI: Digoxin metabolism in the elderly. Circulation 39:449, 1969
18. Fann WE: Pharmacotherapy in older depressed patients. J Gerontol 31:304, 1976
19. Feldman RD, Limbird LE, Nadeau J, Robertson D, Wood AJJ: Alterations in leukocyte beta-receptor affinity with aging. N Engl J Med 310:815, 1984
20. Fogel BS: Letter: Caution in the use of drugs in the elderly. N Engl J Med 308:1600, 1983
21. Gomolin IH, Chapron DJ: Rational drug therapy for the aged. Comp Ther 9:17, 1983
22. Greenblatt DJ, Allen MD, Shader RI: Toxicity of high-dose flurazepam in the elderly. Clin Pharmacol Ther 21:355, 1977
23. Greenblatt DJ, Koch-Weser J: Clinical pharmacokinetics: I and II. N Engl J Med 293:702, 964, 1975
24. Hayes MJ, Langman MJS, Short AH: Changes in drug metabolism with increasing age: I. Warfarin binding and plasma proteins. Br J Clin Pharmacol 2:69, 1975
25. Hodkinson HM: Mental impairment in the elderly. J Coll Physicians Lond 7:305, 1973
26. Hull SM, Mackintosh A: Discontinuation of maintenance digoxin therapy in general practice. Lancet 2:1054, 1977
27. Hurd PD, Blevins J: Aging and the color of pills. N Engl J Med 310:202, 1984
28. Hurwitz N: Admissions to hospital due to drugs. Br Med J 1:539, 1969
29. Hurwitz N, Wade OL: Intensive hospital monitoring of adverse reactions to drugs. Br Med J 1:531, 1969
30. Johnston GJ, McDevitt DG: Is maintenance digoxin necessary in patients with sinus rhythm? Lancet 1:567, 1979
31. Kaiko RF: Age and morphine analgesia in cancer patients with postoperative pain. Clin Pharmacol Ther 28:823, 1980
32. Kampmann J, Siersbaek-Nielsen K, Kristensen M, Molholm-Hansen J: Rapid evaluation of creatinine clearance. Acta Med Scand 196:517, 1974
33. Kiernan PJ, Isaacs JB: Use of drugs by the elderly. J R Soc Med 74:196, 1981
34. Kitanaka I, Ross RJ, Cutler NR, Zavadil AP, Potter WZ: Altered hydroxydesipramine concentrations in elderly depressed patients. Clin Pharmacol Ther 31:51, 1982

35. Klotz, U, Avant GR, Hoyumpa A, Schenker S, Wilkinson GR: The effects of age and liver disease on the disposition and elimination of diazepam in adult man. J Clin Invest 55:347, 1975

36. Kragh-Sorensen P, Larsen N-E: Factors influencing nortriptyline steady-state kinetics: Plasma and saliva levels. Clin Pharmacol Ther 28:796, 1980

37. Law R, Chalmers C: Medicines and elderly people: A general practice survey. Br Med J 1:565, 1976

38. Murray TG, Chiang ST, Koepke HH, Walker BR: Renal disease, age, and oxazepam kinetics. Clin Pharmacol Ther 30:805, 1981

39. Ogilvie RI: An introduction to pharmacokinetics. J Chronic Dis 36:1, 1983

40. O'Malley K, Crooks J, Duke E, Stevenson IH: Effect of age and sex on human drug metabolism. Br Med J 3:607, 1971

41. Owen JA, Sitar DS, Berger L, Brownell L, Duke PC, Mitenko PA: Age-related morphine kinetics. Clin Pharmacol Ther 34:364, 1983

42. Piafsky KM: Disease-induced changes in the plasma binding of basic drugs. Clin Pharmacokinet 5:246, 1980

43. Pomara N, Stanley B, Block R, Guido J, Russ D, Stanley M: Letter: Caution in the use of drugs in the elderly. N Engl J Med 308:1600, 1983

44. Rowe JW, Andres R, Tobin JD, Norris AH, Shock NW: The effect of age on creatinine clearance in man: A cross-sectional and longitudinal study. J Gerontol 31:155, 1976

45. Salem SAM, Rajjayabun P, Shepherd AMM, Stevenson IH: Reduced induction of drug metabolism in the elderly. Age Ageing 7:68, 1978

46. Schentag JJ, Cerra FB, Calleri GM, Leising ME, French MA, Bernhard H: Age, disease, and cimetidine disposition in healthy subjects and chronically ill patients. Clin Pharmacol Ther 29:737, 1981

47. Segal HJ, Bornstein NS: Drug use by the elderly in long-term facilities. Ont Med Rev 51:15, 1984

48. Shocken DD, Roth GS: Reduced beta-adrenergic receptor concentrations in ageing man. Nature 267:856, 1977

49. Skoll SL, August RJ, Johnson G: Drug prescribing for the elderly in Saskatchewan during 1976. Can Med Assoc J 121:1074, 1979

50. Thompson TL II, Moran MG, Nies AS: Psychotropic drug use in the elderly: I and II. N Engl J Med 308:134, 194, 1983

51. Twum-Barima Y, Finnigan T, Habash AI, Cape RDT, Carruthers SG: Impaired enzyme induction by rifampicin in the elderly. Br J Clin Pharmacol 17:595, 1984

52. Vestal RE, Wood AJJ, Shand, DG: Reduced beta-adrenoceptor sensitivity in the elderly. Clin Pharmacol Ther 26:181, 1979

53. Wade, OL: Drug therapy in the elderly: Age Ageing 1:65, 1972

54. Wallace S, Whiting B, Runcie J: Factors affecting drug binding in plasma of elderly patients. Br J Clin Pharmacol 3:327, 1976

55. Wandless I, Davie JW: Can drug compliance in the elderly be improved? Br Med J 1:359, 1977

56. Williamson J, Chopin JM: Adverse reactions to prescribed drugs in the elderly: A multicentre investigation. Age Ageing 9:73, 1980

57. World Health Organization: Use of medicaments by the elderly. Drugs 22:279, 1981

SUGGESTED READINGS

Bochner F, Carruthers SG, Kampmann J, Steiner J: Medication in the elderly. In Handbook of Clinical Pharmacology, 2nd ed. Boston, Little, Brown & Co, 1983

Crooks J: Rational therapeutics in the elderly. J Chronic Dis 36:59, 1983

Crooks J: Aging and drug disposition—pharmacodynamics. J Chronic Dis 36:85, 1983

Greenblatt DJ, Sellers EM, Shader RI: Drug disposition in old age. N Engl J Med 306:1081, 1982

Ouslander JG: Drug therapy in the elderly. Ann Intern Med 95:711, 1981

Ramsay LE, Tucker GT: Clinical pharmacology: Drugs and the elderly. Br Med J 282:125, 1981

Sjoqvist F, Alvan G: Aging and drug disposition—metabolism. J Chronic Dis 36:31, 1983

Vestal RE: Drug use in the elderly: A review of problems and special considerations. Drugs 16:358, 1978

Wilkinson GR: Drug distribution and renal excretion in the elderly. J Chronic Dis 36:91, 1983

8

Special Hazards of Illness in Later Life

John Agate

Most young people who are ill can be expected to have ample bodily reserves, and as a rule they only have to fight their illness. Older invalids have fewer reserves but suffer in addition the extra penalties of being old. Their social circumstances are often reduced, and they have their illness to contend with as well. It must be accepted that older individuals run the risks of particular complications of their illness that are not usually expected in younger individuals. This means that their disorders may have to be managed along special lines. Thus, a young person may be immobilized for long periods without coming to any harm, but an older person deteriorates rapidly in general mobility and capability, in vigor, and even in spirit if they are kept in bed or forbidden to walk about and do things for themselves. And if this is true for a reasonably able-bodied older person involved in a new illness, it is even more certainly true for those who are already suffering from arthritis or any other sort of impediment to locomotion. The era when rest was believed to be the primary essential principle in treatment is rapidly passing.

Now we can see that rest can be overdone. Indeed, enforced rest can be totally disastrous to an elderly invalid. Even though he may like the comfort of his sickbed, it will ensnare him if he does not get away from it for part of every day. There is a strange misconception among many people, young and more mature alike, that the elderly need rest above all else, and that they should never tire themselves or be expected to make any effort. So when they are ill, it is argued, the need for rest must be all the greater, and they are persuaded into bed at the first opportunity. Geriatric physicians recognize that this is largely fallacious, and their management of a case must be a compromise between allowing enough rest

for a hard-taxed, frail, elderly body, yet not so much that worse damage is perpetrated. There is not much merit in curing an active elderly patient of an illness at the cost of leaving him severely handicapped, immobile, dependent on others, or perhaps a permanent nursing problem in consequence of one of the general complications of illness in old age. The special risks that face the elderly lying in bed are contractures, pressure sores, pneumonia, thromboembolism, dehydration and ionic imbalance, incontinence, constipation, hypothermia, and collapse of morale and of the desire for independence.

SPECIAL RISKS IN BEDRIDDEN PATIENTS

Contractures

Contractures are more or less fixed deformities of joints that result from their being held immobile, usually in unsatisfactory positions. Sometimes this is the result of pain, because of which the patient tries to get the joint into the most comfortable position, regardless of the effect of this on subsequent function. The distortions of old, neglected rheumatoid arthritis are a case in point. A contracture is at first correctable by passive movements, but later fibrosis of periarticular structures takes place. The associated muscles become weak and shorten, often causing their tendons to be as tight as bowstrings across the angle of the contracture. Bony bridging across the joint space may take place in time.

All this is made possible by the well-known immobility of the elderly, and by their tendency to lie in bed or sit for hours at a time with their arms and legs flexed. In certain circumstances, contractures can develop with alarming speed—a matter of 2 or 3 days, rather than the span of months that might be expected. The astonishing speed at which this disaster can take place demands constant vigilance from the doctors and nurses of every elderly patient. It is even possible for very old patients with no joint or neuromuscular pathology whatever to develop 90° contractures at the knees and hips simply by sitting still all day and lying all night without straightening their legs. Sometimes this is the sad end result of their demanding the total personal attention from everyone in sight that they believe is their right because of their seniority. Most commonly, however, behind the development of contracture there is joint disease, a spastic muscle group, or a flaccid paralysis with overaction of antagonist muscles to account for the basic deformity.

Strokes account for many contractures at the wrist, shoulder, and fingers, and also for many instances of footdrop. The characteristic spasticity of severe parkinsonism can lead to multiple flexion contractures of arms and legs and to distortion of the foot into a fixed, inverted equinovarus. Bedfast demented patients sometimes have bizarre contractures because of their general decubitus. They adopt strange positions because they lack all comprehension of their surroundings and cannot guard themselves from the most elementary hazards. At worst, their heels may be pressed tightly and permanently against their buttocks. Patients kept strictly in bed under tight bedclothes are very likely to develop disastrous plantar-flexed fixity of the ankles, even when there is no neurologic deficit. This is a form of footdrop unmistakably caused by mismanagement.

But the most common contracture in the elderly is at the knee joint, with secondary flexion at the hip, or vice versa. A person affected in this way may be able to stand and walk only with great difficulty. It follows that if correction of a contracted knee is being contemplated, it is essential to know if the hip can be well extended. Otherwise, the proposed maneuver may leave the patient worse off than he was before.

Contracture prevention is vital because treatment is difficult and sometimes risky and painful. Results will not come from long-term traction methods. However, in the first stages, passive movements by physiotherapists and nurses can help to keep gradually flexing joints straight. Once a contracture is established, it may be necessary to excise the fibrous structures, lengthen short tendons, or perform tenotomies. Good results can be obtained by encasing the limb, extended as far as possible, in plaster of Paris, then waiting some days. The plaster is then half cut through at the angle of the contracture, the limb within it is straightened further, and more plaster is applied across the gap.

After three or four of these wedging procedures, the limb may be straight; but it is a tedious and painful procedure that would be unnecessary if contractures were foreseen and prevented. It is a hazardous maneuver if the circulation of the limb is already impaired, and the medicolegal implications of this must be considered. Once a limb has been straightened, it may be necessary to hold it straight by using a lightweight removable plastic splint with lacing, buckle, or Velcro fastening. Many totally disabled individuals with contractures at the knee have been rescued and made ambulant again by these means, but with good initial management this would not have been necessary.

Pressure Sores

Anyone lying in bed for long is a potential candidate for pressure sores (decubitus ulcers), but an elderly patient is more prone to them than most. In Denmark it has been suggested by Petersen[27] that there are 43 patients with pressure sores per 100,000 of the total population, but estimates from elsewhere have been even higher.[2,10] From the logistical standpoint it is reckoned that a sore adds 50% to the nursing time a patient requires, as well as the extra cost of much longer occupation of beds in hospitals. There is a well-established relationship between the development of large pressure sores and a poor prognosis. This may of course be interpreted variously: acquisition of a large sore endangers life, but patients with the gravest illnesses and therefore the worst prognoses are also most liable to the severest pressure manifestations.

The predisposing factors are many. Sensory deficit from traumatic paraplegia typically puts its victim at immediate risk because no warning of the danger comes from his own nervous system; but this similarly applies to any elderly patient who is in coma or stupor or is totally inert or just too confused to heed the warnings from his sore skin. Additional factors are obesity, anemia, abnormally low blood pressure, peripheral circulatory problems, and faulty nutrition, either in a general respect or occasionally because of therapeutic dietary restrictions, as in the case of a low protein diet ordered because of renal failure, which can cause major tissue breakdown overnight at a pressure point. This can also happen in a case of thrombosis of the inferior vena cava, although no doubt for different reasons. Again, apart from general vitamin deficiency, particularly that of vitamin C, major surgery in the elderly depletes ascorbic acid stores, so that special supplementation before surgery is only common sense. Additionally, the use of sedatives inhibits spontaneous movements, intramuscular injections often cause local tissue damage in pressure areas, while skin that is regularly wet and contaminated by excreta becomes highly vulnerable. It has been suggested by Lowthian[22] that incontinence alone increases the risk of sores by a factor of five.

However, unrelieved pressure is the overriding cause of sores. Much work has been done on the assessment of pressure locally and on methods of relieving it by support systems.[7,15,19,20,29] The greatest risk is when a high proportion of the body weight is applied through a small skin area, particularly where a bony prominence is close beneath the skin. The most common site, as Petersen[26] confirmed, is the sacrum, followed by the greater trochanter, but the heel, ischium, and lateral malleolus are often involved. In very vulnerable patients there can be danger to the skin over the dorsal spine, especially if there is kyphosis or angulation, or over the scapular spines or elbows and even the knees, while the weight of the head can endanger the pinnae of the ears. Some "pressure" sores are aggravated by friction of restless limbs or initiated by shearing stress when heavy patients slide down the bed on wet sheets or are dragged rather than lifted clear of the bed by their attendants.

Thirty years ago, Husain[18] showed that high pressure for a short time is safer than low pressure for a long time, and the damage done is a function of pressure multiplied by time.[30] Experimentally, sensing devices have shown what wide differences of pressure result from using various mattresses and beds, and incidentally how hazardous some operating tables are.[29] Valuable early studies by Exton-Smith and Sherwin[13] showed that paucity of nocturnal movements puts some older patients particularly at risk, and this work led to a simple rating system,[14] needing only clinical observations and no apparatus, by which patients who are especially at risk can be identified. This rating has often proved its worth in practice. It was established by the same investigators that the risk of sores was high in the first week after admission to a hospital and that two thirds of sores appeared during the first 2 weeks.[14]

In well-run geriatric wards it is a matter of pride that conditions that cause pressure sores should seldom if ever be allowed to arise. Even so, the combination of disease, profound inertia, and the patient's final disintegration sometimes defeats the best efforts. Sores only become less common if all concerned believe that their occurrence might reflect adversely on their skills and vigilance: besides the nurses, physicians have a positive role to play, for they must recognize the risk factors, allow as much activity to patients as possible, and prescribe appropriately in order not to increase those risks. Occasionally an extremely old and cachectic patient, perhaps with multiple major disorders, develops signs of pressure at every point of contact with the bed, despite all countermeasures. Except in such circumstances one should avoid ascribing sores just to the patient's "poor general condition," and talking of their inevitability.

Unrelieved pressure on skin and underlying tissues deprives them of blood supply, and tissue death soon threatens. The pathology of sores and the changes in the microcirculation have been explored by Barton,[3] as have the possibilities of thermographic and other monitoring of vulnerable areas.[4] This suggested various pathologically based classifications of pressure sores. Clinicians, however, usually prefer a grading based on their own observations. A fourfold scale of severity is appropriate to most circumstances: (1) discoloration of the skin over a pressure area, (2) superficial skin loss, (3) full-thickness skin loss, and (4) skin loss with loss of deeper structures plus cavitation. In the latter category it is often observed that necrosis of the muscle and fat layers, which may be more vulnerable than the integument, takes place beneath apparently intact skin (although thermography might suggest it was endangered); a sterile ischemic abscess forms and bursts dramatically through, resulting in a large cavitating ulcer with overhanging edges. Often a black necrotic base develops and may become infected,[25] as indeed one would expect from the nature and site of the majority of pressure sores, although the infected wound can drain readily. Superficial sores naturally are less dangerous and heal much more quickly than deep sores with cavities: the latter can only heal by granulation and scarring and may call for surgical intervention. Superficial sores usually are painful; deep ones seldom are.

To prevent sores pressure must be regularly relieved and some activity in the patient encouraged despite other considerations. First then, the patient should be allowed out of bed and should move about as much as possible: at the very least half the day should be spent sitting in a chair taking weight on the ischial tuberosities, which are manifestly the best parts for the purpose. There are remarkably few illnesses in old age in which some sitting in a chair cannot be allowed. Second, if bed rest is obligatory, the patient *must* be turned regularly by her nurses from side to side, back to side as appropriate, and at intervals that depend on the patient's condition. It may have to be hourly in those most at risk, the turning continuing day and night even if the patient or relatives protest. It is better to lose a little sleep than the integrity of one's skin and to be turned is often a welcome relief. The vulnerable areas must be kept clean and dry and gently massaged with powder. All the skill of the patient's nurses is needed in propping him up with suitable pillows, using foam or other kinds of supports to keep his heels clear of the bed, and lifting, not dragging him up the sheets. It is most important that a cradle be used to keep the weight of the covers from pressing on the legs: this should be standard practice in nursing geriatric patients. Meanwhile the physician must be as watchful as the nurses and must correct anemia, malnutrition, or low blood pressure; request passive movements from the physical therapy staff; and encourage active rehabilitation at the earliest opportunity. If the physician unnecessarily insists that the patient stay in bed, he is likely to make the nurses' task harder, as he will also do if he relies on sedatives, since they are seldom essential if the general management of an elderly patient is otherwise correct. Catheterization is sometimes justifiable when trying to preserve intact the skin of a very inert, heavy, and incontinent subject. However the various local applications and elaborately formulated "protective" creams are of no certain value and may simply lull nurses into a false sense of security.

It has been said that the patient has an obligation to help prevent his own sores, by regularly relieving the pressure through spontaneous movement, especially, for example, while sitting in a wheelchair. However much this may be true for an alert young paraplegic, it is usually quite unrealistic to expect an old person to assume such responsibility for himself during major illness.

Physical supportive methods, the outcome of much research and ingenuity over the past 10 to 20 years, are now available both for prevention and as an aid to the management of sores. Valuable as many of them are, they must never be allowed to take the place of fundamental skilled nursing care, for which there is really no substitute. Special mattresses, beds, and mechanical systems generally are an aid and an adjunct to nursing and may take some of the physical effort out of a heavy but necessary nursing maneuver. Yet using special equipment requires special skills and training and good maintenance and is costly. Cost-effectiveness may depend on the equipment preventing the sores, and the consequential cost of these, or reducing the duration of treatment of an established sore, which are difficult matters to evaluate.

Static support systems include many kinds of special mattresses, ranging from the widely used simple polyurethane variety, to an incised variant of this, to mattresses filled with silicone-coated materials, polystyrene globules, and so on that are often supplemented by an upper layer of real or synthetic sheepskin to improve the local microenvironment. Before these systems appeared there had been those who advocated plaster beds, sand-tray beds, multiple feather pillows, and even piles of sawdust. A multiple "spinal pack" mattress of 9 to 12 separate thick sorbo-rubber components proved of value in distributing weight appropriately yet avoiding particular at-risk skin areas. Prolonged lying in a prone position or suspension from an overbed frame has sometimes had to be used. More recently modern adjustable contouring hospital-type beds have come into widespread use: these, with suitable mattresses, make safe positioning and repositioning of frail elderly people much easier. Alongside them have appeared various special suspension, turning, and tilting beds and frames, either mechanically or power-operated, that facilitate the turning of very vulnerable patients, such as those who are comatose. However, they are likely to alarm conscious elderly patients and may restrict their general activity unacceptably. A great many so-called dynamic supporting systems have also been evolved in the past 20 years. The simplest were basic water mattresses, or air-filled mattresses that later evolved into the alternating pressure air mattresses ("ripple mattresses"),[5,6] which have had widespread application and are most useful in contributing to prevention and treatment. They are also relatively cheap. In essence they consist of a series of interdigitating cells differentially inflated in cycles by an air pump to relocate the patient's weight every few minutes. Pumping pressures should be variable to accommodate different patients' weights, and the breadth of the cells should be about 15 cm for reliable results. True deep water beds are specially designed frames allowing vulnerable patients to lie freely floating on a plastic envelope that is a deep water container. These are highly effective for exceptional cases; however, they are bulky, are very heavy, have to be thermostatically controlled, and cause new handling problems for the nurses dealing with these semi-submerged recumbent and helpless patients.

Finally, much inventiveness has been shown by biomechanical engineers in evolving special air support systems such as the low-air-loss (LAL) bed,[17] which comprises a system of small sectional vertical mattresses kept constantly inflated with warm air that supports the patient and provides a controlled environment locally. Originally designed for treatment of burns, these beds are sometimes used now in the fight against pressure sores; however, these beds and other types embodying a supporting medium of myriad minute dry beads kept fluidized by upward currents of air are complex, bulky, and cost more than $15,000. It is surely beyond reasonable expectation that such an apparatus should be available for nursing all the geriatric patients who might at any one time be at risk.

The multiplicity of support systems suggests that no generally applicable solution has yet been found. The interest of engineers and other colleagues from the sphere of biomechanics is most welcome.[20] However, their proposed solutions are often ingenious and elaborate, whereas it is known that prompt and correct management of illness in the elderly by well-trained, conscientious medical and nursing teams using basic skills rather than mechanical methods can prevent all but the minority of pressure sores. Clearly, our aim must always be prevention rather than cure, and simple means must be better than high technology.

Treatment of established sores can appropriately be discussed at this point. Techniques aimed at prevention must be used as unremittingly as before with special support systems perhaps employed in particular cases. General measures must include the correction of fluid and protein loss, which from large sores is considerable, and maintenance whenever possible of a diet high in protein and vitamins, particularly ascorbic acid. Anemia must be corrected, so commonly blood or plasma transfusion is called for. Anabolic corticosteroids are sometimes used, but their value is not necessarily proven. Zinc sulfate in capsules of 220 mg three times a day is often advised, following the discovery that zinc salts accelerate healing in persistent skin ulceration.[28] The local treatment of a pressure sore should be that of a surgical wound in a potentially contaminated field. Pressure on it must be relieved totally or it will never heal. Debridement of dead tissue may not necessarily involve full surgical facilities or anesthesia: local enzyme applications on swabs are often helpful in

this respect. It is generally accepted that the sore should be kept covered as protection against contamination and infection, but the type of dressing is probably not critical in any way. Over the years a vast number of local applications and nostra have been advocated, including ultraviolet light, ultrasound, hyperbaric oxygen, metallic elements, oils, vegetable preparations, and innumerable drugs as solutions, powders, or ointments. Most have had enthusiastic advocates but little critical evaluation, and effective trials have hardly ever been attempted. In 1975, Morgan[24] reviewed the literature on topical applications for pressure sores since the turn of the century, and since that review many more have been suggested, including, now, inert synthetic substances in powder or fluid form, setting as a rubbery, conforming, and inert absorbent dressing that perhaps accelerates healing by a mechanical cleansing action. It may be true, as wise colleagues in the past have suggested, that it matters little what is applied to a sore provided it is not the weight of the patient's body!

Infection must be counteracted, but this should not be by local antibiotic applications, although antiseptic preparations and dyes are sometimes advised. Sepsis locally does not make the work of surgical repair any easier. This has to be the treatment of last resort in some cases of large cavitating lesions that will not heal in any other way. Surgery may indeed be advocated as the treatment of choice for sores (to save time and avoid the later hazards), but to those dedicated to prevention, such a general policy would be an admission of failure. Surgical indications and methods are discussed in the text edited by Constantian,[9] and I have also reviewed the subject of pressure sores at greater length than is possible here.[1]

Thromboembolism

Thrombosis of deep leg veins and its consequences may strike patients of all ages, but perhaps none are so susceptible as the elderly when they are kept in bed. Very occasionally, a spontaneous thrombosis takes place, without neoplastic or any other obstruction, in an arm vein of an elder patient.

These older patients are even less active in bed than younger patients. They are frequently the victims of major paralysis of limbs and consequently have impaired venous return. They are particularly liable to conditions such as cardiac infarction, congestive heart failure, and peripheral vascular insufficiency, all of which reduce the rate of the venous circulation in the legs.

The clinical appearance of a deep vein thrombosis is too well known to require description here. However, there are many patients in whom there are no apparent swelling and no calf tenderness, but autopsy yields the truth after a subsequent sudden cardiovascular catastrophe. Swelling of the legs is also very widespread in the elderly. Some cases are due to congestive cardiac failure, but many are not. In bilateral leg swelling, the diagnostician may not give due regard to venous thrombosis, even though there are cases in which bilateral thrombosis does occur. In a few cases, caval thromboses occur. Unilateral leg swelling is of course highly suspect, and an unexpected asymmetric increase in swelling of one of a heart-failure patient's legs is equally significant, particularly because venous thrombosis with pulmonary embolism is a most frequent complication of heart disease in the elderly.

The clinical and electrocardiographic signs of pulmonary embolism after deep vein thrombosis are discussed elsewhere (see Chapters 11, 14). It is sufficient here to remind the reader of the very high death rate of pulmonary embolism in the older age-group as a whole and of the great difficulty in distinguishing this condition clinically from cardiac infarction. So great is this hazard that all efforts must be made to prevent the venous stasis that initiates the whole malign sequence. There is, naturally, no better way of preventing stasis than making one's patient active. If he cannot get up on to his feet, then regrettably there is not much to be hoped for from breathing exercises and leg exercises in bed, unless these can be repeatedly done under supervision of a therapist.

Patients with paralysis of the legs must have regular passive movements of both limbs from their nurses and all others involved in their treatment, as well as from therapists. Regular inspection and measurement of the girth of the leg are as important as inspection of the pressure areas. When evidence of thrombosis is found, anticoagulant therapy is feasible. Age *per se* is not a bar to using this form of prophylaxis, although there are several contraindications, and appropriate dosage under laboratory control may be very difficult to maintain, except in the wards of a hospital.

Modern technology, using radioactively labeled fibrinogen or the Doppler principle, makes the early diagnosis of thrombosis more simple and more certain. These methods are time consuming and expensive, however, and it seems unlikely that they could be used routinely for the prophylactic management of the generality of elderly invalids

in hospitals and nursing homes who might be prone to thromboembolism.

After due consideration, the geriatric physician will discover far fewer contraindications to his patient's sitting in a chair, and even walking, than will some of his more cautious colleagues, who may look on the elderly as pathetically frail and therefore never to be encouraged to be active. Being perhaps preventable, a death from pulmonary embolism serves as the best possible example of the hazards of bedfastness to an elderly patient; compared with this, the risks of making him active too soon are as nothing.

Dehydration

Many invalids admitted to geriatric wards are seriously dehydrated. Most of them are admitted not so much because of their basic illness but because their fluid balance and sometimes their electrolyte balance have become disturbed. It is not difficult to discover the reasons. Renal function declines with age, as more and more whole nephrons are lost from the kidneys, although if elderly individuals take enough fluid, excretion of waste is still adequate. However, a great many elderly patients, especially women, regularly restrict their fluid intake. Some have always done so, and some are afraid of accidental urinary incontinence and believe that fluid restriction decreases the risk—whereas it may increase it by encouraging infection and decreasing bladder distensibility.

Some of the elderly are inhibited by primitive sanitary arrangements and drink very little, hoping to have to make fewer trips outside. This is a real factor in cold climates, in country districts without water-carriage sewerage systems, and when elderly patients are very restricted in movement. Often, when one of them, living alone, falls ill and goes to bed without enough fluid within reach and then gets no attention from anyone, he finally must be admitted to a hospital severely dehydrated because of simple water deprivation. If diarrhea or vomiting is part of the illness, his plight is all the worse. Even when elderly patients are being nursed at home, the relatives sometimes do not seem to realize the vital need for adequate fluids; perhaps they are also afraid of incontinence. In the hospital, much time must be spent coaxing frail, listless, apathetic patients to take sufficient fluid. This is an aspect of caring that must be impressed on nurses. A jug of water and a tumbler at the bedside is not a sufficient answer to this problem. The water must pass the patient's lips.

The clinical picture of dehydration—a dry brown tongue, sunken cheeks, inelastic skin, and high blood urea level—is all too commonly seen. In the elderly the syndrome is much more often due to simple water depletion than to true uremia from chronic renal disease. Fortunately, it is quickly rectified once detected. In later decades, the upper limit of normal for blood urea estimations may be taken as 60 mg/dl. A remarkable number of geriatric patients are found to have higher levels than this without renal failure; dehydration is the usual reason.

In simple water depletion, the patient has a normal serum sodium level, and water can be readily absorbed by way of the gastrointestinal tract. When the patient cannot or will not drink as he should, intubation is needed.

Combined electrolyte and water depletion is more serious. This can result from overenergetic use of diuretics, or in diabetes and in conditions causing diarrhea or vomiting. The clinical picture is much the same, but lassitude is a special feature here. In advanced cases, acidosis with hyperventilation may be present, and the patient may lapse into coma.

This is not the place for a detailed discussion of the differential diagnosis of disturbed fluid and electrolyte balance and the treatment appropriate to each syndrome. The standard techniques used at other ages are just as appropriate and just as necessary for the elderly, save that intravenous therapy must always be used with great care because the patient may lapse into cardiac failure.

Hypokalemia requires special mention because it is so common. It may occur unexpectedly. Potassium is not well conserved at any age. Unusual losses may accompany acidotic states, as they do in uncontrolled diabetes, in the regular administration of diuretics and corticosteroids, and in diarrhea, vomiting, fistulas, and colostomies. All these are common accompaniments of illness in old age.

The risk is that hypokalemia will go unrecognized or even be attributed to a psychologic disorder because the symptoms are malaise, lassitude, profound weakness, and even general paralysis. The diagnosis naturally is made by detecting a low serum potassium level, below 3.5 mEq/liter, but electrocardiographic signs such as inverted T waves, depressed ST segments, and a prolonged QT interval are especially indicative. The degree of prostration is quite remarkable, and so is the speed by which it can be overcome by the administration of potassium salts, preferably by mouth. It is advisable to suspect potassium depletion in any patient showing lassitude, weakness, or prostration when there is also doubt about his fluid balance. Such conditions as this, when detected, are readily treated; when missed, they are rapidly fatal.

Constipation

Constipation is a persistent problem in a certain group of the elderly. In many more it is a worry that exists largely in the imagination. In their cases, it may have evolved from faulty childhood habits and perhaps was implanted in their minds by parents who were themselves overanxious in this respect. Whatever the reason, these unfortunate individuals have a bowel fixation. They always wonder whether they will have the hoped-for daily bowel movement and are fearful of the consequences of failing, even though a lifetime of experience should tell them that this failure is of little consequence and can be corrected by aperients used judiciously. Some of them are not content with one bowel movement daily, or they forget they have had it and are constantly dosing themselves. In hospitals, they are a trial to their nurses, and "constipation" takes precedence among all their symptoms.

Nevertheless, real constipation is a common consequence of immobility or bedfastness, as anyone who has been ill in bed a few days will understand. In adaptable young patients with no fear of prolonged inactivity, this can be largely ignored, but the elderly are prone to certain happenings in consequence of genuine constipation. Special care must therefore be exercised to keep the bowels of elderly invalids clear. Constipation otherwise may become so severe and persistent that it can only be relieved by regular enemas or manual removal. In a small proportion of cases, actual lower bowel obstruction takes place, and surgery must be used to relieve it. Many more develop fecal impaction at the rectum, which causes pain and distress, incontinent leaking of matter through the sphincter, or more commonly, a form of spurious mucous diarrhea owing to prolonged irritation of the mucosa by a large immovable fecal mass. This may additionally precipitate urinary incontinence.

Many mentally confused elderly patients disregard or are unaware of the natural demands of a distended rectum and become chronically constipated. And some whose intellectual integrity is already suspect seem to be precipitated into confusion and hyperactivity by a full bowel or bladder that they do not recognize as such; yet when they are relieved, their behavior quickly becomes normal again.

The proof of the reality of constipation in elderly patients, especially those confined to bed, comes if one regularly palpates the abdomen, in which it is so often possible to feel a fecal-filled colon, or if one routinely examines the rectum. A contributing cause is likely to be a faulty diet, since many dislike fruit and vegetables, some cannot chew them, and some cannot afford them. Their fluid intake is often too low, as well. Other likely causes are general muscular weakness, especially of the abdominal musculature, lack of exercise in those who could be active, persistent laziness in answering the call to defecate, and daunting lavatory arrangements in old houses—or outside them, in some country districts. The subject and its treatment is further discussed in Chapter 16.

Incontinence

Incontinence is one of the most challenging problems of geriatric medicine. Of all patients entering geriatric hospital wards, one third are likely to develop incontinence at some time during their stay. It comes on commonly when they are for the moment gravely ill or in a state of disturbed consciousness. This can be readily understood and sympathized with. It is established incontinence that causes such difficulty, and this is likely to be present in nearly two thirds of those who must occupy hospital and nursing home beds on a long-term basis, especially if the incidence of mental aberration is high.

Incontinence is not found in bedfast patients alone, but because confining an elderly patient to bed materially increases the risk, the matter is considered here among the hazards of being ill and immobile. Many private households are able to care for elderly invalids indefinitely, provided no excretory problems are involved. Yet once incontinence supervenes, devoted friends and relatives often find it more than they bargained for. Incontinence therefore is the main factor causing the admission of many patients to hospitals or nursing homes. In some of these cases, earlier admission for assessment and diagnosis might have prevented incontinence from occurring, or at least from becoming permanently established.

Incontinence is not easy to define. Broadly, the passing of urine or feces inappropriately is incontinence. Yet many elderly patients are continent if they are reminded of their social duty at regular intervals and given the means of keeping clean and dry by attentive nurses. These patients would probably become incontinent if left to their own devices. Patients in this category could hardly be called continent. Nor, perhaps, would anyone who had to depend entirely on others to keep himself so. Also, many patients are continent and able to attend to their own needs during their waking hours but are incontinent at night.

There is a great deal of difference between a patient who is incontinent but knows it and is distressed by it, and another who is unaware of the malfunction or, worse still, who seems quite indifferent to the trouble he is causing. In these latter cases, the doctor and nurses must beware of thinking the patient has normal volition and insight. In most instances he has not, and he could no more be considered responsible for his excretory actions than he could for managing his own business affairs. The neurophysiology of excretion comprises a nicely balanced system of reflexes that control the motor functions and the relaxation of the sphincters and the muscular coats of the bladder and the bowel. Except in infancy, cortical control is always exercised. However, in many cases of incontinence in the elderly, the reason lies in the loss of cortical inhibition of the act of excretion, either because the neural pathway is interrupted or because the cortex itself is ineffective. Urologic aspects of this problem are discussed in Chapter 43.

Fecal Incontinence

Because fecal incontinence is almost entirely preventable, much depends on the physician's attitude toward it. It always requires the fullest investigation, and nurses must report it and not simply accept it as inevitable. The local causes include proctitis, carcinoma of the rectum, prolapse of the anus, which is often seen in the very aged, and major neurologic lesions of the spinal cord. It is also possible for an old person to be so debilitated and inert that he is unable to exert muscular effort to control the sphincter voluntarily against a normal gastrocolic reflex. Thus, the whole rectum will be full of soft, unformed fecal matter that is neither properly retained nor properly voided.

However, the most common local cause of fecal incontinence is gross constipation. Hard masses cause distention or impaction in the anal canal, and there is overflow incontinence of formed stool. Or fecal impaction may be accompanied by a type of mucous diarrhea owing to irritation of the mucosa by hard or breaking-down fecal masses. Thus, the cause of diarrhea is in reality constipation, which seems a contradiction. Nevertheless, fecal impaction and its sequelae are a widespread clinical reality and are first to be excluded in any case of fecal incontinence or diarrhea at this age. In geriatrics, rectal examination is so rewarding as to be worth making routine. Incontinent patients who are mentally normal and have normal anal sensation are of course fully aware of their predicament and deeply embarrassed by it. The distress of elderly patients, who are slowed up by age or disability and who are rendered incontinent by overenthusiastic use of aperients, is extreme.

There is also a large group of elderly patients who are incontinent because of disturbed consciousness (stupor or coma) or who lack normal cortical control because of physical or vascular brain damage or established dementia. The stools of these patients are usually formed, but the patients are often not in the least aware that they are incontinent. Some of them, regrettably, cannot learn to leave their excreta alone. However, patients who soil their hands, their beds, and themselves, should not be accused of dirty habits as if this were willful misbehavior. Very often it is evidence that they feel uncomfortable in the anal region, although they do not understand why, and their hands constantly stray there with inevitable consequences.

In the management of fecal incontinence, it is first essential to detect and remove if possible the local causes, and the need to control constipation cannot be overemphasized. It may require several days of daily enemas to achieve a clear result, after which the patient can make a fresh start.

Even when incontinence is due to a lack of cortical control, it is often possible to inculcate more reasonable habits by careful habit training, much as an infant is trained to the potty. Otherwise, it is sound practice to cause constipation by giving regular doses of kaolin and opium derivatives by mouth and then to control the bowel by regular aperients or enemas. The incontinence is then predictable and manageable; in institutional surroundings, this is a good method, but it is not without risk in the domestic situation.

In summary, fecal incontinence is preventable; it is less frequent and less serious than urinary incontinence, even if it is temporarily the more embarrassing of the two.

Dependence

Many of the elderly depend on their friends or on social services, to a greater or lesser degree. For some, their cherished independence is more imaginary than real. However, it should be part of geriatric practice to preserve the fact or the illusion as long as possible. Any major illness increases dependence on others. If prolonged immobility or confinement to bed is then allowed or insisted on, the feeling of dependence grows rapidly. Some elderly individuals fight against it, but some rejoice in it, being basically dependent personalities who like nothing better than to be physically cared for and protected from psychologic stress and decision making. Either way, the longer it persists the easier it will be to accept this state of dependence.

Incentives to full recovery and independent living may be few, and this is a fundamental difference between practice with old and other ill patients. The first step in the campaign is undoubtedly to get the patient out of bed, dressed in his own day clothes, and into a sitting room away from the area of illness and sick rooms. It is important that the physician in charge should let it be understood that the current illness, even in a very old and frail patient, is expected to have a limited length and that resumption of the earlier level of activity is also to be expected, or at least hoped for. Many elderly patients themselves, and their relatives, consider that whatever the type of illness, resumption of the former way of living is not possible just because these patients are old. To believe this is to deny most of what modern geriatrics stands for.

When it comes to the time for discharge from hospital, many of the elderly, although talking optimistically, are in fact resistant to the idea. They develop fresh symptoms, plan unrealistically to ''have someone in at home,'' or want to go to live with relatives whom they have not even consulted in the matter—anything rather than resume their own responsibilities. In countries where the cost of being in an institution does not fall directly on the patient or his relatives, the latter sometimes encourage continued dependence on the hospital from ulterior motives.

Kindhearted nurses may have to be shown that their instinct to go to the help of an elderly invalid may in fact hinder his recovery and make him increasingly dependent. Many older patients resent being helped and react adversely to it. Some others accept it all too readily and gradually increase their demands, ending up permanently in bed, being literally spoon-fed by exasperated but overconscientious supporters. A good rule is that no elderly patient should ever be helped to do something he can manifestly do for himself. This is not lack of sympathy for old age and disability; it is therapeutic realism.

In the broader view, it must be accepted that no country will have sufficient medical, nursing, and hospital resources to measure up to the problems of an aging population unless invalids who can care for themselves cease to consume services needed for others.

HYPOTHERMIA

People of all ages, when exposed for long periods to intense cold without being able to take countermeasures, may have a severe reduction of body temperature that endangers them. For example, this is a well-known hazard of warfare in Arctic waters. However, only recently has it been shown how commonly this dangerous state occurs in the elderly and infants. The heat-regulating mechanism of the victims seems in adverse circumstances to have been unable to protect them. There are several reasons why the elderly have difficulty in maintaining normal body heat; these include a reduced basal metabolic rate, inability to shiver in some, and failure to discern temperature fluctuations quickly. An up-to-date review of the subject of heat regulation and hypothermia, for general as well as medical readers, is provided by Collins.[8]

In Great Britain, attention was drawn to the dangers of hypothermia in 1958 by Emslie-Smith,[12] and again in 1961 by Duguid and colleagues,[11] writing from Scotland about 23 elderly patients exposed to cold. They were not out-of-doors, but nevertheless 70% of them died. A very severe winter in 1963 led a year later to the publication of several other series, all reporting a high mortality. In retrospect, there seems little doubt that many cases must previously have been missed, perhaps because the clinical thermometers in regular use did not register below 35°C (95.0°F). Many doctors and nurses did not realize that a reading of 35°C on a standard clinical thermometer may in reality mean any temperature whatever below that figure.

In 1965 the Royal College of Physicians of London[31] instituted a hospital survey simultaneously in ten cities in Great Britain. All patients newly admitted to the selected hospitals had their temperatures checked immediately on arrival, and any oral reading at or below 35°C was confirmed with a rectal reading. During the 3 months of a mild winter in 1965, 0.68% of more than 18,000 patients were found to have temperatures below 35°C, although in most cases this had not been suspected clinically. The highest incidence was in infants under 1 year of age and in individuals aged

75 and over. The overall mortality in these hypothermic patients was 37%.

Simple calculation suggested that there would probably have been 9000 patients with low temperatures admitted to all hospitals in Great Britain in that same period. Hypothermia is therefore no small matter in certain climates and under certain living conditions.

The level at which hypothermia can be said to occur has still to be decided: 35°C has often been taken as a convenient dividing line. However, research in the elderly living in their own homes in London suggested that with low ambient temperatures, mouth temperatures of the elderly were frequently below 35°C without any distress being apparent. The range of normality may thus be much wider than is generally understood. Mouth temperatures can be most misleading, and in any case of doubt a rectal reading should be obtained also.

Hypothermia often results from a fall on the ice, with the elderly victim lying some hours without being able to move. Even more frequently, the fall occurs in a cold bedroom. In such circumstances, the label "accidental hypothermia" is appropriate. Many elderly patients, however, are hypothermic when lying in bed and being ministered to by relatives. Some patients have even been discovered in this state when in adequately heated hospital wards. It seems as if, undramatically, their temperature ceases to be maintained. Often, there is an associated long-term disability that interferes with active movement. The condition is found in the course of coma from any cause and in mentally disturbed individuals who are inert and unable to appreciate common dangers.

Hypothermia can occasionally occur in the late stages of hypothyroidism, but in the reported series of hypothermia cases, examples of hypothyroidism have been uncommon. A further group of patients become hypothermic because of chlorpromazine and similar drugs, alcohol, and barbiturates. Finally, in old age, a considerable number of hypothermic patients present with low temperature at the onset of a major illness such as pneumonia, pulmonary embolism, cardiac infarction, and stroke. In some of these patients, fever might have been expected but serious heat loss is found instead, perhaps being a measure of the severity of the illness.

The complications of hypothermia are pneumonia, pancreatitis, multiple infarctions of organs including the heart, and, occasionally, peripheral gangrene. Death is often quite sudden and unexplained, just at the stage when treatment seems to be successful, and the patient's temperature is nearly normal again. This is perhaps due to sudden cardiac arrhythmia.

Clinically, the elderly hypothermic patient often reaches a dangerous state quite gradually, never presenting symptoms or even complaining of being unusually cold. Characteristically, he seems unable to shiver. His consciousness is clouded, and his speech slurred; stupor is followed later by coma, usually when the temperature has reached 26°C to 27°C. His face may be puffy, temporarily resembling myxedema; there are muscular rigidity and a slow pulse, slow respiratory rate, and a decreased blood pressure. The cardinal sign of fully developed hypothermia is skin that feels like cold marble in an area such as the abdominal wall, which is normally always warm. In appearance, contrary to expectation, hypothermic elderly patients are usually not white or ''blue with cold,'' but pink and even ruddy-complexioned.

Hypothermia is never self-reported: its recognition depends on physicians and paramedical workers understanding the social and medical conditions that give rise to this state, recognizing its clinical picture, and being provided with clinical thermometers that range from 24°C to 41°C. This is a vital tool when the practice includes elderly patients or infants in cold climates. Once detected, hypothermia at a level of 32°C or less calls for rapid action, and most cases require hospital admission if the patient can safely be taken there.

The treatment of hypothermia in elderly subjects is still far from satisfactory, and a high mortality persists. In younger individuals, hypothermia induced for surgery can be safely counteracted by active rewarming and so, usually, can hypothermia due to exposure if the victim is young. However, early experience with this method in the elderly resulted in a high death rate, and there followed a sharp reaction toward slow rewarming at not more than 0.5°C per hour, coupled with therapy with such supportive measures as oxygen, intravenous fluids, antibiotics, and hydrocortisone every 6 hours. The use of hydrocortisone has been rejected more recently by a number of workers. The rationale of slow rewarming is that there is reduced risk of sudden loss of the high vasomotor tone already present, which would lead to vasomotor collapse, a fall in blood pressure, and an even further drop of internal temperature—the so-called after drop. However, the cautious rewarming method has not itself resulted in a much better recovery rate. The whole history of clinical hypothermia from its first recognition, including the arguments for and against various regimens of treatment, including methods of artificial rewarming, was reviewed in a major monograph by Maclean and Emslie-Smith in 1977.[23] In 1973, Gregory and Doolittle,[16] reviewing some 200 patients treated by various means, reported an overall mortality of 48.8%. It seems clear throughout that the brisker methods sometimes used for the young are hazardous for the old. We must hope that the greater availablity for elderly patients of intensive care with monitoring and cardiopulmonary resuscitation, perhaps combined with special active rewarming techniques, will eventually give better results.

Because hypothermia in old age responds disappointingly to treatment, it is all the more important to prevent it from happening. This can be achieved by better housing, better heating and storm windows, more suitable clothing, ample hot food and drinks, and the avoidance of alcohol and tranquilizers. It is particularly important that the elderly should keep active and generate heat from within. They must also avoid cold bedrooms. A regular visit by observant friends would help detect the first stage of a decline into hypothermia. Above all, more information is needed about what happens when body temperatures drop to 33°C to 25°C.

HYPERTHERMIA

Isadore Rossman

When environmental temperatures rise above body temperature and are sustained for one or more days, hyperpyrexic episodes may occur in some elderly patients. Direct exposure to the sun need not necessarily precede the attack. In one outbreak I observed, 12 of some 300 elderly patients residing in nursing homes developed hyperpyrexia. None had been out-of-doors. The attacks occurred in summer after a succession of days in which temperatures had exceeded 38°C in facilities that were not air-conditioned.

Premonitory symptoms included apathy, weakness, faintness, and headache. With the onset of hyperthermia, fevers of 39.5°C were observed, associated with tachycardia and weakness and dryness of the skin. There was one death in the group, but most responded promptly to ice packs and intravenous fluids. Most patients showed no significant electrolyte abnormality, indicating that loss of sodium chloride or potassium did not precede the fever.

Hyperthermia is most likely to occur in elderly patients with cerebral atherosclerosis or with diabetes, which indicates that circulatory changes involving thermoregulatory centers in the brain may be of some importance. Because the elderly have a diminished capacity for sweating, they suffer from an impaired capacity to lower body temperature by sweating. Many of them have notably dry skins compared with younger individuals, even on hot, humid days.

Observations on a large number of elderly patients have been reported by Levine.[21] He observed 25 deaths in a group of more than 200 patients who presented to the emergency ward of the Queens County Hospital in New York City during an intense heat wave in 1966. Their average age was 78; only three were under age 70. The average rectal temperature in the fatal cases on admission was 106.4°F. Twenty-one of them were anhidrotic, and five were in shock. Eighteen were comatose and completely unresponsive, even to painful stimuli. Nineteen patients had clinical signs of pulmonary consolidation with radiographic confirmation of pneumonia in seven. Nine patients had a hemorrhagic diathesis; two had meningitis; four were anuric.

The patients were treated with ice water–alcohol sponging, which was as effective as ice baths for rapid lowering of body temperature. Those in shock were improved by infusion with isoproterenol and intravenous fluid therapy, but Levine warns that hypotension or anuria is not necessarily a sign of water depletion in this group.

The high mortality indicates the gravity of heat stroke in the elderly. Half of those whose cases proved fatal had diabetes, again pointing up the disproportionate percentage of patients with diabetes or cerebral atherosclerosis who develop hyperpyrexia. Other predisposing factors include parkinsonism, especially when treated with anticholinergic medications, and cardiovascular disease with or without congestive failure. Extensive reviews of the subject are available.[32]

REFERENCES

1. Agate JN: Pressure Sores. In Brocklehurst JC (ed): Textbook of Geriatric Medicine and Gerontology, 3rd ed. Edinburgh, Churchill Livingstone, in press
2. Barbenel JC, Jordan MM, Clark MO: Incidence of pressure sores in the Greater Glasgow area. Lancet 2:548, 1979
3. Barton AA: Pressure sores: An electron microscope and thermographic study. Mod Geriatr 3:8, 1973
4. Barton AA, Barton M: The clinical and thermographic evaluation of pressure sores. Age and Ageing 2:60, 1973
5. Bedford PD, Cosin L, McCarthy JF, Scott BO: The alternating pressure mattress. Gerontol Clin 3:68, 1961
6. Bliss MR: The use of ripple beds. Age Ageing 7:25, 1978
7. Bliss MR: Clinical research in patient support systems. Care Sci Prac 1:7, 1981
8. Collins KJ: Hypothermia: The Facts. Oxford, Oxford University Press, 1983
9. Constantian MB (ed): Pressure Ulcers. Boston, MA, Little, Brown & Co, 1980
10. David J: The size of the problem of pressure sores. Care Sci Prac 1:10, 1981
11. Duguid H, Simpson RG, Stowers JM: Accidental hypothermia. Lancet 2:1213, 1961
12. Emslie-Smith D: Accidental hypothermia: A common condition with a pathognomonic electrocardiogram. Lancet 2:492, 1958
13. Exton-Smith AN, Sherwin RW: Prevention of pressure sores: Significance of bodily movements. Lancet 2:1124, 1962
14. Exton-Smith AN, Norton D, McClaren R: An investigation of geriatric nursing problems in hospital. London, National Corporation for the Care of Old People, 1962. Reprinted: Edinburgh, Churchill Livingstone, 1975
15. Ferguson-Pell MW, Bell F, Evans JH: In Kenedi RM, Cowden JM, Scales JT (eds): Bedsore Biomechanics. London, Macmillan, 1976
16. Gregory RT, Doolittle JF: Accidental hypothermia: II. Clinical implications of experimental studies. Alaska Med 15:48, 1973
17. Greenfield RA: The L.A.L. bed system. Nursing Times 68:711, 1972
18. Husain T: An experimental study of some pressure effects in tissues, with reference to the bedsore problem. J Pathol Bacteriol 66:347, 1953
19. Jenied P: Static and dynamic support systems: Pressure differences in the body. In Kenedi RM, Cowden JM, Scales JT (eds): Bedsore Biomechanics. London, Macmillan, 1976
20. Kenedi RM, Cowden JM, Scales JT (eds): Bedsore Biomechanics. London, Macmillan, 1976
21. Levine JA: Heat stroke in the aged. Am J Med 47:251, 1969
22. Lowthian PT: Pressure sores: Practical prophylaxis. Nursing Times 72:295, 1976
23. Maclean D, Emslie-Smith D: Accidental Hypothermia. Oxford, Blackwell, 1977
24. Morgan JE: Topical therapy for pressure ulcers. Surg Gynecol Obstet 141:945, 1975
25. Peromet M, Labbe M, Yourassowsky E, Schoutens E: Anaerobic bacteria isolated from decubitus ulcers. Infection 1:205, 1973
26. Petersen NC: The development of pressure sores during hospitalization. In Kenedi RM, Cowden JM, Scales JT (eds): Bedsore Biomechanics. London, Macmillan, 1976
27. Petersen NC, Bittman S: The epidemiology of pressure sores. Scand J Plast Reconstr Surg 5:12, 1971

28. Pories WJ, Herzel JH, Rob CG, Strain WH: Acceleration of wound healing in man with zinc sulphate given by mouth. Lancet 1:121, 1967
29. Redfern SJ, Jenied PA, Gillingham NE, Lunn HF: Local pressures with ten types of patient support systems. Lancet 2:277, 1973
30. Reswick JB, Rogers JE: Experience with devices and techniques to prevent pressure sores. In Kenedi RM, Cowden JM, Scales JT (eds): Bedsore Biomechanics. London, Macmillan, 1976
31. Royal College of Physicians of London: Report of Committee on Accidental Hypothermia, 1966
32. Shibolet S, Lancaster MC, Danyon Y: Heat stroke: A review. Aviat Space Environ Med 47:280, 1976

9 Common Symptoms and Complaints

John Agate

The natural history of diseases may be considerably altered in old age. It should be expected that any modifications would arise not so much from variations in the potency of infecting organisms or pathologic processes, or even the invasiveness of tumors, but from the altered physiology of aging humans, their less flexible homeostatic mechanisms, and the reduced preparedness of their defensive mechanisms.

It is becoming clear that there is a changing incidence, with respect to age, of a number of infections. Infective diseases that some decades ago were most often found in children or young adults, such as bacterial meningitis, are being discovered more in older patients.[3] Bacteremia or septicemia secondary to established infections, notably of the lungs or genitourinary or gastrointestinal tracts, are menacing the elderly increasingly, and bacterial endocarditis is moving in this direction, too.[2] How much these trends are the consequence of the widespread modern use of antibiotics and altered bacterial responses to them, and how much to the frailty of old age and its altered immune responses, is a matter for debate.

Clinically, a decline in the vigorousness of defensive response is usually manifested by fewer findings and complaints. As an example, temperature-regulating mechanisms are less reliable in the elderly, and their heat-generating activity is reduced. Indeed, one of the most common variants in the natural history of disease is the finding that an older patient cannot work up the high temperature usually expected in acute infection. Pyrexia may be late in appearing, or it may never appear at all. Even when it does, the level is seldom higher than 39.5°C. A physician who waits for pyrexia before diagnosing pneumonia risks losing his patient while he waits. Tachycardia and tachypnea

are far more sensitive indicators of chest infection and must be acted on with promptness. Similarly, rigors are quite exceptional in older patients, even in the presence of such a disorder as acute pyelonephritis. A high, swinging fever, which offers so many diagnostic possibilities earlier in life, most often indicates in an old person a hidden localization of pus such as a lung or perinephric abscess. By contrast, several conditions result in an uncontrollable decrease in body temperature rather than a rise. The conventional temperature chart is of limited use to a geriatric physician; he has much more need of one that covers the subnormal range. Good physicians and experienced nurses in this field develop a special sensitivity to changes in facial appearance and color and to small increases in respiratory rate, which arouse their suspicions before the usual instrumentation and charting does.

Other variants are legion. It is, for example, rare for sepsis to evoke regional lymphadenopathy; yet in certain conditions such as the recticuloses and secondary carcinomatosis, regional lymph nodes may enlarge with astonishing rapidity, even in a nonagenarian. Disorders in which pain is usually expected are often found to be surprisingly pain-free in the elderly. The most outstanding examples are cardiac infarction and various acute abdominal conditions. Thus, Pathy,[4] in an excellent analysis of the presentations of cardiac infarction in the elderly, found chest pain was felt in only 19% of cases. Conversely in numbers of cases in which there is complaint of chest pain, the cause turns out to be a hiatal hernia, diverticulum, or other esophageal or high gastric disorder. In old age, the gullet is a notorious mimic. As for the acute abdomen, it is well recognized to be "silent" in old age, and many cases of perforated appendix or diverticulum, mesenteric infarction, or other catastrophes are misdiagnosed because pain is not evident and the textbook signs are absent.

In this chapter some of the more common symptoms are discussed, not from the systematic standpoint of causation and treatment, but from the viewpoint of a physician who must consider them in special ways when he is dealing with elderly patients. Many of these symptoms are wrongly regarded by philosophically minded patients as the natural consequence of aging and therefore not worth mentioning to a busy physician. These symptoms, indeed all symptoms, may have to be positively sought by questioning, for as Williamson and co-workers[7] showed, self-reporting of illness is notoriously unreliable.

BLINDNESS

Aside from presbyopia, poor vision is not so inevitable as many of the elderly expect. However, if blindness does come on gradually, many patients do not regard it as other than something requiring a change of glasses. Some, who are mentally very active, are depressed at the final realization of this new disability, but few have enough insight to learn their way about safely or to learn braille while they still have some sight left. After going blind the elderly find braille too hard to learn. Gradually failing sight may be the underlying reason for gradually decreasing mobility and domestic capability, poor orientation, and even the occurrence of frightening visual impressions that are so bizarre as to seem like hallucinations. People who live with older relatives sometimes entirely fail to realize how bad their eyesight has become, and so, occasionally do their physicians. Elderly patients in whom cataracts are developing may say that direct light in their eyes causes a glare, so they sit with their backs to windows, and some wear lightly tinted spectacles. Others, however, persist in using dramatically dark glasses, even indoors, or a green eyeshade, claiming that daylight is too much for them. Sadly, this is usually just a histrionic attention-seeking gesture.

The sudden onset of blindness in one eye may indicate retinal detachment, hemorrhage, or retinal vein thrombosis, but in old age consideration must urgently be given to this being retinopathy from giant-cell arteritis; if it is, really prompt treatment with corticosteroids may sometimes save the patient's vision. This condition may be bilateral or may spread quickly to the other eye. Patients struck by this disease say they are suddenly afflicted as if "a blind had been drawn across the eye." Sometimes much more blindness is present than would be expected from an examination of the optic fundus.

Many elderly patients have had no vision in one eye for many years and subsist on the other, which when it also loses sight, is a major disaster for them. Sudden apparent loss of vision in two previously healthy eyes is seldom hysterical in old age unless there is already a history of gross hysterical reactions. It is, however, not uncommonly due to an occipital cortical lesion from a stroke. Some older people with this essentially cortical blindness persist in saying they can see various objects when they are looking in quite a different direction and obviously cannot see at all. This denial is a particular characteristic of cortical blindness in the aged.

Even though blindness is common and a serious handicap, the more so if it comes on too late in life to be accepted and compensated for, it is sometimes remediable, as by lens extraction. This is an entirely justifiable operation at almost any age if the ophthalmic indications are good, especially if it will restore freedom of movement and independence to a "go-ahead" personality. Characteristically, a blind old person who may be lost and apparently dependent in a strange environment such as a hospital ward, is often far safer and more active when restored to his usual home surroundings.

DEAFNESS

Impaired hearing is not inevitable in old age, but some degree of loss is very common, especially that for high-pitched sounds. Although audiograms reveal this high-tone loss also, it is quite common for elderly patients to be able to hear female voices better than male voices. Significant loss may not extend down as far as 3500 cycles per second, so conversational ability may not be affected, even though an older person may not be able to hear the song of birds, orchestral piccolos, or the tick of his watch. In later life, deafness is usually perceptive or nerve deafness, although conduction deafness is not rare. Conduction deafness may have occurred earlier in life, with nerve deafness adding to the disability in old age. With each succeeding decade, there is an increase in the proportion of deaf people, and men are more often affected than women. Deafness is more often noticed in general than personal conversation, or at committee tables, and it causes the victim to withdraw from public work and often to become less sociable.

At any age, deafness is a sad symptom; it elicits little sympathy because it involves other people in effort and frustration. This is particularly true when the victim is aged. The attitudes of others often cause bitterness in elderly deaf people, who feel excluded, become suspicious, may be less and less well oriented, and may even become paranoid in their reactions. Many older sufferers fail to appreciate how severe their deafness is until a late stage, by which time it may be too late to learn lipreading or sign language.

Many extremely deaf elderly patients are so egocentric that they pay no attention to the efforts being made to get through to them; many are already too old or ineducable to take up the use of an electronic hearing aid, although some of them can hear through an old-fashioned ear trumpet or the modern equivalent, which has a flexible tube. But no one can claim to have done his best for a deaf patient until some sort of aid has been suggested and given a trial. A hearing aid requires some manual dexterity in use, besides an understanding of the instrument itself.

Highly efficient, small, portable amplifiers, used with a hand-held microphone and high-grade earphones for the listener, are now available for straight person-to-person interviews, and these sometimes allow very deaf individuals at last to communicate after years of not hearing anything.

Sometimes when a deaf person suffers a stroke and needs rehabilitation, there is no progress whatever until someone thinks of providing a hearing aid; then the physiotherapist begins to succeed dramatically. Because strokes are common in later life, the physician often must determine whether the patient's apparent lack of response to what he says is due to deafness, to receptive or even motor aphasia, or to clouded consciousness. Similarly, an elderly person who is totally deaf and responds to all questions with a blank expression or a polite smile is dismissed occasionally as being mentally abnormal, even though one written question might have revealed the truth. Such mistakes are avoided if a relative is available at the interview. Deafness is naturally a serious added disability when a patient is already mentally abnormal. Some demented patients are entirely mute, so one can only guess whether they can hear.

In all cases of deafness, it is important to help the patient as much as possible by speaking face-to-face and at the correct height, using simple phrases and exaggerated lip movements, in the hope that he will see what he cannot hear or get the meaning of what is going on from the play of facial expression. Some patients who have a reputation for being uncooperative also show selective deafness—they hear what is advantageous to them but apparently cannot hear anything else. Sometimes this is blatant and inexcusable. Much apparent deafness is not deafness at all but failure to properly attend to what the other person is saying.

The speech of those individuals who have been deaf a long time is usually loud, harsh, and badly articulated, affecting their relationships with others. The elderly deaf deserve much more general sympathy; they are seldom as serene as the elderly blind.

FATIGUE

Elderly patients attempting strenuous sustained effort are easily fatigued; they cannot produce maximum effort or rapid movements for very long. This differs however, from the subjective symptom of general fatigue of which the elderly person often complains. Later in life, many routine tasks can only be performed slowly and laboriously, and at a very advanced age every commonplace activity seems to call for great effort. The loss of vigor is only too apparent to the patient himself. There is, in addition, an unfounded general notion that the elderly somehow ought to be tired and so should have everything done for them while they themselves take the "rest" that is said to be their main requirement. Anyone who really believes this fails to understand the essence of modern geriatric practice, in which graded return to activity after illness alone spells success. Some very old people remain full of bustling activity, but most spend the greater part of their days relatively inactive and so have little reason to feel fatigued.

Among younger patients, fatigue often points to psychosomatic disorders, anxiety, and unresolved stressful situations. This type of illness is relatively uncommon in older people, who are not subject to quite the same pressures. However, fatigue coupled with marked inactivity and negativism may strongly suggest depression. Sometimes fatigue is a symptom of boredom in a patient who has no occupation and few contacts or who is isolated by blindness or deafness. For such patients, the days are long and empty, whereas for the active-minded, the greater their age the faster time seems to pass.

Persistent or recurrent fatigue is commonly a symptom of organic disease. Naturally it is to be expected in cachexia and wasting illnesses generally, but it should also suggest a search for anemias of gradual onset. It is a prominent symptom in heart disease, in which it may be complained of as much as dyspnea. It accompanies congestive heart failure and states of low blood pressure, but in particular left ventricular failure and cases of ischemic heart disease in which the heart is very large and close to failing. Fatigue and lassitude, sometimes appearing dramatically, can be symptoms of severe hypokalemia. Finally, many elderly people spend a great deal of time dozing and complaining of supposed tiredness, when in fact they are victims of overenthusiastic sedation, perhaps from the mistaken idea that they need so much more rest than younger people. Nonagenarians often sleep a lot but are not necessarily unduly fatigued.

HEADACHE

In young and middle-aged adults headache is a ubiquitous symptom reflecting, no doubt, the many tensions of a competitive existence. Later in life, headache seems to be less common. If it is true that old age is full of problems, then it is odd that this reaction of the overwrought parent and worried breadwinner should be less a problem to the grandparent. It follows from this that when severe headache does occur in an older patient, it is something that ought not to be ignored.

Many physicians believe that migraine disappears later in life. In some patients, it is modified, or the attacks are reduced in frequency, but many patients continue to suffer as they always did. Elderly patients may sometimes experience typical occipital, muscle-tension headache. When they do, it may be the result of their habit of stooping and inclining forward, with the inevitable muscular and ligamentous strains; or it may be associated with the cervical spondylosis so common in old age. Conversely, the pain associated with coryza and acute infection of paranasal sinuses seems to be rare. Severe periodic headache of a preoccupying type should lead one to suspect a space-occupying lesion within the skull, and a chronic subdural hematoma in particular, because this is common and remediable, if recognized in time.

Finally, severe temporal headache or facial pain in an elderly person makes the geriatric physician search for any evidence of giant-cell arteritis. This is not excluded by the failure to find signs of in-

flammation and tenderness in the temporal vessels themselves, for other vessels can be affected similarly. A raised sedimentation rate and a disturbed electrophoretic pattern may point more certainly to this diagnosis.

SLEEP AND INSOMNIA

We are in the early phase of research on the normal sleeping habits of the elderly. However, certain trends appear from observation of aged patients at home and in hospitals. There is obviously much variation in their individual sleep requirements, just as there is at all ages. It is not true, however, that old people necessarily need more sleep because they are old. If they allow themselves more sleep than active younger people do, it is often because of boredom or because they take sedatives that they may not even need. Often persistent drowsiness is a symptom of disease such as uremia, heart failure, or respiratory insufficiency.

The quality of sleep may change with age. The young adult, working, playing hard, and getting properly tired, sleeps well. The older person, not working, perhaps not employing his mental faculties fully, being too physically handicapped to exert much real muscular effort, and seldom going into the open air, is lacking the best inducements to sound sleep. This difference in quality of sleep also makes itself felt in intelligent middle-aged people who are working hard, often late at night, and have too little physical exercise and relaxation. Besides, the older person's sleep is often interrupted by pain of various kinds, especially rheumatic pains, the distressing ischemic pain of peripheral vascular disease affecting the feet and legs, leg cramps that are not necessarily ischemic, and above all by the need to urinate at night. The latter is a common preoccupation, even in the absence of bladder or kidney disease or diabetes. In men aged 60, about one in four needs to rise to urinate at night, but at 85 the proportion is nine in ten.

Most insomnia is a consequence of various discomforts, or else it is evidence of a psychiatric upset. In the presence of anxiety, there is usually some difficulty in falling asleep at night. With depression, the tendency is for the patient to wake early and to toss and turn. Both these disorders are common in elderly people. Unfortunately, the elderly are often without strong intellectual interests, or they have bad eyesight and poor concentration, so it is not so easy for them to while away the sleepless hours with a book or handwork.

The attitudes of elderly patients to supposed sleeplessness are instructive. Some of them, even when under observation in the hospital, claim that they "hardly sleep a wink" all night, even though their nurses report that these patients have had several hours of intermittent sleep. Many more of them are convinced they must above all things have a great deal of extra repose, and in this they are often encouraged by their relatives. These elderly patients, along with another group who are lonely, bored, or cold, tend to go to bed at 6:00 or 7:00 PM, having perhaps slept during the afternoon as well. They then cannot understand why they wake early and cannot get to sleep again. When this point is made, most elderly patients and their relatives acknowledge that they should not sleep in the daytime and expect to take a full quota at night. They may even accept that an older person who is active to the point of fatigue will sleep better.

Many patients have taken regular hypnotic drugs for alleged insomnia for years and cannot contemplate a night without their help. Some of them take such large doses that they are drowsy all next morning, not to say a little muddled. By this means, they may develop a reversed sleep rhythm in which finally they become restless and confused at night, disturbing their family and neighbors, but sleep all through the next day instead. This can be the outcome of the present widespread tendency to give sedative drugs. Therefore, in any case of obstreperous behavior and wandering at night, all drug treatment should be stopped to determine if a normal sleep rhythm will reestablish itself. In geriatric work, it is generally necessary for doctors and nurses to resist the temptation to use hypnotics, not only for these reasons but because they increase the chances of pressure sores, pneumonia, incontinence, general amnesia, disorientation, and falls on rising from bed. Barbiturates are particularly harmful when they are used in this way and are usually best avoided.

In the management of insomnia, it is essential to eliminate pain and discomfort first, and it is especially unforgivable to allow a dying patient to suffer insomnia and nocturnal pain for lack of appropriate drugs. This whole subject has been reviewed by Saunders and associates, and in particular by Twycross.[6] Next, reassurance is vital, although at least by the time they are old, those individuals with extensive experience of insomnia know it does not threaten their lives or sanity. Many are helped by a regular nightcap of an alcoholic drink. Some need to be told to restrict their fluid intake in the latter half of the day to reduce the need for night rising, but at the same time they must be warned to take enough fluid in the morning to compensate. Patients with heart failure or who are taking diuretics are helped to get the sleep they need by catheterization. Some patients can relax with the help of an electric blanket, with suitable safeguards.

If drugs are needed, in place of barbiturates it is better to use chloral (in the form of dichloralphenazone tablets, 0.6 g to 1.2 g), glutethimide (250 mg to 500 mg), or methaqualone (250 mg). Methaqualone is now out of favor because it has been abused by younger people. Alternative hypnotic preparations with few side-effects for geriatric patients are chlormethiazole edisylate (250–500 mg, tablet or a syrup) and nitrazepam (5 mg), but occasionally as small a dose as 2 mg of diazepam will suffice. Some restless and hyperactive elderly patients respond well to drugs of the phenothiazine group at night, given as a syrup—for example, 250 mg to 100 mg of chlorpromazine or promazine. When there is no response to these drugs, but when sleep is urgent for both patient and those near him, paraldehyde (5 ml to 10 ml given intramuscularly) is as effective as, but less dangerous than, most other powerful drugs.

DYSPHAGIA

A common complaint of elderly patients, dysphagia, must not be ignored, because it is seldom a functional symptom, and it is very rarely simulated. Localization by the patient of the point of difficulty in swallowing is often remarkably accurate, but this cannot be completely relied on because the elderly are often poor historians and even worse observers of their own functions. There are many grades and types of dysphagia. Sometimes the patient attempts to swallow and finds that solid food sticks at a certain point on the way, although fluids are swallowed more easily. Some patients appear to swallow but regurgitate undigested food soon afterward. Some very frail subjects seem to chew for many minutes without being able to get the bolus past the root of the tongue. Eventually they reject it, the effort of swallowing seeming too great even when the normal swallowing reflex is intact.

It is common for the patient to be terrified of swallowing because he fears food will be aspirated. This is seen in stroke patients with involvement of the mechanism of deglutition and particularly in pseudobulbar palsy of cerebrovascular origin. Here the picture is of dysphagia, dysarthria, emotionalism, and impaired locomotion, even though individual limb function is affected very little, if at all. In this state, the patient and everyone else concerned are caused untold anxiety because the risk of choking or aspirational pneumonia is very real and long-lasting. This form of dysphagia is remarkably common among geriatric patients; some of them thus afflicted must put up with long-term nasogastric intubation, although eventually a fair degree of recovery of normal swallowing can be expected. Very occasionally, such a patient must rely on the tube for the rest of his life.

Globus hystericus and the dysphagia of Plummer-Vinson syndrome in iron deficiency states are very occasionally seen in the elderly, but diagnosis of these disorders should only be made by exclusion of other causes. Compared with these, the organic causes of dysphagia are many and varied. They are best considered according to the level at which they seem to cause difficulty. Thus, they include, at the upper end of the tract, abnormalities of the root of the tongue, the fauces, and the pharynx, including at that point pouches, carcinoma, and abscess formation.

Carcinoma of the larynx sometimes manifests itself as dysphagia. Postcricoid carcinoma is particularly found in women, and midesophageal carcinoma is somewhat more common in men. However, it would not be correct to assume that all obstruction at the upper end or midpoint of the esophagus is neoplastic, because in old age there frequently are benign diverticula and various conditions involving involuntary muscle spasm that produce pain and dysphagia: they even mimic angina pectoris. It is common to find on fluoroscopy that the elderly esophagus is tortuous and like a corkscrew in appearance, and it may have traction diverticula that fill and empty and cause pain as this happens.

It is just as true of old people as of younger people that bronchial carcinoma rarely causes dysphagia, and even gross unfolding of the aorta from atheroma, which is very common, is also symptomless. When there are swallowing difficulties at the lower end of the esophagus, neoplasia is naturally suspected first. Achalasia is uncommon in the elderly. On the other hand, hiatal hernia is widespread and often leads to reflux esophagitis if it is of the sliding type, with dysphagia being the most common symptom. Occasionally, elderly patients, especially those who are muddled and disoriented, swallow large pieces of bone or even their own dentures and are not clear about what happened. Before long, severe dysphagia appears.

In dysphagia of sudden onset, a quick digital examination of the lower pharynx is worthwhile, indeed obligatory.

ANOREXIA

The appetites of elderly people are quite variable. Some eat voraciously, almost to the point of gluttony, and as a result are obese: food is perhaps their sole remaining pleasure. This sort of habit has probably persisted throughout their lives. Others, again governed by habit, have very small appetites. It is common to find thin, wiry old people who claim to have always been small and eaten little, and it is tempting to relate their longevity to their specially temperate behavior. When considering the food to be offered during illness, therefore, it is advisable to have the particular patient's usual appetite in mind. If the illness is of a toxic or pyrexial nature, old patients lose their appetites completely and are content to exist for days or weeks on fluids only. Appetite is probably the last thing to recover. In the meantime, fortunately, fortified casein hydrolysates and other balanced fluid preparations can be used. If the appetite lags, convalescence in such cases is likely to be prolonged because strength and vitality take longer than usual to be rebuilt.

Patients who have had a partial gastrectomy usually complain of poor appetite. Anorexia also occurs, although not as the presenting symptom, in renal failure and uremia, and with liver disease. By contrast, anorexia is often the initial symptom of which older patients with gastric carcinoma complain, and it is also a significant early finding in depressive states, being part of the general picture of nihilism and hopelessness.

Anorexia nervosa is not found in elderly women. True, certain old people are determined not to eat and are not anxious even to survive. They do not try to outwit their nurses; they simply refuse food, or having taken mouthfuls, spit it out again. It is an ethical problem to decide how far they should be pressed in the matter. There is also a group of very thin, frail, but apparently mentally normal old people, mostly women, whose appetites remain very poor at all times and who have to be coaxed to take every mouthful of food. Sometimes no cause for this ever appears, but some are found to be under long-term therapy with sedatives or digitalis preparations without very clear indications.

Before the stage of vomiting and bradycardia, anorexia is a useful indication of digitalis overdosage, to which so many older patients are unexpectedly sensitive. Some women patients without good appetites must be suspected of having gastritis caused by swallowing their sputum. Bronchitis and pneumonia affect them very commonly, but it is nevertheless unusual to find older women spontaneously expectorating; some need to be encouraged to do so, and some seem constitutionally incapable of it.

In geriatric nursing practice, lack of appetite is an important and frustrating matter. It affects many patients with small reserves at the height of their illnesses, making it difficult to maintain proper nutritional levels just when they are most needed. It causes their nurses hours of extra work in coaxing and in the slow business of spoon-feeding. If the appetite of these elderly invalids is fickle, there is all the more reason to present their food appetizingly, hot, and in portions of reasonable size. Institutional catering is often at fault in this respect. Activity is a stimulus to appetite, but generally drugs are not. Sometimes a glass of sherry or dry white wine helps a patient who is used to an appetizer. Older patients generally like strongly flavored food, perhaps because their senses of smell and taste have become blunted over the years. So often invalid diets are made insipid and do nothing to help them in their difficulty.

DYSPNEA

As a symptom and sign in geriatric practice, breathlessness can be both helpful and misleading. With increasing age and in the absence of disease, there is a steady decline in lung function. Vital capacity (a crude but simple measurement) falls, and so do diffusing capacity and maximum voluntary ventilatory capacity, whereas the residual volume of the lung rises. These factors must progressively increase breathlessness in aging subjects when they are making any effort at all. More of the elderly would be quite breathless except that they naturally tend to limit their physical exertions. Many seem to expect that old age will make them breathless and so do not bother to comment on it. Whether for this reason or for others, it often happens that the elderly are dyspneic at rest, yet they have either failed to report it or actually deny it.

Dyspnea is a clear symptom of obesity in old age and is regrettably common; equally, it may point to anemia. More specifically, it is a symptom

of lung disease of all kinds and of heart disease. In the course of respiratory tract infections, an increase in the resting respiratory rate is of fundamental and sometimes urgent significance. It may be followed soon afterward by a rise in pulse rate, but it usually appears before there is any fever. In fact, contrary to what is found in younger people, there may be no rise or even a fall of temperature as a chance finding; therefore, dyspnea is all the more important. The ability to detect quickly a slight upward trend in respiratory rate is a most valuable asset in doctor, nurse, or administrator of a home caring for the elderly.

In heart disease, especially in right ventricular failure, the dyspnea that might be expected is often made light of by the older patient. Perhaps he has been leading a very sedentary life at best. Perhaps by instinct and experience he has learned to live within his limitations; perhaps he thinks it is the natural accompaniment of his years. However, in straightforward left ventricular failure in older subjects, urgent dyspnea at night is a very real, common, and distressing symptom, calling for urgent treatment. Many elderly sufferers have learned to sleep well propped up on their pillows without understanding why they do this. Many patients with chronic cardiopulmonary insufficiency are permanently breathless even at rest; but this syndrome has its beginnings in middle age, and it is not conducive to a very long life.

Pulmonary embolism causing acute dyspnea occurs in patients of all ages, but it is not as common in the elderly as the very high incidence of the condition would make one expect. In older people, pulmonary embolism is frequently a cause of sudden death, but otherwise the dramatic cardiac collapse with tachycardia, color change, and catastrophic fall of blood pressure may be seen without much increase in respiratory rate. On the other hand, sudden dyspnea may indicate inhalation of a foreign body, or else acute collapse of a lobe of the lung from a plug of mucus. This calls for urgent postural drainage or bronchoscopic suction.

A few elderly patients are obsessed with the idea of not being able to breathe, a condition amounting to a neurosis, and they either complain of being smothered or display deep, long, sighing respirations and talk about "not getting enough air in." They show no abnormal physical signs, have an excellent color, and can usually be induced to hold their breath voluntarily for long periods.

Hysterical overbreathing, leading sometimes as

far as tetany, can sometimes be observed in both old men and old women. On the other hand, persistent deep, panting respirations in an ill-looking patient on the verge of coma strongly suggest acidosis. Finally, it is quite common for the relatives of elderly invalids to speak of their many "dreadful attacks of breathlessness" when it turns out that these patients are having periodic Cheyne-Stokes respiration. This is very common in old age: sometimes it is as serious a matter as it would be in a younger patient, but very often it can come and go intermittently over a matter of weeks or months without any noteworthy change in the patient's state. Some such patients are even capable of some physical activity while still subject to periodic breathing. In old age, periodic breathing might be due to some coarseness or inaccuracy of acid–base control; there is a link here with cerebral disease and perhaps with variable cardiac output caused by myocardial ischemia.

VERTIGO

A complaint of giddiness or dizziness is one of the most widespread spontaneous symptoms among the elderly, even when they are apparently well. Sheldon,[5] in his classic monograph on the status of older people in Wolverhampton, England, who were well enough to be in their own homes, found that over half spoke of symptoms suggesting vertigo. It is not helpful to try to define too closely what dizziness, giddiness, and vertigo might mean to an old person. These are subjective sensations that are always unpleasant and sometimes frightening. They indicate instability of posture, some immediate spatial disorientation, and in severer forms a sensation of rotation and extreme distress.

The fear of recurrence may haunt the sufferer and seriously undermine his self-confidence, even when he has never fallen during an attack. This fear may make him give up walking altogether, even with canes. Occasionally, an elderly patient with a liking for inactivity who knows that a claim to suffer from "giddiness" is a symptom no doctor can absolutely identify will use it for an excuse for never walking. Most complaints of vertigo, however, are real.

There are innumerable possible causes, including a simple syncopal tendency, severe progressive anemia, acute gastrointestinal hemorrhage, carotid sinus syndrome, postural hypotension, hypertension, changes of cardiac rhythm, episodes of cardiac infarction, and minor cerebrovascular insuf-

ficiency including that of the basilar system. More localized causes are wax in the ears, middle-ear disease, acoustic neuroma, acute labyrinthitis, and paroxysmal labyrinthine vertigo (Ménière's disease). The latter is fairly common in elderly patients, causing them most urgent distress as they cling to their beds in an agony of rotational vertigo, nausea, and vomiting. Patients with persistent vertigo should certainly have the benefit of an otorhinolaryngologist's advice and of a complete examination by a physician with particular reference to neurologic and cardiologic pathology and to the possibility of hypotension.

One particular cause of giddiness can quickly be remedied—the overenergetic use of drugs. Salicylates and quinidine in high dosage are notorious in this respect; so are even normal doses of barbiturates (although this is less recognized) and antihypertensive drugs. Barbiturates are generally unsuitable hypnotics for the elderly, often causing considerable mental confusion, nocturnal giddiness, and falls. Antihypertensive drug therapy is often more distressing and attended by more risk than the hypertension it is used for. Many patients recognize that this group of drugs makes them dizzy and stop taking them, although they sometimes do not tell their physician for fear of hurting his feelings.

When inquiry and investigation have all been completed, there remains a baffling group of patients whose vertigo has no apparent cause, and who in their attacks may not even display nystagmus. Senile degeneration of the labyrinth has been suggested, but until this can be proved or disproved histologically it cannot be offered as a satisfactory explanation.

Those who suffer from vertigo are only too willing to cooperate in its treatment. They must be particularly careful not to precipitate sudden changes in the general or the cerebral circulation, so they must rise slowly from their beds or chairs and not make fast rotational movements of their heads. A cane or stable walking aid is necessary. Treatment with antihistamine drugs used for travel sickness may also help them.

FAINTING, FITS, AND ATTACKS

The elderly are prone to a great variety of happenings that are described in various ways but most often simply as "my attacks." Because patients are alarmed or have disturbed consciousness at the time and because they are often in the company of equally elderly friends or relatives, the physician seldom obtains a clear history of what took place. Even in hospital wards, a completely objective account of the happening is rarely obtained from the experienced nursing staff, nor are immediate observations of pulse, color, blood pressure, and focal signs that could establish the diagnosis obtained. Nonprofessional observers are often too emotionally involved to be objective.

Nevertheless, these attacks, whatever their nature, may result in profound feelings of insecurity on the part of the patient and his friends, for they might occur again in embarrassing circumstances or be a danger to the patient. Many of the victims therefore are kept in chairs or confined to bed for safety's sake, or the relatives may be advised never to let them live alone again for fear of what might happen. Conversely, the relatives themselves may demand that the patient be admitted to a hospital or nursing home. These attacks may therefore assume a pressing medicosocial importance, and the need for a positive diagnosis and prophylactic measures if possible is overwhelming. If, as seems likely from various sorts of evidence, the elderly organism has some difficulty in maintaining good cardiac output and adequate peripheral circulation, and if in particular the cerebral circulation is already at a critical level, it is not surprising that small adverse happenings cause disturbed consciousness, fainting, or unexpected falls.

Major fits or epilepsy are certainly seen in old age, and quite often they appear then for the first time in the patient's life. This may be the initial sign of a stroke or of a serious cardiac infarction. Many other possibilities suggest themselves, but when they have been explored by routine investigations, including lumbar puncture, it often turns out that the epilepsy is simply evidence of local cerebral ischemia from an atheromatous plaque. Also, epileptoid incidents in old age are often of the focal Jacksonian type and are also due to cerebral atheroma.

Simple syncope occurs in older people, although it must not be taken too easily at face value. Vasomotor instability may be an acceptable explanation of the event in an adolescent, but in an older patient full investigation including electrocardiography is necessary. Some fainting is due to a sudden fall in blood pressure, to anemia, and, in particular, to the cerebral anoxia that results from severe melena that has yet to manifest itself.

A sudden attack of vertigo, weakness, and perhaps a convulsion on turning the neck suggest increased sensitivity of the carotid sinus. The carotid sinus syndrome can be positively reproduced sometimes by making the patient do exactly what precipitated his first attack. A rather similar occurrence is the sudden loss or disturbance of consciousness that results from hyperextension of the neck because the vertebral vessels, already atheromatous and tortuous, have been temporarily occluded in their bony canals. This may explain why some elderly patients fall dramatically when they reach up to high shelves or climb onto high chairs to shut upper windows.

A form of falling commonly observed in the elderly is the so-called drop attack. Attacks of this kind have not as yet been adequately explained. They happen while the patient is standing up, perhaps at the kitchen sink. Then suddenly, without warning but without disturbed consciousness, the patient's legs give way, and he finds himself on the floor. At this point, there apparently is a condition of complete muscular flaccidity in the legs, and the patient cannot get up no matter how hard he tries. This loss of normal tonus may last from a minute to hours. However, if he can get the soles of his feet against some firm object, tone and power return at once, and he can get up and continue as if nothing had happened. This syndrome may explain why some people fall and continue to lie on the ground in danger of exposure and hypothermia, even though they are rational and conscious.

Another form of attack is a hypoglycemic episode. Spontaneous hypoglycemia occurs even in old age, but in most cases it takes place during the treatment of diabetes. True, the diabetes of old age is usually mild and readily controlled, but the elderly are unreliable in the matter of dieting, and their appetites are fickle. They are often forgetful and muddled, and the physician may be faced with a patient who is in a hypoglycemic attack, although there is no evidence that he is diabetic. A blood glucose estimation is the first step in the investigation of any unexplained coma in old age, the more so because the state of unrelieved hypoglycemia is so liable to precipitate cardiac infarction or a cerebrovascular accident in these patients. Oral antidiabetic agents are particularly helpful to the elderly diabetic who cannot administer insulin to himself, but such patients are often unexpectedly sensitive to these drugs, which are as capable of producing hypoglycemic coma as insulin is.

Sudden attacks of cardiovascular causation are very common in old people. Some of them precipitate a sudden drop in blood pressure. Some may have done so, and yet the blood pressure has returned to normal only a few minutes later. So, fainting, fits, and falling may be evidence of cardiac infarction without pain, a very common happening indeed. If, after such an event, a triple rhythm is found on auscultation that was not present before, and for which no cause such as hypertension can be found, then electrocardiography is needed. Attacks of paroxysmal atrial tachycardia or paroxysmal fibrillation may be profoundly disturbing to an older patient and may result in collapse, near panic, prostration, and sometimes sudden diuresis. A high pulse rate suggests the diagnosis; however, this may in reality be caused by a new cardiac infarction. Adams-Stokes attacks from conduction defects, with or without a changing degree of block, are probably much more common in geriatric patients than in other age-groups, and these attacks are an indication for insertion of a pacemaker, even in old age. The diagnosis is established if at the moment of the attack a cool-headed observer gets a finger to the pulse. Even very aged patients can subsist for months or years in spite of atrioventricular dissociation if they are given appropriate treatment. Twenty-four-hour electrocardiographic monitoring of the pulse has taught us much about the "attacks" to which the elderly are subject.

There remains a group of happenings that by exclusion of other causes must be attributable to functional illness. Overbreathing, with consequent alkalosis tetany, is not uncommon in old women and some old men, although the classic carpopedal spasms and Chvostek's sign may be hard to elicit. The spectacle of dramatic dyspnea in a mute patient may be terrifying to equally elderly relatives, and the situation must be handled with great tact, for an elderly husband or wife and even a devoted offspring may not like to be told that this illness has no organic basis. So, likewise, one must tread carefully in the face of any of the hysterical manifestations—bizarre histrionic twitchings, gross intermittent bed-shaking, tremors, sprawling on the floor, and strange fits. Thus, the patient, growing self-centered, may believe that he is neglected, underestimated, or unloved; so he brings attention to himself in this fashion. It is often the last resort of someone who realizes he cannot meet the situation by verbal or physical remonstrance.

Hysterical episodes may be directed against the authority of a particular nurse or may appear when the physician declares that time has come to leave the hospital for home when the patient prefers the security of the ward. While it is best and kindest to give an elderly, insecure patient the

benefit of any initial doubt, it is important to recognize hysteria for what it is and act firmly. Otherwise, the effect on relatives and nursing staff morale may be serious and ineradicable, and the patient, having thus achieved his ends, will be in a commanding position ever afterward. Most geriatric departments have a patient or two who cannot be dislodged because of dramatic attacks that are hysterical but that were not recognized and firmly handled years ago.

Finally, it is necessary to consider what attitude ought to be adopted toward these various attacks. If a diagnosis can be made, prophylactic treatment can sometimes be given and a reasonable prognosis made. In some attacks, such as overbreathing, hysterical outbursts, and even drop attacks, it is not expected that the patient will injure himself. In others, such as Adams-Stokes attacks and grand mal that cannot be fully controlled, there is certainly a risk of injury. If the patient normally lives alone, it is correct to consider if he should be placed where help is likely to be prompt. However, it is not realistic to insist that under no circumstances must the patient be left alone, as some physicians attempt to do. The price a member of the family has to pay to obey this order strictly is too great. All living is a risk, and the elderly should accept some risks rather than stultify the life of someone else. Many independent-minded individuals know of the risks they might run, living alone in such circumstances, and gladly accept them, even against the judgment of their families. We should salute their courage and do what we can to support them.

Two conditions are essential if older subjects are to live alone: first, that they should not by this independence be allowed to put anyone else occupying the same premises into any danger; second, that they should be protected as far as possible in the home environment by living on the ground floor only, rather than risk a fall on the stairs, and by having fires and cooking arrangements made as safe as possible. The insistence of some families that elderly patients who are at risk ought to be placed in institutions may have to be countered with an explanation that hospitals and homes are not the safe refuges they usually are believed to be. There is not always staff at hand to prevent a fall. The morbidity and mortality from falls and from cross-infection in elderly persons' wards are quite high, even in well-conducted establishments. Besides, most elderly individuals, given the choice, prefer to be at home, and their wishes should be respected as much as possible.

HYPOTENSION

Physicians and even patients have grown accustomed to the idea that blood pressure tends to rise with age; no doubt it does in many people. High blood pressure takes its toll of life and limb. In a sense, geriatrics is practiced among the group who have managed to survive its bad effects, who have come to terms with hypertension, or who never were affected by it. However, a decrease of blood pressure is also common in old age and gives rise to immediate problems and to difficulties of long-term management.

A sudden decrease in blood pressure is frequently a sign of some severe circulatory disturbance, either from a gross gastrointestinal hemorrhage or a major cardiac or cardiopulmonary incident. Most physicians are now aware that cardiac infarction in old age only rarely takes the classic form of chest pain but manifests itself in a variety of other ways instead, collapse with low blood pressure being a common one. Similarly, pulmonary infarction strikes suddenly and causes collapse with cyanosis, perhaps with minimal respiratory distress, although with a catastrophic fall of blood pressure. It is notoriously difficult to distinguish between these two dangerous conditions, even with the help of electrocardiography. A sudden collapse, usually with fall of blood pressure, and particularly after instrumentation of the bowel or bladder, should give rise to a suspicion of septicemia (bacteremia) caused by a gram-negative or another type of organism, a subject reviewed by Denham.[1] Repeated blood cultures are necessary to establish the fact, but in old age the outlook is so grave that treatment with a likely antibiotic cannot safely be delayed pending clear laboratory confirmation.

Another cause of low blood pressure is the overenthusiastic use of antihypertensive drugs. The elderly are often highly susceptible to the effects of these, and the real indications for using them in geriatric practice are relatively few. It seems that once the body is well-accustomed to higher tension than normal, it functions less well when this hypertension is artificially reduced. Patients on such a regimen often feel far less well than before. This could be a more important consideration than striving for some theoretical increment in the life expectancy of the elderly. Addison's disease from malignant or other forms of destruction of the adrenals is possible in old age but very uncommon. It is a diagnosis often suggested but seldom substantiated by laboratory results. However, low blood pressure is sometimes an indication of hypokalemia from various causes, and a normal blood pressure usually is restored as soon as the electrolytes are brought back to correct levels.

Postural Hypotension

The symptoms of hypotension are limpness and dizziness or even fainting on standing up. Some patients with extremely low blood pressure cannot even sit up because they feel so ill, and when this symptom is talked of, it really must not be ignored.

Profound giddiness, vertigo, and even syncope similarly suggest hypotension, but such symptoms may be transient and related to posture. A general hypotensive tendency and marked lability of the blood pressure further suggests that diagnosis, which then has to be firmly established by comparing the patient's blood pressure at rest and supine with the pressure taken 1 or 2 minutes later standing upright or seated.

Wollner[8] and others showed that perhaps one in ten of elderly hospital patients tends to have postural hypotension and suggested that this is an indication of cerebrovascular disease. When specifically tested, a group of these patients were found to have deficient baroreceptor reflexes, with venous pooling of blood and an uncompensated decrease in cardiac output. Their responses to Valsalva's maneuver were correspondingly altered. More recently it was found that a significant proportion of patients with symptoms of postural hypotension have serum sodium levels at or below the normal lower limit.

No doubt hypotension of this kind is responsible for many falls in elderly patients when no other direct cause can be shown, and it afflicts some of the many who have to rise at night. These patients are particularly susceptible to drugs such as reserpine and chlorpromazine.

The treatment of acute, dangerous hypotension is primarily that of its cause. Postural and other long-term hypotensive tendencies are often hard to combat. A good sodium chloride intake is essential, and the patient may have to be given additional salt tablets. The patient must be made fully aware of his proclivity and should always get up slowly and carefully, being ready to sit down again or lower his head abruptly to counter his symptoms. Getting out of bed should be a routine in three stages—sitting up, sitting with the legs dangling, and finally getting on to the feet with great care. Tight abdominal binders or elastic stockings may perhaps help, but vasoconstrictor drugs seldom do.

A regimen of gradual changes of posture from

the horizontal to the vertical, repeated as a series of exercises over a number of days, helps in this otherwise intractable condition. Progressive raising of the head off the bed or using a tilting couch may gradually improve the patient's baroreceptor reflexes sufficiently for him to remain up and even fairly active. However, some unfortunate patients regularly remain so distressed by faintness and vertigo from this cause that they have to stay permanently recumbent. Such a decision is anathema to any modern geriatric physician.

REFERENCES

1. Denham MJ: Septicaemia. In Coakley D (ed): Acute Geriatric Medicine. London, Croom Helm, 1981

2. Garvey GJ, Neu HC: Infective endocarditis: An evolving disease. Medicine 57:105, 1978

3. Gleckman RA, Gantz NM (eds): Infections in the Elderly. Boston, Little, Brown & Co, 1983

4. Pathy MS: Clinical presentation of myocardial infarction in the elderly. Br Heart J 29:190, 1967

5. Sheldon JH: The Social Medicine of Old Age. London, Oxford University Press, 1948

6. Twycross RG: Relief of pain. In Saunders CM (ed): The Management of Terminal Disease. London, Arnold, 1978

7. Williamson J, Stokoe IH, Gray S, Fisher M, Smith A, McGhee A, Stephenson E: Old people at home: Their unreported needs. Lancet 1:1117, 1964

8. Wollner L: Postural Hypotension in the Elderly. In Agate JN (ed): Medicine in Old Age. London, Pitman Medical, 1966

10　Radiologic and Other Imaging Aspects of Aging

Kakarla Subbarao

One of the radiologist's ideals would be maintaining a file of a person's roentgenograms and other imaging procedures from cradle to grave. This would have a number of important values and applications. It would document the normality of growth processes during the formative years and the later involutionary changes at cellular levels that lead to the gross alterations observed in the roentgenography of the elderly. There is good reason to believe that these seemingly disparate processes may be interrelated. For instance, the appearance of osteopenia as an age-related involution in the bony skeleton undoubtedly has an inverse relationship with the mineral content of the bone at maturity. An early onset of this phenonomen might well be a warning to institute appropriate measures to conserve the declining bone mass. Availability of previous imaging records may also be crucial to diagnosis. A single encounter by the unwary physician with the film of an elderly patient has led to an interpretation of a serious pathologic lesion for an anatomical variant, a physiologic change, or a longstanding benign abnormality. An example of the latter might be an unvarying ''coin'' lesion present on roentgenograms of the chest for many years.

Many changes of aging are widespread and uniform throughout the body, but some proceed at a variable rate. These are determined by such systemic disorders as atherosclerosis, and diabetes or the use and abuse of joints. Calcification of vessels, bone and joint changes, dystrophic calcium deposits in soft tissues, and structural weakening manifested by diverticula of large bowel are among the age-related changes that contribute to the radiologist's interpretation that he is dealing with an aging patient. Many technologic advances have added to this. Computed tomography (CT

scanning) of the head can rapidly reveal atrophic changes in the brain or the existence of ventricular dilatation. The introduction of nuclear magnetic imaging can clearly delineate the pathologic metabolic changes encountered in the brain and other organs of the body. Ultrasonography is able to identify asymptomatic renal cysts as small as 2 cm in diameter. Radionuclide scanning is playing a major role in measuring coronary circulation and left ventricular outputs.

MUSCULOSKELETAL SYSTEM

Osteopenia is a common radiologic finding encountered in an older group of patients. It is manifested as a generalized lucency of bones, owing to a combined loss of mineral and matrix of the bone. When mineral loss alone is pronounced, the process is called osteomalacia; when the proteinaceous matrix is deficient, it is called osteoporosis. Often, a combination exists, and hence the general term *osteopenia* is appropriate. Osteopenia, early on, is chiefly reflected in the axial skeleton. The cortex of the vertebral body is thinner than normal but appears more prominent in contrast to the spongiosa, which is lucent due to resorbed secondary bone trabeculae. In the thoracic spine, wedging of the mid-thoracic bodies is observed, and in the lumbar spine, biconcave deformities are often encountered, resulting in the bulging of the intervertebral disk material into the thin vertebral end plates. A granular appearance to the skull may develop together with persistent intradiploic vascularity and multiple venous lakes.

Senile osteoporosis may also be reflected in the bones of the extremities. Cortical thinning with endosteal resorption and resorption of the trabec-

150

ulae in the spongiosa of metaphyseal ends of tubular bones is characteristic. The primary trabeculae attempt to reorient, reorganize, and reinforce themselves and hence appear thickened. The strength of bone is related to several factors, which include endocrine activity, state of nutrition, and activity of the attached muscles. Declines in these factors aggravate osteoporosis, so that fractures are common in the aged, even with minor trauma. Common sites for such fractures are the femoral necks, the lower end of the radius, and the upper end of the humerus.

Degenerative Changes In the Joints

Degenerative changes in the joints, a poor expression for stress changes, is radiologically inferred by the narrowing of joint spaces resulting from atrophy of the cartilages. Additional features include eburnation of the articular ends, osteophyte formation at the edges, and buttressing at the margins as though nature is trying to support weakened structures.

One of the sophisticated methods of quantitatively assessing the skeleton so that osteoporosis can be detected early is by computed tomography.

CT scans of the spine provide a measure of pure trabecular bone of the vertebral spongiosa, an area more sensitive and responsive to metabolic stimuli. Quantitative measurements by computed tomography are done in the few medical centers where there are high-resolution CT scanners. Subarticular cystic areas may develop as a result of intake of synovial fluid and may contain fibrous tissue and shredded synovium (Fig. 10-1). Para-articular osteoporosis does not develop, but instead, perhaps as a result of ischemia, sclerosis and thickening of the underlying subchondral bone are observed (Fig. 10-2). This lack of para-articular osteoporosis differentiates degenerative joint disorders from the inflammatory and infective joint diseases also encountered in the elderly. The severity and extent of osteophyte formation depends on the degree of stress and degradation of the cartilage (Fig. 10-3). In the vertebral column, these osteophytes originate at the margins of the vertebral bodies and occasionally form bridges in between the bodies. This intervertebral bridging should be differentiated from the inflammatory group of spondyloarthropathies such as ankylosing spondylitis, psoriasis, Reiter's syndrome, arthropathy associated with enterocolic diseases,

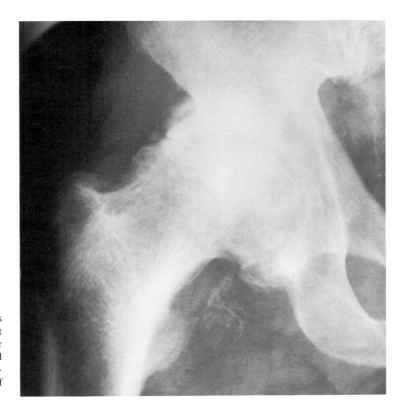

FIG. 10-1. Degenerative changes of the hip. Narrowing of the joint space, eburnation of the articular margins, subarticular lucencies, and osteophyte formation at the weight-bearing margins are characteristic of this entity.

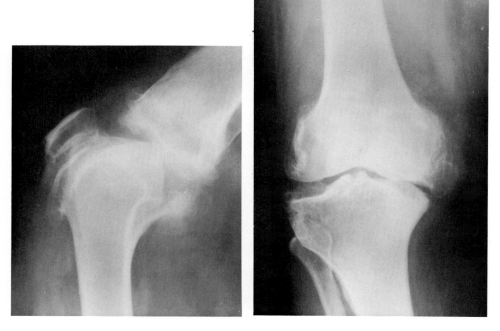

FIG. 10-2. Degenerative joint disorder of the knee. Note the medial space narrowing with sclerosis of articular margins and osteophytes.

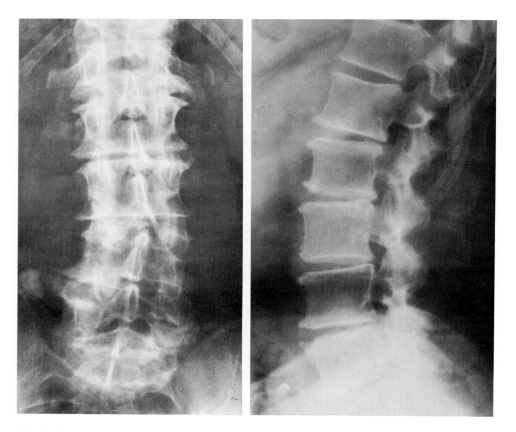

FIG. 10-3. Degenerative changes in the lumbar spine. Narrowing of several of the joint spaces with osteophytosis is diagnostic of degenerative disk disease. Also note the sclerosis particularly of facet articulations.

and, finally, diffuse idiopathic skeletal hyperostosis. Experience has shown that the degree of degenerative changes or osteophyte formation is poorly related to clinical symptoms. In the aged, osteophytosis and the hyperostosis encountered in the spine are common incidental findings observed in various radiographic procedures.

Some specifics as to type and degree of involvement of the joints may relate to occupational history. A manual laborer may develop more severe changes in the joints of the hand and wrist, while one who carries heavy weights on his back may have more pronounced changes in the thoracolumbar spine. Athletic activities also leave their marks on joints, depending on the type of sport. Disseminated idiopathic sclerosing hyperostosis (DISH) is a form of extensive osteophytosis with calcification and ossification at the sites of attachments of ligaments, tendons, and muscles. This disorder also favors old age and should be differentiated from the usual degenerative form of spondylitis. The intervertebral and other joint spaces in DISH are well preserved (Fig. 10-4).

Calcific tendinitis is frequently encountered in the elderly owing to dystrophic calcifications present in the muscular and tendinous attachments as well as in the underlying bursae. When associated with inflammation of the bursa, or fragmentation of the calcareous deposit, a great deal of pain and limitation of movement of the involved joint can result. The crystal deposition is calcium hydroxyapatite (Fig. 10-5). This should be differentiated from pseudogout, in which the crystal deposition is generally intra-articular and composed of calcium pyrophosphate dihydrate crystals. The hyaline and fibrocartilages demonstrate calcification and the joints involved include the knee, hip, shoulder, and wrist.

Decrease in height in old age is a universal phenomenon, and several factors play a role in the process. Osteoporosis with decrease in the vertebral body heights is a major factor, and degenerative changes in the intervertebral disks also contribute. In some, kyphosis and scoliosis play a role. In general, the weight-bearing joints bear the brunt and exhibit major change. Spondylosis deformans, coxa malum senilis, genu varum, and hallux valgus are among the deformities of the joints observed in old age, some of which also contribute to the loss of stature.

Paget's Disease

The average onset of Paget's disease is between 30 and 50 years. It can be monostotic but is generally polyostotic and is seen more often in men than

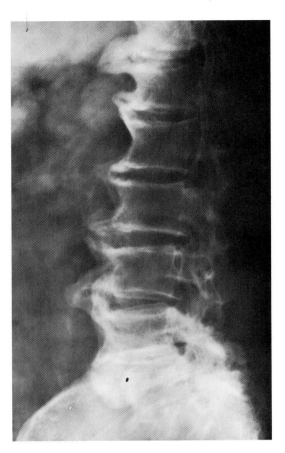

FIG. 10-4. Disseminated idiopathic skeletal hyperostosis (DISH). Note the joint spaces are well preserved despite extensive osteophytosis.

women. The pelvis, forearm, skull, tibia, vertebra, shoulder girdle, and rib are generally involved, although any bone in the body may be affected. Radiologic features depend on the stage of the disease. In the early osteolytic form, areas of lucency with a sharply demarcated border are observed. In the skull, this typical appearance is termed *osteoporosis circumscripta cranii*. In the long bones, one end of the lesion extends all the way to the joint and the other end resembles a blade of grass with a sharply outlined normal bone. In course of time, the areas of osteolysis are interspersed with islands of new sclerotic bone and this represents the mixed phase of Paget's disease. In the skull and innominate bones, the patchy sclerosis presents an appearance of cotton wool (Fig. 10-6). The third phase is the sclerotic form, characterized by thickening and sclerotic cortex, reinforced and prominent trabeculae in the spongiosa, and overall enlargement of the bone. The complications encountered in Paget's disease include

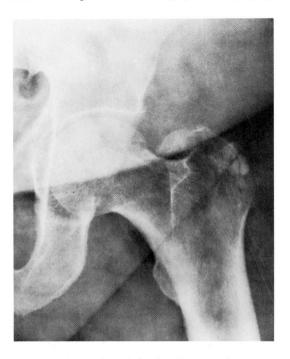

FIG. 10-5. Nodular calcific densities over the greater trochanter representative of calcium hydroxyapatite crystal deposition disease. The calcific tendinitis is in the gluteus medius tendon.

fractures (stress and traumatic), deformities (in the skull basilar invagination), infection, degenerative changes in the contiguous joint, and neoplastic transformation. Giant cell tumors may be encountered particularly in skull and facial bones, and malignant transformation is not unusual. Osteosarcoma, fibrous histiocytoma, and chondrosarcoma are the usual types of malignant lesions. In the spine and pelvis, Paget's disease has to be differentiated from osteosclerotic metastases such as those produced by carcinoma of the prostate. Radionuclide bone scanning with technetium salts reveals "hot areas" and helps in outlining the bones affected by Paget's disease. Radioisotope study, although highly sensitive, is not specific since it does not differentiate this from any other reactive new bone produced by such disorders as metastases or infections.

Neoplasms of Bone

Primary malignant neoplasms encountered in the elderly are myeloma, chondrosarcoma, fibrosarcoma, lymphoma, and osteosarcoma. In any individual case when a suspicion of malignant bone lesion has arisen, myeloma and metastases are to be thought of first, and in these instances radio-

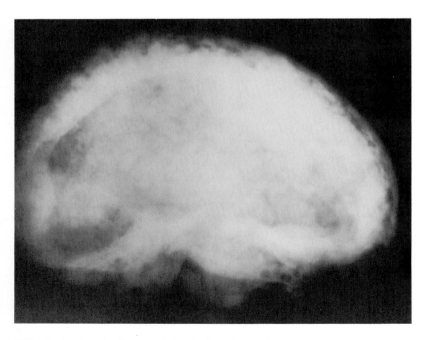

FIG. 10-6. Paget's disease of the skull. Diffuse sclerosis with thickening of the calvaria is the sclerotic form of this entity. Note also the basilar invagination.

nuclide scanning followed by skeletal survey should be done to identify the silent lesions involving the skeleton.

Multiple myeloma is a disease of the aged, and the radiologic manifestations range from mild osteopenia, localized permeative destruction of bones, and multiple punched-out lytic areas to large blow-out lytic lesions. A sclerotic form of myeloma may occur and is often associated with peripheral neuropathy and diabetes. The isolated lesion of myeloma (plasmacytoma) presents as an expanding lytic area, but eventually the majority of these patients develop multiple myeloma. Myeloma may simulate osteolytic metastases radiologically. The common primary malignant lesions that can produce such lytic metastases are from breast, thyroid, kidney, lung, and melanoma. However, any malignant lesion arising from gastrointestinal and genitourinary tracts or from soft tissues can produce osteolytic metastases (Fig. 10-7).

Infections of Bones and Joints

Osteomyelitis and pyogenic arthritis are observed in elderly patients who have a chronic underlying disorder such as arteriosclerosis, diabetes, or other neurologic disorders. The foot is a common site for diabetic osteopathy. The changes in the bones and joints of a diabetic patient's foot are mainly due to the following factors: small vessel occlusion leading to ischemia, peripheral neuropathy with sensory loss leading to unrecognized trauma, and superimposed infection. The latter leads to soft tissue abscess, osteomyelitis, gangrene, and autoamputation of the toes (Fig. 10-8). In diabetic patients, the ankle and foot are the common sites for neuropathic changes. The classic radiologic manifestations of neuropathic skeletal disorder include microfractures at the articular ends, eburnation of the articular margins, fragmentation, cartilage destruction, soft tissue calcification, and marked disorganization of the joint.

In chronically bedridden patients with neurologic problems, the calcanei, ischial tuberosities, greater trochanter, and sacrum are common sites for osteomyelitis, owing to overlying decubitus ulcers and infections. In paraplegics, infection of hip joints with pathologic fractures and abundant callus with extensive dystrophic soft tissue calcifications is a characteristic feature. Para-articular and soft tissue calcifications due to prolonged immobilization with ankylosis of joints are commonly encountered in paraplegics and hemiplegic patients.

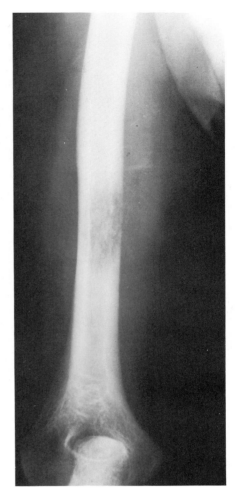

FIG. 10-7. Metastatic osteolytic lesion of midshaft of humerus. The primary lesion was a bronchogenic carcinoma.

Rheumatoid Arthritis

Rheumatoid arthritis is another entity often encountered in the older patient generally with classic deformities of the hands, feet, and knees. The radiologic features of rheumatoid arthritis include para-articular osteoporosis, narrowing of the joint spaces, and erosions of the subarticular bone with subluxations and dislocation (Fig. 10-9). The shoulders are also common sites of involvement and are often associated with a chronic tear of the rotator cuff (Fig. 10-10). Subluxations at the upper cervical spine may lead to severe neurologic problems. In longstanding cases, ankylosis of the deformed joints may necessitate the insertion of joint prostheses.

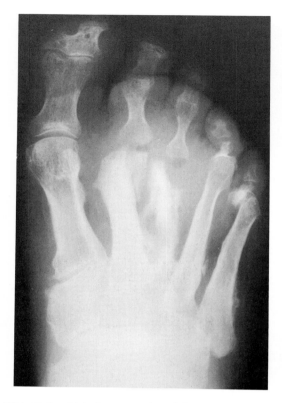

FIG. 10-8. Diabetic osteopathy of the foot. Irregular osteolysis of the heads of the second and third metatarsals with periosteal new bone indicates osteomyelitis. The lucencies at the second and third metatarsophalangeal joints indicate ulceration and infection. Note the partial resorption of the proximal phalanges of the fourth and fifth toes.

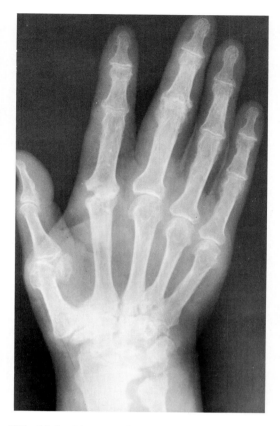

FIG. 10-9. Rheumatoid arthritis. Narrowing of the joint spaces at the wrist, carpus, and metacarpophalangeal joints with subarticular erosion indicate longstanding changes of rheumatoid arthritis.

Chronic gout is another arthritic process mostly affecting men and involving the joints of feet, hands, and knees. Eccentric erosions, calcific tophi in the soft tissues and bones, and lack of para-articular osteoporosis are the major radiologic features. When recurrent and chronic, degenerative joint changes often superimpose.

Osteonecrosis

Several factors lead to osteonecrosis of the articular end of bones in the elderly. The common sites include femoral and humeral heads, lower end of the femur, and, occasionally, small bones of the hands and feet. Besides small vessel disorders, alcoholism and iatrogenic causes produce ischemic necrosis and occasionally infarctions of bone. Since the elderly often ingest pain-killing drugs such as aspirin, butazolidin, indocin, and corticosteroids, ischemic necrosis of the articular ends of bones is not uncommon. Connective tissue disorders such as rheumatoid arthritis and systemic lupus erythematosus may produce osteonecrosis and bone infarcts. A bone infarct is diametaphyseal in location and when healed produces a typical radiologic finding with an oblong, well-demarcated calcification located in the medullary cavity extending into the spongiosa of the metaphysis. This appearance simulates an enchondroma radiologically, which may show central, punctate, nugget, or ringlike calcifications but which lacks the peripheral fibro-osseous membrane typical of a healed infarct. Osteonecrosis of the femoral and humeral heads should be recognized early in order to institute adequate conservative therapy. Radionuclide bone scanning often helps to detect early lesions. The radiologic features of osteonecrosis of femoral or humeral heads include loss of normal rounded contour followed by irregular dense areas in the subarticular portion with areas of fibrosis interspersed simulating cystic appearance (Fig. 10-11). In the lower end of the femur, the medial condyle is a common site for spontaneous osteo-

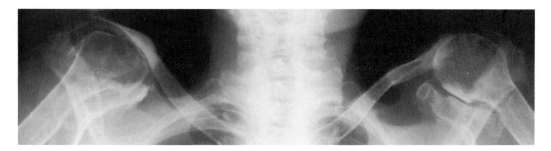

FIG. 10-10. Chronic rheumatoid arthritis of both shoulders. Note the resorption of the lateral ends of the clavicles. The high riding of the humeral heads, the narrowing of the joint spaces, and the changes in the acromion indicate associated chronic tears of the rotator cuffs.

necrosis, and again the loss of normal contour with increased density and a positive radionuclide bone scan are the diagnostic features. When neglected, osteonecrosis leads to degenerative joint disorder.

The skull in the elderly exhibits sclerosis of the cranial sutures that stand out predominantly in a roentgenogram, contrasting to the osteoporosis of the rest of the bones. Marked parietal bone thinning involving the outer tables is often encountered (Fig. 10-12). As a result of osteoporosis, the floor of the sella appears thinned, and this should not be mistaken for raised intracranial pressure. Hyperostosis frontalis interna is a common radiologic finding in elderly women. This has no particular significance except that on occasion, hyperostosis due to underlying meningioma may be mistaken for normal physiologic changes in the skull. Calcification in the pineal, the choroid plexus (particularly the glomus), the falx, the tentorium, the diaphragma sellae, the petroclinoid ligaments, the dura, and the internal carotid artery specifically at the site of the carotid siphon are common in the aged, with increasing incidence found with advancing age. Any shift of these structures from their normal anatomical site may give a clue to the presence of space-occupying lesions in the brain. The increased diploic vascularity and the venous lakes present in the aging skull should not be mistaken for pathologic processes.

CHEST

In the thorax, the tracheobronchial tree, the costal cartilages, the aorta, the mitral annulus (Fig. 10-13), and the coronary arteries show some degree of calcification as age advances. Calcification of the laryngeal and thyroid cartilages and vascular calcification at the bifurcation of the carotid arteries are commonly observed in the neck roentgenograms of the elderly. Arteriosclerosis of the aorta increases its density due to thickening of the wall, and the loss of elasticity in old age leads to elongation and tortuosity of the aorta. Tortuosity and buckling of the brachiocephalic vessels may simulate a superior mediastinal mass. The walls of the alveoli in the lung lose their elasticity. Hyperven-

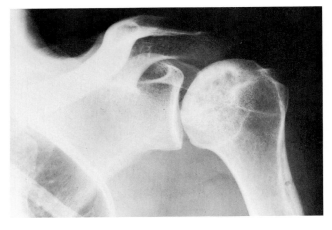

FIG. 10-11. Osteonecrosis of the head of the humerus with areas of sclerosis and lucencies and loss of smooth contour. This patient has systemic lupus erythematosus. Osteonecrosis is encountered with or without corticosteroid therapy.

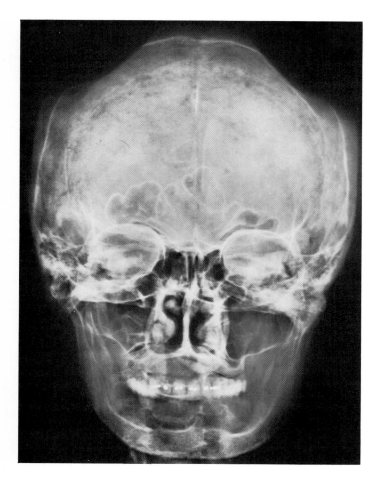

FIG. 10-12. Bilateral symmetrical thinning of parietal bones in an asymptomatic 75-year-old man. Note also calcified falx in the midline.

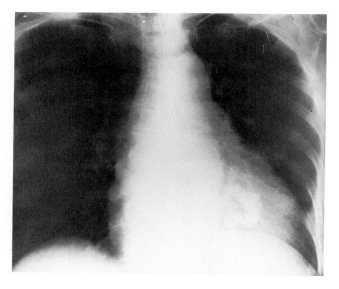

FIG. 10-13. Calcified mitral annulus in the form of inverted C indicates atherosclerosis.

tilation of the lungs with loss of tonicity of the diaphragmatic muscle and decreased intra-abdominal pressure may simulate obstructive pulmonary disease, but these are all physiologic changes in the senile chest. The domes of the diaphragm often show mamillation in the aged. Residual pulmonary scars of old healed inflammatory disease, particularly in the apical pleura, of old emboli, or of thrombosis of small vessels in the lung should be studied with utmost care before any malignant lesions are diagnosed or thoracotomy is contemplated to remove a benign process.

As age advances, the cardiac configuration changes, the silhouette gradually assumes a horizontal position from the vertical position in young age. This change to horizontal configuration together with pericardial fat pads is often mistaken for cardiomegaly.

GASTROINTESTINAL TRACT

The films of the abdomen, in spite of proper preparation to avoid the gas in the intestinal tract, very often demonstrate a nonspecific type of ileus owing to loss of tone in the wall of the intestinal tract. The large bowel is often distended with gas and fecal material. Proper evaluation of intestinal gas shadows and differentiation from mechanical obstruction or paralytic ileus owing to inflammatory disease, or ischemia and low flow, should be made cautiously. When a doubt arises regarding the presence of mechanical intestinal obstruction, a barium enema of the colon should be performed even as an emergency procedure. An upper gastrointestinal examination with barium should be avoided. Cathartics such as castor oil should not be administered in cases of suspected mechanical intestinal obstruction, ischemic disease, diverticulitis, and perforated viscus. A complete obstructive series, which includes supine, erect, and lateral decubitus views, and a chest roentgenogram should be performed. Since as little as 1.5 cc of free air can be detected in instances of perforated viscus, the results of this examination should be carefully studied. In cases of active gastrointestinal bleeding, radionuclide study followed by abdominal angiography should be performed. In certain cases, the angiographer can occlude the vessel that is producing hemorrhage. Calcifications in the abdominal aorta (Fig. 10-14), splenic artery, renal arteries, and iliac vessels are often encountered in plain films of the elderly, and often aneurysms of these vessels are detected by plain films alone. Calcified phleboliths in the pelvis are a common observation and should be carefully evaluated and differentiated from ureteral and vesical stones.

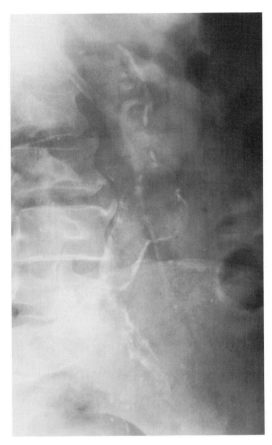

FIG. 10-14. Calcified wall of the abdominal aorta is seen in this oblique view of lumbar spine. A small aneurysmal bulge is also present.

Uterine arteries and fibroids often show calcification, while vas deferens (Fig. 10-15) and corpora amylacea of the prostate frequently calcify.

Examination of the colon by barium enema and air contrast in the elderly is a time-consuming procedure, but a patient, persistent, and meticulously performed examination results in good dividends. Diverticular disease with or without inflammatory changes, premalignant lesions such as polyps and villous tumors, carcinoma, ischemia, and various colitides are often detected by a barium enema procedure. Although right-sided colonic diverticula and angiodysplasia of the cecum are common causes of bleeding, abscesses, sinus tracts, and fistulous tracts are frequent complications of left-sided diverticula.

Chronic constipation and atonicity promote redundancy of the sigmoid and may lead to volvulus. The colon is also distended with gas and feces in chronic systemic disorders such as diabetes, parkinsonism, and certain connective tissue dis-

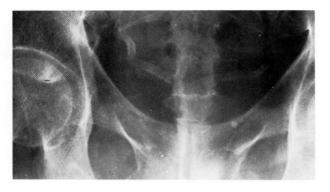

FIG. 10-15. Calcified vas deferens bilaterally. Note the tubular calcification emerging from the seminal vesicles. This type of calcification is more often encountered in the elderly diabetic.

orders. Indiscriminate use of laxatives and other over-the-counter drugs also promote chronic colonic ileus.

In the upper gastrointestinal tract, swallowing disorders are not uncommon. Diverticula of the esophagus, particularly at the pharyngoesophageal junction, at the site of the aortic pulmonary window, at the bifurcation of the trachea, and in the epiphrenic area, are commonly encountered with advancing age. Peristalsis of the esophagus often becomes disorganized and irregular, leading to either tertiary contractions or presbyesophagus. The tertiary contractions are a spontaneous, corkscrew pattern type of contractions of the esophagus oc-

casionally giving rise to symptoms of dysphagia. In presbyesophagus, a moderate degree of dilatation of the esophagus with delay in emptying of the barium, particularly in the horizontal position, is encountered. In all cases of dysphagia, administration of a barium pill that measures 1.2 cm in diameter and spot filming or even cineradiography should be done to detect early organic lesions such as carcinoma. Hiatal insufficiency or hiatal hernia, a common feature in the aged, is often an incidental finding in the routine radiologic examination of the chest and is observed as a viscus containing air or air and fluid in the retrocardiac area (Fig. 10-16). The size of the herniated stomach

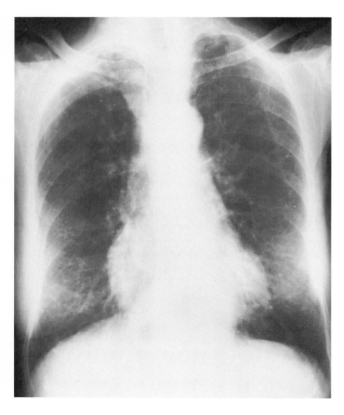

FIG. 10-16. Hiatal hernia. A well-circumscribed retrocardiac opacity observed in a routine roentgenogram of the chest.

has no bearing on symptomatology, but evidence of barium reflux during fluoroscopy is significant in evaluating symptoms.

In the stomach, atony, atrophic gastritis, peptic ulceration, polyps, and carcinoma are detected earlier by properly performed air contrast studies. Although gastric carcinoma is on the decline, esophageal malignancy is on the rise (Fig. 10-17). The reasons for this have not been determined. Volvulus of the stomach is encountered occasionally. Radiologic differentiation as to whether the volvulus is complete or incomplete, whether or-

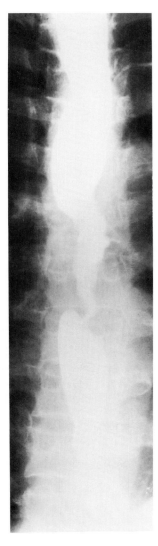

FIG. 10-17. Carcinoma of the middle third of the esophagus. The "apple core" deformity in the barium-filled oseophagus with mucosal loss and overhanging margins is typical.

ganoaxial, mesenteroaxial, or a combination of both types, cannot be readily done. The duodenum and small bowel may demonstrate atony, and nonspecific dilatation and diverticula may be demonstrated. The chief significance of small bowel diverticula is the malabsorption syndrome observed in some patients. The common cause of upper gastrointestinal bleeding is erosive gastritis, although peptic ulcer and esophageal varices also contribute.

In the biliary tract, asymptomatic calculi are often observed as an incidental finding when abdominal and spine films are interpreted for some unrelated complaint. About 20% of all biliary calculi show some degree of calcification and are observed in the films of the abdomen. In elderly women, gallstone ileus is a common cause of small bowel obstruction with air observed in the biliary tree. The stone may impact at the ligament of Treitz or ileocecal valve and produce partial or complete small bowel obstruction. Oral cholecystography is the method of investigating the gallbladder disease, but ultrasonography has almost replaced it (Fig. 10-18). Radionuclide scanning with hepatoiododiacetic acid (HIDA) supplements the examination of the biliary tract. In the presence of severe obstructive jaundice due to a mass either at the porta hepatis or at the distal segment of the common duct, transhepatic cholangiography with a thin needle is the investigation of choice.

Masses in the pancreas, metastases in the liver, and other intra-abdominal masses are best studied by computed tomography (Fig. 10-19). Introduction of the modality of nuclear magnetic imaging has further helped in outlining the structural abnormalities of the body, including the brain.

GENITOURINARY TRACT

In routine scout films of the abdomen, the sizes of the kidneys may be estimated and as age advances, the quantity of functioning renal tissue diminishes and hence the kidneys appear small. The function and morphology of the upper urinary tract are better studied by large-dose infusion pyelography in the aged instead of routine intravenous urography. Retrograde pyelography is rarely performed and is replaced by well-performed infusion pyelography with tomographic techniques. Ultrasonography and CT scanning better demonstrate urinary tract pathology, including early inflammatory and neoplastic lesions. The incidence of benign renal cysts increases with age, and ultrasonography and CT scanning help in determining the nature of cystic lesions. As the kidney parenchyma

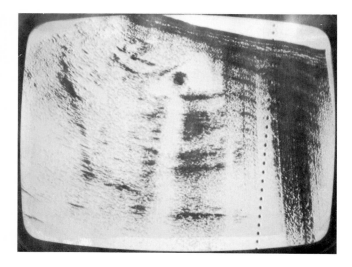

FIG. 10-18. Ultrasonography of the right upper quadrant demonstrates a large calculus in the gallbladder with "shadowing."

undergoes atrophy due to arteriosclerosis or inflammatory processes, the renal sinuses fill with fat, best demonstrated by nephrotomography. Adrenal masses are elucidated by CT and similar techniques so that presacral insufflation of air to study retroperitoneal masses has become anecdotal.

Uterine fibroids may degenerate and calcify and in elderly women show as calcific masses in the pelvis (Fig. 10-20).

Atony of the bladder, cystitis, prostatic hypertrophy, and masses in the bladder and prostate are diagnosed earlier with direct cystograms and CT scanning. Carcinoma of the prostate prior to its extension into the capsule is easily diagnosed by nuclear magnetic imaging. Cystoceles in women, bladder diverticula, and herniation of the bladder into femoral and inguinal canals are identified easily by taking oblique and standing films with cys-

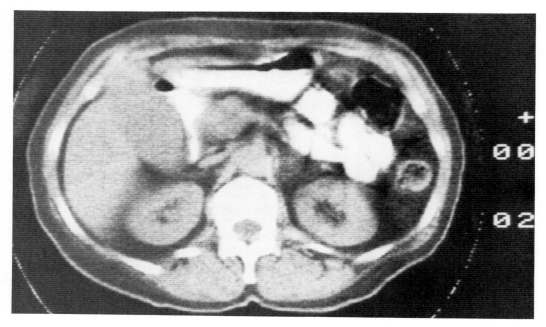

FIG. 10-19.   Computed tomography of the abdomen with Gastrografin swallow. Note the mass in the head of the pancreas with pressure over the concave aspect of the duodenal loop.

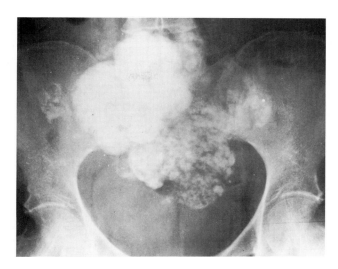

FIG. 10-20. Calcified fibroids of the uterus. The spongelike amorphous calcifications above the bladder are characteristic.

tography. Chain cystograms are useful to study the degree of stress incontinence in women. Gas in the urinary bladder may be due to diabetes with *Escherichia coli* infection (Fig. 10-21) or to a fistulous communication from diverticula or carcinoma of the colon. Crohn's disease may produce fistulous tracts between the small bowel and urinary bladder. Women treated with radiation for malignant lesions in the pelvic cavity may develop fistulous tracts into the bladder years later.

ROLE OF NONINVASIVE DIAGNOSTIC IMAGING METHODS IN GERIATRIC PRACTICE

Advances in diagnostic imaging have added a new dimension in the investigation of diseases in the aged. They are mainly ultrasonography, radionuclide scanning, computed tomography and magnetic resonance imaging.

CT scans are used with increasing accuracy in

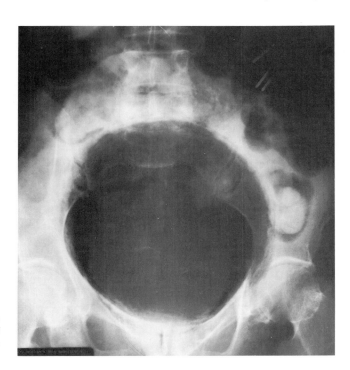

FIG. 10-21. Distended urinary bladder with gas in a diabetic patient with *Escherichia coli* infection observed in a scout film of the abdomen.

the investigation of cerebral, pulmonary, abdominal, and musculoskeletal disorders. Involution of the brain with cortical atrophy in the aged is dramatically demonstrated with magnetic resonance imaging. Herniated disks in the spine, lumber canal stenosis (Fig. 10-22 and 10-23), and extradural and intradural masses are diagnosed early with CT scanning and magnetic resonance imaging. Retroperitoneal masses, metastasis to the liver, evaluation of the mediastinum, and pulmonary nodules are better studied with computed tomography.

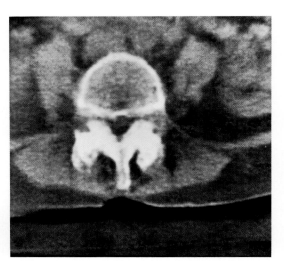

FIG. 10-23. Computed tomographic scan at the level of L3-4 of same patient in Figure 10-22. The triangular spinal canal with osteophytic ridges at the facet joints is characteristic of lumbar canal stenosis.

With nuclear radiology, alterations in regional blood flow and functional changes in the heart, biliary tract, brain, and kidneys are demonstrated easily and better than by other investigative studies.

Positron emission tomography (PET) combines the advantages of nuclear radiology and computed tomography. A functional cross-sectional image is obtained in cerebral disorders, such as Alzheimer's disease. This modality yields an important insight into various disorders of the central nervous system, including cerebrovascular disease, seizures, and degenerative diseases.

Major advances in ultrasonography in geriatric patients with both benign and malignant disorders have been of benefit and thus avoid interventional methods.

Interventional radiology is playing a major role in alleviating many ailments of the elderly. Biliary and urinary tract obstructions are treated with percutaneous drainage procedures and insertion of stents, and percutaneous transluminal angioplasties are performed efficiently to relieve vascular stenoses, including those in coronary arteries. Preoperative embolization of vessels supplying tumors promises to be successful in reducing bleeding before or during surgical procedures.

SUGGESTED READINGS

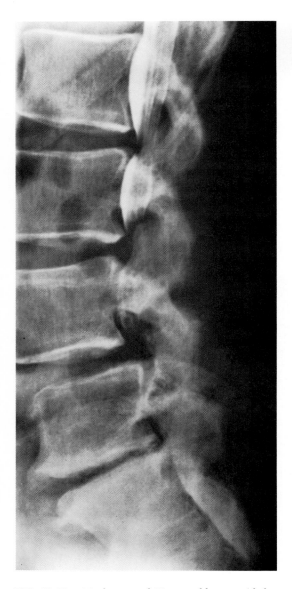

FIG. 10-22. Myelogram of 52-year-old man with leg cramps reveals complete block at the level of L3. Note the narrow canal with posterior scalloping of vertebrae.

Brant-Zawadski M et al: NMR demonstration of cerebral abnormalities: Comparison with CT. AJNR 4:117, 1983

Donner MW, McAfee JG: Roentgenographic manifestations of diabetes mellitus. Am J Med Sci 239:622, 1960

Edeiken J, and Hodes PG: Bone ischemia. Radiol Clin North Am 5:515, 1967

Emmett JL, Witten DM: Clinical Urography, 3rd ed. Philadelphia, WB Saunders, 1971

Fraser RG, Peterpare JA: Diagnosis of Diseases of the Chest, 2nd ed. Philadelphia, WB Saunders, 1977

Herfkens RJ et al. Nuclear magnetic resonance imaging of arteriosclerotic disease. Radiology 148:161, 1983

Jaffee HL: Metabolic Degenerative and Inflammatory Diseases of Bones and Joints. Philadelphia, Lea & Febiger, 1972

Lee JKT, Sagel SS, Stanley RJ (eds): Computed Body Tomography. New York, Raven Press, 1983

McAfee JG, Donner MW: Differential diagnosis of calcifications encountered in abdominal radiographs. Am J Med Sci 243:609, 1952

Margulis AR, Higgins CB, Kaufman L, Crooks LE (eds): Clinical Magnetic Resonance Imaging. San Francisco, Radiology Research and Education Foundation, 1983

Moss AA, Gamsu G, Genant HK: Computed Tomography of the Body. Philadelphia, WB Saunders, 1983

Murray RO, Jacobson HG: The Radiology of Skeletal Disorders, 2nd ed. London, Churchill Livingstone, 1977

Shehadi WH: Radiologic examination of the biliary tract: Plain film of the abdomen; oral cholecystography. Radiol Clin North Am 4:463, 1968

III

The Aged Patient and Clinical Specialties

11 Cardiovascular Disease in Old Age

Jerome L. Fleg and Edward G. Lakatta

As the proportion of elderly Americans continues its upward surge, their disease patterns become increasingly representative of the entire country. Thus, as the percentage of Americans aged 65 years or older rose from 8.2% to 10.7% between 1950 and 1976, cardiac deaths in this age-group grew from 64.9% to 75.8% of all cardiac deaths.[6] Indeed, most of the common cardiovascular disorders (*e.g.*, hypertension, coronary artery disease, congestive heart failure, chronic atrial fibrillation) are seen predominantly in old age. The economic and sociologic costs of cardiovascular disease in the elderly defy estimation.

The presentation of cardiovascular disorders in the elderly is the product of aging changes *per se* in the heart and blood vessels superimposed on disease-induced alterations in their structure and function. The current discussion will begin by delineating our current concepts of normative age-related cardiovascular changes before reviewing the common presentations of cardiac disease in the elderly.

CARDIOVASCULAR FUNCTION AND AGING IN THE ABSENCE OF DISEASE

Methodologic Considerations

The information available to us regarding age-related changes in cardiovascular function has been derived largely from cross-sectional studies, that is, those in which different individuals of different ages have been screened with variable "filters" to exclude disease and differences in life-style variables. The variability in the "filters" from one study to the next has resulted in a literature that exhibits substantial interstudy differences but that also demonstrates many interstudy similarities as well. It is important to bear in mind that virtually all of these studies have been concerned with subjects who are 80 years or less in age. Thus the perspectives gained from this information need not apply to the "old old," that is, those 85 years of age and older.

Most early investigations suggested that progressive functional declines in the cardiovascular system occur inexorably with advancing age. On a casual review of the literature that describes this functional decline, one is struck with the fact that the rate of decline varies dramatically among populations. This implies that some additional factor(s) are potent modulators of cardiovascular function as we age (Fig. 11-1). One such factor is the development of specific disease processes. We might wonder whether we could classify the "aging process" as a disease as well since, like specific pathologic entities, it, too, may result in functional decline and eventually death. However, regardless of what play on language we choose, the two processes (*i.e.*, disease and aging) must be specifically delineated in order to identify and characterize the latter. This task is not so difficult when a disease process is overt; however, the presence of occult disease (*e.g.* coronary artery disease) can cause marked impairments in cardiovascular function during stress and confound characterization of normative aging changes.

In addition to disease, changes in "life-style" occur concomitantly with advancing age. These life-style variables such as physical exercise, eating, drinking, smoking, recreational pursuits, and so on, which are determined by education, socioeconomic status, and character traits, are particularly important because they are subject to change and potentially can alter an "aging process" or

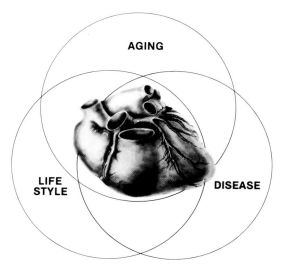

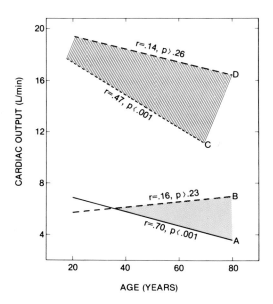

FIG. 11-1. Age-related changes in cardiac structure and function interact to alter the presentation of cardiovascular disease in the elderly. (Lakatta EG: Health, disease and cardiovascular aging. In National Academy of Sciences Institute of Medicine (ed): The Aging Society: The Burden of Long-Term Illness and Disability. Washington DC, National Academy Press. In press)

FIG. 11-2. The best fit linear regression of cardiac output on age at rest (lines A, B) and during bicycle exercise (lines C, D). Note that regression lines B and D, derived from healthy, active, community-dwelling volunteers[82] screened to exclude coronary artery disease by exercise ECG and thallium scintigraphy, are not significant. In contrast, the subjects depicted by line A were hospitalized patients recuperating from noncardiac illness,[8] and those comprising line C were ambulatory volunteers who did not undergo prior screening to exclude coronary disease.[53] (Lakatta EG: Age-related changes in the heart. Geriatr Med Today 4(7) 86, July 1985.)

prevent disease. Indeed, although our understanding is very far from complete, over the past 2 decades we have become aware of the impact of smoking, dietary, behavioral, and possibly physical activity "habits" on the development of coronary artery disease. The impact of life-style on cardiovascular aging, on the other hand, is presently less well defined, and it is likely that many changes in cardiovascular function that are often attributed to an "aging process" were in part due to the sedentary life-style that accompanies aging.

Studies of age-related changes in cardiac output, both at rest and during peak exercise, have provided varying results.[8,35,53,82] Figure 11-2 depicts the best fit linear regression of cardiac output as a function of age at rest and during exercise as measured in three different populations.[8,53,82] The shaded area between the curves can be considered to be due to differences in the filters used to screen subjects in these studies; while all of the determinants of this shaded area cannot at the moment be accounted for or quantitated, certainly the presence of occult disease, and differences in life-style variables (*e.g.*, smoking, nutrition, physical conditioning status) would appear to be the most prominent factors involved. The main message that emerges from the figure, however, is that age *per se* need not be accompanied by the decline in function depicted in lines A and C, and one is

therefore hard pressed to hypothesize the presence of an "aging process" based on measurements of cardiac output.

Measurements of some parameters of cardiovascular function that determine cardiac output, made in subjects of the Baltimore Longitudinal Study of Aging (BLSA) who had been screened to exclude occult coronary disease by prior treadmill stress testing with ECG and/or thallium scintography, are listed in Tables 11-1 and 11-2.[34,82] The average values in each age-group serve as useful functional norms both at rest and during vigorous exercise. Some salient features of these tables are discussed below.

Cardiovascular Function at Rest

When sufficient numbers of subjects are studied, resting heart rate is not altered with aging; basal systolic blood pressure increases *within* the "normal" range, while diastolic pressure tends to increase from approximately 120 mm Hg at age 20

TABLE 11-1 M-Mode Echocardiographic Parameters in Normal Subjects

Parameter	Group I (25–44 yr)*			Group II (45–64 yr)*			Group III (65–84 yr)*		
Mitral valve EF slope (mm/sec)	102.3	± 3.7	(52)	79.0	± 3.8	(35)	67.1	± 5.2	(18)
Aortic root diastolic (mm)	30.9	± 0.6	(45)	32.0	± 0.6	(34)	32.9	± 0.8	(17)
LV wall thickness (mm)									
Systolic	15.4	± 0.5	(33)	17.6	± 0.7	(15)	18.8	± 0.6	(12)
Diastolic	8.7	± 0.3	(33)	9.8	± 0.5	(16)	10.7	± 0.5	(13)
Systolic/m^2	7.6	± 0.3	(33)	9.2	± 0.3	(15)	10.0	± 0.4	(12)
Diastolic/m^2	4.3	± 0.1	(33)	5.0	± 0.2	(16)	5.7	± 0.2	(13)
LV dimension (mm)									
Systolic	34.4	± 1.1	(37)	32.1	± 0.89	(17)	32.1	± 1.4	(11)
Diastolic	51.8	± 1.03	(37)	50.8	± 1.3	(17)	51.2	± 1.4	(11)
Systolic/m^2	17.3	± 0.5	(37)	16.7	± 0.5	(17)	16.8	± 0.6	(11)
Diastolic/m^2	26.0	± 0.5	(37)	26.4	± 0.6	(17)	27.0	± 0.7	(11)
Fractional shortening of the minor									
semi-axis	0.34	± 0.01	(37)	0.36	± 0.01	(17)	0.37	± 0.02	(11)
VCF (circ/sec)	1.17	± 0.04	(37)	1.23	± 0.04	(17)	1.30	± 0.08	(11)

*The number of subjects is given in parentheses next to the mean and SEM. (LV, left ventricle; Vcf, velocity of circumferential fiber shortening)

(Gerstenblith G et al: Echocardiographic assessment of a normal adult aging population. Circulation 56:273, 1977)

TABLE 11-2 Radionuclide Ventriculographic Assessment of Cardiac Performance in Normal Subjects

Parameter	Age (25–44 yr)	Age (45–64 yr)	Age (65–79 yr)
Rest			
Age	35 ± 1 (22)*	56 ± 1 (23)*	71 ± 1 (16)*
Heart rate	73 ± 2	70 ± 2	69 ± 3
Systolic blood pressure	121 ± 3	124 ± 3	138 ± 5
Diastolic blood pressure	82 ± 2	84 ± 2	86 ± 3
End-diastolic volume	132 ± 8	146 ± 9	143 ± 10
Stroke volume	84 ± 6	93 ± 5	96 ± 7
End-systolic volume	48 ± 4	54 ± 5	47 ± 4
Ejection fraction	64 ± 1	64 ± 2	67 ± 2
Cardiac output	6 ± 0.4	6 ± 0.3	6 ± 0.4
Total systemic vascular resistance	17 ± 1	16 ± 1	17 ± 1.3
Upright bicycle exercise (100 watts)			
Heart rate	139 ± 4	122 ± 3	122 ± 5
Systolic blood pressure	183 ± 7	186 ± 5	190 ± 9
Diastolic blood pressure	94 ± 4	99 ± 3	103 ± 5
End-diastolic volume	146 ± 8	165 ± 10	180 ± 14
Stroke volume	117 ± 6	124 ± 7	140 ± 11
End-systolic volume	29 ± 3	40 ± 4	39 ± 6
Ejection fraction	81 ± 2	76 ± 2	79 ± 3
Cardiac output	16 ± 1	15 ± 1	17 ± 1
Total systemic vascular resistance	8 ± 0.5	9 ± 0.5	8 ± 1

The number in parentheses is the number of each age-group. Values represent mean ± SEM.

(Rodeheffer RJ et al: Exercise cardiac output is maintained with advancing age in healthy human subjects: Cardiac dilatation and increased stroke volume compensate for diminished heart rate. Circulation 69:203, 1984)

to 160 mm Hg at age 80 and then level off by the sixth to seventh decade (Fig. 11-3). The large arteries stiffen, as manifested in an increase in pulse wave velocity.[3] This seems to be attributable to changes that occur within the vascular media (*e.g.*, calcification) and changes in the nature and content of collagen and elastin, rather than to atherosclerosis. The increase in systolic blood pressure, which itself seems to be attributable to the vascular stiffening, imposes an increased work load on the heart, resulting in a moderate age-related increase in left ventricular (LV) wall thickness that has been detected via ultrasound techniques in most populations studied (see Table 11-1).[61] This increase in left ventricular thickness with age, which on the average is about 25% from age 20 to 80, like blood pressure, is still within the normal clinical range.[34]

The early diastolic filling rate of the left ventricle, as judged from the mitral valve excursion measured in the echogram, exhibits about a 50% decline between the ages of 20 and 80 years (see Table 11-1).[34] This has been found to be the case in every population studied and can be attributed to a decrease in compliance (an increase in the stiffness properties of the ventricular wall) due to the mild LV thickening or to a prolonged isometric relaxation time that has been observed in noninvasive time-interval measurements in humans and directly measured in isolated cardiac muscle in several animal models.[61] In these studies it has been shown that cellular mechanisms that govern the duration of the cardiac contraction are altered with aging.[63] Specifically, the rate of Ca^{2+} seques-tration of sarcoplasmic reticulum, a major regulator of the duration of the myoplasmic Ca^{2+} transient, declines by about 50% with advancing adult age; the transmembrane action potential that initiates the Ca^{2+} release that causes contractile force is markedly (*i.e.*, twofold) prolonged in muscles from senescent versus younger adult rat hearts; and the myosin isozyme composition shifts to a predominantly slow form.

The slowed early diastolic filling rate at rest in humans is not of functional significance, since the end-diastolic filling volume is not reduced with advancing age (see Table 11-2). Thus, filling in the later part of diastole must increase in elderly subjects, and this might require a more forceful atrial contraction, explaining the clinical observation that an S_4 heart sound is common in the elderly and considered by many physicians to be a normal finding, whereas its presence in younger adults is rare and regarded as abnormal.[95] Although end-diastolic diameter, area, or volume as measured by the echocardiogram or by gated blood pool scans does not differ with age when different individuals are compared, longitudinal studies within the same individuals have shown that aging is associated with a slight (5%) increase in cardiothoracic ratio on the chest roentgenogram, although still well within the clinically normal range.[21] Aortic dilatation with aging has also been demonstrated by echocardiography[34] (see Table 11-1) and chest roentgenography.[21] Systolic pump function at rest assessed by the ejection fraction or velocity of ejection is not altered with adult aging (see Tables 11-1 and 11-2).[34,82]

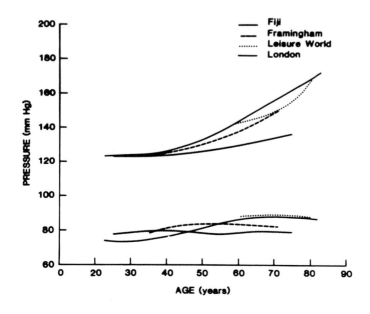

FIG. 11-3. Age-related changes in blood pressure. It is of interest that the rise in systolic blood pressure with age is much greater in the three industrialized cultures shown than in the nonindustrialized island of Fiji. (Berman ND: Geriatric Cardiology. Lexington, MA, DC Heath & Co, 1982)

Cardiovascular Stress Response

In both the young adult and elderly cohorts listed in Table 11-2, high levels of cardiac output were achieved during exercise, and in fact, cardiac output in the elderly group even at peak exercise was maintained at the level observed in the younger age-groups (curve D in Fig. 11-2). By selection of highly screened elderly subjects who could achieve high work loads, it was found that the mechanism used to augment cardiac output was different in the elderly than in the younger subjects (Fig. 11-4 and Table 11-2).[82] To achieve a high level of cardiac output during exercise, younger subjects had higher heart rates (panel A of Fig. 11-4) and exhibited less cardiac diastolic dilatation (panel B)

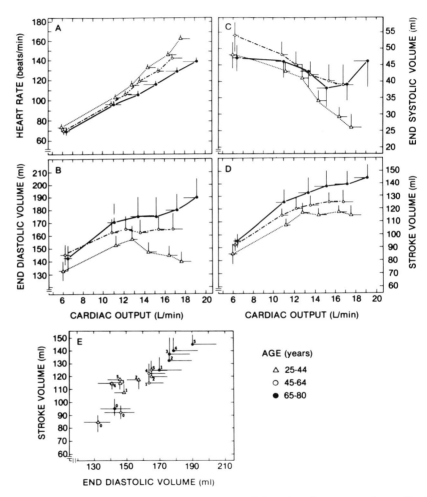

FIG. 11-4. The relationship of heart rate (*A*), end-diastolic volume (*B*), end-systolic volume (*C*), and stroke volume (*D*) to cardiac output at rest and during graded upright bicycle exercise in rigorously screened BLSA volunteers (see lines B and D in Figure 11-2). The major point is that a *unique* mechanism for augmentation of cardiac output during exercise does not exist in all subjects; to achieve the same high output as younger subjects, older subjects increase heart rate to a lesser extent but increase stroke volume to a greater extent than the younger subjects; this is not accomplished by a greater reduction in end-systolic volume but rather by an increase (as much as 30%) in end-diastolic volume. The relationship between stroke and end-diastolic volume is depicted in *E*. This hemodynamic profile is an example of Starling's law of the heart. (Redrawn from Rodeheffer RJ et al: Exercise cardiac output is maintained with advancing age in healthy human subjects: Cardiac dilatation and increased stroke volume compensate for diminished heart rate. Circulation 69:302, 1984)

than older subjects; specifically, in older subjects end-diastolic volume increased as much as 30% above the resting levels. For a given cardiac output, stroke volume in the elderly subjects was greater than that in younger subjects (panel D). Since end-systolic volume in elderly subjects (panel C) did not decline substantially with exercise, the enhanced stroke volume in these subjects is attributable to the Frank-Starling mechanism. Although stroke volume was maintained or increased in elderly subjects due to the increased end-diastolic volume, failure of end-systolic volume to decrease to the extent that it did in younger subjects (panel C), and the failure for ejection fraction to increase during exercise to the extent that it did in younger subjects (Fig. 11-5*B*) may indicate some element of pump dysfunction. However, the magnitude of this deficit in the increase in ejection fraction is substantially less than observed in other presumably normal populations, screened by different filters (Fig. 11-5*B*).[80,89]

The changing hemodynamic profile with advancing age in Fig. 11-2 is similar in many regards to that produced experimentally by β-adrenergic blockade (Fig. 11-6).[81] Thus the finding that cardiac dilatation maintains cardiac output in elderly subjects supports the hypothesis that perhaps the most pronounced age effect on cardiovascular function is a diminished effectiveness of adrenergic modulation during stress.[62] A substantial number

of additional types of studies report this concept. Infusion of catecholamines into either humans or animals results in blunted cardiovascular responses (*e.g.,* the increase in heart rate or stroke index or aortic vasodilation declines with advancing age).[62] The direct response to catecholamines in isolated myocardial and vascular tissue is also diminished with aging.[63] Plasma catecholamine levels are higher in elderly than in younger adult subjects during aerobic exercise[102]; given the negative feedback aspects of hormonal modulation, this finding is consistent with the diminished responsiveness of target organs to the secretion of catecholamines.

Although adrenergic stimulation of cardiovascular target organs is a potent modulator on their function, it is not the unique determinant of performance. Indeed, in the healthy elderly subjects shown in Figure 11-4, enhanced diastolic fiber stretch was able to increase myocardial function and prevent a decline in cardiac output that would have otherwise been encountered due to their lesser increase in heart rate and lesser reduction in end-systolic volume compared with their younger counterparts (*i.e.,* when β-adrenergic modulation was reduced).[82] Thus cardiac output was not significantly affected by age in these subjects. In other human subject studies, however, owing to the impact of occult disease, physical deconditioning and/or other variables that are pres-

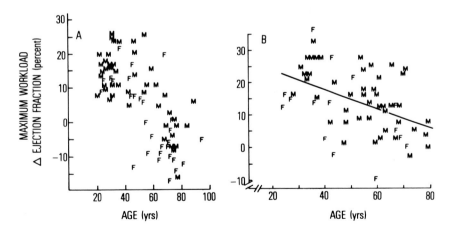

FIG. 11-5. (*A*) The effect of age on the change of left ventricular ejection fraction from the resting level to that at maximum voluntary exercise in apparently healthy subjects. (Port E, Cobb FR, Coleman RE, Jones RH: Effect of age on the response of the left ventricular ejection fraction to exercise. N Engl J Med 303:1133, 1980) (*B*) The effect of age on the change of left ventricular ejection fraction from the resting level to that at maximum voluntary exercise in BLSA subjects. (Rodeheffer RJ, Gersterblith G, Becker LC, Fleg JL, Weisfeldt ML, Lakatta EG: Exercise cardiac output is maintained with advancing age in healthy human subjects. Cardiac dilatation and increased stroke volume compensate for diminished heart rate. Circulation 69:203, 1984)

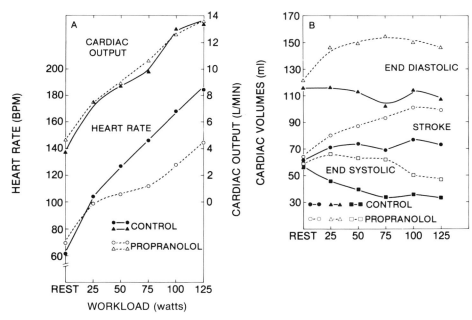

FIG. 11-6. The effect of β-adrenergic blockade (propranolol IV, 0.15 mg/kg) on cardiac output and heart rate (*A*) and on cardiac volumes (*B*) during graded upright bicycle exercise. (Lakatta EG: Altered autonomic modulation of cardiovascular function with adult aging: Perspectives from studies ranging from man to cell. In Weglicki WB (ed): Advances in myocardiology, Vol 7, Pathobiology of Cardiovascular Injury. Boston, Martinus Nijhoff, 1985. In press)

ently uncharacterized, a diminished peak heart rate during exercise in elderly subjects has not been accompanied by a maintained or an increased stroke volume but rather by a decreased stroke volume.[35] In these instances, either end-diastolic volume failed to increase, the deficit in catecholamine modulation of cardiovascular target organs may have been more severe, a greater intrinsic stiffening of the vasculature caused a greater impedance to ejection during exercise, or the effect of stretch to enhance cardiac contraction was compromised owing to deficits in the intrinsic excitation–contraction process or energy supply. However, given the result in Figure 11-4, to imply that the diminution in stroke volume in these earlier studies is due to aging *per se* would be strictly incorrect.

In summary, given the fact that with advancing age the prevalence of coronary artery disease increases sharply and that major changes in life-style occur, and considering that aging, disease, and life-style are intertwined, elucidation of the presence and nature of an "aging process" in the cardiovascular system is a formidable task. An entire spectrum of cardiovascular "aging" changes has been observed, depending on the procedure used

to screen the subjects for study. When individuals with evidence of either clinical or occult disease have been excluded, and when active, community-dwelling subjects' life-style variables are studied, a picture of how aging affects cardiovascular function emerges that is similar to our earlier perspectives in some ways but differs substantially in others.

Between the ages of 20 and 80 years in such a population, arterial stiffening causes systolic blood pressure to increase within the normal range by 25% to 30% and the left ventricle thickens to a similar degree in an apparently adaptive manner. However, pump function and cardiac output at rest are not altered by the aging process. During aerobic exercise, maximal heart rate is diminished but stroke volume is maintained due to an increase in end-diastolic filling volume so that a significant decline in cardiac output does not occur in the elderly; end-systolic volume also fails to decrease from resting values as much as in younger subjects. Thus, maintenance of stroke volume is attributable to use of the Frank-Starling mechanism, which may be considered a successful adaptation to a diminished effectiveness of catecholamines in modulating cardiovascular function. Whether any of these age-related changes in humans can be modified by changes in life-style (*e.g.,* routine physical exercise) is presently unknown.

HYPERTENSION

Epidemiologic Considerations

In addition to an increase in casual resting systolic blood pressure within the clinically normal range with advancing adult age, the prevalence of mixed hypertension, defined as systolic blood pressure greater than 160 mm Hg and diastolic greater than 95 mm Hg, also increases with age. Because of the vascular stiffening that occurs with advancing age, elderly hypertensives are likely to have a disproportionate rise in systolic pressure. Thus, disproportionate systolic hypertension, defined as systolic pressure greater than (diastolic − 15) × 2, was present in 43% of elderly patients in hypertension clinics, and 45% of those had isolated systolic hypertension (ISH), defined by systolic pressure greater than 160 mm Hg and diastolic pressure less than 90 mm Hg.[73]

The decisive impact of both systolic and diastolic blood pressure as a risk factor for cardiovascular disease is clearly evident in Figure 11-7 taken from the Pooling Project Report.[79] The figure depicts the interaction of blood pressure and age on the risk of developing the *first* evidence of the following endpoints: myocardial infarction; sudden death due to coronary disease; angina pectoris; cerebrovascular accident; or intermittent clau-

dication. Several important facts emerge on study of this figure, which is based on pooled data collected in over 8000 individuals in eight different outcome studies. First, at any given age the chance of experiencing a cardiovascular event within the next 5 years increases with the level of systolic and diastolic blood pressures even when they are within the normal range defined by usual clinical criteria. In this respect the clinical definition of normal and abnormal blood pressure range is misleading; rather, the risk of a cardiovascular event is a continuous function of blood pressure, and the exponential nature of this relationship is indicated by the unequal vertical separation of the points at a given age. In fact, the clinically designated abnormal (upper quintile) range separates out from the other quintiles, particularly at younger ages.

Although the risks of systolic and diastolic pressure in this study were not examined independently, other studies have demonstrated that isolated systolic hypertension is at least as potent a risk factor in elderly patients as is diastolic hypertension.[37,73] A second important point is that the curve for any quintile (looking horizontally) is not flat but slopes upward with advancing age and that this slope is not linear but increases exponentially across the age range studied. Thus, the relative risk of an event for a blood pressure in the lowest quintile at age 60 is the same as that of the upper quintile at age 40! This illustrates that age (or time) itself is as potent as blood pressure (or any other known risk factor) as a predictor of a cardiovascular endpoint.

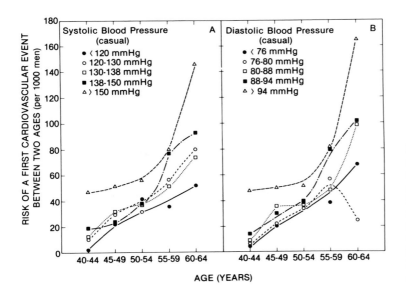

FIG. 11-7. The risk of a first cardiovascular event as a function of age and blood pressure. (*A*) Systolic. (*B*) Diastolic. (Redrawn from Pooling Project Research Group: Relationship of blood pressure, serum cholesterol, smoking habit, relative weight and ECG abnormalities to incidence of major coronary events: Final report of the Pooling Project. J Chronic Dis 31:201, 1978)

The third point made by Figure 11-7 is that the risk associated with *systolic* hypertension is substantial and, in fact, carries at least as much risk as elevations in diastolic pressure. Another important point is that blood pressure and age only account for a fraction of the total variance. In other words, neither a knowledge of the blood pressure, age, nor both can predict the risk of an event in a *given* individual with acceptable accuracy. Nonetheless, like many other areas of clinical medicine in which neither the precise pathophysiology of disease is known nor the precise antidote is available, the rationale for treatment is based on the relative chance of success in the population treated. Because the number of events that can be attributed to hypertension increases with age, it is possible that effective therapy would have a greater short-term impact in older patients.

Therapeutic Considerations

It has been scientifically documented without particular reference to age that effective treatment of "classic" diastolic hypertension significantly reduces the risk of the associated complications of cardiovascular death, congestive heart failure, and stroke.[48–50,104,105] But the question arises as to whether treatment of hypertension similarly reduces the risk of cardiac morbidity and mortality in elderly subjects. Valuable information concerning the effectiveness of antihypertensive therapy in older individuals has been provided by the Hypertension Detection and Follow-Up Program (HDFP) sponsored by the National Institutes of Health.[48–50]

In the HDFP trial both men and women across a broad age range were studied. Entry diastolic

pressure was 90 mm Hg or above. The patients were randomized into two groups, one of which was given antihypertensive therapy in special centers (SC) where every effort was made to treat the patient as effectively as possible and the other group was referred to usual sources of care (UC). Over 10,000 patients aged 30 to 69 years were entered and 5-year follow-up results have been reported. A higher proportion of the SC group received antihypertensive therapy and experienced success in achieving and maintaining long-term control of hypertension.[48] In particular, in the patients aged 60 to 69 years, the reduction in mortality was 16%[49] and the reduction in the incidence of stroke was 45.5% (Fig. 11-8)[50] compared with patients in the UC group. Other cardiovascular endpoints have not been reported to date. Although these results are extremely encouraging, it should be remembered that because of the study design, the physicians were not blinded as to the treatment received and the SC group obtained more frequent and facilitated contact with medical care. Nevertheless, these results indicate that carefully administered antihypertensive therapy has the potential for decreasing the morbidity and mortality of large numbers of elderly patients.

It would seem reasonable that treatment of isolated systolic hypertension would have the same beneficial result. However, it has been argued that the increase in morbidity and mortality from elevated systolic pressure results from the underlying generalized arterial disease rather than the elevated systolic pressure *per se.* In the latter situation, the impact of antihypertensive treatment might be questionable and possibly detrimental.[37] Our understanding of the potential benefits and possible risks of treating isolated systolic hypertension in

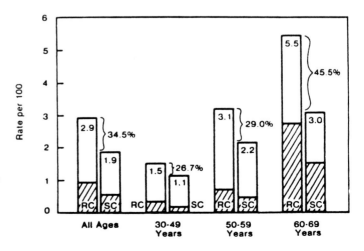

FIG. 11-8. Five-year incidence of fatal and nonfatal stroke by age for stepped care (SC) and referred care (RC) participants in the HDFP study. Data are adjusted for race, sex, and entry diastolic blood pressure. Shaded portion indicates fatal stroke; white portion, nonfatal stroke. (Hypertension Detection and Follow-up Program Cooperative Group: Five year findings of the hypertension detection and follow-up program: III. Reduction in stroke incidence among persons with high blood pressure. JAMA 247:633, 1982)

the elderly is uncertain and awaits the outcome of further studies such as the ongoing Systolic Hypertension in the Elderly clinical trial.

The age-related cardiovascular changes that occur in normotensive subjects are present in hypertensive subjects as well; they often begin to occur at an earlier age, and some are more exaggerated than in normotensives. In elderly (> 65 years of age) patients with hypertension, the cardiac output, heart rate, stroke volume, intravascular volume, renal blood flow, and plasma renin activity were significantly lower than in younger (< 42 years of age) hypertensive patients.[68] Conversely, total peripheral resistance and LV wall thickness were elevated. These and other effects of aging such as diminished creatinine clearance, altered renal sodium retention and potassium conservation, decreased glucose tolerance, diminished β-adrenergic reserve, and a greater tendency to orthostatic hypertension may necessitate closer monitoring of pharmacologic antihypertensive therapy in the elderly than in young patients.[12] Despite these aging changes, the choice of antihypertensive agents is generally similar to that in younger patients.

In the European Working Party Study on High Blood Pressure in the Elderly (EWPHE),[2] 119 hypertensive patients were followed for 1 year and 48 for 2 years in a double-blind, randomized, controlled trial in which they received either placebo or a combination of 25 mg to 50 mg hydrochlorothiazide and 50 mg to 100 mg of triamterene daily. Half of the active treatment group also received 250 mg to 2 g of methyldopa daily. After 2 years the active treatment group had an average increase in the fasting blood glucose level of 9.6 mg/dl compared with an average fall of 3.1 mg in the placebo group (*p* < .001). Blood glucose rose by an average of 26.6 mg/dl in the active group when determined 1 hour after 50 g oral glucose for 2 years (*p* < .05). The hyperglycemic effect of diuretics appeared to be related to potassium loss since, in both groups, impairment of glucose tolerance was most marked in those in whom the serum potassium level decreased over the 2 years. The balance between an increased risk of a small rise in blood glucose and the decreased risk brought about by blood pressure reduction remains to be determined. The overall result of the EWPHE trial should provide this information, but it can be expected that the reduction in blood pressure will more than offset the theoretical risk of a small increase in blood glucose.

β-blocking agents may be less useful in the elderly possibly due to decreased tissue binding[103] or because renin levels tend to decrease in the elderly.[9,68] However, other studies indicate that age *per se* is not a determinant of the ability of propranolol to effect β-blockade. Decreased overall sympathetic responsiveness may also limit the value of β-blockade therapy.[62] Because of the elevated peripheral resistance in elderly hypertensives, it has been suggested that vasodilators may be more useful than β-blocking agents.[12] However, controlled studies are required to substantiate this hypothesis. Attenuated sympathetic responsiveness, decreased total body water, varicose veins, and increased dependence on the Frank-Starling mechanism to augment stroke volume during upright exercise stress may render the elderly more susceptible than their younger counterparts to orthostatic hypotension resulting from the administration of diuretics, ganglionic blocking drugs, and vasodilators. Significant orthostatic hypotension is not uncommon in elderly patients. A decline in systolic pressure of 20 mm Hg on standing has been reported to occur in 10% to 20% of institutionalized elderly individuals, and a decrease of 40 mm Hg occurred in 5%.[10,51,83] Orthostatic hypotension has been associated with numerous conditions, including varicose veins, anemia, hyponatremia, hypokalemia, administration of drugs, and various neurologic defects. The treatment depends on the underlying cause; frequently me-

PHYSIOLOGIC ALTERATIONS IN ELDERLY HYPERTENSIVE PATIENTS THAT MAY INFLUENCE THE THERAPEUTIC EFFICACY AND TOXICITY OF ANTIHYPERTENSIVE THERAPY

Changes in cardiac function at rest
  Decreased cardiac output
  Increased peripheral vascular resistance
  Decreased left ventricular filling rate
Diminished efficacy of β-adrenergic system
  Unopposed α-adrenergic modulation
  Decreased cardiac reserve
  Orthostatic hypotension
Diminished activity of renin–angiotensin "system"
  Decreased plasma renin
  Decreased plasma aldosterone
Renal changes
  Decreased renal blood flow
  Decreased creatinine clearance
  Decreased ability to conserve sodium
Tendency for hyperglycemia, hyperuricemia
Tendency for depression

Coronary Artery Disease   **179**

chanical means to lessen peripheral venous pooling may be sufficient. Peripheral vasoconstricting drugs or blood volume expanders (*i.e.*, mineralocorticoids) should be used with caution in the elderly.

In summary, hypertension continues to exert a potent influence on cardiovascular morbidity and mortality as it does in the young. Available evidence suggests that treatment of diastolic hypertension effects a major reduction in incidence of strokes and a substantial reduction in overall mortality; the benefits of treatment for isolated systolic hypertension are as yet unproven. Despite the well-known decline in plasma renin and β-adrenergic responsiveness and increase in total peripheral resistance in elderly versus young hypertensives, in our opinion none of these age-related changes contraindicates or favors the use of a particular pharmacologic therapeutic regimen in a given subject. In fact, thiazide diuretics, triamterene, methyldopa, and β-blockers all have been used successfully in clinical trials to treat hypertension in the elderly. An important therapeutic guideline to bear in mind, however, is that dosages required to lower pressure in elderly patients may be less than in younger patients, and any of these agents should be prescribed, initially at least, in a lower dosage.

CORONARY ARTERY DISEASE

Epidemiologic Considerations

Despite the widely publicized 37% decline in mortality from coronary artery disease (CAD) that has occurred in the United States over the past 2 dec-

ades,[55] CAD continues to account for approximately half of all deaths in the elderly. The prevalence of coronary atherosclerosis and how often it is likely to be severe enough to be diagnosed clinically can be ascertained by considering the combined results of studies implemented both during life and at autopsy.

The prevalence of fibrous plaques, calcific lesions, and stenosis in coronary arteries in a sample from the New Orleans white population is presented in Figure 11-9.[99] The first point of interest in the figure is that an early manifestation of this disease (*i.e.*, the fibrous plaque) is present in 30% of hearts from individuals between the ages of 15 to 24 years and that by ages 35 to 44, more than 85% of hearts demonstrated this abnormality. Note also that the presence of calcification increases with age and that by age 55 to 64, over 60% of hearts exhibit vascular calcification.

Clinically, the most important vascular abnormality is vessel narrowing or stenosis. Figure 11-9 illustrates that the prevalence of vessel narrowing also increases with age such that by ages 55 to 64, half of all hearts studied had 50% or more occlusion in at least one of the three major coronary arteries. In similar autopsy studies in Rochester, Minnesota, performed in the mid 1950s and again in the late 1970s it was found that 60% to 70% of subjects in this age range or older who died from all causes had significant (> 50% to 60%) narrowing of at least one major coronary artery.[1,20,108] Although significant coronary stenosis is present in a high percentage of elderly individuals, a much smaller percentage has clinical symptoms, that is, the disease is in an occult stage during life in perhaps the majority. However, it is imperative to detect occult CAD in order to deter-

FIG. 11-9. Manifestations of atherosclerosis in coronary arteries from a New Orleans white male population. The data for fibrosis and calcific lesions were derived from those individuals who died of accidents, infections, and miscellaneous causes other than heart disease. Data for stenotic lesions were derived from individuals of this population who died of any cause. (Lakatta EG: Health, disease and cardiovascular aging. In National Academy of Sciences Institute of Medicine (ed): The Aging Society: The Burden of Long-Term Illness and Disability. Washington, DC, National Academy Press. In press)

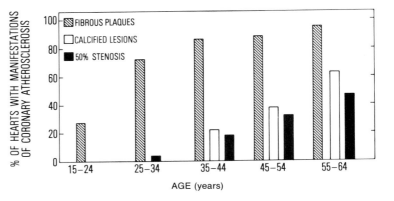

mine whether pharmacologic or life-style interventions will have an impact on its progression.

Recent technologic advances have been made in radionuclide imaging of the myocardium, and this technique, coupled with electrocardiographic monitoring during an exercise stress on the cardiovascular system, has helped to identify many individuals with "occult" CAD. The potential effectiveness of these two relatively noninvasive techniques, employed during exercise in screening for occult CAD, is demonstrated in Figure 11-10.[33] The lower shaded area indicates the prevalence of CAD in community-dwelling volunteers as estimated by the usual epidemiologic criteria (*i.e.,* history of myocardial infarction or angina pectoris and/or Q waves on the resting electrocardiogram). Addition of stress criteria (*i.e.,* ECG or thallium scan abnormalities during exercise) doubles the estimate of prevalence of CAD in these men of middle and advanced age (hatched area), and this approaches that prevalence that is known to exist on the basis of autopsy studies (Fig. 11-11).

Although occlusive CAD connotes atherosclerosis, prominent changes also occur in vascular media in *all* individuals with advancing age even in those populations that do not exhibit atherosclerosis.[3] These include changes in the amount or character of elastin (elasticlike fibers) and collagen (connective tissue) as well as an accumulation of calcium. The precise relationship of these changes to those occurring in the vascular intima has not yet been established. Over the past several decades, attention has focused on the lipid-diet theory as a major causal factor in intimal atherosclerotic process. However, since the intimal processes are paralleled by those in the media it has been suggested by some that the two may be a common manifestation of vascular aging. Although the three major presentations of CAD—angina pectoris, myocardial infarction, and sudden death—occur in the elderly and younger populations alike, important differences in their clinical features do exist.

Clinical Manifestations

Angina Pectoris

Although angina pectoris is a useful marker for the presence of significant CAD in elderly patients as in younger ones, certain factors peculiar to the elderly may create diagnostic difficulty.

If an older person's activities are limited by orthopedic, respiratory, or other problems, he may not be able to exercise sufficiently to be aware of anginal symptoms. Memory deficits, diminished awareness of pain, or the existence of gastrointestinal or musculoskeletal chest pain may similarly obscure the diagnosis. Conversely, aortic valvular stenosis and hypertrophic cardiomyopathy, two cardiac diseases seen commonly in the elderly, may cause anginal pains indistinguishable from CAD; careful auscultation and echocardiography can usually exclude these conditions.

Acute Myocardial Infarction

Even in this age of sophisticated coronary care units and prehospital advanced life support, acute myocardial infarction (MI) continues to present a diagnostic and therapeutic challenge in old age. In an often-quoted study of 597 chronically institutionalized patients aged 65 and older with acute MI, only 19% presented with classic chest pain symptoms.[76] Sudden dyspnea or exacerbation of previously controlled heart failure was the most common presenting complaint (20%); acute confusion (12%), sudden death (7%), syncope (7%), hemiplegia (6%), peripheral arterial occlusion (5%), vertigo (5%), and palpitations (4%) were also common presentations. The high prevalence of dyspnea in the elderly compared with younger

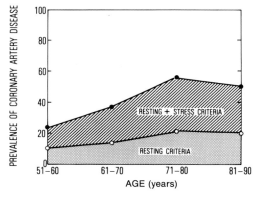

FIG. 11-10. An estimate of the prevalence of coronary artery disease in men aged 51 to 90. Subjects were participants of the BLSA. Resting criteria are history of angina pectoris, myocardial infarction, or an abnormal ECG: stress criteria are the presence of an abnormal ECG (J point depression of at least 1 mm and flat ST segment for at least 0.08 second) and/or a thallium scan perfusion defect during exercise. (Lakatta EG: Health, disease and cardiovascular aging. In National Academy of Sciences Institute of Medicine (ed): The Aging Society: The Burden of Long-Term Illness and Disability. Washington, DC, National Academy Press. In press)

FIG. 11-11. Incidence of CHF in men (Δ) and women (○) from the Framingham Study[67] and the prevalence of CHF reported from physicians' offices in Caledonia County, Vermont in 1963 (●).[58] The diagnosis was established from a well-defined system of major and minor criteria in the Framingham population and from practicing physicians' office assessments in the latter study. In both populations, a striking age-related increase in CHF frequency is observed. (Fleg JL, Lakatta EG: How useful is digitalis in patients with congestive heart failure and sinus rhythm? Int J Cardiol 6:295, 1984)

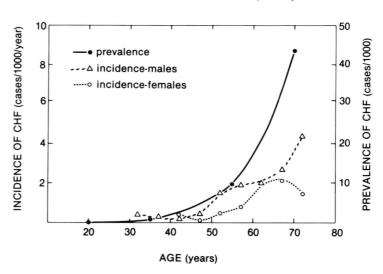

populations with acute MI may relate to the superimposition of the increased LV stiffness accompanying infarction on the heart, which is already stiffer by virtue of age alone,[96] resulting in higher pressure being transmitted to the lung. Although such a high percentage of atypical presentations for MI in the elderly has not been found by others,[111] the message remains clear: because the majority of arrhythmic deaths from MI occur within the first few hours, a high index of suspicion for infarction in geriatric patients should exist so that life-threatening delays in hospitalization can be avoided. Among 2788 patients with suspected MI, the prehospital fatality rate accelerated from 4% of those younger than 35 years to 45% of those 85 or older[110] despite no age-related difference in duration of symptoms before medical attention was sought.

The mortality from acute MI rises dramatically with age, averaging about 40% in those older than 70 years,[19,71,111] a rate at least twice that of younger individuals. This increase in mortality appears to be both an independent effect of age[57,71] as well as a function of the higher incidence of pump dysfunction in elderly patients with infarction. The elderly, for example, are much more likely to present with heart failure, pulmonary edema, or cardiogenic shock. Discriminant analysis applied prospectively to 757 patients with acute MI identified admission systolic blood pressure and age as the most powerful independent prognostic factors for hospital mortality.[71] The reasons for this potent effect of age on mortality in MI are unclear but may include larger infarct size, prior myocardial damage, diminished cardiac reserve in uninfarcted muscle, or more coexistent noncardiac disease in

geriatric than in younger patients. In contrast to pump dysfunction, the incidence of ventricular fibrillation is not age related[19,111]; whether advanced heart block occurs more frequently in older patients is uncertain. Cardiac rupture, a uniformly fatal complication of MI, has a striking predilection for the elderly, particularly in women with antecedent hypertension and suffering their first MI. In a home for the aged, cardiac rupture was the cause of death in 20% of patients with acute fatal MIs.[114]

Therapeutic Considerations in Ischemic Heart Disease

Treatment of angina pectoris in the elderly follows the same general principles as in younger patients. A search for treatable contributing factors such as hypertension, congestive heart failure, "masked" hyperthyroidism, or anemia should always be made. Drug therapy for angina consists of nitrates, β-blockers, and calcium channel antagonists. It remains an open question as to whether there is an effect of age on the benefit or toxicity of these agents. Altered pharmacokinetics of propranolol in the elderly[103] as well as their higher incidence of severe adverse reactions such as bradycardia, heart block, and congestive heart failure[41] dictate careful patient selection. Cardioselective β-blockers may have advantages over propranolol in patients with diabetes, peripheral vascular disease, or mild obstructive lung disease. Altered cardiovascular reflexes and venous varicosities often present in elderly patients may potentiate the hypotensive effects of nitrates and calcium blockers, especially during upright posture. Of the calcium antagonists, diltiazem appears to have the lowest incidence of side-effects and may represent a useful alternative to nitrates or β-blockers in patients intolerant of these agents.[98] For all antianginal drugs, a low starting dose is a good general rule.

Although the dose of some drugs may have to be decreased if renal or hepatic clearance is diminished, there are no qualitative changes in the choice of medical therapy for infarction that depend on the age of the patient. The well-documented increase in lidocaine toxicity in the elderly,[78] frequently manifested by mental confusion, dictates that smaller infusion rates be employed. Early mobilization of geriatric patients with MI is particularly useful in light of their high risk of thromboembolic events and poor tolerance of anticoagulants. Despite their high short-term mortality in acute MI, elderly patients actually have a more favorable long-term prognosis relative to age-matched controls, than do younger patients with infarction.[7] Furthermore, in three recent large randomized trials of β-blockers in survivors of acute MI, patients older than 60 years had a reduction of mortality as large or larger than in younger ones over the subsequent 1 to 2 years.[31]

In the past decade we have witnessed the widespread application of coronary artery bypass surgery and, more recently, percutaneous transluminal coronary angioplasty to the treatment of refractory angina pectoris. In the Multicenter Coronary Artery Surgery Study (CASS), major morbidity and mortality from coronary angiography in patients older than 65 years were low but significantly higher than in younger patients.[32] Mortality from bypass surgery was 1.9% among 7827 patients younger than 65 years and 5.2% in 1086 patients older than 65; elderly women tended to have a higher mortality than their male counterparts, 6.9% versus 4.7%.[32] The increase in mortality with age was independent of other risk variables. The efficacy of such surgery in the elderly is confirmed by relief or attenuation of angina in 89% and a 5-year survival of 81% among 1275 patients aged 70 or older.[18] Due in part to more extensive coronary disease and left ventricular dysfunction, patients aged 65 or more who underwent transluminal angioplasty had a mortality rate (2.2%) and a need for elective bypass surgery (25.4%) each three times as high as in younger individuals; respective success rates in the younger and older patients were 62% and 53%.[70] Thus, despite their modest increase in risk with advancing age, both coronary artery bypass surgery and transluminal angioplasty represent attractive therapeutic approaches for the elderly patient with medically refractory angina pectoris.

VALVULAR HEART DISEASE

Aortic Valve Disease

Systolic murmurs in the aortic area occur in 30% to 55% of institutionalized elderly subjects.[113] The majority of these murmurs are due to fibrous thickening and/or early calcification of the aortic valve cusps. Dilatation of the ascending aorta, a frequent finding in the aged, is thought by some to be a major contributor to these murmurs. These benign basal murmurs usually have the following characteristics: grade 1 or 2/6 in intensity, short, early systolic timing, well-preserved A_2 with normal splitting of S_2, and normal carotid upstroke. In over half, the systolic murmur is also heard at the apex and/or left sternal border. The greatest danger posed by these murmurs is their frequent misdiagnosis as aortic stenosis, which in turn may result in unnecessary invasive diagnostic studies. Significant valvular aortic stenosis (AS) can usually be excluded on M-mode or 2-dimensional (2D) echocardiography by the presence of near-normal leaflet separation, presence of systolic leaflet fluttering, and absence of left ventricular hypertrophy; pulsed Doppler examination may be useful in selected cases.

Degenerative calcification of a previously normal aortic valve accounts for nearly all cases of isolated AS after 75 years of age; in individuals between 55 and 70 years of age, calcification of a congenitally bicuspid valve is the most common etiology. Although a harsh, late-peaking basal systolic ejection murmur with a diminished A_2 is characteristic of this lesion as in younger subjects, the age-related stiffening of the central arteries may mask the expected slowly rising carotid pulse and diminished pulse pressure. Such additional clues as ECG or echocardiographic evidence of left ventricular hypertrophy (LVH) and chest roentgenographic or echocardiographic evidence of significant valvular calcification are helpful. Recently, pulsed Doppler examination has been successful in predicting the aortic valve gradient in elderly as well as younger subjects and may soon become the technique of choice for quantifying the severity of AS.[5] The major differential diagnostic entity, obstructive hypertrophic cardiomyopathy, can be excluded by m-mode, or better yet, 2D echocardiography. The importance of prompt, accurate diagnosis of AS is underscored by the eminent curability of this lesion by aortic valve replacement. Although angina, syncope, and congestive heart failure, followed by death within 3, 2, and 2 years, respectively, represent the natural history of this disorder, aortic valve replacement can be performed with low mortality into the ninth decade and results in excellent long-term survival, even in patients with decreased preoperative ejection fraction.[16,45]

Incompetence of the aortic valve or aortic regurgitation (AR) in the elderly is usually due to calcific degeneration, rheumatic heart disease, or so-called isolated aortic incompetence, possibly attributable to age-related dilatation of the aortic root. Luetic aortitis, formerly the major cause of severe AR in the aged, is an uncommon cause today. Although the clinical prevalence of aortic diastolic murmurs is markedly lower than that of systolic murmurs in old age, the relative difficulty in detecting such murmurs and the prolonged symptom-free survival even with significant AR, certainly contribute to an underestimation of the prevalence of this lesion. Clinical presentation is similar to that in younger patients; echocardiography will reveal significant LV dilatation with relatively normal LV function unless heart failure has supervened. Valve replacement should be considered for symptomatic patients without marked impairment of LV function. The use of end-systolic LV dimension on M-mode echocardiography has been used successfully to determine the optimal timing for aortic valve replacement in chronic AR.[43]

Mitral Valve Disease

Mitral stenosis (MS) in the aged is nearly always rheumatic in origin; MS is the dominant lesion in about one third of rheumatic mitral valve disease cases in this population. There are no distinctive physical findings of MS in the elderly. Whether due to chest wall deformity, a heavily calcified mitral valve, or superimposed atrial fibrillation, the classic auscultatory features of MS may be obscured in old age and the patient's dyspnea attributed to a pulmonary origin. Commissurotomy, the preferred surgical approach to MS in younger patients, is rarely feasible in the elderly due to the presence of valvular calcification and associated mitral regurgitation. Thus mitral valve replacement is usually necessary as well as long-term anticoagulation with warfarin (Coumadin); in the elderly, antiplatelet drugs such as aspirin, dipyridamole, or sulfinpyrazone may represent a more benign alternative to Coumadin.

In contrast to mitral stenosis, mitral regurgitation (MR) in the elderly has numerous etiologies: rheumatic, papillary muscle disfunction due to CAD, mitral valve prolapse, annular dilatation due to LV enlargement, and annular calcification are

the most common. Rheumatic mitral valve disease is seen in 2% to 3% of the geriatric population; MR is the dominant lesion in two thirds.[11] Due to its ubiquitous nature, mitral valve prolapse (MVP) probably represents the most common cause of MR in all age-groups, including the elderly. Non-ejection systolic clicks, mid-to-late systolic murmurs and echocardiographic signs of prolapse remain the diagnostic hallmarks. Although MVP is generally associated with a benign prognosis, two recent series of elderly patients with MVP have emphasized the high frequency of severe MR and congestive heart failure (25% to 40%) in the elderly, especially among men.[60,101] Endocarditis was seen in 10%, none of whom had been instructed in the prophylactic use of antibiotics.[101] Mitral valve replacement in elderly patients with severe MR or MS has been achieved with excellent clinical and hemodynamic results and an operative and long-term (54 month) mortality essentially identical to that in younger patients.[44]

Calcification of the mitral annulus, a condition peculiar to the elderly, is more common in women than men.[87] It is recognized by the "inverted C" pattern of calcification on the chest roentgenogram and the prominent submitral echoes seen on echocardiography. Although frequently without clinical consequences, in extreme cases such calcification may interfere with the proper closure or opening of the mitral valve, resulting, respectively, in regurgitation or, less commonly, stenosis. It may also be a focus for endocarditis or extend into the His bundle or bundle branches, causing conduction disturbances.

Isolated tricuspid or pulmonic valvular disease is rare in the elderly. As in the young, tricuspid regurgitation may accompany right ventricular failure from any cause, due to dilatation of the tricuspid annulus.

Acute Rheumatic Fever

Elderly patients account for approximately 10% of clinically recognized cases of acute rheumatic fever.[11] The diagnosis is difficult in this group because the common features (malaise, fever, and arthralgia or arthritis) have many more common causes in the aged. Evidence of an antecedent streptococcal infection is usually absent, and only about a third have a prior history of rheumatic fever or rheumatic heart disease. Although polyarthritis occurs in the majority of cases, carditis and other major manifestations are usually absent. A trial of salicylates is both diagnostic and therapeutic.

Infective Endocarditis

Infective endocarditis, formerly a condition associated with youth, is now most commonly seen in patients older than 60 years.[106] Although underlying rheumatic heart disease still represents an important predisposing condition in old age, valvular disorders such as calcific aortic stenosis, mitral valve prolapse, mitral annular calcification, and prosthetic valves represent increasingly common foci for endocarditis in the elderly. This diagnosis is often overlooked in old age because of at least three factors: (1) the failure to even consider endocarditis in the elderly, (2) the absence of typical features in most geriatric patients, and (3) the frequent presence of confounding pathologic processes. Genitourinary and gastrointestinal sources of infection are more common in the elderly than in younger patients. Fever, although present in 93% in one geriatric series,[100] is usually low grade, and murmurs are often soft, therefore failing to arouse suspicion. Treatment of endocarditis should be based on the results of blood cultures and sensitivities as in the young, with at least 4 weeks of intravenous antibiotic therapy. As in younger patients, valve replacement should be reserved for patients with secondary congestive heart failure or persistent infection.

PRIMARY MYOCARDIAL DISEASE

Primary myocardial disease (*i.e.*, cardiomyopathy), although not common in old age, probably occurs considerably more often than is clinically recognized. However, as indicated previously, there is no evidence that age-related changes in myocardial function *per se* can cause significant myocardial dysfunction; thus the concept of a "senile cardiomyopathy" in a clinical sense is strictly incorrect. The most common classification scheme for cardiomyopathy is based on the pathophysiology: congestive, restrictive, or hypertrophic. Despite this classification system, congestive symptoms and arrhythmias are common features of all three types. Failure to diagnose cardiomyopathy in the elderly stems from both a failure to entertain such a diagnosis and a tendency to automatically ascribe unexplained chest pain and congestive symptoms to CAD, owing to the high prevalence of CAD in the geriatric population.

Congestive Cardiomyopathy

As compared with heart failure in younger patients, congestive heart failure in the elderly is less likely to be due to primary myocardial disease and more likely to be due to an identifiable cause, particularly CAD. Although strictly speaking, the entity "ischemic cardiomyopathy" is a contradiction in terms, the not uncommon presentation of geriatric patients in heart failure without either chest pain or a prior clinically recognized infarction justifies the use of this expression. The possibility of a toxic and potentially reversible cause of congestive myopathy, particularly ethanol, should always be sought just as in younger patients.

Hypertrophic Cardiomyopathy

Hypertrophic cardiomyopathy describes a nonphysiologic hypertrophy of the LV myocardium. Although several distinct patterns of hypertrophy have been recognized by 2D echocardiography, the interventricular septum is usually more involved than the LV free wall—hence the synonym of asymmetric septal hypertrophy (ASH). ASH may exist in an obstructive form, characterized by a harsh systolic murmur caused by an abutment of the anterior mitral leaflet against the thickened septum, thereby obstructing the LV outflow tract. Such a murmur may be separated from that of aortic valvular stenosis by the former's accentuation with the Valsalva maneuver; echocardiography, which demonstrates the markedly thickened and hypodynamic septum and sometimes systolic anterior motion of the anterior mitral leaflet, is diagnostic. In recent series, the elderly have constituted one fourth to one third of patients with this condition.[42,109] The common presentation as dyspnea coupled with the presence of pathologic Q waves that occur in some 25% of patients with ASH may lead to an erroneous diagnosis of CAD with resultant congestive heart failure. Such a misdiagnosis may lead to treatment with digoxin, which may actually exacerbate symptoms.

The cornerstone of therapy for symptomatic patients with hypertrophic cardiomyopathy is β-adrenergic blockade, as in younger patients. Such agents decrease LV contractility and thereby diminish outflow tract obstruction; perhaps more importantly, they improve diastolic relaxation, which ameliorates dyspnea. The calcium antagonist verapamil has been shown to result in even greater hemodynamic and symptomatic improvement than propranolol in this condition.[84] In elderly patients who remain symptomatic despite high-dose drug therapy, surgical myectomy of the hypertrophied septum may be accomplished with similar benefits and risk as in the young.[59] Neither medical nor surgical therapy has been shown to reduce the risk of sudden death in patients with hypertrophic myopathy.

Restrictive Cardiomyopathy

Restrictive cardiomyopathy is a rare diagnosis in any age-group and is usually due to an infiltrative process such as amyloidosis or to a malignancy arising elsewhere in the chest. It should be emphasized that despite the common presence of amyloid in senescent hearts, usually in the atria, heavy deposits in ventricular myocardium occur in only 5%. Clinical cardiac dysfunction from amyloidosis may be somewhat more common in the very old, as suggested by their implication in fatal cardiac dysfunction in 4 of 40 autopsied patients in their tenth decade.[107] The diagnosis of a restrictive myopathy should be suspected by the presence of a normal-sized, poorly contracting left ventricle with thickened walls and dilated atria. The presence of highly refractile or "granular sparkling" LV echoes on 2D echocardiography strongly suggests the presence of amyloid. One clinicopathologic report of four elderly patients with restrictive cardiomyopathy in the absence of any recognizable cause is noteworthy.[92]

PERICARDIAL DISEASE

Pericardial disease is not uncommon in old age and has a significantly different etiologic spectrum than in younger patients. Posterior echo-free spaces on M-mode echocardiography become more prevalent with increasing age, exceeding 15% in subjects older than 80 years in the Framingham population.[86] Such spaces may represent subepicardial fat rather than fluid in some cases. Viral or idiopathic causes of acute pericarditis are uncommon in the elderly; instead, malignancy, collagen vascular disease, uremia, and acute or recent myocardial infarction are the most likely etiologies. As with younger patients, chest pain aggravated by breathing and attenuated by sitting up is characteristic. Such chest pain and widespread ST-segment elevation occurring in an elderly patient may cause an erroneous diagnosis of acute MI. A normal plasma level of MB-CK, the myocardial-specific isoenzyme of creatine kinase, helps to exclude infarction. The presence of a friction rub, although often soft and evanescent, is pathognomonic of pericarditis. Treatment is that of the underlying disease plus anti-inflammatory agents for relief of pain.

Cardiac tamponade may arise from any of the causes of pericarditis mentioned previously as well as from cardiac rupture post myocardial infarction or from aortic dissection into the pericardial sac. As in the young, pulsus paradoxicus greater than 10 mm Hg is the most reliable clinical sign of tamponade; echocardiography will confirm the presence of an effusion and may also demonstrate right atrial or right ventricular diastolic collapse. Emergency pericardiocentesis and subsequent surgical creation of a pericardial window constitute the definitive treatment as in the young.

Constrictive pericarditis, like tamponade, is a disorder of diastolic filling; common symptoms include dyspnea, fatigue, peripheral edema, and ascites. A peripheral knocking sound in early diastole, low ECG voltage, pericardial calcification on chest roentgenography, and pericardial thickening or duplication on echocardiography are helpful diagnostic clues. As in younger patients, pericardiectomy is the only definitive treatment although operative risk is high.

CONGENITAL HEART DISEASE

Lesions Compatible with Prolonged Survival

Improved diagnostic techniques and perhaps more effective medical therapy have resulted in a growing recognition of congenital heart disease in the elderly. The most common congenital abnormality in old age as in younger adults is a bicuspid aortic valve, occurring in 2% of adults.[77] Such valves usually cause no symptoms until middle age, by which time sufficient calcification has occurred to create aortic stenosis and less frequently aortic regurgitation. Endocarditis is a not uncommon complication in these patients. Valvular pulmonic stenosis is often associated with survival into old age, perhaps because of the tendency for the orifice area to grow in size in parallel to the increase in body size. Atrial septal defect, another common congenital abnormality seen in the elderly, will be discussed below. Coarctation of the aorta may occasionally be associated with prolonged survival; congestive heart failure superimposed on arterial hypertension constitutes the usual presentation.[77] A bicuspid aortic valve occurs in over 25% of patients with coarctation. Survival to old age with patent ductus arteriosus or ventricular septal defect is uncommon, occurring in association with a narrow communication and thence a small left-to-right shunt.

Atrial Septal Defect

Atrial septal defect (ASD) is one of the most common forms of congenital heart disease found in the elderly, usually presenting as congestive heart failure with or without atrial arrhythmias. The hallmarks of diagnosis are as in the young: a wide fixed splitting of S_2, incomplete right bundle branch block on ECG, increased pulmonary blood flow on chest roentgenography, and an enlarged right ventricle with paradoxic septal motion on m-mode echocardiography. In a series of 498 consecutive patients with ASD, severe mitral regurgitation occurred in 15% of those older than 50 years but in only 2% of those between 21 and 49 years.[65] Although it has been taught that surgery is rarely indicated in elderly patients with ASD, a study of 66 patients aged 60 years and older with secundum ASD documented symptomatic benefit in the majority, regardless of preoperative pulmonary artery pressure, pulmonary vascular resistance, or functional class; actuarial analysis confirmed increased longevity at 5 and 10 years postoperatively compared with that predicted for age-matched medically treated patients.[97] All 4 patients (6%) who died had undergone additional operations. Ostium primum ASD may also be seen in old age; such patients aged 60 years and older represented 12% of those seen at the Mayo Clinic with primum ASD without appreciable interventricular communication.[47] The widespread application of corrective or palliative surgery for a broad array of congenital cardiovascular abnormalities has created a large group of adults whose long-term care will be in the hands of internists and geriatricians.

CONGESTIVE HEART FAILURE

Epidemiology

Congestive heart failure (CHF), defined as inability of cardiac output to match metabolic needs despite adequate filling pressure, affects an estimated 3 to 4 million Americans, of whom at least 75% are older than 60 years. The prevalence of CHF rises 200-fold between the second and eighth decades, most of this increase occurring after 65 years of age (Fig. 11-11).[29,58] It is of interest that despite the widely publicized decline in cardiac morbidity and mortality over the past 15 years, the hospital discharge rate for CHF has increased 132% between 1970 and 1980.[39] Hypertension was the most common precursor to the development of CHF in the Framingham study, occurring in 75%

of cases, followed by coronary artery disease in 39% and rheumatic heart disease in 21%.[66]

Given that CHF is primarily a condition of the elderly, it is ironic that minimal information exists regarding the specific precipitants of CHF, hymodynamic response to individual therapeutic agents, or prognosis in elderly versus younger patients with heart failure. Furthermore, the current medical literature on CHF is skewed toward younger patients with relatively severe failure and a disproportionately high prevalence of primary myocardial disease.

Precipitating Factors

No reliable data exist for the relative frequency of specific precipitants of CHF in old age. Noncompliance with complicated medical regimens or with dietary sodium restriction certainly constitute significant and preventable precipitating factors. The common use of nonsteroidal anti-inflammatory drugs for arthritis is undoubtedly a more frequent contributor to CHF exacerbations in the elderly than in younger patients. Atrial fibrillation may be more likely to cause congestive failure in the senescent heart because of the age-related increasing dependence on the atrial contribution to ventricular filling. Tachycardia of any type will decrease diastolic filling time and increase myocardial oxygen demand; these alterations would be expected to cause a greater rise in LV filling pressure in the hypertrophied, stiffer LV of senescence than in that of a younger individual. Anemia, thyrotoxicosis, or systemic infection, particularly of pulmonary origin, may precipitate CHF because of the associated increase in metabolic demands. Myocardial infarction or, less commonly, pulmonary emboli may present as acute CHF with little or no pain.

Diagnostic Pitfalls

The diagnosis of CHF may be elusive in the elderly for several reasons. Poor historical ability due to an unrelated chronic brain syndrome or confusion and memory impairment due to CHF itself may obscure the diagnosis. Breathlessness and fatigue may be due to generalized deconditioning, obesity, or chronic lung disease. Right-sided failure may cause anorexia or nausea, symptoms that may also be caused by cardiac medications or noncardiac illness.

Physical findings may be similarly difficult to interpret in old age. Rales are a frequent finding in the elderly owing to atelectasis or chronic lung disease. Ankle edema is common owing to venous varicosities; a low diaphragm due to obstructive lung disease may cause a palpable liver and erroneously suggest hepatomegaly. Finally, an elongated unfolded aortic arch may compress the left-sided neck veins against the sternum, causing factitious jugular venous distention.

Therapy

Treatment of CHF has undergone significant evolution in recent years. Although prolonged periods of bed rest have been advocated in the past for a wide variety of cardiac disorders including CHF, the efficacy of such therapy is poorly documented. In contrast, the deleterious effects of prolonged bed rest on aerobic capacity, venous stasis, mineral balance, and various metabolic processes have been amply demonstrated. The baseline impairment in these functions among the elderly dictates that complete or prolonged bed rest be particularly avoided in geriatric cardiac patients, regardless of their specific diagnosis.

Digitalis has been the therapeutic cornerstone in chronic heart failure for two centuries, but a growing literature suggests that many, if not most, elderly patients with CHF can be managed without this drug.[29] Unfortunately, in some of these studies of digitalis efficacy, it is unclear whether the patients ever had heart failure. Two studies, however, comprising a total of 54 predominantly elderly clinically stable subjects with documented CHF and sinus rhythm, showed the feasibility of withdrawing digoxin without clinical deterioration.[27,36] Given the expanding armamentarium of diuretics and vasodilators and the well-known long-term risk of digitalis toxicity in the elderly due in large part to their reduced renal drug clearance,[4,23,90] a closely supervised therapeutic trial without digitalis may be warranted in every patient with compensated heart failure and normal sinus rhythm. When employed for CHF, digitalis should be started in maintenance doses without a loading dose.

Diuretics are the mainstay of therapy for CHF. Small doses should be given initially, especially to patients not previously on these drugs. A thiazide rather than a loop diuretic appears preferable for those with mild CHF and preserved renal function. Furosemide starting at 20 mg to 40 mg should be reserved for those with more severe failure. Both thiazide and loop diuretics can cause hypokalemia, hyponatremia, hyperuricemia, and hyperglycemia. Among 200 hospitalized medical and surgical pa-

tients averaging 70 years old, furosemide caused 70% of all drug-induced biochemical abnormalities and 49% of all drug-induced complications.[94] Patients refractory to large doses of furosemide often diurese when an aldosterone antagonist is added. The age-related reduction in plasma renin[22] increases the risk of hyperkalemia from such drugs. Furthermore, blood levels of antidiuretic hormone (ADH) are elevated in the elderly in response to stress[17] and do not respond appropriately to agents that inhibit ADH secretion; this may result in hyponatremia.

The employment of vasodilators for the treatment of severe or refractory CHF has gained widespread acceptance over the past few years. Although most such studies of vasodilators include some elderly patients, the mean age is usually in the 50s. The effect of age *per se* on the response to these drugs has not been specifically addressed. Major unanswered questions in both elderly and younger patients include the need for invasive monitoring when initiating therapy, the development of tolerance, and the effect on long-term mortality. Studies suggest that of all currently used vasodilators, long-term symptomatic benefit occurs most often with captopril, approaching 70% of patients.[74] The propensity of all vasodilators to cause hypotension necessitates caution in the elderly, with frequent monitoring for orthostasis.

ARRHYTHMIAS AND CONDUCTION DISTURBANCES

Normative Data

The prevalence of supraventricular and ventricular arrhythmias increases with age, both in unselected populations and those ostensibly free of cardiac disease. Pooled data from 2482 ECGs in elderly patients demonstrated supraventricular ectopic beats (SVEB) in 10% and ventricular ectopic beats (VEB) in 6%; atrial fibrillation was noted in 8% of patients.[25] Because the standard ECG usually represents less than 1 minute of cardiac activity, 24-hour ambulatory ECG monitoring is a much more sensitive and quantitative technique. In 98 healthy subjects aged 60 to 85 years old who were carefully screened to exclude CAD, such 24-hour monitoring disclosed isolated SVEB in 88% and isolated VEB in 78% of subjects (Table 11-3).[28] Frequent SVEB and VEB ($\geq$ 100 in 24 hours) were found in 26% and 17%, respectively. Short asymptomatic episodes of paroxysmal atrial tachycardia occurred in 13%, ventricular couplets in 11%, and ventricular tachycardia (VT) in 4%. The prevalence of each of these arrhythmias greatly exceeded that found in healthy young subjects studied by others. On the other hand, atrial flutter and fibrillation, sinus bradycardia less than 40 beats/min, sinus pauses exceeding 1.6 seconds and high-degree atrioventricular (AV) block were rare or nonexistent in these highly screened individuals.

In apparently healthy adults undergoing treadmill exercise, the prevalence of both SVEB and VEB has been shown to increase with age. Asymptomatic runs of VT, none exceeding six beats in duration, were seen in nearly 4% of apparently healthy subjects aged 65 or older, a prevalence 25 times that of younger subjects.[30] Over a mean follow-up of 2 years, none of these elderly individuals experienced angina, myocardial infarction, syncope, or cardiac death. From these studies, it should be apparent that the mere presence of SVEB or VEB in geriatric patients, even if frequent or complex, is by no means an accurate marker for organic heart disease. Such ectopic activity, therefore, may require no specific treatment.

Although rigorous data are lacking, it might be anticipated that the hemodynamic consequences of various arrhythmias would be accentuated in old age. As previously noted, the thicker, less compliant senescent left ventricle, in which early diastolic filling is impaired at rest, might suffer a greater compromise than a younger ventricle during any tachycardia, due to the abbreviated diastole. Arrhythmias are also potentially more serious in the elderly because they may further compromise vital organs whose intrinsic function has been reduced by aging and disease. Thus, the 40% to 70% reduction of cerebral flow accompanying ventricular tachycardia might be well tolerated by a young patient but result in syncope in an elderly patient with extensive cerebrovascular disease.

Alterations in Pharmacology of Antiarrhythmic Drugs

The pharmacology of several commonly used antiarrhythmic drugs is altered with aging. The half-life of digoxin is prolonged in elderly subjects owing to their reduced glomerular filtration and generally smaller body size, compared with younger subjects.[24] Despite the widespread availability of serum drug levels, digitalis toxicity continues to be a relatively common occurrence in the elderly, owing to the frequent use of this drug for heart failure and atrial arrhythmias.[46] The clearance of quinidine is reduced by 34% and elimination half-life is prolonged to 9.7 hours in subjects 60 to 69 years

of age compared with 7.3 hours in those 23 to 29 years of age.[72] The demonstration that quinidine therapy increases serum digoxin levels approximately 100%[64] may have particular relevance to the elderly, in whom this drug combination is frequently prescribed. Because hepatic flow is reduced with age, the infusion rate of lidocaine should be reduced in the elderly to avoid the central nervous system toxicity so commonly seen with this agent. Similar considerations pertain to propranolol and other β-blockers handled by first-pass hepatic metabolism.

Specific Arrhythmias

Atrial Tachycardia

Isolated SVEBs, even when frequent, rarely require specific treatment. Paroxysmal supraventricular tachycardia (PSVT) is usually due to a reentrant mechanism and can often be terminated by vagal maneuvers, such as Valsalva, gagging, or carotid sinus massage. The latter maneuver should be performed in the elderly patient only after significant carotid stenosis has been excluded by physical examination. If these vagal stimuli are unsuccessful, verapamil 5 mg to 10 mg should be given intravenously over 2½ to 5 minutes. Digoxin is the preferred prophylactic therapy for PSVT, owing to its documented efficacy[112] and once-daily dosage. Atrial tachycardia with block is usually due to digitalis toxicity; treatment consists of withholding the drug and correcting hypokalemia. Multifocal atrial tachycardia is commonly seen in elderly patients with obstructive lung disease. The lack of effective drug therapy dictates that treatment be directed toward the predisposing condition. Accelerated junctional rhythm, although not usually a cause of hemodynamic impairment, is usually a sign of a serious underlying disorder. In the elderly, the most common causes are digitalis toxicity and acute inferior MI. Sudden regularization of the ventricular rate in a geriatric patient on digitalis for chronic atrial fibrillation should suggest this diagnosis; again, treatment is directed toward the underlying disorder.

Atrial Flutter

Atrial flutter should be suspected when a regular tachycardia occurs at a ventricular rate close to 150 beats/min. Carotid massage may be diagnostic, causing an abrupt slowing of the ventricular response and the emergence of "sawtooth" flutter

TABLE 11-3 Supraventricular and Ventricular Arrhythmias Observed in 98 Healthy Subjects Aged 60 to 85

Arrhythmias	No. Subjects	Percentage of Total
Supraventricular		
Any	86	88
Isolated ectopic beats	86	88
≥ 30 beats in any hour	22	22
≥ 100 beats in 24 hours	25	26
Benign slow atrial tachycardia	27	28
Paroxysmal atrial tachycardia	13	13
Atrial flutter	1	1
Accelerated junctional rhythm	1	1
Ventricular		
Any	78	80
≥ 5 in any hour	76	78
≥ 30 in any hour	37	38
≥ 60 in any hour	12	12
≥ 100 in 24 hours	17	17
Multiform	34	35
Ventricular couplets	11	11
Ventricular tachycardia	4	4
R on T phenomena	1	1
Accelerated idioventricular rhythm	1	1

(Fleg, JL, Kennedy HL: Cardiac arrhythmias in a healthy elderly population: Detection by 24-hour ambulatory electrocardiography. Chest 81:302, 1982)

waves. Common etiologies in the elderly are CAD and obstructive lung disease. Digoxin is the drug of choice if hemodynamic status is stable; otherwise low-level DC cardioversion (25 to 50 joules) converts flutter to sinus rhythm in nearly all cases.

Atrial Fibrillation

In contrast to the other atrial tachyarrhythmias mentioned, atrial fibrillation (AF) is much more likely to be chronic than acute. As in middle age, hypertension, CAD, and mitral valve disease are the most common predisposing conditions; additional considerations in the elderly include amyloidosis, sick sinus syndrome, and thyrotoxicosis. Data from the Framingham study confirm the marked age-related increase in the incidence of AF as well as the high cardiovascular morbidity and

mortality associated with this arrhythmia, even in so-called lone AF.[54] As in younger patients, initial treatment is directed toward slowing the ventricular response to 60 to 100 beats/min with digoxin, verapamil, or propranolol given intravenously. Because of the frequent presence of AV nodal disease, geriatric patients with AF often present with a controlled ventricular response and require no specific therapy. The decision to attempt electrical cardioversion for chronic AF requires consideration of the etiology and duration of AF, atrial size, and risk of anticoagulation. Given the poor prognosis of chronic AF noted previously, an initial attempt at cardioversion is probably warranted in most elderly patients.

Ventricular Ectopic Beats

Although the presence of ventricular ectopic beats (VEB), whether isolated or frequent and complex, does not appear to adversely affect prognosis in clinically healthy elderly individuals, even simple VEBs are associated with increased long-term cardiovascular mortality in patients with documented CAD. Nevertheless, it has yet to be shown that treatment of isolated VEBs in these patients actually reduces their long-term risk of death. These considerations, coupled with the generally higher risk of reactions to the commonly used antiarrhythmic drugs in the elderly, should dictate a conservative approach to long-term therapy of the older patient with isolated VEBs. As with SVEBs, treatment should be directed toward such underlying or exacerbating factors as electrolyte disturbances, hypoxia, or CHF.

Ventricular Tachycardia

In contrast to the relatively benign nature of isolated VEBs, sustained ventricular tachycardia (VT) requires immediate attention. Common precipitants in the elderly are severe myocardial ischemia, acute MI, digitalis intoxication, or CHF. If VT is well tolerated hemodynamically, a bolus of 50 mg to 75 mg lidocaine followed by another 50 mg 2 minutes later may be given initially. Recurrent VT or VT resistant to lidocaine may be treated successfully with intravenous administration of procainamide or with β-blocking drugs. Current data, derived largely from younger patients, suggest that bretylium is the most effective treatment for VT refractory to lidocaine. As in the young, VT associated with hypotension or syncope requires immediate electrical cardioversion.

VT precipitated by an acute event such as MI

or digitalis toxicity has a low recurrence rate and does not require chronic prophylaxis. On the other hand, such arrhythmias occurring without an obvious precipitant, so called primary VT, have approximately a 35% recurrence rate in 1 year and therefore require aggressive prophylactic management. In a recent series, patients with out of hospital cardiac arrest due to a primary arrhythmic event averaged 68.5 years of age and had a 1 year mortality of 29%.[38]

The most promising approach to such patients appears to be intracardiac programmed electrophysiologic stimulation, in which the malignant arrhythmia is induced and the efficacy of various antiarrhythmic agents in preventing VT is determined in a special catheterization laboratory. A marked reduction in 1- to 2-year mortality has been demonstrated in patients whose drug therapy for recurrent VT was thus determined.[67,85] An alternative less invasive but similarly labor-intensive approach using ambulatory ECG monitoring has also been employed successfully.[40] Elderly patients in whom neither of the above medical approaches is successful should be considered for an automatic implantable defibrillator[69] or endocardial resection guided by intraoperative mapping.[52]

BRADYARRHYTHMIAS AND CONDUCTION DISORDERS

Normative Histologic Conduction System Changes with Aging

With advancing age, widespread histologic changes in the conduction system occur. An exaggeration of these normative aging changes may help to explain the striking age-related increase in bradyarrhythmias and conduction disturbances. A progressive decrease in the number of pacemaker cells in the sinoatrial (SA) node begins by the age of 60 years; only about 10% of the number of cells found in young adults remain by 75 years.[15] The SA node is also enveloped by fat, which may cause a partial or complete separation of the node from the atrial musculature. In the bundle of His, aging is associated with a loss of cells, an increase in fibrous and adipose tissue, and amyloid infiltration. The left side of the cardiac skeleton, which includes the central fibrous body, the mitral and aortic annuli, and the proximal interventricular septum, undergoes some degree of fibrosis in senescence. The AV node, bundle of His, and proximal left and right bundle branches may be in-

volved in this process, owing to their proximity to these structures. In extreme cases, the resultant "idiopathic" fibrosis may cause AV block and is, in fact, the most common cause of chronic AV block in the elderly.[15]

Normative Age-related Changes in the ECG

The standard ECG demonstrates several manifestations of these age-related histologic alterations in the conduction system. Although most studies have not demonstrated a significant age-related change in resting heart rate, the respiratory variation in resting sinus rate known as sinus arrhythmia decreases with aging.[14] Small age-associated prolongation of the PR and QT intervals also occur, but QRS duration is unchanged.[93] High-resolution surface electrocardiography in healthy volunteers has localized the increase in PR interval to a delay proximal to the bundle of His; conduction time from the bundle of His to the ventricle was unrelated to age.[13]

The QRS frontal plane axis shifts leftward over time, probably reflecting the combined effects of fibrosis in the anterior fascicle of the left bundle branch and mild age-related LV hypertrophy. Such left axis deviation was the most common abnormality in a survey of nearly 2500 ECGs from elderly subjects' occurring in 51%.[25] Neither first-degree AV block nor axis deviation leftward of −30° is associated with increased cardiac morbidity or mortality in the absence of organic heart disease. An age-associated increase in the prevalence of bundle branch block also occurs. Although left bundle branch block (LBBB) is usually associated with ischemic or hypertensive cardiac disease, complete right bundle branch block (RBBB) is not infrequently seen in apparently healthy older men; 24 such men, of mean age 64 years, who were without clinical heart disease experienced no increase in cardiac events or decline in aerobic capacity compared with age-matched controls over an 8.4 year follow-up.[26] Data from the Framingham study indicate that in women RBBB has the same high likelihood of indicating underlying cardiac disease as does LBBB.[88]

Due to the higher prevalence of intrinsic conduction disease as well as acute processes such as MI and digitalis intoxication, bradyarrhythmias are more common in old age than in the young. Nevertheless, it should be reemphasized that sinus bradycardia less than 40 beats/min, sinus pauses greater than 1.6 seconds, and high-degree AV block were rare or nonexistent in the sample of

98 healthy subjects older than 60 years previously described.[28] Such conduction disturbances are frequently associated with ischemic, hypertensive, and amyloid heart disease. The most common bradyarrhythmias are discussed in the following section.

Specific Bradyarrhythmias

Sinus Bradycardia

Sinus bradycardia, defined by a sinus mechanism at less than 60 beats/min, may just be a sign of excellent physical conditioning, but in the elderly it frequently indicates intrinsic sinus node disease. Inferior MI, hypothermia, myxedema, and increased intracranial pressure may cause this arrhythmia.

Sinoatrial Block

Sinoatrial block occurs when sinus node impulses fail to depolarize the atria. Such block is often 2:1, resulting in a ventricular rate exactly half the sinus rate. Common etiologies in old age are intrinsic conduction disease, ischemia, and digitalis toxicity.

Second-Degree AV Block

Second-degree AV block may present in two distinct patterns. *Mobitz type I,* also called Wenckebach, is recognized by a progressive prolongation of PR interval until a ventricular complex is dropped. Because such block is usually proximal to the His-Purkinje system, the QRS complex is typically normal in appearance. Digitalis intoxication and acute inferior MI are common precipitants. This arrhythmia is usually transient and thus rarely requires specific therapy.

In *Mobitz type II* block, the PR interval is fixed but QRS complexes are dropped. Because the site of block is at or below the bundle of His the QRS complex is usually wide. Mobitz type II block is most frequently associated with acute anterior MI, myocarditis, and advanced sclerodegenerative conduction system disease. Patients with this arrhythmia are usually symptomatic, often presenting with syncope due to inadequate cerebral perfusion (Stokes-Adams attack). Because of its symptomatic presentation and frequent progression to complete heart block, Mobitz type II block usually warrants the insertion of a permanent cardiac pacemaker.

Third-Degree AV Block

Third-degree or complete AV block is characterized by the inability of any atrial depolarizations to activate the ventricle. Block within the AV node is usually associated with normal QRS complexes and an escape rate close to 60 beats/min. Common etiologies are acute inferior MI and digitalis toxicity; in most instances such block is transient. Block within the ventricles, by contrast, is accompanied by wide QRS complexes and a slow escape rate, often less than 40 beats/min. Such block may occur in severe sclerodegenerative conduction system disease or extensive acute anterior MI. These patients usually respond poorly to atropine and isoproterenol, necessitating insertion of a pacemaker.

Sick Sinus Syndrome

The sick sinus syndrome (SSS) encompasses a variety of rhythm disturbances reflecting dysfunction of the SA node and is often associated with dysfunction elsewhere in the conduction system. Although SSS may occur in association with a wide variety of cardiac diseases, CAD or a primary sclerodegenerative process is most often responsible. Patients may present with bradyarrhythmias (sinus bradycardia, sinus pauses or arrest, SA exit block, or AF with a slow ventricular response) or with the so-called bradycardia–tachycardia syndrome, in which a supraventricular tachycardia terminates in a long period of asystole. Symptoms may therefore consist of palpitations or chest pain during tachycardia and dizziness or syncope during bradycardia. The tachycardia—PSVT, atrial flutter or atrial fibrillation—is treated as outlined previously; bradycardia associated with syncope should be treated by permanent pacing.

Acute Therapy of Bradyarrhythmias

Acute therapy for bradyarrhythmia is required in the presence of hypotension, cerebral or cardiac ischemia, and CHF, and in the case of VEB in acute MI. Placement of the patient supine with the legs elevated often ameliorates hypotensive sequelae acutely. Atropine in a 0.5-mg intravenous bolus constitutes initial pharmacotherapy and may be repeated at 3- to 5-minute intervals until 0.04 mg/kg has been given. If atropine is ineffective or causes intolerable side-effects, an isoproterenol drip is begun at 1 μg to 4 μg/min and titrated to produce a ventricular rate of 60 beats/min. When neither drug is successful, or in a setting of acute ischemia or infarction, when isoproterenol is generally contraindicated, temporary transvenous pacing is employed.

Pacemakers

Probably no cardiovascular therapeutic modality is more strongly associated with the elderly than pacemakers. In a series of 707 pacemakers implanted in patients at Toronto Western Hospital in the 1970s, two thirds were implanted in patients 70 years old or older.[6] Approximately a third were implanted for complete heart block and another third for SSS. Data show that SSS now accounts for 48% of all implants.[75] Permanent ventricular pacing has eliminated the accelerated mortality formerly associated with complete heart block (Fig. 11-12).[91] On the other hand, permanent pacing for SSS should be on the basis of documented symptomatic bradyarrhythmia since such pacing does not affect survival. Asymptomatic elderly patients with chronic bifascicular block, with or without PR interval prolongation, do not warrant pacemaker implantation, in light of their infrequent progression to complete heart block. Advances in pacemaker technology, such as rate programmability and dual-chamber AV synchronous pacing, may be extremely useful in selected elderly patients, although their merits in the general population of pacemaker recipients appear to have been oversold.

The decision to insert a permanent pacemaker must be made in full awareness of the small but significant rate of pacemaker-induced complications. Abrupt loss of pacing due to battery failure, fibrosis around the catheter site, myocardial perforation, lead fracture, or electrode dislodgement may result in marked bradycardia or asystole. Catheter perforation of the right ventricle may cause a pericardial friction rub or rarely tamponade. Geriatric patients with little overlying subcutaneous tissue may experience extrusion of the pulse generator or erosion of the pacing wire through the skin. Other nonmedical considerations include the need for regular follow-up and the occasional patient with a psychologic maladjustment to pacemaker therapy.

FUTURE DIRECTIONS IN GERIATRIC CARDIOLOGY

What developments in geriatric cardiovascular disease can be expected to appear or continue in the foreseeable future? It is certain that the age of our

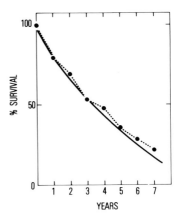

FIG. 11-12. Survival of 139 patients older than 80 years who were paced for complete heart block is shown by the dotted line. The solid line indicates the survival curve for age- and sex-matched members of the general population. The two lines are essentially identical. (Lakatta EG, Gerstenblith G: Cardiovascular system. In Rowe JW, Besdine RW (eds): Health and Disease in Old Age, pp 185–209. Boston, Little, Brown, 1982)

population will continue to increase; most dramatic will be the continued rise in the percentage of very elderly citizens; the group over 85 years of age increased by 40% from 1970 to 1980.[56] The elderly will undoubtedly continue to be plagued by a high prevalence of organic heart disease, especially CAD. Advances in diagnosis such as Doppler ultrasound, radionuclide imaging, computed tomography, and magnetic resonance imaging will allow earlier, less invasive, yet more complete evaluation of heart disease, while advances in pharmacotherapy, surgery, and angioplastic techniques will perpetuate the recent decline in overall cardiovascular mortality, allowing it to be enjoyed by elderly and younger patients alike. The growing appreciation that the deconditioning that accompanies both the aging process and the development of cardiac disease can be ameliorated by aerobic training, even in geriatric patients, will allow the morbidity as well as mortality of such disease to decrease. Finally, the greatest promise for the future of geriatric cardiovascular medicine lies in the recognition that by the optimization of life-style variables such as diet, tobacco use, and exercise, a large proportion of cardiovascular disease will never be allowed to develop.

REFERENCES

1. Ackerman RF, Dry TJ, Edwards JE: Relationship of various factors to the degree of coronary atherosclerosis in women. Circulation 1:1345, 1950

2. Amery A et al: Glucose intolerance during diuretic therapy: Results of Trial by the European Working Party on Hypertension in the Elderly. Lancet 1:681, 1978

3. Avolio AP et al: Effects of aging on changing arterial compliance and left ventricular load in a Northern Chinese urban community. Circulation 68:50, 1983

4. Beller GA, Smith TW, Ablemann WH, Haber E, Wood WB Jr: Digitalis intoxication: A prospective clinical study with serum level correlations. N Engl J Med 184:989, 1971

5. Berger M, Berdoff RL, Gallerstein PE, Goldberg E: Evaluation of aortic stenosis by continuous wave Doppler ultrasound. J Am Coll Cardiol 3:150, 1984

6. Berman ND: Geriatric Cardiology, pp 1, 111, 205. Lexington, MA, The Collamore Press, DC Heath & Co, 1982

7. Biorck G et al: Studies on myocardial infarction in Malmo 1935–1954: III. Follow-up studies from a hospital material. Acta Med Scand 162:81, 1958

8. Brandfonbrener M, Landowne M, Shock NW: Changes in cardiac output with age. Circulation 12:447, 1955

9. Bühler FR et al: Antihypertensive beta blocking action as related to renin and age: A pharmacologic tool to identify pathogenic mechanisms in essential hypertension. Am J Cardiol 36:653, 1975

10. Caird FI, Andrews GR, Kennedy RD: Effect of posture on blood pressure in the elderly. Br Heart J 35:527, 1973

11. Caird FI, Dall JLC: The Cardiovascular System. In Brocklehurst JC (ed): Textbook of Geriatric Medicine and Gerontology, 2nd ed., p 125. New York, Churchill Livingstone, 1978

12. Chobanian AV: Pathophysiologic considerations in the treatment of the elderly hypertensive patient. Am J Cardiol 52:490, 1983

13. Das DN, Fleg JL, Lakatta EG: Effect of age on the components of atrioventricular conduction in normal man. Am J Cardiol 49:1031, 1982

14. Davies HEF: Respiratory change in heart rate: Sinus arrhythmia in the elderly. Geron Clin 17:96, 1975

15. Davies MJ: Pathology of the conduction system. In Caird FI, Dall JLC, Kennedy RD (eds): Cardiology in Old AGe, p 57. New York, Plenum Press, 1976

16. De Bono AHB, English TAH, Milstein BB: Heart valve replacement in the elderly. Br Med J 2:917, 1978

17. Deutch S et al: Postoperative hyponatremia with the inappropriate release of antidiuretic hormone. Anesthesiology 27:250, 1966

18. Elayda MA, Hall RJ, Gray AG, Mathur VS, Cooley DA: Coronary revascularization in the elderly patient. J Am Coll Cardiol 3:1398, 1984

19. El Sherif N, Samad A, Mascarenhas E, Cann D, Schoenfeld C, Samet P: Acute myocardial infarction in the elderly: Influence of coronary care unit on mortality. Chest 66:541, 1974

20. Elveback L, Lie JT: Continued high prevalence of coronary artery disease at autopsy in Olmstead County, Minnesota 1950 to 1979. Circulation 70:345, 1984

21. Ensor RE, Fleg JL, Kim YC, deLeon EF, Goldman SM: Longitudinal chest x-ray changes in normal men. J Gerontol 38:307, 1983

22. Epstein M, Hollenberg NK: Age as a determinant of renal sodium conservation in normal men. J Lab Clin Med 87:411, 1976

23. Evered DC, Chapman C: Plasma digoxin concentrations and digoxin toxicity in hospital patients. Br Heart J 33:540, 1971

24. Ewy GA, Marcus FI: Digitalis therapy in the aged. Gen Pharmacol 1:81, 1970

25. Fisch C: Electrocardiogram in the aged: An independent marker of heart disease? Am J Med 70:4, 1981

26. Fleg JL, Das DN, Lakatta EG: Right bundle branch block: Long-term prognosis in apparently healthy men. J Am Coll Cardiol 1:886, 1983

27. Fleg JL, Gottlieb SH, Lakatta EG: Is digoxin really important in treatment of compensated heart failure? A placebo-controlled crossover study in patients with sinus rhythm. Am J Med 73:244, 1982

28. Fleg JL, Kennedy HL: Cardiac arrhythmias in a healthy elderly population: Detection by 24-hour ambulatory electrocardiography. Chest 81:302, 1982

29. Fleg JL, Lakatta EG: How useful is digitalis in patients with congestive heart failure and sinus rhythm? Int J Cardiol 6:295, 1984

30. Fleg JL, Lakatta EG: Prevalence and prognosis of exercise-induced nonsustained ventricular tachycardia in apparently healthy volunteers. Am J Cardiol 54:762, 1984

31. Frishman WH, Furberg CD, Friedwald WT: β-adrenergic blockade for survivors of acute myocardial infarction. N Engl J Med 310:830, 1984

32. Gersh BJ et al: Coronary arteriography and coronary artery bypass surgery: Morbidity and mortality in patients aged 65 years or older. Circulation 67:843, 1983

33. Gerstenblith G et al: Stress testing redefines the prevalence of coronary artery disease in epidemiologic studies. Circulation 62(suppl 3):308, 1980

34. Gerstenblith G et al: Echocardiographic assessment of a normal adult aging population. Circulation 56:273, 1977

35. Gerstenblith G, Lakatta EG, Weisfeldt ML: Age changes in myocardial function and exercise response. Prog Cardiovasc Dis 19:1, 1976

36. Gheorghiade M, Beller GA: Effects of discontinuing maintenance digoxin therapy in patients with ischemic heart disease and congestive heart failure in sinus rhythm. Am J Cardiol 51:1243, 1983

37. Gifford RW: Management of systolic hypertension

in the elderly. In Vidt D (ed): Cardiovascular Therapy, p 69. Philadelphia, FA Davis 1982

38. Goldstein S et al: Characteristics of the resuscitated out-of-hospital cardiac arrest victim with coronary heart disease. Circulation 64:977, 1981

39. Gorlin R: Incidence, etiology and prognosis of heart failure. Cardiovasc Rev Rep 4:765, 1983

40. Graboys TB, Lown B, Podrid PJ, DeSilva R: Long-term survival of patients with malignant ventricular arrhythmia treated with antiarrhythmic drugs. Am J Cardiol 50:437, 1982

41. Greenblatt DJ, Koch-Weser J: Adverse reactions to propranolol in hospitalized medical patients: A report from the Boston Collaborative Drug Surveillance Program. Am Heart J 86:478, 1973

42. Hamby RI, Aintablian A: Hypertrophic subaortic stenosis is not rare in the eighth decade. Geriatrics 31:71, 1976

43. Henry WL et al: Observations on the optimum time for operative intervention for aortic regurgitation: I. Evaluation of the results of aortic valve replacement in symptomatic patients. Circulation 61:471, 1980

44. Hochberg MS et al: Mitral valve replacement in elderly patients: Encouraging postoperative clinical and hemodynamic results. J Cardiovasc Thorac Surg 77:422, 1979

45. Hochberg MS et al: Aortic valve replacement in the elderly: Encouraging postoperative clinical and hemodynamic results. Arch Surg 112:1475, 1977

46. Houry DA, Lawson DH, Lowe JH, Whiting B: The changing pattern of toxicity to digoxin. Postgrad Med J 358, 1981

47. Hynes JK et al: Partial atrioventricular canal defect in adults. Circulation 66:284, 1982

48. Hypertension Detection and Follow-up Program Cooperative Group: Five year findings of the hypertension detection and follow-up program: I. Reduction in mortality of persons with high blood pressure, including mild hypertension. JAMA 242:2562, 1979

49. Hypertension Detection and Follow-up Program Cooperative Group: Five year findings of the hypertension detection and follow-up program: II, Mortality by race, sex and age. JAMA 242:2572, 1979

50. Hypertension Detection and Follow-up Program Cooperative Group: Five year findings of the hypertension detection and follow-up program: III. Reduction in stroke incidence among persons with high blood pressure. JAMA 247:633, 1982

51. Johnson RH, Smith AC, Spalding JMK, Wollner L: Effect of posture on blood pressure in elderly patients. Lancet 1:731, 1965

52. Josephson ME, Harken AH, Horowitz LN: Long-term results of endocardial resection for sustained ventricular tachycardia in coronary disease patients. Am Heart J 104:51, 1982

53. Julius S, Antoon A, Whitlock LS, Conway J: Influence of age on the hemodynamic response to exercise. Circulation 36:222, 1967

54. Kannel WB, Abbot RD, Savage DD, McNamara PM: Epidemiologic features of chronic atrial fibrillation: The Framingham Study. N Engl J Med 306:1018, 1982

55. Kannel WB, Thom TJ: Declining cardiovascular mortality. Circulation 70:331, 1984

56. Kirkendall WM, Hammond JJ: Hypertension in the elderly. Arch Intern Med 140:1155, 1980

57. Kitchen AH, Pocock SJ: Prognosis of patients with acute myocardial infarction admitted to a coronary care unit: I. Survival in hospital. Br Heart J 39:1163, 1977

58. Klainer LM, Gibson TD, White KL: The epidemiology of cardiac failure. J Chronic Dis 18:797, 1965

59. Koch JP, Maron BJ, Epstein SE, Morrow AG: Results of operation for obstructive hypertrophic cardiomyopathy in the elderly: Septal myotomy and myectomy in 20 patients 65 years of age or older. Am J Cardiol 46:963, 1980

60. Kolibash AJ et al: Mitral valve prolapse syndrome: Analysis of 62 patients aged 60 years and older. Am J Cardiol 52:534, 1983

61. Lakatta EG: Alterations in the cardiovascular system that occur in advanced age. Fed Proc 38:163, 1979

62. Lakatta EG: Age-related alterations in the cardiovascular response to adrenergic mediated stress. Fed Proc 39:3173, 1980

63. Lakatta EG, Yin FCP: Myocardial aging: Functional alterations and related cellular mechanisms. Am J Physiol 242 (Heart Circ Physiol 11):H927, 1982

64. Leahey EB Jr et al: Interaction between quinidine an digoxin. JAMA 240:553, 1978

65. Liberthson RR, Boucher CC, Fallon JT, Buckley MJ: Severe mitral regurgitation: A common occurrence in the aging patient with secundum atrial septal defect. Clin Cardiol 4:229, 1981

66. McKee PA, Castelli WP, McNamara PM, Kannel WB: The natural history of congestive heart failure in the Framingham Study. N Engl J Med 285:1441, 1971

67. Mason JW, Winkle RA: Ability of induced ventricular tachycardia to predict long-term efficacy of antiarrhythmic drugs. N Engl J Med 303:1073, 1980

68. Messerli FH et al: Essential hypertension in the elderly: Haemodynamics, intravascular volume, plasma renin activity, and circulating catecholamine levels. Lancet 2:983, 1983

69. Mirowski M: Prevention of sudden arrhythmic death with implantable defibrillators. Ann Intern Med 95:88, 1981

70. Mock MM et al: Percutaneous transluminal coronary angioplasty (PTCA) in the elderly patient:

Experience in the National Heart, Lung and Blood Institute PTCA Registry. Am J Cardiol 53:89C, 1984

71. Norris RM, Brandt PWT, Caughey DE, Lee AJ, Scott PJ: A new coronary prognostic index. Lancet 1:274, 1969

72. Ochs HR, Greenblatt DJ, Woo E, Smith TW: Reduced quinidine clearance in elderly persons. Am J Cardiol 42:481, 1978

73. O'Malley K, O'Brien E: Management of hypertension in the elderly. N Engl J Med 302:1397, 1980

74. Packer M: Vasodilator and inotropic therapy for severe chronic heart failure: Passion and skepticism. J Am Coll Cardiol 2:841, 1983

75. Parsonnet V, Crawford C, Bernstein AD: The 1981 United States Survey of Cardiac Pacing Practices. J Am Coll Cardiol 3:1321, 1984

76. Pathy MS: Clinical features of ischemic heart disease. In Caird FI, Dall JLC, Kennedy RD (eds): Cardiology in Old Age, p 193. New York, Plenum Press, 1976

77. Perloff JK, Lindgren KM: Adult survival in congenital heart disease: I. Common defects with expected adult survival. Geriatrics 29:94, 1974

78. Pfeifer HJ, Greenblatt DJ, Koch-Weser J: Clinical use and toxicity of intravenous lidocaine. Am Heart J 92:168, 1976

79. Pooling Project Research Group: Relationship of blood pressure, serum cholesterol, smoking habit, relative weight and ECG abnormalities to incidence of major coronary events. Final report of the Pooling Project. J Chronic Dis 31:201, 1978

80. Port E, Cobb FR, Coleman RE, Jones RH: Effect of age on the response of the left ventricular ejection fraction to exercise. N Engl J Med 303:1133, 1980

81. Renlund D, Gerstenblith G, Rodeheffer RJ, Fleg JL, Lakatta EG: Potency of the Frank-Starling reserve in normal man. Am J Cardiol (in press)

82. Rodeheffer RJ et al: Exercise cardiac output is maintained with advancing age in healthy human subjects: Cardiac dilatation and increased stroke volume compensate for diminished heart rate. Circulation 69:203, 1984

83. Rodstein M, Zeman FD: Postural blood pressure changes in the elderly. J Chronic Dis 6:581, 1957

84. Rosing DR, Kent KM, Maron BJ, Epstein SE: Verapamil therapy: A new approach to the pharmacologic treatment of hypertrophic cardiomyopathy: II. Effects on exercise capacity and clinical status. Circulation 60:1208, 1979

85. Ruskin JM, DiMarco JP, Garan H: Out-of-hospital cardiac arrest. Electrophysiologic observations and selection of long-term antiarrhythmic therapy. N Engl J Med 303:607, 1980

86. Savage DD et al: Prevalence and correlates of posterior extra echocardiographic spaces in a free-living population-based sample: The Framingham Study. Am J Cardiol 51:1207, 1983

87. Savage DD et al: Prevalence of submitral (anular) calcium and its correlates in a general population-based sample (The Framingham Study). Am J Cardiol 51:1375, 1983

88. Schneider JF et al: Newly acquired right bundle branch block—the Framingham Study. Ann Intern Med 92:37, 1980

89. Schocken DD, Blumenthal JA, Port S, Hindle P, Coleman RE: Physical conditioning and left ventricular performance in the elderly: Assessment by radionuclide angiocardiography. Am J Cardiol 52:359, 1983

90. Shapiro S, Stone D, Lewis GP, Jick H: The epidemiology of digoxin: A study in three Boston hospitals. J Chronic Dis 22:361, 1969

91. Siddons H: Death in long-term paced patients. Br Heart J 36:1201, 1974

92. Siegel RJ, Shah PK, Fishbein MC: Idiopathic restrictive cardiomyopathy. Circulation 70:165, 1984

93. Simonson E: The effect of age on the electrocardiogram. Am J Cardiol 29:64, 1972

94. Spino M, Sellers EM, Kaplan HL, Stapleton C, MacLeod SM: Adverse biochemical and clinical consequences of furosemide administration. Can Med Assoc J 118:1513, 1978

95. Spodick DH, Quarry VM: Prevalence of the fourth heart sound by phonocardiography in the absence of cardiac disease. Am Heart J 87:11, 1974

96. Spurgeon HA, Thorne PR, Yin FCP, Shock NW, Weisfeldt ML: Increased dynamic stiffness of trabeculae carneae from senescent rats. Am J Physiol 232:H373, 1977

97. St. John Sutton MG, Tajik AJ, McGoon DC: Atrial septal defect in patients ages 60 years or older: Operative results and long-term postoperative follow-up. Circulation 64:402, 1981

98. Strauss WE, McIntyre KM, Parisi AF, Shapiro W: Safety and efficacy of diltiazem hydrochloride for the treatment of stable angina pectoris: Report of a cooperative clinical trial. Am J Cardiol 49:560, 1982

99. Tejada C, Strong JP, Montenegro MR, Restropo C, Solberg LA: Distribution of coronary and aortic atherosclerosis by geographic location, race and sex. Lab Invest 18:49, 1968

100. Thell R, Martin FH, Edwards JE: Bacterial endocarditis in subjects 60 years of age and older. Circulation 51:174, 1975

101. Tresch DD, Siegel R, Keelan MH Jr, Gross CM, Brooks HL: Mitral valve prolapse in the elderly. J Am Geriatr Soc 27:421, 1979

102. Tzankoff SP, Fleg JL, Norris AH, Lakatta EG: Age-related increase in serum catecholamine levels during exercise in healthy adult men. Physiologist 23:50, 1980

103. Vestal RE, Wood AJJ, Shand DG: Reduced β-adrenoceptor sensitivity in the elderly. Clin Pharmacol Ther 26:181, 1979

196 *Cardiovascular Disease in Old Age*

104. Veterans Administration Cooperative Study Group on Antihypertensive Agents: Effects of treatment on morbidity in hypertension: Results in patients with diastolic blood pressures averaging 115 through 129. JAMA 202:1028, 1967

105. Veterans Administration Cooperative Study Group on Antihypertensive Agents: Effects of treatment on morbidity in hypertension: Results in patients with diastolic blood pressures averaging 90 through 114 mm Hg. JAMA 213:1143, 1970

106. Von Reyn CF, Levy BS, Arbeit RD, Friedland G, Crumpacker CS: Infective endocarditis: An analysis based on strict case definitions. Ann Intern Med 94:505, 1981

107. Waller BF, Roberts WC: Cardiovascular disease in the very elderly: Analysis of 40 necropsy patients aged 90 years or over. Am J Cardiol 51:403, 1983

108. White, NK, Edwards JE, Dry TJ: The relationship of the degree of coronary atherosclerosis with age in men. Circulation 1:645, 1950

109. Whiting RD, Powell WJ Jr, Dinsmore RE, Sanders CA: Idiopathic hypertrophic subaortic stenosis in the elderly. N Engl J Med 285:196, 1971

110. Wilcox RG, Hampton JR: Importance of age in prehospital and hospital mortality of heart attacks. Br Heart J 44:503, 1980

111. Williams BO et al: The elderly in a coronary care unit. Br Med J 2:451, 1976

112. Winniford MD, Fulton KL, Hillis LD: Long-term therapy of paroxysmal supraventricular tachycardia: A randomized, double-blind comparison of digoxin, propranolol and verapamil. Am J Cardiol 54:1138, 1984

113. Wong M, Tei C, Shah P: Degenerative calcific valvular disease and systolic murmurs in the elderly. J Am Geriatr Soc 31:156, 1983

114. Zeman FD, Rodstein M: Cardiac rupture complicating myocardial infarction in the aged. Arch Intern Med 105:431, 1960

12

The Peripheral Vascular System

Henry Haimovici

As a result of the prolonged life span with corresponding prevalence of arteriosclerosis and greater susceptibility to thromboembolism in the geriatric population, vascular problems are encountered with ever-increasing frequency. Current diagnostic methods and the available reconstructive surgical procedures have greatly improved the outlook for the vascular problems of the elderly patient.

The most common vascular disorders to be dealt with in this chapter are occlusive arterial diseases, aneurysms, and acute venous thromboembolism.

OCCLUSIVE ARTERIAL DISEASES

Acute Occlusions

Arterial Embolism

Cardiogenic Origin. The most common etiologic factors in arterial embolism are arteriosclerotic heart disease, myocardial infarction, and atrial fibrillation. Atrial fibrillation may or may not coexist with the two other conditions. Rheumatic heart disease is less often encountered in the elderly as a cause of embolism.

Mural thrombi resulting from a silent myocardial infarction may sometimes embolize long before clinical and electrocardiographic evidence of their origin. Peripheral embolism associated with silent myocardial infarction is not infrequent and is present in about 11% of the cases.[12]

Limb emboli occur predominantly in the lower extremities. Their incidence, including the aortoiliac segment, ranges between 77% and 84%.[12] In the upper extremities, most emboli lodge in the

brachial arteries and more rarely in the subclavian or axillary arteries.[20]

The common belief that an arterial embolism is always characterized at onset by severe pain may be misleading. Haimovici noted that sudden onset was found in only 81% of cases, of which 60% displayed sudden pain and the remainder only sudden numbness and coldness without initial pain. Progressive onset was noted in 12% of the cases, and silent arterial occlusion owing to embolism was seen in 7%.[12]

Although peripheral arterial emboli do not always lead to irreversible ischemic changes, it is significant that about half these patients may end up with gangrene of the extremity or die shortly after the onset of the acute arterial occlusion. Because no criteria are entirely reliable at the onset of an arterial embolism to forecast its outcome, management without delay is essential.

Diagnosis of a peripheral arterial embolism is usually simple, its clinical picture being that of an acute arterial occlusion occurring in a patient generally suffering from heart disease. Nevertheless, in some instances a differential diagnosis between arterial embolism and arterial spasm, phlegmasia cerulea dolens, acute arterial thrombosis, and dissecting aneurysm may be necessary.

Although localization of emboli may be achieved by clinical findings alone, in some patients arteriography is indicated, especially in those with preexisting occlusive arterial disease. Preoperative as well as intraoperative arteriography would then provide optimal information, thus facilitating the procedure.[17]

Upper extremity embolism incidence ranges between 16% and 32.6%, with an average of 23.2%. Being generally small, these emboli lodge in the majority of cases in the brachial (61%), followed in decreasing order by the axillary (23.4%), subclavian (11.7%), and radial-ulnar (3.9%).[20]

Differential diagnosis of upper limb emboli in the absence of a cardiopathy includes thromboemboli secondary to a thoracic outlet syndrome, acute thrombosis associated with trauma or arteriosclerosis, or atheroemboli.

Visceral emboli occur with greater frequency than generally is recognized. It is well known that considerable discrepancy exists between their clinical and necropsy diagnosis. Visceral emboli, if small, are often clinically overlooked or remain unsuspected, whereas major embolic occlusions display significant and often rapidly irreversible and lethal changes. Cerebral, mesenteric, and renal emboli are not uncommon, and they are often the cause of serious complications or death.[12].

Noncardiogenic Origin. *Atheroembolism* may occur in two distinct forms: (1) as *microemboli* following a release of cholesterol crystals or other debris of atheromatous components from an ulcerated plaque and (2) as *macroemboli* resulting from major plaques usually mixed with thrombi and cholesterol crystals and lodging in major systemic arteries.[29]

These emboli may occur spontaneously from an abdominal aneurysm or a nonaneurysmal lesion of the aorta, following surgical manipulation of the latter, or during aortic catheterization. The incidence ranges between 1.4% and 3%. The clinical spectrum of problems associated with microemboli includes cyanotic or blue toes, livedo reticularis, and ulcerations or gangrene (especially of toes, but rarely of the fingers or hand). Myalgia or simple muscle tenderness is frequent. Peripheral pulses are usually present with microembolization, except in cases of preexisting distal occlusive disease. Awareness of the existence of such emboli may help in their detection. In a microembolism of a major artery the clinical picture is no different from that of an embolism of cardiac origin. Aortograms or peripheral arteriograms are often necessary to identify the source of the embolic nature of the vascular lesions. The treatment consists of nonsurgical or operative measures.

Acute arterial thromboembolism of the upper extremity associated with a *thoracic outlet syndrome* differs in many ways from a cardiogenic embolism, particularly in its pathophysiology and management. This process is brought about by a damaged subclavian artery due to compression by congenital or acquired anomalous anatomical structures at the thoracic outlet. They are associated with cervical ribs and scalenus anticus, costoclavicular, and hyperabduction syndromes. These entities either alone or in combination are responsible for the vascular complications described under this title.[21]

Treatment. Management of arterial emboli includes two phases: (1) immediate treatment of the ischemia of the extremity and (2) treatment of the underlying heart disease.

As a first measure, the patient should be placed in the head-up position with the ischemic extremity on a pillow to protect it from any pressure. Elevation of the extremity and application of local heat are the two most ill-advised procedures encountered and should be scrupulously avoided. Heparin should be administered intravenously as soon as possible. There is no contraindication to its administration, even if surgery is being contemplated within 2 or 3 hours. Use of fibrinolysin and low-molecular-weight dextran generally are of limited value. Vasodilator drugs, preferably papaverine, when given intra-arterially, may be of some help. Epidural anesthesia offers greater advantage because it may induce vasodilatation and at the same time it can be used in subsequent surgery. If all measures prove ineffective, surgery should be performed without delay.

Embolectomy is the method of choice for managing arterial emboli.[22] Few contraindications exist except in patients who are in very serious general condition. Because the procedure can be carried out most of the time under local anesthesia, an embolectomy can be performed in almost every case. Use of the Fogarty catheter has simplified the operation because it allows surgery to be carried out with ease, safety, and completeness, thus usually restoring patency of the arterial tree. Its application to aortic and iliac emboli obviates the abdominal procedure and has lowered considerably operative morbidity and mortality.[9]

One of the essential differences between arterial embolectomy in the elderly patient and in the younger person with rheumatic heart disease is the presence of preexisting arteriosclerosis. The associated arterial disease usually renders the procedure more difficult and more incomplete than would otherwise be the case in a relatively normal arterial tree.

Late arterial embolectomy (beyond 10 to 12 hours) can be successfully carried out, provided the limb is still viable, although at a borderline level.[22] In cases of associated venous thrombosis, concomitant aspiration of the adjacent vein may be necessary, especially in a delayed case of embolectomy. When the muscles have become edematous as a result of prolonged ischemia, fasciotomy is indicated to decompress the vascular compartments that otherwise would become gangrenous in spite of patency of the arterial tree.

In primary embolic gangrene of the extremity, or after failure of embolectomy, amputation may be deferred until adequate collateral supply develops. However, if toxemia secondary to muscle necrosis occurs, immediate amputation is indicated.

The patient's cardiac status must be assessed before and after management of peripheral emboli and attention directed toward its correction. Arterial embolism, although a serious condition, no longer justifies the pessimism previously attached to it if prompt recognition and treatment are applied.[6,24]

However, in the geriatric patient, in spite of recent progress, peripheral arterial embolism still must be regarded as a serious challenge to both cardiologists and vascular surgeons because of the potential significant risks to life and limb owing to multiple atherosclerotic lesions. Systemic complications resulting from late revascularization of an ischemic limb may adversely affect the prognosis of both limb and life. The resulting muscle ischemia may lead to metabolic complications with myoglobinuria, renal shutdown, and a high mortality rate. If recognized early, the revascularization syndrome usually can be forestalled by adequate alkalinization and hydration of the patient and fasciotomy of the involved limb.[19]

Acute Arterial Thrombosis

Acute arterial thrombosis, as distinct from arterial embolism, may occur as a result of a number of local arterial factors or as a consequence of associated systemic diseases. Although these arterial occlusions are sudden, causing serious tissue ischemia, the clinicopathologic features and management are distinct from those of an acute arterial embolism.

Acute Atherosclerotic Thrombosis. Atherosclerosis is the most common predisposing cause of an acute thrombosis, which may occur in an asymptomatic ulcerated atherosclerotic plaque or be superimposed on a preexisting incompletely occlusive process, with a longstanding clinical history of intermittent claudication.

The majority of cases occur in the lower extremity. The overall relative incidence of acute thrombosis and arterial embolism is variable, although the latter is more prevalent than the former

(56.6% vs. 43.4%, respectively). The most common clinicopathologic forms are *acute aortoiliac thrombosis*, which usually carries a very serious prognosis, especially if unrecognized early, and *acute femoropopliteal thrombosis*, which is by far more frequent.

Management is by immediate intravenous heparin injection and bypass graft. Use of a thrombolytic agent may offer an alternative.

Iatrogenic Acute Arterial Thrombosis. Postcatheterization arterial thrombosis may pose various threats to limb or life. This may follow retrograde catheterization of brachial, radial, or femoral arteries. Early recognition and immediate management may forestall irreversible changes leading to gangrene of digits or limb.[4]

Chronic Occlusions

Arteriosclerosis Obliterans

Arteriosclerosis is the largest cause of arterial disease responsible for ischemic lesions of the extremities.[18] Although arteriosclerosis is a diffusely distributed process involving the intima, wider use of arteriography has disclosed that arteriosclerosis obliterans quite often involves a single segment of the arterial tree. As the disease progresses, two or more segments may become occluded. Whether monosegmental or polysegmental, a patent distal arterial lumen (runoff or outflow tract) is often present and is of great surgical significance.

Clinical manifestations and surgical management of arteriosclerosis obliterans may vary according to the location and extent of the occlusive process.

Aortoiliac occlusion (Leriche syndrome) is usually characterized by slow progression of occlusion of the terminal abdominal aorta and of the common iliac arteries. Although it occurs in younger subjects, aortoiliac occlusion may also be seen in the elderly. This syndrome is well tolerated for quite a number of years before ischemic changes occur. Rest pain and gangrene may occur late in its evolution and may be precipitated by some form of trauma.

Aortoiliac occlusive disease may be well tolerated in many patients. By contrast, involvement of the femoral or popliteal and tibial arteries by arteriosclerosis may lead to severe ischemia and gangrene. The relative incidence of aortoiliac occlusion and occlusion of the femoropopliteal segment varies with the reported studies.[7,14]

Occlusion of the superficial femoral artery, either as an isolated lesion or associated with the popliteal or tibial arterial tree, is one of the most frequently encountered locations of arteriosclerosis in the lower extremities. The popliteal and leg arteries may be involved either independently or in association with the proximal arterial tree. A study of the various occlusive patterns has been reported elsewhere[17]

Although the natural course of arteriosclerosis obliterans has not been entirely elucidated, various statistical studies show that most of these patients have only intermittent claudication—slightly over 70%.[18] Ischemic rest pain, ischemic neuropathy, or both are seen in 16% of patients; ischemic ulceration, gangrene, or both are seen in about 10%. Most published reports indicate that arteriosclerosis obliterans naturally tends to progress at rates that vary from patient to patient and from location to location. Diabetes mellitus seems to accelerate the process and impart a more serious prognosis.[15,18,38]

Peripheral Arterial Disease in Diabetes Mellitus

Vascular manifestations associated with diabetes today represent the gravest single factor underlying the morbidity and mortality of diabetic patients. The gravity of the vascular process stems from the wide involvement of virtually all arterial areas, peripheral as well as visceral (retina, kidney, coronary, and cerebral; Fig. 12-1).

The vascular lesions encountered in diabetes vary with the size and location of the vessel. Basically, two major histologic types have been differentiated: arteriosclerotic, involving primarily the large and medium-sized arteries; and microangiopathic, involving arterioles and capillaries. Atherosclerosis is more diffuse in the diabetic. The site and extent of the initial atherosclerotic disease in larger arteries differ in diabetic and nondiabetic patients. In diabetes, the initial lesions involve the tibial and popliteal arteries, and less frequently the femoral artery (Fig. 12-2).

Clinical manifestations of peripheral arterial disease in diabetes is often associated with, and sometimes dominated by, two other important features: diabetic neuropathy and local infection. Their association, in variable degrees, lends to the lesions a truly characteristic clinical picture, often referred to as the "diabetic foot." The clinical manifestations may thus be conveniently classified under the following four headings: (1) arteriosclerosis obliterans, (2) peripheral neuropathy, (3) infection, and (4) combined lesions.

Accurate diagnosis and prompt treatment of circulatory disturbances seen in the extremities of diabetic patients rest on the fact that such disturbances often may be ascribed to a combination of occlusive arterial disease, neuropathy, and infection. The degree of participation of each of these three major etiologic factors is difficult to assess statistically. Thus, evaluation of each diabetic patient from this triple point of view is essential before deciding on the course to follow.

Evaluation of the Patient

The major clinical manifestation in noncomplicated cases is intermittent claudication, whereas in advanced cases, rest pain, color changes of the skin, ulcerations, and gangrene associated with absent or diminished arterial pulsations are cardinal manifestations.

In attempting to evaluate the degree of arterial insufficiency, clinical criteria may provide much desired information. Whether onset is acute or chronic often determines the extent of ischemic manifestations. The patency of major arteries is determined by palpation and checked with Doppler ultrasound velocity detector. In the absence of functioning major arteries, the vascularization of the tissues depends on the degree of collateral circulation. Elevation-dependency tests and skin temperatures at different levels determined under basal conditions are helpful guides in assessing the collateral arterial supply. Rapid blanching of the toes and foot on elevation and marked rubor on dependency suggest poor collateral circulation. A sharp difference in skin temperature between the proximal and distal areas of the extremity indicates recent arterial occlusion.

Vascular Examination

Although the clinical history and physical findings of peripheral arterial problems provide an overall estimation of the arterial insufficiency, a more quantitative estimate of the extent of arterial disease and an objective method of assessing therapeutic results can be obtained by noninvasive methods and by arteriography.

Noninvasive Methods

At present there are a number of well-established tests available for clinical use to provide objective assessment of vascular insufficiency.[3,42] Essentially, these tests are designed to measure the arterial

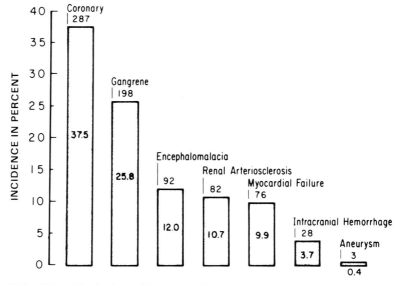

INCIDENCE OF MORTALITY DUE TO SEVERE
VASCULAR DISEASE IN DIABETICS
(766 CASES OF 1555 PATIENTS)

FIG. 12-1. Distribution of incidence of various vascular lesions in diabetics. (Based on statistics from Bell EF: A post-mortem study of vascular disease in diabetes. Arch Pathol 53:444, 1952 and from Haimovici H: Peripheral arterial disease in diabetes mellitus. In Ellenberg M, Rifkin H: Diabetes Mellitus: Theory and Practice. New York, McGraw-Hill, 1970)

pressures at various levels of the extremity and to provide flow measurements. The information thus obtained may indicate the extent and the approximate location and whether single or multilevel occlusive disease exists. The oscillometer, useful for recording pulsations objectively, is a nonstandardized instrument and may be used only in an office setting where no other, more sensitive instruments are available. Of the latter, the Doppler ultrasonic velocity detector can be used in the office, as well as in a vascular laboratory. The pulse volume recorder is used to measure limb systolic pressure and, at the same time, to record the pulse contour. The arterial evaluation can be performed before and after exercise and can provide information about the hemodynamics in the extremity. Other noninvasive techniques, such as radio-isotopes, in assessment of arterial insufficiency are more suitable in a vascular laboratory than in an office setting.[3,34]

Arteriography

Arteriography should be performed only if surgery is being contemplated. It then plays a decisive role in the evaluation and selection of patients for operation. The site, number, and extent of the arterial occlusions, the state of the proximal and distal arterial tree, and the degree of collateral circulation can only be determined by this means. A good arterial outline and comprehensive visualization of the entire tree are prerequisites for a good angiographic study. Two methods of visualization are used: (1) abdominal aortography, either by the translumbar technique or by the Seldinger method, and (2) femoral arteriography. To achieve complete evaluation of arterial lesions of the extremities, it is necessary to carry out comprehensive arteriography from the aorta down to the foot. This may provide the correct indications for surgical management of arterial lesions.[14]

Treatment

The degree of arterial impairment and its clinical manifestations are important in deciding on treatment. Classification of clinical manifestations is divided into three stages: stage I, intermittent claudication; stage II, rest pain without lesions; and stage III, ischemic lesions (ulcers or gangrene).

In the elderly, intermittent claudication rarely requires active treatment. The oft-prescribed vasodilator drugs are of little or no value. By contrast, walking a few miles a day may promote

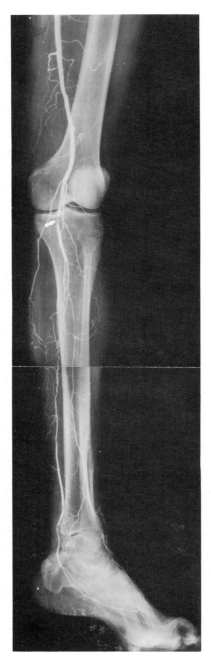

FIG. 12-2. Transfemoral arteriogram of left lower extremity of a diabetic patient. It shows (1) patent femoral and proximal popliteal; (2) a nearly complete block of the distal popliteal (*arrow*); (3) absence of the anterior tibial artery; (4) complete occlusion of the proximal posterior tibial artery and marked stenosis of the proximal peroneal artery; and (5) patency of the distal two thirds of these tibial and peroneal arteries with visualization of the pedal vessels. The patient had gangrene and infection of three toes and marked diabetic neuropathy. A successful transmetatarsal amputation was performed.

collateral circulation and thus may improve intermittent claudication. These patients sometimes also suffer from angina pectoris, which may be brought on by rapid or prolonged walking. Under these circumstances, intermittent claudication might be considered as a blessing in disguise.

In the presence of severe ischemia of the extremities (stages II and III), the scope of medical management is necessarily limited. Relief of rest pain usually requires moderate to large amount of analgestics or narcotics. Failure to achieve this is an indication for surgery.

Care of Ischemic Foot Lesions. Management of ischemic foot lesions, especially in the elderly, has remained poorly defined, and the maneuvers designed to carry out this treatment are generally even more poorly understood. The major objectives of such treatment are avoidance of any trauma to the ischemic foot, control of infection, control of pain, and preservation of muscle strength and joint motion (rehabilitation).

Local care is essential to adequate drainage from the necrotic lesions. Interdigital ulcers often are overlooked. The source of an abscess with minimal opening in these areas is not detected unless one has examined methodically the various parts of the foot. A subungual infection, associated with an ingrowing toenail, is often the precipitating cause of gangrene. The black eschars should be elevated at the corners to allow adequate drainage of the purulent material often trapped under them. The débridement of such scabs should be gentle to avoid bleeding and further trauma to ischemic tissues. In the presence of an infected lesion, use of a wet dressing with normal saline concomitantly with antibiotics for several days is helpful.

Control of pain, especially in patients sitting during the day and most of the night in order to obtain some relief, is essential. This is particularly necessary in the preoperative period to reduce dependency edema and render the tissues more amenable to surgery.

Anesthesia due to diabetic neuropathy deprives the patient of the perception of pain accompanying infection and necrosis. Superficial lymphangitis and cellulitis, not responding promptly to systemic antibiotics, most often mask underlying abscesses, either in subcutaneous tissue or in the subfascial layer. As a rule, infection and necrosis are more extensive than the appearance of the skin would lead one to believe. If antibiotics are ineffective, incision, débridement, and wide drainage, followed by a continuous wet dressing with an antibiotic solution for a week or 10 days, may arrest the septic process.

Salvage of the Ischemic Limb. In patients with intractable rest pain and ischemic lesions, salvage of the limb can be achieved by various operative methods in many cases.[44,45,49]

Percutaneous transluminal angioplasty consists of inducing dilatation of stenosed or occluded arteries by means of special catheters. Introduced as early as 1964, practical application did not occur until 1975 when instrumentation and techniques were improved. In the peripheral vessels this method is mostly applicable in the management of iliac, femoral, and popliteal short arterial stenoses and occasionally even occlusions. In contrast to these arteries, the tibial vessels are the least suitable in most instances for this approach. The overall most durable results are achieved in cases of iliac stenosis. This technique, which has yielded encouraging results, can be used either alone or in combination with bypass grafts or other vascular surgical procedures.[8,11]

Reconstructive arterial surgical procedures (thromboendarterectomy, arterial grafts), lumbar sympathectomy, or a combination of these are yielding gratifying results.

Thromboendarterectomy. Thromboendarterectomy consists of removal of the occluding block through the cleavage plane of the arterial wall. Indication for the procedure usually should be confined to short segmental occlusions. The greatest successes obtained with this procedure are for lesions localized to the common iliac or common femoral arteries (Fig. 12-3), whereas thromboendarterectomy in the superficial femoral or popliteal arteries is rarely as successful in long-term follow-up.

Reestablishment of arterial flow is achieved in most instances by means of *bypass grafts*. Both synthetic and autogenous vein grafts are used, with indication for their use being different according to the location of the arterial lesions. In the aortoiliac segment Dacron grafts are almost universally used, except when thromboendarterectomy can be used. In the femoropopliteal area, the present trend is toward the use of autogenous vein grafts, especially if the distal anastomosis is to be carried out below the knee joint.

Recently introduced grafts, the *expanded polytetrafluoroethylene* (PTFE),[45,46] and the human umbilical cord vein, are being used as substitutes for vein grafts below the inguinal ligament and below the knee in the popliteal as well as in the leg arteries (anterior and posterior tibials, and peroneal). The results indicate that these grafts are of value in arterial reconstruction, especially in cases below the knee for limb salvage (Fig. 12-4).[46]

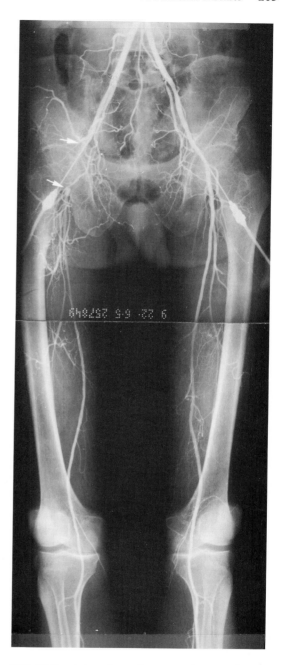

FIG. 12-3. A transfemoral aortoarteriogram of a nondiabetic patient whose chief complaints were rest pain and intermitten claudication of the right lower extremity. This angiogram disclosed a complete occlusion of the right common femoral artery (extent indicated by two arrows). Following a thromboendarterectomy, arterial flow was restored to the entire lower extremity, with complete relief of symptoms.

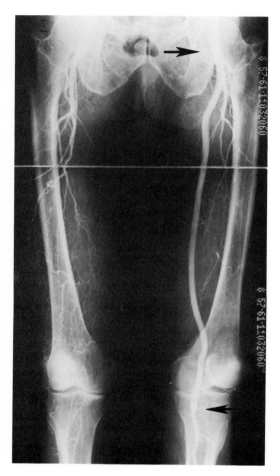

FIG. 12-4. Left femoral arteriogram of a 71-year-old nondiabetic man with a PTFE graft implanted between the common femoral and popliteal below the knee (*arrows*). This graft was carried out for acute thrombosis of the entire superficial femoral artery and four fifths of the proximal popliteal. Patency of the graft was maintained from July 1976 to date.

Since the advent of direct arterial surgery, *lumbar sympathectomy* is obviously considered as only the second best type of revascularization procedure because its objective is more limited. Sympathectomy is designed only to promote development of collateral circulation. Despite these limitations, lumbar sympathectomy is definitely indicated in advanced peripheral arterial occlusive disease where there is an obviously poor or absent runoff that precludes direct arterial surgery but where a potential adequate collateral network exists.[13]

Combined procedures may often be necessary to overcome the multiplicity and great extent of arterial lesions. Thromboendarterectomy or arterial grafts may be combined with lumbar sympathec-

tomy, especially in polysegmental occlusions or in diffuse obliterative disease of the distal arterial tree. These procedures are not competitive, but rather, they supplement each other. The proximal procedures achieve their therapeutic effect by increasing the head pressure into the major collateral branch of the lower extremity, the profunda femoris in this case, while vasodilatation of the available collateral network is achieved distally by lumbar sympathectomy. This combined therapy, in our opinion, is always indicated when the popliteal-tibial system is diffusely or completely occluded. Relief of rest pain and healing of minor toe lesions are obtained in most cases.

Amputations

Six possible levels of amputation for ischemic gangrene are at the toes, the transmetatarsal level, the ankle joint (Syme amputation), the supramalleolar level, midleg (below the knee), and thigh (above the knee; Fig. 12-5). The decision as to which level to use can be made only after careful study of each patient.[36,37,48] Such a choice requires proper evaluation of both local factors and the patient's general condition. Chief among the local factors are the extent of gangrene or ulceration, the degree of infection, the condition of adjacent areas, the degree of arterial impairment, and the severity of the pain.

Single toe amputation is indicated in the presence of well-demarcated necrosis of the distal end of the digit. *Transmetatarsal amputation* is indicated for limited gangrene or ulcerations of two or more toes. The advantages of transmetatarsal amputation cannot be overemphasized (Fig. 12-6). The *Syme* and *supramalleolar* are generally not suitable levels of amputation for ischemic lesions of the foot. *Midleg or below-knee amputation* is indicated in gangrene of several toes that extends into the metatarsal region with or without infection but with no tendency to demarcate. Preservation of the knee joint is an important consideration, especially in the elderly. Every effort should be made to avoid loss of the knee joint. However, in the presence of extensive gangrene and infection of the leg associated with flexion contracture of the knee joint and poor prospect for rehabilitation, an *above-knee procedure* is unavoidable. Below-knee amputation possesses two major advantages over the thigh amputation: (1) a better prospect of rehabilitation owing to the presence of the knee joint and (2) minimal or absent stump pain.

A new concept in the management of the lower extremity amputee by early or immediate fitting of prostheses has been used in the past few years. The results obtained with this method promise to change the outlook of the geriatric amputee by expediting his rehabilitation.

ANEURYSMS OF THE ABDOMINAL AORTA AND MAJOR LIMB ARTERIES

Aneurysms can be caused by a variety of agents that weaken the arterial wall. Most, if not all, aneurysms of the abdominal aorta and of the major limb arteries are caused by arteriosclerosis. Mycotic, traumatic, and luetic aneurysms in these regions are extremely rare.

Aneurysms of the Abdominal Aorta

These aneurysms have been encountered with greater frequency in the past 3 decades essentially because of two factors: increase in life span with a parallel increase in arteriosclerosis and a greater awareness of the diagnosis of abdominal aortic aneurysms. Most patients are elderly and exhibit varying degrees of cardiovascular disease. In our own experience, 75% of patients were in the seventh and eighth decade, and 87% of the entire group were males.[19,49] Cardiovascular disease is often associated with abdominal aortic aneurysm and requires proper evaluation before surgical correction of the abdominal lesion is undertaken. Old myocardial infarction, angina pectoris, and congestive heart failure are often found in these patients. In addition to cardiac involvements, other arteriosclerotic lesions such as occlusive arterial disease of the lower extremities or aneurysms at other levels than the aorta are frequently encountered.[23]

Clinically, an abdominal aortic aneurysm is characterized by an expansile and pulsatile mass in the umbilical region, often accompanied by varying degrees of pain (Fig. 12-7). Because of the significance but inconstancy of pain, abdominal aneurysms are generally classified as symptomatic and asymptomatic. This classification implies that surgical indications are mandatory in the former group but are not valid in the latter. Unfortunately, such implications are misleading, often with disastrous results. When an abdominal aneurysm is symptomatic, pain is an important and sometimes ominous symptom, because it usually indicates rapid, progressive enlargement of the lesion and may signify impending or even actual rupture. In these cases, indications for surgery are obvious. In

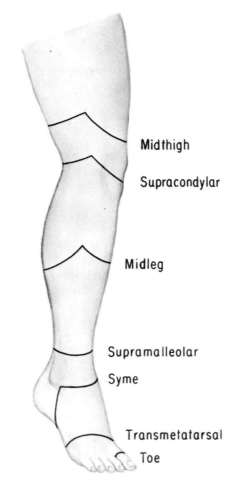

FIG. 12-5. The levels of amputation for ischemic gangrene.

contrast to these cases requiring immediate surgery, the surgical treatment of the so-called asymptomatic aneurysm has evoked controversy in a few recent reports. The vast experience accumulated in recent years shows that absence of pain and the size of the aneurysm are not reliable prognostic indexes. Rupture, the greatest hazard of an aneurysm, may be the first manifestation of an asymptomatic aneurysm. Rupture of an aneurysm may occur either in the retroperitoneal space or into another adjacent organ such as the inferior vena cava or duodenum.

Diagnostic Tests

In most instances the diagnosis of an uncomplicated abdominal aortic aneurysm can be made by clinical findings. Recent advances using noninva-

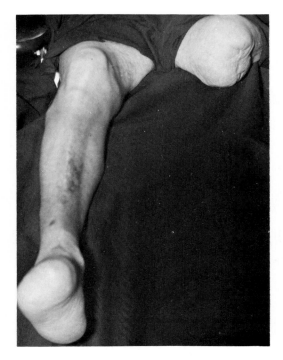

FIG. 12-6. Bilateral amputation in a diabetic 72-year-old man. The left midthigh amputation was performed 3 years before the right transmetatarsal. In both instances the patient had only gangrene of toes. Selection of the level and performance of the procedures reflect two widely different approaches to the management of ischemic gangrene of toes.

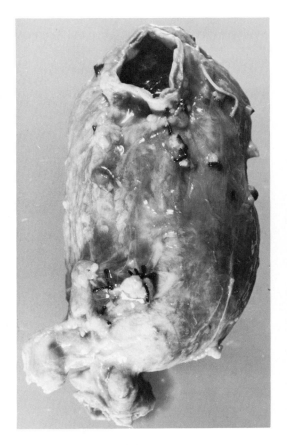

FIG. 12-7. Specimen of abdominal aortic aneurysm of a 70-year-old man. The lesion involved infrarenal abdominal aorta, its bifurcation, and the proximal segment of both common iliac arteries.

sive procedures may facilitate an evaluation of the aneurysm in doubtful diagnosis. Echography may obviate the use of angiography and provide enough information both for the diagnosis of the lesion and its extent. However, associated intra-abdominal vascular lesions may require contrast visualization of the aorta and visceral arteries, as well as of the distal arterial tree in the lower extremities.[25]

Prognosis

The natural course of an untreated abdominal aortic aneurysm has been fairly well documented in recent years.[49] From an overall survey of various studies, it is clear that the prognosis in untreated abdominal aneurysm is poor. Although some patients survive for years, and some die of unrelated causes, most patients will die of rupture within 1 or 2 years of diagnosis. Above all, these studies of the natural course of unrelated cases have disclosed a few important facts:

The survival rate of patients with abdominal aortic aneurysms is much lower than that of the normal population, especially after the age of 65.

There are no absolute criteria for predicting which patient will suffer an aortic aneurysmal rupture, because of a substantial number of the so-called asymptomatic type eventually do rupture.

Regardless of age, abdominal aneurysmectomy can successfully be performed for any patient in reasonable health, including octogenarians.[33]

Prognosis for patients after resection of an unruptured aneurysm is unquestionably better than that for untreated patients. With greater technical competence, operative mortality has decreased uniformly. Of the fatal complications following surgery, the most frequently encountered are myocardial infarction, cerebrovascular accident, acute renal insufficiency, and hemorrhage from the operative site. Preoperative hypertension and cardio-vascular-renal disease are the most significant factors influencing survival after operation. In ruptured aneurysms, the operative mortality is vastly different and ranges from 30% to 76%.[23,47] Among the chief factors that influence survival are duration and severity of the hypovolemic shock and acute renal shutdown. For the surgery to be successful, prompt recognition of these complications and immediate surgical intervention are essential.

Peripheral Aneurysms

The most common peripheral aneurysms involve the femoral and popliteal arteries.[24] Their diagnosis can usually be made by palpation along the course of the femoral or popliteal axis. Physical examination often permits accurate assessment of location and extent along with the patency of the vessel. Arteriography is not always necessary and is reserved only for accurate visualization of the distal vessels when palpation indicates that arterial flow is diminished distal to the aneurysm.

More than other aneurysms of the peripheral arteries, those of the popliteal carry a high rate of amputation if complications are allowed to occur. The main cause is thrombosis of the aneurysm and the distal arterial tree (Fig. 12-8).

As in other aneurysms, there is a high incidence of coexisting cardiovascular disease in patients with femoral and popliteal aneurysms. Of these, arterial hypertension is present in almost 50% of patients. Arteriosclerosis obliterans of the distal arterial tree is another coexisting lesion that may complicate the reconstruction of the arterial tree or may lead to gangrene owing to extension of thrombosis from the aneurysm. Another important feature is the frequent presence of bilateral lesions and associated aneurysms in other locations of the arterial tree (abdominal or thoracic aorta).

Management of femoral or popliteal aneurysms consists in resection or exclusion of the lesion with reestablishment of continuity of the arterial tree, either with a prosthetic material or with a vein. Occasionally, a lumbar sympathectomy may be indicated in the presence of associated occlusive disease of the leg. To be successful, surgery must be undertaken before the aneurysm becomes large and causes complications.

In recent years, false aneurysms owing to disruption of an anastomotic line of a graft or secondary to trauma have been frequently encoun-tered. The clinical manifestations vary with the location and the presence or absence of sepsis. In the septic group, a false aneurysm is rather an early postoperative manifestation (a few weeks), consisting of intermittent bleeding from the affected areas, formation of a hematoma, pus drainage, and lymphorrhea, all of which precede the appearance of the aneurysm. Presence of sepsis is a very serious, if not ominous, prognostic factor.[23,24,43]

The exact incidence of anastomotic false aneurysms is not entirely known and has been variously estimated as ranging between 2.9% and 16%. Their management is somewhat more difficult than that of a spontaneous aneurysm of the femoral or popliteal arteries. It consists of either simple resuture at the site of disruption if the edge of the arteriotomy is in good condition or excision of a distal portion of the graft and of the anastomotic area, with regrafting at a more distal level.

Whereas the gravest complication of abdominal aortic aneurysms is rupture, in peripheral aneurysms the greatest hazard remains thrombosis with consequent loss of limb. Both hazards are equally serious. They can be easily prevented by prompt diagnosis and management. Reconstructive arterial surgery has proven successful, even in advanced age.

VENOUS THROMBOEMBOLISM

Venous thrombosis and pulmonary embolism are encountered with increasing frequency in geriatric patients.[41,42] Reasons for the increased incidence of these complications are a longer survival of critically ill patients and more extensive surgical procedures carried out in the elderly. It is well known that in both medical and surgical patients age has a profound influence of the susceptibility to thromboembolism.

The increased frequency of vein thrombosis of the leg and pulmonary embolism seems to be directly correlated with a progressive enlargement of the intramuscular calf veins, which occurs with advancing years.[26]

Clinical Manifestations

There are several areas of predilection for the occurrence of thrombophlebitis in the lower extremities. One of the most common sites is the calf muscle veins, referred to often as sural thrombophlebitis. It is most frequently seen as a postoperative complication or in patients bedridden as a

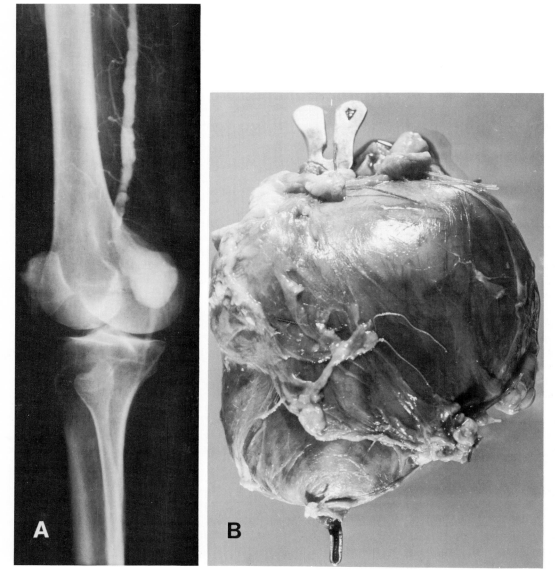

FIG. 12-8. *(A)* Arteriogram showing the residual lumen of a popliteal aneurysm, the remainder being filled with laminated thrombi. *(B)* Size of popliteal aneurysm excised, which shows a great disparity with that seen on the arteriogram. As usual, the aneurysmal sac was almost completely occluded by old and recent thrombi, leaving only a small lumen in the center.

result of a chronic ailment (*e.g.,* infectious diseases, neoplasms, cardiac decompensation) or during convalescence from myocardial infarction. More rarely, it may occur as a result of prolonged sitting in a car or airplane. Occasionally, it may occur without apparent cause. Because of the paucity of symptomatology, the classification of venous thrombosis of the sural veins has been the topic of considerable discussion. The term *phle-*

bothrombosis was coined to designate a condition characterized by thrombosis in the vein as a primary phenomenon and inflammatory process of the venous wall as secondary to it. In contradistinction, thrombophlebitis was used to indicate that the inflammatory reaction of the wall was primary and thrombosis secondary. These definitions have not been unanimously accepted as a valid explanation for the thrombophlebitic process. Clinically, however, they have served the purpose of reminding the physician of the silent form of venous thrombosis, the first sign of which may be a fatal pulmonary embolism.

Examination of a patient suspected of having calf thrombophlebitis may disclose mild to moderate edema of the involved leg or ankle and pretibial area. Cyanosis is usually mild or absent. Engorgement of the superficial veins over the anterior surface of the leg is an unreliable diagnostic sign in most instances. Homans' sign, often credited as reliable index of the presence of venous thrombosis of the calf, has been shown to be present in only a small percentage of the cases. Likewise, pain from the blood pressure cuff is equally unreliable. Therefore, the positive findings of calf thrombophlebitis are unfortunately often not conclusively demonstrable. Tenderness, induration, edema, or cyanosis may not always be present or may be only minimal. Under these circumstances, a presumptive diagnosis based on one's experience and comprehension of the problem is often the only alternative. This is especially valid from a statistical standpoint in the postoperative state during heart disease, anemia, carcinoma, very advanced age, obesity, and varicose veins.

The second location of thrombophlebitis is the iliofemoral segment. It usually offers no diagnostic problems because the clinical manifestations are obvious. The patients complain of swelling that involves the entire lower extremity, including the thigh. The manifestations consist of general aching of the lower extremities, diffuse enlargement owing to edema, cyanosis of mild to severe degree, tenderness of the upper thigh over the femoral vein, especially in the fossa ovalis, and engorgement of the superficial veins. Arterial pulsations in iliofemoral thrombophlebitis are usually unaffected. Arterial spasm may occur rarely, leading to pain of the entire leg, some pallor, coolness, and diminution or absence of arterial pulsations in the involved limb. Therefore, this may be confused with an arterial embolism.

In contrast to the common form of iliofemoral thrombophlebitis referred to as phlegmasia alba dolens, in a certain number of cases the circulatory disturbances associated with acute thrombophlebitis may range from severe anoxemia of the tissues to gangrene, all of which are secondary to venous thrombosis without arterial participation.[16] Because the dominant manifestation is ischemia of tissues, we have proposed the comprehensive term *ischemic venous thrombosis* for this entity, subdivided into two clinical forms: (1) phlegmasia cerulea dolens, or blue thrombophlebitis, which is a reversible ischemic form, and (2) venous gangrene, in which the changes are by definition irreversible. These two forms are part of the same clinicopathologic entity. The distinction between them is a significant difference of degree of extent of the underlying venous occlusion. Recognition and management of phlegmasia cerulea dolens is of the utmost importance in order to prevent its progression to venous gangrene, the prognosis of which is often not only loss of limb but also death of the patient.[16]

Thrombophlebitis involving the *inferior vena cava* may represent a primary condition or an extension of iliofemoral thrombophlebitis. It may occur first on one side, especially on the left, and then involve the inferior vena cava and the right side. The symptomatology and physical findings of inferior vena cava thrombosis are the same as for iliofemoral thrombophlebitis except that they are bilateral.

Thrombophlebitis of the *superficial veins* in the lower extremity is simple to diagnose in most instances (Fig. 12-9). It may involve the greater or lesser saphenous veins, whether normal or varicose. Occasionally, this diagnosis may be difficult and may have to be differentiated from acute cellulitis and lymphangitis. Most patients with lymphangitis have a fever ranging from 101°F to 104°F. Many have a shaking chill at the onset of their illness. Those with superficial thrombophlebitis never have such a significant temperature elevation or chill.

A frequently encountered superficial thrombophlebitis in the elderly is that affecting varicose veins. The diagnosis is usually simple. The only question is the extent of the process. Occasionally, the thrombosis extends toward the groin or affects the communicating veins linking the superficial to the deep venous system. Under these circumstances, thromboembolic manifestations may occur and may require urgent ligation of the saphenous vein at its junction with the femoral or popliteal veins, as the case may be.

Thrombophlebitis involving the veins of the upper extremities is rare. It may occur as a result of extension from superficial veins into the deep system, in patients who have intrathoracic neoplasms or aneurysms compressing the subclavian vein, or following trauma. Clinical manifestations of the upper extremity involvement are basically the same as for deep thrombophlebitis in the lower extremities.

There are many precipitating factors causing thrombophlebitis in the elderly. Any cause that leads to stasis and coagulation of blood in the calf

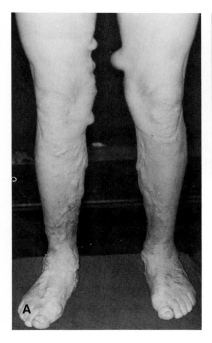

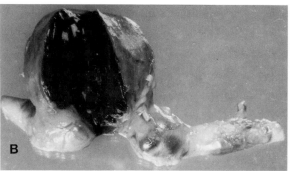

FIG. 12-9. (*A*) Lower extremities of a 74-year-old patient with large protruding varicose veins. Apparently, they were asymptomatic up to his admission to the hospital for a thromboembolic episode. (*B*) Specimen of the left greater saphenous vein with a large thrombosed aneurysmal varicosity. Surgery consisted of bilateral saphenofemoral ligation and multiple excisions of protruding thrombosed veins.

veins or in the iliac system is associated with an increased risk of pulmonary embolism, and that risk increases with age. Rest in bed is the most potent immediate cause. The incidence of calf vein thrombosis is known to rise with increasing length of bed rest. Postoperative states are major precipitating factors because of the operative trauma to tissues mobilizing several clotting factors and because of patient immobility. The effect of a specific type of operation on the risk of thromboembolism is difficult to determine. It seems, however, that exploratory laparotomies for gastric, biliary, and prostate operations are most often related to this complication.

Fractures of the lower limbs and pelvis in elderly patients are often followed by venous thrombosis and embolism. In a study of patients over 55 years of age, it was found that of patients who died after such a fracture, 80% had thrombosis of the lower limbs, and 40% to 50% had pulmonary embolism.[26] Heart disease, especially heart failure, and malignant disease figure prominently in the etiology of thromboembolism.

The poor position of the bedridden patient often causes stasis and subsequent thromboembolic phenomena. Prophylaxis may be achieved by promoting venous drainage of the lower extremities in raising the foot of the bed and using the head-down position. It has been calculated that a 10° head-down position promotes venous drainage of the legs at a rate almost double that in the horizontal position. In severe thrombophlebitis and

edema, a 30° to 40° elevation of the bed may be necessary to promote greater and faster drainage of the venous blood (Fig. 12-10 and 12-11).

Although most thrombi are in the venous plexus of the lower extremities, many are in the pelvis, and a few may be in the right heart. The embolus detached from a venous thrombus occasionally migrates to the right heart and from there to the lungs in two stages. Even the most careful search for any source of emboli sometimes proves futile, and it is estimated that in more than half the patients the source of embolism is unknown at the time of the attack.[26] As pointed out by de Takats[41] it is possible that some subclinical signs may have been overlooked in the evaluation of these patients. Among these signs, the most important to look for are pain in the sole of the foot, especially on pressure; pain at the inner malleolus or around the Achilles tendon, with minimal edema; tenderness on ballottement of the calf muscles, with or without a tight feeling on deep pressure, and increased temperature of the calf compared with the other side. These and a few other minor signs, if properly evaluated, may provide an index of suspicion of deep thrombophlebitis of the leg veins.

Diagnosis

The clinical recognition of a deep venous thrombosis is often difficult. False-positive or false-negative clinical signs occur quite often in these pa-

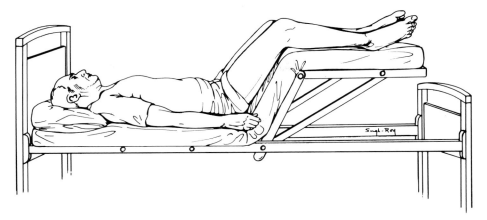

FIG. 12-10. Correct leg-elevation and head-down position for unimpeded venous return and drainage. The bed is broken at the popliteal space in order to provide a comfortable position of the lower extremity.

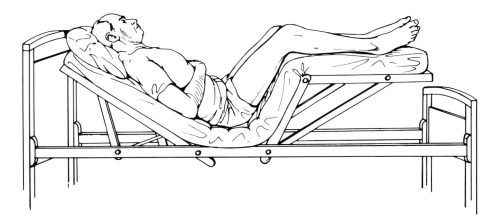

FIG. 12-11. Elevation of lower extremities with head-up position is incorrect method inasmuch as it causes iliac venous stasis and possible thrombosis. (For further discussion see text.)

tients. Recent development of screening tests that can reveal venous thrombi before they become evident clinically has facilitated recognition of this process.

Contrast venography will provide direct evidence of both occlusive and nonocclusive venous thrombi. The disadvantages of venography are that it usually requires movement of the patient to the x-ray table and occasionally may result in local complications.

Noninvasive screening tests are being used extensively in many vascular centers. They consist of the ultrasonic technique, using the Doppler effect,[1,31,34,40] radioactive-labeled fibrinogen, impedance plethysmography, and phleborheography.[1] While the noninvasive techniques are most often useful in detecting the presence of thrombi, ven-

ography remains most accurate in confirming the diagnosis and the extent of the disease.

Laboratory testing for hypercoagulability of the blood has been disappointing because it has been unable routinely to provide evidence for altered clotting factors responsible for this state. Indeed, most hematologists have denied existence of such a state of hypercoagulability, and only recently has its significance been acknowledged.

Pulmonary Embolism

Four recognizable forms of pulmonary embolism occur, although transition from one form to another readily occurs.[2,13,28,35] The four forms are (1) the fatal pulmonary embolus without any evidence of a source of thrombosis, (2) the massive sublethal pulmonary embolus that is still amenable to salvage if measures are taken without delay, (3) the small pulmonary infarct, and (4) a subclinical pulmonary embolism. Diagnostic tests for pulmonary embolism do not always provide adequate information. Radioactive scanning of the lung may provide information concerning the vascularity of the lungs and may have to be correlated with pulmonary angiography, which is the most important diagnostic tool available to determine the presence of major pulmonary emboli. Plain radiography of the chest quite often fails to elucidate diagnostic features even when pulmonary infarction is present, not to mention their unreliable features concerning pulmonary embolism.

Enzymatic studies of the blood in patients with pulmonary emoblism have provided in recent years information that may be valuable if properly interpreted. Essentially, these studies have disclosed a triad of normal serum glutamic oxaloacetic transaminase (SGOT), elevated serum lactic dehydrogenase (LDH), and elevated serum bilirubin. This triad indicates the presence of infarction in about 93% of cases. However, the triad may be present in many necroses of visceral organs, and it is not present during the first 6 to 24 hours. It is absent in embolism without infarction, in which a specific test is most needed because infarction is comparatively easy to diagnose.

TREATMENT OF THROMBOEMBOLISM

Medical Treatment

Management depends on the location and extent of thrombophlebitis. Superficial segmental involvement of the saphenous veins or of the upper extremity rarely, if ever, requires bed rest and elevation. In the absence of spreading thrombosis, and lack of edema or pain, application of an Ace bandage and use of an anti-inflammatory agent (*e.g.,* phenylbutazone [Butazolidin] or oxyphenbutazone [Tandearil]) may overcome the local process within a few days to 2 weeks. If the superficial thrombophelbitis extends above the knee and has a definite tendency to spread up to the groin, bed rest, elevation of the extremity, anticoagulation, and possibly surgery are indicated. The use of surgery depends on whether edema and embolic phenomena are associated with the superficial thrombophlebitis. Fatal emboli may even arise from either following injection of sclerosing agents for varicose veins or as a result of prolonged intravenous infusions. Although such complications are extremely rare, they should nevertheless be borne in mind as possibilities.

In deep thrombophlebitis involving either the sural veins or the iliofemoral segment, the therapeutic approach may vary·sharply, depending on the preceding type of venous involvement.

Bed rest is advisable as a concomitant measure with other methods of management. Elevation of the extremity is essential in order to provide venous drainage. The correct procedure consists of leg elevation and head-down position (Fig. 12-10). A hospital bed is the best means for achieving adequate elevation of the lower extremities with effective venous drainage. In the absence of a hospital bed, especially for patients treated at home, this may be best accomplished by raising the foot of the bed by blocks 12 to 15 inches high. Use of pillows alone too often interferes with proper venous drainage. Elevation of lower extremities associated with head-up position should be avoided as a rather hazardous method because the dependent part of the body—the iliac area—will be the site of venous stasis and a source of possible iliac thrombosis (Fig. 12-11). If the head-up position is necessary because of cardiac decompensation, the legs should be in the horizontal position as a compromise solution, thus avoiding stasis at the iliac level. Local application of either dry heat or ice bags has largely been superseded by application of moist hot packs for the full length of the involved extremity. Hydration of the patient is important to prevent hemoconcentration, which predisposes to thrombosis of the veins. Avoidance of deep breathing and straining should be emphasized, especially at the acute phase of venous thrombosis. This should especially be observed if embolic phenomena are suspected. Too frequently when the patient has chest pain and hemoptysis, he is subjected to a thorough examination of the chest, which may put strain on the thrombosed venous areas and be a further source of embolization. Likewise, roentgenograms taken at the bedside should be carefully carried out by slipping a cassette under the patient rather than moving him in various positions or taking him to the radiology department, where technicians may not be completely versed in the hazards of mobilizing the patient too much.

Anticoagulant Therapy

In geriatric patients it is often desirable to use anticoagulant drugs as a prophylaxis of venous thromboembolism, especially in those undergoing surgical procedures. Under these circumstances, to minimize potential complications of anticoagulant drugs, low or mini doses of heparin have been recommended so as not to alter the laboratory clotting profile.[28]

In established venous thromboembolism, the usefulness of anticoagulation therapy is generally accepted by most workers in this field.

Heparin, preferably administered intravenously, should be started without delay using 5,000 to 7,500 USP units every 4 to 6 hours, or less preferably, by the subcutaneous route, 7,500 to 12,500 units every 12 hours. With the heparin, oral anticoagulant therapy with warfarin sodium (Coumadin) is started in almost all instances. The initial dose of warfarin varies with the method used and ranges from 10 mg to 40 mg. Subsequent maintenance doses range from 2.5 mg to 10 mg a day, adjusted to keep the prothrombin time between 20% and 30% of normal. Oral therapy should be continued 3 to 6 months, especially if the patient has a chronic condition predisposing him to embolism or has had a previous thromboembolic episode. Fibrinolysins have been used in recent years with variable degrees of effectiveness.[32] Their usefulness is still questionable. Low-molecular-weight dextran may likewise be administered in certain cases for 3 to 4 days. In the elderly, it must be given cautiously to prevent cardiac overload.

Surgical Treatment

The rationale for vein interruption in the treatment of thrombophlebitis is that of a mechanical barrier provided to prevent extension of thrombosis and pulmonary emboli. Ligation, plication, or transvenous interruption of the inferior vena cava is indicated only if anticoagulant therapy is ineffective or contraindicated.[27,30,39] Plication may be achieved by suture or, rather, by clips specially designed to divide the lumen of the cava into small compartments.

In recent years, venous thrombectomy has been advocated both in phlegmasia alba dolens and phlegmasia cerulea dolens. Results in the former in terms of persistent patency have not been encouraging. Indications for thrombectomy in the latter condition to prevent pulmonary emboli or the further extension of the thrombosis that may lead to actual gangrene of the limb are more compelling. Balloon catheters specially designed for venous thrombectomy have facilitated this procedure in most instances. To be successful, the procedure should be carried out in the first 2 or 3 days after onset.[16]

Pulmonary Embolectomy

Until a few years ago before the use of cardiopulmonary bypass for pulmonary embolectomy, this procedure carried a forbidding high mortality. Even the current method embolectomy with bypass is not entirely a benign procedure. The operative mortality for all patients undergoing pulmonary embolectomy was 57%. Based on the most recent experience in this field, indications formulated for pulmonary embolectomy are restricted to major embolism with shock, associated with central venous pressure exceeding 30 cm of saline, with an angiogram positive for a filling defect in either or both pulmonary arteries and showing more than 50% obstruction. If the patient's condition is critical, partial venoarterial bypass in the groin improves the situation greatly, and it may render the patient operable.

An alternative approach to open pulmonary embolectomy has been suggested by Greenfield and co-workers and consists of a transvenous removal of pulmonary emboli.[10] This procedure is still in an experimental stage.

REFERENCES

1. Barnes RW: Noninvasive evaluation of venous disease. In Haimovici H (ed): Vascular Surgery: Principles and Techniques, 2nd ed, chap 57. Norwalk, CT, Appleton-Century-Crofts, 1984
2. Bell WR, Simon TL, DeMets DL: The clinical features of submassive and massive pulmonary emboli. Am J Med 62:355, 1977
3. Bergan JJ et al: Medical instrumentation in peripheral vascular disease (Report of the Inter-Society Commission for Heart Disease Resources). Circulation 54:A-1, 1976
4. Brener BJ, Couch NP: Peripheral arterial complications of left heart catheterization and their management. Am J Surg 125:521, 1973
5. Dardik H, Baier RE et al: Morphologic and biophysical assessment of long-term human umbilical cord vein implants used as vascular conduits. Surg Gynecol Obstet 154:17, 1982
6. Darling RC, Austen WG, Linton RR: Arterial embolism. Surg Gynecol Obstet 1·24:106, 1967
7. DeBakey ME, Crawford ES, Morris GC Jr, Cooley DA, Garret HE: Late results of vascular surgery in the treatment of arteriosclerosis. J Cardiovasc Surg 5:473, 1964
8. Dotter CT, Judkins MP: Transluminal treatment of arteriosclerotic obstruction. Circulation 30:654, 1964
9. Fogarty TJ, Cranley JJ: Catheter technic for arterial embolectomy. Ann Surg 161:325, 1965
10. Greenfield LJ, Peyton JD, Brown PP, Elkins RC: Transvenous management of pulmonary embolic disease. Ann Surg 180:461, 1974
11. Gruntzig A, Hopff H: Perkutane Rekanalisation chronischer Arterieller Verschlusse miteinem neuen Dilatation: Modification der Dotter-Technik. Dtsch Med Wochenschr 99:2503, 1974

12. Haimovici H: Peripheral arterial embolism. Angiology 1:20, 1950

13. Haimovici H, Steinman C, Karson IH: Evaluation of lumbar sympathectomy in advanced occlusive arterial disease. Arch Surg 89:1089, 1964

14. Haimovici H: Patterns of arteriosclerotic lesions of the lower extremity. Arch Surg 95:918, 1967

15. Haimovici H: Peripheral arterial disease in diabetes mellitus. In Ellenberg M, Rifkin H (eds): Diabetes Mellitus: Theory and Practice. New York, McGraw-Hill, 1970

16. Haimovici H: Ischemic Forms of Venous Thrombosis: Phlegmasia Cerulea Dolens, Venous Gangrene. Springfield, IL, Charles C Thomas, 1971

17. Haimovici H, Moss CM, Veith FJ: Arterial embolectomy revisited. Surgery 78:409, 1975

18. Haimovici H: Atherogenesis. Recent biological concepts and clinical implications. Amer J Surg 134:174, 1977

19. Haimovici H: Muscular, renal, and metabolic complications of acute arterial occlusions: Myonephropathic-metabolic syndrome. Surgery 85:461, 1979

20. Haimovici H: Cardiogenic embolism of the upper extremity. J Cardiovasc Surg 23:209, 1982

21. Haimovici H: Arterial thromboembolism of the upper extremity associated with the thoracic outlet syndrome. J Cardiovasc Surg 23:214, 1982

22. Haimovici H: Arterial embolism and techniques of embolectomy. In Haimovici H (ed): Vascular Surgery: Principles and Techniques, 2nd ed, chap 23. Norwalk, CT, Appleton-Century-Crofts, 1984

23. Haimovici H: Abdominal aortic aneurysm. In Haimovici H (ed): Vascular Surgery: Principles and Techniques, 2nd ed, chap 42, p 685. Norwalk, CT, Appleton-Century-Crofts, 1984

24. Haimovici H: Peripheral arterial aneurysms. In Haimovici H (ed): Vascular Surgery: Principles and Techniques, 2nd ed, chap 44, p 745. Norwalk, CT, Appleton-Century-Crofts, 1984

25. Hertzer NR, Beven EG: Ultrasound aortic measurement and elective aneurysmectomy. JAMA 240:1966, 1978

26. Hume M, Sevitt S, Thomas DP: Venous Thrombosis and Pulmonary Embolism. Cambridge, MA, Harvard University Press, 1970

27. Hunter HA et al: Permanent transvenous balloon occlusion of the inferior vena cava: Experience with 60 patients. Am Surg 186:491, 1977

28. Kakkar VV, Carrigan TP, Fossard DP: Prevention of fatal pulmonary embolism by low doses of heparin. Lancet 2:45, 1975

29. Kempczinski RF: Lower extremity arterial emboli from ulcerating atherosclerotic plaques. JAMA 241:807, 1979

30. Mobin-Uddin K et al: Transvenous caval interruption with umbrella filter. N Engl J Med 286:55, 1972

31. Mozersky DJ, Sumner DS, Barnes RW, Strandness DE Jr: Intraoperative use of a sterile ultrasonic flow probe. Surg Gynecol Obstet 136:279, 1973

32. National Cooperative Study: The urokinase-streptokinase pulmonary embolism trial. JAMA 229:1606, 1974

33. O'Donnell TF Jr, Darling RC, Linton RR: Is 80 years too old for aneurysmectomy? Arch Surg 111:1250, 1976

34. Raines JK et al: Vascular laboratory criteria for the management of peripheral vascular disease of the lower extremities. Surgery 79:21, 1976

35. Sabiston DC: Pathophysiology, diagnosis and management of pulmonary embolism Am J Surg 138:384, 1979

36. Silbert S, Haimovici H: Criteria for the selection of the level of amputation for ischemic gangrene. JAMA 155:1554, 1954

37. Silbert S, Haimovici H: Results of midleg amputations for gangrene in diabetes. JAMA 144:454, 1950

38. Silbert S Zazeela H: Prognosis in arteriosclerotic peripheral vascular disease. JAMA 166:1816, 1958

39. Silver D, Sabiston DC: The role of vena caval interruption in the management of pulmonary embolism. Surgery 77:1, 1975

40. Strandness DE Jr, Sumner DS (eds): Hemodynamics for Surgeons. New York, Grune & Stratton, 1975

41. Strandness DE Jr, Thiele BL (eds): Selected Topics in Venous Disorders: Pathophysiology, Diagnosis and Treatment. New York, Futura Publishing, 1981

42. Strandness DE Jr, Ward K, Krugmire R Jr: The present status of acute deep venous thrombosis. Surg Gynecol Obstet 145:433, 1977

43. Szilagyi DE, Smith RF et al: Anastomotic aneurysms after vascular reconstruction: Problems of incidence, etiology, and treatment. Surgery 78:800, 1975

44. Tyson RR, Reichle FA: Femorotibial bypass for salvaging of an ischemic leg. Geriatrics 25:203, 1970

45. Veith FJ, Haimovici H: Limb Salvage for Severe Ischemia of the Lower Extremity. In Haimovici H (ed): Vascular Surgery: Principles and Techniques, 2nd ed, chap 32, p 533. Norwalk, CT, Appleton-Century-Crofts, 1984

46. Veith FJ, Moss CM, Fell SC, Rhodes BA, Haimovici H: Comparison of expanded PTFE and vein grafts in lower extremity arterial reconstructions. J Cardiovasc Surg 19:341, 1978

47. Vorhees AB Jr, McAllister FF: Long-term results following resection of arteriosclerotic abdominal aortic aneurysms. Surg Gynecol Obstet 117:355, 1963

48. Warren R, Kihn RB: A survey of lower extremity amputations for ischemia. Surgery 63:107, 1968

49. Wright IS, Urdaneta E, Wright B: Reopening the case of the abdominal aortic aneurysm. Circulation 13:754, 1956

13

Renal Disease in the Elderly

Eben I. Feinstein

The kidney undergoes anatomical and physiologic changes with advancing age. In this respect, it is no different from most other organs. Some alterations reflect degenerative cardiovascular processes; others reflect intrinsic renal changes. In the vast majority of otherwise healthy people, the progressive loss of renal mass and function with age is of little significance, causing neither signs nor symptoms. Knowledge of the aging kidney will assist in diagnosis and proper treatment of the sick patient. New advances, particularly hemodialysis and transplantation, have improved the prognosis for the older patient whose kidneys have failed, and these advances have increased tremendously the importance of geriatric nephrology. It is increasingly common to find patients over age 60 being treated with maintenance hemodialysis.

ANATOMICAL CHANGES IN THE AGING KIDNEY

In 1931 Moore counted the number of glomeruli per kidney in 29 persons ranging in age from 1 to 73 years.[41] Between birth and 40 years each kidney contains 500,000 to 1.2 million glomeruli, although most often the number falls between 800,000 and 1 million. A continuing loss of glomeruli occurs with age. By the seventh decade the number may be reduced by one third to one half. Of interest is Moore's observation that 5 of 20 persons under 40 years of age had between 500,000 and 700,000 glomeruli while 3 of 9 over 40 years had more than 700,000 glomeruli. There was no evidence of postnatal nephrogenesis.

Darmady and co-workers studied 105 subjects who had suffered sudden or relatively sudden death.[10] None had a history or anatomical evidence of hypertension or renal disease. Ages ranged from birth to 101 years. Renal mass declined continuously with advancing age. The progressive nature of the aging process was best demonstrated in the basement membranes of glomeruli and tubules and the arterial tree. In arteries there was gradual, age-related development of medial hypertrophy, intimal proliferation, reduplication of elastic tissue, and some hyalinization in vessels less than 100 μm in diameter. No accurate measurements of tubular lumens could be made. Electron microscopy showed a gradual but patchy thickening of the glomerular and tubular basement membranes. Microdissection techniques were used to determine tubule length and volume and to calculate surface area of glomeruli. Gradual reductions were found in all three: for the group 20 to 39 years old, the mean proximal tubule length was 19.36 mm, proximal tubule volume was 0.076 cu mm, and glomerular surface was 0.254 sq mm; for the 60- to 69-year age-group, 17.38 mm, 0.067 cu mm, and 0.222 sq mm; and for the group 80 to 101 years old, 12.50 mm, 0.052 cu mm, and 0.155 sq mm, respectively. No sex differences were detected.

Changes in nephrons also reflected alteration in heterogeneity with aging; thus, the percentage of tubular volume comprised by juxtamedullary nephrons decreased from 15% of total tubular volume at age 20 to 9% at age 84. Interstitial fibrosis increased gradually, especially in the renal pyramid. The number of diverticula of the distal convoluted tubules, varying from side pouches to pedunculated sacs, rose linearly with age. As many as 200 to 300 diverticula per 100 tubules were present in some kidneys from cadavers over the age of 70. Their etiology is unknown. Some diverticula contain casts, epithelial debris, or clumps of organisms. It was not possible to attribute the renal parenchymal changes observed directly to arteriolar changes as the correlation between the two was inconstant. They seemed to occur concurrently and not sequentially.[10]

Following injection of contrast material, Ljungqvist and Lagergren described an increase in spiraling of renal afferent arterioles after age 50.[34] Such spiraling could be a result of interstitial fibrosis with shortening of the vessels. Cortical arterioles not connected to glomeruli increase with age, reflecting the end result of glomerular degeneration, which makes the arterioles appear to end blindly. In contrast, the juxtamedullary arterioles associated with obsolescent tufts do not end blindly, maintaining the continuity of afferent and efferent vessels. In the older kidney, blood supply to the medullary region is preserved proportionately better than the cortical circulation. Reynes and co-workers confirmed the amputation of a portion of the glomerular bed with age and associated the location of terminal aglomerular arterioles with triangular cortical scars. Cortical aglomerular arteries carry blood toward the capillary beds around tubules while medullary blood is supplied by arterioles derived from the cortical juxtamedullary network. An increase in aglomerular juxtamedullary arterioles was found as a correlate of aging.

Further confirmation of the increasing presence of aglomerular arterioles with age was provided by Takazakura and co-workers.[58] A continuity index was devised that related the number of arterioles with obsolescent or no glomerular tufts to the total number of juxtamedullary units. The continuity index increased linearly with age in normal subjects. It became predominant, that is, greater than 50% after age 45. In diseased kidneys, no correlation with age was found, and in kidneys with chronic glomerulonephritis the index was over 90%, regardless of age.

The aging kidney may show changes related to racial background. Tauchi and co-workers compared Japanese and white autopsy cases and found comparable rates of weight loss with advancing age in kidneys of both groups.[59] The kidneys of white subjects weighed significantly more than those of the Japanese, and their glomeruli were significantly larger and more cellular. When sclerosis of middle-sized arteries (interlobar arteries) and smaller vessels (interlobular) was compared, this change appeared earlier in the Japanese and increased more markedly with age. Earlier renal arterial sclerosis, although of unknown etiology, is consistent with systemic vascular changes and a higher incidence of cerebrovascular and coronary arterial disease in Japanese.

Renal Hypertrophy

In assessing the loss of renal mass with age, the role of compensatory hypertrophy of remaining functioning units must be considered. Verzar described a series of rat experiments using animals between 1 and 22 months of age.[60] The hypertrophy quotient* of the remaining kidney, 30 days after unilateral nephrectomy, was 140 in young male animals, decreasing to 122 at 26 months of age. In advanced senescence (29 to 31 months) the quotient rose to 138. Thus, the capacity for hypertrophy exists in old rats. The biochemical correlates of this hypertrophy will be considered in the discussion of physiologic changes.

In the human, the use of live-donor kidneys for transplantation has made possible an assessment of contralateral renal hypertrophy in donors. Boner and co-workers studied 49 donors for up to 4 years after nephrectomy, including 7 who were between the ages of 51 and 63 at the time of nephrectomy.[6] Although mean glomerular filtration was significantly lower in donors over 40 years of age (105 ± 4.1 ml/min as compared with 115 ± 2.9 ml/min, inulin clearance); at 3 weeks post nephrectomy, the percentage of the original value attained by both groups was similar (66.2 ± 2.4 ml/min for over 40 and 66.3 ± 1.7 ml/min for under 40). Using multiple linear regression analysis, the effect of age on subsequent increases in rate was plotted. From their nomograms, a 20-year-old person with a rate of 120 ml/min preoperatively would have a rate of 86 ml/min 3 years later, and a 60-year-old donor starting at 120 ml/min would have a value of 76 ml/min indicating diminished but persistent capacity for renal hypertrophy in older humans. After an initial large increment in renal function owing to compensatory hypertrophy at 3 weeks, any subsequent increase in function varies inversely with increasing age of the subject.

Disturbances in Renal Function

The anatomical changes in the kidney can be expected to affect renal function. Degenerative changes in other organs may have an additive effect. A failing heart, for example, will reduce

---

* Hypertrophy quotient =

$$\frac{\text{weight of hypertrophied kidney}}{\text{weight of normal kidney}} \times 100$$

renal perfusion and have a deleterious effect on already compromised renal function.

Glomerular filtration rate begins a gradual fall from peak values in the second decade of life, declining continuously through the tenth decade.

Davies and Shock[11] studied glomerular filtration in 70 males from the third to the ninth decades who were free of hypertension and renal and heart disease. In the fifth decade, mean inulin clearance was 121.2 ml/min/1.73 sq m; the mean for the sixth decade was 99.3 ml/min/1.73 sq m; and for the ninth it was 65.3 ml/min/1.73 sq m. The average fall in inulin clearance between the ages of 20 and 90 was 46%. Over the same period iodopyracet (Diodrast) clearance dropped from 613 ml to 289 ml plasma/min/1.73 sq m (43.5%) Olbrich and co-workers studied a group of 50 elderly subjects aged 60 years or more (36 men and 14 women) and compared their renal function with that of younger patients and of hypertensive elderly patients.[44] Compared with healthy young men, the elderly showed a mean decrease of about 30% in Diodrast clearance, inulin clearance, and tubular excretory capacity. Urea clearance also fell with age, 82.4 ml/min to 62.3 ml/min. Diastolic hypertension was associated with a further significant decline of 12%.

Sixteen years after the report of Davies and Shock, the Gerontology Research Center, National Institute on Aging (NIA) in Baltimore, reported the results of a longitudinal study of creatinine clearance in 584 men.[50] These were volunteer subjects studied at 12- to 18-month intervals. Determinations of true creatinine concentrations in serum and urine were made (*i.e.*, noncreatinine chromogens were removed). The ratio of creatinine to inulin clearance was:

$$\frac{\text{creatinine clearance}}{\text{inulin clearance}} = $$
$$1.22 + 0.0012 \cdot (\text{age in years})$$

As in previous reports, a significant decline in filtration rate was found, beginning at age 34. Mean serum creatinine concentration rose slowly from 0.813 mg/dl (ages 25 to 34) to 0.843 mg/dl (ages 75 to 84). This relatively small increase may at first appear less impressive than the corresponding fall in creatinine clearance. However, the lesser muscle mass in aged subjects would have decreased mean serum creatinine had renal function remained constant. A linear equation describes the relationship:

true creatinine clearance
(ml/min/1.73 sq m) =
$$165.57 - 0.80 (\text{age in years})$$

Routine laboratory creatinine clearance times 1.25 equals true creatinine clearance. Surprisingly, hypertension and prostatic enlargement did not significantly alter renal clearance in this select group of upper middle class, well-educated subjects. This was interpreted as a reflection of good medical management during the course of this study. The longitudinal nature of the NIA study also allowed the rate of decline by age decade to be measured. A minimally significant acceleration of the rate of decline was measured in the later decades of life[50]

Wesson compiled the results from many studies and prepared graphic representation of the serial decline in glomerular filtration and renal plasma flow.[62] His plots show a decline in renal blood flow from 670 ml/min in the second decade to 350 ml/min in the eighth. Changes in the rates of glomerular filtration and renal plasma flow may not be parallel as reflected in the filtration fraction: glomerular filtration rate per renal blood flow. For example, in the sixth decade, the ratio was 20.5, rising to 26.24 in the 70- to 79-year age-group.[11] Diastolic hypertension in one report was associated with a further increment in filtration fraction from 24.3 to 27.7.[44] Brenner and co-workers[8] have suggested that the decline in glomerular filtration rate and the increasing incidence of glomerular sclerosis seen with normal aging may be due to the effects of a chronically elevated dietary protein intake. From data in rats, they argue that high protein intake produces alterations in the pressure and flow in the glomerulus that leads to eventual sclerosis. If substantiated in the human, this hypothesis would have profound implications.

The factors responsible for decreased blood flow in aging kidneys are not completely settled. The anatomical changes enumerated above are not considered by some to be sufficient to explain the fall in perfusion. Alteration in vascular tone has been postulated as an alternative explanation. Infusion of pyrogen will induce vasodilatation of renal vasculature in elderly subjects, a result interpreted as evidence of an increase in resting vascular tone.[36] Hollenberg and co-workers have explored the role of vascular tone in careful experiments on kidney transplant donors ranging in age from 17 to 76.[25] Radioactive xenon washout studies indicated a decline in cortical blood flow with age. Acetylcholine-induced increases in blood flow were significantly smaller in aged subjects; the response to increments in dosage of the drug was greater in younger subjects. Vasoconstrictor response, however, assessed by the infusion of angiotensin, showed no significant age-related changes. Several conclusions regarding intrarenal blood flow were drawn: (1) the observed fall in outer cortical perfusion results in proportionately better perfusion of juxtamedullary nephrons (anatomical correlates of this inference have already been noted); (2) these inner nephrons are known to have a higher filtration fraction and may account for the disproportionate change in glomerular filtration and blood flow; (3) diminished renal blood flow may relate to histologic changes in the small vessel wall, not active vasoconstriction, because the responses to acetylcholine do not support a rise in resting vascular tone; and (4) the angiotensin study demonstrates that despite mural changes, smooth muscle in arteries is capable of contracting normally.

Hollenberg's group has also investigated the response of aging kidneys to variations in sodium intake.[16] Increased sodium intake results in volume expansion and renal vasodilatation in subjects of all ages. As in the acetylcholine study, however, renal vasodilatation was blunted in aged subjects placed on a 200 mEq/day sodium intake. Age also impairs the sodium-conserving ability of the kidney when sodium intake is decreased to 10 mEq/day. On a sodium-restricted diet, the half-time to achieve a urine sodium concentration as low as 20 mEq/liter was significantly longer in subjects over 60 compared with a group between 30 and 60 years old (30.9 ± 2.8 hours as compared with 23.5 hours). The explanation for this reduction in sodium-conserving ability likely involves both a decrease in nephron mass and the diminished aldosterone secretion rate in response to acute stimuli in the elderly as reported by Flood and co-workers.[20]

Tubular Function

Clinically, tubular function can be measured in the basal resting state or after physiologic maneuvers. The transport maximum (Tm) for glucose, a proximal tubular function, declines with age.[39] The rate of decline is identical to that of the glomerular filtration rate and, when expressed as a percentage of baseline level (Tm glucose at age 20), is identical to the decline in Tm for Diodrast.[11]

Urinary Concentration and Dilution

The subject of water metabolism and aging has been extensively reviewed.[56] Maximum urinary concentrating ability decreases with age.[13,34] In a study of healthy subjects, the mean maximum urinary osmolality after dehydration was 882 ± 49 mOsm/kg in subjects 60 to 79 years old compared

with 1109 ± 22 mOsm/kg in young adults (20 to 39 years old).[38,51] One explanation for this observation is that the solute load per nephron rises as nephrons are lost during aging. However, there is no correlation between the decrease in creatinine clearance and the urinary osmolality.[51] A reduced renal tubular response to antidiuretic hormone[40] may contribute to the impairment in concentration. Also, elderly patients with bacteriuria exhibit impaired concentrating ability to a greater degree than nonbacteriuric patients.[14]

The renal response to a water load demonstrates an impaired diluting capacity. Following a water load the mean minimum urinary osmolality was 52 ± 3 mOsm/liter in young subjects and 92 ± 11 mOsm/liter in old subjects.[33] Impaired urinary dilution may be due to changes in glomerular filtration rate and renal blood flow and to distal tubular defects.

Renal Acid–Base Regulation

Acid excretion by the kidney is also affected by aging.[1,2] To assess this function, an acute acid load is given in the form of ammonium chloride. Elderly subjects excreted 18 ± 5% of the acid load in 8 hours (59 ± 5% of which was ammonium) compared with 35 ± 6% excreted in a younger population (72 ± 7% in the form of ammonium).[1] The defect in acid excretion does not appear to be due to a reduction in glomerular filtration rate but rather to diminished ammonia excretion.[2] This then is another perturbation in tubular function associated with increasing age.

CLINICAL ASPECTS OF RENAL DISEASE IN THE AGED

The clinical implications of these basic alterations can now be understood. In treating the patient without renal disease, it is essential to know age-related alterations to interpret laboratory data intelligently and to prescribe medications appropriately. For the diagnosis of renal disease, a knowledge of differential diagnostic criteria is needed. Finally, treatment requires awareness of the suitability of older patients for the various modes of modern nephrologic therapy.

The blood urea nitrogen (BUN) increases with age. Of 100 normal subjects, average age 81.7, 65 had BUN values greater than 20 mg/dl, and 14 were greater than 30 mg/dl.[47] The serum creatinine value, also an important screening test of renal function, rises with age (see above). It is important to remember that the creatinine clearance may be markedly decreased to as little as 30% of predicted normal while the serum creatinine concentration remains within the normal limits for most laboratories.

Along with a reduced glomerular filtration rate, the decrease in concentrating ability may make certain diagnostic tests particularly hazardous in the elderly. Overnight dehydration for radiologic studies may profoundly injure an older patient. The osmotic load of contrast material will further stress the kidneys, and an adverse reaction to the contrast material could result in hypotension and acute renal failure. This can be lethal in the elderly, and any steps that might prevent this iatrogenic complication should be taken, including avoidance of unnecessary intravascular volume contraction.

ACUTE RENAL FAILURE

If acute renal failure (ARF) develops, the older patient is treated similarly to the young. Attention must be paid to electrolyte imbalance, particularly hyperkalemia; volume overload, which could precipitate pulmonary edema; and infections, which exacerbate an existing catabolic state. Hemodialysis should not be withheld because of age. Reliance on conservative (nondialytic) management of an elderly patient with ARF could prove disastrous. I have performed both acute peritoneal and hemodialysis without difficulty in octogenarians and nonagenarians.

ARF is a sudden, often precipitous, fall in glomerular filtration rate that occurs in diseases involving the renal vasculature, the glomeruli, and

INTRINSIC RENAL DISEASES THAT CAUSE ACUTE RENAL FAILURE

Vascular Disease

Cholesterol atheroembolism
Malignant nephrosclerosis
Renal artery thrombosis

Glomerular Disease

Postinfectious glomerulonephritis
Systemic lupus nephritis

Tubulointerstitial Disease

Acute interstitial nephritis
Acute tubular necrosis due to nephrotoxic agents
    or ischemic injury

the tubules and interstitium. Acute tubular necrosis due to hypotension, sepsis, or nephrotoxins is the leading cause of reversible ARF due to intrinsic renal disease. It is important to consider other causes in the elderly, especially if the diagnosis is not clear cut. In one series,[43] about half of the patients over 60 years old with a clinical diagnosis of acute tubular necrosis were found to have other diseases such as bilateral renal infarction, myelomatosis, hypersensitivity angiitis, cortical necrosis, or atheromatous embolization.

Compromise of the renal circulation from embolism or thrombosis is more frequent in older patients. They are more likely to have atherosclerotic disease and may develop renal failure from the underlying vascular disease or the angiography and surgery they may undergo. A good example of ARF seen mostly in the elderly is atheroembolism to the kidneys from atherosclerotic plaques in the aorta. Most patients reported with this syndrome were over 60 years of age.[26] This disease may occur during angiography or during aortic surgery, but improved techniques of aortography and careful handling of the aorta during surgery should minimize it.

The diagnosis of atheroembolic renal failure requires a high index of suspicion especially in the old patient with acute oliguria superimposed on known aortic atherosclerotic disease. Renal failure results when atheromatous material dislodges from the aorta and occludes the lumens of involved vessels. The emboli can be recognized by the characteristic clefts in the lumens after the cholesterol has been dissolved in fixing the tissue (Fig. 13-1). The vessel reacts to the emboli with macrophages, giant cells, and later, intimal fibrosis. Acute uremia and hypertension are the most common clinical manifestations of massive bilateral arteriosclerotic embolization. Without a biopsy of the kidney, a definite diagnosis cannot be made. Evidence of pancreatitis and gastrointestinal bleeding from diffuse atheroembolism supports the diagnosis. The discovery of cholesterol emboli in a muscle biopsy of the thigh provides strong presumptive evidence for the diagnosis. No diagnostic urinary sediment findings are described. Some erythrocytes and leukocytes and granular and hyaline casts may be present but will not distinguish atheroemboli from acute tubular necrosis.

Although often thought of as a disease of children and young adults, acute glomerulonephritis does occur in the elderly. In the older patient atypical features may predominate.[52] Dyspnea and edema are the most common initial symptoms; only one of seven cases in the report of Samiy and

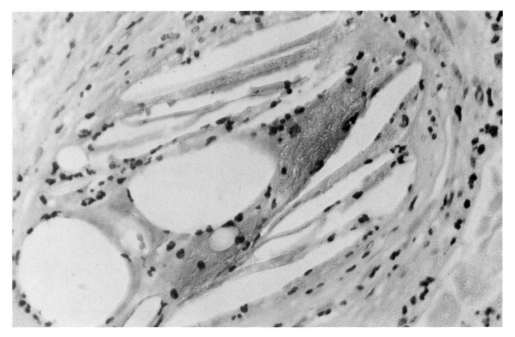

FIG. 13-1. Renal arteriole showing atheroembolic disease. Characteristic cholesterol clefts remain as clear areas after dissolving during fixation. This example from a failed renal transplant is morphologically identical to the changes observed after aortic surgery or catheterization in recipients with previously normal renal function. Relentless progress of renal failure is the rule.

his colleagues presented with hematuria, while only two of seven had erythrocyte casts, a ubiquitous finding in younger patients. β-Hemolytic *Streptococcus* was cultured from the throat of one patient, while three patients gave a history of prior sore throat. The correct diagnosis was made in only one case on admission. Vascular obstruction of the renal arteries and ureteric or prostatic obstruction were considered more likely diagnoses before the correct diagnosis was made. Other types of acute glomerulonephritis that may be seen in an elderly population are idiopathic crescentic glomerulonephritis and Wegener's granulomatosis.[42]

In addition to intrinsic renal disease, a reduction in renal function may be seen when there is volume depletion, hypotension, or impaired renal perfusion from other causes. It is important to make the diagnosis of prerenal azotemia because treatment of the predisposing condition may lead to recovery of renal function. Some of the clinical circumstances frequently seen leading to dehydration with azotemia are the nursing home resident, too weak to provide himself with adequate water, who may continue to receive potent diuretics; the victim of a cerebrovascular accident also unable to

CAUSES OF PRERENAL AZOTEMIA

Hypotension

Hemorrhage
Sepsis

Volume Depletion

Vomiting
Diarrhea
Thermal injury
Third space loss (*e.g.*, pancreatitis, intestinal obstruction)
Excessive use of diuretics

Impaired Cardiac Function

Congestive heart failure

Increased Renal Vascular Resistance

Hepatorenal syndrome

get enough oral fluid intake; and the diabetic patient who does not require insulin, with an intercurrent acute illness, who develops hyperosmolar nonketotic coma. Indeed, anorexia may occur with any acute infection and result in inadequate fluid intake. These patients present with elevated blood urea nitrogen and serum creatinine (as high as 200 mg/dl and 8 mg/dl, respectively), which is reversible with intravenous fluid therapy.

Congestive heart failure is important to bear in mind when prerenal azotemia exists. Heart failure may cause decreased renal perfusion. The kidney responds by avid sodium retention, and extracellular fluid volume expansion results. Improvement in myocardial function after therapy with digitalis glycosides and diuretics is generally accompanied by improvement in renal function. Nonetheless, it is not uncommon to see prerenal azotemia develop in patients receiving diuretic drugs for heart failure. The intravascular volume depletion that follows diuretic administration may lead to azotemia without complete elimination of edema. A balance must be struck; the patient may need to tolerate some edema if renal functional deterioration is to be avoided.

As noted, azotemia may occur with a febrile illness owing to increased insensible losses, hypercatabolism, and impaired fluid intake. When a definite cause of fever is not apparent, particularly in a patient in whom azotemia has developed, blood cultures are imperative to exclude bacterial endocarditis. This entity can produce parenchymal renal disease either by embolization to the kidneys or by glomerulonephritis with deposition of immune complexes in the glomerular capillary basement membrane.[24]

The catabolic effects of corticosteroids will cause increased serum urea concentration. This rise in BUN is disproportionate to any rise in serum creatinine (*i.e.,* the BUN-to-creatinine ratio is equal to or greater than 20:1), and this is helpful in differentiating renal insufficiency from prerenal azotemia. In the patient receiving steroids who develops renal insufficiency, the serum creatinine should be relied on to assess intrinsic renal function.

A third category of extrarenal disorders that may cause ARF are those associated with urinary tract obstruction or post-renal azotemia. Obstruction may occur at any level of the urinary tract, but common sites in the elderly are the prostate gland in men and the lower ureter (due to pelvic carcinoma) in women.

Differentiating acute oliguric renal failure owing to acute tubular necrosis from volume depletion is a common problem. The usual criteria include a urine sodium concentration greater than

CAUSES OF POST-RENAL AZOTEMIA

Neoplastic Diseases

Bladder and prostate carcinoma
Cervical carcinoma
Retroperitoneal lymphoma

Renal Calculi

Renal Papillary Necrosis

Analgesic abuse nephropathy
Diabetes mellitus

Passage of Blood Clots

20 mEq/liter and a urine to plasma (U/P) creatinine ratio of less than 20 (Table 13-1). Sporn and coworkers make the point that the decreased concentrating ability of the older patient may interfere with the interpretation of a fixed U/P osmolality ratio.[57] However, in two elderly patients with acute renal failure that they describe, the U/P osmolality ratios were only slightly above 1.1; while in three old patients with volume depletion the ratios were well above that figure. Urine sodium concentrations followed expected courses in the two groups. In my experience both a high urinary sodium concentration and a U/P creatinine ratio of less than 20 are reliable clues to the diagnosis of acute tubular necrosis in the elderly.

A U/P ratio of greater than 1.1 does not exclude other causes of oliguria besides volume depletion.[7] Two examples of this are the hepatorenal syndrome (in which ascites and edema are present, while urine output is low, and urine sodium concentration is decreased) and acute poststreptococcal glomerulonephritis with oliguria.

TABLE 13-1   Differential Diagnosis of Pre-Renal Azotemia and Acute Tubular Necrosis

	Prerenal Azotemia	Acute Tubular Necrosis
Creatinine U/P	>40	<20
Osmolality U/P	>1.1	1.0–1.1
Urine Sodium	<20 mEq/liter	>20 mEq/liter
BUN/Serum Creatinine	≥20:1	10:1

Management

The management of patients with ARF depends on the extent of their loss of renal function and on the degree of their protein catabolism. Many patients, particularly those with nephrotoxin-induced acute tubular necrosis, have nonoliguric ARF (daily urine volume of 500 ml or more). They do not exhibit increased protein breakdown. As a result, urea production and the rate of rise in BUN is not rapid (30 mg/dl/day or less). Frequently, such patients can be managed without dialysis or with one or two peritoneal dialyses.

In contrast, patients with ARF due to shock or sepsis frequently have marked increases in protein breakdown.[18] The BUN rises at a rate of 50 mg/dl or greater. Oliguria is usually present. In such cases, hemodialysis is usually required. Often, provision of adequate nutrition via the gastrointestinal tract is not possible and parenteral hyperalimentation is needed. When total parenteral nutrition is prescribed, hypokalemia, hypophosphatemia,

---

NONDIALYTIC MANAGEMENT OF ACUTE RENAL FAILURE

Monitor serum electrolytes and hemoglobin daily.
Diet:
    Protein: 0.5 g/kg/day
    Potassium: 2 g/day or less
    Calories: 30 Kcal/kg/day
Catheterization of the bladder should be avoided.
Infections should be treated with appropriate antibiotics at dosages adjusted for the renal impairment.

MANAGEMENT OF ACUTE RENAL FAILURE IN THE CATABOLIC PATIENT

Dialysis

To treat hyperkalemia, azotemia, acidosis, fluid overload, and other uremic manifestations such as bleeding and encephalopathy

Nutrition—Parenteral hyperalimentation

Calories: 30–35 Kcal/kg/day using hypertonic dextrose and lipid emulsions
Amino acids: Up to 1 g/kg/day of essential and nonessential amino acids
Electrolytes: May require potassium, phosphorus, and magnesium

---

and hypomagnesemia may occur, requiring administration of these electrolytes.

Prevention

Certain precautions may prevent the development of ARF. Correction of hypovolemia is important since this may cause renal failure and may render the patient more prone to ARF from other insults. When use of a nephrotoxic drug is necessary it should be given with caution. Since renal function declines with age, dosage adjustments of drugs such as the aminoglycoside antibiotics are usually required. Awareness of the level of renal function is important if renal damage is to be avoided and adverse reactions from drugs requiring renal excretion (*e.g.,* digoxin) are to be minimized. If serum drug levels are available they should be used to monitor dosing intervals (drug dosing guidelines should be consulted for detailed information on individual drugs).[5] Other drugs to be used with caution are the nonsteroidal anti-inflammatory agents that can produce ARF, especially in patients with congestive heart failure or chronic liver disease.

Even with the benefits of modern dialytic therapy, the overall mortality in ARF has not changed dramatically and remains about 50%.[28] It should be appreciated that, in recent years, vigorous treatment with crystalloid and colloid solutions to maintain the extracellular fluid volume may have prevented ARF in patients who sustained nephrotoxic or ischemic insults. On the other hand, modern therapy for burns, advanced cardiovascular surgery, and highly nephrotoxic drugs have maintained the lives of many patients who subsequently developed ARF. Therefore, the current patient population with ARF may consist of pa-

---

PREVENTION OF ACUTE RENAL FAILURE

Maintain adequate extracellular fluid volume, especially before surgical procedures.
Exercise caution with nephrotoxic agents such as the following:
    Radiocontrast agents
    Aminoglycoside antibiotics
    Nonsteroidal anti-inflammatory agents
    Certain cytotoxic agents (*e.g., cis*-platinum)
If oliguria is present, rule out the presence of prerenal azotemia and urinary tract obstruction.

tients who are older and more critically ill than patients of several decades ago. It is well established that survival is lower in patients with ARF who are over 50 years of age as compared with younger patients. This difference may be due to the higher prevalence of arteriosclerotic cardiovascular disease in the elderly.[19]

Nephrotic Syndrome

A major concern of the nephrologist is the diagnosis and treatment of the nephrotic syndrome. Criteria for diagnosis are proteinuria of 3.5 g/day or greater, usually accompanied by a serum albumin level of less than 3 g/dl, edema, and hyperlipidemia. There are many diseases associated with this syndrome whose incidence varies with age. Lipoid nephrosis or minimal change nephropathy is common in children, while membranous nephropathy[9] and nephrotic syndrome secondary to systemic illnesses are more common in adults.

The clinical implications of these differences in disease incidence are important. Minimal change nephropathy is a disease of unknown etiology. It is associated with normal or minimally abnormal light microscopic findings on renal biopsy specimens. There are no immune deposits seen by immunofluorescent techniques, but fusion of foot processes of epithelial cells is seen on electron microscopic examination. The disease is highly responsive to steroid therapy, a large proportion of cases being cured by one course of prednisone for 8 weeks.

In contrast, membranous nephropathy exhibits findings indicative of an immune complex pathogenesis, follows a more chronic course, and is not as amenable to treatment. Renal biopsy reveals diffuse thickening of the glomerular capillary basement membrane. Deposition of immune complexes on the subepithelial surface of the membrane can be shown by immunofluorescence. Membranous nephropathy may occur without associated illness (the idiopathic form), or it may be associated with a variety of illnesses, particularly chronic infections and solid tumors. It has been postulated that the antigenic component of the immune complex may be derived from an infectious agent or tumor cell.

An associated clinical condition seen particularly with membranous nephropathy is renal vein thrombosis. The thrombi may be unilateral or bilateral and may extend into the inferior vena cava. The reason for the association of these clinical entities is not known, but it seems certain that the glomerular disease is the primary condition and that the venous thrombosis does not cause proteinuria.[35]

There is no specific set of clinical findings diagnostic of membranous nephropathy. Microscopic hematuria, casts, and hypertension may be present initially but less frequently than in the other primary forms of nephritis. The diagnosis must be made by renal biopsy and should alert the physician to the possibility of either renal venous thrombosis or a solid tumor.

Renal vein thrombosis may be heralded by onset of flank pain, hematuria, or sudden deterioration in renal function. Pulmonary embolism may occur. The lack of these findings should not deter selective renal venography because the thrombosis may be found without any associated clinical changes.[35]

A 10% incidence of adult membranous cases associated with neoplasms has been reported.[49] The tumor may be diagnosed only months after onset of proteinuria. Search for a tumor is mandatory because it may lead to early diagnosis of cancer, and successful control of the malignant process may lead to remission of the proteinuria. Return of proteinuria may herald recurrence of the tumor.

The natural history of membranous nephropathy is varied. Spontaneous remission may occur in 25% of cases. In the majority of cases, the nephrotic syndrome persists with chronic renal failure developing in up to one third of patients.[17]

In addition to neoplasms, other systemic illnesses may be associated with the nephrotic syndrome. These include multiple myeloma, diabetes mellitus, chronic inflammatory conditions, and systemic lupus erythematosus.

Chronic Renal Failure

Chronic renal failure (CRF) refers to the decline in glomerular filtration rate seen in a variety of diseases affecting the kidney. Aging, as already

---

COMMON CAUSES OF CHRONIC RENAL FAILURE

Chronic glomerulonephritis
Diabetes mellitus
Hypertension
Congenital or familial disease (*e.g.,* polycystic kidney disease)
Obstructive uropathy

---

mentioned, is itself a cause of CRF. There are various stages of CRF, from mild renal insufficiency (loss of 25% to 30% of renal function) to advanced renal failure (loss of 80% to 90%). End-stage renal failure denotes that stage of CRF that requires dialysis or transplantation (usually less than 5% of normal renal function).

The diagnosis of CRF can frequently be made from the history and assessment of renal size. A reduction in renal size is an indication of a chronic irreversible disease process. However, in CRF due to diabetes mellitus, amyloidosis, polycystic kidney disease, and obstructive uropathy, the kidney size may be normal or even increased. If obstruction is considered a likely diagnosis, further evaluation should be performed to find a correctable cause. When the cause of obstruction is not treatable (*e.g.,* inoperable pelvic carcinoma), then diversion of the ureters may preserve renal function and delay the need for dialysis.

Radiologic techniques are very helpful in the diagnosis of CRF, particularly for assessment of renal size and determination of obstruction. Intravenous pyelography, radioisotope scanning, and renal ultrasonography are the most commonly used procedures. Age may have an important bearing on the interpretation of the pyelogram and scan. Friedman and associates[21] studied 35 patients with a mean age of 75 years who had no evidence of renal disease. Most patients had normal pyelograms, but there was a high incidence of abnormal scans. Thus, in the presence of a normal serum creatinine value and normal pyelogram, many patients had evidence of anatomical defects as determined by isotope scanning. In recent years, the ultrasound examination has become the primary tool for assessing size and contour of the kidneys, not only in the elderly but in all age-groups.

Several causes of CRF are of particular importance in the elderly.

Multiple Myeloma

Multiple myeloma deserves special attention because of its increased incidence in the elderly, its frequent involvement of the kidneys, and the possibility of preventing or treating some of its renal complications. Faced with an elderly patient with nephrotic syndrome or acute or chronic renal failure, the clinician should consider myeloma as a major diagnostic possibility. Tubular dysfunction (such as renal tubular acidosis) and tubular obstruction leading to oliguric renal failure may result from the effects of myeloma proteins on tubule cell function and urine flow. Hypercalcemia will impair concentrating and may lead to nephrocalcinosis. Suppression of the immune response is a feature of myeloma and is compounded by antineoplastic agents. Pyelonephritis can be the renal expression of susceptibility to infection.[23]

The kidneys are affected in one half the cases of myeloma. Heptinstall found severe renal failure in 30% of sixty patients.[24] In older patients with unexplained renal disease, the possibility of myeloma should lead to a search for Bence Jones proteinuria. Certainly this should be done to prior to intravenous pyelography. Maintenance of a normal calcium level and aggressive treatment of urinary tract infection are obviously desirable.

Interpretation of serum electrolytes may be affected by myeloma. Increase in serum chloride concentration owing to renal tubular acidosis has been mentioned. Spurious hyponatremia is seen when the plasma protein concentration is so high as to replace a significant amount of plasma water.

Diabetes Mellitus

Diabetes mellitus is an increasingly common cause of end-stage renal failure leading to maintenance hemodialysis or peritoneal dialysis. In agreement with the experience of others,[55] about one fourth of the patients whom I place on maintenance dialysis have diabetes mellitus. The mechanisms for renal failure in the diabetic patient include glomerulosclerosis (most commonly diffuse glomerulosclerosis), renal infection, papillary necrosis, and obstruction from a neurogenic bladder. Renal failure is the cause of death in about one half of juvenile-onset diabetic patients; this is lessened in older patients because of the rising mortality from atherosclerosis. The outlook for the young adult or the elderly diabetic patient with renal failure although improving is still poorer than that of the nondiabetic of a similar age. Atherosclerosis is the leading cause of death in both age-groups during dialysis therapy. Retinopathy may progress and severe visual impairment may result. Vascular access for hemodialysis is difficult to maintain owing to peripheral vascular disease. Severe neuropathy may make a useful life impossible.[29]

OBSTRUCTION

Prostatic obstruction is, of course, a very important consideration in the older man with renal insufficiency, especially because it is potentially reversible. Urinary tract obstruction predisposes to urinary tract infection, especially following instrumentation, which will further exacerbate renal insufficiency.[38] Women may also develop urinary tract obstruction or incomplete bladder emptying. Weakening of the pelvic and bladder musculature may decrease bladder emptying, leading to urinary retention and infection. Prolapse of the uterus may cause bilateral ureteric obstruction.[15]

Olbrich and co-workers[45] studied renal function in chronic urinary obstruction owing to prostatic hypertrophy and carcinoma. Almost one half (28 of 60) of cases had urine infection, although none were hypertensive. The inulin clearance and renal plasma flow were reduced to two-thirds that of younger men. Infection was associated with an even greater fall (50%) in clearance and renal plasma flow. Repeat study after prostatectomy in 12 patients showed a consistent increase in plasma flow to a mean of 29% above preoperative values. Tubular function (measured by Tm for Diodrast) was impaired only in the infected cases. The lack of improvement in glomerular filtration rate after relief of obstruction was attributed to irreversible renal damage.

MANAGEMENT OF CHRONIC RENAL FAILURE

The management of CRF before end-stage is reached requires control of hypertension, relief of urinary tract obstruction, treatment of infection, if present, and dietary modifications to control azotemia, hyperkalemia, hyperphosphatemia, and

NONDIALYTIC MANAGEMENT OF CHRONIC RENAL FAILURE

1. Control of hypertension
2. Relief of urinary tract obstruction
3. Treatment of urinary tract infection
4. Dietary
   a. Protein restriction with glomerular filtration rate below 25 ml/min[32]
   b. Potassium restriction usually with glomerular filtration rate below 10 ml/min
   c. Salt restriction usually not required until advanced CRF
5. Medications
   a. Aluminum hydroxide to bind phosphate in the intestine
   b. Shohl's solution to treat acidosis
   c. Vitamin D (1,25-dihydroxycholecalciferol) to treat vitamin D deficiency and hypocalcemia

acidosis. Protein restriction early in the course of CRF has been advocated to slow the progressive loss of renal function.[8] Research based on this hypothesis is now being done and a definitive answer should be available in the next 5 years.

There are three types of treatment for end-stage renal failure: (1) hemodialysis, (2) peritoneal dialysis, and (3) transplantation. The two dialytic procedures are most pertinent for the elderly. Each can be performed at home or in a professionally staffed center. A minor surgical procedure is required for both treatments to allow access either to the vascular system or the peritoneal cavity.

Maintenance Hemodialysis

Hemodialysis requires repetitive access to the circulation. This is usually accomplished with an external shunt (now used mostly for temporary access), a subcutaneous arteriovenous fistula, or an arteriovenous graft. The creation of vascular access may be very difficult in some patients, particularly those with impaired arterial flow due to arteriosclerotic narrowing. In such cases, peritoneal dialysis provides the only feasible alternative.

From its inception, hemodialysis has been used with success in older patients. The first case in which hemodialysis is credited with saving a patient's life dates back to the experiences in World War II of Kolff, who in 1945 treated a 67-year-old woman with cholecystitis and acute glomerulonephritis with anuria. After one 11-hour treatment she recovered. She was the 17th patient to have been dialyzed by Kolff. ''It is significant,'' wrote Kolff, ''that this 67-year-old patient was not considered to be a very useful member of society.''[31]

Kolff also described the course of dialytic therapy in a 77-year-old woman with systemic lupus erythematosus and acute uremia. On the tenth day of anuria, dialysis was performed. The patient recovered and left the hospital. ''Neither the age of a patient nor the severity of his disease need stand in the way of dialysis for the treatment of uremia if there is a chance for recovery or hope for prolongation of an enjoyable span of life,'' wrote Kolff in 1959.[27] I hold Kolff's view to be just as appropriate and timely now.

The advent of the Scribner shunt in 1960 allowed the end-stage renal disease patient to be maintained indefinitely with intermittent hemodialysis. It was not initially appreciated that the older patient would be suitable for maintenance hemodialysis. Shaldon, in describing his ideal candidate for chronic dialysis, specifically dismissed those patients over age 55: they ''stand little chance of adequate rehabilitation and tend to do badly . . . one reason for this is the disequilibrium effect of dialysis on these patients which is exaggerated in the elderly."[54] Patients with a multisystem cause for renal failure, such as diabetes mellitus, vascular thrombotic disease, or other chronic diseases likely to cause death, were excluded as candidates for maintenance hemodialysis because of the extraordinary cost of this therapy and the fear that high morbidity and mortality would limit rehabilitation.

The watershed for maintenance dialysis therapy for those over 50 years old in the United States was the passage in 1972 of P.L. 92-603, which extended Medicare coverage to all end-stage renal failure patients. Yet even before this act, older patients were being treated successfully in several centers. In Los Angeles 26% were over 50 years old before 1968, and 63% were 50 years or older in 1973.[53]

How well the older dialysis patient performs on a maintenance hemodialysis program can be judged from the report of Ghantous and co-workers, who treated 60 patients over 50 (mean 57.3 years) for 4½ years.[22] Half the patients were treated by home hemodialysis. There were 20 deaths—the majority owing to infection. Three of four patients with diverticulosis died after colonic rupture. Seven of the 20 deaths followed transplantation. Cardiovascular disease was present in 20, including myocardial infarction in 4, cerebral ischemia in 1, diabetes mellitus in 1, and severe atherosclerosis in 3 patients. Forty percent of the patients were fully rehabilitated to gainful employment; one third of the patients were able to do household chores.

As more older patients are dialyzed, the success of the therapy increases. Sellers and Gral describe a drop in annual mortality from 28.3% to 11.1% when comparing their post-1971 experience with that gained before 1968.[53]

In my view, the best regimen is self-dialysis at home. A retrospective analysis of 10 years' experience in Nashville, Tennessee, confirms that age is not a medical contraindication to home dialysis and, furthermore, that the necessary psychological and social adjustments are often accomplished more easily in older patients.[61] It was only after 3 years on dialysis that a significant difference in survival developed between the under- and over-50 age-groups. The length of time on dialysis before death in the 65- to 69-year age-group was similar to that of the 50- to 55-year age-group. Older patients spent less time in the hospital: 0.93 day per patient month (under age 50) and 0.74 day per patient month (over age 50). This was attributed to a greater number of nephrectomized

young patients and to better adherence to a strict medical regimen by the older patients. Greater social stability and maturity underlie the latter difference. Formal education was not correlated with performance of home treatment.

Rehabilitation was also very good in a group of 41 patients 50 to 80 years old undergoing maintenance hemodialysis in Boston.[3] Eighty-four percent of patients returned to previous activities after completion of training (only nine were retired). (The mortality rate per year of dialysis, however, was not given in this report.) In one report of hemodialysis patients over the age of 75, both home and in-center patients did equally well in terms of quality of life and adjustment to their chronic illness.[63] The 1-, 3-, and 5-year survival rates were 28%, 47%, and 22%, respectively.

Chronic Peritoneal Dialysis

Chronic peritoneal dialysis in recent years has expanded from a treatment performed usually only in hospital to an increasingly popular form of outpatient therapy. This change has been made possible by the use of plastic bags instead of glass bottles to contain dialysis fluid, the Tenckhoff and other indwelling permanent peritoneal catheters, and the automatic dialysate cyclers that reduce the number of repetitive changes of dialysis fluid containers. Continuous ambulatory peritoneal dialysis (CAPD) is a treatment in which the patient exchanges dialysis fluid usually four times/daily. Because the dialysis is carried out around the clock, there is less fluctuation of the concentrations of uremic metabolites and electrolytes, and reduced weight gain due to fluid accumulation. For patients who cannot perform exchanges four times/day, the use of an automatic cycling machine allows them to have intermittent dialysis while they sleep at night. The major drawback to chronic peritoneal dialysis is peritonitis; however, newer techniques promise to reduce the incidence of this complication. Many patients are willing to accept the risk of peritonitis because of the greater freedom that chronic peritoneal dialysis allows them. The experience with chronic intermittent peritoneal dialysis in the elderly indicates that their mortality rate is higher than hemodialyzed patients, which reflects the fact that more patients with severe cardiovascular disease are treated with peritoneal dialysis.[37]

Transplantation

Replacement of lost renal function with a kidney transplant is certainly the most dramatic and desirable way of fully reversing the uremic syndrome. In the view of several of the largest transplant centers, advanced age has not been a contraindication to surgery. The National Transplant Registry recorded 800 transplant recipients over age 50 as of 1975. At the Massachusetts General Hospital between 1963 and 1974, 13.2% of transplants (25 of 189) were in the over 50-year age-group, 2.1% (four grafts) were in those over 60 years old.[12]

Only three living, related-donor grafts were transplanted. A high proportion of cadaveric grafts in older patients (75%) was also reported by Bailey and co-workers.[3] The Najarian group in Minnesota, however, was able to obtain living donors in 36 of their 69 patients over age 50.[30] As might be expected, survival of cadaver grafts and recipients in older transplant recipients has been much less than in recipients of the living, related-donor kidneys. Valid comparisons are difficult to make because of the different ways of expressing survival rates. In Minnesota, the cumulative 5-year survival was 81% (related) and 52% (cadaver), but only 16 patients were in the 5-year or longer survival groups.[30] In Boston, a 66.7% survival at 1 year was reported in the overall group of cadaver graft recipients.

In the older transplant recipient, as is true for all ages, infection is the leading cause of death.[4] Particularly important in the older recipient, however, is the incidence of fatal rupture of colonic diverticula. Twenty-five percent of deaths in Bailey's series were due to this complication. The increased incidence of diverticular disease with age, the use of adrenal steroids, and the induction of steroid diabetes mellitus contribute to the importance of infectious complications in aged transplant recipients. Steroid diabetes may become a major risk factor in old age; 67% of Bailey's patients developed elevated fasting blood glucose levels, and 6 of the 16 patients died.

A number of factors must be considered in choosing a therapy for the elderly patient with end-stage renal disease; these include medical, dialysis-related, psychological, social, and ethical concerns.[46] Of the medical problems faced by these patients, cardiovascular disease is most important, since it may make hemodialysis too dangerous. Peritoneal dialysis will be the treatment of choice for such patients. Dialysis therapy at home is possible in all age-groups, but the unwillingness of the patient and the lack of suitable assistance in the home limits acceptability of this choice. Depression and dementia also affect the choice of therapy, making an in-center facility with professional staff almost obligatory. If severe dementia is present before chronic dialysis is required, the advisability of starting the treatment should be discussed with the family. Once chronic dialysis is begun, physicians and family members are reluctant to discontinue it.

In conclusion, most elderly patients with CRF will be treated with hemodialysis or peritoneal dialysis, both of which are effective in maintaining a productive life. Despite current attention to rising health care costs, it is imperative that the largest segment of the population requiring dialysis, those over 60 years old, not be denied the treatment to which they are entitled.

REFERENCES

1. Adler S, Lindeman RO, Yiengst MJ, Beard E, Shock NW: Effect of acute acid loading on urinary acid excretion by the aging kidney. J Lab Clin Med 72:278, 1968
2. Agarwal BM, Cabebe FG: Renal acidification in elderly subjects. Nephron 26:291, 1980
3. Bailey GL et al: Hemodialysis and renal transplantation in patients of the 50-80 age group. J Am Geriatr Soc 20:421, 1972
4. Barnes BA: The report of the human transplant registry. Transplant Proc 9:9, 1977
5. Bennett WM, Singer L, Golper T, Feig P, Coggins CJ: Guidelines for drug therapy in renal failure. Ann Intern Med 86:754, 1977
6. Boner G, Shelp WD, Neton M, Rieselbach RE: Factors influencing the increase in glomerular filtration rate in the remaining kidney of transplant donors. Am J Med 55:169, 1973
7. Bricker NS: Acute renal failure. In Beeson P, McDermott W (eds): Textbook of Medicine. Philadelphia, WB Saunders, 1975
8. Brenner BM, Meyer TW, Hostetter, TH: Dietary protein intake and progressive nature of kidney disease: The role of hemodynamically mediated glomerular injury in the pathogenesis of progressive glomerular sclerosis in aging, renal ablation and intrinsic renal disease. N Engl J Med 307:632, 1982
9. Churg J, Ehrenreich T: Membranous nephropathy. In Kincaid-Smith P, Mathew TH, Becker EL (eds): Glomerulonephritis, Morphology, Natural History and Treatment, Part I. New York, John Wiley & Sons, 1973
10. Darmady EM, Offer J, Woodhouse MA: The parameters of the aging kidney. J Pathol 109:195, 1973
11. Davies DF, Shock NW: Age changes in the glomerular filtration rate, effective renal plasma, and tubular excretory capacity in adult males. J Clin Invest 29:496, 1950
12. Delmonico FL, Cosimi AB, Russell PS: Renal transplantation in the older age group. Arch Surg 110:1107, 1975
13. Dontas AS, Marketos S, Papanayiotou P: Mecha-

nisms of renal tubular defects in old age. Postgrad Med J 48:295, 1972

14. Dontas AS, Papanayiotou P, Marketos SG, Papanicolaou NT: The effect of bacteriuria on renal functional patterns in old age. Clin Sci 34:73, 1968

15. Elkins M, Goldman SM, Meng CH: Ureteral obstruction in patients with uterine prolapse. Radiology 110:289, 1974

16. Epstein M, Hollenberg NK: Age as a determinant of renal sodium conservation in normal man. J Lab Clin Med 87:411, 1976

17. Erwin DT, Donadio JV, Holley KE: The clinical course of idiopathic membranous nephropathy. Mayo Clin Proc 48:697, 1973

18. Feinstein EI, Blumenkrantz MJ, Healy M, Koffler A, Silberman H, Massry SG, Kopple JD: Clinical and metabolic responses to parenteral nutrition in acute renal failure—a controlled double-blind study. Medicine 60:124, 1981

19. Finn WF: Recovery from acute renal failure. In Brenner BM, Lazarus JM (eds): Acute Renal Failure. Philadelphia, WB Saunders, 1983

20. Flood C et al: The metabolism and secretion of aldosterone in elderly subjects. J Clin Invest 46:960, 1967

21. Friedman SA, Raizner AE, Rosen H, Solomon NA, Sy W: Functional defects in the aging kidney. Ann Intern Med 76:41, 1972

22. Ghantous, WN, Bailey GL, Zschaeck D, Hampers CL, Merrill JP: Long-term hemodialysis in the elderly. Trans Am Soc Artif Intern Organ 17:125, 1971

23. Glassock RJ, Friedler RM, Massry SG: Kidney and electrolyte disturbances in neoplastic diseases. Contrib Nephrol 7:2, 1977

24. Heptinstall RH: Pathology of the Kidney, 2nd ed. Boston, Little, Brown & Co, 1974

25. Hollenberg NK et al: Senescence and the renal vasculature in normal men. Circ Res 34:309, 1974

26. Kassirer J: Atheroembolic renal disease. N Engl J Med 280:812, 1969

27. Kelman WA, Kolff WJ: Use of artificial kidney in the very young, the very old, and the very sick. JAMA 171:530, 1959

28. Kennedy AC et al: Factors affecting the prognosis in acute renal failure. Q J Med 42:73, 1973

29. Kjellstrand CM: Dialysis in Diabetics, In Friedman EA, (ed): Strategy in Renal Failure. New York, John Wiley & Sons, 1978

30. Kjellstrand CM el al: Kidney transplants in patients over 50. Geriatrics 31:65, 1976

31. Kolff WJ: First clinical experience with the artificial kidney. Ann Intern Med 62:608, 1963

32. Kopple JD: Nutritional management. In Massry, SG, Glassock RJ (eds): Textbook of Nephrology. Baltimore, Williams & Wilkins, 1983

33. Lindeman RD: Age changes in renal function. In Goldman R, Rockstein M (eds): The Physiology and Pathology of Human Aging. New York, Academic Press, 1975

34. Ljungqvist A, Lagergren C: Normal intra-renal arterial pattern in adult and aging human kidney. J Anat 26:285, 1962

35. Llach F, Arieff AI, Massry SG: Renal vein thrombosis and nephrotic syndrome: A prospective study of 36 adult patients. Ann Intern Med 83:8, 1975

36. McDonald, RK, Solomon KH, and Shock NW: Aging as a factor in the renal hemodynamic changes induced by a standardized pyrogen. J Clin Invest 30:457, 1951

37. Marai A, Rathaus M, Gibor Y, Bernheim J: Chronic dialysis in the elderly: Intermittent peritoneal dialysis or hemodialysis. Perit Dialy Bull 3:183, 1983

38. Marketos S, Papanayiotou P, Dontas AS: Bacteriuria and non-obstructive renovascular disease in old age. Gerontol 24:33, 1969

39. Miller JH, McDonald RK, Shock NW: Age changes in the maximal rate of renal tubular reabsorption of glucose. J Gerontol 7:196, 1952

40. Miller JH, Shock HW: Age differences in the renal tubular response to antidiuretic hormone. J Gerontol 8:446, 1953

41. Moore RA: Total number of glomeruli in the normal human kidney. Anat Rec 50:709, 1931

42. Moorthy AV, Zimmerman SW: Renal disease in the elderly clinicopathologic analysis of renal disease in 115 elderly patients. Clin Nephrol 14:223, 1980

43. Oken DE: Mannitol and the prevention of vasomotor nephropathy. Proceedings of the 6th International Congress of Nephrology, Florence. Basel, S Karger, 1976

44. Olbrich O, Ferguson MH, Robson JS, Stewart CP: Renal function in aged subjects. Edinburgh Med J 57:117, 1950

45. Olbrich O, Woodford-Williams E, Irvine RE, Webster D: Renal function in prostatism. Lancet 1:1322, 1957

46. Oreopoulous DG: Geriatric nephrology. Perit Dialy Bull 4:197, 1984

47. Pelz KS, Scottfired SP, Paz E: Kidney function studies in old men and women. Geriatrics 20:145, 1965

48. Reynes M, Coulet T, Diebold J Jr: Microvascularization of normal and aging kidney. Pathol Biol 16:1081, 1968

49. Row PG et al: Membranous nephropathy: Long-term follow-up and association with neoplasia. Q J Med 44:207, 1975

50. Rowe JW, Andres R, Tobin JD, Norris AH, Shock NW: The effect of age on creatinine clearance in man: A cross sectional and longitudinal study. J Gerontol 31:155, 1976

51. Rowe JW, Shock NW, DeFronzo RA: The influence of age on the renal response to water deprivation in man. Nephron 17:270, 1976

52. Samiy AH, Field RA, Merrill JP: Acute glomerulonephritis in elderly patients. Ann Intern Med 54:603, 1961

53. Sellers AL, Gral R: Morbidity and mortality in patients undergoing maintenance hemodialysis. In Massry SG, Sellers AL (eds): Clinical Aspects of Uremia and Dialysis. Springfield, IL, Charles C Thomas, 1975

54. Shaldon S: Hemodialysis in chronic renal failure. Postgrad Med J 42:669, 1966

55. Shapiro FL, Leonard A, Comty CM: Mortality, morbidity and rehabilitation results in regularly dialyzed patients with diabetes mellitus. Kidney Int 6:5, 1974

56. Shannon RP, Minaker KL, Rowe JW: Aging and water balance in humans. Semin Nephrol 4:346, 1984

57. Sporn IN, Lancestremere RG, Papper S: Differential diagnosis of oliguria in aged patients. N Engl J Med 267:130, 1962

58. Takazadura E et al: Intrarenal vascular changes with age and disease. Kidney Int 2:224, 1972

59. Tauchi H, Tsuboi K, Okutomi J: Age changes in the human kidney of the different races. Gerontologia 17:87, 1971

60. Verzar F: Compensatory hypertrophy in old age. In Nowinski WW, Goss RJ: Compensatory Renal Hypertrophy. New York, Academic Press, 1969

61. Walker PJ et al: Long-term hemodialysis for patients over fifty: A symposium. Geriatrics 31:55, 1976

62. Wesson LG: Physiology of the Human Kidney. New York, Grune & Stratton, 1969

63. Westlie L, Umen A, Nestrud S, Kjellstrand CM: Mortality, morbidity and life satisfaction in the very old dialysis patient. Trans Am Soc Artif Intern Organs 30:21, 1984

14 Pulmonary Disease in the Elderly

William M. Anderson, Gene G. Ryerson, and James W. Wynne

THE AGING LUNG

Anatomical changes in the lungs and chest wall with advancing age have long been recognized.[124,173,177] On opening the chest at autopsy, the lungs of the elderly individual collapse normally but more slowly than those of the younger individual. The alveolar ducts and sacs enlarge progressively with age, and the cut surface appears coarser. Alveoli join to form cystic areas with dilation and disruption of adjacent walls and associated capillaries, without fibrosis.[177] As a consequence, there are fewer alveoli and less total alveolar surface area for gas exchange.[41] In addition, the collagen content decreases without associated change in the amount of elastic tissue.[7]

The more proximal bronchi remain unchanged with age except for some calcification of cartilage, but more distal bronchioles (*e.g.,* less than 2 mm) decrease in diameter. A loss of elastic recoil is the postulated mechanism of this reduced airway diameter.[80,192] Studies have demonstrated increased resistance to airflow in bronchioles with tendency for early airway closure in progressively more distal bronchioles with advancing age (depicted in Figure 14-1 by the rise in airway closing capacity).[80,108] To what extent these changes are due to aging or reflect the effects of smoking, air pollution, or infection is still unclear.

Other age-related changes affecting lung function involve the chest wall and respiratory muscles. Progressive calcification of chondral cartilages and kyphoscoliosis may lead to a steady decline in chest wall compliance and limit thoracic expansion.[144] Dorsal kyphosis, prominence of the sternum, and an increase in the ratio of anteroposterior to lateral chest diameters have been termed the *barrel chest deformity.* Its similarity to the findings in patients with the emphysematous form of chronic obstructive pulmonary disease (COPD) has suggested an association of this disease with aging. Physiologic testing, however, has shown the barrel chest abnormality to be nonspecific and by itself is not associated with airway obstruction.[173] Further limitation of chest excursion can occur with decreased respiratory muscle strength, as evidenced by a decrease in maximal inspiratory and expiratory pressures in the older population.[25]

Postmortem morphologic studies of lung elastic recoil and chest wall compliance help to elucidate the abnormalities in flow measurement (see Fig. 14-1).[156] Maximum voluntary ventilation (MVV), forced vital capacity (FVC), forced expiratory volume in 1 second (FEV_1), and the ratio of the forced expiratory volume in 1 second to the forced vital capacity (FEV_1/FVC) are all reduced.[145,149,192] The FEV_1 decreases 30 ml/year with increasing age, while the FVC decreases 20 ml to 30 ml/year.[149] Total lung capacity (TLC) was originally thought to decrease with age; however, when adjustments for height and weight are made, this parameter is not altered by the aging process.[145,149,192] Despite the loss of lung elastic recoil, TLC remains unchanged due to the opposite effect of loss of chest wall compliance and weakened respiratory muscles. Variable increase in alveolar diameter and the tendency for distal airways to collapse leads to an increase in residual volume (*i.e.,* the amount of air remaining in the lungs after a maximal expiration) and functional residual capacity (*i.e.,* the amount of air remaining in the lung at the end of normal expiration).[80,108,120,145]

Alteration in alveolar-capillary gas exchange is related to the decline in alveolar surface area. This can be measured by the decrease in the carbon monoxide diffusing capacity ($D_{L}CO$).[41,50,145] Al-

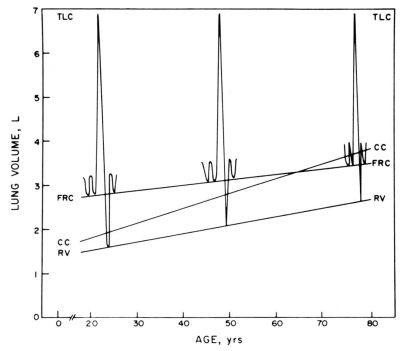

FIG. 14-1. Changes in static lung volumes and closing capacity in the upright position with age. (*TLC,* total lung capacity; *FRC,* functional residual capacity; *CC,* closing capacity; and *RV,* residual volume) (Peterson DD, Fishman AP: The lungs in later life. In Fishman AP (ed): Update: Pulmonary diseases and Disorders, pp 123–126. New York, McGraw-Hill, 1982)

though a 0.20- to 0.32-ml/min/mm Hg decrease occurs per year of adult life, this does not appear to be clinically relevant in the healthy individual. However, the changes noted in ventilation and perfusion are more significant. With the diffuse changes in alveoli and a tendency toward collapse of airways during exhalation, a mismatch of lung perfusion to ventilation is created. Poorly ventilated alveoli may receive a significant amount of blood supply. For this reason, arterial oxygen tension progressively decreases with age. In contrast, carbon dioxide tension remains unchanged.[50,120] A clinically useful formula for the expected Pao_2 from healthy nonsmoking supine subjects ranging in age from 14 to 84 has been derived.[203]

$$Pao_2 = 109 - 0.43 \text{ (age)} \pm 4$$

Similar calculations have been derived for the seated subject at any age.[139]

EXERCISE

With advancing age, the rate of maximum oxygen consumption (Vo_{2max}) progressively declines. Although the exact rate of decline is variable, a decrease of 0.04 ml/min/kg after age 40 is a good estimate.[57,97] Although this decline may be decreased by physical conditioning, a fixed rate of

decline in maximum oxygen consumption occurs despite training. In Figure 14-2 the rate of decline in exercise capacity with age for subjects with differing levels of daily activity is shown. A well-

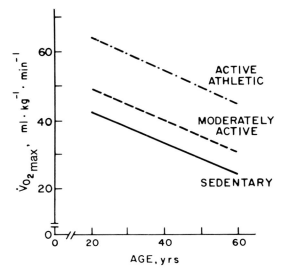

FIG. 14-2. Decrease in maximum oxygen consumption with age for subjects with differing levels of daily activity. (Hodgson JL, Buskirk ER: Physical fitness and age, with emphasis on cardiovascular function in the elderly. J Am Geriatr Soc 25:385, 1977)

trained sexagenerian can obtain a higher maximum oxygen consumption than a subject 10 years younger or nearly equivalent to a sedentary subject 40 years of age.[57,185] Importantly, once exercise conditioning is stopped, the maximum level of oxygen consumption returns to sedentary levels within a short period of time.

Although many factors are involved, the decline in maximum oxygen consumption is primarily related to a decrease in the maximum cardiac output. Although the resting heart rate shows little change with advancing age, a decline occurs in the maximal heart rate achieved during exertion. This reduction is often estimated by the formula:

$$220 - \text{age in years} = \text{maximum heart rate}$$

Furthermore, stroke volume, both at rest and during heavy exercise, is decreased.[168] Despite changes in cardiac performance, older individuals obtain benefits from physical conditioning similar to younger patients. With endurance training, sedentary elders can increase work capacity or the maximum rate of oxygen consumption.[59,97,197] Exercise protocols attempt to have the subject perform at 60% to 80% of a predicted heart rate for three to four half-hour sessions per week.[168,226]

ALTERED CONTROL OF VENTILATION AND SLEEP-DISORDERED BREATHING

The integrative factors involved in controlling ventilation are extensive and well reviewed elsewhere.[22] Normal elderly subjects 65 to 80 years of age subjected to progressive hypoxemia with an oxygen saturation of 70% to 75% may increase ventilation to only 50% of that of healthy subjects 19 to 30 years of age. Similar results have been shown for hypercapnia. These blunted responses appear independent of chemoreceptor function, respiratory muscle strength, or other mechanical properties. The decreased ventilatory response in the elderly may be due to altered central processing or altered perception of the chemical stimulus.[169] Damped response is believed to be a factor contributing to Cheyne-Stokes breathing (a cyclical breathing pattern of slowly increasing then decreasing tidal volumes interspersed with periods of apnea), which is noted with increased prevalence in the elderly population. Heart failure and cerebrovascular disease further contribute to this breathing pattern.[48]

Another group of patients with altered responses to hypercapnia, not restricted to the elderly population, are those with the pickwickian syndrome or obesity hypoventilation.[38,88] Research into their sleep disorders led to the discovery of upper airway obstructive apneas associated with oxygen desaturation. Despite nocturnal hypoxia, upper airway obstruction and obesity prevent normal respiratory mechanical compensation.[127]

Sleep apnea has been shown to exist in apparently normal males and postmenopausal females with incidence increasing with age, COPD, as well as obesity.[26,28,88] Three general types of apneas have been described. Central apnea is defined as a cessation of airflow at the nose and mouth of greater than 10 seconds' duration accompanied by cessation of chest and abdominal respiratory movements. Obstructive apnea occurs when there is no airflow in spite of persistent respiratory efforts. Mixed apnea involves cessation of airflow and an absence of respiratory effort early during an episode followed by resumption of unsuccessful respiration later in the episode. The three forms of sleep apnea become clinically significant when associated with a drop in arterial saturation of 4%. Severity of symptoms vary with the frequency and severity of the apneic episodes.[88]

CLINICAL FEATURES OF THE SLEEP APNEA SYNDROME

Hypersomnolence
Noisy snoring
Abnormal motor activity during sleep
Morning headaches and disorientation
Intellectual and personality changes
Impotence
Hypnagogic hallucinations
Enuresis
Pulmonary hypertension
Cor pulmonale, heart failure
Polycythemia
Cardiac arrhythmias
Nocturnal sudden death

Sleep-disordered breathing occurred in 37% of patients 61 to 81 years of age with the presenting symptom of excessive somnolence.[186] Narcolepsy should be differentiated from sleep apnea in the older patient by the characteristic findings of sleep attacks lasting less than 15 minutes, cataplexy, sleep paralysis, and hypnagogic hallucinations without disordered breathing.[109]

Disorders associated with sleep apnea are noted in Table 14-1. Treatment of patients with mild sleep apnea (*i.e.*, without severe hypoxemia or

TABLE 14-1 Disorders Associated with Sleep Apnea

Type of Apnea	Disorder
Central apnea	Poliomyelitis, encephalitis
	Brain stem infarction
	Brain stem neoplasm
	Cervical cordotomy
	Spinal surgery
	Primary (idiopathic) hypoventilation syndrome
Obstructive apnea	Obesity
	Hypertrophy of tonsils and adenoids
	Lymphoma of tonsils and adenoids
	Hemangioma of oropharynx
	Acromegaly
	Myxedema
	Micrognathia
	Temporomandibular joint disease
	Goiter
	Myotonic dystrophy
	Shy-Drager syndrome
	Testosterone administration

cardiac abnormality) may correct the etiology. Weight loss by diet alone has been poorly studied but is the mainstay of therapy in obese patients. Large amounts of weight loss improve oxygen desaturation as well as symptoms of somnolence.[90,209] Medications such as protriptyline and medroxyprogesterone appear to be effective in certain cases. For patients with obstructive sleep apnea when other measures have failed, the surgical removal of excess oropharyngeal tissue (uvulo-palatopharyngeoplasty [UPPP])as well as removal of hypertrophied tonsils and adenoids may be effective. Another therapy circumvents the upper airway obstruction by the application of airway pressure. This can be applied to the nose, as in nasal continuous positive airway pressure (CPAP) or by mask with expiratory positive airway pressure (EPAP).[27]

When apneic episodes are accompanied by severe oxygen desaturation and cardiac failure with arrhythmias, selected patients may benefit from nocturnal oxygen.[114] On a long-term basis, 100% of patients have improvement or complete relief of clinical symptoms after tracheostomy. Other aspects of apneas and sleep disorders in the elderly are discussed in Chapter 42.

DISEASES CAUSING AIRWAY OBSTRUCTION

The diverse group of illnesses that cause airway obstruction are second only to heart disease as a cause of morbidity and mortality in the elderly. Since the obstruction involves the airways, alveoli, or both, a confusing array of terms have evolved (*i.e.*, chronic obstructive lung disease [COLD], chronic airway obstruction [CAO], or chronic obstructive pulmonary disease [COPD]). COPD, one of the most common terms, is used here to describe a spectrum of diseases. At one end is cystic fibrosis, which specifically involves airways along with bronchiolitis, asthma, and bronchiectasis. Diseases involving predominantly alveoli make up the other end of the spectrum (*i.e.*, chronic bronchitis and emphysema). The term *COPD* is most often applied to patients who have either chronic bronchitis, emphysema, or a combination of the two (with or without asthma). Since cystic fibrosis and bronchiolitis are predominantly diseases of childhood, they will not be considered further.

Pulmonary function tests have become increasingly indispensable in the diagnosis of airway obstruction. Without a reduction in the spirometry values of FEV_1 and the ratio of FEV_1/FVC, it is difficult to attribute an elderly patient's symptoms (*i.e.*, dyspnea) to airways obstruction. Improvement in the spirometry values with inhalation of a bronchodilator is used to document bronchospasm as a component of chronic bronchitis and asthma. This is rarely a component of emphysema. Determination of lung volumes and diffusing capacity for carbon monoxide can further help classification. Lung volumes are increased in COPD, with residual volume and functional residual capacity showing the largest and earliest changes. Patients in whom emphysema predominates have the highest lung volumes of COPD patients. An abnormal diffusing capacity for carbon monoxide also indicates emphysema with loss of effective surface area for gas transfer. This occurs along with the altered spirometry because of loss of lung elastic recoil, peripheral airway narrowing, and increased collapsibility of airways.[165] The degree of emphysema is most correlated with diffusing capacity in COPD patients, reflecting the variable presence of chronic bronchitis and mucus obstructing the airways.[99,143,165]

Cigarette smoking is the major determinant in the development of COPD.[11,103] Heredity, air pollution, occupation, and childhood respiratory infection may increase the damage done by cigarette smoking but seldom cause the disease by themselves.[103]

The natural history of COPD is characterized by a long silent period followed by the insidious onset of symptoms. It is, therefore, a disease of middle and old age, with peak incidence in the fifth decade. Evidence strongly suggests that COPD has its beginnings in the small airways and alveoli and that the pathologic precursors of full-blown disease are present very early.[3,165,178] It is only when a large number of small airways have become diseased or when large airways are involved that symptoms occur. Standard tests of airway resistance are not sensitive enough to detect even large changes in the small airways, making it difficult to diagnose the disease short of its advanced stages. With the expected uniform decline in FEV_1 of 60 ml/year, this value would be less than 80% of predicted for approximately 10 years before it reached a level likely to be associated with clinical symptoms (assumed to be at an FEV_1 of 2.0 liters).[3]

Emphysema

The patient with emphysema has the clinical characteristics of airway obstruction, but the true description is made at autopsy as "a condition of the lung characterized by increase beyond the normal in the size of air spaces distal to the terminal bronchioles, with destructive changes in their walls."[3] In clinical practice, emphysema is diagnosed by compatible clinical and physiologic findings. This term has also been used to describe the change in the lung associated with aging (*i.e.*, senile emphysema), which as discussed earlier, is misleading. The cause of emphysema is obscure, but the current theory describes an increase of locally destructive enzymes (proteases) released from leukocytes or alveolar macrophages in response to inhaled toxins. In addition, there is an imbalance in the amounts of locally protective antiproteases.[103,215]

Clinically, the patient with emphysema is 50 to 70 years old and presents with dyspnea, with or without cough that is minimally productive. The chest is held in an inspiratory position, giving the appearance of a barrel chest. It is hyperresonant to percussion with faint breath sounds and a prolonged expiration. The impulse of the heart is difficult to palpate and may be shifted to the epigastrium. Cyanosis and edema are not usually found since patients remain well oxygenated without heart failure until late in the course of illness. These clinical features are thus characteristic of the "pink puffer."[74]

The chest roentgenogram in emphysema may show hyperinflation with low flat diaphragms and large retrosternal air space, a vertical narrow heart, large pulmonary vessels, tapering in the periphery, and bullae; the latter may appear with such subtle findings as a thick white line or a lucent area with no margin. These findings are not diagnostic or specific for emphysema and cannot be used to associate emphysema with age.[66] In one study of patients with severe emphysema, only 41% were diagnosed by roentgenography as having this disease.[216]

Chronic Bronchitis

Chronic bronchitis is defined clinically by the presence of a productive cough on most days at least 3 months of the year for more than 2 consecutive years. The cough results from excessive production of tracheobronchial mucus, usually because of cigarette smoking. Hyperplasia and hypertrophy of the mucous glands in the submucosa of the large airways are often present. In the small airways, chronic inflammation and edema, plus increased smooth muscle and goblet cell hyperplasia, are noted. These pathologic changes are not specific for chronic bronchitis and may or may not cause the airway obstruction occurring in many patients with chronic bronchitis.[143,180]

The typical patient with chronic bronchitis is middle aged at the time of initial presentation. He may have a moderate level of dyspnea, particularly noted on exertion, with a history of recurring or chronic respiratory tract infections. Frequently overweight and with a cyanotic appearance from chronic hypoxemia, these patients are described as "blue and bloated."[74] Auscultation of the chest reveals moderately decreased breath sounds with variable rales, rhonchi, and wheezing diffusely.[103,165] Evidence of right-sided heart failure and cor pulmonale may be present with distended neck veins, swollen tender liver, and peripheral edema.[74]

In contrast to the patient with emphysema, the chest roentgenogram tends to have normal diaphragmatic position, with cardiomegaly and occasional bronchovascular markings. Electrocardiographic abnormalities include right-axis deviation, right bundle branch block, as well as various atrial arrhythmias. Functional hallmarks in chronic bronchitis are related to airway obstruction with a decrease in FEV_1/FVC and FEV_1 as previously described. Lung volumes may be normal or only slightly increased with a normal diffusing capacity for carbon monoxide. Arterial blood gases are frequently abnormal with hypercapnia and hypoxemia, associated with erythrocytosis and hematocrits greater than 55%. The increased carbon dioxide level relates to altered control of breathing and secondary alveolar hypoventilation. Sleep studies of blue bloaters as compared with pink puffers have shown more serious oxygen desaturation associated with sleep-disordered breathing. This is one explanation for the different clinical characteristics of these two groups.[43]

Asthma

Asthma is a functional, not an anatomical, disorder characterized by "hyperirritable" airways (*i.e.*, they respond abnormally to certain stimuli by constriction of the airway smooth muscle, resulting in bronchial narrowing). Persistence of this stimulation leads to bronchial mucosal edema and hypersecretion of mucus, with resultant obstruction to airflow.[32,140]

Viral or *Mycoplasma* infections are associated with heightened airway reactivity and may actually denude the respiratory epithelium. Nerve receptors and mast cell membranes are thus made accessible to allergens and inhaled irritants.[208] Cellular debris as well as the increased secretions of mucus glands are thought to be associated with increased cross-linking of glycoproteins and binding of water. Subsequent decreased viscosity of secretions leads to fibrin formation and mucus plugging. Cast formation then results in further airway obstruction.[140]

For years, asthma has been classified as extrinsic or allergic and intrinsic or nonallergic. Among the elderly, asthma is usually intrinsic (nonallergic). These patients often present with continuous rather than episodic wheezing as in the younger age-group. Care must be taken to sort out other diseases known to present with the symptom

---

DISEASES ACCOMPANIED BY WHEEZING

Congestive heart failure (so-called cardiac asthma)
Foreign body obstruction
Neoplasm
Acute and chronic bronchitis
Inhalation of irritants (dusts, fumes, chemicals, smoke)
Hypersensitivity reaction (extrinsic allergic alveolitis)
Drug-induced causes (*e.g.*, cholinergic intoxication, β-adrenergic blockade)
Carcinoid syndrome
Exercise-induced wheezing
Aspirin or nonsteroidal anti-inflammatory drug sensitivity
Recurrent aspiration
Systemic diseases (lupus erythematous, polyarteritis nodosa, parasitic infection)

---

of wheezing. Symptoms may not always resemble asthma as when a patient presents with a chronic cough or dyspnea on exertion.[53,128] Recent reports of upper airway obstruction with wheezing must be considered.[62] Infection, especially viral or *Mycoplasma*, is likely to precipitate acute attacks. Vigorous therapy for sinusitis, which frequently accompanies the disease, may improve wheezing. Patients may have a family history of allergy, but their own allergic history is usually not remarkable.

The degree of tachycardia, tachypnea, and diaphoresis, as well as assumption of the upright posture[34] during attacks help assessment of the patient during initial therapy. A pulse rate greater than 120 beats/min, respiratory rate greater than 30/min, pulsus paradoxus greater than 18 mm Hg, peak expiratory flow rate of less than 120 liters/min, moderate to severe dyspnea, accessory muscle use, and wheezing are helpful in determining the need for extended hospital therapy.[73] A total index of these features is not as helpful as the recognition that the illness is severe.[45] The absence of wheezing and breath sounds, an altered state of consciousness, reduction of Pao_2 to less than 60 mm Hg, and pulsus paradoxus are ominous signs of impending respiratory failure.[130,179]

Many elderly patients with chronic asthma show characteristics of both intrinsic and extrinsic disease and are termed *mixed*. Also some subgroups of asthma do not fit into either category. In one such group, asthma forms a triad with nasal polyposis and an abnormal reaction to aspirin and other nonsteroidal anti-inflammatory drugs,[191,201] as well as the tartrazine yellow food dye.[193] The mechanism of induced wheezing does not fit the categories of either intrinsic or extrinsic asthma.[129] Other factors affecting the airway mucosa such as repeated damage by aspiration of gastric contents may be of particular consequence in the older age-groups. A higher incidence of reflux, which may precipitate wheezing, has been demonstrated in patients with asthma, especially the intrinsic type.[84,136]

Diagnosis can be further confirmed by various tests. A consistent improvement in FEV_1 of 15% to 20% on spirometric testing in response to an inhaled bronchodilator is considered a reliable sign.[32,174] Bronchoprovocation tests are used in patients with usually normal spirometry who have symptoms consistent with asthma and in whom the diagnosis is obscure. Inhalation of histamine or methacholine may cause marked airway reactivity, thus confirming the clinical diagnosis.[235]

Serum IgE levels are variable in elderly patients with intrinsic asthma, and blood eosinophil counts may be normal or markedly elevated. These tests are helpful in the diagnosis of bronchopulmonary aspergillosis. Thick, usually brownish sputum production in an asthmatic patient with recurrent infiltrates on chest roentgenography and central bronchiectasis suggests this diagnosis. Confirmation can be made with the finding of blood eosinophilia, increased serum IgE level, presence of serum precipitating antibodies, and a positive immediate skin test to *Aspergillus* antigen.[187] Other skin tests are seldom of benefit in elderly patients with asthma except those with a characteristic allergic history.[123]

Bronchiectasis

Bronchiectasis is an irreversible usually focal dilation of bronchi. The abnormal dilation occurs in the proximal segmental bronchi, associated with chronic inflammation and obliteration of bronchi and bronchioles distally. Destruction of the bronchial wall most commonly results from infection with pneumonia, childhood illness (*i.e.,* pertussis, measles, influenza) as well as tuberculosis.[69,112] The advent of antibiotics has decreased the occurrence of this illness and made the clinical course more indolent than previously reported.[47] In the elderly, bronchiectasis may follow pneumonia due to a variety of organisms, aspiration, and obstruction from a foreign body or neoplasm. Abnormalities in bronchial ciliary function have been shown to be a factor, as in patients with congenital airway abnormalities, such as immobile cilia syndrome, who develop bronchiectasis.[52]

Classically in bronchiectasis, there is persistent cough and production of purulent sputum and occasional hemoptysis. A history of febrile episodes as well as episodic wheezing and shortness of breath is common. Physical examination is frequently normal; however, rales over the involved areas with wheezing may be heard.[158] Digital clubbing and cyanosis with signs of right-sided heart failure appear in severe cases. Radiographic findings include loss of lung volume in the involved area, leading to shifts in the lung fissures, hemidiaphragm, or trachea, with subsequent crowding of bronchovascular markings. Peribronchial "cuffing" with cystic air spaces distally is a common feature. Pulmonary function studies may be normal or show a variable degree of obstruction with or without reversibility on bronchodilator inhalation. Lung volumes may be lower than expected from the degree of obstruction due to fibrosis and scarring.[47,158]

Bronchoscopy is not useful for diagnosis of bronchiectasis but is indicated to rule out a local obstructive lesion when there is hemoptysis, slowly resolving pneumonia, or atelectasis or to evaluate the extent of inflammation of the bronchial tree prior to surgery. In the past, bronchograms were frequently done to document the disease; however, their findings may not be specific and their use should be limited to patients under evaluation for curative lung resection.[8,222]

THERAPY OF DISEASES OBSTRUCTING THE AIRWAYS

Principles of Management

Therapy is aimed at control of symptoms and improved survival. Pulmonary rehabilitation includes a multidisciplinary program of diagnosis, therapy, emotional support, and education to return the patient to as near normal a life-style as possible. With the possible exception of asthma, obstructive lung disease in the elderly can seldom be cured, but morbidity and mortality can be improved with current therapy.[31,61,102,111,175,218] Each aspect of therapy should be appraised critically, in terms of effectiveness, cost, and availability. The importance of discontinuing all tobacco products cannot be overemphasized.

Bronchial Hygiene

Measures promoting good bronchial hygiene are important in lung disease, especially in chronic bronchitis and bronchiectasis, in which airway secretions can lead to further obstruction. Avoidance of irritants, adequate bronchial hydration, postural drainage, exercise, antibiotics, and bronchodilators, are the mainstays of therapy.[75,96,102,171] Evaluation and treatment for gastroesophageal reflux and chronic sinusitis must also be considered. Obstructive lung disease is often aggravated by nonspecific bronchial irritants such as dust, cigarette smoke, and polluted air.[103] Changes in humidity and temperature can worsen airway obstruction, especially in patients with asthma. Patients with lung disease should be advised to stay indoors during periods of high environmental pollution and to avoid dusty areas and smoky rooms. In hot, humid weather, air conditioning may prove invaluable. Heating units that provide hot, dry air may require devices for humidification. Filters in heating and air conditioning units must be changed regularly. During hot humid months or during prolonged periods without use, they can be a source of fungal antigen.

Hydration, Mucolytic Agents, and Expectorants

Hydration of bronchial mucus is believed to lessen its viscosity and may aid in expectoration. Even though there is little scientific evidence to show hydration benefits the patient with COPD, encouraging hydration by mouth seems safe and reasonable. The use of nebulizers, which add water to the bronchial tree in the form of small particles, is of little value. There may even be a potential for contamination by bacteria.

Mucolytic agents and expectorants have been recommended in the past for liquefying and removing mucous secretions, with little evidence to support their use. Acetylcysteine (Mucomyst) has been shown to be irritating to the bronchial mucosa, can induce bronchospasm, and has a foul smell. Glyceryl guaiacolate (guaifenesin) and saturated solutions of potassium iodide (SSKI) are the most widely used expectorants. The clinical efficacy of glyceryl guaiacolate when compared with placebo has been questioned. Iodine preparations have associated hypersensitivity reactions and the potential for alteration in thyroid function is a particular concern in the geriatric patient. Bronchodilator drugs may be more efficacious since they can produce some reversal of airway obstruction and possibly improve mucus transport.

Chest Percussion and Postural Drainage

The techniques of chest percussion and postural drainage are controversial in the therapy of COPD.[15,55,72,75,150,159] In the patient with emphysema with little cough and sputum production, they may be of little benefit.[102] With persistent cough productive of large amounts of sputum, all measures aimed at improving bronchial hygiene may be useful in conjunction with postural drainage. This can be done on rising and again before retiring, since secretions tend to pool in airways at night. More frequent treatments during acute exacerbations are necessary, and performance after a shower may be particularly convenient. A family member should be taught to percuss with the cupped hand sequentially over the ribs, creating a "popping" hollow sound as the hands strike the chest wall. Postural drainage using complicated maneuvers to drain specific lung segments is usually not necessary. The simple knee-in-chest position, or any position that places the tracheobronchial tree in a downward tilt, is sufficient. Patients who are responsive to bronchodilators should use them prior to postural drainage.[55] Repeated productive coughing should be encouraged and may be the most effective component of this therapy.[3]

Exercise and Breathing Techniques

Tests in patients with symptomatic COPD suggest that nonventilatory muscle exercise such as arm and leg cycling does not improve ventilatory function or endurance.[19,102,164] Patients in these programs often feel better subjectively with apparent improvement in various psychological parameters and improved sleep patterns. In patients with severe COPD on a program using inspiratory resistive loading, there is a definite improvement in maximum work capacity as well as respiratory muscle endurance.[162,164,202] A program of increasing resistance could be individualized for patients to perform once daily for 30 minutes, or for two 15-minute periods.[163,164] The resistance devices are easy to use and are currently available.[20] Patients should be evaluated for cardiac illness prior to initiating exercise.

Pursed lip breathing is frequently initiated by patients with COPD on their own. The secondary slowing of expiration has been believed to be of some benefit by maintaining alveolar distention and preventing early airway collapse. This has been shown to improve ventilation and arterial blood gases.[148] When coupled with conscious slowing of respiration, this breathing may also help combat panic associated with severe dyspnea.

Bronchodilators

Bronchodilating drugs are the basic therapy in diseases obstructing the airways. They decrease bronchial muscle tone, inhibit release of chemical mediators of asthma from mast cells, improve clearance of secretions, and improve diaphragm contractility. Since most patients with COPD have some component of bronchospasm, all patients are given a trial of these agents. Decisions on whether to continue the drugs past the trial period are based on subjective improvement in patient symptoms and objective improvement in pulmonary function tests (*i.e.*, 10% to 20% improvement in FEV_1). These factors must be evaluated in view of the toxicity of these drugs, particularly in the elderly population.

The four main classes of bronchodilators are the β-adrenergics, the methylxanthines, the anticholinergics, and the corticosteroids. The action of β-adrenergic drugs is mediated through α-, β_1-, and β_2-adrenergic receptors. Early β-agonist bronchodilators such as ephedrine and epinephrine have some α-adrenergic activity, causing hypertension, urinary retention, and other toxic effects. They should not be used in the elderly, and their use in the over-the-counter metered dose inhalers should be discouraged. The pure β-adrenergic drugs are considered in Table 14-2. Stimulation of β_1-receptors causes chronotropic and inotropic effects on the heart, while stimulation of β_2-receptors causes relaxation of smooth muscle of bronchi and blood vessels in the lung and skeletal muscles. All β-adrenergic drugs have both β_1- and β_2-stimulating action, but new drugs with proportionately more β_2- than β_1-effects have been developed.

The β-adrenergic drugs can be administered by several routes as shown in Table 14-2; however, the aerosol route is preferred due to possible improved bronchodilation and less side-effects of nausea, palpitations, and nervousness.[195,229] Medication can be delivered by pocket metered-dose inhalers, hand-held bulb nebulizers, or power nebulizers. The delivery of medication by intermittent positive pressure breathing (IPPB) devices is of no proven benefit.[60,106] Parenteral administration should be considered contraindicated in the elderly. In terms of relative potency of bronchodilation, albuterol and metaproterenol show some superiority over isoetharine.[21,184] In the patient with minimal symptoms of asthma or chronic bronchitis, the use of two puffs four times a day may be sufficient to provide symptom relief. The patient should wait for 1 minute before taking the second puff.[154] All the β-adrenergic bronchodilators, independent of route of administration, can stimulate the cardiovascular system. Although angina and arrhythmias are relative contraindications to use, these agents may be necessary and should be administered under medical supervision. Other side-effects may be avoided in the elderly patient by beginning with a low dose and increasing it slowly over several days or weeks. It should further be noted that intensity and duration of effect of sympathomimetic bronchodilators may decrease over time; that is, tolerance and tachyphylaxis can develop.[229]

The methylxanthine derivatives in addition to decreasing airway reactivity improve diaphragm contractility, which may be of particular importance to the patient with COPD.[10] These agents should be considered for single or combined use in asthma or chronic bronchitis as initial therapy or when a β-sympathetic agent is not sufficient to control symptoms. Clinical evidence suggests improved bronchodilation with a combination of both agents over either agent alone.[102,121,233]

In this class of medications, of which theophylline is the most active, the need for drug levels stems from unpredictable drug metabolism among patients.[107] Toxicity, including seizures, gastrointestinal irritation, nervousness, agitation, altered mentation, and cardiostimulatory effects does not necessarily correlate with the clinical response.[229] In addition, some patients with a low drug level in the therapeutic "normal" range of 10 μg to 15 μg/ml may benefit from an increase in level to 15 μg to 20 μg/ml. Patients with liver disease, obesity, congestive heart failure, and cor pulmonale and

TABLE 14-2   Dosage Forms Available and Relative Receptor Stimulation of Newer Sympathomimetic Agents

Agent	Dosage Forms*	α	β_1	β_2	Duration of Action After Inhalation (hr)
		\multicolumn{3}{c}{Adrenergic Effects†}	
Isoproterenol	N, M	0	+ + +	+ + +	2–3
Isoetharine hydrochloride	N, M	0	+ +	+ + +	1–5
Metaproterenol sulfate	N, M, O	0	+	+ + +	3–4
Terbutaline sulfate	M, O, S	0	+	+ + +	3–6
Albuterol	M, O	0	+	+ + +	3–6
Bitolterol	M	0	+	+ + +	4–8
Fenoterol	NA	0	+	+ + +	NA

* N indicates nebulizer solution; M, metered dose inhaler; O, oral preparation (*i.e.*, tablet or syrup); S, solution for subcutaneous injection; and NA, not yet commercially available.

† 0, none; +, slight; + +, moderate; and + + +, notable. (Adapted from George RB: Some recent advances in the management of asthma. Arch Intern Med 142:933, 1982)

those taking certain medications such as cimetidine, β-blockers and erythromycin are more likely to become toxic.[51,181,183] Cigarette smoking, current viral infection, or possibly even vaccination and use of medications such as phenytoin (Dilantin) may lead to subtherapeutic drug levels.[46,131,182] In spite of the multiple factors affecting serum drug levels, reduction in theophylline dose on the basis of age is probably not indicated.[17,76]

Long-acting forms of anhydrous theophylline administered twice a day have been adequately tested and shown to maintain a steadier serum concentration than the previous plain tablets or liquids.[230] Current evidence with some once-a-day preparations suggests that increased absorption when the dose is taken with meals (dose dumping) can lead to significant toxicity.[94] Rectal suppositories and enemas are not recommended due to the altered absorption secondary to product formulations.[229]

The third class of bronchodilator drugs are the anticholinergics, which block cholinergic stimulation and decrease intracellular cyclic guanosine monophosphate (GMP). Known to be effective bronchodilators for many years, they are gaining use in combination with other bronchodilators. One of the newer agents, ipatropium, has fewer systemic effects than inhaled atropine.[81,121] Atropine, however, should not be routinely used in the elderly population, because of the increased incidence of side-effects.

Corticosteroids as bronchodilating drugs are most efficacious in asthma. This is particularly true in asthma associated with allergic pulmonary aspergillosis. Recent clinical evidence suggests that patients with COPD, whether airway hyperreactivity or wheezing are present, should be given a trial of prednisone at 40 mg/day for 2 weeks. If a greater than 15% increase in FEV_1 can be demonstrated, the patient is tapered to every-other-day steroids or to inhaled beclomethasone or triamcinolone. If the FEV_1 does not improve 15% over the 2-week trial, then steroids should be discontinued.[102,118,190] Inhaled steroids have been most effective in reducing or eliminating the need for systemic steroids in steroid-dependent patients with asthma.

Cromolyn sodium is a medication used to help prevent bronchoconstriction by stabilization of the mast cell membrane. It is not a bronchodilator but is included here because it is frequently used in conjunction with the above medications. Long-term studies have shown that about 50% of adults with severe asthma will respond to cromolyn therapy; however, it has not been evaluated in the elderly. Newer medications are being evaluated

with properties similar to cromolyn, such as lodoxamide for oral use and thiazinamium for inhalation.[44]

Antibiotics

Benefit from antibiotic therapy in acute exacerbations of COPD has been difficult to demonstrate using well-designed, placebo-controlled studies.[210] Nonetheless, clinical experience suggests that they may be used to treat, reduce severity of, and possibly prevent exacerbations of COPD owing to infection. Prophylactically, antibiotics can be given at the first sign of chest infection or used in continuous rotating regimens as in the patient with bronchiectasis. Most exacerbations caused by infection are probably initiated by viruses or mycoplasma,[199] with flare-up of bacterial infection. The bacteria most likely to be present during exacerbations are *Hemophilus influenzae* and *Streptococcus pneumoniae*, for which ampicillin and tetracycline are commonly used. Other antibiotics such as first-generation cephalosporins and the combination of sulfamethoxazole-trimethoprim are also effective. Sputum cultures are not a prerequisite for initiating prophylactic antibiotic therapy because the tracheal flora of patients with COPD is generally predictable, and the success of antibiotic therapy does not necessarily correlate with culture results. Annual prophylaxis against influenza and pneumococcal vaccination at least once are recommended for all COPD patients.[119]

Oxygen

Long-term home oxygen therapy has been shown to be of significant benefit to selected patients with COPD. The NIH-sponsored multicenter nocturnal oxygen therapy trial reported better survival and greater reduction in pulmonary vascular resistance with continuous (24 hours/day) as compared with nocturnal (12 hours/day) oxygen therapy in patients with severe resting hypoxemia (Pao_2 less than 55 mm Hg).[157] Patients selected for study also showed improvement in neuropsychological testing, as manifested by improved mood, personality, and quality of life.[93] Improvement in cardiac function, as well as reversal of compensatory mechanisms such as elevated hematocrit values, may be demonstrated. In patients with stable COPD, oxygen at 2 liters/min improves their oxygenation, prolongs sleep, and has no apparent ill effects on sleep-disordered breathing.[114]

Diagnostic criteria for institution of home oxygen therapy are presented below:

1. Persistent hypoxemia (Pao_2 of 55 mm Hg or less as measured at rest in the sitting position)

2. $Pao_2 > 55$ mm Hg with evidence of hypoxic organ dysfunction:
   a. Pulmonary hypertension
   b. Cor pulmonale
   c. Secondary erythrocytosis
   d. CNS dysfunction
3. $Pao_2 < 55$ mm Hg during exercise, when oxygen therapy improves exercise tolerance
4. Sleep hypoxemia, when documented improvement is shown in the hospital

Once patients have been identified as needing chronic oxygen therapy, they should have an established current diagnosis; an optimal medical regimen, including a trial of bronchodilators (and possibly steroids for 30 days); completely recovered from any exacerbation of their illness for 1 month; and documentation that oxygen therapy can improve hypoxemia or provide overall clinical benefit. The dosage of oxygen should alleviate hypoxemia (*e.g.*, to increase the Po_2 to above 60 mm Hg) and/or alleviate the deleterious effects on end organ dysfunction. This can usually be accomplished with the use of a nasal cannula at 1 to 4 liters/min continuous flow or by the use of an intermittent demand nasal cannula system.[6] Patients receiving oxygen therapy should be clinically evaluated and have arterial blood gases or ear oximetry sampling of oxygen saturation at 1, 6, and 12 months to document the need for oxygen; thereafter, at least once yearly is adequate in the stable patient. The clinician should also be aware that at altitudes used for commercial aircraft, patients with chronic hypoxemia may require supplemental oxygen. Since the patient will not be allowed to take his own equipment on the plane, information concerning the patient's diagnosis and oxygen flow rate must be given to the airline prior to travel.[2]

In a high-risk patient scheduled to undergo elective surgery, a program that includes cessation of smoking, administration of bronchodilators and antibiotics, and postural drainage is necessary. Identification of patients needing this advance preparation, as well as prediction of postoperative course, is aided by standard spirometric tests.[85] After surgery, appropriate pulmonary toilet including the use of incentive spirometry should be performed frequently. Intermittent positive-pressure breathing (IPPB) devices are of no benefit and bronchodilators can be easily administered by nebulizers.[60,106] Although there are no pulmonary contraindications to emergency surgery, the same general precautions should be used whenever possible.

Diagnosis and Treatment of Complications of COPD

Some of the important complications of COPD are listed below:

Hypoxemia and hypercarbia
Cor pulmonale
Secondary erythrocytosis
Left ventricular heart failure
Arrhythmias
Nocturnal oxygen desaturation
Pulmonary embolism
Pneumothorax
Peptic ulcer disease
Acute respiratory failure

Arterial blood gases are important in defining the degree of hypoxemia and hypercarbia and can be followed yearly with spirometry in the stable outpatient. Cor pulmonale signifies that disorders affecting either the structure or function of the lungs have resulted in right ventricular enlargement.[74] Standard criteria for right ventricular hypertrophy have been met in only one third of patients with chronic bronchitis and emphysema at autopsy. An associated erythrocytosis is frequent; its absence may signify gastrointestinal bleeding. Appropriate treatment for cor pulmonale includes the overall therapy of COPD as well as the administration of supplemental oxygen as previously described. Erythrocytosis will also improve with this therapy. In the nonsmoking patient with headaches, dizziness, and visual changes with a hematocrit above 60%, phlebotomy may be helpful.[238]

Left ventricular dysfunction complicating COPD has been well described; however, the mechanism is controversial in patients without concomitant coronary artery disease.[135] Whether right ventricular pathology leads to left ventricular failure is probably not as important as the long-standing effects of hypoxia, acidosis, and possibly the large swings in intrathoracic pressures. Diagnosis is often difficult since the physical examination, chest roentgenogram, and electrocardiogram are occasionally misleading in the COPD patient with heart failure.[74] 2D-echocardiography and cardiac imaging by radionuclear techniques may aid the clinician in difficult cases. Treatment is often instituted with diuretics, which reduce the excess lung fluid causing abnormal gas exchange. In addition, peripheral blood pooling as an effect of loop diuretics such as furosemide and bumetanide leads to a further decrease in central fluid overloading.[82] Use of digitalis in patients with heart failure and COPD is controversial. Current recommendations suggest its use should be restricted to patients with cor pulmonale and coexistent left ventricular failure. Supraventricular arrhythmias are frequent in COPD patients and are another indication for digitalis therapy once hypoxemia and electrolyte imbalances have been corrected.

Pulmonary embolus may go unnoticed because of lack of specific clinical findings. Incidences ranging from 18% to 60% are reported in COPD patients.[125] Certain clinical characteristics may aid in the diagnosis: precipitous worsening of dyspnea that is unresponsive to bronchodilators, a reduction in Pa_{CO_2} in a previously hypercapnic patient, severe tachypnea of greater than 30 breaths/min, and cor pulmonale and right-sided heart failure. These risk factors are especially helpful in the patient with an FEV_1 greater than 1.5 liters.[71,125] Angiography should be the diagnostic procedure of choice since ventilation and perfusion scans are frequently abnormal in these patients.

Sponataneous pneumothorax and peptic ulcer disease also occur with increased incidence in COPD. Their diagnosis is usually fairly straightforward and if therapy is delayed, serious morbidity and mortality may result.

Respiratory failure is one of the more common complications of COPD. Contributing factors include infection, oversedation, and overuse of oxygen. Diagnosis is made from the presentation of worsening symptoms with abnormal arterial blood gases (Pa_{O_2} less than 50 mm Hg and a Pa_{CO_2} greater than 50 mm Hg and sufficiently elevated to cause acidosis with pH less than 7.3). The change in symptoms as well as development of acidosis is used to help differentiate acute from chronic respiratory failure.

The immediate goal in treating respiratory failure is to correct hypoxia with oxygen-air mixtures. This is not without some risk since elimination of the hypoxic ventilatory drive may cause a decrease in ventilation with an associated respiratory acidosis and altered sensorium. In the chronically hypercapnic patient in respiratory failure, inspired oxygen concentration can be controlled by use of the Venturi face mask. This is not usually necessary in the eucapnic patient in whom nasal prongs can be used safely at 1 to 2 liters/min. The cannula has the added advantage of not requiring removal to eat.

The next objective in management of acute respiratory failure is the improvement in airway obstruction by treatment of bronchospasm, removal of secretions, and management of infection. Inhalation of β_2-sympathomimetic drugs such as

metaproterenol in a 5% solution should be instituted. Doses of 0.3 ml to 0.5 ml diluted in 2.5 ml normal saline may be given at 3- to 4-hour intervals. Intravenously administered aminophylline is also effective in respiratory failure. Dosage adjustment must be made as shown in Table 14-3, and note that this need not be changed because of age. Serum theophylline levels should be determined due to the potential 50% variation between individual patients even with careful dosing.[176] The combination of sympathomimetics with the infusion of aminophylline has been shown to have an additive effect. The theophylline drug level should be maintained at between 10 mg and 20 mg/liter since the cardiac toxicity may also be additive.

The benefit of corticosteroids in patients with COPD and respiratory failure is no longer considered controversial. Intravenous methylprednisolone, 0.5 mg/kg, or hydrocortisone, 2.5 mg/kg, given every 6 hours should provide optimum patient benefit.

Antibiotic therapy should be directed at specific organisms identifiable on Gram's stain or in sputum and blood cultures when pneumonia is present. When multiple organisms are present on Gram's stain, therapy with a penicillin or cephalosporin with an aminoglycoside is adequate until culture results are available. Acute respiratory failure associated with bronchitis may be treated with either ampicillin or tetracycline, 500 mg orally every 6 hours. In patients with an acute exacerbation of COPD with no clear evidence of infec-

TABLE 14-3 Recommended Doses of Intravenous Aminophylline*

Condition	Loading Dose (mg/kg)†	Maintenance Dose (mg/kg/hr)
Adult smoker	6	0.8
Adult nonsmoker	6	0.5
Severe obstructive pulmonary disease	6	0.4
Heart failure, pneumonia, or liver disease	6	0.2

* To achieve a serum level of 10 mg/liter based on ideal body weight.
† Eliminate if patient was receiving therapeutic doses of oral theophyllpine.
(Adapted from Powell JR, Voseth S, Hopewell P et al: Theophylline disposition in acutely ill hospitalized patients. Am Rev Respir Dis 118:229, 1978)

tion, antibiotic therapy has been shown to be of no benefit over placebo.[155]

Adjunctive therapy, which is often referred to as "vigorous pulmonary toilet," involves hydration, suctioning of secretions, postural drainage, and chest percussion. This terminology is misleading in that much of it is without proven benefit. Inspissated secretions may possibly be cleared more easily after hydration; however, too vigorous hydration should be discouraged since it may increase total lung water and affect lung compliance. Postural drainage and chest percussion have not been shown to decrease morbidity or mortality in acute exacerbations of COPD. Nasotracheal suctioning of patients who are unable to clear secretions may be of benefit.

When these measures fail to improve alveolar ventilation and correct respiratory acidosis and hypoxemia, intubation and mechanical ventilation should be instituted. An example would be the patient with progressive hypoxemia, hypercarbia, and acidosis (particularly less than a pH of 7.25) who is becoming somnolent and exhausted from an increased work of breathing.

The prognosis in acute exacerbation of COPD with or without respiratory failure has greatly improved. Burk and George reported that in acute episodes treated conservatively, 86% resulted in recovery and discharge from the hospital, while only 58% of the episodes requiring mechanical ventilation resulted in survival.[37] Two-year survival after an acute exacerbation of COPD is now reported to be 72%.[133] These results should encourage an aggressive approach in management of these patients. However, the elderly patient is more adversely affected. A follow-up study of elderly patients discharged from the hospital after an exacerbation of COPD revealed prolonged disability with depression and inability to perform prehospitalization household chores or social activities.[166]

CANCER OF THE LUNG

Lung cancer has been rapidly increasing during this century and is now responsible for 100,000 deaths a year in the United States.[42] It is the most common fatal malignancy in males and will soon replace breast cancer as the most common malignancy in females. Although cigarette smoking is by far the greatest predisposing factor, other carcinogenic materials to consider are uranium, asbestos, fluorspar, chromates, arsenic, and chloromethyl ether. Since cancer of the lung occurs later in life, with peak incidence in the fifth and sixth decades, the elderly are at risk.

In patients with lung cancer, the overall 5-year survival rate remains at 8% to 10%. One would expect that periodic screening of high-risk patients (*i.e.,* smokers) with yearly chest roentgenograms and sputum cytology would enhance early detection and thus reduce mortality. However, results have been controversial and not cost effective. Early screening has been shown to detect a number of asymptomatic cancers in which 5-year survival after resection is 70% or higher.[138] Currently, surgical resection of all types of bronchogenic carcinoma, except the small cell group, is the treatment of choice.[54] Small cell cancer is considered unresectable if the cell type is identified before thoracotomy because silent metastases occur early in lymph nodes, bone marrow, liver, kidneys, or adrenals. Fortunately, this type of tumor responds to chemotherapy.

Clinical Picture

The patient with lung cancer may present with an asymptomatic lesion found on a routine chest film. More commonly, however, the patient will have symptoms relative to the site of the tumor or its metastasis. With an endobronchial location, the patient may have cough with sputum production, obstructive pneumonia, or hemoptysis. Weight loss is another common complaint. There are no neural fibers involved in the sensation of pain from the lung, hence complaint of pain can signify spread beyond the confines of the lung (*i.e.,* pleura, pericardium, or chest wall). Progressive enlargement of a pleural effusion may cause dyspnea, and pericardial involvement may lead to tamponade. Mediastinal involvement may be represented by hoarseness (recurrent laryngeal nerve paralysis), raised diaphragm (phrenic nerve paralyses), or dysphagia if the esophagus is involved or compressed. Superior vena cava obstruction may present with facial swelling, venous dilation, and headache. When the apical segments of the lung are involved with tumor (Pancoast's tumor), a syndrome can occur with an ipsilateral Horner's syndrome and pain in the upper chest and shoulder from brachial plexus compression. Secondary muscle weakness and neuropathy of the involved extremity may also occur.[141]

Many paraneoplastic syndromes have been described[153] and endocrine abnormalities include inappropriate antidiuretic hormone secretion (SIADH), Cushing's syndrome, and gynecomastia. Hypercalcemia with altered mental status, nausea, and vomiting results from secretion of a parathyroidlike hormone or some other osteolytic hormone. Another manifestation is hypertrophic pulmonary osteoarthropathy, with pain and periosteal proliferation of the distal ends of long bones and digital clubbing. Various neurologic manifestations not due to metastasis include corticocerebellar degeneration, spinocerebellar degeneration, peripheral neuropathy, myasthenia (Eaton-Lambert syndrome), and myopathy. Skin manifestations may include acanthosis nigricans. Clotting abnormalities such as nonbacterial thrombotic endocarditis and recurrent thrombophlebitis (Trousseau's syndrome) may be difficult to treat with anticoagulants.

Diagnosis

The diagnosis is usually established by a combination of clinical history and examination coupled with chest roentgenograms, sputum cytology, bronchoscopic examination, and thoracotomy. The chest roentgenogram may reveal hilar or perihilar masses as well as peripheral nodules which occur with all cell types but particularly squamous cell carcinoma. Cavitation is also noted, and enlargement of the tumor, which obstructs a bronchus, may produce distal pneumonia, atelectasis, or abscess.[40] Adenocarcinomas arising out of a previous scar in the periphery of the lung are being reported with increased frequency. Computed tomography of the chest has nearly replaced whole lung tomograms for further evaluation of roentgenographic abnormalities.[220] Further diagnosis requires tissue. The acquisition of sputum for cytology is the initial step in evaluating the patient with abnormal clinical and roentgenographic findings. If the cytology is positive for malignancy and the patient demonstrates no evidence of local spread (mediastinum or chest wall) or distant metastasis, then bronchoscopy is performed to determine the extent of involvement with transbronchial aspiration of mediastinal nodes as indicated.[40] If cytology is negative, bronchoscopic examination is indicated with mucosal or transbronchial biopsy or needle aspiration[196] of the suspected lesion. Evaluation of elderly patients undergoing bronchoscopy has shown that it is safe, well tolerated, and helpful in providing a diagnosis.[91] In the absence of clinical signs, liver and brain scans are uniformly negative and bone scans are positive in only about 4%.[100] They should not, therefore, be routinely ordered in all patients.

Determination of mediastinal node involvement and tumor cell type may prevent unnecessary thoracotomy for inoperable disease. Mediastinoscopy or limited mediastinotomy is then recommended for patients with proven or suspected bronchogenic carcinoma who have hilar or mediastinal lymphadenopathy on the thoracic roentgenogram or who have peripheral lesions greater than 2 cm to 3 cm in diameter.[116,134] Gallium-67 imaging for detection of mediastinal metastasis has been only marginally useful.[98,227] Hematoporphyrin derivatives injected intravenously may help localize occult tumor or metastasis as it is selectively taken up by neoplastic cells. These techniques in the future may allow localization of areas for biopsy and for localized resection with high-intensity laser coagulation.[92]

Treatment

Surgical Resection

Surgical resection is still the primary therapy in non-oat-cell cancer of the lung. Five-year survival rates approaching 69% are reported[232] with tumors less than 3 cm diameter in size and without metastasis. These rates have also been reported in patients older than 70 years of age in selected cases.[91,237] Resection is usually planned when the tumor is localized with only ipsilateral hilar node involvement and no distant metastasis. Selected patients with more extensive tumor involvement are sometimes considered for surgery: Pancoast tumors after radiation therapy, tumors involving the chest wall that can be removed en bloc, squamous cell cancers with ipsilateral mediastinal involvement, and certain cancers that impinge on the phrenic nerve. Contraindications to surgery include recurrent laryngeal nerve involvement, obstruction of the superior vena cava or proximal main pulmonary artery, most cases with subcarinal involvement, and pleural effusion with positive cytology or positive pleural biopsy. In patients over 70 years of age, lung-sparing procedures must be considered during pulmonary resection for carcinoma (*i.e.*, sleeve lobectomy, segmental resection, wedge resection). An in-hospital mortality of 4% has been reported, which is an improvement over previous combined reports revealing 17% mortality. Long-term follow-up in these elderly patients reveals overall survival rates of 27%, ranging from 13% for patients having pneumonectomy to 42% for those having segmental resection.[35,237]

We use an approach based on easily obtainable physiologic data that predicts ability to withstand pneumonectomy. All candidates for pulmonary resection undergo pulmonary function testing and arterial blood-gas analysis. Patients with an arterial oxygen less than 45 mm Hg at rest or during exercise or with an elevated arterial carbon dioxide tension are excluded from surgery. If pulmonary function tests reveal: an FEV_1 of less than 50% of the FVC, FEV_1 of less than 2 liters, an MVV of less than 50% of predicted, a ratio of residual volume to total lung capacity greater than 50% predicted or DL_{co} less than 50% predicted; a split-function lung scan study is performed. The number of counts over each lung is recorded, and a predicted postoperative FEV_1 is calculated multiplying the preoperative FEV_1 by the fraction of the total perfusion constituted by the uninvolved lung. If the predicted postoperative FEV_1 is greater than 800 ml, our studies show that pneumonectomy can be performed with an acceptable mortality rate.[160] This approach permits consideration for pneumonectomy in patients who would otherwise not be considered. Exercise studies of oxygen consumption may prove to be an accurate predictor of postoperative complications. In one study, a Vo_{2max} greater than 20 ml/kg/min implied minimal risk while patients with a preoperative value less than 15 ml/kg/min implied nearly 100% complication rate in a small group of patients tested.[200]

Radiation Therapy

Radiation therapy is used as an adjunct to surgery and for palliation. In Pancoast's tumor its adjunctive role is well established. Radiation therapy preoperatively and postoperatively in other situations is being investigated. Most studies indicate little benefit, with claims of radiation therapy for "cure" considered unproven at this time.[33,172] Selected patients undergoing irradiation after resection of squamous cell carcinoma with mediastinal involvement have shown some encouraging increased survival rates.[116]

Palliative irradiation of painful bone metastasis and of tumors occluding bronchi, obstructing the superior vena cava, or producing hemoptysis can often be of benefit. Further palliation of obstructing tumors can be provided by laser therapy, which is currently under investigation.[64]

Chemotherapy

The limited role of chemotherapy is changing most dramatically in the treatment of small-cell undifferentiated oat cell carcinoma. Patients with this type of lung cancer had a median survival of 3 months. With polychemotherapy and thoracic irradiation for disease that is limited, 72% of patients experienced complete remission with no evidence of residual disease and 23% remained free of detectable cancer for 2 or more years. Unfortunately, this limited form of the disease is not

common. Metastasis to the brain and other sites in the lung occur early with oat cell carcinoma such that in extensive disease the median survival is 10 months.[86,126] Chemotherapy has been administered to patients with inoperable carcinoma of types other than oat cell. Results vary widely, and it is not clear that treatment of asymptomatic patients significantly prolongs or improves the quality of life.

TUBERCULOSIS

While the overall incidence and mortality from infections with *Mycobacterium tuberculosis* has been decreasing since 1900 (Table 14-4), the elderly now comprise the largest group with active infection.[152] This increase in the elderly results from an age-related decline in cell-mediated immunity.

Other contributing factors include illnesses known to alter cell-mediated immunity such as alcoholism, malnutrition, diabetes, neoplasia, renal dialysis, and treatment with immunosuppressive drugs. Most geriatric cases appear to be due to reactivation of latent infection from the breakdown of dormant granulomas persisting from a primary infection at an earlier age. Latent infection is a state in which the tubercle bacillus has become established in the body but symptoms, roentgenographic abnormalities, and sputum positive for acid-fast bacilli, as seen in active infection, are not found. This clinical state can thus be diagnosed by positive tuberculin skin testing or suggested by the appearance of apical scarring on the

TABLE 14-4   Tuberculosis Mortality Rates in the United States*

| | Year | | |
Age (Years)	1900	1950	1973
0–4	413.4	14.8	0.5
5–14	36.2	1.8	0.05
15–24	205.7	11.3	0.1
25–34	294.3	19.1	0.3
35–44	253.6	26.1	1.2
45–54	215.6	35.9	2.5
55–64	223.0	47.8	4.5
65–74	256.1	58.2	7.3
75–84	279.3	63.2	11.6
85+	204.5	47.7	15.2

* Death rates per 100,000 population.
(Myers JA: A tapering off of tuberculosis among the elderly. Am J Public Health 66:1101, 1976)

chest roentgenogram. Active infection occurs within the first 5 years of exposure in only 15% of individuals with latent infection. There is then a decline in cumulative risk over the next 50 patient-years such that the overall reactivation rate is about 4%.[113]

Primary infection also represents active disease. Formerly a disease of childhood and adolescence, primary tuberculosis is being reported with increasing incidence in adulthood as a larger segment of the population grows older without exposure to tuberculosis. This becomes significant in the geriatric population, as evidenced by the recent report of an epidemic in a nursing home.[206] Forty-nine (30%) of 161 previously tuberculin-negative residents became infected and eight (17%) developed progressive primary tuberculosis, with one death. There were 138 tuberculin-negative employees who were infected without developing active disease. Other manifestations of early infection and disease occur when a subpleural caseous focus breaks into the pleural space with resulting pleurisy and pleural effusion. The patient may present with a paucity of clinical findings and may be tuberculin skin test negative, making diagnosis difficult in the geriatric population.[22] Extrapulmonary tuberculosis appears to have an unchanged or slightly increased incidence in the United States. It was 7% to 8% in 1964 and 13.7% in 1976. This includes miliary tuberculosis (multiple organs affected from hematogenous spread). A lower frequency of accompanying cavities or diffuse "miliary" infiltrates on chest roentgenogram and the presence of concomitant disease with nonspecific signs and symptoms have made diagnosis more difficult. This is particularly worrisome in the geriatric population since patients over age 60 make up the majority of both undiagnosed and fatal cases of miliary tuberculosis. A delay in diagnosis of up to 15 to 16 weeks is reported in some series.[1]

Diagnosis

The typical patient with tuberculosis may present with fever, chills, night sweats, weight loss, and anorexia. He may have a cough with some hemoptysis. When the sputum is collected and smears reviewed, acid-fast bacilli are seen. The chest roentgenogram in these patients usually reveals an infiltrate or cavitation in the apical and posterior segments of the right upper lobe. Mantoux skin testing with 5 units of purified protein derivative (PPD) is positive at 10 mm of induration (not erythema) or more. This presentation may not occur in many patients with tuberculosis in the elderly population.[152] Clinicians frequently fail to recognize the other many varied clinical and roentgenographic abnormalities found in the elderly, leading to further morbidity and mortality. Multiple studies have revealed tuberculosis as the primary cause of death, which was undiagnosed until necropsy.[9,30,67,70,142,205] In one study of 21 patients, 15 were over the age of 60, with alcoholism, renal failure, diabetes, and gastrectomy representing other underlying diseases in the younger patients reported.[30] Even when tuberculosis is considered in the initial diagnosis, there may be a 10-day interval prior to diagnosis that lengthens to 23 days when tuberculosis is not initially considered.[205] Factors that contribute to delay in diagnosis include a paucity of clinical and radiographic findings, particularly when miliary disease is present. The geriatric patient may present with weight loss, anorexia, altered mental status, or fever of unknown etiology. The PPD may be indeterminate, making diagnosis even more difficult. Misinterpretation of the chest roentgenogram as not consistent with tuberculosis can occur in up to 43% of patients who have findings not considered diagnostic for disease. Radiologic patterns quite unusual for tuberculosis might include masslike densities resembling carcinoma, chronic infiltrates in a lower lobe, pleural effusion, and miliary tuberculosis either superimposed on diffuse interstitial lung disease or associated with a diffuse lung pattern atypical for miliary disease.[9,142]

The tuberculin skin test may be negative in persons infected with *Mycobacterium tuberculosis.* This has been shown to occur in active disease when there is extensive cavitary pulmonary involvement or miliary disease.[79] Many of these PPD negative patients will usually respond with a reactive skin test once therapy has been initiated or malnutrition has been corrected.[152] This points again to the altered cell-mediated immunity in tuberculosis patients. Tuberculin sensitivity may be low in the geriatric patient, even in the face of dormant infection acquired in the past. A borderline PPD, when repeated, may show a greater than 6-mm increase in induration in patients with a remote tuberculous infection or sensitization to atypical mycobacteria.[214] This indicates a previously diminished skin hypersensitivity has been activated by exposure to tuberculous protein. This booster effect occurs as soon as 1 week following the initial skin test, may last for over a year, and appears most frequently in the elderly. In 200 elderly persons given skin tests at the time of entry into a nursing home, 6% showed a positive skin test initially and another 6% became positive on reapplying the test 10 to 14 days later.[206] Negative tuberculin skin tests should, therefore, be repeated at 1 week in the elderly to detect a waned response. This will also prevent unnecessary therapy at some later date for a boosted routine skin test with conversion.

Further diagnosis after the above measures have taken place requires obtaining sputum and/or tissue. In patients unable to cough productively, heated saline aerosol-induced sputum is culture positive in 28% to 57% of untreated patients with pulmonary tuberculosis and fasting gastric aspirates, neutralized with sodium bicarbonate, are culture-positive in 10% to 30%. This latter procedure should be performed on awakening the patient prior to getting up or eating.[16] When these measures are unsuccessful and the diagnosis of tuberculosis is still strongly suspected, then bronchoscopy with transbronchial biopsy should be performed. This procedure when coupled with bronchial brushings and washings with three post bronchoscopy sputum specimens yields the diagnosis of tuberculosis in 20% of a group of 56 culture-negative patients and yielded other diagnoses in 32%.[224] When all evaluations are negative and there are no contraindications to therapy, a diagnostic trial of drug treatment is indicated with follow-up. Therapy can then be discontinued if cultures remain negative and there is no clinical or roentgenographic improvement.

Treatment

Treatment of the elderly patient with tuberculosis must take into account the possibility of adverse reactions to the drug, patient compliance, and other underlying disease.[152] Short-course chemotherapy for non-drug-resistant pulmonary tuberculosis has been well studied in a large group of elderly patients in Little Rock, Arkansas, and consists of isoniazid, 300 mg, and rifampin, 600 mg, daily for 9 months.[4] An equally effective regimen is isoniazid, 300 mg, and rifampin, 600 mg, daily for 1 month, followed by rifampin, 600 mg, and isoniazid, 15 mg/kg (usually 900 mg), twice weekly for another 8 months for a total 9-month treatment period.[65,207] The addition of ethambutol and streptomycin probably adds nothing to the effectiveness of either of these regimens in the absence of isoniazid resistance.[207] Furthermore, the renal, auditory, and vestibular toxicities of streptomycin and the ocular toxicity of ethambutol make use of these drugs more risky in the elderly population. In patients with other underlying diseases such as diabetes mellitus and silicosis, those

postgastrectomy, and those with immunosuppressive diseases, the American Thoracic Society and Centers for Disease Control (CDC) do not currently recommend short-course chemotherapy,[152] even though it has been shown to be effective.[207] Streptomycin and ethambutol are also effective; however, their toxicity in the elderly must be considered. Since neither drug has liver toxicity, substitution for rifampin may be considered.

Chemoprophylactic Therapy

Individuals who should receive chemoprophylactic treatment are listed below[5]:

Household and close contacts of patients with active infection
Newly infected persons (skin test conversion within the past 2 years)
Patients with abnormal chest roentgenograms (*i.e.,* stable parenchymal lesions and not isolated calcifications or pleural thickening)
Patients with special clinical situations (silicosis, diabetes, immunosuppressive therapy, hematologic malignancies, chronic hemodialysis)
Patients with clinical situations associated with malnutrition (postgastrectomy, chronic ulcer disease, malabsorption, and certain gastrointestinal malignancies)
Tuberculin skin test reactors under 35 years of age

The currently accepted regimen for therapy in skin test reactors includes isoniazid, 300 mg/day for 1 year. Other drugs and shorter regimens are under evaluation but are not approved. In the over 35-year age-group risk of isoniazid-induced hepatitis rises to 1.2% by age 49 and to 2.3% by age 64 without apparent further increase thereafter. Since this adverse effect approaches the actual risk of developing active tuberculosis in the elderly skin test converter, prophylaxis is not usually recommended except in those clinical situations listed previously.

The hepatotoxicity of isoniazid appears to develop early in the course of therapy (*i.e.,* within the first 3 months); however, chronic hepatitis and death may rarely occur late without antecedent clinical symptoms. Patients who consume alcohol daily, those who have concomitant liver disease, and possibly those over 50 years of age should receive periodic transaminase determination (SGOT or SGPT). A transient rise in these values occurs after initial isoniazid therapy and should not lead to discontinuance of medication. Should the patient develop nausea and vomiting or the transaminase level rise above three times normal, then the isoniazid should be stopped. Other effects of isoniazid include peripheral neuropathy, which may be prevented or treated with pyridoxine, 50 mg/day, taken by mouth. Hyperexcitability is sometimes noted in the elderly patient and can be managed by dividing the dose at 100 mg, three times a day. Other effects include dry mouth, constipation, optic neuritis and atrophy, lupuslike syndromes, exfoliative dermatitis, and delay in maturation.[152]

Rifampin when combined with isoniazid has an additive but not synergistic hepatotoxic effect. Factors that may predispose to this include advancing age and previous hepatic disease. Other effects of rifampin include "flu-like" symptoms, and occasionally thrombocytopenia, shock, hemolytic anemia, and renal failure, which occur rarely at doses of 600 mg a day or twice weekly. In spite of these adverse reactions, rifampin appears to be well tolerated in the elderly.[65,207]

PULMONARY EMBOLISM

The incidence of pulmonary embolism is estimated to be 500,000 embolic events per year. Of these, 10% are thought to be fatal, thus resulting in 50,000 deaths per year. Predisposing factors include those listed in Table 14-5, which represents coexisting illnesses in 167 patients with angiographically proven pulmonary emboli.[18] In addition, congenital deficiencies of certain proteins involved in lysis of clots, use of oral contraceptives, and advancing age must be considered as predisposing factors.[36,83,146,212] In the elderly, underlying pulmonary or cardiovascular disease often makes pulmonary embolism more devastating.

The majority of these emboli arise from the deep venous system of the lower extremities. Emboli can originate in the right atrium or ventricle and in the pelvic or renal veins. They seldom result from thrombosis of the upper extremities or from superficial venous thrombosis unless there is extension to the deep venous system.

Diagnosis

The diagnostic findings associated with pulmonary embolus reflect the size of the embolus and subsequent obstruction to flow of blood, hemorrhage, and infarction. Whether infarction (death of parenchymal tissue distal to the obstruction) occurs appears related to the presence of preexisting cardiopulmonary disease.[18,56] The classic symptoms

TABLE 14-5 Coexisting Conditions and Their Incidence in 167 Patients with Pulmonary Embolism

Condition	% Total
Thrombophlebitis	39.5
Venous varicosity and insufficiency	15.0
Peripheral arterial disease	4.8
Recent immobilization from fracture (casting)	15.0
Bed rest	32.4
Recent surgery	32.4
Recent termination of pregnancy	1.2
Pelvic disease	6.0
Obesity	30.0
Cerebrovascular disease	6.6
Hypertension	10.2
Myocardial infarction	12.0
Angina	5.4
Congestive heart failure	17.4
Arrhythmia	16.2
Rheumatic heart disease	1.2
Other heart disease	9.0
Primary pulmonary disease	7.8
Dehydration	3.6
Diabetes mellitus	8.4
Malignancy	7.2
Hemoglobinopathy	1.2
Polycythemia	0.0
No predisposing etiology	6.0

(Bell WR, Simon TL, DeMets DL: The clinical features of submassive and massive pulmonary emboli. Am J Med 62:355, 1977)

have included pleuritic chest pain, sweats, and hemoptysis, which actually appear in only 82%, 23%, and 40%, respectively, of patients with submassive pulmonary emboli. Dyspnea occurs in approximately 80% of all patients having pulmonary emboli with a lesser frequency of symptoms such as apprehension and cough.[18,221] Massive pulmonary embolus (significant filling defects or obstruction of two or more lobar arteries) usually involves more proximal obstruction to blood flow with less incidence of pleuritic pain or hemoptysis. Patients presenting with this abnormality are more likely to present in shock or have a history of syncope prior to arrival at a hospital. While syncope is likely to occur secondary to obstruction of blood flow to the brain, other etiologies have been postulated, such as sinus bradycardia due to a parasympathetic reflex.[198,213]

A third clinical syndrome different from massive and submassive pulmonary embolism involves recurrent small pulmonary emboli. Occlusion of progressively more of the pulmonary vasculature leads to the symptoms associated with cor pulmonale. Diagnosis is made by association of symptoms of fatigue and dyspnea on exertion, usually in a young female patient with progressive right-sided heart failure. This uncommon disorder is difficult to document without open lung biopsy and is considered by some to be a cause of primary pulmonary hypertension.[68]

Physical examination reveals a normal blood pressure unless massive embolism has taken place. The most common abnormality is a respiratory rate greater than 16 breaths/min. Its frequency (92%) is so striking that the absence of tachypnea should rule against the diagnosis with either massive or submassive embolism. Other signs common to both forms are rales, pulse greater than 100/min, temperature above 37.8°C (100°F), phlebitis, and edema. Findings more frequent with massive emboli include an increase in the pulmonic component of the second heart sound, gallop rhythm, diaphoresis, and cyanosis.[18] The electrocardiogram generally reflects nonspecific findings, with sinus tachycardia and nonspecific ST or T wave abnormalities occurring most frequently. With massive emboli, evidence of right-sided heart dysfunction occurs with the presence of right bundle branch block, right axis deviation, p-pulmonale and an $S_1Q_3T_3$ (S wave in lead 1, Q wave in lead 3, and an inverted T wave in lead 3). The chest roentgenogram is frequently abnormal with areas of consolidation and atelectasis, usually located peripherally in the lower lung fields. These reflect early hemorrhage or infarction as in submassive emboli. A pleural effusion may be bloody in 65% with greater than one half showing characteristics of an exudate.[39] Those patients with massive emboli may present with a normal chest roentgenogram or show an elevated hemidiaphragm, distended pulmonary arteries, or an area of decreased lung markings referred to as regional oligemia. Laboratory studies in the past have been of limited value as evaluation of increased lactic dehydrogenase, SGOT, and bilirubin are not specific for pulmonary emboli. Arterial blood gases are quite helpful in that 88% of patients with pulmonary embolus of either type have a PaO_2 of less than 80 mm Hg. It should further be noted that these patients frequently hyperventilate and a reduction in $PaCO_2$ should be noted particularly if found in a patient with previously known chronic hypercapnia.[221]

Although clinical and laboratory findings can strongly indicate pulmonary embolism, it can be confirmed only by special diagnostic procedures.

A normal perfusion lung scan properly performed (*i.e.,* with an anterior, posterior, and two lateral views) virtually rules out a diagnosis of pulmonary embolism. A follow-up study in patients suspected of having a pulmonary embolus but with a normal scan revealed no further morbidity or mortality from pulmonary emboli.[115] An abnormal lung scan requires interpretation, since many other diseases besides pulmonary emboli can cause disturbances in regional blood flow.

The diagnostic accuracy of perfusion lung scans can be improved by considering only lobar or segmental perfusion defects as indicative of pulmonary embolism. Improving the diagnostic accuracy of the perfusion study is the presence of a normal xenon gas ventilation scan in the area of a perfusion defect. Unfortunately, when there is infiltrate present on the chest roentgenogram in the area of the perfusion scan defect, even the addition of the ventilation scan will not improve the accuracy of these nuclear medicine studies.

If ventilation-perfusion scanning is not indicated or available, and if the perfusion scan is nondiagnostic, pulmonary arteriography should be performed. This should also be done in patients with high risk of bleeding from anticoagulation as well as when embolectomy or thrombolytic therapy is contemplated. A pulmonary arteriogram showing vessel cut-off and intraluminal defects will confirm the presence of embolism. Arteriography also allows determination of the patient's hemodynamic status.[132]

The extent to which one should carry the diagnostic evaluation varies from patient to patient. Elderly patients have a high risk of complications from anticoagulation and, in our opinion, require a higher degree of diagnostic certainty. When any doubt exists, proceed with anteriography, the risks of which are low, even in older patients. The information gained is invaluable in planning the patient's care, and a negative study eliminates the need for anticoagulation.

Treatment

The best way to reduce death and disability from pulmonary embolism is to prevent thrombi in the venous system of the lower extremities. Approaches that have been used include "mechanical" methods such as early ambulation, elastic stockings, electric calf muscle stimulation, and external, periodic calf compression; anticoagulant drugs such as warfarin and heparin; other potential antithrombotic agents such as dextran and "antiplatelet drugs" (aspirin, dipyridamole, and others). Unfortunately, early ambulation and standard elastic stockings have not been shown to offer prophylactic effect. "Graded" elastic stockings (which apply a decreasing pressure from ankle to thigh) may be effective, but additional proof is necessary in view of their cost. Electrical stimulation is seldom acceptable to the patient. External calf compression devices have been shown to be quite effective in preventing emboli especially in neurosurgical and urologic patients. There appears to be no apparent risk to this therapy. Cost and patient acceptance of long-term use must be considered.[147]

Heparin given subcutaneously in doses of 5000 units 2 hours before surgery and every 8 or 12 hours until ambulation reduces deep venous thrombosis, embolism, and lethal emboli in most surgical subpopulations. However, it has lacked efficacy in most patients with hip fracture and replacement as well as those undergoing urologic procedures. The risk of hemorrhage from this regimen in surgical patients is quite low.[105,147] In a study of 1358 medical patients with a predominance of cardiopulmonary disorders, there was an estimated 31% decrease in mortality in the group randomized to receive low dose heparin.[89] The majority of patients in this study were older than 65 years of age.

Warfarin has been studied extensively in surgical populations and its effectiveness has been debatable. Due to the risk of bleeding and its prolonged half-life, it is probably not the best agent in the geriatric population. The efficacy of low molecular weight dextran, given on the day of surgery and at intervals thereafter, is not universally accepted. Potential fluid overload and allergic and bleeding reactions may limit its use in the elderly. Other antiplatelet agents, especially aspirin, have not been demonstrated to be efficacious as prophylactic agents and are not recommended.[147]

Whether or not the above measures are undertaken, when pulmonary embolism is suspected, documentation and then appropriate treatment should begin. Heparin is the drug of choice in the patient not at risk for bleeding. We recommend the intravenous route with a continuous infusion of approximately 1000 units/hour. Intermittent intravenous infection at 4- to 6-hour intervals is also acceptable but more difficult to monitor owing to peaks and troughs in the level of anticoagulation. Subcutaneous regimens are also used and often require about 30,000 units/day administered in two to six equal doses.

Monitoring of heparin administration appears to be controversial, and we use the activated partial thromboplastin time (APTT). An initial test is performed to rule out coagulopathy and then repeated after 8 to 12 hours of therapy. Performance of the repeat test soon after the initial bolus of heparin may give misleading APTT elevation. A loading dose of approximately 10,000 units of heparin is recommended. The APTT can then be monitored with adjustment in dosage to maintain the values at twice normal levels.[14] Although many physicians do not recommend repeating APTT testing during therapy, we have found it helpful especially in elderly and critically ill patients. Therapy should be continued for 7 to 10 days with initiation of oral anticoagulation prior to the discontinuance of the heparin infusion. (Subcutaneous heparin twice a day is an acceptable but expensive alternative to oral anticoagulation.) A 3-month course of therapy with anticoagulants is arbitrarily believed to be adequate. This can be shortened if the underlying factors leading to embolus have been corrected. Long-term anticoagulation should be considered in certain patients (*i.e.,* those that are immobile, obese, or have underlying diseases such as cancer or cardiomyopathy).[147]

Thrombolytic therapy with either streptokinase or urokinase has emerged in recent years as an alternative. Expense has limited the use of urokinase, which is produced from human renal parenchymal cells, as opposed to the less expensive but more antigenic streptokinase.[194] This thrombolytic therapy has been shown to bring about more rapid resolution of emboli. Rapid resolution has not been shown, however, to reduce mortality or reduce the long-term extent of thrombosis following therapy. One group of patients who may especially benefit are those with prolonged hypotension secondary to emboli. Rapid resolution of the obstructing embolus with thrombolytic therapy is thus the only recommended use of these agents in pulmonary embolus.

Other therapy for massive pulmonary embolism with associated hypotension includes embolectomy. This may be preferred when an experienced cardiothoracic team with bypass facilities is available. Another surgical therapy in patients with pulmonary emboli is vena caval interruption. The technique of choice (plication, Mobin-Uddin umbrella, Hunter balloon, Greenfield filters)[29] depends on the experience of the surgeon and should be limited to the patient with angiographically proved embolism in whom recurrence of an embolus is anticipated to be lethal.[147] An example might include a patient who has sustained a pulmonary embolus following hospitalization for intracerebral hemorrhage or who had neurosurgery several days previously. In this situation, anticoagulation would be hazardous and yet recurrent embolization would be equally as lethal.

THE ASPIRATION SYNDROMES

Aspiration is common of gastric contents and oropharyngeal secretions, which generally pass without sequelae and later are cleared from the lung of the healthy individual.[104] In the elderly, however, aspiration of foreign material into the airways represents a debilitating and life-threatening problem. This appears to be due to underlying conditions that predispose the older patient to develop pulmonary complications. Principal conditions include alcoholism, seizure disorders, cerebrovascular accidents, tracheal intubation, sedative medications, general anesthesia, esophageal disease, and nasogastric tube feeding.[13,223] The significance of these predisposing factors, and their relationship to the severity of bronchopneumonia, has been documented in a nursing home population. Of 57 patients who were found to have bronchopneumonia at autopsy, 49% had underlying congestive heart failure while 72% had chronic brain damage with the severest disease present in this latter group.[189]

Applying the term *aspiration pneumonia* to all forms of possible consequences from aspiration may be misleading, since there are three separate syndromes: (1) aspiration of toxic fluids, (2) aspiration of bacterial pathogens, and (3) recurrent aspiration.

Aspiration of Toxic Fluids

The first of these syndromes involves aspiration of certain fluids that can initiate an inflammatory reaction that is independent of bacterial infection. Examples include acids, animal fats, mineral oil, alcohol, and hydrocarbons. Of these, gastric acid is the most frequently encountered and most completely studied. The most important factors determining the degree of lung injury appear to be the low *p*H and volume of fluid aspirated as documented by Mendelson.[223] Atelectasis occurs almost immediately and is followed by peribronchial exudate and hemorrhage, pulmonary edema, and areas of necrosis.

Clinical features include the acute onset of dyspnea, usually within 2 hours of the observed event. This is associated with bronchospasm and production of frothy, nonpurulent sputum, with

chest roentgenography showing widespread dense alveolar and interstitial infiltrates. Hypoxemia becomes prominent with determinations in the 35 mm Hg to 50 mm Hg range associated with a normal or low $Paco_2$. Such values indicate a large right-to-left intrapulmonary shunt owing to underventilated areas of the lung.

Treatment calls for aggressive ventilatory support, fluid management, and general supportive care. With aspiration of large food particles, manual removal from the hypopharynx should be performed or the Heimlich maneuver tried. Food particles more distal in the airway that do not respond to the above methods may require rigid bronchoscopy. Otherwise repeated tracheal suction may be necessary to clear the airway. The early initiation of ventilatory support based on blood-gas determinations, along with the appropriate application of continuous positive airway pressure (CPAP), appears to be one of the most important modes of supportive care. This offers the advantage of maintaining oxygenation without the risk of oxygen toxicity. Other modes of therapy such as lavage with saline or alkaline solutions are unnecessary since the acid is rapidly neutralized by tracheobronchial secretions. Likewise corticosteroids are of no proven benefit.[223] Antimicrobial therapy is controversial; its use as prophylaxis against infection when aspiration is diagnosed has not been documented. Early use may predispose the patient to development of more resistant infections following the initial lung injury from the effects of acid. Appropriate antibiotics should be employed if and when bacterial infection occurs.

Fluid management becomes of paramount importance in aspiration in the elderly. The large outpouring of fluid in the lung and hypovolemia is difficult to manage in these patients with underlying cardiac illness. Therefore, fluid management may require right-sided heart intracardiac pressure monitoring with a Swan-Ganz catheter.

Another toxic substance causing lung injury particularly in the elderly is mineral oil. Injudicious use may lead to lung injury with acute pneumonitis with basilar infiltrates on the chest film. Other patients may be relatively asymptomatic except for progressive dyspnea and may develop lower zone interstitial markings or pulmonary nodules that pathologically are lipoid granulomas.[13]

Aspiration of Bacterial Pathogens

The second syndrome of aspiration injury is caused by aspirates contaminated by oropharyngeal bacteria. This may also occur from aspiration of gastric contents that have become colonized. Although not uncommon in elderly persons with atrophic gastritis, this syndrome may become more common with the increased use of cimetidine, ranitidine, and antacids.[236] The initiating aspirate is usually small, and patients present not with respiratory failure but with infection. Evidence for infection is subtle, however, with nonspecific symptoms such as tachypnea, tachycardia, nocturnal dyspnea, and wheezing. Fever may not be present in the chronically aspirating elderly patient. Pneumonia may be found on the chest film with location in the dependent lung zones, that is, the posterior segments of the upper lobes and superior segments of the lower lobes, particularly on the right. The pneumonia may continue unnoticed with this paucity of symptoms, with subsequent development of an abscess or empyema.

Treatment involves adequate drainage of the affected area and appropriate therapy with antibiotics as well as correction of any predisposing factors. Empyemas are best drained by chest tube, while vigorous chest percussion and postural drainage will usually drain a lung abscess. In certain cases, however, bronchoscopy may be indicated to rule out an obstructing lesion such as tumor or foreign body.

Antibiotic therapy should be directed toward coverage of infection by organisms colonizing the oropharyngeal area, and expectorated sputum may show mixed gram-positive and gram-negative organisms on smear. Anaerobes are present in high quantity, with increased numbers noted in patients with poor oral hygiene. Organisms with the greatest pathogenic potential include anaerobic streptococci and *Fusobacterium* and *Bacteroides* species as well as aerobes such as pneumococcus. Hospitalized patients are likely to be colonized with enteric gram-negative bacilli (*e.g., Escherichia coli, Klebsiella*) *Pseudomonas,* or *Staphylococcus aureus.*[13] Therapy directed toward anaerobic infection such as lung abscess should include penicillin G, begun parenterally in doses of from 2 to 10 million units/day and continued after several days or weeks on an oral basis.[231] An equally effective regimen would include clindamycin, which has recently been suggested to be superior to penicillin.[122] Metronidazole has not been shown to be as effective.[167] It is important to emphasize that in these mixed infections, specific therapy for all organisms cultured is not necessary and some organisms may even be resistant to the drug used. For infection acquired in the hospital, there should be adequate coverage for gram-negative and gram-positive organisms, including *Straphylococcus* until

culture results are confirmed. A combination of an aminoglycoside with oxacillin, clindamycin, or a cephalosporin is recommended. Therapy, particularly for lung abscess, may continue for a prolonged period before resolution. Surgery is seldom if ever necessary, despite older literature describing its role.

Recurrent Aspiration

The third form of aspiration injury results from repeated small-volume aspirations and may present different clinical pictures. This is particularly a problem in the patients with alteration of the mechanical properties of the hypopharynx and esophagus either structurally or by altered neurologic control. Recurrent pulmonary infiltrates in dependent lung segments, adult-onset asthma, or changes in the lower lung field resembling miliary tuberculosis may all be clinical expressions of aspiration. Occasionally, recurrent and small aspirations, particularly with hiatal hernia, can result in pulmonary fibrosis in the lower lung fields without the history of recurrent pneumonia.[137]

PNEUMONIA

Lower respiratory tract infections are a major cause of morbidity and mortality among the elderly. Pneumonia and influenza together constitute the leading infectious cause of death in this older age-group and the fourth most common cause of death overall. Complications from pneumonia are also more common, such as bacteremia, empyema, and meningitis; all lead to increased mortality. The reasons for this appear to be age-related declines in immunologic defense systems.[78,101]

A second factor causing such high incidence of pneumonia is the prevalence of underlying disease, which is higher in this population.[223] An 80% to 100% incidence of diseases such as chronic obstructive pulmonary disease, cancer, alcoholism, diabetes mellitus, and arteriosclerotic heart disease appears correlated with pneumonia in the elderly. Chronic disease thus further decreases immunity and impairs respiratory tract clearance. This allows for pharyngeal colonization by pathogens that may be aspirated into the lungs. Institutionalized individuals undergoing treatments for chronic disease or courses of antibiotics have pneumonias more frequently due to gram-negative and other resistant organisms.

Clinical Picture

The clinical picture of pneumonia in the elderly is quite variable. Usual symptoms including chills, sweats, pleuritic chest pain, and sputum production may be present, but the clinician should not rely on these in making the diagnosis. Subtle changes in mental status, exacerbation of underlying chronic illness such as congestive heart failure, or COPD may be the only presenting features. The patient may even have chronic unresolving pneumonia, as in the debilitated nursing home patient with chronic aspiration. On physical examination, two reliable but nonspecific signs are tachypnea and tachycardia. Fever, when present, is a normal response to infection, but there may be extensive pneumonia, with only a nominal increase in temperature. Corticosteroids or infection with gram-negative organisms may further suppress the normal febrile response. Shallow respirations are frequently present in the elderly owing to a decrease in lung compliance, and thus adequate minute ventilation must be maintained by an increase in rate rather than tidal volume. An ineffectual cough may further illness owing to inability to clear secretions. Signs of consolidation on examination of the chest such as dullness to percussion and increased vocal fremitus and bronchial breath sounds may be absent. In one study, only one fourth of patients with radiographic diagnosis of pneumonia had appropriate findings on physical examination.[161] Furthermore, the characteristic finding of lobar or segmental consolidation may be distorted by underlying emphysema, producing a pattern of incomplete consolidation (Swiss cheese pattern). This may be interpreted as abscess or tuberculosis, leading to a delay in the correct diagnosis and treatment.[223]

Treatment

Examination of sputum is imperative in directing appropriate therapy, but it is often difficult to obtain an adequate expectorated sputum sample from the lower respiratory tract.[24,110,204] (See also Chapter 26.) Positive blood or thoracentesis cultures are invaluable in confirming the organism causing infection. When an accurate diagnosis is essential, bronchoscopy with a plugged brush followed by immediate transfer of the brush to quantitative cultures is currently showing promising results.[24] Highly specialized techniques are seldom required for routine therapy, and results can be misleading in the face of prior antibiotic therapy.

With pneumonia in the elderly, consideration

should be directed toward whether the infection is community acquired (Table 14-6) or whether it developed in an institution (hospital or nursing home) (Table 14-7).[78,223] *Streptococcus pneumoniae* remains the leading cause of community-acquired pneumonia with an increasing role of *Hemophilus influenzae* reported currently. Accurate determination of the rate of infection of anaerobic organisms in the elderly is not known. *Legionella* is being considered with increasing frequency since its recognition in 1976.[77] Its prevalence appears to be related to geographic areas, and in England it is considered to be the second most common cause of pneumonia.[239] (See Chapter 26.)

In nosocomial infection, there is a clear difference in causative organisms with the emergence of gram-negative organisms as indicated in Table 14-7. The pneumonia is believed to be acquired by aspiration of oropharyngeal contents, bacteremic spread (especially with *E. coli* pneumonia), and aerosolization equipment such as humidifiers

TABLE 14-6 Frequency of Community-Acquired Bacterial Pneumonias

Bacteria	%
Streptococcus pneumoniae	40–60
Hemophilus influenzae	2.5–20
Gram-negative bacilli	6–37
Staphylococcus aureus	2–10
Legionella	0–22.5
Anaerobic infections	?

(Verghese A, Berk SL: Bacterial pneumonia in the elderly. Medicine 62:271, 1983)

TABLE 14-7 Nosocomial Pneumonias: Frequency of Various Pathogens

Pathogen	%
Klebsiella	13
Pseudomonas aeruginosa	10–12
Staphylococcus aureus	3–10.6
Escherichia coli	4–7.2
Enterobacter	6.2
Group D *Streptococcus*	1.3
Proteus and *Providentia*	6
Serratia	3.5
Pneumococcus	10–20
Legionella	0–15
Aspiration (*i.e.*, anaerobic) pneumonia	?

(Verghese A, Berk SL: Bacterial pneumonia in the elderly. Medicine 62:271, 1983)

and ultrasonic nebulizers. Compressed gas nebulizers (in which the outlet tubing is below water level) have not been shown to lead to increased infection when properly sterilized and frequently changed.

In nonbacterial pneumonia, influenza continues to play a significant role in the elderly. Barker and co-workers[12] reported that 68% of deaths attributable to pneumonia and influenza type A (H_3N_2) occurred in persons over the age of 65. Influenza is considered in greater detail in Chapter 26, as are also the merits of influenza and pneumonia vaccination in the elderly.

REFERENCES

1. Alvarez S, McCabe WR: Extrapulmonary tuberculosis revisited: A review of experience at Boston City and other hospitals. Medicine 63:22, 1984
2. American College of Chest Physicians-National Heart Lung Blood Institute National Conference on Oxygen Therapy. Chest 86:234, 1984
3. American Thoracic Society: Definition and classification of chronic bronchitis, asthma, and pulmonary emphysema: A statement. Am Rev Respir Dis 85:762, 1962
4. American Thoracic Society: Guidelines for short-course tuberculosis chemotherapy. Am Rev Respir Dis 121:611, 1980
5. American Thoracic Society: Treatment of tuberculosis and other mycobacterial diseases. Am Rev Respir Dis 203:790, 1983
6. Anderson WM, Ryerson G, Block AJ: Evaluation of an intermittent demand nasal flow system with a fluidic valve (abstr). Chest 86:313, 1984
7. Andretti L, Bussotti A, Cammelli D et al: Connective tissue in aging lung. Gerontology 29:377, 1983
8. Annest LS, Kratz JM, Crawford FA: Current results of treatment of bronchiectasis. J Thorac Cardiovasc Surg 83:546, 1982
9. Ashba JK, Boyce JM: Undiagnosed tuberculosis in a general hospital. Chest 61:447, 1972
10. Aubier M, DeTroyer A, Sampson M et al: Aminophylline improves diaphragm contractility. N Engl J Med 305:249, 1981
11. Auerbach O, Hammond EC, Garfinkel L, Benante C: Relation of smoking and age to emphysema: Whole lung section study. N Engl J Med 286:853, 1972
12. Barker WH, Mullody JP: Pneumonia and influenza death during epidemics: Implications for prevention. Arch Intern Med 142:85, 1982
13. Bartlett JG, Gorbach SL: The triple threat of aspiration pneumonia. Chest 68:560, 1975
14. Basu D, Gallus A, Hirsh J, Cade J: A prospective study of the value of monitoring heparin treatment with the activated partial thromboplastin time. N Engl J Med 287:324, 1972
15. Bateman JRM, Daunt KM, Newman SP et al: Regional lung clearance of excessive bronchial secreation during chest physiotherapy in patients with stable chronic airways obstruction. Lancet 1:294, 1979
16. Bates JH: Diagnosis of tuberculosis. Chest 76:757, 1979
17. Baur LA, Blouin RA: Influence of age on theophylline clearance in patients wtih chronic obstructive pulmonary disease. Clin Pharmacokinet 6:469, 1981
18. Bell WR, Simon TL, DeMeto DL: The clinical features of submassive and massive pulmonary emboli. Am J Med 62:355, 1977
19. Belman MJ, Kendregan BA: Physical training fails to improve ventilatory muscle endurance in patients with chronic pulmonary disease. Chest 81:440, 1982
20. Belman MJ, Mittman C: Ventilatory muscle training improves exercise capacity in chronic obstructive pulmonary disease patients. Am Rev Respir Dis 121:273, 1980
21. Berezuk GP, Schondelmeyer SW, Seidenfield JJ et al: Clinical comparison of albuterol, isoetharine, and metaproterenol given by aerosol inhalation. Clin Pharm 2:129, 1983
22. Berger AJ, Mitchell RA, Severinghaus JW: Regulation of respiration. N Engl J Med 297:92, 138, 194, 1977
23. Berger HW, Mejia E: Tuberculous pleurisy. Chest 63:88, 1973
24. Berk SL, Holtsclaw SA, Khan A, Smith JK: Transtracheal aspiration in the severely ill elderly patient with bacterial pneumonia. J Am Geriatr Soc 29:228, 1981
25. Black LF, Hyatt RE: Maximal respiratory pressures: Normal values and relationship to age and sex. Am Rev Respir Dis 99:696, 1969
26. Block AJ, Boysen PG, Wynne JW, Hunt LA: Sleep apnea, hypopnea, and oxygen desaturation in normal subjects: A strong male predominance. N Engl J Med 300:513, 1979
27. Block AJ, Faulkner JA, Hughes RL et al: Factors influencing airway closure. Chest 86:114, 1984
28. Block AJ, Wynne JW et al: Menopause, medroxyprogesterone and breathing during sleep. Am J Med 70:506, 1981
29. Bomaloski JS, Martin GJ, Hughes RL, Yao JST: Inferior vena cava interruption in the management of pulmonary embolism. Chest 82:767, 1982
30. Borrowitz JD: Active tuberculosis undiagnosed until autopsy. Am J Med 72:650, 1982
31. Bosse R, Sparrow D, Rose CL et al: Longitudinal effects of age and smoking cessation on pulmonary function. Am Rev Respir Dis 123:378, 1981
32. Boushey HA, Holtzman MJ, Sheller JR, Nadel JA: Bronchial hyper-reactivity. Am Rev Respir Dis 121:389, 1980

33. Brashear RE: Should asymptomatic patients with inoperable bronchogenic carcinoma receive immediate radiotherapy? No. Am Rev Respir Dis 117:411, 1978

34. Brenner BE, Abraham E, Simon RR: Position and diaphoresis in acute asthma. Am J Med 74:1005, 1983

35. Breyer RH, Zippe C, Pharr WF et al: Thoracotomy in patients over age seventy years. J Thorac Cardiovasc Surg 81:187, 1981

36. Broekmans AW, Veltkamp JJ, Bertina RM: Congenital protein C deficiency and venous thromboembolism. N Engl J Med 309:340, 1983

37. Burk RH, George RB: Acute respiratory failure in chronic obstructive pulmonary disease. Arch Intern Med 132:865, 1973

38. Burwell C, Rubin E, Whaley R, Bikelmann A: Extreme obesity associated with alveolar hypoventilation: A pickwickian syndrome. Am J Med 21:811, 1956

39. Bynum LJ, Wilson JE: Characteristics of pleural effusions associated with pulmonary embolism. Arch Intern Med 136:159, 1976

40. Byrd RB, Carr DT, Miller WE et al: Radiographic abnormalities in carcinoma of the lung as related to histological cell type. Thorax 24:573, 1969

41. Campbell EJ, Lefrak SS: How aging affects the structure and function of the respiratory system. Geriatrics 33:68, 1978

42. Cancer Facts and Figures. New York, American Cancer Society, 1980

43. Carp H, Janoff A: Possible mechanisms of emphysema in smokers. Am Rev Respir Dis 118:617, 1978

44. Case RL, Roger PB et al: The protective effect of lodoxamide on antigen-induced bronchospasm. JAMA 247:661, 1982

45. Centor RM, Yarbrough B, Wood JP: Inability to predict relapse in acute asthma. N Engl J Med 577, 1984

46. Chang KC, Lauer BA, Bell TD et al: Altered theophylline pharmacokinetics during respiratory viral illness. Lancet 2:1132, 1978

47. Cherniak NS, Carton RW: Factors associated with respiratory insufficiency in bronchiectasis. Am J Med 41:562, 1966

48. Cherniak NS, Longobardo GS: Cheyne-Stokes breathing. N Engl J Med 288:952, 1973

49. Chodosh S: Objective sputum changes associated with glyceryl guaiacolate in chronic bronchial disease. Bull Eur Physiopathol Respir 9:452, 1973

50. Cohn JE, Carroll DG, Armstrong BW et al: Maximal diffusing capacity of the lung in normal male subjects of different ages. J Appl Physiol 6:588, 1954

51. Conrad KA, Nyman DW: Effects of metoprolol and propranolol on theophylline elimination. Clin Pharmacol Ther 28:463, 1980

52. Corkey CWB, Levision H, Turner JAP: The immotile cilia syndrome. Am Rev Respir Dis 124:544, 1981

53. Corrao WM, Braman SS, Irwin RS: Chronic cough as the sole presenting manifestation of bronchial asthma. N Engl J Med 300:633, 1979

54. Cox JD, Yesner RA: Adenocarcinoma of the lung: Recent results from the Veterans Administration Lung Group. Am Rev Respir Dis 120:1025, 1979

55. Cruz RS, Landa J, Hirsch J et al: Tracheal mucous velocity in normal man and patients with obstructive disease: Effects of terbutaline. Am Rev Respir Dis 109:458, 1978

56. Dalen JE, Haffajee CI, Alpert JS et al: Pulmonary embolism, pulmonary hemorrhage, and pulmonary infarction. N Engl J Med 296:1431, 1977

57. Dehn MM, Bruce RA: Longitudinal variations in maximal oxygen intake with age and activity. J Appl Physiol 33:805, 1972

58. DeMarco Jr JF, Wynne JW, Block AJ et al: Oxygen desaturation during sleep as a determinant of the ''blue and bloated'' syndrome. Chest 79:621, 1981

59. DeVries HA: Physiologic effects of an exercise training regimen upon men aged 52. J Gerontol 25:325, 1970

60. Dohi S, Gold MI: Comparison of two methods of postoperative respiratory care. Chest 73:592, 1978

61. Doll R, Petro R: Mortality in relation to smoking: 20 year's observations on British doctors. Br Med J 2:1525, 1976

62. Downing ET, Braman SS, Fox MJ, Corrao WM: Factitious asthma: Physiologic approach to diagnosis. JAMA 248:2878, 1982

63. DuMoilin GC, Patterson DG, Hedley-White J et al: Aspiration of gastric bacteria in antacid-treated patients: A frequent cause of postoperative colonization of the airway. Lancet 1:242, 1982

64. Dumon JF, Shapshay S, Bourcerray J et al: Principles of safety in application of neodymium-YAG laser in bronchology. Chest 86:163, 1984

65. Dutt AK, Jones L, Stead WW: Short-course chemotherapy for tuberculosis with largely twice-weekly isoniazid-rifampin. Chest 75:441, 1979

66. Edge JR, Millard FJC, Reid L, Simon G: The radiographic appearances of the chest in persons of advanced age. Br J Radiol 37:769, 1964

67. Edlin GP: Active tuberculosis unrecognized until necropsy. Lancet 1:650, 1978

68. Edwards WD, Edwards JE: Clinical primary pulmonary hypertension: Three pathologic types. Circulation 56:884, 1977

69. Ellis DA, Thornley PE, Wightman AJ et al: Present outlook in bronchiectasis: Clinical and social study and review of factors influencing prognosis. Thorax 36:639, 1981

70. Enarson DA, Grzybowski S, Dorken E: Failure of diagnosis as a factor in tuberculosis. Can Med Assoc J 118:1520, 1978

71. Fanta CH, Wright TC, McFadden EF: Differentiation of recurrent pulmonary embolism from chronic obstructive lung disease as a cause of cor pulmonale. Chest 79:92, 1981

72. Feldman J, Traver GA, Taussig LM: Maximal expiratory flows after postural drainage. Am Rev Respir Dis 119:239, 1979

73. Fischl MA, Pitchenik A, Gardner LB: An index predicting relapse and need for hospitalization in patients with acute bronchial asthma. N Engl J Med 305:783, 1981

74. Fishman AP: Chronic cor pulmonale: State of the art. Am Rev Respir Dis 114:775, 1976

75. Fishman DB, Petty TL: Physical, symptomatic, and psychological improvement in patients receiving comprehensive care for chronic airway obstruction. J Chron Dis 24:775, 1971

76. Fox RW, Samaan S, Bukantz SC et al: Theophylline kinetics in a geriatric group. Clin Pharm Ther 34:60, 1983

77. Fraser DW, Tsai TR, Orenstein W et al: Legionnaires' disease: Description of an epidemic of pneumonia. N Engl J Med 297:1189, 1977

78. Garb JL, Brown RB, Garb JR, Tuthill RW: Differences in etiology of pneumonias in nursing home and community patients. JAMA 240:2169, 1978

79. Gelb AF, Leffler C, Brewin A et al: Miliary tuberculosis. Am Rev Respir Dis 108:1327, 1973

80. Gelb AF, Zamel N: Effect of aging on lung mechanics in healthy nonsmokers. Chest 68:538, 1975

81. George RB: Some recent advances in the management of asthma. Arch Intern Med 142:933, 1982

82. Gertz I, Hedensterirna G, Wester PO: Improvement in pulmonary function with diuretic therapy in the hypervolemic and polycythemic patient with chronic obstructive pulmonary disease. Chest 75:146, 1979

83. Goldhaber SZ, Savage DD, Garrison RJ et al: Risk factors for pulmonary embolism: The Framingham study. Am J Med 74:1023, 1983

84. Goodall RJR, Earis JE, Cooper DN et al: Relationship between asthma and gastroesophageal reflux. Thorax 36:116, 1981

85. Gracey DR, Divertic MB, Didier EP: Preoperative pulmonary preparation of patients with chronic obstructive pulmonary disease. Chest 76:123, 1979

86. Greco FA, Oldham RK: Small-cell lung cancer. N Engl J Med 301:355, 1979

87. Guilleminault C, Simmons FB, Motta J: Obstructive sleep apnea syndrome and tracheostomy. Arch Intern Med 141:985, 1981

88. Guilleminault C, Tilkian A, Dement WC: The sleep apnea syndromes. Annu Rev Med 27:465, 1976

89. Halkin H, Goldberg J, Modan M et al: Reduction of mortality in general medicine in-patients by low dose heparin prophylaxis. Ann Intern Med 96:561, 1982

90. Harman EM, Wynne JW, Block AJ: The effect of weight loss on sleep-disordered breathing and oxygen desaturation in morbidly obese men. Chest 82:291, 1982

91. Harviel JD, McNamara CJ, Straehley CJ: Surgical treatment of lung cancer in patients over the age of 70 years. J Thorac Cardiovasc Surg 75:802, 1975

92. Hayata Y, Kato H, Konaka C et al: Photoradiation therapy with hematoporphyrin derivative in early and stage 1 lung cancer. Chest 86:169, 1984

93. Heaton RK, Grant I, McSweeny AJ et al: Psychologic effects of continuous and nocturnal oxygen therapy in hypoxemic chronic obstructive pulmonary disease. Arch Intern Med 143:1941, 1983

94. Hendeles L, Weinberger M, Milavetz G et al: Food-induced "dose-dumping" from a once-a-day theophylline product as a cause of theophylline toxicity. Chest 87:758, 1985

95. Hirsch SR, Viernes PF, Kory RC: The expectorant effect of glyceryl guaiacolate in patients with chronic bronchitis: A controlled *in vitro* and *in vivo* study. Chest 63:9, 1973

96. Hodgkin JE: The scientific status of chest physiotherapy. Respir Care 26:657, 1981

97. Hodgson JL, Burskirk ER: Physical fitness and age, with emphasis on cardiovascular function in the elderly. J Am Geriatr Soc 25:385, 1977

98. Hoffer P: Status of gallium-67 in tumor detection. J Nucl Med 21:394, 1980

99. Hogg JC, Williams J, Richardson JB et al: Age as a factor in the distribution of lower-airway conductance and in the pathologic anatomy of obstructive lung disease. N Engl J Med 282:1283, 1970

100. Hooper RG, Beechler CR, Johnson MC: Radioisotopic scanning in the initial staging of bronchogenic carcinoma. Am Rev Respir Dis 118:279, 1978

101. Howells CHL, Vesselinova-Jenkins CK, Evans AD: Influenza vaccination and mortality from bronchopneumonia in the elderly. Lancet 1:381, 1975

102. Hudson LD, Pierson DJ: Comprehensive respiratory care for patients with chronic obstructive pulmonary disease. Med Clin North Am 65:629, 1981

103. Hugh-Jones P, Whimster W: The etiology and management of disabling emphysema. Am Rev Respir Dis 117:343, 1978

104. Huxley EJ, Viroslav J, Gray WR et al: Pharyngeal aspiration in normal adults and patients with depressed consciousness. Am J Med 64:564, 1978

105. International Multicenter Trial. Prevention of fatal postoperative pulmonary embolism by low doses of heparin. Lancet 12:45, 1975

106. IPPB Trial Group. Intermittent positive pressure breathing therapy of chronic obstructive pulmonary disease: A clinical trial. Ann Intern Med 99:612, 1983

107. Jacobs MH, Seniro RM, Kessler G: Clinical experience with theophylline: Relationships between dosage, serum concentration and toxicity. JAMA 235:1983, 1976

108. Jones RL, Overton TR, Hammerlindl DM, Sproule

BJ: Effects of age on regional residual volume. J Appl Physiol 44:195, 1978

109. Kales A, Kales JD: Sleep disorders. N Engl J Med 290:487, 1974

110. Kalinske RW, Parker RH, Brandt D: Diagnostic usefulness and safety of transtracheal aspiration. N Engl J Med 276:694, 1969

111. Kanner RE, Renzetti AD Jr, Klauber MR et al: Variables associated with changes in spirometry in patients with obstructive lung diseases. Am J Med 67:44, 1979

112. Kaschula ROC, Druker J, Kipps A: Late morphologic consequences of measles: A lethal and debilitating lung disease among the poor. Rev Infect Dis 5:395, 1983

113. Kasik JE, Schudt S: Why tuberculosis is still a health problem in the aged. Geriatrics 35:63, 1977

114. Kearley R, Wynne JW, Block AJ et al: The effect of low flow oxygen on sleep disordered breathing and oxygen desaturation. Chest 78:682, 1980

115. Kipper MS, Moser KM, Kortman KE et al: Long-term follow-up of patients with suspected pulmonary embolism and a normal lung scan. Chest 82:411, 1982

116. Kirsh MM, Rotman H, Argenta L et al: Carcinoma of the lung: Results of treatment over ten years. Ann Thorac Surg 21:371, 1976

117. Laforet EG: Surgical management of chronic obstructive lung disease. N Engl J Med 278:175, 1972

118. Lam WK, So SY, Yu DYC: Response to oral corticosteroids in chronic airflow obstruction. Br J Dis Chest 77:189, 1983

119. Landesman SH, Smith PM, Schiffman G: Pneumococcal vaccination in elderly patients with COPD. Chest 84:433, 1983

120. Leblanc P, Ruff F, Milic-Emili J: Effects of age and body position on "airway closure" in man. J Appl Physiol 28:448, 1970

121. Lefcoe NM, Toogood JH et al: The addition of an aerosol anticholinergic to an oral β-agonist plus theophylline in asthma and bronchitis. Chest 82:300, 1982

122. Levison ME, Manguna CT, Lorber B et al: Clindamycin compared with penicillin for the treatment of anaerobic lung abscess. Ann Intern Med 98:466, 1983

123. Lichtenstein LM: An evaluation of the role of immunotherapy in asthma. Am Rev Respir Dis 117:119, 1978

124. Liebow AA: Biochemical and structural changes in the aging lung (summary). In Cander L, Moyer JH (eds): Aging of the Lung: Perspectives, p 97. New York, Grune & Stratton, 1964

125. Lippmann M, Fein A: Pulmonary embolism in the patient with chronic obstructive pulmonary disease. Chest 79:39, 1981

126. Livingston RB: Small cell carcinoma of the lung. Blood 56:575, 1980

127. Lopata M, Onal EM: Mass loading, sleep apnea, and the pathogenesis of obesity hypoventilation. Am Rev Respir Dis 126:640, 1982

128. McFadden ER Jr: Exertional dyspnea and cough as preludes to acute attacks of bronchial asthma. N Engl J Med 292:555, 1978

129. McFadden ER Jr, Ingram RH Jr: Exercise induced asthma: Observations on the initiating stimulus. N Engl J Med 301:763, 1979

130. McFadden ER, Lyons HA: Arterial blood gas tension in asthma. N Engl J Med 278:1027, 1968

131. Marquis JF, Carruthers SG, Spence JD et al: Phenytoin-theophylline interaction. N Engl J Med 307:1189, 1982

132. Marsh JD, Glynn M, Torman HA: Pulmonary angiography: Application in a new spectrum of patients. Am J Med 75:763, 1983

133. Martin TR, Lewis SW, Albert RK: The prognosis of patients with chronic obstructive pulmonary disease after hospitalization for acute respiratory failure. Chest 82:310, 1982

134. Martini N, Flehinger BJ, Zaman MB, Beattie EJ: Prospective study of 445 lung carcinomas with mediastinal lymph node metastasis. J Thorac Cardiovasc Surg 80:390, 1980

135. Matthay RA, Berger HJ: Cardiovascular performance in chronic obstructive pulmonary disease. Med Clin North Am 65:489, 1981

136. Mays EE: Intrinsic asthma in adults: Association with gastroesophageal reflux. JAMA 236:2626, 1976

137. Mays EE, Dubois JJ, Hamilton GB: Pulmonary fibrosis associated with tracheobronchial aspiration. Chest 69:512, 1976

138. Melamed MR, Flehinger BJ, Zaman MB et al: Screening for early lung cancer: Results of the Memorial Sloan-Kettering study in New York. Chest 86:44, 1984

139. Mellemgaard K: The alveolar-arterial oxygen difference: Its size and components in normal men. Acta Physiol Scand 67:10, 1966

140. Middleton E Jr, Atkins FM, Fanning M, Georgitis JW: Cellular mechanisms in the pathogenesis and pathophysiology of asthma. Med Clin North Am 65:1013, 1981

141. Miller JI et al: Carcinoma of the superior pulmonary sulcus. Ann Thorac Surg 28:44, 1979

142. Miller WT, MacGregor: Tuberculosis: Frequency of unusual radiographic findings. AJR 130:867, 1978

143. Mitchel RS, Stanford RE, Johnson JM et al: The morphologic features of the bronchi, bronchioles and alveoli in chronic airway obstruction: A clinicopathologic study. Am Rev Respir Dis 114:137, 1976

144. Mittman C, Edelman NH, Norris AH et al: Relationship between chest wall and pulmonary compliance and age. J Appl Physiol 20:1211, 1965

145. Morris JF, Koski A, Johnson LC: Spirometric stan-

dards for healthy nonsmoking adults. Am Rev Respir Dis 103:57, 1971

146. Moser KM: Pulmonary embolism. Am Rev Respir Dis 115:829, 1977

147. Moser KM, Fedullo PF: Venous Thromboembolism: Three simple decisions. Chest 83:117, 256, 1983

148. Mueller RE, Petty TL, Filley GF: Ventilation and arterial blood gas changes induced by pursed lip breathing. J Appl Physiol 28:784, 1970

149. Muiesan G, Sorbini CA, Grassi V: Respiratory function in the aged. Bull Eur Physiopathol Respir 7:973, 1971

150. Murry JF: The ketchup-bottle method. N Engl J Med 300:1155, 1979

151. Myers JA: Tapering off of tuberculosis among the elderly. Am J Public Health 66:1101, 1976

152. Nagami PH, Yoshikawa TT: Tuberculosis in the geriatric patient. J Am Geriatr Soc 31:356, 1983

153. Nathanson L, Hall TC: Lung tumors: How they produce their syndromes. Ann NY Acad Sci 230:367, 1974

154. Newman SD, Clarke SW: The proper use of metered dose inhalers. Chest 86:342, 1984

155. Nicotra MB, Rivera M, Awe RJ: Antibiotic therapy of acute exacerbations of chronic bronchitis. Ann Intern Med 97:18, 1982

156. Niewoehner DE, Kleinerman J: Morphologic basis of pulmonary resistance in the human lung and effects of aging. J Appl Physiol 36:412, 1974

157. Nocturnal oxygen therapy trial group: Continuous or nocturnal oxygen therapy in hypoxemic chronic obstructive lung disease: A clinical trial. Ann Intern Med 93:391, 1980

158. Nogrady SG, Evans WV, Davies BH: Reversibility of airways obstruction in bronchiectasis. Thorax 33:635, 1978

159. Oldenburg FA Jr, Dolovich MB, Montgomery JM et al: Effects of postural drainage, exercise and cough on mucus clearance in chronic bronchitis. Am Rev Respir Dis 120:739, 1979

160. Olsen GN, Block AJ, Swenson EW et al: Pulmonary function evaluation of the lung resection candidate: A prospective study. Am Rev Respir Dis 111:379, 1975

161. Osmer JC, Cole BK: The stethoscope and roentgenogram in acute pneumonia. South Med J 59:75, 1966

162. Paez PN, Phillipson EA et al: The physiologic basis of training patients with emphysema. Am Rev Respir Dis 95:944, 1967

163. Pardy RL, Rivington RN, Despas PJ et al: The effects of inspiratory muscle training on exercise performance in chronic airflow limitation. Am Rev Respir Dis 123:426, 1981

164. Pardy RL, Rivington RN, Despas PJ et al: Inspiratory muscle training compared with physiotherapy in patients with chronic airflow limitation. Am Rev Respir Dis 123:421, 1981

165. Park SS, Janis M, Shim CS et al: Relationship of bronchitis and emphysema to altered pulmonary function. Am Rev Respir Dis 102:927, 1970

166. Peach H, Pathy MS: Follow-up study of disability among elderly patients discharged from hospital with exacerbations of chronic bronchitis. Thorax 36:585, 1981

167. Perlino CA: Metronidazole vs. clindamycin treatment of anaerobic pulmonary infections. Arch Intern Med 141:1424, 1981

168. Peterson DD, Fishman AP: The lungs in later life. In Fishman AP (ed): Update: Pulmonary Diseases and Disorders, p 123. New York, McGraw-Hill, 1982

169. Peterson DD, Pack AI, Silage DA, Fishman AP: Effects of aging on ventilatory and occlusion pressure responses to hypoxia and hypercapnia. Am Rev Respir Dis 124:387, 1981

170. Petty TL, Brink GA, Miller MW et al: Objective functional improvement in chronic airway obstruction. Chest 57:216, 1970

171. Pham QT et al: Pulmonary function and rheologic status of bronchial secretions collected by spontaneous expectorations and after physiotherapy. Bull Eur Physiopathol Respir 9:293, 1973

172. Phillips TL, Miller RJ: Should asymptomatic patients with inoperable bronchogenic carcinoma receive immediate radiotherapy? Yes. Am Rev Respir Dis 117:405, 1978

173. Pierce JA, Ebert RV: The barrel deformity of the chest, the senile lung and obstructive pulmonary emphysema. Am J Med 25:13, 1958

174. Pierson RN Jr, Grieco MH: Isoproterenol aerosol in normal and asthmatic subjects. Am Rev Respir Dis 100:533, 1969

175. Postma DS, Burema J, Gimeno F et al: Prognosis in severe chronic obstructive pulmonary disease. Am Rev Respir Dis 119:357, 1979

176. Powell JR, Vozeth S, Hopewell P et al: Theophylline disposition in acutely ill hospitalized patients. Am Rev Respir Dis 118:229, 1978

177. Pump KK: The aged lung. Chest 60:571, 1971

178. Pump KK: Emphysema and its relationship to age. Am Rev Respir Dis 114:5, 1976

179. Rebuck As, Read J: Assessment and management of severe asthma. Am J Med 51:788, 1971

180. Reid L: Measurement of the bronchial mucous gland layer: A diagnostic yardstick in chronic bronchitis. Thorax 15:132, 1960

181. Reitberg DP, Bernhard H, Schentag JJ: Alteration of theophylline clearance and half life by cimetadine in normal volunteers. Ann Intern Med 95:582, 1981

182. Renton KW, Gray JD, Hall RI: Decreased elimination of theophylline after influenza vaccination. Can Med Assoc J 123:288, 1980

183. Renton KW, Gray JD, Hung OR: Depression of theophylline elimination by erythromycin. Clin Pharmacol Ther 30:422, 1981

184. Riker JB, Cacace LG: Double-blind comparison of metaproterenol and isoetharine-phenylephrine solutions in intermittent positive pressure breathing in bronchospastic conditions. Chest 78:723, 1980
185. Robinson S, Dill DB et al: Physiologic aging of champion runners. J Appl Physiol 41:46, 1976
186. Roehrs T, Zorick F et al: Age-related sleep-wake disorders at a sleep disorder center. J Am Geriatric Soc 31:364, 1983
187. Rosenberg M, Patterson R, Mintzer R et al: Clinical and immunologic criteria for the diagnosis of allergic bronchopulmonary aspergillosis. Ann Intern Med 86:405, 1977
188. Rossman I: True incidence of pulmonary embolization and vital statistics. JAMA 230:1677, 1974
189. Rossman I, Rodstein M, Bornstein A: Undiagnosed diseases in an aging population. Arch Intern Med 133:366, 1974
190. Sahn SA: Corticosteroids in chronic bronchitis and pulmonary emphysema. Chest 73:389, 1978
191. Samter M, Beers RF Jr: Intolerance to aspirin: Clinical studies and consideration of its pathogenesis. Ann Intern Med 68:975, 1968
192. Schmidt CD, Dickman ML et al: Spirometric standards for healthy elderly men and women. Am Rev Respir Dis 108:933, 1975
193. Settipane GA, Pudapukam RK: Aspirin intolerance: III Subtypes, familiar occurrence, and cross-reactivity with tartrazine. J Allergy Clin Immunol 56:215, 1975
194. Sharma GVRK, Cella G, Parisi AF, Sasarana AA: Thrombolytic therapy. N Engl J Med 306:1268, 1982
195. Shim C, Williams MH Jr: Bronchial response to oral versus aerosol metaproterenol in asthma. Ann Intern Med 93:428, 1980
196. Shure DA, Fedullo PF: Transbronchial needle aspiration of peripheral masses. Am Rev Respir Dis 128:1090, 1983
197. Sidney KH, Shephard RJ: Frequency and intensity of exercise training for elderly subjects. Med Sci Sports 10:125, 1978
198. Simpson RJ Jr, Podolak R, Mangano CA et al: Vagal syncope during recurrent pulmonary embolism. JAMA 249:390, 1983
199. Smith CB, Golden CA, Kanner RE et al: Association of viral and *Mycoplasma pneumoniae* infections with acute respiratory illness in patients with chronic obstructive pulmonary diseases. Am Rev Respir Dis 121:225, 1980
200. Smith TP, Kinasewitz GT, Tucker WY et al: Exercise capacity as a predictor of post-thoracotomy morbidity. Am Rev Respir Dis 129:730, 1984
201. Snyder RD, Siegal GL: An asthma triad. Ann Allergy 25:377, 1967
202. Somme LJ, Davis JA: Increased exercise performance in patients with severe COPD following inspiratory resistive training. Chest 81:436, 1982
203. Sorbini CA, Grassi V, Solinas E et al: Arterial oxygen tension in relation to age in healthy subjects. Respiration 25:3, 1968
204. Spencer CD, Beaty HN: Complications of transtracheal aspiration. N Engl J Med 276:304, 1972
205. Stack BHR: Diagnosis of tuberculosis in a general hospital. Br Med J 4:610, 1971
206. Stead WW: Tuberculosis among elderly persons: An outbreak in a nursing home. Ann Intern Med 94:606, 1981
207. Stead WW, Dutt AK: Chemotherapy for tuberculosis today. In Green GM, Daniel TM, Ball WC Jr (eds): Koch Centennial Memorial. Am Rev Respir Dis 125:94, 1982
208. Stempel DA, Boucher RC: Respiratory infection and airway reactivity. Med Clin North Am 65:1045, 1981
209. Sugerman HJ, Fairman RP, Linderman AK et al: Gastroplasty for respiratory insufficiency of obesity. Ann Surg 193:677, 1981
210. Tager I, Speizer FE: Role of infection in chronic bronchitis. N Engl J Med 292:563, 1975
211. Tarham S, Moffitt A, Sessler AD et al: Risk of anesthesia and surgery in patients with chronic bronchitis and chronic obstructive pulmonary disease. Surgery 74:720, 1973
212. Thaler E, Lechner K: Antithrombin III deficiency and thromboembolism. Clin Haematol 10:369, 1981
213. Thames MD, Alpert JS, Dalen JE: Syncope in patients with pulmonary embolism. JAMA 238:2509, 1977
214. Thompson NJ, Glassroth JL, Snider DE, Farer LS: The booster phenomenon in serial tuberculin testing. Am Rev Respir Dis 119:587, 1979
215. Thurlbeck WM, Ryder RC, Sternby N: A comparative study of the severity of emphysema in necropsy populations in three different countries. Am Rev Respir Dis 109:239, 1974
216. Thurlbeck WM, Simon G: Radiographic appearances of the chest in emphysema. AJR 130:429, 1978
217. Toshihiko S, Martin CJ, Hildebrandt J: Length-tension properties of alveolar wall in man. J Appl Physiol 30:874, 1971
218. Traver GA, Cline MG, Burrows B: Predictors of mortality in chronic obstructive pulmonary disease. Am Rev Respir Dis 119:895, 1979
219. Turner JM, Mead J, Wohl ME: Elasticity of human lungs in relation to age. J Appl Physiol 25:664, 1968
220. Underwood GH Jr, Hooper RG, Axelbaum SP et al: Computed tomographic scanning of the thorax in the staging of bronchogenic carcinoma. N Engl J Med 300:777, 1979
221. Urokinase Pulmonary Embolism Trial Study Group: The urokinase pulmonary embolism trial: A national cooperative study. Circulation 47(suppl II):1, 1973

222. Vejlsted H, Hjelms E, Jacobsen O: Results of pulmonary resection in cases of unilateral bronchiectasis. Scand J Thorac Cardiovasc Surg 16:81, 1982

223. Verghese A, Berk SL: Bacterial pneumonia in the elderly. Medicine 62:271, 1983

224. Wallace JM, Deutsch AL, Harrell JH, Moser KM: Bronchoscopy and transbronchial biopsy in evaluation of patients with suspected active tuberculosis. Am J Med 70:1189, 1981

225. Wang KP, Terry PB: Transbronchial needle aspiration in the diagnosis and staging of bronchogenic carcinoma. Am Rev Respir Dis 127:344, 1983

226. Wasserman K: Physiologic basis of exercise testing. In Fishman AP (ed): Assessment of Pulmonary Function, p 131. New York, McGraw-Hill, 1980

227. Waxman Ad, Julien PJ, Brachman MB et al: Gallium scintigraphy in bronchogenic carcinoma. Chest 86:178, 1984

228. Weill H, Ferrans VJ, Gray RM, Ziskind MM: Early lipid pneumonia. Am J Med 36:370, 1964

229. Weinberger M, Hendeles L, Ahrens R: Pharmacologic management of reversible obstructive airways disease. Med Clin North Am 65:579, 1981

230. Weinberger M, Hendeles L, Bighley L: The relation of product formulation to absorption of oral theophylline. N Engl J Med 299:852, 1978

231. Weiss W, Cherniak NS: Acute nonspecific lung abscess: A controlled study comparing orally and parenterally administered penicillin G. Chest 66:348, 1974

232. Williams DE, Pairolero DC, Davis CS et al: Survival of patients surgically treated for stage I lung cancer. J Thorac Cardiovasc Surg 82:70, 1981

233. Wolfe JD, Tachkin DP, Calvarese B et al: Bronchodilator effects of terbutaline and aminophylline alone and in combination in asthmatic patients. N Engl J Med 298:363, 1978

234. Woolner LD, Fontana RS, Sanderson DR et al: Mayo Lung Project: Evaluation of lung cancer screening through December 1979. Mayo Clin Proc 56:544, 1979

235. Workshop proceedings on bronchoprovocation technique for the evaluation of asthma. J Allergy Clin Immunol 64:563, 1979

236. Wynne JW, DeMarco FJ, Hood CI: Physiological effects of corticosteroids in foodstuff aspiration. Arch Surg 116:46, 1981

237. Yellin A, Benfield JR: Surgery for bronchogenic carcinoma in the elderly. Am Rev Respir Dis 131:197, 1985

238. York EL, Jones RL, Sproule BJ et al: Management of secondary polycythemia with hypoxic lung disease. Am Heart J 100:267, 1980

239. Yu VL, Kroboth FJ, Shonnard J, Brown A et al: Legionnaire's disease: new clinical perspective from a prospective pneumonia study. Am J Med 73:357, 1982

240. Ziment I: Respiratory Pharmacology and Therapeutics. Philadelphia, WB Saunders, 1978

15 Gastrointestinal Disorders in the Elderly

Lawrence J. Brandt

It is increasingly appreciated that the elderly patient reacts to disease processes in the digestive system in a different fashion than in earlier years. A few clinical examples borrowed from an extensive text[5] can illustrate this fact:

There are important disorders chiefly found in senescence, including preeminently presbyesophagus, atrophic gastritis, diverticulosis, and mesenteric vascular ischemia.

For any given symptom, the differential diagnosis may be very different in an elderly patient. What is routinely diagnosed as heartburn in a 30-year old may reflect esophageal candidiasis in an octogenarian. Severe rectal bleeding may suggest Crohn's disease in a 20-year old, whereas vascular ectasias or diverticulosis are of greater concern in patients over age 65.

The same disease process may be markedly different at extreme ends of the age spectrum. Celiac sprue in a youngster typically manifests itself with foul smelling diarrhea or growth retardation, whereas in an elderly patient, osteoporosis and hip fracture may be the sole expression of intestinal malabsorption.

What appears to be the same disease process in disparate age-groups may reflect totally different causes. Examples include the achalasia-like presentation of gastric carcinoma and the "atypical" behavior of ulcerative colitis in the elderly. It is now recognized that most colitis beginning after the age of 50 years is probably not idiopathic inflammatory bowel disease but rather (ischemic) colitis of vascular origin.

Complications that occur only after many decades of disease are therefore more commonly seen in the elderly. The neoplastic complications of celiac sprue and postgastrectomy carcinoma are illustrative.

ESOPHAGUS

Dysphagia

Patients ultimately diagnosed as having esophageal disease usually complain of "trouble swallowing," or dysphagia. Dysphagia is not a diagnosis but only a symptom and is conveniently classified by its location.[22]

Patients with oropharyngeal dysphagia usually complain that food seems to "stick on the way down"; elderly patients, especially when depressed, may also occasionally complain of inability to initiate swallowing, probably in part due to cortical inhibition. Lesions at the cardioesophageal junction notoriously present as symptoms localized to the sternal notch, and when a patient complains of dysphagia, apparently confined to the cervical region, a more general evaluation of the esophagus is needed. Cervical dysphagia is only infrequently accompanied by pain, and odynophagia should alert one to the possibility of a foreign body or infection in the oropharynx.

Incoordination of the swallowing mechanism may result in food being aspirated or regurgitated through the nose. Thus, oropharyngeal dysphagia is associated with postdeglutitive coughing, wheezing, recurrent pulmonary infections, and exacerbation of chronic pulmonary disease. Unexplained or recurrent pulmonary infection warrants evaluation of the swallowing mechanism and esophageal function. Patients with neurologic disorders have greater difficulty swallowing liquids than solids, and a complaint of nasal regurgitation following ingestion of liquids should prompt a search for a neurologic disorder. Less common but more specific complaints of oropharyngeal dysphagia are halitosis and "noisy" swallowing, both

DYSPHAGIA IN THE ELDERLY

Oropharyngeal Dysphagia

Malignancy
Central nervous system disease (*e.g.,* Parkinson disease, cerebral accident)
Peripheral nervous system disease (*e.g.,* diabetes mellitus)
Motor end-plate disease
Myopathy (thyroid disease), metabolic (polymyositis), autoimmune, inflammatory
Mechanical—intrinsic (carcinoma, stricture, webs); extrinsic (*e.g.,* cervical spine disease)
Postoperative (laryngectomy, tracheostomy)
Medication induced

Midesophageal Dysphagia

Malignancy—primary, contiguous
Motility disorder—presbyesophagus (esophageal spasm)
Stricture—Barrett's
Infectious—(*Candida,* herpes)

Distal Esophageal Dysphagia

Malignancy—gastric > esophageal
Reflux—esophagitis, stricture
Webs, rings, diverticula
Hernia—paraesophageal

of which may be seen with pharyngeal or esophageal stasis as in Zenker's diverticulum or achalasia.

Zenker's Diverticulum and Cricopharyngeal Dyschalasia

First described by William Hunter in 1769 as "obstructed deglutition from a preternatural dilatation of a bag found in the pharynx," this abnormality is usually documented after age 50. Symptoms develop insidiously and are those of oropharyngeal dysphagia in general; more specific complaints are "noisy" swallowing and postcibal or nocturnal regurgitation of undigested food because the diverticulum may empty in a retrograde direction when the patient is recumbent. Such diverticula are seen on upper gastrointestinal series projecting posteriorly through an area of potential weakness at the back of the pharynx. An associated incoordination or incomplete relaxation of the upper esophageal sphincter with pharyngeal contraction supports the controversial theory that cricopharyngeal dysfunction leads to high pharyngeal pressures, which in turn result in formation of a pulsion (Zenker's) diverticulum proximally.

In the management of oropharyngeal dysphagia any underlying disease should be treated with specific medication. In severely symptomatic patients with a documented abnormality of pharyngoesophageal motor function and without gastroesophageal reflux, cricopharyngeal myotomy is usually beneficial and a "good" result can be expected in about two thirds of patients; when the muscular dysfunction is due to preexisting vascular, degenerative, or neurologic disease, however, results are less predictable. Small diverticula usually disappear spontaneously after cricopharyngeal myotomy, but diverticulectomy or diverticulopexy may also be performed if the diverticulum is large.

Sideropenic Dysphagia (Plummer-Vinson, Paterson-Kelly syndrome)

Sideropenic dysphagia refers to the association of dysphagia and iron deficiency that is variably accompanied by glossitis, cheilosis, anemia, achlorhydria, splenomegaly, and koilonychia.[24] Its etiology is probably nutritional (especially iron deficiency), but possibly it is autoimmune. The condition is quite rare in the United States now and is usually seen in association with secondary iron deficiency (*e.g.,* after gastrectomy). Most commonly, the dysphagia is associated with a postcricoid web, although upper esophageal strictures, thickened folds, and ulcers have also been seen. About half the patients are older than 50, and of further importance in the elderly is its association with autoimmune diseases (*e.g.,* myxedema) and pernicious anemia because of the subsequent development of oropharyngeal or esophageal carcinoma. Treatment consists of nutritional repletion and dilatation of the web; periodic surveillance for supervening carcinoma is mandatory.

Presbyesophagus

Presbyesophagus refers to alterations in esophageal motility thought to be due to degenerative aging changes of esophageal muscle.[38] A normal complete esophageal response to swallowing (*i.e.,* a relaxation phase), followed by a contraction phase and ultimately a return to baseline, is seen less frequently in subjects over 60 years of age. Resting esophageal pressures are generally higher in older patients and may reflect incomplete emptying of the esophagus because of weak and disordered esophageal pressure contractions. Peristaltic contractions appear to be relatively weaker and their velocity may be slower in older individuals, especially in the upper esophagus. The distinction between age-related changes in esophageal function and disease seems to lie in the degree rather than in the nature of the motility changes.[26]

Symptomatic Diffuse Esophageal Spasm

Dysphagia and chest pain with high amplitude, nonperistaltic, simultaneous and spontaneous contraction waves is referred to as symptomatic diffuse esophageal spasm. In some cases, there are striking abnormalities on barium esophagography. Patients may present with anginal-type chest pain indistinguishable from that of coronary artery disease and relieved by nitroglycerin.[4] Thus, esophageal motility testing is an integral part of the evaluation of patients having "atypical" chest pain. The keystone in managing esophageal hypermotility disturbances is the use of smooth muscle relaxants such as nitroglycerin, long-acting nitrates, or perhaps the newer calcium channel blocking agents such as nifedipine and verapamil. Diffuse esophageal spasm can be effectively managed with long-acting nitrites over extended periods in the absence of reflux. If there is a reflux, the use of nitrites is unpredictable and less effective. For selected patients with severe symptoms not responsive to medical therapy, esophagomyotomy may be advisable.

Lower Esophageal Ring

The lower esophageal or "Schatski" ring is a thin, membranous, annular ridge of mucosa projecting perpendicularly into the lower esophageal lumen and located at or near the squamocolumnar junction.[18] The most common symptom is acute dysphagia, typically occurring when the patient is eating a hurried meal; hence the rubric "steakhouse syndrome." After an initial episode, there frequently are not further difficulties for an extended period of time. However, as the lumen of the ring diminishes to less than 12 mm, recurrent and progressive attacks are characteristic. Total obstruction of the esophagus secondary to food impaction may bring the patient to the emergency department. Immediate therapy may be administering a solution of "meat tenderizer" to "digest" enough of the impacted food to allow it to pass. The solution is made by adding a tablespoon of commercially available crude papain powder to 250 ml of warm water. One ounce is administered every 30 minutes. If the impacted bolus does not pass, it must be removed by esophagoscopy. The ring is best diagnosed by roentgenographic study. Multiple endoscopic biopsies to disrupt the ring, dilatation with mercury-weighted bougies, or even pneumatic dilatation are techniques used to treat symptomatic rings. Surgical resection is rarely required.

Diaphragmatic Hernias

The incidence of esophageal hiatal hernias increases progressively with each decade from less than 10% in those under 40 years to approximately 40% in those in the sixth and seventh decades and finally to 70% in patients older than 70. Direct hernias are usually small and commonly "slide" back and forth between the thoracic and abdominal cavities. Many of the symptoms formerly attributed to the hiatal hernia itself (*e.g.*, pyrosis and regurgitation) are now ascribed to lower esophageal sphincter dysfunction, which is independent of the hernia. The paraesophageal hernia is an uncommon hernia that occurs most often in patients between the ages of 60 and 70 years. Paraesophageal hernias are of major importance because significant complications are frequent. They may be present for many years with few or no symptoms and, if untreated, usually enlarge until the bulk of the stomach lies within the thorax. As the parahiatal defect enlarges and herniation occurs, the stomach usually undergoes an organoaxial volvulus, the so-called upside down stomach. The volvulus tends to be recurrent as the gastric anchoring attachments progressively stretch. Paraesophageal hernias are frequently asymptomatic or cause only nagging discomfort until mechanical entrapment of the hernia. Such a catastrophe is associated with progressive distention of the incarcerated segment, vascular embarrassment, hemorrhage, gangrene, and perforation. In the absence of contraindications the "mere" presence of a parahiatal hernia is enough to warrant surgical repair.[19]

Reflux Esophagitis

The lower esophageal sphincter is the most important and most studied physiologic barrier to gastroesophageal reflux. The only deviation in the manometric characteristics of the "old" sphincter is reduction in amplitude of the postdeglutitive contraction. The relative normalcy of the sphincter and the observations that (1) gastrin, a hormone that increases the strength of the lower esophageal sphincter, tends to rise with aging, (2) the sphincter demonstrates supersensitivity to gastrin, and (3) gastric acid secretion diminishes with advancing age explain the infrequent complaint of reflux for the first time in advanced age. Thus, when an aged individual complains of new-onset substernal burning, other disorders must be excluded before assuming the presence of reflux esophagitis. However, the complications of chronic and asymptomatic reflux such as stricture may be the initial presentation of esophagitis in approximately 20% of affected elderly patients. Thus, not all elderly patients with dysphagia and a distal esophageal stricture have carcinoma.

Therapy of gastroesophageal reflux in the elderly is the same as in the younger group. It consists of such simple measures as elevating the head of the bed, dietary restrictions (avoidance of fats, chocolate, and alcohol), avoidance of certain drugs (theophylline, anticholinergics, β-adrenergic agonists, α-adrenergic antagonists, dopamine, diazepam, and the calcium channel blocking agents), and the use of antacids. Therapeutic agents for reflux symptoms include bethanechol, metoclopramide, and cimetidine. Bethanechol is a cholinergic agent that increases lower esophageal sphincter pressure and improves the acid-clearing capacity of the esophagus. This agent may produce dangerous hypertension and reflex tachycardia, and it is contraindicated in the presence of organic obstruction of the urinary tract (*e.g.,* prostatic hypertrophy). Patients who fail to respond to medical therapy may require surgical intervention to create an antireflux barrier or to dilate or resect a distal stricture. Advanced age is no longer considered an obstacle to surgery. However, with evolving nonoperative techniques for dilatation of strictures (*e.g.,* the use of Eder-Puestow olives, mercury bougies, and more recently, inflatable balloon catheters), the need for operative procedures may diminish.

Columnar Epithelium-Lined Esophagus (Barrett's Esophagus)

In Barrett's esophagus the lower esophagus is lined for a variable distance by columnar rather than the usual stratified squamous epithelium. Its importance lies in its association with deep esophageal ulcers, high esophageal strictures, and adenocarcinoma of the esophagus.[32] The columnar lining is believed to be a consequence of gastroesophageal reflux, in which damaged esophageal squamous epithelium is replaced by an overgrowth of gastric columnar cells. Most cases occur between ages 50 and 70, although the exact incidence is unknown. The most common symptoms

are those of reflux itself, and the entity is diagnosed by barium roentgenography, radionuclide scanning with ^{99m}Tc pertechnetate, manometrically guided suction biopsies, esophageal potential difference measurements, and esophagoscopy with biopsy. Stricture and neoplasia are important long-term complications of Barrett's esophagus. By careful periodic screening using esophagoscopy with directed biopsy and cytology, premalignant dysplastic changes can be detected. The development of severe dysplasia or carcinoma *in situ* mandates resection of the involved esophagus. Antacids and cimetidine therapy usually result in symptomatic improvement, but regression of the columnar epithelium has not been reported.

Dysphagia Aortica

Impingement on the mobile upper esophagus by a thoracic aortic aneurysm or compression of the anatomically restricted distal esophagus between the rigid atherosclerotic aorta posteriorly and the heart anteriorly is known as dysphagia aortica. Most patients respond to conservative measures (*e.g.,* avoiding bulky and solid foods), although occasionally the obstruction is severe enough to warrant surgical mobilization of the esophagus at the hiatus.

Esophageal Diverticula

Mid-esophageal as well as epiphrenic diverticula occur with increased frequency in elderly patients. The former are usually asymptomatic, but the latter are frequently associated with thoracic symptoms. The epiphrenic diverticulum is almost invariably associated with an esophageal motility disorder or hiatal hernia, thus the need for analyzing the actual cause of the patient's complaints. Treatment for reflux or a structural motility disorder may totally relieve complaints of dysphagia and chest pain.[11] With large diverticula, surgical resection may be necessary. Complications of large diverticula include halitosis and local problems of infection, abscess, perforation with mediastinitis, and recurrent aspiration and pulmonary infections.

Esophageal Neoplasms

Esophageal cancer occurs most frequently between the ages of 50 and 70 years and is two to six times more common in the male. In the United States it accounts for approximately 2% of all reported cancers. The cause is unknown, although the following carcinogenic factors have been implicated:

thermal irritation, poor intraoral hygiene, esophageal stasis, and exogenous toxins including alcohol and tobacco. An association has also been noted with certain acquired esophageal diseases, especially achalasia, lye stricture, Plummer-Vinson syndrome, and previous gastric surgery. Approximately 95% of esophageal malignancies are squamous cell carcinoma. Most "esophageal" adenocarcinoma represents cancer of the gastric fundus that has spread proximally. However, true cases of primary adenocarcinoma usually arise in columnar epithelium–lined (Barrett's) esophagus. Esophageal cancer most commonly involves the middle third of the esophagus. Local spread occurs early, and because the esophagus dilates so readily, dysphagia, the most common complaint at the time of diagnosis, is a late symptom. An important presentation of esophageal cancer in the elderly is that of an achalasialike syndrome. Primary achalasia is uncommon in patients past age 50, and the diagnosis should be made with caution in this age-group. Such patients with symptoms for less than 1 year and with marked weight loss should be considered to have achalasia secondary to malignancy, most often gastric adenocarcinoma. The pathogenesis of secondary achalasia is unknown; possibly this motility disorder reflects a paraneoplastic neuropathic state.

Prognosis for esophageal cancer is usually dismal. Surgical extirpation of the lesion and radiation therapy are the accepted primary modes of therapy. Chemotherapy may result in symptomatic improvement but little change in the survival time. Fewer than half of all patients presenting with esophageal carcinoma have operable conditions. Even in this highly selected group, postoperative mortality rates from pooled statistics approximate 25%, with a cumulative 5-year survival rate after resection of slightly less than 10%.

Palliative therapy with endoscopically placed esophageal stents has been gaining in popularity. Tytgat reviewed part of the European experience, comprising 2,683 patients with an age range of 54 to 69 years. Early and late procedure-related complications totaled only about 5%, with just four procedure-related deaths.[43a] Although survival was not altered by insertion of the prosthesis, the quality of life improved.

Medication-Induced Esophageal Injury

Esophageal injury can occur due to the local caustic effects of medications. The most frequent offenders are antibiotics, especially of the tetracycline class, potassium chloride, ferrous sulfate, quinidine, and a variety of steroidal and nonsteroidal anti-inflammatory preparations.[27] Most patients with medication-induced esophageal injury have no underlying esophageal disorders; some have preexisting esophageal compression due to either valvular heart disease with left atrial enlargement or to mediastinal adhesions following thoracic surgery. The most frequent symptoms are odynophagia and retrosternal pain. Of note is the appearance on single contrast barium esophagography of a lesion resembling malignancy with esophageal irregularity, narrowing, and intraluminal polypoid defects caused by quinidine injury. Symptoms of medication-induced esophageal injury usually resolve within 6 weeks. Continuing the medication may result in worsening symptoms and even death. Patients should be advised not to take pills at bedtime when esophageal retention is promoted by recumbency and the decrease in salivation and swallowing during sleep. Furthermore, pills should never be taken dry but with sufficient water to ensure their passage into the stomach.

Miscellaneous Forms of Esophagitis

Candidiasis

Esophageal candidiasis is a disease of the elderly, perhaps because of diminution in esophageal peristalsis, reduction in gastric acid secretion, and the age-related alterations in both cellular and humoral immunity. Other predisposing conditions in the elderly include malignancy, endocrine disorders (hypoadrenalism, hypothyroidism, hypoparathyroidism), malnutrition, surgery, longstanding venous and urinary bladder catheterization, and antibiotic and drug use.

Symptoms of esophageal candidiasis are nonspecific, but in the clinical settings mentioned dysphagia, odynophagia, or substernal burning should suggest it. Even in the presence of infection, up to one half of patients may be asymptomatic. The absence of oral thrush does not guarantee the lack of esophageal involvement. The diagnosis may be suggested by an abnormal barium esophagogram and can be confirmed by esophagoscopy, biopsy, and cytologic smears. On esophagoscopy, the candidal lesions typically appear as raised white plaques associated with hyperemia, ulceration, and friability. Serum *Candida* agglutinin titers of less than 1:160 militate against the diagnosis of *Candida* esophagitis, while a titer of 1:160 may be due to *Candida* infection in other organs or reflect a past infection. In the presence of esophageal symptoms, such an elevated titer suggests the diagnosis.

Most patients respond to oral therapy with either nystatin troches or ketoconazole. Failure to respond, with continuing symptoms and documentation that the fungus is invasive, necessitates systemic therapy with antifungal agents.

Irradiation

One of the major limiting side-effects of intrathoracic radiation is development of acute esophagitis. Symptoms of radiation esophagitis usually begin within 3 weeks of the initiation of therapy and continue for several weeks after the completion. Esophagoscopy may be necessary to differentiate radiation esophagitis from candidiasis superimposed on a radiated esophagus. Radiation esophagitis usually resolves without sequelae, however, stricture formation and tracheoesophageal fistulization have been reported. A study in the opossum demonstrated that indomethacin significantly reduces the severity of acute radiation esophagitis; it is hoped that this may be applicable to the human.

Esophageal Involvement in Systemic Diseases

The esophagus is rarely involved in systemic diseases that occur in old age. Esophageal involvement has been documented with connective tissue diseases (polymyositis), skin diseases (pemphigoid and pemphigus), and endocrine and metabolic disorders (diabetes mellitus, myxedema, and amyloid).

Abnormal esophageal motility is found in approximately half of patients with diabetes mellitus. It is characterized by an absence or a decrease in the primary peristaltic wave, reduced lower esophageal sphincter pressures, delayed esophageal emptying, and esophageal dilatation. A close correlation exists between the frequency and severity of the esophageal motor abnormalities and peripheral neuropathy. However, esophageal symptoms in the diabetic patient should not be attributed to a neuropathy until other causes have been excluded by appropriate studies.

STOMACH

It is generally accepted that gastric secretion diminishes with advancing age, although the methods used to establish this belief are not considered sensitive enough today. Most older studies were performed on fractional gastric samples withdrawn after a test meal. "Free acid" denoted the amount of acid that could be titrated up to the change in color of Topfer's reagent, a reaction that occurs at pH 2.8 to 3.5. However, "absence of free acid" is not synonymous with true achlorhydria. Furthermore, in some studies the gastric secretory maximum was not achieved because of an inadequate stimulus. The classic Ewald test meal was demonstrated by Bockus and Bank[2] to be just such an inadequate stimulus, since 47% of those who did not show "free acid" in response to the test meal showed a secretory response to histamine. In the elderly, the gastric secretagogue pentagastrin is preferred to histamine or histalog. The latter in a dosage sufficient for maximal parietal cell stimulation may produce potentially hazardous side-effects (flushing, hypotension, nausea, and cramps). With these reservations in mind, almost all studies show a reduced acid secretion with aging both in normal subjects and those with ulcer disease and also that relative hypochlorhydria is more common than absolute anacidity.[44] As gastric acid secretion diminishes with aging, the basal gastrin concentration increases.

In 1933, Sagal and associates[36] speculated that the presence of "high acid" in old age might be an index to longevity. Vanzant and her colleagues showed that there was a decrease in the incidence of achlorhydria after age 65, possibly because patients with achlorhydria were not "hardy or long lived" as were those with "strong acid gastric juice."[45] Is it possible that a 65-year-old patient with achlorhydria is actually biologically older than a patient of similar age whose stomach still produces acid? The histologic appearance of the aged stomach has been correlated with gastric secretion especially in atrophic gastritis and gastric atrophy.

Atrophic Gastritis and Gastric Atrophy

In atrophic gastritis there is a variable amount of inflammation accompanied by an equally variable degree of atrophy. Atrophic gastritis tends to be progressive and may eventuate in gastric atrophy. Gastric atrophy is a more diffuse disorder characterized by a reduction in the number of chief and parietal cells in the mucosa of the gastric body and fundus with atrophy of the deeper antral mucosal glands. In general, there is an increased frequency of these atrophic changes with advancing age and a close correlation between gastric secretory function and the histologic appearance.[1] In superficial gastritis, gastric secretion is lessened, and with development of atrophic gastritis or gastric atrophy, the ability to secrete acid is progressively reduced.[25] Atrophic gastritis is classified into two types.[42] Type A is characterized by antiparietal cell antibody in the serum and is a diffuse process with relative antral sparing. Acid secretion is markedly reduced with resultant hypergastrinemia and eventually impaired vitamin B_{12} absorption (i.e., pernicious anemia). Type B lacks serum antiparietal cell antibody and is a more focal antral process with less reduction of acid secretion, normal gastrin levels, and only rare malabsorption of vitamin B_{12}. Type A disease also has a greater frequency of associated autoimmune disease including thyroiditis, hyperthyroidism and hypothyroidism, diabetes mellitus, hypoadrenalism, and hypoparathyroidism.

Atrophic gastritis and gastric atrophy are usually asymptomatic, but dyspepsia, abdominal pain, distention, nausea, and vomiting may develop. Intermittent diarrhea has been noted in approximately 10% of achlorhydric patients ("gastrogenous diarrhea") and may justify a search for parasitic infestation or bacterial overgrowth. Gastric ulcer occurs with increased frequency in atrophic gastritis and may be symptomatic. It is believed that the gastritis is a cause rather than a result of the ulcer. Hypochromic microcytic anemia and iron deficiency are also associated with atrophic gastritis. The incidence of cancer in atrophic gastritis is similar to that in pernicious anemia and approximates 10% in patients observed for up to 20 years.[46] An etiologic role for intestinal metaplasia has been postulated for some gastric cancers, and occasionally a clear transition is seen between the metaplastic and neoplastic epithelia. Once a patient with atrophic gastritis or gastric atrophy has been identified periodic surveillance for carcinoma with endoscopic cytology and biopsy techniques is advisable.

Pernicious Anemia

The adult form of pernicious anemia is a distinct variety of atrophic gastritis selectively involving the parietal cell and the synthesis of gastric acid and intrinsic factor. The intrinsic factor is a specific binder of cyanocobalamin that protects it from bacterial destruction. Without it, only about 2% of the vitamin is absorbed.

Pernicious anemia has an insidious onset and is most often diagnosed by the discovery of a profound anemia out of proportion to the patient's complaints. The classic triad consists of weakness, sore tongue, and paresthesias. Laboratory investi-

gation reveals a typical peripheral blood smear with macro-ovalocytosis and hypersegmented granulocytes, and a megaloblastic bone marrow; a slight unconjugated hyperbilirubinemia due to destruction of erythrocyte precursors within the bone marrow (i.e., "ineffective" erythropoiesis); high levels of lactic dehydrogenase activity in the serum; histamine-fast achlorhydria, with the scant gastric juice containing a reduced pepsin concentration and being devoid of intrinsic factor; elevated levels of gastrin in the serum because of the achlorhydria; and the hallmark of the disease, greatly reduced vitamin B_{12} levels in the serum.

Many disorders in the elderly can produce a low serum vitamin B_{12} level so that the diagnosis of pernicious anemia usually relies on tests, the most popular of which is the Schilling test. The differential diagnosis of pernicious anemia in the elderly includes small bowel bacterial overgrowth, infestation by fish tapeworm (*Diphyllobothrium latum*), pancreatic insufficiency, Zollinger-Ellison syndrome, small intestinal disorders such as Crohn's disease, intestinal or gastric surgery, folate deficiency, and drug-induced cyanocobalamin malabsorption. The reader is referred elsewhere for a further discussion.[5]

Treatment with parenteral vitamin B_{12} has completely changed the "pernicious" prognosis formerly described. Overtransfusion of an otherwise stable patient with a low hematocrit and acute hypokalemia due to massive reticulocytosis after therapy are the major causes of death. The most serious long-term complication is carcinoma of the stomach, which is found in up to 10% of patients. The gastric cancers in pernicious anemia typically are bulky and slow growing. A postulated immunologic etiology for adult pernicious anemia is based on the high frequency of autoantibodies in the serum, on aberrations in cellular immunity, and on the association with other immunologic disorders.

Peptic Ulcer Disease

The number of elderly patients hospitalized with peptic disease, especially with duodenal ulcer, is on the increase. Ulcer disease in the elderly frequently exhibits a virulent course with more complications and a higher mortality than in the young.[33] Duodenal ulcer occurs two to three times more frequently than gastric ulcer, but the latter is responsible for two of every three deaths. The incidence of ulcer-related deaths seems unchanged in those older than 60 years, and the death rate increases with advancing age.

A history of exposure to drugs capable of precipitating ulcer disease is common in elderly patients. Anticoagulants and drugs used in the treatment of rheumatoid disorders, including corticosteroids and the nonsteroidal anti-inflammatory agents (*e.g.,* aspirin, indomethacin, phenylbutazone), are especially notorious.

The presentation late in life tends to be rather acute, often with bleeding or perforation, but it is not uncommon for symptoms to be more variable and subtle than in younger years; this is especially true for gastric ulcers. So-called geriatric ulcers high in the cardia may cause misleading symptoms, such as dysphagia mimicking esophageal neoplasm or substernal pain mistaken for angina. Chronic blood loss is more common with gastric than duodenal ulcers. The resultant anemia may lead to cardiac or cerebral symptoms, which can further confuse the clinical picture. Profound weight loss and poor health may be the only complaints and suggest a malignancy, a presentation characteristic of giant gastric and giant duodenal ulcers.

The complication rate rises progressively from 31% in patients 60 to 64 years of age to 76% in those 75 to 79 years of age.[28] *Bleeding* is the most common complication, accounting for one half to two thirds of all fatalities.[28] In a surgical series reporting patients with exsanguinating hemorrhage, the age distribution peaked during the seventh decade, with 40% over 65.[6] Surgery should not be withheld nor delayed solely because of advanced age. The first episode of persistent or massive bleeding in an elderly patient, especially from a gastric source, should prompt surgical intervention. In a patient whose condition is unstable, endoscopic therapy or angiographic therapy with intra-arterial vasoconstrictors or embolic agents may be lifesaving.

Perforation is the second most frequent complication. Signs and symptoms attending this catastrophe may differ from the classic picture of acute severe pain and rapidly developing boardlike abdominal rigidity seen in younger patients. The less dramatic or subtle presentation associated with atypical signs and symptoms often leads to an inordinate delay in diagnosis and a needlessly high mortality rate.[39]

Gastric outlet *obstruction* complicates ulcer disease in 10% to 15% of patients over 60 and almost exclusively in those with a long history of peptic disease[39]; the symptoms are similar to those of younger patients. Since gastric carcinoma not infrequently causes antropyloric obstruction in the advanced years, coexistence of a malignant lesion must be excluded. The initial therapy of gastric outlet obstruction includes correction of fluid and electrolyte balances and nasogastric intubation to decompress the stomach. In selected cases, stenosis of the pylorus may be treated endoscopically, using dilating balloon catheters.

Intractability is an uncommon problem among elderly patients with peptic disease and rarely necessitates surgical intervention. Intractable pain usually indicates a superimposed complication or the presence of a particularly virulent form of ulcer disease, such as giant duodenal ulcer or giant gastric ulcer.

Giant Duodenal Ulcer

When an ulcer exceeds 2 cm in diameter or involves much of the surface area of the bulb, it often behaves so dissimilarly from the smaller more usual ulcer that it should be considered a different entity. Giant duodenal ulcer presents most frequently in the seventh decade predominantly in men, many without a history of ulcer disease. Abdominal pain is the most frequent symptom, and often it radiates to the back or right upper quadrant and mimics pancreatic or gallbladder disease. It is variably relieved by antacids and may be worsened by eating. Significant weight loss often accompanies the pain and may raise the specter of malignancy. Gastrointestinal bleeding occurs in most patients, and serum albumin levels are usually below normal, probably due to protein loss from the ulcer bed. The diagnosis is usually established by roentgenologic means, although a large ulcer may be mistaken for the duodenal bulb. Giant duodenal ulcers are frequently complicated by bleeding, penetration, pyloroduodenal obstruction, perforation, and inflammatory masses. Surgical therapy has been considered preferable but in an individual who is stable and without pressing need for emergent surgery, a course of medical therapy is reasonable. Twenty-five years ago giant duodenal ulcers were uniformly fatal, but one recent report consisting of medically and surgically treated patients demonstrated a giant ulcer–related mortality rate of only 8%.[12]

Giant Gastric Ulcer

A giant gastric ulcer is one with a diameter of 3 cm or more. It is slightly more common in males, with a peak incidence at age 60 to 70 in men and 70 to 80 in women. Pain is not a major complaint, but only about 10% are totally pain free. In about 20% the pain is typical with radiation to the chest, periumbilical region, or lower abdomen and with high complication and mortality rates.[41] Hemorrhage is the most common complication. Many of these ulcers penetrate outside the stomach wall, resulting in severe hemorrhage from the splenic or left gastric arteries. Perforation and obstruction are much less frequently encountered. Giant gastric ulcers are much more likely to be benign than malignant. Nonetheless, achlorhydria is presumptive evidence that the ulcer is malignant. In the absence of hemorrhage or perforation, an intensive program of medical therapy with H_2 blockers is warranted; the healing process must be carefully monitored by periodic roentgenographic and endoscopic studies. One unusual complication is colonization with *Candida;* the ulcer may not heal with the usual medical therapy until an antifungal agent is given.

Therapy of Peptic Ulcer Disease

Medical therapy is a double-edged sword, especially in the elderly, and its risks must be carefully weighed. Rigorous administration of antacids is associated with increased salt load sufficient to upset the delicate balance in renal disease or congestive heart failure. Further problems include change in bowel habits and drug interactions. The aluminum hydroxide compounds have been shown to adsorb drugs (*e.g.,* digoxin and quinidine) and to interfere with their absorption. Side-effects of the H_2 blocker cimetidine of particular concern in the elderly are mental obtundation or confusion, sinus node dysfunction, and drug interactions; ranitidine may be safer. Anticholinergic agents may precipitate gastric stasis, intestinal atony, obstructive uropathy, and acute glaucoma. Gastric irradiation, a safe technique to temporarily reduce gastric acid secretion, is an alternative mode of therapy for selected patients.[8]

Long-Term Consequences of Partial Gastrectomy in the Aged

The most important of these include bezoar formation, nutritional deficiency states, and gastric-pouch cancer.

Phytobezoars develop from foods with a high content of insoluble and indigestible fiber in the presence of abnormal gastric emptying and diminished gastric secretion. Phytobezoars are most common in the edentulous patient who has had a Billroth I or II operation, but they are also seen after vagotomy and gastrojejunostomy, antral resection, pyloroplasty, and even simple gastroenterostomy. Patients are commonly asymptomatic, although abdominal fullness or discomfort, nausea, vomiting, and bleeding may occur. Results of

a physical examination are usually normal but there may be signs of a gastric outlet obstruction. Diagnosis is not difficult if borne in mind when a large mass is seen on upper gastrointestinal series in a patient who has had gastric surgery. Oral administration of cellulase, either alone or in a commercial preparation combined with papain and other enzymes, occasionally results in bezoar digestion. If this technique is not satisfactory, endoscopic disruption is usually successful. Metoclopramide is best used as an adjunct to prevent bezoar formation, rather than to help them pass once formed.

The most common metabolic consequences of partial gastrectomy are metabolic bone disease and anemia due to deficiencies of iron, folate, or cyanocobalamin. If a diagnosis of osteomalacia is made, therapy with calcium and vitamin D is usually curative. A quantitative stool fat examination may be helpful in determining patients at risk since in fat malabsorption excessive fecal losses of calcium and vitamin D occur.

Patients who have had a partial gastrectomy or gastroenterostomy have a distinct increase in hyperplastic polyps, adenomas, epithelial dysplasia, and carcinoma within the remaining gastric pouch beginning 10 to 15 years after operation.[34] It has been estimated that the risk of such "stump cancer" approximates 3% at 15 years after the initial surgery. This special group of cancer-prone patients would benefit from periodic endoscopic screening.

Gastric Motility

Studies show that liquids empty more slowly from the elderly stomach, whereas solids are emptied at the same rate as in a young population.[31] In achlorhydric patients with pernicious anemia or atrophic gastritis, gastric emptying for liquids is essentially normal but for solids is markedly delayed; the latter is improved by instillation of acid into the stomach. Studies of age-dependent physiologic slowing of gastric emptying may lead to a better understanding of why orally administered drugs may have diminished pharmacologic effect in aged patients.

Volvulus of the Stomach

Volvulus of the stomach is more common in the elderly and results from relaxation of the ligamentous supports of the stomach, thus enabling the organ to roll or twist. Two basic types are defined by the axis on which the stomach rotates. In the more common organoaxial type, the stomach twists on its longitudinal axis (*i.e.,* the line connecting the cardia and the pylorus); this is the type usually seen in patients with an ''upside-down stomach.'' With mesenteroaxial volvulus, rotation is about a vertical axis passing through the middle of the lesser and greater curvatures.

Acute gastric volvulus is rare and almost always presents as abrupt onset of severe epigastric pain that may radiate to the back or left chest. Early vomiting is followed by retching and an inability to vomit or belch. This characteristic history is soon followed by rapidly increasing upper abdominal distention, and, typically, there is an inability to pass a nasogastric tube into the stomach. Acute gastric volvulus usually requires emergency surgical treatment.

Chronic gastric volvulus is more frequent and often asymptomatic. The usual history is of intermittent epigastric pain precipitated by eating a large meal and is accompanied by regurgitation or vomiting and abdominal distention. An erect film may show an intragastric air–fluid level, and a barium examination reveals tapering of the distal esophagus. Therapy usually consists of elective reduction of the volvulus and a gastropexy.

Gastric Mucosal Webs or Diaphragms

These lesions either are congenital or produced by scarring from an annular ulcer. Gastric webs occur exclusively in the distal antrum and are 2 mm to 3 mm in thickness. They usually present as postcibal vomiting, variably accompanied by pain. Attacks are often precipitated by intake of food and relieved by the vomiting. Episodes are intermittent and associated with long periods of remission. Webs may be diagnosed by barium study or by endoscopy and appear as thin, lucent bands that divide the stomach into a larger proximal and a smaller distal chamber. Endoscopic resection or surgical removal of the web is curative.

Benign Gastric Tumors

The incidence of benign gastric tumors increases with advancing age.

The hyperplastic polyp, the most common epithelial polyp seen in the stomach, comprises 75% to 90% of such growths. It is usually found as a single, small, ''pencil eraser'' lesion at the junction of the gastric body and the antrum. The histologic appearance suggests excessive regeneration after inflammatory destruction of the gastric mucosa. The lesion is not considered a true neoplasm nor

premalignant, but independent carcinoma in the same stomach has been reported in up to one fourth of the patients.[43]

Adenomatous polyps are true neoplasms and comprise 10% to 25% of gastric polyps. The surrounding gastric epithelium shows chronic atrophic gastritis with prominent intestinal metaplasia. The mean incidence of malignant change in gastric adenomas is reported as 41%, with a range of 6% to 75%. The danger of malignant degeneration seems to be greater the older the patient is at the time of diagnosis.

Gastric polyps may occur in some gastrointestinal polyposis syndromes, but the only one to occur in older individuals is the Cronkhite-Canada syndrome. This syndrome is not hereditary and is characterized by diffuse gastrointestinal polyposis, protein-losing enteropathy, and ectodermal abnormalities, including pigmentation, alopecia, and dystrophic nail changes.

Mesenchymal tumors comprise a large percentage of benign gastric tumors and include leiomyomas, fibromas, and neural tumors. In general, symptoms of benign gastric tumors are more closely related to their size than to histologic type. Pain is the most common symptom followed by gastrointestinal bleeding.

Malignant Gastric Tumors

Gastric cancer is inexplicably decreasing in frequency, and relatively more cases are being diagnosed in younger patients. Certain gastric lesions are accepted as precancerous (*e.g.,* gastric adenomas, mucosal atrophy with intestinal metaplasia, and pernicious anemia). Individuals who have had a subtotal gastrectomy or gastroenterostomy are also at increased risk. Achlorhydria is considered precancerous, although tests of gastric secretion cannot be used to establish nor exclude the existence of gastric cancer.

Carcinoma of the stomach is usually incurable by the time symptoms appear, in part because symptoms are not produced until late and initially are frequently mild and nonspecific. The temptation to prescribe antacids for symptomatic relief in elderly patients without investigation must be avoided, for as Sir Heneage Ogilvie stated in 1938, ''In carcinoma of the stomach, alkalis are the undertaker's best friend.'' Vague epigastric discomfort, anorexia, early satiety, and weight loss are the most frequent ''early'' symptoms. Physical examination may reveal abnormalities that usually connote far-advanced disease. Lymph nodes in the left axilla or supraclavicular space, an umbilical nodule, and an enlarged left hepatic lobe are characteristic. The infrequent velvety pigmentation of acanthosis nigricans or the development of dermatomyositis should also raise the suspicion of a visceral neoplasm.

Laboratory abnormalities are nonspecific and include iron deficiency anemia, leukemoid reactions with eosinophilia, and achlorhydria. The most common roentgenologic expressions of gastric cancer are a mass, a mass with an ulcer, and infiltration of the gastric wall. Gastroscopy is indispensable in permitting direct observation of the extent of the lesion and for histologic and cytologic studies.

Surgical excision is the only potentially curative treatment. Only 70% to 90% of patients with gastric cancer are considered suitable for laparotomy. Of these only half are eligible for potentially curative resections. Even in such selected patients, death occurs in the majority within 1 year. Five-year survival rates are generally between 5% and 15%. Objective responses have been reported in about 25% of patients for an approximate median duration of 4 to 5 months with several chemotherapeutic regimens including 5-fluorouracil,[30] doxorubicin (Adriamycin), and the nitrosoureas. Combined with chemotherapy, irradiation may be of some benefit. Roentgen therapy alone is ineffective except for symptomatic palliation of bone pain due to metastases.

Other Gastric Malignancies

Gastric myosarcoma is a rare tumor that usually occurs in patients between 50 and 70 years. Characteristically the tumor has a large exogastric and a small intragastric component. Resection is the only effective treatment.

Carcinoid tumors of the stomach are uncommon, but an increased incidence has been noted in patients with severe chronic gastritis and with pernicious anemia. Urinary excretion of histamine is increased, and 5-hydroxytryptophan and 5-hydroxytryptamine levels are often elevated. Levels of 5-hydroxyindoleacetic acid are usually not elevated, because gastric carcinoids frequently lack L-aromatic acid decarboxylase. Treatment is wide surgical excision with removal of local metastases.

Kaposi's sarcoma may involve the viscera. The nodules resemble those in the skin, and gastrointestinal bleeding usually results. An unusually high incidence of second primary cancers (approaching 37%) has been observed in patients with Kaposi's sarcoma, particularly lymphomas and leukemias.

The stomach is the most frequent site of primary extranodal *lymphoma* and accounts for one half to three fourths of reported patients with gastrointestinal tract lymphoma. Gastric lymphoma produces no specific symptoms, but epigastric pain with weight loss and a palpable mass in a patient who seems in generally good condition is typical. There is fasting achlorhydria in about one half of patients, and anemia is usual. Roentgenologically in up to two thirds of cases, lymphoma resembles carcinoma. Large ulcerated masses, hyperrugosity, polypoid lesions, and antral narrowing are suggestive of lymphoma and unusual with carcinoma. Definitive diagnosis may elude gastroscopic biopsies and brush cytology and require a large particle biopsy or even laparotomy. The generally accepted therapy of wide surgical resection, followed by radiation therapy results in a crude 5-year survival rate of 40 to 50%.

Vascular Lesions of the Stomach

Very rarely in the elderly, a large dilated and tortuous gastric artery may be responsible for massive bleeding, typically 2 cm distal to the cardioesophageal junction. These large vessels usually have a small mucosal defect overlying them referred to as "exulceratio simplex," or the ulcer of Dieulafoy. Conceivably, focal pressure from the enlarged vessels leads to superficial erosion of the overlying mucosal membrane.

Telangiectasias of the Osler-Weber-Rendu (hereditary, hemorrhagic) type, which are responsible for recurrent gastrointestinal bleeding, have been seen in the elderly. There is usually no history of childhood epistaxis nor a family history of similar occurrences. Such lesions occur in association with other vascular lesions marking senescence, including sublingual varices (caviar lesions) and capillary phlebectasias of the scrotum. Until a definitive classification is developed it is probably preferable to consider all of them under a broad descriptive category such as "degenerative vasculopathy associated with aging."

Systemic Diseases

Diabetes Mellitus

Gastric motor abnormalities are being increasingly recognized with new techniques of study. Patients with symptoms of motor dysfunction and normal cinefluorographic studies on retesting with radio-labeled mixed solid and liquid meals reveal profound abnormalities in the gastric emptying of the solid phase of the meal. In diabetes mellitus such abnormalities are often without clinical manifestations. The development of gastric atony is usually insidious and presents as upper abdominal fullness, early satiety, and vomiting. Difficulty in controlling the underlying metabolic disorder may be a more subtle presentation of gastroparesis due to inconstant and unpredictable gastric emptying. Gastric bezoar formation and bacterial and fungal overgrowth are additional complications of long-standing diabetes, probably because of the accompanying hypochlorhydria. It is generally accepted that diabetic gastroparesis results from an abnormality in the autonomic nervous system almost always associated with peripheral or autonomic neuropathy. Metoclopramide and bethanechol have each been successfully used to normalize the abnormal gastric motility pattern.[29]

Gastric secretion is diminished in diabetes mellitus, which may explain the reduced incidence of peptic ulcer disease. However, when peptic ulcer develops, the course is frequently more complicated than in nondiabetics.

Hypothyroidism

Hypothyroidism like thyrotoxicosis is usually associated with a decrease in gastric acid secretion and a high incidence of atrophic gastritis. There is a further association with pernicious anemia. Gastric problems in hypothyroidism tend to be clinically silent.

Amyloidosis

The gastrointestinal tract is involved in 50% to 75% of patients with amyloidosis, and in approximately one half of cases the stomach is affected. It is unusual that signs and symptoms of gastrointestinal involvement are directly attributable to the amyloidosis *per se*. Amyloidosis can closely mimic carcinoma and appear as an isolated tumor, usually in the distal stomach. Outlet obstruction may be caused by an obstructing mass lesion or infiltration of the gastric wall. Amyloidosis is another cause of giant gastric ulcer that does not heal with medical therapy. Treatment is usually overshadowed by the need to care for the primary disease. Surgical therapy should only be used to treat life-threatening complications, since postoperative complications (*e.g.,* anastomatic leaks) occur when the gastric wall is heavily infiltrated.

SMALL INTESTINE

The weight of the human intestine decreases after the fifth decade of life, and the jejunal villi of elderly subjects are broader and shorter with a greater population of leaf-shaped and convoluted forms than is found in normal young subjects. Barium studies of the small intestine reflect these morphologic changes and show a coarser mucosal pattern in patients over 60 years of age. It is probable that such senescent changes result from diminished cell turnover and that there is an "ineffectual enteropoiesis" in the aged gut.[20]

Absorption and Malabsorption

The functional capacity of the small intestine decreases with aging. The diminished ability to absorb carbohydrates with aging is subtle and is not accompanied by clinical evidence of undernutrition. The validity of D-xylose testing to document intestinal malabsorption in the elderly is controversial. With breath hydrogen analysis, a progressive reduction in absorptive capacity with advancing age has been demonstrated.[15]

Fat absorption is also altered or diminished; abnormal intestinal and pancreatic function seem to play a role, but the contribution of delayed gastric emptying, achlorhydria, and diminished blood flow remain to be established.

Vitamin deficiencies in the elderly generally reflect diminished intake or disease states such as malabsorption syndrome; the concept of "physiologic avitaminosis" should be disregarded. However, the aged gut seems to absorb calcium and vitamin D poorly despite an apparently greater need for these micronutrients. The diets of the elderly are frequently deficient in calcium, and the adaptive response of the intestine to increase absorptive capacity with low intake is blunted; perhaps this contributes to the progressive loss of bone with advancing age. When iron deficiency occurs, gastrointestinal blood loss must be excluded, although some factors that may adversely influence iron absorption in the elderly include hypochlorhydria and the increased ingestion of cereal grains from which iron is poorly absorbed.

The differential diagnosis of malabsorption syndrome in the elderly encompasses a large number of disorders. Some entities cause symptoms by interfering with the intraluminal digestion of nutrients (pancreatic insufficiency); others alter the mucosa (celiac sprue); and still others interfere with intestinal blood flow (irradiation). Elderly individuals may also suffer from systemic disorders that directly involve the intestine (amyloidosis) or affect it as an innocent bystander (congestive heart failure).

One of the more common causes of malabsorption in the elderly is bacterial overgrowth or the blind loop syndrome, in which bacteria colonize the upper small bowel and interfere with the absorption of micronutrients and macronutrients. Also, it is known that bacterial counts are increased and coliforms and *Bacteroides* species are more prominent in small bowel cultures of achlorhydric patients. Bacterial overgrowth develops because of local or general stasis. Examples of local stasis include small bowel diverticulosis, enteroenteric anastomoses or fistulas, and partial small bowel obstruction. General stasis within the small bowel is more common and can be seen with endocrine disorders (diabetes mellitus, hypothyroidism), neuromuscular disorders (Parkinson's disease), renal or metabolic disorders, and collagen vascular disorders and in association with drug therapy (anticholinergic compounds and tranquilizers).

Weight loss, anemia, steatorrhea, and diarrhea are frequent with bacterial overgrowth, and osteomalacia, vitamin A deficiency, and even hypocalcemic tetany may occur as a consequence of lipid malabsorption. Tests for bacterial overgrowth include the 24-hour urinary excretion of indican (low), determination of serum folate level (high), and the timed analysis of metabolic products ($14CO_2$ and H_2) produced by bacteria and excreted in the breath after an oral load of substrate. Use of the Schilling test is based on the common occurrence of cyanocobalamin malabsorption with bacterial overgrowth. Most patients cannot be surgically cured of the intestinal stasis, and long-term treatment with antibiotics (*e.g.*, tetracycline, ampicillin) is often helpful.

Adult Celiac Disease (Celiac Sprue)

In one large series[9] about 7% of patients with celiac sprue presented during the seventh decade, and in another series[35] celiac disease was the most common cause of steatorrhea in patients older than 50 years of age. Many elderly patients do not have any symptoms referable to the gastrointestinal tract, but exhibit anemia, metabolic bone disease, edema, neurologic disorders, or cachexia. Sometimes the disease is precipitated by a bout of antibiotic-associated or ''traveler's'' diarrhea, and occasional cases present acutely after abdominal surgery, especially vagotomy and partial gastrectomy for peptic ulcer disease.

Because they develop only after a long inter-val, complications such as osteomalacia and malignancy[40] are more common in the elderly. Lymphoma typically develops 2 decades and carcinoma develops 4 decades after diagnosis of celiac sprue. Sprue is typically a painless disorder, and when it is accompanied by pain, the diagnosis of lymphoma must be excluded. Patients with celiac disease are at increased risk of carcinoma in many sites, including the lung, ovaries, skin, and especially the esophagus. Failure to respond to gluten withdrawal or the return of symptoms on a gluten-free diet strongly suggests the development of malignancy.

Intestinal Pseudo-Obstruction Syndromes

In intestinal pseudo-obstruction the signs and symptoms of obstruction exist without a demonstrable obstructing lesion.[14] It may be isolated to a segment of intestine or be part of a more generalized process involving most or all of the gastrointestinal tract and other organs including the urinary bladder. Acute pseudo-obstruction is a transient disorder mainly in elderly patients who are chronically ill. Typically it presents as nausea, vomiting, abdominal discomfort, and distention; and in contrast to organic obstruction, constipation, failure to pass gas, fever, and leukocytosis are not prominent. Causes include infections (sepsis, pneumonia), inflammatory conditions (pancreatitis, cholecystitis), electrolyte abnormalities (hypokalemia, hypocalcemia), congestive heart failure, neoplasms, and medications (anticholinergics, tranquilizers). Chronic pseudo-obstruction has been described with renal failure, diabetes mellitus, myxedema, hypoparathyroidism, neurologic disorders (Parkinson's disease), collagen vascular disorders (scleroderma), laxative abuse, and jejunal diverticulosis.

Initial management consists of excluding organic obstruction, defining and correcting any underlying metabolic disturbances or systemic illnesses, decompressing the intestine, and in general, supporting the patient's needs. With the first episode it may be very difficult to distinguish between organic obstruction and an acute pseudo-obstruction; again, the absence of fever and leukocytosis is helpful. Mechanical bowel obstruction shows little or no gas in the distal colon and rectum whereas ileus and pseudo-obstruction usually do. Barium enema may be of help, and if no obstruction is demonstrable, decompression with a long or nasogastric tube and careful monitoring of fluid balance and electrolytes is advisable. Obviously, sepsis should be rapidly treated. Subsequent evaluation can be directed at excluding associated systemic disorders.

Intestinal Obstruction

Small bowel mechanical obstruction at all ages is usually caused by hernia and adhesions; carcinoma is rarely responsible.[17] Other causes in the elderly infrequently encountered in the young are gallstones, intestinal ulcers, and strictures.

Gallstone Ileus

Gallstone ileus is a mechanical intestinal obstruction caused by impaction of one or more gallstones within the lumen of the bowel.[10] The disease is more common in women and is responsible for 20% of intestinal obstructions in patients older than 65 years. Half the patients have a history of gallbladder disease, and a previous episode of jaundice has been observed in up to 15% of patients.

Symptoms of intestinal obstruction are more prominent than symptoms of biliary tract disease, and cramping abdominal pain and vomiting are usual. A classic but rare presentation is two-phase pain (*i.e.*, biliary colic followed after a pain-free interval by colicky pain in another location). The abdominal roentgenogram is diagnostic if it reveals the triad of air in the biliary tree, a gallstone in the intestine or changing position of a previously observed stone, and small intestinal obstruction. The calculus is usually at least 2.5 cm in diameter and most commonly impacts in the distal ileum. The stone may lodge at various levels, producing a "tumbling obstruction," which may delay prompt diagnosis and therapy. Cholecystectomy and repair of the biliary-enteric fistula constitute definitive therapy and may be performed at the same time as enterolithotomy or as a second-stage procedure.

Intussusception

Intussusception is an unusual condition in adults and is almost always caused by an organic lesion. Malignant lesions are more common causes of the disorder than benign lesions in the 60 to 80-year age-group.

Small Intestinal Ulcers and Strictures

Small bowel ulcers distal to the duodenum are rare. In adults, commonly suggested causes include ischemia, medications (enteric-coated potassium chloride and indomethacin), neoplasia, inflammation, irradiation, trauma, and, most commonly, "idiopathic." Potassium marketed in slow-release wax matrices has been reported to cause ulcers proximal to areas of anatomical restriction. The "potassium ulcer" probably results from the release and absorption of high concentrations of potassium within a short segment of bowel. This causes spasm of the intramural and mesenteric vessels, especially the veins, with subsequent infarction of varying extent. Patients present with obstruction, perforation, and bleeding. In the reversible stage of ischemic injury, discontinuation of the drug may be sufficient to allow resolution of symptoms.

Indomethacin which is known for its potential to cause gastric ulcer, has also been associated with ulceration and stricture of the small intestine. Severity seems to be dose related and varies from superficial ulceration to full-thickness necrosis and perforation. A contributory role for the intestinal flora has been postulated, and, experimentally, antibiotics seem to be protective.

Nonspecific ulcers of small intestine without a clearly defined etiology seem to increase progressively with each decade of life, and most are found in patients older than 50 years.[3] Obstruction is the most common presentation, whereas hemorrhage and perforation occur as isolated features. While three fourths of these ulcers are located in the ileum, perforation is more common in the jejunum.

Aortoenteric Fistula

The average age at which aortoenteric fistula occurs is about 62, and the vast majority of affected patients are males.[7] Symptoms of primary aortoenteric fistula are similar to those of an uncomplicated aortic aneurysm and usually include abdominal or back pain. Aortoenteric fistulas usually present with hematemesis or melena. In more than half of the patients, the initial hemorrhage occurs more than 24 hours before the final exsanguination and so there is adequate time for definitive surgical correction.

Successful management depends on early recognition, which is accomplished only if the diagnosis is suspected in all elderly patients with an abdominal mass and gastrointestinal bleeding. With endoscopy the visualization of friability, a clot, or the fistula itself in the distal duodenum is sufficient to commit the patient to abdominal exploration. Angiography rarely demonstrates the fistulous communication, although it may be valuable in planning the operative approach. The operation of choice is resection of the aneurysm with interposition of an aortic graft, and survival approaches 60% in those highly selected cases in which this can be performed.

Aortic Graft-Enteric Fistula

The incidence of aortic graft-enteric fistula after reconstructive aortic surgery ranges from 0.6% to 4% and occurs most frequently when surgery is performed for a ruptured abdominal aneurysm.[13] Most cases present because of gastrointestinal hemorrhage, and just as in patients who have not had reconstructive surgery, a brisk hemorrhage typically occurs, followed by a massive uncontrollable bleeding episode 12 to 18 hours later. Sepsis heralds the development of an aortic graft-enteric fistula almost as frequently as does hemorrhage, and sepsis or fever of obscure origin, occurring any time after placement of an aortic graft, should raise suspicion of communications between the aorta and the bowel.

Radiation Damage

Because of its mobile mesentery, the amount of radiation the small intestine receives is substantially less than if it were fixed. Any process rendering the bowel less mobile (*e.g.,* previous abdominal surgery, adhesions, or intra-abdominal inflammatory processes) increases the possibility of radiation damage. The ileum is most often injured because of its relatively fixed position and its location in the pelvis to which radiation is frequently directed. Also, any disease associated with vascular damage such as hypertension, arteriosclerosis, or diabetes mellitus reduces the tolerance to radiation of the bowel. Most clinically significant radiation damage to the small intestine manifests months to years after therapy as intestinal ulceration with obstruction, hemorrhage, or perforation; malabsorption; or mesenteric vascular insufficiency. Roentgenologic changes include separation, matting, and adhesions of the bowel loops that may be difficult to distinguish from recurrent or metastatic disease. A "malabsorption pattern" may require differentiation from lymphoma, and a rigid "formless" fibrotic loop perhaps associated with fistulas may mimic Crohn's disease, ischemic enteritis, or lymphoma. Medical therapy has little to offer to ameliorate the underlying disorder; treatment of associated bacterial overgrowth with antibiotics and cholorrheic enteropathy with bile-sequestering resins may result in dramatic resolution of symptoms. The use of

medium-chain triglycerides and elemental diets may reduce steatorrhea and diarrhea.

Neoplasms of the Small Intestine

The small intestine is the digestive organ least likely to develop cancer, a remarkable fact in view of the high frequency of cancer in the neighboring stomach and colon. Most benign small bowel tumors are incidental findings, and the vast majority of tumors that produce clinical symptoms are malignant. Symptoms from each of the major types of intestinal neoplasms are similar and include abdominal pain, gastrointestinal bleeding, intestinal obstruction, and an abdominal mass.

The most common benign neoplasms of the small bowel, in order of decending frequency are leiomyoma, adenomatous polyp, lipoma, and hemangioma. None of these occurs with particularly increased frequency in the elderly population, although they tend to be more common in the later years.

Carcinoid tumors, the most common malignancy of the small intestine,[37] increasingly found from the duodenum to the terminal ileum, are most frequent in the appendix. Duodenal carcinoids usually produce symptoms (duodenal or common bile duct obstruction or bleeding), whereas carcinoids in the jejunum or ileum are ordinarily silent. Carcinoid tumors are typically small, most of the obstructive symptoms are due to an associated desmoplastic reaction that produces retraction of the mesentery and kinking of the bowel. The desmoplastic reaction in the mesentery may also produce intestinal ischemia and infarction. A history of chronic intestinal obstruction, weight loss, diarrhea, and a right-sided abdominal mass should point to the diagnosis. Other striking features are their tendency to multicentricity and their association with second primary malignancies, most commonly adenocarcinoma of the colon, stomach, breast, and lung. A history or observation of a typical flush and high levels of 5-hydroxyindoleacetic acid in the urine are diagnostic but almost always observed with advanced disease. All visible tumor should be removed, since even in the presence of nodal or peritoneal metastases 5-year survival rates approach 70%.

Adenocarcinoma is the most common symptom-producing malignant lesion of the small bowel. Within the duodenum, the signs, symptoms, and prognosis of cancer vary with its relationship to the ampulla of Vater. Adenocarcinomas of the duodenum tend to be more virulent, but in one series 50% of the tumors were resectable for cure and the 5-year survival rate for patients with resectable lesions was 46%.[23]

Jejunal and ileal carcinomas are rarer. Five-year survival rates vary from 5% to 25%, although when "curative" resections are performed a 5-year survival rate approaching 50% has been reported.

Leiomyosarcoma is the third or fourth most frequent malignancy of the small bowel and is most commonly found distally. Treatment consists of generous resection of the involved bowel. The prognosis varies widely, but survival is generally less than 50% at 5 years.

The small bowel, although infrequently involved by primary carcinoma, is commonly involved by *metastases* from other sites, such as the breast and lung, or by direct extension from adjacent organs such as stomach, pancreas, kidney, uterus, and ovaries. Partial small bowel obstruction is the most common presentation. Management may include palliative bypass resection and chemotherapy.

Lymphoma

Small intestinal *lymphomas* are commonly manifested by abdominal pain usually due to intestinal obstruction but also to perforation. Diarrhea and steatorrhea may be due to obstruction of the mesenteric lymphatics, diffuse spread of tumor throughout the mucosa, or even bacterial overgrowth proximal to an obstructing neoplasm. The usually treatment is wide segmental resection including the involved lymph nodes; adjuvant radiation therapy is used if lymph nodes are involved, the disease is complicated by perforation of fistula, or the resection was incomplete. Five-year survival rates vary greatly (10% to 50%) and may be correlated with cell type.

Leukemia

Gross involvement of the gastrointestinal tract is especially observed in the acute varieties of leukemia in which the incidence approaches 20%. The ileum is the most common site involved, and the most common symptom is massive hemorrhage. In most cases, bleeding is due to ulceration, coexistent ulcer disease, gastric erosions, and coagulation abnormalities.

Waldenström's Macroglobulinemia

Small intestinal involvement in Waldenström's macroglobulinemia is uncommon and is not usually accompanied by the characteristic features of the disease (*i.e.,* enlargement of the liver, spleen, and lymph nodes with retinal abnormalities and cutaneous pathology). Affected patients usually present with diarrhea, and a small bowel series reveals dilatation, thickening of the folds, and nodularity. In addition to other usual laboratory parameters there may be evidence of malabsorption, including steatorrhea and a diminished D-xylose excretion in the urine.

APPENDIX

The appendix undergoes involutional change with aging and is an uncommon cause of problems in the elderly.

Acute Appendicitis

Appendicitis in patients older than 60 years of age accounts for 6% to 8% of all appendectomies performed and in one series was responsible for 5% of acute abdominal diseases in patients older than 70 years of age.[16] Signs and symptoms in the elderly are similar to those in children. However, appendicitis in the elderly tends to progress to perforation more rapidly with less evidence of advanced disease than ordinarily expected. Thus, perforation is at least two to three times more frequent in patients older than 60 years of age. Furthermore, delay in diagnosis because of meager findings is four times as common in patients over 60 years of age compared with control subjects between the ages of 30 and 40.[47] In addition, the initial diagnosis is incorrect in about half of elderly patients in whom operation is so delayed.

Elderly patients may harbor far-advanced disease within the abdomen yet show a paucity of signs and symptoms. Guarding is not as pronounced as in younger patients, and temperatures beyond 102°F (37.9°C) and white blood cell counts of more than 20,000/cu mm are unusual. A right lower quadrant or rectal mass is appreciated in about one third of elderly patients and usually indicates abscess or phlegmon formation. Abdominal distention and constipation are also quite common presentations. Chills portend an ominous prognosis because of their frequent association with peritonitis and sepsis. Hypothermia usually implies abscess formation and generalized peritonitis. A "shift to the left" despite a minimal leukocytosis also implies an advanced stage of disease. The presence of hypochromic microcytic anemia or blood in the stool should arouse suspicion that the appendicitis is secondary to neoplastic obstruction.

Prompt surgical therapy is advisable in patients of advanced age with appendicitis and a mass. In view of the virulence of clinical appendicitis in the elderly, appendectomy during the course of abdominal operations for unrelated disorders is recommended.

Neoplasms

Primary noncarcinoid malignant epithelial neoplasms of the appendix are quite rare and are generally discovered during appendectomy for appendicitis. There seems to be an association between carcinoma of the appendix and other colonic neoplasms (most commonly adenomatous polyps or synchronous carcinoma). Thus, it becomes important to follow such patients with barium studies or colonoscopy to exclude the development of other neoplasms. Five-year survival is 29% when treated with simple appendectomy and 50% for those having a right hemicolectomy.

Mucocele: Benign Versus Malignant

Mucocele results when the drainage of mucus from the appendix to the cecum is blocked. Such obstruction may be caused by granulation tissue or hyperplastic or neoplastic mucosa. Benign epithelial neoplasms of the appendix are complicated by mucocele formation much more often then malignant lesions and are not uncommonly associated with synchronous colonic neoplasms. If the tumors are confined to the appendix, the distinction between a benign and a malignant lesion is of little importance since appendectomy is usually curative. In pseudomyxoma peritonei, benign or malignant cells appear on the peritoneal surface and actively secrete mucus into the peritoneal cavity. When caused by an appendiceal lesion, pseudomyxoma peritonei is most often produced by rupture of a cystic neoplasm. Therapy consists of operative removal of the gelatinous material and instillation of chemotherapeutic agents in the malignant variety. Appendectomy is performed for diagnostic and therapeutic purposes, and if an obvious malignant appendiceal tumor is present, right hemicolectomy is advisable.

REFERENCES

1. Bock OAA, Richards WCD, Witts LJ: The relationship between acid secretion after augmented histamine stimulation and the histology of the gastric mucosa. Gut 4:112–114, 1963

2. Bockus HL, Bank J: The value of histamine as a test for gastric function. Arch Intern Med 39:508–519, 1927

3. Boydstun JS Jr, Gaffey TA, Bartholomew LG: Clinicopathologic study of nonspecific ulcers of the small intestine. Dig Dis Sci 26:911–916, 1981

4. Brand DL, Martin D, Pope CE II: Esophageal manometrics in patients with angina-like chest pain. Dig Dis 22:300–304, 1977

5. Brandt LJ: Gastrointestinal Disorders of the Elderly. New York, Raven Press, 1984

6. Brooks JR, Eraklis AJ: Factors affecting the mortality from peptic ulcer: The bleeding ulcer and ulcer in the aged. N Engl J Med 271:803–809, 1964

7. Champion MC, Sullivan SN, Coles JC, Goldbach M, Watson WC: Aortoenteric fistula: Incidence, presentation, recognition and management. Ann Surg 195:314–317, 1982

8. Cocco AE, Mendeloff AI: Effects of gastric irradiation in duodenal ulcer patients: Gastric secretory response to maximal histamine stimulation during a three-year period. Johns Hopkins Med 126:61–68, 1970

9. Cooke WT, Asquith P (eds): Clinics in Gastroenterology. Philadelphia, WB Saunders, 1974

10. Day EA, Marks C: Gallstone ileus. Am J Surg 129:552–558, 1975

11. Debas HT, Payne WS, Cameron AJ, Carlson HC: Physiopathology of lower esophageal diverticulum and its implications for treatment. Surg Gynceol Obstet 151:593–600, 1980

12. Eisenberg RL, Margulis AR, Moss AA: Giant duodenal ulcer. Gut 11:592–599, 1978

13. Elliot JP Jr, Smith RF, Szilagyi DE: Aortoenteric and paraprosthetic-enteric fistulas. Arch Surg 108:479–490, 1974

14. Faulk DL, Anuras S, Christensen J: Chronic intestinal pseudo-obstruction. Gastroenterology 74:922–931, 1978

15. Feibusch JM, Holt PR: Impaired absorptive capacity for carbohydrate in the aging human. Dig Dis Sci 27:1095–1100, 1982

16. Fenyo G: Acute abdominal disease in the elderly: Experience in two series in Stockhom. Am J Surg 143:751–754, 1982

17. Fraser WJ: Intestinal obstruction by gallstone. Br J Surg 42:210–212, 1954

18. Goyal RK, Glancy JJ, Spiro HM: Lower esophageal ring. N Engl J Med 282:1298–1305, 1970

19. Hill LD: Incarcerated paraesophageal hernia: A surgical emergency. Am J Surg 126:286–291, 1973

20. Holt PR, Pascal RR, Kotler DP: Ineffectual enteropoiesis in aging rat gut (abstr). Gastroenterology 82:1086, 1982

21. Hurwitz AL, Duranceau A: Upper esophageal sphincter dysfunction: Pathogenesis and treatment. Am J Dig Dis 23:275–281, 1978

22. Hurwitz AL, Duranceau A, Haddad JK: Disorders of esophageal motility. XVI Series. In Smith LH Jr

(ed): Major Problems in Internal Medicine, pp 1–79. Philadelphia, WB Saunders, 1979

23. Joesting DR, Beart RW Jr, van Heerden JA, Weiland LH: Improving survival in adenocarcinoma of the duodenum. Am J Surg 141:228–231, 1981

24. Jones RFMcN: The Paterson-Brown-Kelly syndrome—its relationship to iron deficiency and post cricoid carcinoma: I. J Laryngol Otol 75:529–543, 1961

25. Joske RA, Finckh ES, Wood IJ: Gastric biopsy: A study of 1000 consecutive successful gastric biopsies. Q J Med 24:269–294, 1955

26. Khan TA, Shragge BW, Chrispin JS, Lind JF: Esophageal motility in the elderly. Am J Dig Dis 22:1049–1054, 1977

27. Kikendall JW, Friedman AC, Oyewole MA, Fleischer D, Johnson LF: Pill-induced esophageal injury: Case reports and review of the medical literature. Dig Dis Sci 28:174–182, 1983

28. Leverat M, Pasquier J, Lambert R, Tissot A: Peptic ulcer in patients over 60: Experience in 287 cases. Am J Dig Dis 11:279–285, 1966

29. Malagelada J-R, Rees WW, Mazzotta LJ, Go VLW: Gastric motor abnormalities in diabetic and postvagotomy gastroparesis: Effect of metoclopramide and bethanechol. Gastroenterology 78:286–293, 1980

30. Moertel CG: The stomach. In Holland JF, Frei E (eds): Alimentary Tract Cancer, pp 1760–1774. Philadelphia, 1982

31. Moore JG, Tweedy C, Christian PE, Datz FL: Effect of age on gastric emptying of liquid-solid meals in man. Dig Dis Sci 28:340–344, 1983

32. Naef AP, Savary M, Ozzello L: Columnar-lined lower esophagus: An acquired lesion with malignant predisposition: Report on 140 cases of Barrett's esophagus with 12 adenocarcinomas. J Thorac Surg 70:826–835, 1975

33. Narayanan M, Steinheber FU: The changing face of peptic ulcer in the elderly. Med Clin North Am 60:1159–1172, 1976

34. Orlando R, Welch JP: Carcinoma of the stomach after gastric operation. Am J Surg 141:437–491, 1981

35. Price HL, Gazzard BG, Dawson AM: Steatorrhoea in the elderly. Br Med J 1:1582–1584, 1977

36. Sagal Z, Marks JA, Kantor JL: The signficance of gastric acidity: A study of 6679 cases with digestive symptoms. Ann Intern Med 7:76–88, 1933

37. Sanders RJ, Axtell HK: Carcinoids of the gastrointestinal tract. Surg Gynecol Obstet 114:369–380, 1964

38. Soergel KH, Zboralski F, Amberg JR: Presbyesophagus: Esophageal motility in nonagenarians. J Clin Invest 43:1472–1479, 1964

39. Stafford CE, Joergenson EJ, Murray GC: Complications of peptic ulcer in the aged. Calif Med 84:92–94, 1956

40. Stokes PL, Holmes GKT: Malignancy. Clin Gastroenterol 3:159–169, 1974

41. Strange SL: Giant innocent gastric ulcer in the elderly. Gerontol Clin 5:171–189, 1963

42. Strickland RG, Mackay IR: A reappraisal of the nature of chronic atrophic gastritis. Dig Dis Sci 18:426–440, 1973

43. Tomasulo J: Gastric polyps: Histologic types and their relationship to gastric carcinoma. Cancer 27:1346–1355, 1971

43a. Tytgat GN: Endoscopic methods of treatment of gastrointestinal and biliary stenosis. Endoscopy 12 (Suppl): 57–68, 1980

44. Van Liere EJ, Northup DW: The emptying time of the stomach of old people. Am J Physiol 134:719–722, 1941

45. Vanzant FR, Alvarex WC, Eusterman GB, Dunn HL, Berkson J: The normal range of gastric acidity from youth to old age. Arch Intern Med 48:345–359, 1932

46. Walker IR, Strickland RG, Ungar B, Mackay IR: Simple atrophic gastritis and gastric carcinoma. Gut 12:906–911, 1971

47. Wolff WI, Hindman R: Acute appendicitis in the aged. Surg Gynecol Obstet 94:239–247, 1952

16

The Colon and Retroperitoneum

Lawrence J. Brandt

ABNORMALITIES OF DEFECATION

One of the most common bowel disturbances of older individuals, constipation, is much more frequent with immobility. In one survey 70 to 80% of patients over 60 years of age had five to seven bowel movements per week.[45] In another, most mobile elderly subjects evacuated 80% of radiodense capsules within 5 days after ingestion, while immobile subjects had a very long transit time.[17]. The markers in the immobile patients seem to accumulate in the left side of the colon and in the rectum, a condition referred to by Brocklehurst and Kahn[17] as the "terminal reservoir syndrome." In healthy subjects, the elasticity of the rectal wall has been shown to diminish with advancing age,[35] supporting the "terminal reservoir" concept.

Hard stools may impact in the rectum and cause local abnormalities, proximal or diffuse colonic disturbances, or systemic derangements, such as angina, myocardial infarction, or arrhythmias. Local complications of fecal impaction include stercoral ulceration, proctitis, rectal prolapse, hemorrhoidal bleeding, anorectal infection, and even mechanical obstruction of the urinary tract. Ischemic colitis, cecal rupture, and volvulus may develop more proximally in the colon. Fecal incontinence may result and produce recurrent genitourinary and skin infections with sepsis. Chronic use of laxatives may be associated with many other problems.

Stercoral ulceration refers to an ulcer that is intimately associated with and underlies an adherent mass of stool.[32] Such ulcers occur at the same locations fecalomas are found, namely, the rectosigmoid, followed by the transverse colon. There is usually a sharp demarcation between the margins of the ulcer and the adjacent mucosa, and

COMPLICATIONS OF CONSTIPATION AND FECAL IMPACTION

Cardiovascular sequelae (angina, myocardial infarction, arrhythmias)
Megacolon
    Volvulus—sigmoid
    Ischemic proctocolitis
    Cecal rupture
Rectal prolapse
Fecalith formation
    Stercoral ulcers
Fecal incontinence
    Urinary tract infection and sepsis
    Decubitus ulcers
Hemorrhoids
    Bleeding, anemia
    Anorectal infection
Laxative use and abuse

the involved intestinal segment is consistently stretched and thinned so that perforation may occur in the central portion of the lesion. Stercoral ulcers are said to occur in almost 5% of consecutively autopsied adults with an average age of 68.6 years, and although occasionally asymptomatic, massive hemorrhage and perforation are common complications. Periodic disimpaction is usually effective in preventing stercoral ulcers and their complications, but occasionally hemorrhage and perforation are produced by vigorous disimpaction.

When fecal matter stagnates in the colon and acquires characteristics of a tumor the term *fecaloma* is used. Fecalomas may complicate chronic constipation of any cause and may be initiated by antidiarrheal medication, confinement to bed, or colonic neoplasia. Their presence is suggested by the association of constipation, meteorism, and an abdominal mass. Most fecalomas occur in the rectum. The mass must be removed, either manually or by careful catharsis, or rarely by operative extirpation.

Fecal impaction is the most commonly identified cause of diarrhea in elderly patients.[48] In such cases, the static stool proximal to an obstructing fecal mass is liquefied and oozes out of the rectum. Because of the longstanding nature of these impactions, the rectum usually develops a high maximal tolerable volume with a diminished awareness of rectal filling and urge to defecate. Hence, the overflow runs out the anal canal because of sphincteric dysfunction. Treatment is directed to removing the impaction and treating any underlying disorders.

Rectal prolapse may occur as a complication of constipation because of anorectal muscle dysfunction or the associated straining of stool. Prolapse is much more common in women than in men. In the absence of a neuromuscular disorder, treatment of constipation is the keystone of rectal prolapse therapy, and operative repair of the prolapse is done in severe cases.

Laxative use is prevalent in the elderly, but only in a few cases must laxatives be taken chronically. An acute episode of fecal impaction or constipation can usually be treated safely with a saline enema. Soapsuds enemas are irritating and may cause a severe colitis. Once acute constipation has been relieved, dietary manipulation using prunes and high-fiber foods such as bran, suppositories, and even weekly enemas may be used. Mineral oil should be used with great caution since it may cause lipid pneumonia. Use of mineral oil with a surface active "stool softener" is contraindicated because enhanced absorption of the mineral oil may cause systemic lipid granulomatosis. Obviously a careful distinction must be made between constipation of functional and organic etiology. The most common causes for constipation are bad habits and improper diet. Simple measures such as heeding the call to stool and setting aside the time necessary to have an undisturbed bowel movement are usually rewarding. Simple exercise such as a daily walk is to be encouraged.

Bran has been used successfully alone and in combination with a laxative/stool softener to regulate bowel function in the elderly. During the first 2 weeks of bran supplementation, bowel habits often become erratic and patients complain of abdominal discomfort and "gas." Such complaints are transient. With prolonged administration of wheat bran, hypocalcemia and reduced serum levels of iron may result. Bran and high fiber supplements are also relatively contraindicated in the bed bound and in patients with intestinal strictures lest an intestinal obstruction be precipitated.

Acute constipation may be treated with small volume saline enemas or perhaps a stimulant suppository such as Bisacodyl. Therapy of chronic constipation consists primarily of correcting any improper dietary and toilet habits. Patients who frequently become impacted should be maintained on stool softeners, perhaps combined with periodic low volume saline enemas. If the need arises for a saline or stimulant cathartic, the choice varies for each patient. Senna derivatives, phenolphthalein products, and Bisacodyl are usually safe and well tolerated by the elderly; the more potent stimulant cathartics such as castor oil are best avoided.

Between 15% and 30% of the population older than 60 years of age take at least one dose of laxative per week, so that complications of these agents are often seen in the elderly.[20] Chronic laxative abuse usually presents as diarrhea and is variably accompanied by weakness, abdominal pain, distention, nausea, vomiting, and weight loss. Other manifestations include hypokalemia and abnormal renal function. Less commonly, chronic laxative abuse will be manifested by steatorrhea, hypocalcemia, or achlorhydria.

When the colon is damaged by chronic laxative abuse, the term *cathartic colon* is used. The right colon is most often involved, and occasionally the abnormalities are confused with those of "burned out" ulcerative colitis or Crohn's disease. Clinically, the paradox of a barium enema suggesting chronic ulcerative or Crohn's colitis in a patient complaining of constipation should raise suspicion of laxative abuse. Cathartic colon is seen only with laxatives of the stimulant class. Although the mechanism by which colonic damage results is unclear, fortunately the roentgenologic abnormalities may reverse after discontinuation of ingestion of the laxative.

Pathologically, *melanosis coli* is virtually diagnostic of recent and prolonged cathartic ingestion. This entity is associated with laxatives of the anthraquinone group; on their discontinuation the melanosis disappears within 4 to 12 months. Melanosis coli is frequently found in association with colonic neoplasms. Interestingly, the neoplasms are never pigmented. Melanosis coli is almost always visible on sigmoidoscopy and is usually darker the more distal in the bowel it is located.

VOLVULUS OF THE LARGE BOWEL

Volvulus accounts for 10% to 13% of all large bowel obstruction in the United States. Inexplicably, in Eastern Europe and the Scandinavian countries, volvulus is much more common and is responsible for 30% to 50% of intestinal obstructions. Volvulus of the sigmoid colon is more common than torsion of other segments and is predominantly a disorder of elderly men. In one representative series,[2] sigmoid volvulus peaked during the eighth decade and the mean age of the first episode was 66 years. Neuropsychiatric disorders are reported in 25% to 75% of patients. Presenting symptoms include crampy abdominal pain followed by obstipation, vomiting, diarrhea, and abdominal distention. The initial physical examination will usually reveal visible peristalsis, tympany, abdominal tenderness or a mass, and empty rectum, and a feculent odor to the breath. A plain abdominal roentgenogram is diagnostic in most instances, and barium enema usually confirms the diagnosis with visualization of the characteristic ''bird-beak'' at the site of the volvulus. Nonoperative techniques to reduce the volvulus are recommended initially and include proctosigmoidoscopy, insertion of a rectal tube, therapeutic barium enema examination, and, recently, decompression using the flexible colonoscope. These methods are successful in 75% to 100% of cases and have a mortality of about 2%.[57] Recurrence ranges from 30% to 90%, which in view of a mortality rate of 40% is unacceptable. Unsuccessful attempts at conservative therapy must be followed by some operative procedure. In general, detorsion and fixation procedures have higher mortality and recurrence rates than resection with anastomosis. Thus surgery is the procedure of choice after nonoperative methods fail or is used to treat recurrent volvulus.

Cecal volvulus exhibits more of a female predominance and a more diffuse age distribution; about one third of these patients have had a prior abdominal operation. Hypofixation of the cecum is a prerequisite for torsion, and a freely mobile cecum is found in all patients. Sufficient mobility of the cecum to allow for volvulus is present as an anatomical variant in 11% of adults at autopsy.[60] However, hypofixation of the cecum does not suffice to produce volvulus, and precipitating factors must be invoked such as distal colon obstruction, previous operation, associated medical illnesses, or use of positive pressure respirators.[47] Surgery should be undertaken as soon as is practicable; the mortality rate approximates 18%.[1]

DIVERTICULOSIS

The incidence of diverticular disease increases from approximately 5% during the fifth decade to 50% during the ninth decade.[28] Progression more often occurs within the segment initially involved than by spread to one segment after another; thus, recurrent segmental colonic resections are rarely required for diverticulosis. Abdominal pain is the most common symptom requiring hospitalization, caused by inflammatory complications or colonic muscular dysfunction. Occasionally it is difficult to distinguish between these two entities, and correlation between clinical features and pathologic findings is poor.

Complications include diverticulitis, peridiverticulitis, and diverticular hemorrhage. Diverticulitis and a perforation results in peridiverticulitis. Pain is usually localized to the left lower quadrant; diffuse abdominal discomfort usually signifies peritonitis. A tender mass with guarding is typically found in the left lower quadrant. Leukocytosis is common, and white blood cells and erythrocytes may be seen in the urine because of contiguous involvement of the urinary bladder by a pericolic abscess. The serum alkaline phosphatase may be elevated as a result of the systemic effect of sepsis and bacterial toxins on liver cell function or secondary hepatic abscesses. Diverticulitis may be complicated by a pericolic abscess, peritonitis, intestinal obstruction, or fistula formation.

Diverticulitis is a clinical diagnosis requiring treatment with parenteral antibiotics. Barium enema examination or colonoscopy is usually unnecessary and potentially dangerous. After the inflammatory process has been adequately treated, these techniques are appropriate to exclude associated diseases.

Hemorrhage more commonly occurs with diverticulosis than diverticulitis. Bleeding typically begins without warning and is severe; in most instances it stops spontaneously. Mild and persistent bleeding in a patient with diverticulosis should always suggest another cause, such as a polyp, carcinoma, or a cecal vascular ectasia. Diverticular hemorrhage is claimed to the most frequent cause of lower intestinal bleeding in the elderly, although recent experience suggests that cecal ectasias (angiodysplasias) are as important or even more important.[7] In most patients diverticular hemorrhage stops spontaneously with conservative management; if not, mesenteric angiography should locate the site of bleeding and allow infusion of vasocontrictor agents (*e.g.,* vasopressin). Athanosoulis and associates found diverticular bleeding to stop in 92% of cases with such infusion therapy.[3] Segmental colectomy is advised for uncontrollable or recurrent diverticular bleeding, and subtotal colectomy should be used only if the bleeding site cannot be found.

Current views on the pathogenesis of diverticular disease make it rational to prescribe a high-fiber diet and spasmolytic agents. Despite symptomatic improvement, it has not been shown whether such treatment has any effect on the natural history of existing diverticular disease or offers any protection against diverticulitis.

One unusual complication, giant diverticulum, usually occurs in the sigmoid colon, and 90% of patients are older than 50 years of age. Abdominal pain is the most common symptom. Examination usually reveals a soft, mobile, often slightly tender abdominal mass that may rapidly change in size with changes in intra-abdominal pressure. It is believed that inflammation with narrowing of the diverticular neck results in a ball-valve mechanism whereby gas may enter but not exit. Therapy consists of elective surgical resection.

INFLAMMATORY BOWEL DISEASE

Many of the so-called atypical features described by previous authors for "ulcerative colitis" in the elderly are now recognized as characteristic of ischemic colitis. These include segmental distribution of the disease, the less frequent involvement of the rectum, the high incidence of spontaneous resolution, and the frequent progression to a fibrotic stenosis with a delayed presentation of colonic obstruction. In a retrospective study of patients with colitis whose symptoms began after the age of 50 years,[14] 75% were considered to have ischemic colitis, 14% to have ulcerative colitis, and 5% to have Crohn's colitis. Half the cases classified retrospectively as ischemic colitis had previously been diagnosed as having ulcerative or granulomatous colitis. Such incorrect diagnosis might explain why colitis has been reported to behave differently in the elderly than in the young.

The clinical course of true ulcerative colitis beginning after 50 years varies considerably.[15] All my patients had intermittent exacerbations, and only half responded promptly to standard medical therapy. The remaining half had a more complicated or protracted course and often required surgical therapy or died, making the prognosis worse than in the young.

Onset of Crohn's disease after age 50 is infrequent, accounting for about 5% of the reported cases. Ileitis as the sole lesion is more common in the elderly, colonic involvement is less common, and ileocolonic disease is the least frequent. This is a contrast to the previous teaching that disease confined to the colon and rectum is usually seen in patients older than 60 years and that left-sided colonic Crohn's disease is a disorder of older women. In elderly patients with new onset Crohn's disease, surgery tends to be required after fewer years of disease and more commonly for hemorrhage rather than for fistulous, obstructive, or septic complications. Also, the incidence of emergency operations seems to increase with the age at which the diagnosis is made.

In any elderly patient with what appears to be new-onset Crohn's disease, other colitides that may resemble inflammatory bowel disease, such as ischemic and infectious colitis, must be excluded.

Radiation Proctocolitis

The rectosigmoid is damaged more frequently than any other segment of bowel because it is relatively fixed in the pelvis and most radiation for gynecologic or prostatic malignancy is directed to this region.

When more than 4000 rad is given, most patients develop transient diarrhea accompanied by tenesmus, mild abdominal cramps, and a mucoid or occasionally bloody discharge. Whether chronic bowel injury will subsequently develop cannot be judged by the severity of the acute symptoms or the appearance of the rectal mucosa. Roentgenographically, changes of acute ischemic colitis are usually found, with "thumbprinting" (representing submucosal edema and hemorrhage) and spasm predominating. In more severe cases, the appearance resembles that of acute idiopathic ulcerative proctocolitis.

About 10% of these patients develop complications including chronic proctitis or colitis, fistulation (especially to the vagina or bladder), stricture formation with colonic obstruction, and ulcer disease of the anterior rectal wall. Constipation that develops following radiation therapy should always raise suspicion of a rectal stricture. Abdominal cramps are unusual in pure rectal injuries and generally imply the presence of more proximal colonic disease. Chronic proctocolitis with bloody diarrhea or hematochezia usually presents after the acute proctitis has apparently resolved and there has been a symptom-free interval of months to years. Less commonly, there is no recognizable hiatus between the acute onset and the development of chronic disease.

Most patients with proctocolitis, rectal ulcers, and mild stenosis improve on medical therapy. Spasmolytics, anticholinergics, and antidiarrheal agents such as diphenoxylate hydrochloride with atropine sulfate (Lomotil) or ioperamide (Imodium) are helpful, and serotonin antagonists (*e.g.*, cyproheptidine [Periactin]) may aid in relieving tenesmus and rectal pain. Rectal administration of corticosteroids is the keystone of management for severe distal disease; oral corticosteroids have been used for more extensive disease. Experimentally, the long-term use of sulfonamides has been shown to diminish the damaging effects of bowel radiation, but only meager clinical evidence exists that sulfasalazine (Azulfidine) helps control symptoms or progression. Patients with distal stenosis can usually be managed with dilatation and low-residue diet.

Surgery for relatively minor complaints should be avoided because of the problems with wound healing in irradiated tissue. A proximal defunctionalizing colostomy is the key to the successful management of tight rectal strictures, severe and unrelenting proctitis, and rectovaginal fistulas. Reconstructive surgery can be attempted when healing is maximal and an adequate opportunity has been allowed to determine whether the primary cancer has been controlled.[16]

Antibiotic-Associated (Pseudomembranous) Colitis

In association with the use of all antibiotics (except vancomycin, parenteral aminoglycosides, and antituberculosis drugs), some patients, mostly beyond middle age, develop diarrhea and a colitis characterized by pseudomembranes and caused by a toxin of *Clostridium difficile*.[4] Pseudomembranous colitis associated with clindamycin therapy can occur after both oral and parenteral administration of the drug, although it appears three to four times as often with oral usage.[56] The onset is usually marked by watery diarrhea, cramps, and fever and may occur while the patient is still on therapy or up to 1 month after the drug has been stopped. Bloody diarrhea is very unusual. In about 20% of patients, abdominal pain is accompanied by rebound tenderness, fever, and leukocytosis. On proctosigmoidoscopy typical grayish green or yellow plaquelike pseudomembranous lesions are seen. Their absence, however, does not exclude diagnosis. The most reliable criterion on which the diagnosis should be based is one of the specific laboratory assays for *C. difficile* toxin. Once the putative antibiotic is discontinued, the disease is usually self-limited. If antibiotic therapy is continued, a mortality of 20% and significant morbidity has been reported.

Cholestyramine, which binds the toxin (and also binds certain antimicrobial agents, *e.g.*, clindamycin and vancomycin), appears to be rapidly effective in some patients. Constipating agents such as Lomotil or Imodium are contraindicated because they prolong the toxin's contact with the bowel. Vancomycin, which has been considered the treatment of choice, is quite expensive, must be given orally, and has a relapse rate of about 20%. Metronidazole and bacitracin have been used successfully both as primary therapy and for cases that have relapsed on therapy with vancomycin.[19]

LOWER INTESTINAL BLEEDING AND VASCULAR ECTASIAS

The first step in the diagnosis of severe lower intestinal bleeding is aspiration of gastric contents.[7,11] The absence of blood and the presence of bile in the aspirate virtually exclude a source of bleeding proximal to the ligament of Treitz. A clear but nonbilious aspirate eliminates only a lesion in the esophagus or stomach and is an indication for upper gastrointestinal endoscopy prior to colonoscopy or angiography. Standard proctosigmoidoscopic examination is done to exclude anorectal pathology, and appropriate hematologic tests are performed to rule out an underlying clotting defect.

In patients with bleeding from the lower intestinal tract that has stopped, total colonoscopy is the initial diagnostic procedure. If this reveals no explanation for the bleeding other than diverticulosis, barium studies are indicated. If both colonoscopy and barium opacification studies are normal or show only the presence of diverticula, selective mesenteric angiography is performed. Angiography can diagnose or exclude many vascular lesions, even in the absence of extravasation.

In patients who are unstable or bleeding massively, selective angiography, rather than colonoscopy, is the initial diagnostic procedure. It also provides an access for the intra-arterial infusion of vasoconstrictors.

In patients thought to be actively but not massively bleeding, the initial study is abdominal scintigraphy performed with both technetium Tc 99m sulfur colloid and ^{99m}Tc-labeled red blood cells.

Radionuclide imaging agents can detect bleeding at rates as low as 0.1 ml/min and can determine whether the patient is actively bleeding or merely passing old intraluminal blood. These agents are complementary in their diagnostic usefulness. Sulfur colloid, cleared by the liver and spleen, is not accurate for detection of bleeding sites in the upper abdomen. Imaging with ^{99m}Tc-labeled red blood cells detects sites in the upper and lower tracts, and repeat scanning can be performed over a 24-hour interval without reinjection of tracer; thus, intermittently bleeding sites can be detected. If scintigraphy demonstrates a bleeding site and the patient's condition is neither unstable nor is there massive bleeding, colonoscopy is performed.

VASCULAR ECTASIAS (ANGIODYSPLASIAS)

The vascular ectasia, or angiodysplasia, also referred to as an arteriovenous malformation or angioma, is by far the most common vascular lesion of the large bowel. It is probably the most frequent cause of recurrent lower intestinal bleeding after 60 years of age.[7] Ectasias are not associated with angiomatous lesions of the skin or other viscera, almost always occur in the cecum or proximal ascending colon, are usually multiple and less than 5 mm in diameter, rarely can be identified by the surgeon at operation or the pathologist in the laboratory using standard techniques, and usually can be diagnosed clinically only by angiography but occasionally by colonoscopy.[9]

Most patients are over 55 and two thirds of our patients were over 70.[9] A history or clinical diagnosis of heart disease is present in almost half the patients, and in 20% to 25% of all patients with ectasias, aortic stenosis has been said to be present; these patients may bleed from ectasias at an earlier age than patients without aortic disease.

Bleeding from ectasias is most often recurrent and low grade, although about 15% of patients present with acute massive hemorrhage. Patients may have bright red blood, maroon stools, and melena on separate occasions. In 10% to 15% of the patients, bleeding is evidenced by iron-deficiency anemia with stools that are intermittently positive for occult blood. In contrast to diverticular hemorrhage, the bleeding stops spontaneously in more than 90% of patients with vascular ectasias.

Structurally, these tiny lesions appear to be ectatic veins, venules, and capillaries. We believe their distinct cause is chronic, partial, intermittent, low-grade obstruction of the submucosal veins, especially where they pierce the muscle layers of the colon.

Histologically, the most consistent and earliest abnormality is a dilated, often huge, submucosal vein. Later lesions show increasing numbers of dilated and deformed vessels traversing the muscularis mucosa and involving the mucosa. In the most severe lesions, the mucosa is replaced by a maze of distorted, dilated vascular channels. An ectasia visualized colonoscopically has already progressed beyond the stage in which only the submucosal vasculature is affected. Colonoscopy is useful to identify and treat only advanced ectasias; criteria exist to diagnose vascular ectasias angiographically in all stages of their development.[12]

The usual therapy for vascular ectasias proven or strongly suspected as the cause of lower intestinal bleeding has been right hemicolectomy. Colonoscopic electrocoagulation or laser obliteration are alternate therapeutic options in selected patients.

BENIGN TUMORS

Benign Polyps

It has been estimated that 5% to 10% of a random adult population in the United States would have polyps on proctosigmoidoscopy and that this figure would double or triple if flexible sigmoidoscopy or barium enema examination were used. The older the population, the greater is the frequency of polyps. Hyperplastic (or metaplastic) polyps are so common in elderly subjects that some authorities consider them a normal aging change in the colonic mucosa. In this lesion, the cells grow more slowly and live longer than normal epithelial cells so the cells at the base of the crypts appear "hypermature." The hyperplastic polyp has no malignant potential and is not a neoplastic growth.

Adenomas are the most common neoplastic polyp in the colorectum. There appears to be an increased involvement of the ascending colon in patients 60 to 80 years of age.[54] Adenomas are precancerous lesions; an "adenoma-carcinoma sequence" is supported by the frequency with which adenomas and carcinomas are found concurrently and by histologic studies showing actual transition from adenoma to carcinoma.

The risk of finding cancer in a given polyp is related to its size and histologic type.[25] The prevalence of cancer in adenomas less than 1 cm in size is about 1%; in those over 2 cm in size, it is about 50%. The risk of malignancy is greatest in the villous type of adenoma. Ninety-five percent of polyps are beyond the reach of the rigid sigmoidoscope, and almost one third are beyond the reach of the 60 cm flexible sigmoidoscope.

Benign colonic polyps infrequently cause symptoms, and even bleeding is usually occult. Acute and severe hemorrhage requires exclusion of another cause. Villous adenomas, especially when large and distal, commonly cause constipation or mucoid diarrhea and occasionally prolapse. Profuse mucorrhea may result in hypokalemia. With proximal lesions, the colon can absorb the fluid secreted by the tumor and the patient may do well for many years. When the tumor becomes large, a syndrome of volume depletion, electrolyte imbalance (especially hypokalemia and hyponatremia), hypoalbuminemia, azotemia, and circulatory collapse may eventuate. This clinical picture may resemble adrenal insufficiency, diabetic coma, sprue syndrome, or laxative abuse. Villous adenomas are soft and may be easily missed by perfunctory rectal examination.

The advent of colonoscopy has revolutionized the therapeutic approach. Colonoscopy, with polypectomy, has a 0.05% risk of mortality and a 2.4% risk of morbidity; localization of the polyp and its removal is successful in up to 97% of cases.[59] Removal of colonic adenomas may reduce the subsequent incidence of colorectal carcinoma to as low as 15% of the expected rate.[30] Hyperplastic and adenomatous polyps need no further immediate treatment, although repeat inspection of the colon in 1 year is advisable. A completely excised "benign" polyp that contains a focus of intramucosal carcinoma superficial to the muscularis mucosae (*i.e.*, carcinoma *in situ*) requires more frequent surveillance but no further immediate therapy. The management of polyps with foci of microscopically invasive carcinoma is controversial.

Cronkhite-Canada Syndrome

The Cronkhite Canada syndrome is the only one of the multiple polyposis syndromes to affect middle-aged and elderly patients. It consists of polyposis of the esophagus, stomach, small bowel, and colon associated with alopecia, cutaneous hyperpigmentation, and atrophic changes of the nailbeds. All cases appear spontaneously (*i.e.*, without familial transmission). The clinical course is characterized by watery diarrhea, weakness, severe weight loss, hypoalbuminemia, and electrolyte losses. The polyp in this syndrome is an in-flammatory lesion with features resembling a juvenile polyp. It does not appear to have a malignant potential. In females the disease runs a progressive deteriorating course, while in males there is a tendency for spontaneous remission. There is no known specific therapy for this disorder.

Lipomas

Most lipomas are located in the colon at or near the ileocecal valve, and in later life are usually incidental findings. When therapy is required, operative removal is standard; but on occasion, especially when the tumors are pedunculated, they may be removed colonoscopically.

Hemangiomas

The colorectum is a frequent site for vascular tumors, most common of which is the hemangioma. Hemangiomas usually present with bleeding. Roentgenographically, especially with cavernous hemangioma of the rectum, typical clusters of calcifications (phleboliths) may occur. The usual therapy is surgical resection, although symptoms may be controlled with endoscopic fulguration, laser coagulation, or local sclerosis.

MALIGNANT TUMORS

Carcinoma

Cancer of the large bowel afflicted approximately 120,000 residents of the United States in 1981 and was exceeded as a cause of death only by lung cancer in the male and by breast cancer in the female.[46] Its incidence appears closely associated with the consumption of high-meat, high-fat, and low-fiber foodstuffs. Certain underlying disorders such as ulcerative colitis are known to be associated with a higher than usual incidence of colonic cancer. In the elderly, underlying disorders that more often cause concern are dermatomyositis, multiple adenomas, ureterosigmoidostomy, and radiation colitis.

The incidence of carcinoma of the colon rises progressively with advancing age and peaks in the eighth decade. In one study [54] there was a significantly greater percentage of patients over the age of 70 years with cancer in the right colon and in whom the colonic cancer was indolent, progressing slower than in a younger population.[18] Occult blood loss sufficient to cause symptoms of anemia occurs in about one third of patients with right-sided carcinomas, and only later do alteration of bowel habits, obstruction, and weight loss occur. In the left colon, the clinical presentation is usually more obvious, with increasing obstruction and occasionally rectal bleeding.

Carcinoma of the rectum most often presents as bleeding and a change in bowel habits. Patients may manifest a so-called morning-diarrhea or dyschezia syndrome in which there is an urgent desire to defecate on arising. Tenesmus, or a harassing sense of incomplete evacuation, is common. Rectal cancers are within reach of the examining finger in about three fourths of instances compared with left colon lesions in which the tumor mass itself is palpable in fewer than half of cases. Palpable lymphadenopathy is unusual with metastatic colon cancer, although a sentinel lymph node is occasionally present in the left supraclavicular space. Hepatomegaly usually indicates spread to the liver.

Routine laboratory studies are rarely helpful in establishing the diagnosis. Anemia, leukocytosis, and an elevated serum alkaline phosphatase level usually suggest advanced disease. A single examination of the feces for occult blood is often negative, even when the subject is anemic. To be reliable, such an examination should be performed on successive days with the patient on a meat-free, vegetable-free, high-fiber diet. Hemoccult slide positivity and predictive value for neoplasia increased from 27% for ages 40 to 49 to 52% for patients older than 69 years.[58] It has been demonstrated that flexible sigmoidoscopy is superior to conventional rigid sigmoidoscopy as a routine diagnostic procedure.

An association between colonic carcinoma and septicemia with *Streptococcus bovis* has been described.[39] This organism is a part of the normal fecal flora in 10% to 16% of healthy human subjects, but an increased fecal carriage rate in patients with carcinoma of the colon has been described. In most patients, no gastrointestinal signs or symptoms are present and the stools are without occult blood. Bacteremia with *S. bovis* demands a thorough gastrointestinal evaluation to exclude the presence of neoplasia, especially in the colon.

The only curative therapy for cancer of the large bowel is surgical. Colonoscopic resection of pedunculated adenomas bearing cancer is considered adequate if the malignant change is confined to the head of the polyp and is within the mucosa. Age-corrected survival rates in the elderly, as computed by actuarial methods, reveal a more favorable prognosis for elderly patients with surgically treated disease than for the young.[36,37]

Most studies of preoperative adjunctive radiation therapy indicate some increase in patient survival without an increase in complication rate.[40] Regional lymph node involvement seems to be diminished, and some lesions are rendered resectable by the therapy. Postoperative adjuvant radiation therapy is less studied but has the advantage of treating the patients after staging, so that those for whom such treatment would be of little or no benefit are spared. Radiation therapy also has a role with locally unresectable or recurrent rectal cancer and may ease bleeding, mucorrhea, tenesmus, and pain. Occasionally radiation therapy may be used to supplement locally destructive measures. Some patients who have nonresectable low-lying lesions may be benefited by local measures to destroy the tumor. Such procedures include electrofulguration, laser therapy, and radiation therapy. The precise role of chemotherapy alone or as an adjuvant to colorectal cancer surgery and/or radiation therapy is yet to be identified.

Carcinoid Tumors of the Colorectum

Carcinoid tumors of the large bowel tend to occur at the rectal and cecal ends, infrequently involving the intervening bowel. Cecal carcinoids are invariably malignant and have the highest incidence of metastases compared with carcinoids in any other area of the gastrointestinal tract. Colon carcinoids do not have an association with second malignancies and rarely cause either the carcinoid syndrome or elevations of urinary 5-hydroxyindoleacetic acid. Because of the high incidence of malignancy, colonic carcinoids should be treated by hemicolectomy.

Carcinoids in the rectum are usually less than 1 cm in size and are clinically silent. Their prognosis, because of small size and low incidence of overt malignancy, is good. Multicentricity and second malignancies are also unusual. Proctosigmoidoscopically, these lesions usually appear as small slightly yellowish or tan nodules or as submucosal tumors. Local excision or fulguration is the preferred therapy.

Lymphoma

Malignant tumors of lymphoid tissue usually involve the large bowel as part of a generalized lymphoma. Primary lesions of the colon and rectum are much less common. They usually affect patients over the age of 50 years and most often involve the cecum followed by the rectosigmoid.

Treatment of primary colorectal lymphoma is surgical, and 5-year survival rates of 55% or more can be expected. The role of radiation therapy in treating unresectable tumor is well established, but that of radiation therapy as an adjuvent to surgical therapy is in need of further study.

Anal Malignancies

A variety of malignant processes occur in the anal region because of its histologic complexity and because of the varied types of epithelial surfaces and soft tissues that share this small area. The three most commonly encountered lesions are squamous cell cancer, cloacogenic carcinoma, and malignant melanoma.

Squamous cell cancers account for more than 90% of all primary cancers of the anus and are slightly more common in women. Bleeding is the most common symptom, followed by anal discomfort, complaints frequently erroneously attributed to hemorrhoids. As the tumor grows, it restricts the anal passage and causes constipation and diminished stool caliber. In women, anal cancers are associated with second cancers of the adjacent squamous epithelium—lined structures (*i.e.*, vagina, vulva, cervix).

Anal cancers spread by local invasion into the adjacent and surrounding structures and then into the lymphatics. Treatment involves local excision for early lesions and abdominoperineal resection for the more extensive tumors. Radiation therapy is perhaps most appropriate as a palliative measure when operation is considered unwise.

The anus is the third most common site for malignant melanoma after the skin and eye. Most such patients present with rectal bleeding or an anal or inguinal mass. Melanoma may resemble a thrombosed hemorrhoid; however, pigmented nevi are seldom seen in this area and any pigmented lesion should be considered a melanoma until proven otherwise. About half of the lesions will be amelanotic and grossly may resemble hemorrhoidal "tags." Lymphogenous and hematogenous spread occur early, and prognosis is dismal.

Malakoplakia

Malakoplakia is an inflammatory granulomatous disorder usually involving the urinary tract but also affecting the genital and gastrointestinal tracts and retroperitoneum. In adults, malakoplakia occurs with a peak age incidence of 57 years.

The rectosigmoid is most often involved, and in 15% to 20% of cases a carcinoma of the colon or rectum is associated. Clinical symptoms usually consists of diarrhea, abdominal pain, and rectal bleeding.

Lesions may resemble cancers grossly but microscopically are characterized by dense aggregates of large histiocytes (von Hanseman cells) in a scanty connective tissue stroma infiltrated with lymphocytes and plasma cells. Characteristic Michaelis-Gutmann bodies, also referred to as siderocalcific bodies or calcospherules, are found. The disorder is believed to represent defective phagocytosis of bacteria or other foreign bodies. The association with carcinoma, immune diseases, corticosteroid therapy, and immune deficiency syndromes has led to the supposition that the disease reflects an acquired abnormality of intraphagosomal digestion.

The first line of therapy should include a combination of an intracellularly active antibiotic such as sulfonamides, trimethoprim-sulfamethoxazole, or rifampin in conjunction with bethanechol and ascorbic acid to improve leukocytic function.

PSEUDO-OBSTRUCTION OF THE COLON

Pseudo-obstruction of the colon and its management have previously been considered. A variant of colonic pseudo-obstruction is the "megasigmoid syndrome," which is observed in psychotic patients.[41] Its etiology remains obscure, although a causative role has been suggested for both neglect to respond to defecation stimuli and psychologically evoked diminution of vagal tone. In some cases, the dilatation is seen both proximal and distal to the sigmoid, which helps differentiate this entity from volvulus; in others, the enlargement is confined just to the rectosigmoid. Patients with the megasigmoid syndrome are usually in the seventh decade of life and confined to neuropsychiatric hospitals. Characteristically there is a paucity of symptoms despite severe constipation and bowel distention, a relaxed anal sphincter with fecal incontinence, chronic proctosigmoiditis, and stercoral ulcers with fecal concretions. Serious complications are frequent and may be prevented by early diagnosis and appropriate medical or surgical therapy, including a decompressive colostomy, a sigmoid resection, or, in some cases, a subtotal colectomy and ileoproctostomy.

SYSTEMIC DISORDERS

Systemic disorders interfering with normal colonic motility cause constipation and occasionally pseudo-obstruction. Three such disorders are diabetes mellitus. Parkinson's disease, and myxedema.

Constipation is the most frequent bowel complaint in these disorders. In diabetes it is believed to reflect an autonomic neuropathy. In Parkinson's disease, constipation tends to be aggravated by the medications. Massive colonic dilatation may be indistinguishable from mechanical bowel obstruction. Additional problems in differential diagnosis may arise when large bowel dilatation is associated with small bowel ileus and abdominal pain mimicking an "acute abdomen." Antiparkinsonian drugs should be discontinued during the acute phase of management.

Megacolon can develop as a complication of longstanding thyroid deficiency or can be the initial and dominant manifestation of the disease. Reversibility of the colonic ileus is unpredictable and variable despite replacement of thyroid hormone.

INTESTINAL GAS

The composition of intestinal gas varies with its site, but in any location nitrogen is the most plentiful and is believed to be derived essentially from swallowed air. Hydrogen, methane, and carbon dioxide, all of which are odorless, are the three gases produced in appreciable quantities in the human gut. Hydrogen and methane are produced solely by bacteria, while carbon dioxide may be produced by bacterial action and human metabolic processes.

Most gaseousness is caused by aerophagia or the excessive swallowing of air. With each swallow, 2 cc to 3 cc of air normally enters the digestive tract. Aerophagia may be a manifestation of nervous tension or depression in the elderly patient who, having previously been productive, is now beginning to question his role in society. Aerophagia is common in elderly patients who complain of gaseousness for the first time. It is often explained by poorly fitting dentures with hypersalivation or habitual sucking on candies. Both lead to frequent swallowing and aerophagia, often without the patient's knowledge. Aerophagia may be produced by nausea or by the willful desire of the patient to cause belching to relieve the uncomfortable feelings associated with hiatal hernia, peptic ulcer, or gallbladder disease. If a patient is not depressed and is not an "air-swallower," a dietary history should consider increased ingestion of starches and vegetables often believed by the elderly to be "better tolerated." Disease states enabling bacteria to thrive and multiply in the proximal bowel or maldigestive and malabsorptive disorders bringing undigested food substances into

the distal bowel should also be excluded. Gastric hyposecretion may cause excess gas production by allowing bacterial overgrowth and parasitic infestation.

The clinical syndromes of excess gaseousness are belching, the magenblase syndrome, flexural (splenic or hepatic) syndromes, and flatulousness. The magenblase syndrome refers to an enlarged gas bubble within the stomach, usually acquired by aerophagia, producing early satiety and postprandial fullness. Occasionally, the magenblase syndrome may present as a sharp or stabbing pain in the left abdomen and chest and be confused with angina pectoris.

Flexural syndromes are similar to the magenblase syndrome; symptoms are due to a collection of gas in the splenic or, less commonly, the hepatic flexure. Sharp abdominal pain and aching discomfort are the most frequent complaints. Symptoms of the hepatic flexure syndrome often prompt an evaluation for cholecystitis, while in the splenic flexure syndrome, the patient is usually concerned about the possibility of cardiac disease.

Flatulence may be caused by excessive ingestion of air or bacterial production of gas within the bowel lumen. Roentgenographic studies are of value in detecting abnormal patterns of gas or underlying disorders. Laboratory studies are important in excluding underlying disorders such as parasitic infestation, blind loop syndrome, and malabsorption, while breath testing may aid in evaluating carbohydrate malabsorption, lactase deficiency, and bacterial overgrowth states.

Successful therapy is based on careful delineation of cause. If aerophagia is prominent, simple explanation of the role of swallowed air is occasionally helpful. Attention to proper chewing, swallowing, and oral hygiene and dietary alteration may have a substantial effect. Foods to be avoided include inadequately cooked starch, high-fiber foods, and certain legumes and vegetables, such as beans, peas, cabbage, Brussel sprouts, cauliflower, broccoli, turnips, onions, many raw fruits, and the juices of apples, grapes, and prunes. Milk products may be transiently withdrawn in a therapeutic trial, or in lactase deficiency they are omitted from the diet and gradually reintroduced to establish the maximum amount tolerated. Establishment of regular bowel habits, use of antacids that do not release carbon dioxide, and the avoidance of stress when possible are desirable. Of course, any underlying bowel disorders should be treated. Anecdotal reports abound of patients who obtained dramatic relief using activated charcoal or simethicone to absorb gas, but to date no carefully controlled trials have validated these hopeful claims.

INTESTINAL ISCHEMIA

Relatively few patients suffer from chronic intestinal ischemia; acute mesenteric ischemia is far more common in the elderly. A practical approach to ischemic bowel disorders considers four broad categories of disease; in three there is a single episode of acute ischemia, and in the fourth, chronic mesenteric ischemia, there are multiple recurrent attacks:

1. Acute mesenteric ischemia—acute ischemia of major portions of the small intestine with or without involvement of the colon
2. Focal mesenteric ischemia—acute ischemia of localized segments of small intestine
3. Colonic ischemia—acute ischemia involving only the colon
4. Chronic mesenteric ischemia—ischemia of small and large bowel but without loss of tissue viability

Acute Mesenteric Ischemia

Nonocclusive mesenteric ischemia and superior mesenteric artery embolus each accounts for 25% to 50% of episodes of acute mesenteric ischemia.[8] Fewer patients with nonocclusive mesenteric ischemia are being reported, possibly because of better monitoring in intensive care units with correction of hemodynamic abnormalities before hypotension occurs and widespread use of systemic unloading (vasodilating) agents in the management of congestive heart failure and myocardial ischemia.

Acute mesenteric ischemia, whether caused by superior mesenteric artery embolus or thrombosis, mesenteric venous thrombosis, or nonocclusive mesenteric ischemia ("low flow" syndrome) is an intra-abdominal catastrophe as lethal today as 50 years ago, with an average mortality of 70% to 80%. In 1972, Boley and colleagues[13] proposed an aggressive plan of management calling for earlier and more extensive use of angiography and the intra-arterial infusion of papaverine to interrupt splanchnic vasoconstriction. This has resulted in an impressive improvement in survival and salvage of compromised bowel.

Early diagnosis depends on recognition of patients at risk. Acute mesenteric ischemia is most likely to develop in patients over 50 years of age with longstanding congestive heart failure, cardiac arrhythmias, recent myocardial infarctions, or hypovolemia or hypotension.

Abdominal pain is present in 75% to 98% of patients with intestinal ischemia but varies in severity, nature, and location. Characteristic of early acute mesenteric ischemia is a disparity between the severity of the abdominal pain and the paucity of significant abdominal findings. Sudden severe pain accompanied by forceful intestinal emptying is strongly suggestive of an acute arterial occlusion. A history of postprandial abdominal pain for several weeks or months preceding the acute episode is common in patients with superior mesenteric artery thrombosis.

Unexplained abdominal distention or gastrointestinal bleeding may be the only indication of acute intestinal ischemia. Pain may be absent in up to 15% to 25% of patients, especially those with nonocclusive mesenteric ischemia. Distention, usually absent early in the course, may be the first sign of impending intestinal infarction. Gastrointestinal bleeding may precede any other symptom, although stools are positive for occult blood in up to 75% of patients.

Early there are usually no abdominal findings. As infarction develops, increasing tenderness, rebound tenderness, and muscle guarding reflect progressive intestinal changes. Significant abdominal findings are strong evidence for the presence of nonviable bowel. Nausea, vomiting, fever, rectal bleeding, hematemesis, intestinal obstruction, back pain, shock, and increasing abdominal distention are other late signs.

Leukocytosis above 15,000 cells/cu mm occurs in approximately 75% of patients with acute mesenteric ischemia, and a metabolic acidosis with increased base deficit is present in about 50%. Elevations in serum and peritoneal fluid amylase, alkaline phosphatase, and inorganic phosphates have been reported, but the consistency and specificity of these findings have not been established. Leukocytosis, especially if out of proportion to the physical findings, an elevated hematocrit, and blood-tinged peritoneal fluid, often with a high amylase content, are signs of advanced intestinal necrosis.

For patients too ill to undergo angiography, laparoscopy is helpful but potentially hazardous, since profound decreases in superior mesenteric arterial flow occur with pressures over 20 mm Hg. Laparoscopy, although useful to diagnose transmural infarction, is not reliable for evaluating earlier stages of mucosal ischemia in which blood is shunted to the serosa and the normal intestinal appearance is preserved.

Angiography has been successfully used to diagnose and manage acute mesenteric ischemia. For example, after the type of occlusion has been identified, intra-arterial papaverine can be used to overcome vasoconstriction. Mesenteric vasoconstriction may occur with hemorrhage, pancreatitis, and other conditions, but in patients with suspected intestinal ischemia not in shock or receiving vasopressors, it is strong evidence for nonocclusive mesenteric ischemia. If angiography is performed sufficiently early, patients with acute mesenteric ischemia of a nonocclusive origin as well as those with surgically correctable occlusive lesions can be identified before bowel infarction occurs.

All patients are promptly treated for associated cardiovascular problems and sent for plain film studies of the abdomen. Abdominal angiography is then routinely performed unless some other intra-abdominal condition is diagnosed on the plain film examination. Based on the angiographic findings and the presence or absence of signs of peritoneal irritation on physical examination of the abdomen, the individual patient is then treated according to the schema outlined in Figure 16-1.

Patients over 50 years of age with any of the predisposing conditions and sudden onset of abdominal pain lasting more than 2 or 3 hours are started on the management protocol. These broad selection criteria are essential for early diagnosis and treatment because the presence of more extensive and specific signs and symptoms usually signifies irreversible intestinal damage.

Even when the decision to operate has been made, an angiogram must be obtained to manage the patient properly at operation. Moreover, the relief of mesenteric vasoconstriction is an integral part of the therapy for emboli and thromboses, as well as for "low flow" states and can best be achieved by intra-arterial infusion of papaverine through the angiography catheter.

Initial treatment is directed to correction of predisposing or precipitating causes. Relief of acute congestive heart failure, correction of cardiac arrhythmias, and replacement of blood volume precede any diagnostic studies. In general, efforts at increasing intestinal blood flow will be futile if low cardiac output, hypotension, or hypovolemia persists. Patients who are hypotensive, hypovolemic, or in shock should not have angiography, since mesenteric vasoconstriction always will be evident even without intestinal ischemia. Such patients should not receive papaverine intra-arterially, since this will increase the size of the vascular bed and aggravate the hypovolemia.

The management of associated congestive heart failure or shock is especially difficult. Digitalis preparations all have a direct vasoconstrictor ac-

tion on superior mesenteric artery smooth muscle. Vasopressors are contraindicated in the treatment of shock if mesenteric ischemia is suspected. A helpful development is increased use of systemic vasodilators in the therapy of congestive heart failure and myocardial infarction. These drugs (*e.g.,* hydralazine, prazosin, nitroglycerin, and nitroprusside) reduce arterial impedance by diminishing preload and/or afterload and theoretically are ideal agents to treat low mesenteric flow syndromes associated with congestive failure.

When intestinal ischemia has progressed to the extent that systemic alterations are present, correction of plasma volume deficits, gastrointestinal decompression, and parenteral antibiotics are essential before any roentgenologic studies. Systemic and locally administered antibiotics are of value in improving the viability of compromised bowel. After these initial measures, roentgenologic studies are undertaken irrespective of the abdominal physical findings or the surgeon's decision whether to operate.

Initially, plain film examination of the abdomen is performed to exclude other diagnosable causes of abdominal pain (*e.g.,* a perforated viscus or intestinal obstruction). Signs of intestinal ischemia on plain film studies occur late and usually indicate bowel infarction. If the plain films do not reveal another cause for the pain, angiography is performed.

Emergency angiography is the keystone of our aggressive approach. Emboli, thrombosis, and mesenteric vasoconstriction can be diagnosed, and the adequacy of the splanchnic circulation can be evaluated; the angiographic catheter also provides a route for the administration of intra-arterial vasodilators. The angiographic technique has been revealed in detail elsewhere.[6]

The use of anticoagulants in the management of acute mesenteric ischemia is controversial. We do not use heparin in the perioperative period, except with venous thrombosis, because of the danger of intestinal hemorrhage. Because of the occurrence of thromboses late in the postoperative period, we start anticoagulation 48 hours postoperatively following embolectomy or arterial reconstruction.

Laparotomy is indicated to restore intestinal arterial flow (*i.e.,* after an embolus or thrombosis) or to resect irreparably damaged bowel. There is no proven reliable objective means of determining the viability of ischemic intestine. Measurements of serosal temperature and pH, electromyography, and the distribution of injected vital dyes or ^{99m}Tc-tagged albumin microspheres have all been used. More recently, direct Doppler determination of ser-

(Text continues on p. 292.)

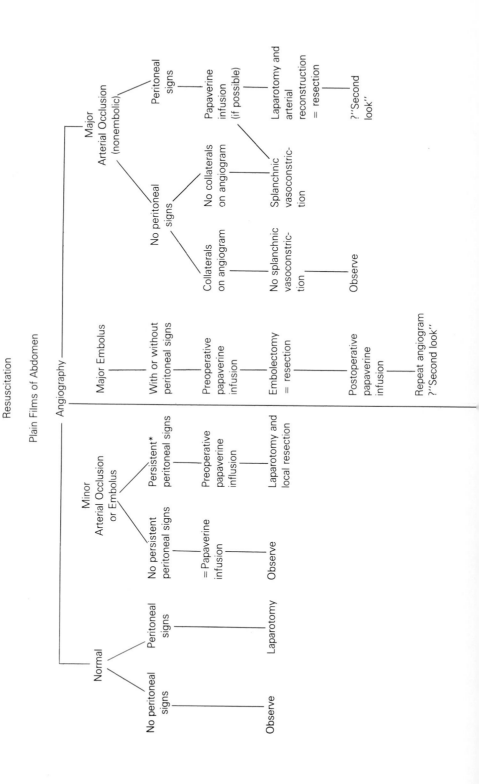

Resuscitation

Plain Films of Abdomen — Angiography

Normal
- No peritoneal signs → Observe
- Peritoneal signs → Laparotomy

Minor Arterial Occlusion or Embolus
- No persistent peritoneal signs → = Papaverine infusion → Observe
- Persistent* peritoneal signs → Preoperative papaverine infusion → Laparotomy and local resection

Major Embolus
- With or without peritoneal signs → Preoperative papaverine infusion → Embolectomy = resection → Postoperative papaverine infusion → Repeat angiogram ?"Second look"

Major Arterial Occlusion (nonembolic)
- No peritoneal signs
  - Collaterals on angiogram → No splanchnic vasoconstriction → Observe
  - No collaterals on angiogram → Splanchnic vasoconstriction
- Peritoneal signs → Papaverine infusion (if possible) → Laparotomy and arterial reconstruction = resection → ?"Second look"

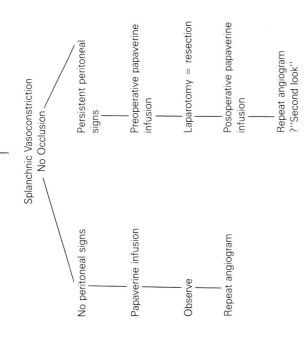

Splanchnic Vasoconstriction
No Occlusion

Persistent peritoneal
signs

Preoperative papaverine
infusion

Laparotomy = resection

Posoperative papaverine
infusion

Repeat angiogram
?"Second look"

No peritoneal signs

Papaverine infusion

Observe

Repeat angiogram

* Peritoneal signs are considered persistent if they are not relieved within 20 minutes by the bolus injection of tolazine.

FIG. 16-1. Protocol of management of patients with acute mesenteric ischemia.

osal blood flow is being evaluated.[21,42] Clinical assessments of the color of the bowel and the presence of pulsations, bleeding, and peristalsis remain the inexact criteria on which judgment of viability usually is made. If there is any question of the viability of any remaining intestine, a planned reexploration or "secondlook" is performed within 12 to 24 hours.

Superior Mesenteric Artery Embolus

Emboli to the superior mesenteric artery, responsible for 40% to 50% of episodes of acute mesenteric ischemia, usually originate from a mural or atrial thrombus associated with arteriosclerotic heart disease. Many patients have a previous history of peripheral arterial embolism, and about 20% have synchronous emboli in other arteries. The artery may be completely occluded, but more often the embolus only partially obstructs blood flow.

Patient management according to the schema in Figure 16-1, is reviewed in detail elsewhere.[6,8] A few patients managed only by papaverine infusions have had compelling medical reasons for avoiding operation and have had good perfusion of the vascular bed distal to the embolus. Thrombolytic agents infused through the angiographic catheters have also been used successfully in a few patients with superior mesenteric artery emboli. Combination of a thrombolytic agent and a vasodilator would appear ideal and various regimens are being investigated.[10]

Acute Superior Mesenteric Artery Thrombosis

Acute thromboses are always superimposed on severe atherosclerotic narrowing, most commonly in the region of the origin of the main artery. Since the acute episode represents the end state of a chronic problem, it is not surprising that 30% to 50% of patients have had abdominal pain during the preceding weeks to months. Most patients have severe diffuse atherosclerotic narrowing, most commonly close to the origin of the main artery. Since the acute episode represents the end state of a chronic problem, it is not surprising that 30% to 50% of patients have had abdominal pain during the preceding weeks to months. Most patients have severe diffuse arteriosclerosis, and a prior history of coronary, cerebral, or peripheral arterial ischemia is frequent.

Identification of a superior mesenteric artery thrombosis is usually made from the flush aorto-gram, which most often shows total occlusion of the artery within 1 cm to 2 cm of its origin. Angiographic differentiation between a thrombosis and an old embolus may be difficult. It is also important to differentiate an acute occlusion from a longstanding one. In such a dilemma, the presence or absence of prominent collaterals is the decisive factor in management (see Figure 16-1).

Nonocclusive Mesenteric Ischemia

Angiographically nonocclusive mesenteric ischemia is diagnosed when signs of mesenteric vasoconstriction are present in a patient who is neither in shock nor receiving vasopressors. Patients are managed according to the protocol in Figure 16-1 and as outlined elsewhere.[6]

Acute Mesenteric Venous Thrombosis

Mesenteric venous thrombosis is responsible for only a few cases of intestinal infarction and can be primary or secondary to a variety of conditions, including hematologic disorders, "hypercoagulable" states such as neoplasms, intra-abdominal sepsis, local venous stasis, and abdominal trauma.[49] In one series[44] 55% of the patients experienced abdominal pain from 5 days to 1 month before admission, and in another series 27% had had symptoms for more than 1 month. On examination, signs of volume depletion are usually pronounced and the abdomen is distended. Because of the marked fluid loss into the bowel, a succession splash may be present. Plain films of the abdomen are usually abnormal since infarction of the bowel has frequently occurred. The angiographic diagnosis of acute mesenteric venous thrombosis is rarely made. Most often the diagnosis is established at laparotomy performed because of peritoneal signs.

Mesenteric venous thrombosis is the one condition in which anticoagulants are used routinely postoperatively after both resection and thrombectomy. Heparin and then warfarin are administered to prevent the frequent recurrence of venous thrombosis.

Prognosis and Results

Although mortalities of 70% to 90% have been reported through 1979 using traditional methods the aggressive approach can reduce the catastrophic figures.[10] Of the first 50 patients so managed, 35 (70%) proved to have acute mesenteric ischemia and 19 (54%) survived. Eighty-five percent of the survivors did not lose any bowel or had excision of less than 3 feet of small intestine, thus enabling normal bowel function.

In 47 patients with intestinal ischemia resulting from superior mesenteric artery emboli,[10] the survival rate was 55% in patients managed according to an aggressive protocol, whereas only 20% of those treated by traditional methods survived.

Complications of the angiographic studies and prolonged infusions of vasodilator drugs have not been excessive. Three of our first 50 patients developed transient acute tubular necrosis. There were several instances of local hematomas at the arterial puncture site. Problems with prolonged papaverine infusions have been minimal.

FOCAL SEGMENTAL ISCHEMIA OF THE SMALL BOWEL

Ischemic insults localized to short segments of the small bowel are most commonly caused by atheromatous emboli, strangulated hernias, collagen diseases, blunt abdominal trauma, and segmental venous thrombosis. With focal ischemia there is usually adequate collateral circulation that prevents transmural hemorrhagic infarction. Hence, the most common lesions are infected infarcts resulting from partial necrosis of the bowel wall and secondary invasion of the intestinal bacterial flora.

Patients with short-segment ischemia may present in one of three clinical patterns:

1. In the acute presentation, seen with transmural necrosis, there is a sudden onset of abdominal pain that often simulates acute appendicitis.
2. Other patients present with signs or symptoms of chronic enteritis (*i.e.,* crampy abdominal pain, diarrhea, weight loss, and occasionally fever). The clinical and roentgenologic pictures may be indistinguishable from that of Crohn's disease of the small bowel. A diagnostic feature of help is the location of the involved segment; Crohn's enteritis usually, but not always, includes the terminal ileum, whereas focal ischemia can occur anywhere in the small bowel.
3. The most common presentation is that of chronic small bowel obstruction. Intermittent abdominal pain, distention, and vomiting results from the obstruction. Bacterial overgrowth in the dilated loop may lead to the "blind loop syndrome," that is, anemia, diarrhea, and steatorrhea. Radiologic studies reveal a smooth, tapered stricture of varying length with an abrupt change to normal bowel distally and dilated bowel proximally.

Treatment is usually surgical. Some patients without signs of peritonitis can be managed expectantly on intravenous fluids, nasogastric suction, and parenteral antibiotics. Both clinical and roentgenographic findings must resolve or the nonoperative approach is abandoned.

COLONIC ISCHEMIA

In our experience, ischemia of the colon is presently the most common vascular disorder of the intestines. Specific forms of colonic ischemia include reversible ischemic colopathy (33%); transient ischemic colitis (16%); chronic ischemic colitis (21%); colonic stricture (12%); and colonic gangrene (18%). Mild ischemia produces morphologic changes that will regress and ultimately disappear. Severe ischemia may result in gangrene, perforation, or persistent colitis; if healing occurs, it may do so with fibrosis and resultant stricture formation. It is impossible to predict the prognosis and progression of the ischemic process from the initial physical, roentgenologic, or sigmoidoscopic evaluation.

In most cases no specific etiology or occlusion is identified. Such "spontaneous" episodes have been attributed to "low flow" states and/or small vessel disease. The greater frequency of colonic ischemic lesions in the elderly suggests a relationship to degenerative changes in the vascular tree, although angiography only rarely has demonstrated a significant occlusion or abnormality. What finally triggers the ischemic episode is still conjectural, but the combination of a normally low blood flow and further diminution during functional activity would seem to make the colon uniquely susceptible to ischemic injury. About 20% of patients have an associated and potentially obstructing colonic lesion; usually this is distal to the ischemic segment of the bowel. In half of these cases the lesion is a carcinoma; in the others, various causes include fecal impaction and diverticulosis.

Most episodes of colonic ischemia produce clinical, radiologic, and pathologic changes that are completely reversible. Typically, colonic ischemia presents with the sudden onset of mild lower abdominal crampy pain, usually localized to the left side. The pain is frequently accompanied by or followed within 24 hours by bloody diarrhea or bright red blood per rectum. With irreversible lesions or accompanying small bowel involvement, the pain is quite severe. Characteristically, blood loss is minimal; massive bleeding militates against a diagnosis of colonic ischemia.

Initially, the only physical finding is mild abdominal tenderness over the involved left colon. Signs of peritoneal irritation have been noted with ultimately reversible lesions; if these persist for more than a few hours, they should be considered evidence of irreparable tissue damage.

The initial problem with colonic ischemia is to differentiate it from acute mesenteric ischemia. Patients with acute mesenteric ischemia appear sicker, have more severe pain, and usually have an acute precipitating disorder (Table 16-1). Patients with colonic ischemia present with only mild to moderate complaints and findings.

If acute mesenteric ischemia is not believed to be present, the elderly patient with sudden abdominal pain and rectal bleeding or bloody diarrhea should have a "gentle" barium enema or possibly colonoscopy within 48 hours. Distending the colon, either by barium or gas, when it has suffered a vascular insult may theoretically worsen an ischemic injury. Rigid sigmoidoscopy is of value only if the segment of involved bowel is within reach of the sigmoidoscope and the typical submucosal hemorrhages are present. Nonspecific inflammatory changes neither establish nor exclude an antecedent ischemic episode.

"Thumbprints," or pseudotumors, which disappear on serial studies are the major criteria for roentgenologic diagnosis. Thumbprints represent submucosal hemorrhages present only in the acute stage of colonic ischemia. A barium enema repeated 1 week after the initial study should reflect the evolution of the ischemic injury. Either the hemorrhages resorb and the study returns to normal or the thumbprints are replaced by a segmental colitis pattern as the mucosa ulcerates.

In mild cases, the symptoms and signs usually subside in 24 to 48 hours, the blood is resorbed and complete clinical and roentgenologic healing occurs within 1 to 2 weeks. In more severe ischemia, areas of mucosa may slough with ultimate, complete healing over 1 to 6 months. Patients with prolonged lesions may be clinically well even in the presence of persistent enema changes.

Irreversible lesions may become obvious in hours when gangrene or perforation occurs or follow a protracted course when chronic colitis or stricture develops. The diagnosis of colonic infarction is made on the basis of abdominal tenderness, guarding, rebound tenderness, a rising fever, leukocytosis, and evidence of paralytic ileus. These signs, not specific for infarction, dictate the need for emergency laparotomy.

Treatment of acute colonic ischemia is based on early diagnosis and continued monitoring of the patient and the roentgenologic appearance of the colon. Systemic antibiotics are administered when indicated, and blood and fluid loss is corrected as necessary. It is best to place the bowel at rest and provide fluids intravenously. Contrary to their efficacy in ulcerative colitis, corticosteroids are of no value. Serial barium studies are essential: they establish the diagnosis definitively, verify the reversibility of the colonic damage, or demonstrate progression to an ischemic colitis or stricture. If deterioration in the clinical course is suggested by increasing abdominal signs, fever, and leukocyto-

---

TABLE 16-1 Differential Diagnosis of Acute Mesenteric Ischemia and Colonic Ischemia

Colonic Ischemia	Acute Mesenteric Ischemia
90% in patients over 60 years	Most in older-age group but more apt to occur in younger patients
Acute precipitating cause rare	Acute precipitating cause usual, *e.g.,* myocardial infarct, congestive failure, arrhythmia, or hypotensive episode)
Predisposing associated lesion present in 20% (*e.g.,* colonic carcinoma, stricture, diverticulitis)	Predisposing lesion uncommon (excluding atherosclerosis)
Do not appear seriously ill	*Uusually appear ill*
Usually have mild abdominal pain with minimal tenderness and guarding	Pain more severe; findings are minimal early in course but become pronounced later
Mild rectal bleeding or bloody diarrhea	Rectal bleeding and diarrahea uncommon until late in the course
Should have barium enema first	*Should have angiography first*

sis, or if the diarrhea, bleeding, or both persist for more than 2 weeks, irreversible damage almost certainly has occurred and surgical intervention is indicated. Operative treatment consists of local resection with primary anastomosis.

CHRONIC MESENTERIC ISCHEMIA (ABDOMINAL ANGINA, INTESTINAL ANGINA)

Patients with chronic mesenteric ischemia experience recurrent acute episodes of insufficient blood flow during periods of maximal intestinal work. The pain is analogous to that arising in the myocardium with angina pectoris or in the calf muscles with intermittent claudication. Intestinal angina is almost always caused by atherosclerosis of the splanchnic vessels, generally in individuals over 45 years of age.[50] The consistent feature is abdominal discomfort or pain. Most commonly pain occurs 10 to 15 minutes after eating, gradually increases in severity, reaches a plateau, and then slowly abates in 1 to 3 hours. The pain most often is crampy, is located in the upper abdomen, and may radiate from the epigastrium through to the back. Some patients find it can be relieved by squatting as assuming a prone position. Initially, the pain occurs only after a large meal, but characteristically the pain pattern progresses such that the patient will reduce the size of his meals ("small meal syndrome") and become reluctant to eat. Weight loss is characteristic and often massive. Bloating, flatulence, and derangements in motility with constipation or diarrhea are also seen. Intermittent episodes of vomiting occur less commonly. Steatorrheic stools are observed by half of the patients. Physical findings are limited and nonspecific. A systolic bruit is heard in the upper abdomen in approximately one half of the patients; similar bruits have been reported in up to 15% of healthy patients.

There is no specific or reliable diagnostic test for abdominal angina. The diagnosis is based on the typically clinical symptoms, the arteriographic demonstration of an occlusive process of the splanchnic arteries, and exclusion of other gastrointestinal disease. Conventional roentgenologic examinations of the gastrointestinal tract usually are unremarkable. Angiographic demonstration of stenosis or occlusions of one or two or all of the major vessels does not by itself establish the diagnosis of arterial insufficiency. In a demanding method described by Hansen and co-workers,[33] splanchnic blood flow and intestinal oxygen con-

sumption is measured before and after a test meal. In their study, patients with abdominal angina failed to increase their splanchnic blood flow after the test meal. After arterial reconstruction, the postprandial increase was similar to that in the control group.

In the past, treatment was some form of operative arterial reconstruction. Today, transluminal angioplasty may afford an alternative approach of lesser magnitude and risk.[29] A patient with classic abdominal angina and unexplained weight loss whose diagnostic evaluation has excluded other gastrointestinal disease and whose angiogram shows occlusive involvement of at least two of the three major arteries should be treated. The issue has been much less clear if only one major vessel is involved.

Although hundreds of cases of elective revascularization of the mesenteric arteries have been reported, long-term follow-up information is limited. In three recently reported series comprising 70 patients, the operative mortality was 7%; 70% of the patients were relieved of their symptoms.[43,51] Late deaths in 21% of patients are a reflection of their generalized arteriosclerotic disease. However, only one patient died of intestinal infarction after the immediate postoperative period. In McCollum and co-worker's series of 33 patients, 83% were alive 5 years after operation and 62% were alive after 10 years.[43] Most patients will be relieved of their pain and malabsorption, although complete relief of the latter may take months.[22,52]

DISEASES OF THE MESENTERY, PERITONEUM, AND RETROPERITONEUM

The Acute Abdomen

The term *acute abdomen* refers to a clinical syndrome of severe abdominal pain usually in the presence of other signs and symptoms of peritoneal irritation and due to a host of intra-abdominal disorders that often require surgical therapy.

Often in the elderly, signs and symptoms are subtle and lull the examiner into a false sense of confidence that a "watchful approach" is reasonable. Elderly patients may not develop the pronounced fever, leukocytosis, or abdominal signs characteristic of younger individuals. Disorders producing acute abdominal pain must be distinguished from the causes of an acute "surgical" abdomen. In a report detailing the Swedish ex-

CONDITIONS COMMONLY ASSOCIATED WITH AN ACUTE ABDOMINAL PRESENTATION TO THE ELDERLY

Acute gastrointestinal obstruction
  Neoplasia
  Adhesions
  Volvulus
  Hernias
Inflammatory disorders
  Cholecystitis (with perforation, gangrene)
  Diverticulitis
  Pancreatitis
  Appendicitis
Peptic ulcer disease (with perforation, penetration)
Intramural and mesenteric hemorrhage (with anticoagulant therapy)
Acute mesenteric ischemia
Aortic aneurysm with leakage, dissection, rupture
Primary peritoneal disorders
  Neoplasia (mesothelioma)
  Infection (*e.g.*, tuberculosis)
Medical disorders
  Cardiopulmonary (acute myocardial infarction, congestive heart failure with hepatic congestion, pulmonary embolus)
  Pneumonia, pneumothorax
Urinary tract infection (stone)
Systemic diseases
  Diabetic ketosis
  Adrenal insufficiency
  Hyperlipemia
  Parkinson's disease
  Herpes zoster

perience with acute abdominal disease in patients older than 70 years,[27] acute cholecystitis was most common and accounted for one fourth of the cases; intra-abdominal malignancy is increasingly the cause of acute abdominal pain in the elderly. In contrast, in a British series reporting on patients older than 75 years who required emergent abdominal surgery,[5] strangulated hernia and intestinal obstruction were the most common causes, each accounting for approximately one third of cases. Large bowel obstruction was more common than small bowel obstruction and was most often caused by carcinoma. Small bowel obstruction was usually due to adhesions but also to carcinoma, gallstone ileus, volvulus, and ischemic stricture. Other problems necessitating emergent surgery in-

cluded acute appendicitis, perforated viscus, biliary tract disease, ruptured aneurysm, and acute mesenteric ischemia.

In the British series, an overall mortality of 32% was reported. Most deaths were divided equally between cardiopulmonary complications and the primary cause for surgery.[5]

Vascular Causes

Abdominal Aortic Aneurysms. Abdominal aortic aneurysms are a lethal disease with a poor, short-term prognosis when symptomatic. Up to 80% of such patients die within 1 year, attesting to the need for early diagnosis.[31] Physical examination is a highly accurate means of diagnosing aortic aneurysms,[53] but even minor suspicion warrants noninvasive evaluation by ultrasonography. Measurement of the size is crucial, for an aneurysm larger than 7 cm in diameter is in imminent danger of rupture and surgery is imperative even if the patient is asymptomatic.

The symptom most suggestive of abdominal aortic aneurysm is lower back pain. When dissection occurs or an aneurysm ruptures or leaks into the retroperitoneum or abdominal cavity, acute abdominal pain develops. Cardiovascular collapse often rapidly follows, although death is not necessarily immediate and there is usually time for emergent operation.

The prognosis for patients with unrepaired abdominal aortic aneurysms is poor, with representative survival statistics approximating 50% at 1 year,[26] 30% at 2 years, and 20% at 5 years. Elective surgery can now be relatively safely performed with an average mortality of 5%. Operation for a ruptured aneurysm carries a mortality rate of about 50%.[51]

Aortic Dissection. Aortic dissection is one of the most dramatic, fulminating, and rapidly fatal catastrophes known. It is more common in men between the ages of 50 and 70 years; over the age of 70, females predominate. Hypertension is an important predisposing cause.

The typical history begins with the sudden onset of severe, tearing chest pain with radiation to the arms, neck, or back. Dissection of the abdominal aorta or its branches is present in 75% of the cases. With occlusion of the visceral arteries, intense searing pain develops and is often accompanied by nausea, vomiting, abdominal tenderness and rigidity, and, rarely, cutaneous ecchymoses over the lower abdomen, flank, or chest. The abdominal picture may be confused with other causes of an acute abdomen, including acute pancreatitis, peptic ulcer with perforation, cholecystitis, appendicitis, mesenteric thrombosis, and intestinal obstruction.[34] Cardiomegaly, aortic insufficiency, congestive heart failure, and disorders of consciousness are often present. Absent or unequal pulses are common with acute dissections.

Roentgenographic findings include changes in the aortic contour, asymmetric enlargement of the aorta, and mediastinal widening. Aortography has traditionally been used to diagnose the dissection, but for elderly patients who have severe renal and cardiovascular disease and may not tolerate angiography well computed tomography is becoming increasingly helpful. Immediate therapy with nitroprusside or other regimens to induce hypotension may be lifesaving while awaiting definitive and emergent surgery.

Aneurysms of the Visceral Arteries. About 40% of visceral artery aneurysms involve the splenic artery, 20% affect the hepatic artery, 10% to 20% occur on the superior mesenteric artery, and the remainder develop on branches of these vessels.[23,54]

Diagnosis of splenic aneurysms is most commonly made in the seventh decade and more often in females. Most patients are asymptomatic, and in two thirds the diagnosis is suspected on the basis of the characteristic left upper quadrant curvilinear calcifications seen on abdominal roentgenograms. The most common complaint is vague pain in the left upper quadrant or epigastrium, occasionally with radiation to the left subscapular region and worsened with physical activity and flexing of the trunk. Expanding splenic artery aneurysms produce more severe symptoms, and rupture causes an acute abdominal catastrophe.

With an incidence of rupture between 5% and 10%, all patients with splenic artery aneurysms, especially when they are large, should be considered operative candidates.

Hepatic artery aneurysms are more common in males and are usually diagnosed after 50 years of age. The most common symptom is right upper quadrant or epigastric abdominal pain, often mimicking cholecystitis. Hemobilia, if the aneurysm leaks or ruptures into the biliary ducts and then into the gastrointestinal tract, presents as melena, often accompanied by biliary colic and transient biliary obstruction with hyperbilirubinemia and a high alkaline phosphatase level.

Aneurysms of the other splanchnic vessels are infrequent and usually due to arteriosclerosis, ex-

cept for *superior mesenteric artery aneurysms*, which are usually mycotic. These aneurysms must be suspected in any patient with subacute bacterial endocarditis who develops epigastric pain and an expanding or tender abdominal mass.

Hemorrhage with Anticoagulant Therapy. An acute abdomen may be seen with anticoagulant-induced hemorrhage into the mesentery and bleeding into the bowel wall. Roentgenographic studies usually reveal a characteristic "picket fence" or "stacked-coins" appearance of the bowel, and treatment consists of correcting the coagulation disturbance.

Systemic and Medical Causes

Systemic and medical disorders must always be excluded as a cause of severe abdominal pain. Cardiopulmonary disorders predominate among the many conditions capable of mimicking an acute abdomen and shortness of breath associated with severe abdominal pain should prompt exclusion of pneumonia, pulmonary embolism, pneumothorax, and congestive heart failure as explanations of the abdominal process.

In any patient with severe lower abdominal or back pain, atypical ureteral colic must be excluded. Acute adrenal insufficiency, especially when precipitated by septicemia and accompanied by disseminated intravascular coagulation, can cause severe abdominal pain. Parkinson's disease has been stressed as a cause of intestinal pseudo-obstruction but also may be associated with abdominal pain and rigidity, mimicking an "acute abdomen." Herpes zoster may closely simulate various intra-abdominal painful disorders over a relatively small segment of the abdomen.

Peritonitis and Causes of Ascites in the Elderly

Bile Peritonitis

Bile peritonitis is uncommon and is caused by the presence of bile and bacteria in the peritoneal cavity.[24] The clinical picture is quite variable; inexplicably, some patients tolerate a substantial amount of free bile lying silently in the peritoneal cavity while others go into shock and have severe pain with only a few milliliters of bilious fluid. In the proper clinical circumstances (cholecystitis, obstructive jaundice, abdominal trauma, or recent biliary surgery), progressive abdominal distention or the sudden onset of abdominal pain with signs of peritoneal irritation should suggest the possibility of bile peritonitis. Management includes removal of the bilious collection, prevention of further bile leakage, use of antibiotics, peritoneal lavage, and biliary decompression if necessary. Mortality increases with the age of the patient and presently approximates 20%.

Acute Chylous Peritonitis and Ascites

The basic factor producing chylous ascites is obstruction or disruption of the thoracic duct or cysterna chyli. In adults, the more common etiologies include inflammatory, neoplastic, and traumatic disorders. Inflammatory conditions such as cirrhosis and pancreatitis are commonly seen in the developed nations, but worldwide, tuberculosis and filariasis are more common causes. Lymphomas more often produce chylous effusions than do carcinomas, and among the latter, breast, pancreatic, and gastric neoplasms predominate. Surgical and nonsurgical trauma is another major cause.

The acute form of chylous ascites usually presents as an acute abdomen, with symptoms often beginning suddenly after a heavy fatty meal. In contrast, most patients with chronic chylous ascites manifest painless accumulation of ascitic fluid; there is a progressive increase in abdominal girth with only mild abdominal discomfort. Late sequelae are the results of a loss of chyle and failure of the thoracic duct to function as the route for the transport of chylomicrons to the venous circulation. This phase is characterized by weight loss, inanition, and hypoproteinemia.

Usually the diagnosis is made on inspection and analysis of the abdominal fluid, which appears milky and odorless. Occasionally, chylous ascites resolves after repeated paracentesis and supportive therapy. On other occasions when surgical therapy is not deemed appropriate and specific medical treatment is not effective, control of effusion formation may be achieved using a low-fat diet supplemented with medium-chain triglycerides that do not depend on the lymphatics for absorption. Peritoneovenous shunting has also been reported to afford relief from chylous ascites in some instances.

Other Cases of Ascites in Elderly Patients

In elderly patients with ascites, just as in younger adults, liver disease, especially cirrhosis, is a common finding. The incidence of neoplastic disorders is greater than in a younger population, and hepatocellular carcinoma, ovarian carcinoma, and malignancy of the stomach, pancreas, uterus, biliary tract, and colon must be carefully excluded. Obstruction of the hepatic veins or portal veins caused by malignancy or hematologic disease become important considerations in this age-group, and of course cardiopulmonary diseases (congestive heart failure, constrictive pericarditis and recurrent pulmonary emboli) may all cause elevated venous pressure and ascites. Unusually, a metabolic disorder such as myxedema will be responsible for ascites in an aged subject. Finally, infections such as tuberculosis must not be forgotten.

Peritoneal Tumors

The peritoneum is frequently involved by metastatic implants from intra-abdominal tumors. Carcinoma of the stomach and ovary are especially prone to seed the peritoneum, and ovarian cancer in particular may stud the peritoneal surface and produce a large amount of ascites in the absence of any hepatic involvement. Pseudomyxoma peritonei from mucinous lesions of the colon, appendix, and ovary has been discussed previously. Malignant ascites usually has the characteristics of an exudate and is present in large amounts that rapidly reaccumulate after drainage. Diagnosis is usually established by cytologic examination of the ascitic fluid, blind peritoneal biopsy, or peritoneoscopy and biopsy. Peritoneal involvement usually occurs late in the growth of the tumor, and little chance for cure exists.

The only primary cancer of the peritoneum is mesothelioma, which, like its pleural counterpart, shows a clear relationship to asbestos exposure. Most patients present with weight loss and ascites and abdominal pains occasionally worsened by urination or defecation. Many patients have coincidental asbestos-related respiratory disease and clubbing of the fingers. There are no specific laboratory or roentgenologic findings, and the diagnosis is usually established at operation or laparoscopy. No effective therapy has been developed against this tumor.

Mesenteric Disease

Benign and malignant tumors are the most common disorders involving the mesentery; fatty change, inflammation, and fibrosis are the respective predominant elements in mesenteric lipodystrophy, mesenteric panniculitis, and retractile mesenteritis.

Tumors

Benign or malignant tumors may arise from each of the seven component tissues within the mesentery, including lymphatic, fibrous, adipose, neural smooth muscle, vascular tissues, and embryonic rests. Benign tumors are twice as common as malignant ones, and of the benign growths, fibromas and lipomas are most prevalent. Malignant lesions are usually fibrosarcomas or leiomyosarcomas. Mesenteric tumors frequently grow to very large sizes before producing symptoms and indeed may be incidental findings during routine examination.

Mesenteric Lipodystrophy (Intestinal Lipodystrophy)

Mesenteric lipodystrophy is a self-limiting condition that produces few symptoms and presents predominantly in elderly men as vague abdominal complaints.

The characteristic physical finding is a deep-seated, poorly defined, firm abdominal mass, usually in the left upper quadrant or epigastrium. This may transmit aortic pulsations and may be mistaken for an aortic aneurysm.

Surgery is frequently performed for diagnosis, but many patients undergo spontaneous recovery, often with complete disappearance of the masses. A major concern in predicting a good prognosis for patients with mesenteric lipodystrophy is the potential for developing malignant lymphomas within a few years of the original diagnosis.[38]

Mesenteric Panniculitis (Mesenteric Weber-Christian Disease)

Mesenteric panniculitis refers to an entity with a mass in the small bowel mesentery composed of inflamed adipose tissue. Patients usually present with low-grade fever, malaise, and recurrent episodes of moderately severe abdominal pain. The long-term prognosis is excellent.

Retractile Mesenteritis

Retractile mesenteritis is characterized by fibrofatty thickening and sclerosis. Progressive scarring and retraction pulls the bowel toward the mesentery, producing an intra-abdominal mass. As loops of bowel typically become fixed and distorted, intestinal obstruction and vascular compromise occur. Patients usually present with abdominal pain and recurrent or progressive constipation. Not infrequently, the matted mass of bowel loops will transmit aortic pulsations and be mistaken for an aortic aneurysm.

The cause of this syndrome is unclear, and treatment is essentially surgical to relieve intestinal obstruction.

Retroperitoneal Fibrosis

Retroperitoneal fibrosis affects middle-aged males and results in a wide variety of symptoms but is typically characterized by entrapment and compression of the ureters.

An elevated erythrocyte sedimentation rate, anemia, and abnormal urinalysis are frequent, and uremia occurs in the late stages. Intravenous pyelography is often diagnostic. Many other fibrotic disorders are associated with retroperitoneal fibrosis and influence the clinical picture, including mediastinal fibrosis, sclerosing cholangitis, Riedel's thyroiditis, episcleritis, and Dupuytren's contracture.

The disease is occasionally self-limiting, although it tends to be progressive and is associated with a substantial mortality rate.

Retroperitoneal Tumors

Primary retroperitoneal tumors are infrequent. The most common, the liposarcoma, which usually occurs in patients 55 years of age or older, may produce abdominal enlargement and a palpable mass. In the retroperitoneum, the tumor usually arises from the peritoneal area and pushes the kidneys forward and laterally. Invasion of renal parenchyma is not generally seen.

Enucleation of the tumor is invariably followed by local recurrence since the "capsule" actually consists of flattened tumor cells attenuated by expansile growth of the tumor. Wide excision with a large margin of healthy tissue is advised.

In general, patients with retroperitoneal liposarcomas do not do as well as those with the same lesion in other sites. Treatment is surgical. Radiation therapy has been employed with some success for incompletely resected lesions, for inoperable tumors, and for metastatic and recurrent disease.

REFERENCES

1. Andersson A, Bergdahl L, Van Der Linden W: Volvulus of the cecum. Ann Surg 181:876–880, 1976
2. Arnold JG, Nance FC: Volvulus of the sigmoid colon. Ann Surg 177:527–537, 1973

3. Athanasoulis CA, Ring EJ, Smith JC Jr, Sugarbaker E, Wood W: Mesenteric arterial infusions of vasopressin for hemorrhage from colonic diverticulosis. Am J Surg 129:212, 1975

4. Bartlett JG, Chang TW, Gurwith M, Gorbach SL, Onderdonk AB: Antibiotic associated pseudomembranous colitis due to toxin-producing clostridia. N Engl J Med 298:531–534, 1978

5. Blake R, Lynn J: Emergency abdominal surgery in the aged. Br J Surg 63:956–960, 1976

6. Boley SJ, Brandt LJ, Veith FJ: Ischemic disorders of the intestines. Curr Probl Surg 15:1–85, 1978

7. Boley SJ, DiBiase A, Brandt LJ, Sammartano RJ: Lower intestinal bleeding in the elderly. Am J Surg 137:57–64, 1979

8. Boley SJ, Feinstein FR, Sammartano R, Brandt LJ, Sprayregen S: New concepts in the management of emboli of the superior mesenteric artery. Surg Gynecol Obstet 153:561–569, 1981

9. Boley SJ, Sammartano R, Adams A, DiBiase A, Kleinhaus S, Sprayregen S: On the nature and etiology of vascular ectasias of the colon. Gastroenterology 72:650–660, 1977

10. Boley SJ, Sammartano R, Brandt LJ, Mitsudo S, Sheran M: Intra-arterial vasodilators and thrombolytic agents in experimental superior mesenteric artery embolus (SMAE) (abstr). Gastroenterology 82:1021, 1982

11. Boley SJ, Sammartano R, Brandt LJ, Sprayregen S: Vascular ectasias of the colon. Surg Gynecol Obstet 149:353–359, 1979

12. Boely SJ, Sprayregen S, Sammartano RJ, Adams A, Kleinhaus S: The pathophysiologic basis for the angiographic signs of vascular ectasias of the colon. Radiology 125:615–621, 1977

13. Boley SJ, Sprayregen S, Veith FJ, Siegleman S: An aggressive roentgenologic and surgical approach to acute mesenteric ischemia. In Nyhus LM (ed): Surgery Annual, p. 355. New York, Appleton-Century-Crofts, 1973

14. Brandt LJ, Boley SJ, Goldberg L, Mitsudo S, Berman A: Colitis in the elderly: A reappraisal. Am J Gastroenterol 76:239–245, 1981

15. Brandt LJ, Boley SJ, Mitsudo S: Clinical characteristics and natural history of colitis in the elderly. Am J Gastroenterol 77:382–386, 1982

16. Bricker EM, Johnston WD, Patwardhan RV: Repair of postirradiation damage to colorectum: A progress report. Ann Surg 193:555–564, 1981

17. Brocklehurst JC, Khan Y: A study of fecal stasis in old age and use of Dorbanex in its prevention. Gerontol Clin 2:293–300, 1969

18. Calabrese CT, Adam YG, Volk H: Geriatric colon cancer. Am J Surg 125:181–185, 1973

19. Cherry RD, Portnoy D, Jabbari M, Daly DS, Kinnear DG, Goresky CA: Metronidazole: An alternate therapy for antibiotic-associated colitis. 82:849–851, 1982

20. Connell AM, Hilton C, Irvine G, Lennard-Jones JE, Misiewica JJ: Laxative-induced diarrhoea: A continuing clinical problem. Br Med J 1:537–541, 1965

21. Cooperman M, Martin EW, Evans WE, Carey LC: Assessment of anastomotic blood supply of Doppler ultrasound in operations upon the colon. Surg Gynecol Obstet 149:15–16, 1979

22. Dardik H, Seidenberg B, Parker JG, Hurwitt ES: Intestinal angina malabsorption treated with elective revascularization. JAMA 194:1206–1210, 1965

23. Deterling RA: Aneurysm of the visceral arteries. J Cardiovasc Surg 12:309–322, 1971

24. Ellis H, Cronin K: Bile peritonitis. Br J Surg 48:166–170, 1960–1961

25. Enterline HT: Polyps and cancer of the large bowel. Curr Top Pathol 63:65–141, 1976

26. Estes JE Jr: Abdominal aortic aneurysm: Study of one hundred and two cases. Circulation 2:258–264, 1950

27. Fenyo G: Acute abdominal disease in the elderly: Experience from two series in Stockholm. Am J Surg 143:751–754, 1982

28. Fleischner FG: Diverticular disease of the colon: New observations and revised concepts. Gastroenterology 60:316–324, 1971

29. Furrer J, Gruntzig A, Kugelmeier J, Goebel N: Treatment of abdominal angina with percutaneous dilation of an arteria mesenterica superior stenosis. Cardiovasc Intervent Radiol 3:43–44, 1980

30. Gilbertsen VA: Proctosigmoidoscopy and polypectomy in reducing the incidence of rectal cancer. Cancer 34:936–939, 1974

31. Gliedman ML, Ayers WB, Vestal BL: Aneurysms of the abdominal aorta and its branches: A study of untreated patients. Ann Surg 146:207–214, 1957

32. Grinvalsky HT, Bowerman CI: Stercoraceous ulcers of the colon. JAMA 171:1941–1946, 1959

33. Hansen HJB, Engell HC, Ring-Larsen H, Raneck L: Splanchnic blood flow in patients with abdominal angina before and after arterial reconstruction. Ann Surg 186:216–220, 1977

34. Hirst AE Jr, Johns VJ Jr, Kime SW Jr: Dissecting aneurysm of the aorta: Review of 505 cases. Medicine 37:217–279, 1958

35. Ihre T: Studies on anal function in continent and incontinent patients. Scand J Gastroenterol 9:5–64, 1974

36. Jensen H-E, Balsley I, Fenger HJ, Kragelund E, Nielsen J: carcinoma of the colon in old age. Acta Chir Scand 139:563–567, 1973

37. Jensen H-E, Nielsen J, Balsley I: Carcinoma of the colon in old age. Ann Surg 171:107–115, 1970

38. Kipfer RE, Moertel CG, Dahlin DC: Mesenteric lipodystrophy. Ann Intern Med 80:582–588, 1974

39. Klein RS, Catalano MT, Edberg SC, Casey JI, Steigbigel NH: *Streptococcus bovis* septicemia and carcinoma of the colon. Ann Intern Med 91:560–562, 1979

40. Kligerman MM: Radiotherapy and rectal cancer. Cancer 39:896–900, 1977

41. Kraft E, Finby N, Egidio PT, Glenn JS: The megasigmoid syndrome in psychotic patients. JAMA 195:1099–1101, 1966

42. Lee BY, Trainer FS, Kavner D, McCann WJ: Intraoperative assessment of intestinal viability with Doppler ultrasound. Surg Gyncecol Obstet 149:671–675, 1979

43. McCollum CH, Graham JM, DeBakey ME: Chronic mesenteric arterial insufficiency: Results of revascularization in 33 cases. South Med J 69:1266–1268, 1976

44. Mathews JE, White RR: Primary mesenteric venous occlusive disease. Am J Surg 122:579–583, 1971

45. Milne JS, Williamson J: Bowel habit in older people. Gerontol Clin 14:56–60, 1972

46. Moertel CG, Thynne GS: Alimentary tract cancer: Large bowel. In Holland J, Frei E (eds): Cancer Medicine, pp 1830–1859. Philadelphia, Lea & Febiger, 1982

47. O'Mara CS, Wilson TH Jr, Stonesifer GL, Cameron JL: Cecal volvulus: Analysis of 50 patients with long-term follow-up. Ann Surg 189:724–731, 1979

48. Pentland B, Pennington CR: Acute diarrhoea in the elderly. Age Ageing 9:90–92, 1980

49. Polk H: Experimental mesenteric venous occlusion. Ann Surg 163:432–444, 1966

50. Reiner L, Jiminez FA, Rodriguez FL: Atherosclerosis in the mesenteric circulation: Observations and correlations with aortic and coronary artherosclerosis. Am Heart J 66:200–209, 1963

51. Reul GJ Jr, Wukasch DC, Sandiford FM, Chiarillo L, Hallman GL, Cooley DA: Surgical treatment of abdominal angina: Review of 25 patients. Surgery 75:682–689, 1974

52. Rob C: Surgical disease of the celiac and mesenteric arteries. Arch Surg 93:21–32, 1966

53. Shafer N: Abdominal aortic aneurysm. NY State J Med 78:1727–1738, 1978

54. Slater G, Papatestas AE, Tartter PI, Mulvihill M, Aufses AH Jr: Age distribution of right- and left-sided colorectal cancers. Am J Gastroenterol 77:63–66, 1982

55. Stanley JC, Thompson NW, Fry WJ: Splanchnic artery aneurysms. Arch Surg 101:689–697, 1970

56. Tedesco FJ: Clindamycin-associated colitis: A review of the clinical spectrum of 46 cases. Dig Dis 21:26–32, 1976

57. Wertkin MG, Aufses AH Jr: Management of volvulus of the colon. Dis Colon Rectum 21:40–45, 1978

58. Winawer SJ, Andrews M, Miller CH, Fleisher M: Review of screening for colorectal cancer using fecal occult blood testing. In Winawer SJ, Schottenfeld D, Sherlock P (eds): Colorectal Cancer: Prevention, Epidemiology, and Screening, pp 159–165. New York, Raven Press, 1980

59. Witt TR, Winawer SJ: Editorial comment. Gastroenterology 81:625–627, 1981

60. Wolfer JA, Beaton LE, Anson BJ: Volvulus of the cecum: Anatomical factors in its etiology: Report of a case. Surg Gynecol Obstet 74:882–894, 1942

17

Pancreas, Liver, and Gall Bladder

Lawrence J. Brandt

THE PANCREAS

Anatomical and Functional Changes in the Pancreas With Aging

The duodenal sweep and the pancreas may be displaced inferiorly with aging; this probably accounts for the supposed nonvisualization of the pancreas in some elderly patients because the scanning field was not sufficiently low to image the organ.[50]

The caliber of the pancreatic ducts progressively increases with advancing age at a yearly rate of 0.8% (*i.e.*, 8% per decade) uniformly throughout the head, body, and tail of the gland. The duct that dilates with aging retains its uniform tapering appearance with smooth margins, in contrast to the sudden and irregular duct dilatation seen in pancreatic carcinoma or the segmental dilatation and stricture formation("chain of lakes") characterizing chronic pancreatitis. Single or conglomerate tiny rounded cystlike collections are also occasionally seen in the periphery of the ductules in the aged pancreas. Cyst formation is more common in association with ducts of greater width and so is usually seen in the older subjects. Rarely, the pancreatic duct may show long narrowed segments that resemble the appearance of neoplasia but that are probably caused by compression of the gland as it crosses the spine.

At autopsy, normal pancreatic morphology is found in only a small percentage of elderly human subjects. Parenchymal fibrosis and fatty change are frequent, and the glands may show lipofuscin deposition and infiltration by a hyaline material with the tinctorial properties of amyloid. Degenerative changes in individual acinar cells are also commonly seen. In a study of degenerative lesions of the pancreas, Wallace and Ashworth[105] showed the most common lesion associated with aging was adipose tissue "invasion," which was present in 79% of patients older than 50 years of age. Such fatty change was followed by increased fibrosis (60%), acinar and ductal dilatation (56%), arteriolar sclerosis (45%), and ductular metaplasia (10.5%).

Proliferation and metaplasia of the ductal epithelial cells may form apparently solid masses of cells, a change followed by lumen formation and expansion leading to epithelial flattening and locule or cavity formation. Occasionally, the walls of adjacent locules break down and large irregular cavities are formed, some of which contain a material resembling keratin.[1]

Senescent pathologic changes in the pancreas are not paralleled by dramatic alterations in the function of the gland,[3] and age-related changes in pancreatic function do not cause any obvious clinical dysfunction or loss of nutrition.

Inflammatory Disorders

Of the usual identified causes for acute pancreatitis in the elderly, gallstones are most common.[33] Sequelae of alcoholic pancreatitis (*i.e.*, pancreatic insufficiency and steatorrhea) may present in the elderly, usually after a long quiescent interval of subclinical disease activity. Less common causes of acute pancreatitis in the older patient are listed in the box on page 303.

The presentation in the elderly may be more subtle than expected even in the presence of severe disease. Females are affected more than males.[33] Epigastric pain is the most common initial symptom; since gallstones are such a frequent cause of acute pancreatitis in the elderly, pain may be

CAUSES OF ACUTE PANCREATITIS IN THE ELDERLY

Biliary tract disease
   Gallstones
   Biliary pigment aggregates
   Sphincter of Oddi dysfunction
Duodenal disorders
   Periampullary diverticula
   "Closed-loop" obstruction
Endocrine and metabolic diseases
   Uremia
   Diabetes mellitus
   Hypercalcemia
Medications
   Thiazides
   Furosemide
   Cimetidine
Postoperative states
Post endoscopy
Vascular (ischemia)
Tumors (primary and metastatic)
Hypothermia
Hypoxemia

sensed more often in the right upper quadrant. Fever, tachycardia, and abdominal tenderness and guarding are characteristic but may be less pronounced in the elderly. Neither a lack of jaundice nor the presence of painless jaundice excludes gallstones as a cause of pancreatitis.

Hyperamylasemia, the key to laboratory diagnosis, may be seen in the elderly with disorders of nonpancreatic origin, including salivary gland lesions, biliary tract disease, peptic ulcer disease with perforation, intestinal obstruction, mesenteric infarction, aortic aneurysm with dissection, afferent loop syndrome, peritonitis, renal failure, cerebral trauma, prostatic disease, pneumonia, and after upper tract endoscopy or operation. Occasionally the magnitude of the amylase elevation may be helpful. For example, in biliary pancreatitis, the degree of hyperamylasemia is usually fivefold to tenfold greater than normal and is beyond the range produced by nonpancreatic disorders and alcoholic pancreatitis.

In an effort to narrow the differential diagnosis of hyperamylasemia, the ratio of the renal clearances of amylase to creatinine has been used. In the absence of burns or diabetic ketoacidosis, a value of greater than 5% is virtually diagnostic of pancreatitis.[44]

During the acute phase of pancreatic inflammation, electrocardiographic changes (usually ST-T wave abnormalities) simulating an acute myo-

cardial infarction may be produced. Electrocardiographic changes tend to resolve quickly unless true myocardial damage occurs or some complication associated with pancreatitis supervenes, such as pericarditis.

Plain films of the abdomen most commonly reveal a localized ileus or "sentinel loop," and occasionally a "colon cut-off" sign is reported. In more than half the cases, chest films demonstrate platelike atelectasis, pleural effusions, or pulmonary infiltrates.

The mortality rate for pancreatitis increases with advancing age and is further increased by the preexistence of cardiovascular disease and diabetes.[73] Pollack noted double the mortality rate in patients older than 60 years as in those under 50 years (29% vs. 15%), and it was 40% in patients over 70 years of age.

Colonic Ischemia and Pancreatitis

Patients usually present with colonic signs or symptoms during a bout of acute pancreatitis when complicated by colonic ischemia.[39] Rectal bleeding is the most common symptom, and a colon "cut-off" sign is frequently seen. The colonic lesions are most often located at or about the splenic flexure because inflammation spreads to the transverse mesocolon and induces a local change in the colonic (micro) vasculature, with resulting bowel ischemia. Management consists of a conservative approach with serial barium enema studies and resection when necessary for gangrene, perforation, or obstruction.

Respiratory Complication of Acute Pancreatitis

Clinical descriptions have noted the early occurrence of cyanosis, agitation, restlessness, dyspnea, or tachypnea.[47] An "early" phase of respiratory insufficiency occurs in most patients with acute pancreatitis, begins during the initial days of illness, and is frequently discovered only by arterial blood-gas measurements when some degree of arterial hypoxemia is observed. Individuals in all age-groups are affected, and such early hypoxemia does not influence mortality.[78] In contrast, the frequency of clinically apparent pulmonary complications is related to the severity of the pancreatitis, occurs more commonly in patients of advanced age, and adversely affects prognosis.[78] The pathogenesis of the respiratory insufficiency is not understood and thus preventive measures cannot be employed. Administration of albumin and diuretics and the early use of assisted ventilation and prompt laparotomy when required have been advised.[78] Periodic assessment of blood-gas values, especially in elderly subjects with severe pancreatitis, should be routine.

Pulmonary Edema of Acute Pancreatitis

A particular and uncommon form of respiratory distress seen in acute pancreatitis is acute pulmonary edema.[107] It is important to distinguish this entity in elderly patients from the more common pulmonary edema on the basis of cardiac disease, because treatments differ. Pulmonary edema of pancreatitis typically develops several days after the onset of a severe episode of acute pancreatitis and appears to develop mainly in those individuals with elevated levels of serum triglycerides. In contrast to the respiratory failure syndrome previously discussed, respiratory status, chest roentgenograms, and arterial blood-gas determinations are of no value in predicting the development of pulmonary edema. Therapy consists of endotracheal intubation with controlled ventilation using positive end-expiratory pressure to keep the small airways open.

Types of Pancreatitis

Gallstone ("Biliary") Pancreatitis. The association of cholelithiasis and pancreatitis is well accepted, although the pathogenesis of the acute inflammation is controversial. In a typical case of acute pancreatitis, the patient is a nonalcoholic with a history of gallbladder disease who develops epigastric pain associated with an amylase level exceeding 1000 Somogyi units and hyperbilirubinemia. However, an oral cholecystogram that does not visualize the gallbladder during or for approximately 2 weeks after an acute bout of pancreatitis cannot reliably be used to support a diagnosis of biliary pancreatitis. Although the pathophysiology is not well understood, it has been amply shown that a normal gallbladder may not be visualized in the presence of acute pancreatitis.

A newer diagnostic modality useful in the presence of acute pancreatitis is hepatobiliary imaging with technetium-labeled analogues of iminodiacetic acid (IDA).[21] Nonvisualization of the gallbladder with these imaging agents in a patient with acute abdominal pain implies the cystic duct is obstructed, and failure to see the nuclide enter the duodenum by 30 to 45 minutes usually signifies common bile duct obstruction.

Endoscopic retrograde cholangiopancreatography (ERCP) and percutaneous transhepatic cholangiography (PTC) play an important role in diagnosis and management. ERCP should be performed promptly in patients with suggested biliary pancreatitis because if an obstructing gallstone is visualized, a papillotomy may be performed and the stone removed. Alternatively, a stent may be inserted into the biliary tree for decompression or the stone may just be disimpacted and pushed proximally. The standard approach to the patient who has not had a cholecystectomy and who has biliary pancreatitis is cholecystectomy and some form of biliary drainage procedure (*e.g.,* choledochoduodenostomy, choledochojejunostomy, or sphincteroplasty).

In a series of 11 "severely ill" patients between the ages of 52 and 85 years with gallstone pancreatitis, Safrany and Cotton[83] reported their results with emergency duodenoscopic sphincterotomy. Stone extraction was accomplished with forceps, balloon catheters, and wire baskets. On performing the sphincterotomy there often followed free flow of pus or putrid bile; dramatic clinical improvement followed within 24 hours.

Routine duodenoscopic sphincterotomy has a success rate of over 90% for removal of bile duct stones, and even in series containing a large proportion of elderly and high-risk patients, the complication rate can be as low as 6% and the mortality rate below 1%.[11,82]

Since most patients with gallstone-related pancreatitis have a benign course, it is reasonable to select for emergency decompression only patients who present with evidence of sepsis and a rapidly deteriorating course. Which operative procedure is best is controversial.[48,77]

In some experts' experience,[77] prompt operation in the presence of severe pancreatitis has resulted in an awesome mortality, and survival was greater when definitive operation was delayed until the acute pancreatitis had resolved. A reasonable approach is to reserve early surgery for patients in whom stone passage does not occur or in whom endoscopic decompression is impossible or has failed and the severity of the pancreatitis increases.

Pancreatitis Associated With (Periampullary) Duodenal Diverticula. Duodenal diverticula are commonly found near the ampulla of Vater, and many reports suggest that such diverticula may cause diseases of the pancreatic and biliary tracts. Both duodenal diverticula and biliary stones are more common with increasing age, and in all patients older than 40 years the incidence of such diverticula is higher for those with biliary calculi than for those without.[71] Most of these stones are of the pigment variety, and stasis of food, mucus, and intestinal secretions, bacterial proliferation, and biliary infection probably all play an important role in their formation.

Ischemic Pancreatitis. Experimentally, embolism of the pancreatic arterial system has resulted in pancreatic necrosis, and edematous pancreatitis has been converted to hemorrhagic pancreatitis by temporary occlusion of the pancreatic blood supply. The role of diminished blood flow in initiating or exacerbating the disorder in the clinical setting remains unproven.

Tumor-Induced Acute Pancreatitis. Acute pancreatitis may occur in association with a primary neoplasm of the pancreas or on the basis of a wide variety of metastatic carcinomas, including carcinoma of the prostate, breast, and lung.[68] Tumor-associated pancreatitis is usually a focal phenomenon demonstrated at operation or at autopsy and is without clinical significance. The presence of pancreatitis may obscure and delay the diagnosis of cancer and in any elderly person with new-onset pancreatitis that fails to resolve or recurs, the possibility of an underlying malignancy should be excluded.

Drug-Induced Pancreatitis. Mallory and Kern[58] classified drugs reported to cause pancreatitis into three groups: (1) drugs definitely causing pancreatitis (thiazides, sulfonamides, furosemide, estrogens, and tetracyclines), (2) drugs probably causing pancreatitis (chlorthalidone, corticosteroids, ethacrynic acid, phenformin, and procainamide), and (3) drugs inadequately documented to cause pancreatitis (cholestyramine, cyproheptidine, propoxyphene, indomethacin, acetaminophen, and cimetidine).

Whenever such a relationship is suspected, it is wise to withdraw the drug; rechallenge with the drug in question should only be attempted if the agent (and no other) is essential for the medical well-being of the patient.

Postoperative Pancreatitis. Most instances of postoperative pancreatitis follow surgery of the stomach or biliary tree and are thought to represent direct trauma to the pancreas or interference with its blood supply. Postoperative hyperamylasemia occurs much more commonly than does pancreatitis and is especially frequent after cardi-

othoracic procedures. The ratio of amylase to creatinine clearance has been shown to rise nonspecifically following a variety of abdominal and nonabdominal operative procedures and thus cannot be used as reliable evidence of pancreatitis in the postoperative period; a normal clearance ratio helps exclude this diagnosis.

In general, pancreatitis developing in the postoperative period is more lethal than other forms of pancreatitis and has a mortality of 25% to 75%.

Chronic Pancreatitis

Chronic pancreatitis is not nearly as common in the elderly as in the young, probably because many patients with alcoholic pancreatitis succumb in earlier years and because pancreatitis due to gallstones and other causes in older subject rarely progresses to chronic disease. Nonetheless, chronic pancreatitis is exceeded only by celiac disease as a cause for steatorrhea in patients older than 65 years of age.[75]

Chronic pancreatitis usually presents with pain, diabetes mellitus, or nutritional and metabolic sequelae caused by inability to digest and absorb fat and protein. Compared with genetic diabetes, the diabetes of chronic pancreatitis has a greater tendency for the serum glucose level to fluctuate and a substantial risk of hypoglycemia from insulin administration or alcohol abuse. Vasculopathy is less common in pancreatic diabetes, perhaps because of the low lipid values due to maldigestion; neuropathy is present in 10% to 30% of cases.

Patients with chronic pancreatitis are said to have a higher incidence of pancreatic cancer than the general population. Recognition of the cancer, even at laparotomy, may be quite difficult. Carcinoma should be suspected in patients with deep jaundice, progressive weight loss, and severe abdominal pain.

Problems in the differential diagnosis of chronic pancreatitis most usually include its distinction from pancreatic carcinoma in a patient with severe abdominal pain, weight loss, and steatorrhea, the differentiation of pancreatic and genetic diabetes, and the differentiation of intestinal malabsorption and pancreatic maldigestion in a patient with steatorrhea. Clues to these differential diagnoses are outlined in Tables 17-1 through 17-3.

Medical therapy for chronic pancreatitis involves removing or reversing any precipitating factors such as alcohol, drugs, stones, and hypercalcemia and treating any complications of the disease such as pain, diabetes, steatorrhea, and weight loss. Surgical therapy is usually reserved

TABLE 17-1   Differential Diagnosis of Pancreatic Cancer and Chronic Pancreatitis

	Pancreatic Cancer	Pancreatitis
History and physical examination	Weight loss, depression, constipation, constant abdominal pain, palpable gallbladder with jaundice, left upper quadrant bruit, metastases (sentinel node), hepatomegaly, thrombophlebitis	Alcohol abuse, diarrhea, recurrent abdominal pain, fat necrosis
Roentgenogram	Vanishing calcification	Calcification
Fecal urobilinogen	Absent in jaundice	Present in jaundice
Secretin test	↓ Volume	↓ Volume, ↓ bicarbonate, ↓ enzyme
ERCP	Ductal cutoff	"Chain-of-lakes" appearance
CT scan	Abnormal	Abnormal
Needle aspiration	Malignant cells	Inflammatory cells
Angiogram	Vessel encasement, obstruction, metastases	

TABLE 17-2   Differential Diagnosis of Intestinal and Pancreatic Steatorrhea

	Intestinal Steatorrhea	Pancreatic Steatorrhea
Fecal fat	> 20 g, monoglycerides and diglycerides, soapy stools	> 20 g, triglycerides, oily seepage
d-Xylose	Low	Normal
Secretin test	Normal	Abnormal
Small bowel series	Abnormal	Normal
Small bowel biopsy	Abnormal	Normal
Lundt meal	Normal	Abnormal
PABA test	Normal	Abnormal
Alkaline phosphatase	Normal or high (bone)	Normal or high (liver)
Vitamin B_{12} and folate	Low	Normal
Treatment with pancreatic enzymes	No change	Improvement

TABLE 17-3 Differential Diagnosis of Genetic and Pancreatic Diabetes

	Genetic Diabetes	Pancreatic Diabetes
Family history	Yes	No
History of pancreatitis	No	Yes
Abdominal pain	No	Yes
Exocrine insufficiency	No	Yes
Ketosis and coma	Yes	No
Vasculopathy	Yes	No
Neuropathy	Yes	Yes

for patients who have persistent jaundice or unrelenting pain.

In the absence of a ductal obstruction, pseudocyst, or abscess formation, treatment of the painful crises associated with chronic pancreatitis is the same as for that in acute pancreatitis: avoidance of pancreatic stimulation, nasogastric suction, nothing by mouth or at least no high protein or fat-containing foods, bed rest, analgesics, and occasionally the administration of pancreatic enzymes.

A variety of pancreatic replacement preparations are available; the best one is the preparation the patient will take regularly.[14] In elderly subjects who have reduced gastric acid secretion, relief of steatorrhea may be more easily achieved and for longer periods of time after a dose of replacement therapy. Prognosis of chronic pancreatitis is highly variable; however, chronic pancreatitis, even when associated with pancreatic insufficiency and diabetes may be associated with a reasonably normal life span.

Neoplasms of the Pancreas

The pancreas may host a wide variety of neoplasms in its exocrine, endocrine, or supporting structures. However, only adenocarcinoma is especially more frequent in the elderly. Inexplicably, its incidence appears to be steadily rising. It now ranks fifth as a cause of cancer death, exceeded only by cancer of the lung, large bowel, breast, and prostate.[63] The disease in males more than 75 years old is eight to ten times that in the general population.[15] Its importance is evidenced by a series in which the cause of jaundice in 80 patients with a mean age of 75.7 years was reviewed; malignant obstruction was more common than benign disease, and pancreatic cancer was the most common neoplasm observed.[15]

Pancreatic cancer should be excluded in any elderly patient who develops new diabetes mellitus or in whom previously well-controlled diabetes becomes unstable.

Pain, weight loss, and jaundice are the predominant symptoms of pancreatic cancer; unfortunately the course of pancreatic cancer is rapidly progressive so that by the time symptoms develop, it is usually too late for curative therapy. Presenting complaints are often vague and nonspecific, and metastatic spread occurs early. In most series, survival from the time of diagnosis to death is usually less than 6 months.

Abdominal pain is the predominant symptom and typically manifests as an insidious dull ache or boring sensation in the epigastrium that becomes steadily progressive; back pain is not uncommon. Weight loss occurs in almost all patients and is usually rapid and progressive despite a relatively well-preserved appetite and adequate food intake. Jaundice is typical and is progressive, unremitting, and painful. Nonspecific bowel symptoms such as constipation, obstipation, diarrhea, bloating, and flatulence are also common.

A few special presentations of pancreatic cancer include depression, migratory and recurrent thrombophlebitis and thromboembolic phenomena, gastrointestinal bleeding with gastric varices, polyarthritis with skin nodules, and the association with diabetes mellitus.

On physical examination, except for jaundice, "early" signs of pancreatic carcinoma are unusual. A reliable sign of malignancy in a jaundiced patient is the presence of a palpable (Courvoisier) gallbladder, since only rarely when a benign obstruction (stone or stricture) causes jaundice is the gallbladder wall pliable enough to allow distension.

There is no routine laboratory test specific to a diagnosis. Reliability must be placed on a high degree of suspicion with confirmation by ERCP, Computed tomography (CT scanning), pancreatic secretory studies, selective angiography, percutaneous needle biopsy, and occasionally laparotomy.

Roentgenographic approaches to the diagnosis of pancreatic cancer were able to detect only advanced disease until the advent of endoscopic cannulation, ultrasound, and CT scanning. Endoscopic retrograde brush cytology may also be performed with a rate of positivity approaching 90% in patients with primary pancreatic cancer.

Both ERCP and PTC are now widely used as therapy to implant stents in the biliary tract for drainage and palliative relief of jaundice, pruritus, and cholangitis. Radiation therapy and chemotherapeutic regimens in advanced pancreatic cancer have not been shown to be of dramatic benefit, although combination chemotherapy regimens have shown some promising results.

Simple therapeutic modalities must not be forgotten in management. Aspirin, perhaps with codeine, is sometimes effective therapy for pain; if not, a splanchnic nerve block can sometimes achieve dramatic results. Caution must be employed in attempting nerve block in the elderly since postural hypotension is a frequent complication. Pruritus may be eased substantially in the presence of an incomplete biliary obstruction by an orally administered bile-sequestering resin such as cholestyramine (Questran). Pancreatic replacement therapy or use of medium-chain triglycerides as a source of nutrition not requiring lipolysis for absorption will diminish steatorrhea and perhaps ease frequent and foul smelling stools. The patient's diabetic status requires the usual monitoring.

THE LIVER

Alteration in the Liver With Aging

The weight of the liver decreases after the age of 50,[7] a change that parallels a reduction in body weight and that is correlated at autopsy with a diminished number of hepatocytes.[99] Better nutrition may lead to earlier maturational and senescent change.[99] There is little age-related alteration in the hepatic lobular architecture, although an increase in portal and periportal fibrous tissue with atrophy of the centrilobular liver-cell plates has been described. The existence of a "senile cirrhosis" has even been postulated, however, these changes probably reflect associated pathologic processes and not physiologic senescence.[19] An age-related diminution in glycogen and increase in the lipid content of the aged liver is also questionable.

The hepatic parenchymal cells of aged subjects tend to be larger and to contain larger or multiple nuclei and nucleoli. Binucleate hepatic cells increase in number with aging up to the seventh decade and decrease thereafter.[98] Many reports suggest a relationship between hepatic nuclear size or binuclearity and the need for hepatic regeneration and cellular differentiation. These nuclear changes are believed to reflect a state of inhibited cellular division that also accounts for the diminished number of hepatocytes in the aged. Ultrastructural cellular changes associated with aging include invaginations of the nuclear membrane containing entrapped masses of cytoplasm, often with mitochondria or endoplasmic reticulum, a decrease in the number of mitochondria per cell, larger mitochondria with more dense crista, an increase in lipofuscin pigment and lysosomes and microbodies (peroxisomes), a diminution in the surface area of the Golgi apparatus, and an increase in the rough and smooth endoplasmic reticulum.[97] The latter is particularly interesting in view of the reduction in hepatic drug-metabolizing enzyme activity that characterizes the elderly liver.

The levels of hepatic enzymes change only little with aging, but the patterns of change are very complex.[108] In general, the activities of respiratory enzymes decrease and those of the hydrolytic enzymes increase, paralleling the observed diminution in mitochondria and increase in lysosomes. More important than any absolute amount of enzyme, however, may be the adaptability or inducibility of the enzyme, and there is evidence that these functions diminish with advancing age.

Age-related changes in pharmacokinetics have been the subject of several reviews.[31,70] Many studies suggest that aging *per se* reduces the drug metabolizing capacity of the liver, especially within the mono-oxygenase (mixed function oxidase) enzyme system. However, many other factors that affect drug disposition may be influenced by aging, including volumes of distribution, protein binding, hepatic blood flow, and renal clearance.

Age is a major factor in determining the healing and regenerative potential of the liver after physicochemical injury or surgical resection. The livers of older animals exhibit a depressed regenerative potential and a longer latent period prior to cellular mitosis and growth. However, the growth potential of regenerating livers is independent of age, and during regeneration there appears to be a temporary rejuvenation of the growing tissue, with morphologic and functional changes resembling those of young animals.

Changes in "Liver Function" Tests

In healthy elderly subjects, standard "liver function" tests such as bilirubin, transaminase, hepatic alkaline phosphatase, and sodium sulfobromophthalein (Bromsulphalein, BSP) are within normal limits. Deviation cannot be attributed to the aging process *per se* and implies the presence of a disorder.[46]

Although serum levels of bilirubin and transaminase are invariably normal in "healthy" aged individuals, about 10% have elevated levels of alkaline phosphatase.[88] This usually represents clinically silent bone disease such as Paget's disease or occasionally osteomalacia. Rarely, an isolated elevation of alkaline phosphatase is the sole manifestation of perforated diverticulitis, sepsis, the functional hepatopathy of hypernephroma, or a focus of intrahepatic tumor or abscess formation.

In the only study in which normality was assured by liver biopsy, Kampmann and his associates could find no change in the serum concentrations of bilirubin, transaminase, alkaline phosphatase, BSP, or rose bengal retention in elderly persons. However, in 10 of 53 elderly subjects with no evidence of congestive heart failure, liver, kidney, or bone disease, alcohol abuse, or treatment with hepatotoxic drugs, pathologic findings in the liver were documented and included fatty degeneration (5), cirrhosis (2), hemosiderosis (2), and chronic persistent hepatitis (1). These patients all had normal values of serum bilirubin, transaminase, and alkaline phosphatase, yet had abnormal retention of BSP and rose bengal; had such apparently healthy subjects not been excluded because of the abnormal liver biopsy, the interpretation of the data would have been severely distorted.

Jaundice

In most series of jaundice affecting the aged,[17,37,67,69] obstructive lesions are far more common than hepatocellular disease (Table 17-4). Malignant obstruction is seen one and one half to two times more commonly than benign calculous obstruction. Carcinoma of the head of the pancreas is the most commonly encountered cause of malignant biliary obstruction, followed by metastatic deposits from the lung, stomach, colon, gallbladder, kidney, breast, and prostate.

One of the most prevalent causes of hepatocellular jaundice in the elderly is drug-induced hepatitis, and in one large series,[17] intrahepatic cho-

TABLE 17-4 Causes of Jaundice in the Elderly

Cause	Percentage
Tumor	15—44
Gallbladder disease (calculi)	14—29
Viral hepatitis	8—15
Cirrhosis	4—26
Drugs	6—21
Alcohol–fatty liver	6—14
Systemic (congestive heart failure, sepsis, pulmonary emboli, shock)	2—4
Hemolysis	4
Obstructive picture	50—80
Extrahepatic	58—73
Intrahepatic	27—42
Benign	36—60
Malignant	40—64

(Data compiled from the following sources: Eastwood HDH: Causes of jaundice in the elderly. Gerontol Clin 13:69–81, 1971; Huete–Armijo A, Exton–Smith AN: Causes and diagnosis of jaundice in the elderly. Br Med J 1:1113–1114, 1962; Naso F, Thompson CM: Hyperbilirubinemia in the patient past 50. Geriatrics 22:206–212, 1967; O'Brien GF, Tan CV: Jaundice in the geriatric patient. Geriatrics 25:114–127, 1970)

lestasis from medications accounted for 20% of the cases of jaundice in patients older than 65 years of age; in that particular series chlorpromazine was the most common offender but in other series, diuretics, oral hypoglycemic agents, and 17-alkyl substituted steroids predominate. It has been stated that the diagnosis of jaundice in the elderly often lies between drugs, neoplastic obstruction, and gallstones; Eastwood[17] showed that hepatitis and cirrhosis accounted for 15% and 10% of cases, respectively.

Unconjugated hyperbilirubinemia is uncommon in the elderly and most frequently is associated with a pulmonary infarction in the presence of chronic congestive heart failure.[40] It may also be seen with bacterial sepsis, shock, fever, hemolysis associated with autoimmune disease, transfusion, neoplasm (leukemia, lymphoma), or drugs (*e.g.*, methyldopa).

Helpful clues to the diagnosis of biliary obstruction are marked pruritus, deep jaundice, clay-colored stools, and jaundice that fluctuates, remains stationary over long periods, or progressively increases. On physical examination, an enlarged gallbladder suggests the presence of malignant obstruction ("Courvoisier" gallbladder), but a palpable spleen should lead to the consideration of systemic disorders such as a lymphoma that may be accompanied by jaundice. An elevation of alkaline phosphatase with minor changes in the serum transaminase level and a high serum cholesterol is characteristic of extrahepatic obstruction or intrahepatic cholestasis.

The initial diagnostic test in excluding an extrahepatic obstruction should be ultrasonography. Ultrasonography is superior to computed tomography in evaluating the biliary tree and diagnosing calculi. If the ultrasound examination reveals dilatation of the common bile duct and/or intrahepatic biliary radicals, endoscopic cannulation of the common bile duct may define the nature of the obstruction. If no dilatation is appreciated, intrahepatic cholestasis is probable and it is safe to observe the patient while searching for the cause of the disorder; liver biopsy should not be performed in the presence of a cholestatic process unless an obstructing lesion and bile duct dilatation have been excluded.

Hepatitis

The spectrum and prognosis of inflammatory and infectious disorders that involve the liver of elderly patients differ from that of a younger population. However, all large studies of hepatitis in the elderly[18,23,45,91] were performed prior to our ability to distinguish between the various hepatotoxic viruses (*i.e.,* hepatitis A virus, hepatitis B virus, cytomegalovirus, Epstein-Barr virus). A particularly virulent epidemic of infectious hepatitis in Scandinavia after World War II exhibited a striking predilection for postmenopausal women.[45] Subsequently, the tendency of viral hepatitis to behave in a ''malignant'' fashion in the elderly was described and the higher incidence of fulminant disease or a chronic course, of anicteric subacute necrosis, and of a fatal outcome was acknowledged.[18] Other features in this elderly population included a long delay between the onset of symptoms and hospitalization, a high incidence of associated medical disorders, a high incidence (42%) of hepatic encephalopathy and, finally, in nearly half of the patients the illness was initially misdiagnosed as extrahepatic obstruction.

More recently, Gabinski and colleagues[23] described nearly 200 Polish patients older than 60 years of age with viral hepatitis and compared them with two groups of younger adults. They found that jaundice was more intense and of longer duration in the elderly patients, with greater depression of serum albumin levels. The period of hospitalization was 20% to 30% longer,

and fulminant hepatitis and hepatic coma both occurred more commonly in the aged. The 26% mortality figure of Fenster's series probably reflected some selection bias, but the 3% mortality in patients older than 60 years reported by Gabinski and colleagues is still ten times greater than the mortality rate in patients 20 to 60 years of age.

Type A hepatitis (''infectious'') is endemic throughout the world. Individuals older than 50 years of age are two to four times more likely to have antibodies to hepatitis A virus (HAV) than are those younger than 20 years, and the prevalence of anti-HAV rises to approximately 75% in this older population.[95] Thus, immunity to hepatitis A increases with age as individuals are continually exposed to the virus.

In general, HAV causes an acute self-limited hepatitis that is usually subclinical. Fatalities from HAV infection are rare but may be more common in the elderly. A chronic carrier state or chronic hepatitis resulting from HAV has not been identified.

Compared with hepatitis A virus, hepatitis B virus (HBV) tends to occur in an older population and in the elderly is more prolonged and more frequently fulminant, with greater morbidity and mortality.

One form reported to occur more often in older patients is the so-called cholangiolitic or cholestatic hepatitis that clinically, and often histologically, may mimic extrahepatic obstructive jaundice; endoscopic visualization can clearly make the distinction between the two entities. Jaundice usually persists for about 2 months in cholangiolitic hepatitis and is often accompanied by significant pruritus, hypercholesterolemia, and, occasionally, a disturbed coagulation mechanism. Recovery is usually complete, and progression to chronic liver disease is unusual, although the older literature did describe progression to a ''cholangiolitic (biliary) cirrhosis.''

Chronic hepatitis has not been described following acute hepatitis A but occurs in 5% to 10% of patients with acute hepatitis B and may occur with an even greater frequency after non-A, non-B disease. It is more likely to develop in the elderly, although most patients with chronic hepatitis are in late middle-age when the diagnosis is established.

For most patients with chronic persistent hepatitis or chronic active hepatitis who also have viral markers for HBV infection, corticosteroid therapy is *not* advisable because the risks of treatment outweigh the benefits; for the treatment of elderly patients who have chronic active disease but who do *not* have HBV markers, corticosteroid therapy may be beneficial especially in the presence of marked symptoms or when the biopsy demonstrates severely active and progressive hepatic necrosis or transition to cirrhosis. In the elderly, corticosteroids should be given only with extreme caution because of the high incidence of side-effects, including osteopenia, bone fractures, hypertension, and diabetes mellitus.

Drug-induced Acute Hepatic Injury

Disordered liver function associated with drug therapy is surprisingly uncommon considering the frequency with which drugs are prescribed in today's society and the essential role of the liver in drug biotransformation. Nonetheless, this iatrogenic disorder accounts for up to 20% of cases of jaundice in elderly patients[17] and is responsible for about 25% of cases of fulminant hepatic failure in the United States. Recognition of drug-induced hepatic injury may be difficult because the diagnosis usually rests on circumstantial evidence and often requires rechallenge with the putative agent for confirmation. Hazardous repeat challenges are not frequently performed especially in view of the wide variety of drug alternatives. Many comprehensive reviews[2,53] and summaries of this problem are available.

Among the more commonly used drugs that may adversely affect the liver are allopurinol, many nonsteroidal anti-inflammatory agents (ibuprofen, naproxen, indomethacin, sulindac, phenylbutazone), anesthetic agents such as halothane and methoxyflurane, antibiotics (erythromycin estolate, nitrofurantoin, the penicillins, sulfonamides) antineoplastic agents (azathioprine, 6-mercaptopurine, methotrexate), isoniazid, rifampicin, methyldopa, procainamide, quinidine, chlorpropramide, and tolbutamide.[5,9,24,61]

Psychotropic drugs are so widely used in the elderly as to deserve special mention since jaundice is estimated to occur in 1% to 2% of patients so treated.[35] Jaundice complicates phenothiazine therapy in 1% to 2% of patients. The prototype for phenothiazine-induced liver injury is chlorpromazine (Thorazine), although similar damage is known to occur with other drugs of this class.[104] A latent period of 1 to 4 weeks and averaging 2 weeks is usual before onset of jaundice. In half the cases, jaundice is preceded by week-long prodrome that commonly resembles an acute febrile illness with fever, chills, malaise, myalgias, and bone aches.

Phenothiazine jaundice is essentially a cholestatic phenomenon, characterized by hyperbilirubinemia, elevated alkaline phosphatase levels, and hypercholesterolemia. A hypersensitivity mechanism is postulated, but since recurrence of hepatic dysfunction is unusual with readministration of the drug and remission occurs in some subjects despite its continued administration, it is believed "desensitization" can occur.

The prognosis for phenothiazine jaundice is generally good with discontinuation of the drug, and most patients recover within 2 to 3 months,[43] although peculiar and prolonged course may be seen in almost 20% of individuals. Even when jaundice persists longer than 6 months, it is believed that complete recovery is usual although not inevitable. During this period, marked hypercholesterolemia, xanthomatosis, osteopenia, and other features of biliary cirrhosis may occur, and in some patients this chronic cholestatic syndrome does indeed eventuate in biliary cirrhosis. Long-term follow-up, perhaps with liver biopsies, may be necessary to establish the prognosis.

Drug-induced Chronic Liver Disease

Hepatic damage associated with drug therapy is acute and usually transient.[57] However, oxyphenisatin, halothane, isoniazid, and methyldopa have caused liver disease that is clinically and histologically indistinguishable from chronic active hepatitis. Phenothiazines are well known to cause a chronic cholestatic syndrome resembling primary biliary cirrhosis, and sporadic reports have also associated chronic hepatic injury with other drugs including sulfonamides, nitrofurantoin, propylthiouracil, and aspirin. In patients with drug-induced chronic liver disease, all evidence of disease usually resolves on withdrawal of the offending agent and self-perpetuation of liver damage after discontinuation of the agent is exceedingly rare.

Cirrhosis

The term *senile cirrhosis* has been used to refer to a cirrhotic process etiologically related to old age; however, most authorities no longer believe in a specific form of cirrhosis due to the hepatic effects of aging.[54]

Cirrhosis in elderly individuals is usually clinically silent and exhibits decreased incidence of active disease and manifestations of portal hypertension.[54] Such patients may succumb to hepatic coma with renal failure, especially postoperatively and less often to sepsis, variceal hemorrhage, or hepatocellular carcinoma.

A practical etiologic classification in the elderly includes autoimmune disease (primary biliary cirrhosis), biliary obstruction (secondary biliary cirrhosis), drugs and toxins (especially alcohol), infectious organisms, metabolic disorders (hemochromatosis), and cardiovascular diseases. The idiopathic and cryptogenic category constitutes a substantial number if not the majority of cases, especially when the liver disease is clinically silent. Alcohol is still the most commonly identified cause of clinically active cirrhosis in patients 70 years of age or older.

Hemochromatosis

Hemochromatosis is a group of disorders in which there is a progressive increase in total body iron stores with iron deposition in the parenchymal cells of the liver, heart, pancreas, and other organs.[74] In most instances idiopathic hemochromatosis is transmitted as an autosomal recessive trait, and for many years the disease remains latent. In most patients the classic triad of skin pigmentation, hepatomegaly, and diabetes mellitus is present, and compared with other forms of cirrhosis there is a relatively high incidence of gonadal atrophy, skin pigmentation, hepatomegaly, and a relatively prolonged and benign course. Liver function is usually well preserved despite the cirrhosis. Cardiac disease in about 15% of patients manifests as arrhythmias and congestive heart failure. In the elderly, diabetes and heart disease are so commonly caused by other disorders that these manifestations of iron overload are usually misdiagnosed. Hepatocellular carcinoma is a complication of hemochromatosis that is increasingly important as the life span of these patients improves. Phlebotomy prolongs life, arrests and perhaps reverses tissue damage, and improves other overt manifestations.

Primary Biliary Cirrhosis (Chronic Non-suppurative Destructive Cholangitis)

Primary biliary cirrhosis, chiefly a disease of middle-aged women, is often detected in an asymptomatic person because of an elevation in the alkaline phosphatase level.[90] The most frequent clinical presentation is the gradual onset of pruritus, followed by jaundice within 6 months to 2 years. Immune disorders associated with primary biliary cirrhosis include Sjögren's syndrome, rheumatoid arthritis, CRST syndrome, and thyroiditis. With the passage of time, increased pigmentation, xanthomas, and splenomegaly gradually develop.

Although the alkaline phosphatese level is particularly high, the bilirubin elevation is usually less than 3 mg/dl and is commonly normal. Hypercholesterolemia is usual. Serologic markers supporting the diagnosis include an elevated IgM level and the presence of antimitochondrial antibody (AMA). A negative AMA test should arouse suspicion that the patient does not have primary biliary cirrhosis; a positive test casts doubt on the diagnosis of an extrahepatic obstruction. Ancillary tests include ultrasonography, to exclude a dilated and obstructed biliary system, and ERCP, which can demonstrate irregular, tortuous, and narrowed bile ducts. The histopathologic diagnosis is more confidently made on a (operative) wedge biopsy than a (closed) needle biopsy.

The course is marked by all the complications of cholestasis, including pruritus, steatorrhea, and malabsorption. Bone changes are common in the older patient with longstanding disease, and fractures involving the back, ribs, and clavicle are not uncommon. Similarly, the lamina dura disappears and the teeth loosen and fall out. These bone changes may be accelerated by prednisone therapy, the results of which may be disastrous.

Advancing age has an unfavorable influence on disease progression. Prognosis is better in patients with granulomas on liver biopsy and, in general, survival bears a relationship to the bilirubin level. Once jaundice occurs, the patient has a 50% chance of surviving 5 years and as the degree of bilirubin elevation increases, survival time diminishes.

Therapy is directed toward relieving pruritus using cholestyramine, phenobarbital, and diphenhydramine and in replacing the nutritional elements lost because of steatorrhea. Calcium and vitamins A, D, and K are important dietary supplements, while medium-chain triglycerides can be used as a source of caloric energy. Clofibrate (Atromid) should not be given for hypercholesterolemia because of possibly irreversible paradoxic elevations in the serum cholesterol level following its administration. The exact role of immunosuppressive therapy has not been clarified, but early reports do not appear promising.

Secondary Biliary Cirrhosis

Biliary cirrhosis may develop as a consequence of longstanding obstruction of the common bile duct. The presence of cholangitis may greatly accelerate the cirrhotogenic process, however, and a full-blown cirrhosis may be produced within only several weeks. Patients are deeply jaundiced, and their skin typically exhibits a greenish hue. Although it is believed by some authors that stone removal and biliary decompression can retard the cirrhosis or relieve pruritus, frequently these patients succumb postoperatively to liver failure accompanied by hepatorenal syndrome, encephalopathy, and coagulation disturbances. Endoscopic papillotomy with stone removal may be a safer technique, although papillotomy in the face of portal hypertension and coagulation disturbances is also hazardous.

Complications of Cirrhosis

Complications of cirrhosis in the elderly are much the same as in younger patients, with the exception that hepatic encephalopathy tends to occur more frequently, is more often overlooked, and has a worse prognosis. The development of refractory ascites or bleeding esophageal varices, indications for a portosystemic shunting procedure in the young, are better treated in the elderly by less heroic measures. Thus, ascites which does not respond to rigorous salt and water restriction or diuretic administration, may show dramatic improvement with peritoneovenous shunting.[51] Esophageal varices can be sclerosed via flexible fiberoptic endoscopy or temporarily obliterated by percutaneous transhepatic technique without the need for general anesthesia. Variceal bleeding may be controlled acutely by the systemic administration of vasopressin, with or without balloon tamponade, while orally administered propranolol has been used to lower portal pressure and reduce the number of bleeding episodes.

Vasopressin is a potentially dangerous drug in elderly individuals. Arrhythmias, ischemic changes on electrocardiography, angina, myocardial infarction, and circulatory collapse have all been reported following vasopressin, usually in high doses and with boluses of the drug.

The transient effect of vasopressin on portal venous pressure and the need to administer it by the intravenous or intra-arterial route precludes its use for long-term control. Continuous oral administration of propranolol produces a sustained decrease in portal venous pressure in cirrhosis and has been used to prevent recurrent gastrointestinal bleeding associated with portal hypertension. Because propranolol decreases cardiac output and causes bronchoconstriction, its use in patients with heart failure or asthma is relatively contraindicated. Atenolol, a cardioselective β-blocker, has also been shown to reduce portal pressure primarily by diminishing cardiac output. Any influ-

ence of these agents on patient survival is yet to be demonstrated.

The Liver in Congestive Heart Failure and Shock

Hepatic abnormalities with heart failure are usually mild and not clinically significant.[16,89] With acute right-sided congestive failure or exacerbation of chronic failure, abdominal discomfort due to stretching of the liver capsule may occur. Nausea and vomiting may reflect hepatic or intestinal congestion, digitalis therapy, or other undefined factors. Overt jaundice, uncommon in congestive heart failure, occurs most often in patients with mitral stenosis, especially when complicated by pulmonary infarction or associated with tricuspid insufficiency.

The most sensitive method of detecting hepatic dysfunction in patients with congestive heart failure is the BSP retention test. The result of this test is frequently abnormal when those of all other "liver function" tests are normal.

Of the routing parameters of hepatic function, the prothrombin time is the most often affected. Prolongation of the prothrombin time, noted in 80% to 90% of patients with "congestive hepatopathy," is not influenced by administration of vitamin K. As might be predicted, these patients are quite sensitive to the effects of coumarin-type anticoagulants; spontaneous bleeding diatheses rarely occur.

Although overt jaundice is uncommon in congestive heart failure, mild unconjugated hyperbilirubinemia has been reported in up to 70% of patients and is usually seen in those with acute right-sided failure. The mechanism for this is not well understood.[89] Serum alkaline phosphatase levels are usually normal. Elevations of serum transaminases seen in about one-third of patients are essentially confined to individuals with acute heart failure. In severe or acute heart failure, if there is substantial hepatic necrosis, serum transaminase levels may exceed 1000 IU/ml and the clinical picture may simulate viral hepatitis.[8]

A common clinical problem is the differentiation of a modest serum glutamic oxaloacetic transaminase (SGOT) elevation due to congestive heart failure from that caused by a myocardial infarction. Serial electrocardiograms are most helpful, but occasionally analysis of the patterns of enzyme abnormality is critical to proper clinical management. An elevation of the serum glutamic pyruvic transaminase (SGPT) favors a diagnosis of liver disease since concentrations of this enzyme are far greater in the liver than the heart. In contrast, creatine phosphokinase (CPK) is more abundant in the myocardium. The hepatic damage even in as advanced a stage as "cardiac cirrhosis" may show almost complete healing if the congestive failure can be controlled and reversed. For this reason, some authors do not consider it to be true cirrhosis but refer to it as cardiac "fibrosis."

Hepatic Infarction

Infarcts of the liver are quite uncommon and are most often reported at necropsy. Infarction of the liver may result from a disturbance in either hepatic arterial or portal venous flow or may occur in the absence of demonstrable vascular compromise. In one series,[87] the most prevalent etiologic factors in hepatic infarction appear to be arteriosclerosis and aneurysms of the hepatic artery.

Clinically, hepatic infarctions present with right upper quadrant or epigastric pain and tenderness, associated with a sharp elevation of the serum transaminase, a delayed rise and fall of the alkaline phosphatase, and mild hyperbilirubinemia. Liver spleen scanning is a reasonable method to follow the course of such lesions. Hepatic infarctions are not usually life threatening.

Budd-Chiari Syndrome and Veno-Occlusive Disease

Occlusion of the hepatic veins, the Budd-Chiari syndrome, is an uncommon and often dramatic illness characterized by abdominal pain, progressive ascites, hepatomegaly, and a poor prognosis.[62] The clinicopathologic features of this disorder closely resemble those of congestive liver disease and the easiest means of differentiating them is by hepatic scintiscanning. In approximately one half the cases of hepatic vein occlusion, a characteristic "bull's-eye scan" occurs in which there is central accumulation of tracer in an enlarged, hypertrophied caudate lobe with diminution or absence of uptake in the remainder of the liver.

Liver biopsy typically reveals sinusoidal congestion and hemorrhage with atrophy or necrosis. While not specific for Budd-Chiari syndrome, its presence in association with normal jugular and right atrial pressures is virtually diagnostic of the entity.

In many cases of Budd-Chiari syndrome, no predisposing cause is found and no etiology is apparent in about one third of cases.[62] Etiologic factors of importance in the elderly include he-

matologic disorders (polycythemia rubra vera, myeloproliferative disorders), tumors (hepatocellular cancer, hypernephroma, and adrenal cancer). and congestive heart failure.

The prognosis is dismal. Therapy of hepatic vein occlusion is devoted toward preventing extension of the thrombus, relieving the hepatic congestion, and managing the ascites and fluid retention; of course, any underlying disorder should be treated definitively.

The Liver in Infection and Sepsis

Pyogenic Abscess

In the elderly, pyogenic abscesses are an important cause of fever, sepsis, and jaundice and if not promptly and fully treated are associated with a mortality rate exceeding 80%. In early series, infection from a distal source that spread to the liver via the portal vein (*i.e.*, pyelophlebitis) was most common. With the advent of antibiotics, portal pyemia has become less common, although it is important to consider the colon as a potential source of infection in any case of fever of unknown origin or hepatic abscesses without an identified etiology. Conversely, if a patient with diverticulitis develops jaundice or abnormal liver function tests, hepatic abscesses must be excluded.

Today, most instances of hepatic abscesses in older patients are due to biliary tract disease.[80] Such hepatic abscesses are usually multiple and result from ascending cholangitis due to partial obstruction of the common bile duct by calculus, inflammatory stricture, or neoplasm. Infections from adjacent organs such as the gallbladder or pancreas usually result in a single large abscess, whereas abscesses in the setting of systemic bacteremia are usually multiple and almost always microscopic. Neoplastic disease also plays an increasingly important role: in one series, malignancy was etiologically implicated in 36% of instances of hepatic abscess due to biliary obstruction, contiguous spread, or sepsis; all but 2 of 18 such patients were "elderly."[80]

Patients with microscopic or large abscesses exhibit a slower paced progression of disease than do those with microabscesses, and symptoms are often of a constitutional nature (*e.g.*, fever, malaise, weakness, anorexia, and weight loss). In contrast, patients with microscopic abscesses have a more acute course with chills and fever. A small group present with symptoms suggesting pulmonary disease, such as chest pain, dyspnea, hemoptysis, or a dry hacking cough—the so-called tussis hepatica of Pel.

Signs of pyogenic hepatic abscesses include hepatomegaly and right quadrant tenderness. Jaundice may be present especially if the patient is septic or has a biliary source for the abscess. Intrathoracic findings may be evident with an abscess adjacent to the right diaphragm or when infection has extended directly into the pleural space or lung parenchyma. Leukocytosis is present in most patients with pyogenic abscess, but the most helpful laboratory test is evaluation of the alkaline phosphatase level, which is elevated in over 90% of cases.

Conventional plain film studies are rarely diagnostic, and chest films generally reveal nonspecific pulmonary findings. Various scintigraphic agents including ^{99m}Tc sulfur colloid and gallium citrate as well as ultrasonography, computed tomography, and angiography are exceedingly helpful in diagnosing and localizing hepatic abscesses prior to operation or percutaneous needle aspiration.[81]

Anerobic bacteria alone or in combination with gram-negative bacilli are responsible for almost half of pyogenic abscesses and probably account for most of the "sterile" abscesses reported in the past. *Escherichia coli* is still the most common single isolate identified. *Staphylococcus aureus* and *Streptococcus* are the most frequently identified gram-positive organisms. The enterobacteriaceae are especially prominent in abscesses of biliary tract origin, whereas when the primary lesion is the intestine, two or more species of bowel flora, often including anaerobes, are usually identified.

Early drainage and prompt antimicrobial therapy are standard for pyogenic hepatic abscesses. Identification of the causative organism(s) is crucial to the proper selection of antimicrobials, but a good broad-spectrum regimen when a biliary or bowel source is suspected includes an aminoglycoside and either cefoxitin or the combination of ampicillin and clindamycin. Antibiotic use alone may be effective in instances of small and multiple hepatic abscesses not amenable to drainage and without biliary obstruction.

Although survival with pyogenic hepatic abscess is no longer a rarity, this disorder is still associated with a prodigious mortality and morbidity. Especially in the elderly with coexistent biliary tract disease or malignancy, clinical findings include jaundice, hypoalbuminemia, elevated serum transaminase levels, leukocytosis, bacteremia (especially with multiple organisms), aerobic infections with multiple abscesses, and significant complications.[72]

Jaundice Due to Bacterial Infections and Sepsis

Cholestatic jaundice is observed in less than 1% of adult bacteremias within a few days of the onset, and hepatomegaly is present in about half the patients.[109] The serum level of bilirubin, usually in the range of 5mg to 10mg/dl, is accompanied in about half the case by an elevated alkaline phosphatase. All biochemical derangements resolve with resolution of the sepsis. Liver biopsy usually reveals simple cholestasis with little or no parenchymal reaction or portal inflammation.

A variety of infections are associated with this cholestatic dysfunction, and the sudden onset of jaundice with high fever should suggest the possibility of sepsis in addition to the usual considerations of cholangitis or liver abscess. The presence of jaundice in a septic patient does not by itself adversely affect prognosis; the high mortality rate reported is a reflection of the severity of the sepsis.

Benign Tumors

The most common benign tumor that affects the liver is the hemangioma. It is found in approximately 5% of autopsies and with few exceptions is clinically silent. Treatment has consisted of either segmental resection or hepatic irradiation. Angiography with Gelfoam embolization or occlusion with various mechanical devices is a recent and potentially useful alternative method of control.

Malignant Tumors

Primary Liver Cancer

The adult liver is commonly involved with malignancy, either by metastatic spread from a distant focus or as a primary site of neoplasia. Of the primary adult hepatic cancers, 90% arise from the liver cells (hepatocellular carcinoma, hepatoma) and 5% to 10% from the bile ductular cells (cholangiocarcinoma); a small number exhibit features of both hepatic and ductal cell lines. Other types of primary liver cancers (*e.g.,* angiosarcoma) are rare lesions.

In the United States, the incidence of primary liver cancer is relatively constant and accounts for about 2500 deaths or 0.75% of all cancer deaths annually. It is more common in males, with an age incidence between 50 and 70 years.

Two well-identified hepatocellular carcinogens with long latent periods and thus of special concern in the elderly are vinyl chloride and Thorotrast. The former produces an angiosarcoma, whereas the latter, a roentgenographic contrast agent used from 1928 to the mid 1950s, causes a variety of primary hepatic tumors. The HBV carrier also has a greatly increased risk of developing primary liver cancer; in the United States, for the male carrier this approximates 5% per year after the age of 50 years.[76] An etiologic association between cirrhosis and primary liver cancer has long been appreciated, and coexistent cirrhosis is seen in 50% to 70% of patients with this tumor. This association is most clear in patients with hemochromatosis and so-called postnecrotic cirrhosis.

Most patients present with right upper quadrant or epigastric pain, accompanied by a right upper quadrant mass or an enlarged hard liver in a setting of weight loss or increasing abdominal girth.[41] A useful diagnostic laboratory test for primary liver cancer is the assay for α-fetoprotein, levels of which are elevated in about 90% of patients. Because of tumor hypervascularity there is a potential danger of hemorrhage after needle biopsy, and some authorities recommend biopsy only under direct vision at laparoscopy or operation.

The failure of surgical therapy for primary liver cell cancer is revealed in an almost zero 5-year survival. Irradiation and chemotherapy are both ineffective. There has been considerable enthusiasm for intrahepatic arterial infusion of chemotherapeutic agents or the angiographic embolization of occluding agents and devices directly into the main tumor vessel. Hepatic tumor devascularization with Gelfoam, Ivalon (polyvinyl alcohol sponge), or stainless steel coils appears effective in management of primary and secondary liver tumors. These techniques have been responsible for symptomatic improvement as well as some prolongation of survival.[10]

Metastatic Tumors

At autopsy 30% to 50% of all patients with carcinoma have secondary spread of tumor to the liver. The most common malignancies metastatic to liver are within the area drained by the portal vein (*e.g.*, stomach, intestine, pancreas, and gallbladder). Metastases via the hepatic artery are most often from primary or secondary cancers of the lung, breast, or kidney. Contiguous spread is most commonly seen with gallbladder tumors.

Many patients with hepatic metastases have complaints easily traceable to the liver, such as abdominal pain and jaundice. The liver is often markedly enlarged, hard and nodular, and commonly tender. A friction rub is sometimes heard because of subcapsular involvement. Anemia is common but usually not severe, and leukocytosis is seen especially with tumors that are necrotic. Liver function tests are too insensitive to reveal metastases early; the most consistent abnormality, an elevated alkaline phosphatase level, does not necessarily constitute evidence of hepatic involvement.

Survival time for patients with untreated hepatic metastases is depressingly brief and most attempts at treatment have not greatly improved survival. The major attempts to prolong survival comprise systemic chemotherapy, irradiation, hepatic resection, and interruption of the arterial blood supply to the tumor alone or combined with intra-arterial infusions of chemotherapeutic agents.[20] Resection of liver metastases in the case of solitary tumors or with multiple nodules in one lobe is not often suggested in the elderly.

The Hepatopathy of Hypernephroma

In 1961, Stouffer described the nephrogenic hepatic dysfunction syndrome or the ''hepatopathy or hypernephroma.'' This syndrome, seen in about 10% of patients with hypernephroma, is characterized by constitutional symptoms (fever, weight loss), hepatosplenomegaly, an elevated serum alkaline phosphatase level, prolongation of the prothrombin time, altered serum protein values (increased α$_2$-globulin and diminished albumin), and BSP retention—all without any metastatic involvement of the liver. Moreover, angiographic studies have revealed findings compatible with metastatic disease, including hypervascularity. The syndrome presumably reflects a reaction of the liver to one or more substances released form the tumor, since with removal of the primary lesion all the manifestations of the syndrome may disappear.[101]

Liver Involvement in Lymphoproliferative Disorders

In the elderly, the lymphoproliferative disorders that most often affect the liver are chronic lymphocytic leukemia, Hodgkin's disease,[6] and multiple myeloma. Chronic lymphocytic leukemia manifests itself in the liver primarily by portal tract infiltration with lymphocytes. Occasionally such infiltration may be massive and result in hepatomegaly, jaundice, and an elevation in serum alkaline phosphatase. Hepatic involvement does not alter treatment of this entity. The major clinical findings when Hodgkin's disease affects the liver are jaundice and hepatomegaly, usually in association with fever, chills, diaphoresis, weight loss, and other evidence of systemic illness. The development of jaundice is a serious prognostic sign and usually heralds the terminal phase. Occasionally jaundice and liver dysfunction indirectly result from the underlying disorder or they are drug or transfusion related.[99] Rarely, the cause of the jaundice is not found; such idiopathic cholestasis may rarely constitute the presenting feature of lymphoma.

Liver function testing is an insensitive and poor predictor of hepatic involvement. Gallium scanning can detect hepatic involvement with Hodgkin's disease, but only liver biopsy is diagnostic.

In a series of 64 individuals with multiple myeloma, 40% had plasma cell infiltration of the liver,[99] but hepatic or splenic enlargement did not always reflect involvement with malignant cells. Ascites and jaundice were each observed in about 15% of cases. Hyperbilirubinemia constitutes a poor prognostic sign, and most such patients succumb within 3 weeks of onset of icterus. Jaundice in myeloma patients is most often due to plasma cell infiltration of the hepatic sinusoids but additionally it may reflect tuberculosis, amyloid, viral hepatitis, hemolysis, and drug reactions.

Liver Involvement in Myeloid Metaplasia and Myelofibrosis

Gastrointestinal and hepatic manifestations of the disorder are well known and may greatly influence its clinical course.[94] Splenomegaly is universal, and hepatomegaly is present in almost three fourths of patients. Liver function is well preserved, and microscopic examination of the liver may fail to reveal abnormalities or satisfactorily account for its increased size. It has been postulated that hepatomegaly may result simply from increased portal flow through a massively enlarged spleen. Abnormalities in liver function and size may also reflect the influence of associated treatment such as transfusion, androgens, or splenectomy with resulting compensatory hepatic extramedullary hematopoiesis. Gastrointestinal bleeding related to duodenal ulcer or portal hypertension with varices has been described.

Liver biopsy in myeloid metaplasia is believed by some authors to be a hazardous procedure attended by inordinate bleeding despite normal coagulation studies prior to biopsy. Extramedullary hematopoiesis, triaditis, portal and periportal fibrosis, and increased iron deposition constitute the major histopathologic findings.

Radiation Hepatitis

The liver is a relatively radioresistant organ but does occasionally develop dose-related functional and histologic abnormalities following radiation therapy for tumors (*e.g.,* hemangiomas or lymphomas).[42] Clinical features vary, but in general, 2 to 6 weeks after completing a treatment schedule of more than 4000 rad, the patient notes the onset of rapid weight gain and an increase in abdominal girth. Physical examination usually reveals hepatomegaly and ascites, and laboratory studies show nonspecific elevations of the liver function tests, most notably the alkaline phosphatase. Microscopically, acute radiation damage to the liver is manifested as centrilobular sinusoid congestion or hemorrhage with atrophy of the hepatocytes and usually resolves within 2 months. Late effects of radiation on the liver are more variable.

The Liver in Systemic Diseases

Amyloidosis

Clinical and laboratory features of hepatic dysfunction are often mild or absent even with extensive hepatic involvement. Hepatomegaly in the presence of anemia, hypoalbuminemia, and azotemia should suggest the diagnosis. The most common liver function abnormality, an elevation of the serum alkaline phosphatase level, does not correlate with the degree of amyloid infiltration. Jaundice is unusual and is a grave prognostic sign.

Diabetes Mellitus

There is no specific liver disease that occurs in the diabetic; here only the changes in liver function and structure that accompany preexisting adult-onset diabetes will be noted.[12]

The older and more overweight a diabetic is, and the milder the diabetes, the more likely there is coexisting fatty liver. The major clinical manifestation is hepatomegaly, perhaps accompanied by a minor elevation of the alkaline phosphatase level and also insulin insensitivity. This condition is not progressive and improves with weight reduction.

Viral hepatitis, especially the "serum" variety, is said to be more common in diabetics, and a prolonged course is said to be characteristic; whether this is because of the predominance of hepatitis B or the diabetic state itself is not yet resolved.

Cirrhosis is found more frequently in diabetics, but in almost two thirds of instances, the abnormality in glucose regulation develops as a consequence of preexisting cirrhosis; it is not believed that the diabetic state *per se* predisposes to a higher incidence of cirrhosis; when diabetes and cirrhosis appear simultaneously, hemochromatosis should be excluded.

Giant Cell (Temporal) Arteritis

The incidence of associated liver dysfunction is unknown, but liver function tests, especially the alkaline phosphatase value, may be elevated in a nonspecific pattern. Liver biopsy may reveal intrahepatic cholestasis, with noncaseating granulomas. Therapy with corticosteroids usually results in rapid improvement.

Polymyalgia Rheumatica

Liver abnormalities may occur in polymyalgia rheumatica and rarely may be the main presenting feature of the illness. Granulomatous hepatitis, portal lymphocytic infiltration, or liver cell necrosis have all been found and are said to return to normal following treatment with corticosteroids. A high incidence of anti-HB$_S$ has been reported in some patients.

Sjögren's Syndrome

Liver disease has been found in 6% of patients with Sjögren's syndrome without rheumatoid arthritis. Conversely, sicca features of this syndrome occur with primary biliary cirrhosis and chronic active hepatitis. Clinical evidence of liver disease is unusual but most often manifested by hepatomegaly. Of the laboratory tests, the alkaline phosphatase value is the most frequently abnormal.

GALLBLADDER AND BILIARY TREE

Anatomic and Physiologic Changes With Aging

The common bile duct dilates slightly with advancing age.[65] In contrast to the pancreatic duct that dilates throughout its length with advancing age, the preampullary portion of the common bile duct becomes progressively narrowed with aging.[66]

In the absence of biliary tract disease, gallbladder emptying does not appear to slow with advancing age, nor does the organ's size appear greatly influenced by aging alone. Ptosis of the gallbladder due to ligamentous laxity, hypertrophy of the gallbladder wall, mucosal atrophy, and sclerosis of the blood vessels have been observed in some elderly individuals, but the functional significance and validity of these observations remain to be clarified.

The lithogenic index of bile increases with age[22,103] because of an increase in biliary cholesterol. The total bile salt pool and turnover of cholic acid do not appear to be altered in elderly subjects, which suggests that the dynamics of the enterohepatic circulation are not influenced by aging.

Milk of Calcium Bile

Milk of calcium bile, caused by the precipitation of calcium carbonate in the gallbladder fluid, almost always occurs in association with cystic duct obstruction, usually in the presence of chronic cholecystitis. Clinical manifestations are similar to those of simple cholelithiasis, and cholecystectomy is recommended. The entity should be suspected if a gallbladder of calcium density is present on plain film examination.

Gallstones

Gallbladder disease is the most common condition requiring abdominal operation in persons older than 60 years. This is in large part due to the progressive increase in the incidence of gallstones with each decade of life after age 20. Representative incidences of gallstones reported for each decade beyond 50 years are 50 to 60 years, 25% to 30%; 60 to 70 years, 40%; 70 to 80 years, 40% to 50%; and beyond 80 years, 55%.[13,27] The incidence of common bile duct stones also increases steadily beyond 50 years of age and is twofold to fourfold greater in patients 60 to 80 years of age than in patients younger than age 50. Problems of special concern to the physician taking care of geriatric patients will be stressed in this section, including the "silent" gallstone and the biliary complications that occur more frequently in the elderly (*e.g.*, gangrene and ischemic necrosis of the gallbladder, biliary-enteric fistulas, and malignancy).

Silent Gallstones

Symptoms eventually develop in half of patients with initially asymptomatic gallstones. This tends to be more sudden in older age patients, in whom the prognosis is frequently unfavorable because cholecystitis is often complicated by gangrene or perforation.[85] Even though the mortality of untreated biliary tract disease gradually increases as age advances,[55] there is no uniformity of opinion as to when or whether an elderly patient with "silent" gallstones should be operated on; the decision depends largely on the relative risks of operation and the dangers of complication from the stones in a particular patient. The single large stone is more frequently associated with acute obstructive cholecystitis and its ischemic complications than are multiple small stones. Obesity and diabetes mellitus increase the risk of "watchful waiting." Advanced age in the absence of severe and debilitating disease does not contraindicate elective cholecystectomy; cardiopulmonary and degenerative processes accompanying senescence are responsible for the increased mortality of operations in older subjects.[32] Most authorities believe that there is little difference in the mortality rate of elective cholecystectomy in the elderly and young but that there is a vastly increased mortality when emergency surgery is performed in the elderly.[25] My personal belief is that a healthy elderly subject with no major associated illnesses who has a solitary gallstone would probably benefit from elective cholecystectomy. For small stones in the gallbladder with a normal alkaline phosphatase level and no suspicion of common bile duct involvement or history of pancreatitis, it is probably reasonable to adapt a watchful attitude. The role of endoscopic papillotomy in the elective management of these patients is yet to be established. Elective cholecystostomy plays no role in the management of the "silent" gallstone. Cholecystectomy remains the only acceptable form of surgical therapy when calculi in the gallbladder are symptomatic. Dissolution therapy (*e.g.*, with chenodeoxycholic acid) is usually not appropriate to treat most "silent" gallstones since they are usually calcified and cannot be dissolved.

A causal relationship has been suggested between calculous disease and carcinoma of the gallbladder. Since the risk of developing gallbladder carcinoma in a patient with stones is less than the mortality rate of elective cholecystectomy, fear of developing carcinoma is not considered a valid indication for cholecystectomy.

Acute Calculous Cholecystitis

Acute cholecystitis is more prevalent with advancing age and is more frequently accompanied by complications such as gangrene and perforation.

Fever, abdominal findings, and leukocytosis are often less pronounced than expected. In a retrospective study of 88 patients older than 60 years of age acutely ill with biliary tract disease,[64] more than one third were afebrile, one fourth had no abdominal tenderness, and frank peritoneal signs were present in less than half. This frequent absence of overt right upper quadrant peritoneal findings resulted in delay in diagnosis of longer than 24 hours in one third of the patients. Jaundice is more common with acute cholecystitis in the elderly than in a younger population because of the greater frequency of common bile duct stones.

Atypical abdominal findings are more common with acute cholecystitis in the elderly probably because of the high incidence of gangrene and perforation of the gallbladder. As necrotic material and purulent bile drain down the paracolic gutters, a picture resembling appendicitis or diverticulitis with lower abdominal finding may be produced.

About 40% of the elderly patients undergoing emergency operation in one series had empyema of the gallbladder, gangrenous cholecystitis, or free perforation, while another 15% had concomitant subphrenic or hepatic abcesses.[64] Silent carcinoma of the gallbladder is also found not uncommonly in elderly patients being operated on for acute cholecystitis.[25] The converse problem in which the picture of acute cholecystitis may be simulated by common nongastroenterologic disorders such as a lower lobe pneumonia, myocardial infarction, or right-sided pyelonephritis must also be kept in mind. Radionuclide scintiscanning with one of the biliary imaging agents may be invaluable.

The elderly patient with acute cholecystitis is much less likely to recover without surgery than a younger individual. Delay in cholecystectomy after the acute inflammatory phase has resolved often results in advanced infection and a high mortality rate. In neglected or complicated biliary tract disease or in patients with associated severe disease, a cholecystostomy with evacuation of the gallbladder contents and establishment of drainage may be all that can be safely accomplished.[59] Additional gallstones develop in about 50% of patients within 2 years after cholecystostomy. Thus, the procedure constitutes definitive treatment only in patients whose life expectancy is severely limited.[30] Mortality rates for cholecystectomy increase in patients older than 60 to 70 years especially when there is associated cardiovascular or debilitating disease,[27] and emergent cholecystectomy has a much higher mortality rate than elective removal of the gallbladder.[64]

Choledochotomy in combination with either cholecystectomy or cholecystostomy is much more frequently performed in the elderly because of the greater incidence of common bile duct stones and jaundice. Siegel performed endoscopic papillotomy in 624 patients older than 65 years of age with choledocholithiasis, with overall mortality and morbidity rates of 0.16% and 8%, respectively.[92] In most patients, the procedure was indicated because of complications of common bile duct stones, including cholangitis and pancreatitis. In almost one third, papillotomy was performed to treat simple choledocholithiasis or biliary tract obstruction. In none of these was cholecystectomy subsequently required. Of 549 patients who had stones retained in the common bile duct after cholecystectomy, papillotomy with stone removal was accomplished successfully in 89%, with a morbidity rate of 9% and a mortality rate of 0.18%. In an additional 8%, retained stones were treated by papillotomy and placement of a permanent endoprosthesis without untoward effects.[93]

Perforation of the Gallbladder

Gallbladder perforation tends to occur primarily in elderly males and is probably caused by ischemia of the gallbladder wall.[79] A mortality rate of 15% to 25% results chiefly from delay in diagnosis and failure to initiate prompt therapy.

The major complications of gallbladder perforation include bile peritonitis, intra-abdominal abscess formation and cholecystoenteric fistula with gallstone ileus, cholerrheic enterocolopathy,[34] bacterial overgrowth and recurrent sepsis. Patients with spontaneous biliary enteric fistulas, especially the cholecystocolonic variety, are prone to develop recurrent cholangitis and sepsis. Antibiotic therapy is helpful in controlling the infections, but operative intervention is usually required. Endoscopic retrograde cannulation of the biliary tree may be very helpful in identifying the precise site of the fistulous communication, although conventional barium studies can usually demonstrate the fistula.

Acute Cholangitis

Acute cholangitis primarily affects the elderly and usually complicates benign biliary tract disease such as choledocholithiasis, postoperative common bile duct stricture, and biliary tract manipulation.[84]

A confusing feature of many published descriptions of cholangitis arises because of the failure of many authors to distinguish between suppurative (obstructive) cholangitis and the much more common nonsuppurative ascending cholangitis. Suppurative cholangitis mandates emergent operative or endoscopic decompression of the common bile duct and is likely when there are manifestations of septicemia such as hypotension or shock, confusion and mental impairment, high fever, leukocytosis, and thrombocytopenia. Nonsuppurative or ascending cholangitis exhibiting "Charcot's triad" of chills, spiking fever, jaundice, and pain or tenderness in the right upper quadrant usually responds promptly to antibiotic therapy. More than 90% of patients with cholangitis have positive biliary cultures at operation, and in more than half of these, multiple organisms are isolated. Both the incidence of biliary infection and the frequency of biliary calculi rise with age.[56]

Not all patients with cholangitis exhibit all the characteristic clinical features, and a high degree of clinical suspicion is necessary to make an early diagnosis and salvage the patient. Once the diagnosis is suspected, blood cultures should be obtained and combination antimicrobial therapy with ampicillin or a cephalosporin and an aminoglycoside begun. Hypovolemia and hypotension should be corrected promptly and a coagulation profile performed since these patients have a high incidence of thrombocytopenia, fibrinolysis, and consumption coagulopathy. For the emergent treatment of a critically ill patient with suppurative cholangitis, endoscopic papillotomy or insertion of large-caliber endoprosthesis to decompress and drain the duct are alternatives to formal operation and may even be preferable, since they can be performed more rapidly and without general anesthesia.

Acute Acalculous Cholecystitis

Acute acalculous cholecystitis, an often misdiagnosed and potentially lethal disorder, is increasing in frequency. It presently comprises 5% to 15% of all patients with acute cholecystitis but accounts for a higher percentage of cholecystitis occurring postoperatively or in a wide variety of critical clinical settings, including bacterial sepsis, major trauma, burns, multiple transfusions, and debilitation.[36] Most cases are in men over 65 years of age.[28]

Signs and symptoms of acute acalculous cholecystitis do not usually differ from those of acute cholecystitis with stones, and even radionuclide scintiscanning may not distinguish between the two. The incidence of advanced disease with gangrene and perforation is greater when acute cholecystitis is not associated with stones, especially when it follows trauma or an operation unrelated to the biliary tract. The critical nature of the patients' illnesses, the high incidence of associated disorders, and the advanced stage of inflammatory process is reflected in the high mortality rate of 6.5% associated with acute acalculous cholecystitis compared with 3.4% when acute cholecystitis with calculi is diagnosed.[52]

Factors identified as contributing to acalculous cholecystitis in the elderly include cystic duct obstruction (*e.g.*, with a neoplasm), concentration of bile (*e.g.*, with dehydration or fasting), narcotic administration and use of positive pressure respirators, and impairment of the blood supply (*e.g.*, with shock, congestive heart failure or arteriosclerosis). Acute acalculous cholecystitis has also been associated with systemic illnesses such as diabetes mellitus and pernicious anemia; cardiovascular disease is presumed to be of etiologic significance in almost one half of the patients.[26] Unless there are contraindications, cholecystectomy is the treatment of choice.

Acute Emphysematous Cholecystitis[60]

The diagnosis of acute emphysematous cholecystitis is made roentgenographically by the presence of gas in the gallbladder lumen or surrounding the wall of the gallbladder. Most cases occur in patients between the ages of 50 and 70 years, and the incidence in men is three to seven times greater than in women. Diabetes mellitus is present in 20% to 30% of cases. Clinically the disease is heralded by the sudden onset of fever and intense right upper quadrant pain. Often the patient appears even more ill and toxic than the physical signs would suggest. Jaundice is rare, and the gallbladder is usually present as a palpable mass in the right upper quadrant.

It is believed an endarteritis obliterans renders the gallbladder ischemic and thus provides the environment necessary for the proliferation of gas-producing organisms, most common of which are *Clostridium perfringens, Escherichia coli* and anaer-

obic gram-positive bacilli. Antibiotic therapy should be initiated promptly, but cholecystectomy is the operative procedure of choice.

Torsion of the Gallbladder

Torsion of the gallbladder, a rare cause of acalculous cholecystitis, is most often reported in elderly women. The condition is possible only when there is a lax mesentery, enabling it to twist and compromise the blood supply of the organ. About half of the patients with torsion do have calculi, and it is assumed that the weight of the organ initiates a twist in the flaccid mesentery. In a group without stones, the mechanism for torsion and rotation is not clear. Gangrene is frequently present, but frank perforation is uncommon. The clinical presentation is not distinctive, and the most frequent preoperative diagnosis is that of an "acute abdomen."

Hemobilia

Hemobilia refers to hemorrhage into the biliary tree and ultimately into the gastrointestinal tract.[4] Minimal and prolonged bleeding causes only occult blood in the stools, perhaps accompanied by anemia, while major bleeding causes a characteristic triad of abdominal pain (biliary colic), jaundice, and gastrointestinal bleeding. Gastrointestinal hemorrhage usually follows the onset of abdominal pain and is often accompanied by a fall in the serum levels of alkaline phosphatase and bilirubin as the biliary obstruction is relieved.

Hemobilia is most often caused by trauma, but other prominent causes, especially in the elderly population, include vascular disease (aneurysms of the hepatic artery), gallbladder disease (cholelithiasis and carcinoma), and primary hepatic neoplasms, especially hepatoma.

The diagnosis should be considered in any jaundiced patient with gastrointestinal hemorrhage or in an individual with occult blood in the stools and no defined source of the bleeding on repeated roentgenographic and endoscopic evaluation. Retrograde cannulation of the biliary tract is often helpful in demonstrating the presence of structurally identifiable disease such as tumor or calculi. Cholecystectomy, aneurysmectomy, vessel ligation, and hepatic resection may each be indicated in selected instances.

The Gallbladder in Diabetes Mellitus

The size of the gallbladder may be increased in diabetes because of autonomic visceral neuropathy. The organ may demonstrate poor visualization and/or poor contraction on cholecystography—in the absence of any inflammatory or calculous disease. Gallstones occur almost twice as commonly in the diabetic population. When cholelithiasis complicates diabetes, gangrene perforation and emphysematous cholecystitis are especially common. A common clinical finding in cholecystitis complicating diabetes is the rather rapid progression to tissue necrosis.[86] Moreover, the mortality of acute gallbladder disease and the incidence of death with emergent surgery in the diabetic beyond age 65 is twice as great as in the nondiabetic of similar age.[100] In contrast, the outcome of elective biliary tract operations in the diabetic is not substantially different from that in nondiabetics, which suggests that gallbladder disease in a diabetic should be treated with a "judicious aggressive" approach.

Biliary Stricture

In the absence of prior abdominal surgery (especially involving the biliary tract, stomach, or pancreas) a biliary stricture, even if it appears benign, should be considered malignant and should be approached operatively both for accurate diagnosis and therapy.[106] A history of prolonged biliary drainage following cholecystectomy, or of postoperative sepsis or jaundice, suggests the possibility of an injury to the biliary tract, while jaundice, chills, and fever several years after biliary tract surgery are the usual indications that a stricture has developed. Features of secondary biliary cirrhosis (*e.g.*, hepatosplenomegaly) and portal hypertension are uncommon but can occur with longstanding obstruction. Laboratory data usually reveal features of pure obstruction (*i.e.*, elevated serum bilirubin and alkaline phosphatase levels) unless secondary hepatocellular damage has occurred. The types of operations have been reviewed elsewhere,[106] but in the past several years, a number of endoscopic and percutaneous nonoperative approaches to the management of biliary stricture have been developed.[49]

Tumors of the Bile Ducts and Gallbladder

Benign tumors of the biliary apparatus are rare and in general do not affect the elderly population with particular frequency.

Malignancy of the Biliary Tract

Cancer of the extrahepatic bile ducts is encountered at operation about one third to one half as frequently as carcinoma of the gallbladder.

Bile duct cancer is more frequent in men and occurs in individuals with a mean age of 62 years.[96] Predisposing causes include chronic ulcerative colitis in Western countries and parasitic infestation with the liver fluke in the Orient. Cholelithiasis accompanies cancer of the extrahepatic biliary tree in fewer than one third of cases.

Progressive jaundice usually accompanied by intense pruritus is the most frequent symptom of cancer of the extrahepatic bile ducts, followed by upper abdominal pain, weight loss, nausea, vomiting, and anorexia. Chills and fever due to associated cholangitis are unusual in the absence of a surgical procedure on the biliary tract. Hepatomegaly is usually present, and about one third of patients have a palpable gallbladder (Courvoisier sign).

Carcinomas of the bile ducts are radioresistant and systemic chemotherapy has not brought about prolonged survival. A practical approach is to attempt resection, usually most successful for lesions in the distal common bile duct or more rarely the middle portion of the duct, and to palliate the remaining lesions using operative or nonoperative percutaneous or endoscopic implantation of a wide variety of internally or externally draining prostheses.[38] Palliation is of particular value in relieving pruritus and in diminishing cholangitic episodes. It also results in an improved quality of life and may be associated with an extended survival, ranging from 2.5 to 14.5 months.

Carcinoma of the Gallbladder

Carcinoma of the gallbladder occurs predominantly in women, with a peak incidence in the seventh decade.[102] An etiologic role for gallstones and inflammatory bowel disease has been postulated but remains unproven. The incidence of gallstones in patients with carcinoma of the gallbladder ranges from 60% to 92% and, conversely, gallbladder cancer is seen in 1% to 4% of gallbladders containing calculi.

Most gallbladder cancer is discovered incidentally during cholecystectomy for chronic biliary symptoms, and in Glenn and Hay's series,[29] approximately 85% of cases in which the presenting complaint was not related to liver metastases were clinically indistinguishable from nonmalignant biliary tract disease. When a change in symptoms occurs, and abdominal pain becomes continuous rather than intermittent, or weight loss, obstructive jaundice, or anorexia develop, carcinoma of the gallbladder is likely.

Treatment is surgical. If the cases of fortuitous cholecystectomy are eliminated, resection of all grossly apparent neoplasm will be possible in only about 10% of cases. In such instances, radical cholecystectomy with excision of the gallbladder and surrounding liver tissue and regional lymph nodes is suggested. Unfortunately, the prognosis is dismal, and even when the carcinoma is found incidentally during simple cholecystectomy, cure rate is less than 5%. Poor survival is explained by the aggressive nature of the lesion and the high incidence of local and distal spread at the time of initial presentation.

REFERENCES

1. Andrew W: Senile changes in pancreas of Wistar Institute rats and of man with special regard to similarity of lobule and cavity formation. Am J Anat 74:97–127, 1944
2. Bagley Jr, Roth JA, Thomas LB, Devita VT Jr: Liver biopsy in Hodgkin's disease: Clinicopathologic correlations in 127 patients. Ann Intern Med 76:119–225, 1972
3. Bartos V, Groh J: The effect of repeated stimulation of the pancreas on the pancreatic secretion in young and aged men. Gerontol Clin 11:56–62, 1969
4. Bismuth H: Hemobilia. N Engl J Med 288:617–619, 1973
5. Black M, Mitchell JR, Zimmerman HJ, Ishak KG, Epler GR: Isoniazid-associated hepatitis in 114 patients. Gastroenterology 69:289–301, 1975
6. Bouroncle BA, Vazques AG: Pathogenesis of jaundice in Hodgkin's disease. Arch Intern Med 110:108–118, 1962
7. Boyd E: Normal variability in weight of the adult human liver and spleen. Arch Pathol 16:350–372, 1933
8. Bynum TE, Boitnott JK, Maddrey WC: Ischemic hepatitis. Dig Dis Sci 24:129–135, 1979
9. Carney FMT, VanDyke RA: Halothane hepatitis: A critical review. Curr Res 51:135–160, 1972
10. Chuang VP, Wallace S: Current status of transcatheter management of neoplasm. Cardiovasc Intervent Radiol 3:256–267, 1980
11. Cotton PB: Nonoperative removal of bile duct stones by duodenoscopic sphincterotomy. Br J Surg 67:1–5, 1980
12. Creutzfeldt W, Frerichs H, Sickinger K: Liver diseases and diabetes mellitus. Prog Liver Dis 3:371–407, 1970
13. Crump C: The incidence of gallstones and gallbladder diseases. Surg Gynecol Obstet 53:447–455, 1931
14. DiMagno EP: Medical treatment of pancreatic insufficiency. Mayo Clin Proc 54:435–442, 1979
15. Doll R, Muir M, Waterhouse J (eds): Cancer Incidence in Five Continents, Vol. 2, International Union Against Cancer. Berlin, Springer, 1970
16. Dunn GD, Hayes P, Breen KJ, Schenker S: The liver in congestive heart failure: A review. Am J Med Sci 265:175–189, 1973
17. Eastwood HDH: Causes of jaundice in the elderly. Gerontol Clin 13:69–81, 1971
18. Fenster LF: Viral hepatitis in the elderly: An analysis of 23 patients over 65 years of age. Gastroenterology 78:535–541, 1965
19. Findor J, Perez V, Bruch Igartus E, Giovanetti M, Fioravantti N: Structure and ultrastructure of the liver in aged persons. Acta Hepato Gastroenterol 20:200–204, 1973
20. Foster JH, Lundy J: Liver metastases. Curr Probl Surg 18:160–202, 1981
21. Frank MS, Weissmann HS, Chun KJ, Sugarman LA, Brandt LJ, Freeman IM: Visualization of the biliary tract with ^{99mm}Tc-HIDA in acute pancreatitis (AP)(abstr). Gastroenterology 78:1167, 1980
22. Fujiyama M, Kajiyama G, Maruhashi A et al: Change in lipid composition of bile with age in normal subjects and patients with gallstones. Hiroshima J Med Sci 28:23–29, 1979
23. Gabinski K, Fojt E, Suchan L: Hepatitis in the aged. Digestion 8:254–260, 1973
24. Geltner D, Chajeck T, Rubinger D, Levij I: Quinidine hypersensitivity and liver involvement: A survey of 32 patients. Gastroenterology 70:650–652, 1976
25. Glenn F: Surgical treatment of acute cholecystitis in the elderly. Geriatrics 20:728–738, 1965
26. Glenn F: Acute acalculous cholecystitis. Ann Surg 189:458–465, 1979
27. Glenn F: Surgical management of acute cholecystitis in patients 65 years of age and older. Ann Surg 193:56–59, 1981
28. Glenn F, Becker CG: Acute acalculous cholecystitis: An increasing entity. Ann Surg 195:131–136, 1982
29. Glenn F, Hays DM: The age factor in the mortality rate of patients undergoing surgery of the biliary tract. Surg Gynecol Obstet 100:11–18, 1955
30. Glenn F, McSherry CK: Calculous biliary tract disease. Curr Probl Surg 12:1–38, 1975
31. Greenblatt DJ, Seller EM, Shader RI: Drug disposition in old age. N Engl J Med 306:1081–1088, 1982
32. Haff RC, Butcher HR Jr, Ballinger WF: Factors influencing morbidity in biliary tract operations. Surg Gynecol Obstet 152:195–203, 1971
33. Hoffman E, Perez E, Somera V: Acute pancreatitis in the upper age groups. Gastroenterology 36:675–685, 1959
34. Hofmann AF, Poley JR: Cholestyramine treatment of diarrhea associated with ileal resection. N Engl J Med 281:397–402, 1969
35. Horst DA, Grace HD, LeCompte PM: Prolonged cholestasis and progressive hepatic fibrosis following imipramine therapy. Gastroenterology 79:550–554, 1980
36. Howard RJ: Acute acalculous cholecystitis. Am J Surg 141:194–198, 1981

37. Huete-Armijo A, Exton-Smith AN: Causes and diagnosis of jaundice in the elderly. Br Med J 1:1113–1114, 1962

38. Huibregtse K, Tytgat GN: Palliative treatment of obstructive jaundice by transpapillary introduction of large bore bile duct endoprothesis. Gut 23:371–375, 1982

39. Hunt DR, Mildenhall P: Etiology of strictures of the colon associated with pancreatitis. Dig Dis 20:941–946, 1975

40. Hyams DE: The liver and biliary system. In Brocklehurst JC (ed): Text of Geriatric Medicine and Gerontology, 2nd ed. Edinburgh, Churchill Livingstone, 1978

41. Idhe DC, Sherlock P, Winawer SJ, Fortner JG: Clinical manifestations of hepatoma: A reveiw of 6 year's experience at a Cancer Hospital. Am J Med 56:83–91, 1974

42. Ingold JA, Reed GB, Kaplan HS, Bagshaw MA: Radiation hepatitis. Am J Roentgenol 93:200–208, 1965

43. Ishak KG, Irey NS: Hepatic injury associated with phenothiazines: Clinicopathologic and follow-up study of 36 patients. Arch Pathol 93:283–304, 1972

44. Jam I, Shoham M, Wolf RO, Mishkin S: Elevated serum amylase activity in the absence of clinical pancreatic or salivary gland disease. Am J Gastroenterol 70:480–488, 1978

45. Jersild M: Infectious hepatitis with subacute atrophy of the liver: An epidemic in women after menopause. N Engl J Med 237:8–11, 1947

46. Kampamm JP, Sinding J, Moller-Jorgensen I: Effect of age of liver function. Geriatrics 30:91–95, 1975

47. Kaye MD: Pleuropulmonary complications of pancreatitis. Thorax 23:297–306, 1968

48. Kelly TR: Gallstone pancreatitis. Arch Surg 109:294–297, 1974

49. Kozarek RA, Sanowski RA: Nonsurgical management of extrahepatic obstructive jaundice. Ann Intern Med 96:743–745, 1982

50. Kreel L, Sandin B: Changes in pancreatic morphology associated with aging. Gut 14:962–970, 1973

51. LeVeen HH, Wapnick S, Diaz C, Grosberg S, Kinney M: Ascites: Its correction by peritoneovenous shunting, pp 1–61. Curr Probl Surg 16, 1979

52. Long TN, Heminback DM, Carrico CJ: Acalculous cholecystitis in critically ill patients. Am J Surg 136:31–36, 1978

53. Ludwig J, Axelson R: Drug effects on the liver: An updated tabular compilation of drugs and drug-related hepatic diseases. Dig Dis Sci 28:651–666, 1983

54. Ludwig J, Baggenstoss AH: Cirrhosis of the aged and senile cirrhosis—Are there two conditions? J Gerontol 3:244–248, 1970

55. Lund J: Surgical indications in cholelithiasis: Prophylactic cholecystectomy elucidated on the basis of long-term follow-up on 526 nonoperated cases. Ann Surg 151:153–162, 1960

56. Lygidakis NJ: Incidence of bile infection in patients with choledocholithiasis. Am J Gastroenterol 77:12–17, 1982

57. Maddrey WC, Boitnott JK: Drug-induced chronic liver disease. Gastroenterology 72:1248–1353, 1977

58. Mallory A, Kern F Jr: Drug-induced pancreatitis: A critical review. Gastroenterology 78:813–820, 1980

59. Malmstrom P, Olsson AM: Cholecystostomy for acute cholecystitis. Am J Surg 126:397–402, 1973

60. May RE, Strong R: Acute emphysematous cholecystitis. Br J Surg 58:453–458, 1971

61. Menard DB, Gisselbrecht C, Marty M, Reyes F, Dhumeaux D: Antineoplastic agents and the liver. Gastroenterology 78:142–164, 1980

62. Mitchell MC, Boitnott JK, Kaufman S, Cameron JL, Maddrey WC: Budd-Chiari syndrome: Etiology, diagnosis and management. Medicine 61:199–218, 1982

63. Moertel CG: Alimentary tract cancer. Exocrine pancreas. In Holland J, Frei E (eds): Cancer Medicine, pp 1792–1804. Philadelphia, Lea & Febiger, 1982

64. Morrow DJ, Thompson J, Wilson ED: Acute cholecystitis in the elderly: A surgical emergency. Arch Surg 113:1149–1152, 1978

65. Nagase M, Kikasa Y, Soloway RD, Tanimura H, Setoyama M, Mukaihara S, Kato H: Surgical significance of dilatation of the common bile duct—with special reference to choledocholithiasis. Jpn J Surg 10:296—301, 1980

66. Nakadi I: Changes in morphology of the distal common bile duct associated with aging. Gastroenterol Jpn 16:54–63, 1981

67. Naso F, Thompson CM: Hyperbilirubinemia in the patient past 50. Geriatrics 22:206–212, 1967

68. Niccolini DG, Graham JH, Banks PA: Tumor-induced acute pancreatitis. Gastroenterology 71:142–145, 1976

69. O'Brien GF, Tan CV: Jaundice in the geriatric patient. Geriatrics 25:114–127, 1970

70. O'Malley K, Kelly J: Recent pharmacokinetic studies of metabolized drugs in the elderly. In Kitani K (ed): Liver and Aging, pp 303–313. New York, Elsevier Biomedical Press, 1982

71. Osnes M, Lotveit T, Larsen S, Aune S: Duodenal diverticula and their relationship to age, sex and biliary calculi. Scand J Gastroenterol 16:103–107, 1981

72. Pitt HA, Zuidema GD: Factors influencing mortality in the treatment of pyogenic hepatic abscess. Surg Gynecol Obstet 140:228–234, 1975

73. Pollock TW, Ring ER, Oleaga JA, Freiman DB, Mullen JL, Rosato EF: Percutaneous decompression of benign and malignant biliary obstruction. Arch Aurg 114:148–151, 1979

74. Powell LW, Basset ML, Halliday JW: Hemochro-

matosis: 1980 update. Gastroenterology 78:374–381, 1980

75. Price HL, Gazzard BG, Dawson AM: Steatorrhea in the elderly. Br Med J 1:1582–1584, 1977

76. Prince AM: The role of viruses in human cancer. In Girald G, Beth E (eds): Proceedings of the 1st International Congress of Viral Oncology, Naples, Italy. New York, Elsevier-North Holland, 1979

77. Ranson JHC, Turner JW, Roses DF, Rifkind KM, Spencer FC: Respiratory complications in acute pancreatitis. Ann Surg 179:557–566, 1974

78. Ranson JHC: The timing of biliary surgery in acute pancreatitis. Ann Surg 189:654–663, 1979

79. Roslyn J, Busuttil RW: Perforation of the gallbladder: A frequently mismanaged condition. Am J Surg 137:307–312, 1979

80. Rubin RH, Swartz MN, Malt R: Hepatic abscesses: Changes in clinical, bacteriologic and therapeutic aspects. Am J Med 57:601–610, 1974

81. Rubinson HA, Isikoff MB, Hill MC: Diagnostic imaging of hepatic abscesses: A retrospective analysis. AJR 135:735–740, 1980

82. Safrany L: Endoscopic treatment of biliary tract disease. Lancet 3:983–985, 1978

83. Safrany L, Cotton PB: A preliminary report: Urgent duodenoscopic sphincterotomy for acute gallstone pancreatitis. Surgery 89:424–428, 1981

84. Salk RP, Greenburg AG, Farris JM, Peskin GW: Spectrum of cholangitis. Am J Surg 130:143–150, 1975

85. Sato T, Matsushiro T: Surgical indications in patients with silent gallstones. Am J Surg 128:368–375, 1974

86. Schein CJ: Acute cholecystitis in the diabetic. Am J Gastroenterol 51:511–515, 1969

87. Seeley TT, Blumenfeld CM, Ikeda R, Knapp W, Ruebner BH: Hepatic infarction. Human Pathol 3:265–276, 1972

88. Sharland DE: Clinical value of serum alkaline phosphatase isoenzyme estimations in the elderly. Age Ageing 4:1–7, 1975

89. Sherlock S: The liver in heart failure: Relation of anatomical functional and circulatory changes. Br Heart J 13:273–293, 1957

90. Sherlock S, Scheuer PJ: The presentation and diagnosis of 100 patients with primary biliary cirrhosis. N Engl J Med 289:674–678, 1973

91. Sherman IL, Eichenwald HF: viral hepatitis: Descriptive epidemiology based on morbidity and mortality statistics. Ann Intern Med 44:1049–1069, 1965

92. Siegel JH: Interventional endoscopy in diseases of the biliary tree and pancreas. Mt Sinai J Med 51:535–542, 1984

93. Siegel JH, Yatto RP: Biliary endoprosthesis for the management of retained common duct stones. Am J Gastroenterol 79:50–54, 1984

94. Silverstein MN, Wolleager EE, Baggenstoss AH: Gastrointestinal and abdominal manifestations of agnogenic myeloid metaplasia. Arch Intern Med 131:532–537, 1973

95. Szmuness W, Dienstag JL, Purcell RH, Harley EJ, Stevens CE, Wong DC: Distribution of antibody to hepatitis A antigen in urban adult populations. N Engl J Med 295:755–759, 1976

96. Takasan H, Kim CI, Arii S, Takahashi S, Uozumi T, Tobe T, Honjo I: Clinicopathologic study of seventy patients with carcinoma of the biliary tract. Surg Gynecol Obstet 150:721–726, 1980

97. Tauchi H, Sato T: Some micromeasuring studies of hepatic cells in senility. J Gerontol 17:254–259, 1962

98. Tauchi H, Sato T: Effect of environmental conditions upon age changes in the human liver. Mech Ageing Dev 4:71–80, 1975

99. Thomas FB, Clausen KP, Greenberger NJ: Liver disease in multiple myeloma. Arch Intern Med 132:195–201, 1973

100. Turrill FL, McCarron NM, Mikkelsen WP: Gallstones and diabetes: An ominous association. Am J Surg 102:184–190, 1961

101. Utz DC, Warren MM, Gregg JA, Ludwig J: Reversible hepatic dysfunction associated with hypernephroma. Mayo Clin Proc 45:161–169, 1970

102. Vaittinen E: Carcinoma of the gallbladder: A study of 390 cases diagnosed in Finland 1953–1967. Ann Chir Gynaecol Fenn 168(suppl):1, 1970

103. Valdivieso V, Palma R, Wunkaus R, Antezana C, Severin C, Contrera A: Effect of aging on biliary lipid composition and bile acid metabolism in normal Chilean women. Gastroenterology 74:871–874, 1978

104. Walker CO, Combes B: Biliary cirrhosis induced by chlorpromazine. Gastroenterology 51:631–640, 1966

105. Wallace SA, Ashworth CT: Histopathology of the senile pancreas. Texas State J Med 37:584–591, 1942

106. Warren KW, Mountain JC, Midell AI: Management of strictures of the biliary tract. Surg Clin North Am 51:711–731, 1971

107. Warshaw AL, Lesser PB, Rie M, Cullen DJ: The pathogenesis of pulmonary edema in acute pancreatitis. Ann Surg 182:505–510, 1975

108. Wilson PD: Enzyme changes in ageing mammals. Gerontologia 19:79–125, 1973

109. Zimmerman HJ, Fang M, Utili R, Seeff LB, Hoofnagle J: Jaundice due to bacterial infection. Gastroenterology 77:362–374, 1979

18   The Neurologic Aspects of Aging

Alan Barham Carter

The physician's approach to illness in the elderly person is often slightly less enthusiastic than it is when he is dealing with younger patients, and this seems to be particularly true in the discipline of neurology. Here the specialist is traditionally thought to be more concerned with the niceties of precise diagnosis than he is with therapy because, according to some, most neurologic treatment is of little value. We are therefore faced with two negative therapeutic views in the consideration of neurology in the elderly. It is probable that both these concepts are false and that a correct evaluation of neurologic symptoms and signs in the elderly may be surprisingly rewarding for both the patient and the physician.

The adjective "elderly" is very difficult to define, because age cannot be measured by years alone. However, because some yardstick is necessary, the present review of neurologic disease in the elderly is based on experience with patients over the age of 65.

NORMAL VARIATIONS

The assessment of a neurologic illness depends to a large extent on physical signs, and it is therefore important to know which of these indicate the presence of organic illness and which are within the normal limits for a particular age-group. Aging is little understood, but a least we know that in the nervous system it is characterized by a steady loss of neurons, which begins surprisingly early, probably at the age of 25. This accounts for the fact that as we grow older we forget people's names, tend to become more rigid and circumscribed in our outlook, experience at times a de-gree of absentmindedness, and wake earlier in the morning.

Because of this loss, which affects both spinal cord and brain, many elderly patients show what in younger people would be considered abnormal physical signs. These comprise irregular pupillary outline; loss of tone in the facial, neck, and spinal musculature; loss of ankle jerks; loss of appreciation of tuning-fork vibrations at the ankle; and some loss of position sense in the toes. In addition, there is a general decrease in muscle bulk, with particular emphasis on the small muscles of the hands, which are not uncommonly found to be wasted, even in patients with no obvious arthropathy. If other abnormal physical signs are present or if these variations produce symptoms, such abnormalities may indicate an organic systemic neurologic disorder, but if not they may safely be considered normal variations owing to the aging process. The elderly often show evidence of peripheral occlusive vascular disease affecting the blood flow in the vasa nervorum so that the general effects of aging are accentuated locally, even though true ischemic neuropathy and myelopathy may be absent. Wasting of the intrinsic muscles of the hands is generalized but is more obvious on the back of the hand, where guttering and loss of the first dorsal interosseus muscle are often marked, although strength is reasonably well preserved. Disuse in old age possibly plays some part, and any arthropathy affecting the wrist joint makes the condition much worse, even to the extent of suggesting motor neuron disease. Another factor is the universal presence of cervical spondylosis in the elderly, which may accentuate wasting of the hands, but care must be taken not to blame coincidental abnormalities for what are in fact normal variants, so that unnecessary treatment may be avoided.

In order to obtain data on this point 100 consecutive patients over age 70 were studied. These patients seemed free from organic disease of the nervous system; were cooperative, well oriented, and reliable in their answers; and were not suffering from diabetes, deficiency states, cancer, or the grosser forms of arthropathy. Most of them were hospital inpatients recovering from respiratory infections, hematemesis, or other general medical disorders. The object was to find how frequently wasting of the interossei, absence of ankle jerks, and diminution of position sense and vibratory appreciation in the lower limbs occurred as a normal variation. Any correlation with increasing age or with obvious occlusive peripheral artery disease was evidenced by absence of the posterior tibial pulse at the ankle. Reinforcement of the ankle jerk was obtained by asking the patient to clench the jaws, and the appreciation of vibration was measured by applying a C tuning fork to the malleoli. Reinforcement is essential in eliciting tendon jerks in elderly patients because limb relaxation is difficult for them, and, because vibratory appreciation is affected by cold, the malleoli were used as the bony points rather than the big toe for application of the tuning fork. Position sense was elicited by inquiry about the position of the big toe—straight or bent—without the patient seeing it. The results are given in the following paragraphs.

Eyes

If cataract and glaucoma are excluded, the only common evidence of aging in the eyes is the presence of arcus senilis (70 patients), some irregularity and inequality of the pupils (33 patients), and fading of iris color (percentage was difficult to determine because blue-eyed patients were more affected than brown-eyed patients). Sluggishness of the light reflex and of the convergence accommodation reflex is considered a normal variant in the elderly, but it was found in only eight patients, thus probably always indicating some local ophthalmic abnormality. In addition a normal variant in external ocular movements in the elderly is a progressive restriction of upward gaze with advancing years.[9] This has been attributed to disuse, and, in my view, this is an attractive hypothesis because a combination of cervical spondylosis and vertebral artery insufficiency make stargazing or viewing cathedral roofs a hazardous occupation for old people. It should therefore be regarded as normal if elderly patients are unable to look upward on condition that they are not complaining of diplopia.

Tendon Reflexes

The tendon reflexes in the upper limbs were present in all but seven patients, in whom the supinator jerks could not be obtained. In three of these patients, the triceps jerks were also unelicitable. In the lower limbs, knee jerks and ankle jerks could not be obtained in 13 patients, and in another 31 the ankle jerks were not elicited even with rigorous reinforcement techniques. One report[19] suggests that ankle jerks are retained rather more frequently in old age, although experienced neurologic opinion[5,11,18,29] agrees with my own findings that they are commonly lost.

Position and Vibration Sense

Fourteen patients had lost their position sense in the big toes, and in another 15 this sense was impaired. Fifty-seven patients were unable to appreciate the vibrations of a tuning fork at the ankles, including 11 very elderly patients in whom no appreciation of vibration was present in the whole of the lower limbs. Probably this particular sensory modality diminishes more steadily with age than others, and it was accompanied in most patients by loss of ankle jerks.

Muscular Wasting

All patients thought that they had lost some muscle bulk and muscle tone, and objective evidence of muscle wasting was obtained by examining the back of the hand. In exactly half the patients (50), there was no clinically discernible wasting—that is, the back of the hand was flat, and the first dorsal interosseus could be seen and felt to contract. In 19 patients, there was just discernible guttering between the metacarpals (slight wasting); in 11 this was quite discernible and accompanied by poor contraction of the first dorsal interosseus (moderate wasting); and in 20 the guttering was very marked, and very little of the first dorsal interosseus could be felt at all (severe wasting). In spite of this, the strength of grip was reasonable, even in the most wasted hand. The impression was that a combination of inactivity, degenerative arthropathy, and advancing age gave the greatest correlation with hand muscle wasting.

No patient was included with rheumatoid arthritis or crippling osteoarthritis.

This small survey suggests that the loss of neurons from the anterior horn cell pool gives rise to clinically recognizable neurologic signs in about half the patients over 70 years old, that peripheral vibratory appreciation is lost in more than half, and in fact some abnormality on neurologic examination was found in 80 of 100 patients.

It is obviously impossible in one chapter to deal with all the neurologic problems that occur in elderly patients, and only the fairly common conditions usually confined to this age-group are described, together with those that change in their presentation with age or that are easily overlooked. Particular attention is paid to treatable illnesses masquerading as incurable degenerative processes because it is in this field that tragedies of misdiagnosis occur.

Some classification is necessary and comprises infections, the effects of trauma, neoplasms, vascular disorders, deficiency states, metabolic disorders and a heterogeneous group of degenerative, systemic or localized neurologic diseases often of unknown etiology.

INFECTIONS

Meningitis

One of the most silent neurologic abnormalities of old age is, surprisingly, pyogenic meningitis, and it is, therefore, commonly missed. Slight headache, disorientation in place and time, a lack of desire to get out of bed, increasing drowsiness, and loss of interest may be the only symptoms. Neck stiffness is often not complained of but is usually present if looked for, affecting flexion of the head but not rotation. It has been suggested that this is an unreliable sign in the elderly because of the natural neck rigidity that some patients in this age-group develop owing to cervical spondylosis. However, the careful elicitation of this sign should involve head flexion mostly at the atlanto-occipital joint, which is spared in spondylosis and, therefore, remains mobile unless subarachnoid hemorrhage or meningitis is present. The temperature may be only slightly elevated, and vomiting with dehydration is a late feature, often too late. In my opinion, lumbar puncture is obligatory in all elderly patients who show mental confusion, disorientation, stupor, dementia, or coma, unless examination of the fundi shows obvious papilledema. Also, meningitis is more common in the

elderly than is meningism, and unless lumbar puncture is performed, differential diagnosis is almost impossible because the usual signs, such as fever, leukocytosis, and neck stiffness, may be absent in the old. If the cerebrospinal fluid supports the diagnosis of meningitis, a blood culture should be taken because some elderly patients have a silent bacterial endocarditis that first shows itself by infected embolism of the brain with subsequent meningeal spread.

Management of these patients includes bed rest in a darkened and quiet room, adequate hydration, sedation for restlessness, analgesics for pain, and, above all, the early administration of parenteral penicillin even before the organism has been identified and its antibiotic sensitivity established.

Because the diagnosis is sometimes difficult and often delayed, the prognosis of pyogenic meningitis in the elderly is bad, with a mortality rate of 50%, and, therefore, it should be obligatory to start antibiotic treatment before organism identification. The most common infecting organism in my experience is *Streptococcus pneumoniae* (pneumococcus), followed by the meningococcus, and present opinion[24] is that benzyl penicillin, 150 mg/kg/day by intravenous infusion, is the initial antibiotic of choice. My regimen is a little different because the infecting organism in some of my patients with pyogenic meningitis is *Hemophilus influenzae*, and, therefore, I use ampicillin, 200 mg/kg/day by intravenous infusion. If the penicillins are contraindicated by known sensitivity or if the patient does not respond to either of the above regimens, chloramphenicol, in doses of 2 g/day by mouth, should be used without hesitation since it is life saving in some patients. Treatment is usually needed in high dosage for a week and at half this level for another week. The dangers to the bone marrow of prolonged use of chloramphenicol must be remembered and its dosage reduced as soon as possible. If penicillin is used intrathecally, the maximum dose is 20,000 units, but if the above regimens are instituted early, intrathecal therapy is seldom justified.

Corticosteroid therapy should not be used routinely in these patients, but there are two indications. The first is circulatory collapse, which will require intravenous hydrocortisone in doses of 100 mg every 6 hours, and the second is evidence of cerebral edema, cerebral infarction, or subarachnoid block as complicating factors. The first two of these can be recognized by the presence of intracranial hypertension and focal neurologic signs and the third by lumbar puncture. Dexamethasone is the corticosteroid of choice under these conditions in doses of 4 mg every 6 hours with reduction to half this dose after 48 hours.

Zoster Infection

The elderly are generally more prone to infection by the herpes zoster virus than are younger patients, probably because they gradually lose their resistance to the varicella virus. In particular, zoster infection of the cranial ganglia is common, with ophthalmic and geniculate zoster predominating, although the cervical, dorsal, and lumbar types also occur. Ophthalmic zoster can be very serious, with severe pain, redness, and swelling of one side of the forehead, around one eye, down the side of the nose, and on the cheek. The eye itself becomes acutely inflamed with a neuropathic keratitis, and orbital edema is often so great that the eyelids cannot be separated.

The edema is followed by a vesicular rash in the area supplied by one or two divisions of the trigeminal nerve, rapidly becoming purulent, and the pain is intense, reaching from the jaw to the vertex of the skull. The rash comes across the midline for about 1 cm, and occasionally zoster vesicles may appear on other parts of the body. Temperature is elevated, there is leukocytosis, and occasionally ipsilateral oculomotor paralysis occurs. The use of specific antiviral agents has mostly replaced the former combination of corticosteroid and antibiotic therapy, although the latter are useful if secondary bacterial infection does occur. Because this is usually staphylococcal, cloxacillin, tetracycline, or erythromycin are the most effective.

Local antiviral therapy consists of painting the skin vesicles with 40% (or in mild cases 5%) idoxuridine in dimethyl sulfoxide, avoiding any contact with mucosal surfaces. If the zoster is particularly severe with evidence of viral spread into the brain or spinal cord, the use of intravenous antiviral agents must be considered.[21,22,38]

Supportive treatment is very important because elderly patients become very dehydrated easily from severe infections and may already be suffering from nutritional deficiencies requiring treatment with vitamins and folic acid. The analgesics used should be powerful because of the severity of the pain; compound codeine tablets; dextropropoxyphene and paracetamol combination (acetaminophen, distalgesic); dihydrocodeinone bitartrate; and dextromoramide are of the greatest value. Meperidine (Demerol), methadone, and morphine should be avoided in this age-group if possible because the pain of postherpetic neuralgia

is chronic, troublesome, and repetitive, and there may be considerable difficulty in weaning the patient from an addictive drug.

Geniculate zoster attacks elderly patients with a vesicular eruption on the external auditory meatus, on the soft palate, on the inside of the cheek, or along the jaw. Loss of taste on the same side is not uncommon. The classic complication is a severe peripheral ipsilateral facial palsy, usually with denervation and, therefore, very slow recovery. Pain is felt in the ear, in the throat, or down the side of the neck. Although called geniculate zoster, the infection is probably more widespread. Antibiotics and corticotropin gel are useful, particularly because there is evidence that the prognosis of facial palsy is improved by early corticosteroid therapy.[36]

Zoster elsewhere is no different from that in the young, except that persistent post-herpetic pain is more common in elderly patients.

Post-herpetic Neuralgia

Herpetic and post-herpetic neuralgia may be very troublesome, particularly in ophthalmic zoster, and once the neuralgia is established very few analgesic drugs work. Most benefit is obtained from a pain-relieving spray followed by vibrator therapy, and often patients are so pleased with this that they carry the vibrator with them on visits and plug in to their hosts' electricity so they can obtain instant pain relief. Use of the rubber pad on the vibrator is preferable to the vulcanite in this condition. The only analgesic of much use is carbamazepine, although even this is not always very effective. Sleep is fortunately not badly disturbed, and any insomnia responds to the usual hypnotic and analgesic combinations used for elderly patients.

Syphilis

The effects of previous syphilitic infection are very rarely seen in elderly patients, because most of those affected die before reaching old age, and the disease seems to be becoming much less common. Dementia paralytica, however, may first show itself after 65 if the primary infection has occurred in middle age, as it frequently did in the war years. It presents in the elderly as epilepsy of late onset, with tremor, particularly of the tongue and extremities, slurred speech, depression, and progressive dementia with delusions that are not always grandiose. The pupils show no reaction to light, the plantar reflexes are usually extensor; the cerebrospinal fluid is abnormal, with increased cells and protein, a first- or second-zone type of Lange curve, and a positive serologic test in all patients. Treatment consists of a 4-week course of intramuscularly administered penicillin, 30 megaunits in all, repeated twice with a 4-week interval between courses.

TRAUMA

The elderly tend to fall more readily than others, owing to loss of youthful balancing reflexes, and perhaps more importantly, they tend to forget that they have had a fall. This makes the diagnosis of the more serious effects of head injury difficult, particularly because classic effects do not occur as often in these patients as in other age-groups.

Subdural Hematoma

Subdural hematoma is the most important and the most overlooked of these effects. It may show itself in the usual way, by a history of head injury followed by an inconstant period of normality, followed by a varying hemiparesis or hemiparesthesia with jacksonian convulsions and a fluctuating level of consciousness. Even in the classic presentation, headache is often not a complaint. If this type of history is obtained, diagnosis should be easy. No such patient, however old, should be denied neurosurgical advice. Diagnosis is more difficult if there is no history of head injury and no localizing neurologic signs are present. The patient may gradually deteriorate, showing a change of personality, confusion, forgetfulness, and loss of judgment, so that the condition is thought to be one of senile dementia or cortical atrophy. If, however, the possibility of a subdural hematoma is borne in mind and a lumbar puncture performed, the presence of xanthochromia and an excess of protein in the cerebrospinal fluid may lead to further investigations and final correct diagnosis. Electroencephalography may show an electrically silent area over the hematoma, but because most of these produce a shift of the midline structures away from the lesion, the use of ultrasound should be considered. The sound echo is reflected back

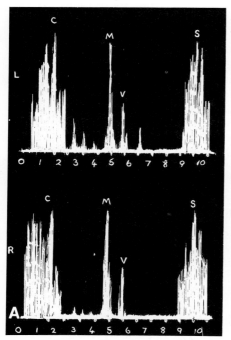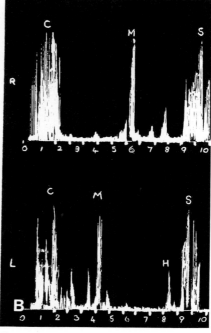

FIG. 18-1.   Tracings from ultrasonic investigations (Scanoscope; Park Ultrasonic Ltd.) (*A*) The normal appearance with the midline echo (*M*) from left to right (*top*), exactly opposite the midline echo from right to left (*bottom*). (*B*) The midline echo shifted from right to left in both records by a subdural hematoma over the right cerebral hemisphere. An echo from the edge of the hematoma can also be seen (*H*) in the left to right record (*bottom*). (*R*, Right-to-left tracing; *L*, left-to-right tracing; *C*, artefacts; *M.* midline; *V,* wall of lateral ventricle; *S*, skull)

from the septum pellucidum to the ultrasonoscope (Fig. 18-1), and if this is done from right to left and then from left to right, any shift of the midline structures to one or the other side can be seen unless the hematoma is bilateral.

Further diagnostic investigations depend on the equipment available. Until recently carotid angiography was the final clincher, showing the hematoma as a large clear area on the convexity of the hemisphere and also demonstrating a shift across the midline away from the lesion in unilateral cases (Fig. 18-2). However, the advent of computed cerebral tomography has given us an excellent and almost infallible noninvasive technique, and this is undoubtedly the investigation of choice from the beginning of diagnostic suspicion if the requisite equipment is available within reasonable distance of the patient (Fig. 18-3).

If neither of these radiologic techniques is possible and if a patient with a suspected subdural hematoma is deteriorating, bilateral parietal bur holes should be made as an emergency measure.

Extradural Hematoma

Extradural hematoma is less common in elderly patients, but if it occurs, the downhill course is rapid, with convulsions, hemiplegia, and coma owing to cerebral compression. Often the lucid interval described in textbooks is absent, but a parietal bone fracture is usually present and craniotomy is a matter of urgency.

Again computed cerebral tomography is the best confirmatory investigation, but it must be remembered that the time margin from the onset of the lesion to operation is critical, and no delay is possible if a good result is to be obtained. This is quite a different situation from that encountered in subdural hematoma in which the sense of urgency is less, and more detailed investigation is possible without affecting the patient's prognosis.

Intracerebral Hematoma

Intracerebral hematoma, if not part of cerebrovascular disease, follows severe head injury; when the patient recovers consciousness, he is found to be hemiplegic. The lesions are often multiple, and surgery is not indicated unless there is evidence of continued expansion of the hematoma with papilledema, slowing of the pulse, and a decreasing level of consciousness.[26,27]

The progress of the lesion can be monitored by computed cerebral tomography, which may also

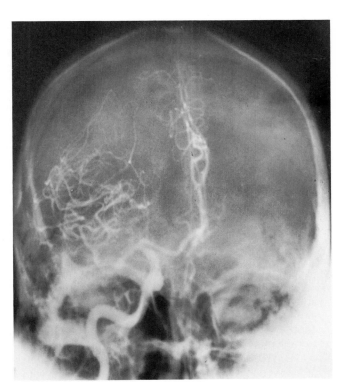

FIG. 18-2. Right carotid angiogram showing right subdural hematoma. Note the clear area devoid of blood vessels on the convexity of the cerebral hemisphere and the displacement of the anterior cerebral artery to the left.

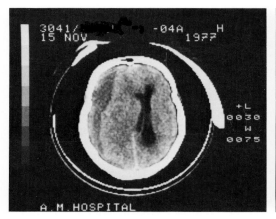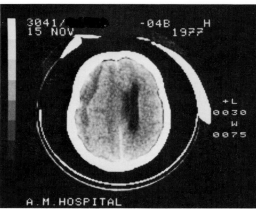

FIG.18-3. CT scan of left subdural hematoma. The lesion is clearly seen as a crescentic low-density (black) area between the left cerebral cortex and the skull. (Courtesy of Dr. James Ambrose)

show a clear area around the hematoma owing to cerebral edema (Fig. 18-3). Many authorities consider this to be an indication for corticosteroid therapy using dexamethasone in doses of 16 mg in 24 hours, but elderly patients are unlikely to tolerate doses of this order, and my own practice is to use much smaller doses, such as 6 mg in 24 hours for no longer than a week if I think cerebral edema is playing any part in the patient's disability.

NEOPLASMS

Diagnosis of neoplasms affecting the brain and spinal cord of elderly patients is not very often made because attention is traditionally directed toward degenerative diseases and because a sense of hopelessness is mistakenly conveyed to the physician when paraplegia, hemiplegia, or status epilepticus is found. No age-group is exempt from benign new growths, and even primary or secondary malignant neoplasms tend to have a slower rate of growth in elderly patients.

If such a patient has a convulsion, focal or general, and has no history of previous cerebral infarction or evidence of an embolic focus elsewhere, the diagnosis is more likely to be cerebral tumor than occlusive cerebrovascular disease, uremia, or accelerated hypertension. Many meningiomas have been successfully removed in patients over 70 years of age; astrocytomas are usually less invasive in the elderly and therefore more amenable to surgery, radiation therapy, or both. Papilledema is late in its appearance, and diagnosis should therefore not be delayed until the triad of headache, vomiting, and blurring of vision occurs because it certainly is too late by then.

Investigation should be by plain skull radiography, isotope brain scanning, and computed cerebral tomography. Lumbar puncture is used only when there is no symptom or sign suggesting increased intracranial pressure. This last investigation is most useful in patients with dementia, disorientation, and forgetfulness, in whom the exclusion of treatable illness is obligatory.

Cerebral metastases may occur some years after removal of a primary tumor, particularly if it was in the breast or colon. Metastases may also show themselves before the primary tumor becomes apparent, notably when it arises in a bronchus. Neuropathy in elderly patients may be the first evidence of neoplasms, again particularly bronchial in origin, and sometimes in patients with multiple myeloma. Wasting of the peripheral muscles is accompanied by loss of the supinator and ankle jerks, and sensory loss follows in the hands and feet. Many growths are slowed by age, so that even a metastasis may be well worth removing if it produces pain or disability in an elderly person.

One word of warning is essential. Pneumoencephalography is dangerous in the elderly and may be followed by dementia or even sudden death. It seems to interfere with cerebral blood flow and with medullary activity, and it is one investigation that should never be performed on elderly patients.

VASCULAR DISEASES

Syncopal Attacks

Syncopal attacks may not be obviously associated with occlusive vascular disease, although it is probably present, and they are due to failure of baroreceptor mechanisms in the neck or to changes in systemic arterial blood flow.

Micturition syncope is the probable diagnosis when an old man gets out of bed at night to pass water and finds himself lying on the bathroom floor, often with head or facial injuries. Many of these patients are referred to the physician with the provisional diagnosis of epilepsy, but if the patient sits down to urinate at night and then gets up slowly to return to bed, the attacks usually clear up.

Cough Syncope

Cough syncope rarely troubles the elderly because emphysematous and bronchitic patients do not have a long life expectancy. Heart block may produce a Stokes-Adams attack, in which sudden loss of consciousness occurs, which is often prolonged. Pulse is usually below 40/min, and there is electrocardiographic evidence of complete atrioventricular dissociation. Prednisone and ephedrine are useful in dealing with these attacks, but in heart block, an artificial pacemaker may be required.

Dizziness

Vertigo, unsteadiness, and loss of equilibrium sometimes occur late in life when there is a change of position. Such patients must get up slowly in the morning and be careful how they rise from a chair following their afternoon nap. Similarly, hospitalized elderly patients must not sit in upright chairs for a long time after a physical illness: diminished cerebral blood flow is common, and syncope with subsequent injury may occur.

Transient Cerebral Ischemic Attacks (TCIA)

Recent interest in geriatric neurology has focused attention on attacks of neurologic disability lasting minutes or hours, followed by complete recovery of function within 24 hours, usually affecting late middle-aged or elderly patients. Occlusive cerebrovascular disease is an important underlying cause, with either intracranial or extracranial arterial atherosclerosis, often complicated by atheromatous ulceration of the intima.[14]

A patient may experience transient attacks of hemiparesis, hemianesthesia, hemianopia, aphasia, or loss of vision in one eye if the lesion is in the territory of the carotid artery. Attacks characterized by falling forward on the knees without

loss of consciousness, accompanied by vertigo, vomiting, dysarthria, dysphagia, visual blurring, and diplopia, suggest hindbrain ischemia in the vertebral artery territory. These transient attacks are often due to atheromatous occlusion of the main neck arteries with diminished blood flow associated with local stenosis, with systemic hypotension, or with platelet, cholesterol, or fibrin microemboli that arise in these vessels and may be carried to the cerebral arteries (Figs. 18-4 and 18-5). The attacks occasionally cease spontaneously, either because of improving collateral circulation through the circle of Willis or because an atheromatous ulcer no longer gives off emboli. This may be due to the occlusion of a stenosed artery becoming complete, and it is paradoxic but true that if collateral circulation is adequate, it is probably better to have complete rather than incomplete occlusion of a neck artery in the elderly.

Possible causes of diminished cerebral blood supply apart from anatomical abnormalities must be looked for. In my experience, drugs are often responsible, particularly the thiazide diuretics, re-

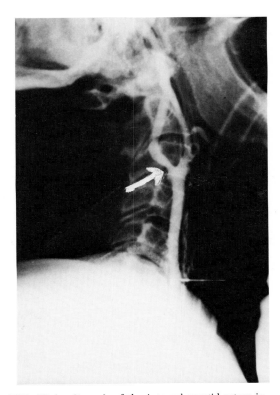

FIG. 18-4. Stenosis of the internal carotid artery in the usual site in an elderly patient with attacks of left hemiparesis.

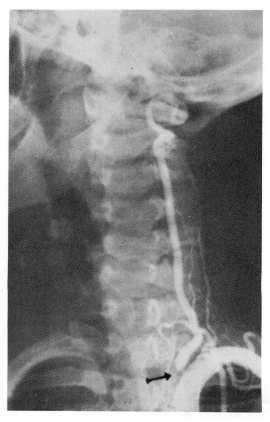

FIG. 18-5. Stenosis of the vertebral artery at its origin from the subclavian artery in an elderly patient who experienced attacks of vertigo and unsteadiness, in which she would suddenly fall forward on her knees.

serpine compounds, and promazine derivatives, because all these have a hypotensive effect.

Personal experience has shown that the hindbrain type of TCIA is more common when hypotension is the cause; the carotid type is more frequently associated with distal embolism from local atheroma and with hypertension.

Anemia is often overlooked in the elderly, and physical exertion or even standing for any length of time produces signs of cerebral ischemia if the hemoglobin is below normal. Apart from this, extension and full rotation of the head interfere with vertebral artery flow if, as is common, cervical spondylosis is combined with degenerative arterial disease.

Similarly, by its vasoconstrictive effects, smoking may cause ischemic attacks, so that before any radical or potentially harmful treatment is contemplated it is advisable to inquire into drugs used by the patient, to check the hemoglobin level, to re-

strict exaggerated neck movements, and to persuade the patient to stop smoking.

The risk factors in TCIA are therefore similar to those in stroke and coronary heart disease, comprising hypertension, hyperlipidemia, smoking, inactivity, obesity, diabetes, and family history among others, and the first aim of treatment must be the attempted prevention of this type of cerebrovascular disease. Hypertension either moderate or severe must be controlled by salt deprivation or drug therapy, and in addition advice must be given encouraging active exercise, a decrease in fat intake, loss of excess weight, and the elimination of smoking.

Obvious other abnormalities such as diabetes, gout, hypothyroidism, nephritis, and anemia must be put right.

Apart from the above preventive measures, treatment of the attacks is divided into medical and surgical. Surgical treatment for TCIA has been controversial at all age levels, as shown in a large controlled trial of carotid endarterectomy compared with medical treatment, which showed no overall benefit unless the mortality and morbidity of the surgical procedure were disregarded.[13] However, the recurrent rate of new strokes after surgery is only 3% per year compared with the expected 6% without surgery.[16,35]

In favor of surgical treatment are youth, a good general vascular state, an experienced vascular surgeon, normotension, and a localized accessible short lesion of the internal carotid artery.[32] In severe vertebral TCIA, surgery is directed to the origin of the artery (see Fig. 18-5) or to the subclavian artery itself.[12]

It seems therefore that in the elderly, who are often fragile and mildly hypertensive, medical treatment is in most cases preferable to surgery. Control of severe hypertension, diabetes, and anemia combined with the mandatory stopping of smoking, as stated previously, are the obvious starting points, and in the absence of hypertension, anticoagulants in the form of warfarin are indicated if the TCIAs are recent and frequent. Treatment is continued for 3 to 6 months after the attacks cease and then replaced by antiplatelet aggregation drugs such as soluble aspirin or dipyridamole or both.[33] It is important to remember the potentiating action of aspirin on anticoagulants, and a combination of these drugs is unwise in the elderly, whose cerebral arteries are often brittle.

Perhaps a word about surgical technique is apposite. For TCIA due to a proven lesion in the neck arteries, carotid or vertebral endarterectomy is performed at the appropriate site, but if the lesion is situated at the origins of the great vessels a bypass technique is usually used with either autogenous vein or Dacron grafting. No truly controlled studies have appeared so far, although I have already mentioned the reduction in recurrence rate compared with expected morbidity.

Extracranial/intracranial anastomosis consists of microvascular surgery joining branches of the superficial temporal artery, which arises from the external carotid artery, to branches of the middle cerebral artery, which arises from the internal carotid. The indications are proximal stenotic lesions of the middle cerebral artery, distal stenosis of the internal carotid artery, and complete carotid occlusion in some cases. The technique is a microvascular side-to-side anastomosis through a bur hole after dissection of a piece of the superior temporal artery. It seems that few of these moderately major operations will apply to our elderly patients, but if the general health and cardiac state are good and if they are combined with alertness of intellect and good motivation age alone should never be a contraindication to active surgical therapy.[4]

Head or Heart

Interest has been aroused by the finding of unsuspected transient cardiac dysrhythmias in elderly patients whose routine resting and exertional electrocardiograms showed sinus rhythm. A series of such patients was studied by fitting them with a single channel cassette tape electrocardiographic recorder, which they wore continuously for 24 hours, and the results were analyzed by an automatic dysrhythmia detector.[15] Seventy-four percent of the 130 patients were found to have dysrhythmias that were considered sufficient to cause their transient cerebral attacks, and they included episodes of asystole, sinus bradycardia, sinoatrial block, atrial fibrillation, runs of atrial and ventricular ectopic beats, ventricular tachycardia, and various degrees of heart block.

Focal cerebral ischemic episodes are more common with cerebrovascular disease than with cardiac irregularities because the latter are more likely to cause episodes of syncope and dizziness. If, however, the two problems are combined and a patient with a focal cerebral low perfusion state is subjected to a general systemic arterial insufficiency, it is very likely that a focal disability will be the result. The index of suspicion that the heart rather than the head is more likely to be the cause of a transient cerebral ischemic attack should be high if the patient complains of palpitations, faint-ness, confusion, dizziness, or loss of balance in addition to his localized neurologic deficit.

If the connection between a cardiac dysrhythmia and cerebral ischemic attacks is strongly suspected, there is a place for the implantation of a pacemaker to relieve the neurologic symptoms.

Minor Strokes

A minor stroke may be defined as a neurologic deficit owing to occlusive cerebrovascular disease lasting more than 24 hours but showing almost complete recovery within a few weeks.[3] The arterial lesion is similar to that producing transient ischemic attacks, but the effects are probably due to ischemic necrosis with small areas of infarction. In North America, these have been given the name "reversible ischemic neurologic deficits" (RIND), but "little strokes" or "minor strokes" seems preferable to underline their difference from temporary ischemic attacks.

Treatment may be more urgent because these are a prelude to major strokes within 1 or 2 years in about half the patients, and, because in many elderly patients anticoagulant therapy is contraindicated, the question of surgery arises. The best results are obtained in short stenotic lesions of the internal carotid artery[37] and in similar lesions of the subclavian artery. The former can be diagnosed clinically in half the patients affected by finding a fairly high pitched pansystolic murmur over the artery on the side opposite the neurologic deficit (Fig. 18-6). Confirmation of the lesion and of the condition of other parts of the cerebral circulation can be obtained only by carotid arteriography, which itself has a morbidity of 1% to 10%, according to the skill of the operator. In my opinion, arteriography is only justified when surgery is contemplated, and in the elderly this should be considered only if recurrent transient ischemic carotid attacks are uncontrolled or if a minor stroke recurs in an otherwise healthy old man or woman. Successful thromboendarterectomy has been performed in patients well over 70 but not very often. In hindbrain ischemia, the best surgical results are obtained in the subclavian steal syndrome, in which subclavian artery occlusion leads to the ipsilateral arm being supplied by a reversed flow in the vertebral artery so that strenuous use of the arm leads to hindbrain arterial insufficiency.[20]

Major Stroke

A major stroke is one in which considerable neurologic deficit remains after a few weeks and may

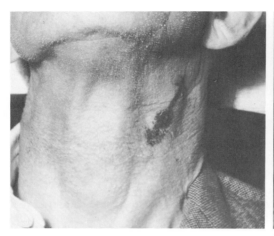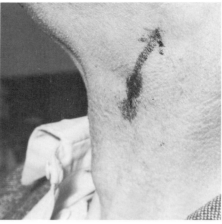

FIG. 18-6. Common site of systolic murmur heard in some patients with internal carotid artery stenosis. (Carter AB: Cerebral Infarction. New York, Pergamon Press, 1964)

be clinically seen either as a progressing or a completed lesion. The clinical picture differs very little from that seen at other ages, but it is more difficult for a very old person to survive a massive cerebral infarction, or if he does, to achieve excellent recovery of function. Mental disturbances, with forgetfulness, loss of interest, inability to persevere, blunting of determination, and failure to understand, are the chief bars to successful rehabilitation. All depends on how much of the former youthful vigorous personality remains at the time of the stroke in old age and how strong the wish is to remain alive and independent. Personal experience suggests that surgery has little part to play in major strokes in spite of some optimistic reports. Apart from anticoagulation in normotensive patients with progressing strokes and a search for associated disease such as anemia, diabetes, gout, hypothyroidism, and silent cardiac infarction, treatment should be confined to early mobilization and activation with enthusiastic physiotherapeutic and social rehabilitation.[8,25,34]

In the immediate treatment of a major stroke affecting an elderly patient, nursing care is more important than any specific medical therapy. The main principles are maintenance of a free airway at all times, adequate hydration and nutrition, and preservation of a good systemic circulation combined with prevention of respiratory and urinary infection, urine retention, burns, injuries, and pressure sores.

Each hospital may have differing techniques for the implementation of these principles, but general experience suggests that the patient be nursed in the anterolateral position with one pillow and that an intragastric tube be passed nasally. A mechanical airway with intermittent pharyngeal suction has obviated the need for tracheostomy in all my patients. Frequent turning and occasional forced respiration help to prevent respiratory infection. Through the intragastric tube is given 1800 ml of fluid in 24 hours, as 5% glucose at first, and then milk, eggs, sugar, salt, and vitamins, until the patient is capable of swallowing. A high-protein or composite food may be used to save time in preparation. Feedings are given every 2 hours, just after the patient has been turned.

I no longer use antibiotic cover prophylactically for respiratory or urinary infection, and results have been just as good if evidence of actual infection is obtained first. Retention of urine is more common in men than in women. Women are more often incontinent. A self-retaining catheter may be used quite safely if aseptic precautions are observed and the catheter not changed too often. Some authorities would disagree, but the saving of the patient's skin and nurses' time may far outweigh any theoretic danger of infection.

Hot-water bottles must be forbidden, and care must be taken with electric blankets. Restlessness requires sedation, particularly at night, but drugs in elderly patients must be much more carefully used. I have abandoned paraldehyde, believing it to be a powerful and outdated sedative and at present use the following drugs in ascending order of potency: dichloralphenazone, 1.3 g; meprobamate, 800 mg; thioridazine, 10 mg to 25 mg; promazine, 25 mg to 50 mg; and chlormethiazole, 0.5 g. All these may be given by mouth in elixir form, and, if agitation and restlessness are so severe that they are ineffective, chlorpromazine 50 mg or haloperidol 5 mg can be given by intramuscular injection with good effect.

Rehabilitation

Although general rehabilitation of the elderly patient is dealt with in Chapter 33, there are some particular aspects of stroke rehabilitation that deserve special mention here. A new dynamism in the approach to this problem has been apparent in the last 30 years, and previous neglect has been replaced by enthusiasm, original ideas, and perseverance in spite of many disappointments.[1,2,25,34] Most major stroke survivors will have some permanent disability. The curve of improvement flattens out considerably after about 6 weeks, and hardly any further recovery can be expected after 6 months.

In stroke rehabilitation a start must be made as soon as the patient recovers consciousness, so that the physician can assess as early as possible the likely quality and extent of recovery. His aim should be to create optimism in the patient and his relatives without promising too much, to evaluate the physical and mental[2] obstacles to success, and to have the patience and perseverance to follow these ideas right through to the final resettlement of the stroke survivor.

The success or failure of this will depend as much on the tenacity of the patient as it will on that of the team, and it is, therefore, important that physicians have some element of dedication and of leadership in their personality. Unless inspiration can be communicated to all concerned, only partial success will be achieved.

Ischemic stroke patients should, if conscious, be gotten into a chair on day 1, practice balancing exercises on the edge of the bed or in the chair on day 2, and stand on their feet fully supported by nurses or physiotherapists on day 3. From then on, active exercises must begin with walking, balancing, and limb and trunk movements, and as soon as possible a provisional discharge date should be given—this enormously cheers up most patients. Many obstacles both mental and physical will have to be overcome, but, eventually, considerable satisfaction is surely to be gained in knowing help is being given to patients who, until comparatively recently, were neglected.

Primary Intracranial Hemorrhage (Apoplectic Stroke)

The two types of nontraumatic intracranial hemorrhage are intracerebral hemorrhage and primary subarachnoid hemorrhage.

Intracerebral Hemorrhage

Apoplexy, as this disorder is also called, occurs mostly in hypertensive patients and is less common in the elderly than other types of stroke. It is probably due to rupture of microaneurysms in the perforating branches of the middle cerebral artery, as originally described by Charcot and recently reviewed.[30] The hemorrhage usually bursts into the lateral ventricle or the subarachnoid space, and the patient complains of headache, vomits, becomes rapidly unconscious, and passes into a deep coma; the disorder is usually fatal within 72 hours. Flaccidity of the limbs and drooping of the face occur on the hemiplegic side and can be recognized even in coma. The eyes are first turned conjugately toward the affected limbs and then away from them. Lumbar puncture shows an evenly blood-stained cerebrospinal fluid with xanthochromic supernatant after centrifuging. Treatment is symptomatic, with good nursing care, an intragastric tube for hydration, and self-retaining catheter for urinary retention and incontinence.

Primary intracerebral hematoma may occur if the hemorrhage is confined locally in the brain substance, but this is uncommon in elderly patients and, until recently, extremely difficult to differentiate from ischemic cerebral infarction. However, computed cerebral tomography will separate these two conditions immediately, the infarct having a low-density appearance (Fig. 18-7), and the hematoma having a very high one (Fig. 18-8). Treatment is similar to that of ordinary stroke pa-

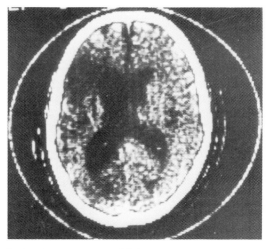

FIG. 18-7. CT scan of left cerebral hemisphere infarction in a man aged 70. The low-density area (black) is clearly seen, and the lateral ventricles are secondarily dilated.

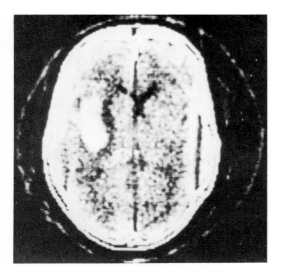

FIG. 18-8. CT scan of left intracerebral hematoma. The lesion is shown as a high-density (white) area in the left hemisphere surrounded by low-density edema.

tients unless the hematoma expands sufficiently to produce cerebral compression when a combination of surgery and dexamethasone will be required.[31] This combination is urgently indicated in the special case of cerebellar apoplexy, which shows itself by nausea, headache, vomiting, ataxia, vertigo, ocular palsies, and dysarthria, rapidly followed by unconsciousness, with periodic breathing and deep coma.[28] Early diagnosis and intervention before loss of consciousness is important if a good result is to be obtained. Otherwise the mortality rate is 75% (Fig. 18-9).

Primary Subarachnoid Hemorrhage

It is not uncommon for a congenital cerebral aneurysm to rupture in later years, although subarachnoid hemorrhage is mistakenly thought of as a young person's disease. The average age of first rupture is 54, and 10% to 15% of patients first bleed later than age 65. The symptoms are often identical to those in other age-groups, although neck stiffness and headache may be unremarkable, coma may be sudden and prolonged, and gastrointestinal symptoms with vomiting and diarrhea may be surprisingly predominant in a stuporous patient. Diagnosis is made by lumbar puncture. Differentiation from ruptured primary intracerebral hemorrhage may be impossible until either necropsy or recovery. Xanthochromic cerebrospinal fluid may be obtained from some confused and demented elderly patients who seem to be quite

unaware of a fairly recent attack of subarachnoid hemorrhage, and also in some alert elderly patients who say they have had a severe headache a few days previously. Unfortunately, the elderly survivors usually show many more permanent physical and mental disabilities than younger patients, and the final result may be very disappointing. Communicating hydrocephalus may occur owing to occlusion of the arachnoid villi. If present, severe dementia is the rule. If the diagnosis is made, a simple bypass from ventricle to subcutaneous tissue is very rewarding.

Hypertensive Encephalopathy

Hypertensive encephalopathy is uncommon in the elderly, but two such patients over 70 have come under my care. The diastolic pressure is over 140 and fits occur—either focal or generalized—with headache, blurring of vision, and hemiparesis. If the fundi can be seen, the diagnosis is easy because retinal hemorrhages and exudates with papilledema are present. The response to a parenteral hypotensive drug such as intravenous diazoxide is dramatic.

Cranial Arteritis (Giant-Cell Arteritis)

Cranial arteritis is a very important vascular disease in the elderly because, if undiagnosed and

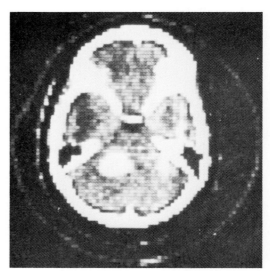

FIG. 18-9. CT scan of left spontaneous cerebellar hemorrhage. The lesion is seen as a well-circumscribed high-density (white) area in the left cerebellar hemisphere.

untreated, half the patients become permanently blind. Temporal arteritis is one of its local manifestations and is often unfortunately used as its descriptive term, thus ignoring its most damaging retinal involvement. The condition presents with persistent and severe headache, often temporal and unilateral, with dimness or loss of visual acuity, and with accompanying pains in the shoulders and hips if the arteritis is widespread. The temporal arteries are always tender, sometimes lose their pulsation, and occasionally stand out as thickened cords under the red and hot overlying skin. Examination of the fundi shows retinal hemorrhage or some degree of optic atrophy or thrombosis of the retinal artery in about half the patients. These abnormalities may be bilateral. The erythrocyte sedimentation rate is raised, usually to above 40 mm in 1 hour, and the patient may run a mild fever with leukocytosis and occasionally eosinophilia. Diagnosis is established by biopsy of an affected segment of the temporal artery.

The condition must be treated by corticosteroid therapy to avoid blindness, and large doses are needed in the first month, at least 40 mg to 80 mg of prednisone being given orally daily until the pain, tenderness, and swelling have gone and the sedimentation rate has decreased. Dosage may slowly be reduced after this, but treatment is usually required for at least 4 to 6 months, and some patients need a maintenance dose of 10 mg/day for much longer.

DEFICIENCY STATES

Old age brings to many a loss of interest in food and an inability to judge what foods are beneficial. In England, many elderly women live on bread and butter and tea, and this problem of dietary intake combined with poor absorption and slow metabolism may produce a situation in which the nervous system maintains normal function with difficulty.

Patients with dementia are often sent to a neurologist before a psychiatrist because of prejudice. Probably they should go first to a general physician, because many diseases with local manifestations are generalized, and because multiple pathology is common in old age. Forty years ago, I was taught to fit all symptoms and signs into one cause, but experience has corrected this error.

Hypothyroidism

Hypothyroidism may present neurologically in the elderly by coma owing to hypothermia, deafness owing to auditory nerve degeneration, cerebellar ataxia, or peripheral neuropathy. This is not the place to deal with the first two, but cerebellar disturbance with loss of balance, unsteadiness, giddiness, and clumsiness may be the presenting syndrome. If looked for, this is accompanied by mental sluggishness, obesity, a deepening voice, deafness, and bradycardia with a characteristic facies. The tendon reflexes are diagnostic with their slow phase of relaxation (Fig. 18-10). The peripheral neuropathy is usually an entrapment effect with the carpal tunnel syndrome predominating, although this is less common in the very old than in the middle-aged. Diagnosis is confirmed by biochemical tests, the protein-bound iodine in the blood being below 3 μg/dl and the free thyroxine concentration below 1 to 1.4 ng/dl. Thyroxine by mouth produces a miraculous change for the better within weeks, but it should be given in small doses at first to elderly patients, starting at 0.05 mg twice daily, slowly increasing to a maintenance dose of 0.1 mg twice a day.

Cyanocobalamin (Vitamin B$_{12}$) Deficiency

In its straightforward form, cyanocobalamin deficiency produces subacute combined degeneration of the cord. This condition starts as a symmetric neuropathy with absent reflexes and peripheral sensory loss, particularly of vibration and position sensibility. The patient complains of tingling in the fingers and toes, difficulty in feeling the ground when walking or standing, clumsiness of hands and in gait, and weakness of ankles. Pernicious anemia can sometimes be demonstrated, the tongue is atrophic, there is almost always complete achlorhydria, the bone marrow is megaloblastic, and the serum cyanocobalamin level is always low, below 80 μg/dl. Treatment is by injection of hydroxocobalamin in doses of 1000 μg every month for life.

In addition to this classic form, cyanocobalamin deficiency can show itself as a slowly increasing dementia, with forgetfulness, confusion of thought, and psychotic reactions such as paranoid, manic, or depressive states. It can also produce primary optic atrophy, particularly in elderly cigarette smokers, and the importance of a simple estimation of the serum cyanocobalamin level in what is a reversible dementia is obvious.

Thiamine (Vitamin B$_1$) Deficiency

Chronic alcoholism is the most common cause of thiamine deficiency in the Western world, producing neuropathy, myelopathy, and encephalopathy.

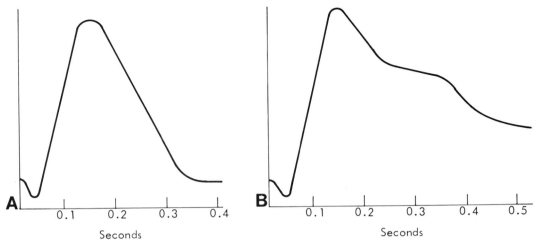

FIG. 18-10. Supinator jerk. (*A*) The normal response finished at 0.35 second. (*B*) The slow relaxation phase in hypothyroidism lasted beyond 0.5 second.

The neuropathy is of the sensory-motor type, with pain in the legs, paresthesias in the hands, and peripheral weakness and wasting. It may be accompanied by heart failure and cardiomyopathy (wet beriberi). The encephalopathy is of two kinds, the first showing itself as Korsakoff's psychosis, with disorientation of time, place, and person; amnesia for recent events; and confabulation. The second is known as Wernicke's encephalopathy, with nystagmus, pupillary abnormalities, ocular nerve palsies, ataxia, tremor, and stupor passing in severe cases into coma. This clinical picture is often of sudden onset and may be mistaken for virus encephalitis, meningitis, or intracranial tumor. An associated neuropathy, a history of high alcoholic intake, cerebrospinal fluid in which there is no abnormality except a modest protein increase, and the response to intravenously administered thiamine should make the diagnosis clear in an elderly patient.

Treatment is parenteral and oral vitamin-B complex with vitamin C (often the deficiency is multiple), a high carbohydrate diet, and avoidance of alcohol. Some of the neurologic changes may be permanent, such as areflexia, tenderness of muscles, disorientation, and amnesia.

Deficiency of other vitamins in the B group may produce acute confusional states in elderly malnourished patients, particularly deficiency of riboflavin and nicotinic acid. Diagnosis is made easier by finding a red raw tongue, fissures at the angles of the mouth, and pigmentation over pressure areas. Nothing is lost, and sometimes something will be gained by treating all confused elderly patients with parenteral vitamin B complex.

METABOLIC DISORDERS

Diabetes is the most important disease producing metabolic neurologic disorders in the elderly, although consideration must be given to the distant effects of carcinoma and to the responses to certain drugs. Drug reactions in the aged are already described in Chapter 7, and the main effects of alcohol on the nervous system have been mentioned already in this chapter.

Diabetes Mellitus

In the elderly, diabetes may present neurologically as a mild peripheral neuropathy, with impaired peripheral circulation, absent tendon reflexes, muscular wasting, peripheral sensory loss with trophic changes, and a flapping gait. The acute neuropathy with peripheral weakness is less common, but diabetic amyotrophy, in which proximal weakness and wasting of the lower limbs are combined with increased cerebrospinal fluid protein, is difficult to diagnose because of the mildness of the diabetes. This is an eminently treatable condition, even in the elderly, by good diabetic control, and it should be watched for. In any patient presenting with proximal weakness of this type, a glucose tolerance curve is mandatory.

Hypoglycemia may show itself in the elderly patient as a manifestation either of insulin therapy or of an intrinsic overproduction of insulin by an islet cell tumor. The former type is relatively benign if the patient is a known diabetic who has been told about or made to experience hypoglycemia, but even in these instances, sudden fainting attacks with convulsion or hemiplegia and sudden episodes of irrational behavior may well be attributed to senile rather than metabolic changes. Islet cell tumors can delay their clinical manifestations for a long time. The last two patients I saw with this condition were aged 68 and 74. Thus, a blood glucose estimation is always worth doing in case of doubt.

One of these two patients was diagnosed by chance because admission to hospital for a hernia repair was followed by two episodes of confusion in the morning, during which the patient wandered out of the hospital into the street in his pajamas. It transpired that he was accustomed to taking three or four lumps of sugar in his early morning cup of tea, and he had been too diffident to ask for this in the hospital.

Carcinomatous Neuropathy

Although many believe that bronchial carcinoma is nearly the most common cause of peripheral neuropathy in England, it seems to be less common in elderly patients, who tend to have other carcinomas rather than bronchial. However, in any patient, no matter how elderly, who develops a neuropathy of uncertain cause, a chest roentgenogram is obligatory. The neuropathy itself may be sensory, motor, or mixed, and a carcinomatous myopathy has been described rather like the amyotrophy of diabetes.

NEUROLOGIC DISEASE OF UNKNOWN CAUSE

A heterogeneous collection of neurologic diseases may affect those who survive into their 70s, and although some are uncommon and irreversible, some can be relieved if diagnosed. Many patients, of course, with chronic neurologic illness fail to reach this age-group, so that the profile of neurology changes with the life span.

Myasthenia Gravis

Myasthenia gravis occasionally starts in elderly patients, but usually not in the classic form of peripheral or ocular weakness that increases as the day progresses. The incidence is mainly bulbar, and loss of voice after talking for a few minutes, difficulty in getting through a meal because chewing and swallowing become weak, and ptosis, often without diplopia, make the diagnosis clear. One patient was forced to go around with his hand holding up his lower jaw, which would not close

in any other way. Later, the disorder affects the respiratory muscles, and in this age-group treatment may be very easy or extremely difficult, according to the severity of the symptoms. The therapeutic test of intravenous edrophonium chloride is always worth doing, and in mild cases neostigmine (30 mg orally three or four times a day) is enough to control the weakness. In others, I have found pyridostigmine bromide more useful (60 mg to 120 mg three times a day) because it has the advantage of a rather more prolonged action and has no tendency to produce refractory myasthenia through overdosage as neostigmine may have. If the myasthenia remains uncontrolled in spite of adequate amounts of these anticholinesterase drugs, other forms of treatment should be considered. Thymectomy has little place in this age-group, but both spironolactone, 75 mg/day by mouth, and oral corticosteroids such as prednisone or intramuscular corticotrophin may help patients who have not responded to the more orthodox therapy. Corticosteroid therapy requires hospital admission as symptoms of myasthenia often worsen from the fourth to tenth day of treatment, and dosage should start low at 10 mg/day with daily increments of 10 mg until a good effect is achieved. The dose of corticosteroids for elderly patients should not exceed 80 mg of prednisone in 24 hours because the ensuing fluid retention and potassium depletion are conducive to congestive failure and cardiac arrhythmias.

Motor Neuron Disease

Motor neuron disease shows itself usually before the seventh decade, but two forms sometimes appear during this period. The medullary form is usually severe, with atrophy of the tongue, rapidly increasing dysphagia, dysarthria, respiratory failure, and a prognosis of 6 months to a year. The peripheral form occurs as progressive, symmetric, muscular atrophy affecting the hands and upper extremities, with the usual wasting, fasciculation, early increase of tendon reflexes, and preservation of sensation. This form is often more benign, and a few patients of mine have kept going for 5 years or more. Wheat-germ oil and physiotherapy are useful for those patients, but they probably come under the heading of placebo therapy and are of considerable importance in maintaining morale.

Trigeminal Neuralgia (Tic Douloureux)

Trigeminal neuralgia mostly affects the elderly, with paroxysms of sudden lancinating pain in one side of the face brought on by talking. washing, eating, or any sensory stimulus to the affected side. The onset of an attack is evident by the sudden screwing up of the patient's face on one side accompanied by obvious pain: the true tic douloureux. Pain is often absent at night, and when asked to show the position of the pain, the patient will point to the spot but never touch the face. No other disorder can be confused with this, although many patients with any sort of facial pain are often wrongly given this label.

Treatment has been transformed by the use of carbamazepine, a drug originally produced as an anticonvulsant but also very useful in trigeminal neuralgia, which the drug will relieve in three of every four patients. From 600 mg to 1000 mg/day in divided doses is given and continued for 3 weeks before the drug is tailed off. Possible side-effects are dizziness, occasional nausea with dyspepsia, and ataxia. One or two patients have been described who have developed aplastic anemia, and treatment should not be given for more than 4 months continuously without checking the white blood cell count. If pain is confined to the infraorbital or supraorbital distribution, injection of the affected nerve with procaine followed by 5% phenol in oil is easy and useful. Ganglion injection is practiced less since the advent of carbamazepine, and many believe that selective section of the sensory root is a more satisfactory form of treatment for those resistant to this drug.

Clonic Facial Spasm

Clonic facial spasm is associated with degenerative changes in the facial nerve nucleus. It is a unilateral abnormality much more common in women than men, and it starts with a slight repetitive twitch in one eye. This spreads without relief to the whole side of the face, and recurrent spasms of increasing severity occur, with tight closure of the eye and an updrawing of the angle of the mouth. The organic nature of this condition is shown by the presence of associated movements of the face between attacks, as occurs after reinnervation in denervating Bell's palsy, so closing the eye is always associated with a twitch of the mouth and cannot be performed as a completely isolated act.

Drug treatment is often disappointing, although anxiety and self-consciousness may be relieved by the benzodiazepine preparations. The use of propranolol in doses ranging from 10 mg to 40 mg twice daily has produced a good effect in many of my patients; the usual contraindications in any elderly patient with a history of bronchial spasm

or with any form of cardiac failure or with peripheral occlusive vascular disease must be remembered.

If this therapy has no effect or if postural hypotension prevents adequate dosage, surgical treatment is indicated.

The accurate injection of phenol in oil, 1 ml of 1% into the branch of the facial nerve supplying the orbicularis oculi or the selective severance of this nerve will relieve the orbital spasm, and if the whole of one side of the face is involved the facial nerve may need injection at the angle of the jaw. Facial palsy may follow this procedure, and although this is not usually permanent the patient should be shown the effects of a complete facial palsy by a procaine injection *in situ*. The possible medicolegal consequences of injection or of surgery involving the facial nerve are obvious, and patients may well prefer to keep their spasm with some hope for relief from propranolol therapy.

Senile Tremor

There are two main forms of senile tremor. It may be an exaggeration of essential or familial tremor, gradually worsening with age, in which the hands are first affected, then the head, and finally the tongue. It is an example of an intention tremor and is made worse by social occasions, stress, and voluntary movement. Drinking, eating, shaving, and writing are the most difficult problems, although patients with this disorder can often dress and undress without much trouble. Characteristically, patients use two hands to drink from a glass and at the same time bend their nodding head forward to reach it, sometimes with surprising success.

Most patients discover for themselves that ethanol is a specific for familial tremor, and although most discipline themselves to use this only for important occasions, alcoholism sometimes becomes their way of life. For this reason, very few patients should be told of its value. If they have already discovered it, a sense of discipline and rationing must be strongly encouraged.

Drug therapy should start with propranolol in similar doses to those used for clonic spasm and with the same conraindications. If propranolol cannot be used, small doses of the benzodiazepines or of the promazine derivatives may be of some help.

The second form of this disorder is true senile tremor with no familial component and no presenile evidence of tremor. It is a slow three to four per second regular tremor with head nodding and tongue protrusion as the main features. Reassurance that this is not parkinsonism (equally important in the treatment of essential familial tremor) and that it is a natural effect of advancing age may be all that is needed, but small doses of chlordiazepoxide (5 mg three times a day) are occasionally beneficial.

Parkinsonism

Parkinsonism, characterized by slowness and weakness of voluntary movement, rigidity, and tremor, affects about one person in 1000 of the total population. In persons over age 55 its incidence rises to about one in 100 so that it is not surprising to find that this condition is the second most common neurologic disorder of the elderly coming some way behind strokes.

In old age the most common cause of parkinsonism is Parkinson's disease (paralysis agitans) followed by drugs given for sedation, particularly haloperidol and the phenothiazines. Cerebrovascular disease as a cause of parkinsonism is much less common than is supposed, and most patients in whom this diagnosis is correct have had bilateral deep cerebral hemisphere infarctions or longstanding hypertensive cerebrovascular disease with status lacunaris of the upper brainstem and corpora striata. The presentation in this type is usually with facial and generalized rigidity, difficulty in initiating voluntary movements, little in the way of tremor, and some accompanying dementia; also the response to antiparkinsonian drugs is poor.

In elderly patients, paralysis agitans differs little with regard to physical signs from that seen at earlier ages, and the main problems are the emotional state of the patient and an undue sensitivity to the drugs commonly used for this condition and to their side-effects. Disorientation, aggressive behavior, ideas of persecution, depression, and frightening hallucinations may be present, producing behavior disorders often difficult to control. For this reason if an elderly patient is showing some of the classic signs of parkinsonism but is not really disabled by his disease, it is often wise to withhold treatment, and this certainly should be the rule in those patients who are confused or demented.

The elderly patient with true Parkinson's disease cannot tolerate large doses of cholinergic blocking drugs, which are used with success in this illness, and the dose of benzhexol should probably not exceed 6 mg in 24 hours. Mental agitation associated with the illness is often not helped by this type of drug and is sometimes difficult to control. Chlordiazepoxide and diazepam usually do not mix well with the cholinergic blocking drugs, and the antihistamines make elderly patients too drowsy to be of much use. Meprobamate in doses of 200 mg or 400 mg with each dose of anticholinergic is useful, and promazine (50 mg) at night is helpful in controlling nocturnal restlessness, aggression, and wandering. Other cholinergic blocking drugs used with success in the elderly are benztropine (2 mg three times daily) or orphenadrine (50 mg three times daily). Once the right drug has been found for each particular patient, it should not be changed. Sudden discontinuing of these drugs results in intense muscular rigidity and often complete immobility and must be avoided.

Surgery has now little part to play in the treatment of parkinsonism, particularly when the patient is older than 65. Occasionally a "young" sexagenarian shows the rigidity and disability of Parkinson's disease without any mental or emotional deficit, without weakness of voice, and without very much tremor. If the usual cholinergic blocking drugs do not improve the situation, stereotactic thalamotomy using cryosurgical techniques may be justified, but surgical success in the elderly is infrequent, and the risk of morbidity from the operation is high.

The fairly recent discovery that parkinsonism is probably due to a deficiency of dopamine[6,7] in the extrapyramidal system has transformed prognosis and treatment. Confirmation has come from autopsy studies[17] in which dopamine was found to be materially depleted in the brains of patients with parkinsonism. In view of this, the therapeutic possibilities of dopamine were investigated in patients with all forms of parkinsonism, but dopamine itself does not cross the blood–brain barrier and is therefore ineffective. However, the level of dopamine in the brain can be raised by giving levodopa or a monoamine oxidas inhibitor that prevents its destruction.

Clinical trials, begun in 1961,[10] have now established that levodopa is the most successful and powerful drug for the treatment of Parkinson's disease but less useful in patients with postencephalitic parkinsonism. It is completely ineffective in drug-induced parkinsonism because such drugs block its effect on the dopamine receptors in the nigrostriatal system, and an anticholinergic drug such as orphenadrine must be used if the offending drug has to be continued for clinical reasons.

The main problem of treatment in these trials was patient intolerance, particularly in the elderly, because large doses up to 2 g daily were often necessary to control the disease, and this dosage produced nausea, vomiting, postural hypotension, hallucinations, cardiac arrhythmias, and involuntary movements in many patients. Fortunately, if a peripheral dopa-decarboxylase inhibitor is given with levodopa, a much smaller dose is needed because, if levodopa is given alone, 80% of it is converted by the body to dopamine before it can reach the brain. Since the inhibitors that are used—carbidopa and benserazide—cannot cross the blood–brain barrier, all the levodopa that reaches the brain can be converted to dopamine at the appropriate site.

Present authoritative opinion is that this combination of levodopa and carbidopa or levodopa and benserazide is the most effective treatment of disabling Parkinson's disease in the elderly. There seems little to choose between the two, and dosage should start low with 100 mg levodopa combined with 10 mg carbidopa or with 25 mg benserazide once daily, increasing by a similar amount every third day until the disability is controlled or side-effects become more disabling than the parkinsonism.

Improvement occurs rapidly once a therapeutic dose has been reached with loosening of the rigidity, speeding up of all voluntary movement, and improvement in gait, in posture, in balance, in dressing, and in handwriting. Speech weakness and tremor may show less or later improvement, and the final appearance does not often change in elderly patients.

Side-effects are entirely dose dependent in most patients, comprising nausea, postural hypotension, and involuntary movements. The nausea responds to taking levodopa with food, and to cyclizine 50 mg; the hypotension is treated by warning the patient to take care on adopting the vertical posture, not to go to sleep in an upright chair, and, in the case of a man, to sit down if he has to get up to urinate at night. Involuntary movements indicate overdosage and require lowering of the dose of levodopa, which must be done slowly, otherwise, a rigid immobility will ensue. The involuntary movements commonly start in the mouth and lips, spreading to the neck, then to the face, and occasionally to the limbs. They are of a choreiform nature with dystonic features in some patients. The onset of these movements is often delayed, and, although they are dose-dependent and usually improve with suitable reduction of levodopa, occasionally, they remain a permanent feature.

Two additional problems are common with long-term treatment. The first is that Parkinson's disease is progressive, and eventually the loss of dopamine receptors is so severe that response to levodopa or to any other dopamine agonist becomes poorer and poorer, and the patient steadily deteriorates. Moreover, the prolongation of life with levodopa highlights the mental and emotional deterioration that was less obvious before because of the naturally reduced life span of untreated patients.

The second problem is the well-documented "on-off" syndrome in which the effects of levodopa seem suddenly to disappear or equally suddenly to be intensified so that disabling oscillations of performance occur. Possibly defective absorption, defective metabolism, changes in cerebral blood flow in the brain stem, or swings in serum levels produce this phenomenon. Some improvement can be obtained by giving the drug more frequently in smaller doses.

In addition to the above, I have encountered two less obvious problems, both connected with the increased mobility that therapy brings to elderly patients previously almost chair-bound by their parkinsonism. The first is aggravation of the symptoms of osteoarthropathy in knees, hips, and shoulders; and the second is the emergence of symptoms of cardiac ischemia owing to the increased work load on the heart. Both of these problems can be treated by conventional methods, and successful hip replacements have been done on some elderly parkinsonian patients.

Contraindications to levodopa therapy are overt cardiovascular disease, especially any persisting arrhythmia, and also the presence of dementia sufficiently severe to cause abnormal behavior. Increased activity would make these patients more difficult to look after, and the levodopa would probably make the symptoms of dementia worse.

Drugs other than levodopa seem to help patients with Parkinson's disease, but none is so effective at present. Amantadine is an antiviral agent that by chance was found to increase the mobility of patients in doses of 100 mg twice daily. It certainly can help mild cases and has some synergistic action with levodopa, but, unfortunately, its effect seem to wear off after some weeks, and, on the whole, it has been disappointing.

Bromocriptine is a dopaminergic agonist with an effect on the presynaptic and postsynaptic receptors and has been shown to be useful in the treatment of Parkinson's disease. It improves all the features of the disease and is at present used in patients who are unable to tolerate levodopa and not helped by amantadine. It seems to be of little use in patients on levodopa in full doses, with persisting disability, and, therefore, it is not very helpful as adjuvant therapy. It remains to be seen whether it will prove useful in patients plagued by the on-off syndrome.

There is no doubt that the dopamine agonist drugs have transformed the treatment of idiopathic Parkinson's disease, and, at first, it was hoped that they would be as useful as insulin in diabetes or thyroxine in hypothyroidism. It has unfortunately become evident that the disease is steadily progressive with continuing neuronal loss, and, although treatment improves the quality and quantity of life, the end is eventually unaltered.

It is the usual practice to continue anticholinergic drugs for some months when starting treatment with these new substances, but usually a slow reduction and, in many patients, complete withdrawal is possible.

Cerebral Atrophy

Among the more depressing neuropsychiatric illnesses of old age is the slowly increasing dementia estimated to affect up to 4% of the population over age 65.

The symptoms are an exaggeration of what happens to all of us as age takes its toll of our neurons with some slowing up of memory recall, particularly with regard to people's names, some hardening of our attitude to changes in society, and some tendency to withdraw from new social contacts. In addition to some general intellectual loss, we find learning more difficult, concentration less dependable, judgment more rigid, attention difficult to maintain, and originality of ideas gradually decreasing.

With dementia these changes are grossly accelerated with loss of memory for recent events, inability to reason and, therefore, the formation of unreliable judgments, lability of affect, loss of interest and of conative drive, and often periods of disorientation. When these lead to behavior disorders, the problem of social care becomes urgent, and few families are prepared to look after an elderly demented relative.

These patients may be brought to the neurologist rather than the psychiatrist at first on account of their difficulty in understanding and in speaking, the appearance of fits for the first time, or because a head injury is suspected as a possible cause. All forms of reversible dementia must be excluded before the diagnosis of cerebral atrophy is accepted, and it is wise to confirm the diagnosis by computed cerebral tomography (Fig. 18-11).

One particular cause, which although infrequent may be reversible, is the presence of communicating normal pressure hydrocephalus associated with the effects of past meningitis, subarachnoid hemorrhage, or head injury. In this condition, dementia is usually combined with urinary incontinence and a disorder of gait, partly ataxic and partly spastic. Computed tomography shows large ventricles with no corresponding enlargement of the subarachnoid space over the hemispheres, and a ventriculoperitoneal shunt may arrest the progress of this condition.

Other forms of dementia under the headings of acute or chronic brain syndromes are the province of the psychiatrist and are dealt with in Chapter 34 of this volume.

Any hope of improving a patient's intellectual capacity by drug therapy is misplaced in my opinion and experience, although aggressive advertising by some drug firms might make patient's relatives and a few physicians think otherwise. Tender, loving nursing or home care is all one can hope for with the emphasis on some daily walking exercise, frequent attention to micturition and bowel function, and the provision of some simple tasks and of some recreation, which may be the playing of some simple indoor games, reading, listening to the radio, or even watching television. It is most important to ensure that adequate amounts of food and drink are both provided and taken because patients of this type tend either to neglect to eat at all or to eat almost anything they can lay their hands on. Drugs for dealing with restlessness, agitation, and insomnia should be prescribed with care, and the most useful are those already mentioned previously in this chapter for patients with completed major stroke.

NEUROLOGIC DISORDERS OWING TO SKELETAL CHANGES

Skeletal abnormalities are likely to occur more often in the elderly patient, and three main conditions are commonly encountered at this time of life.

Paget's Disease

The neurologic complications of this disorder are due to overgrowth and distortion of the skeleton with compression of nerve roots and of the spinal cord. The most common pressure neuropathies owing to bony changes in the skull affect the seventh and eighth cranial nerves with resulting facial palsy and deafness often accompanied by generalized headache, associated with involvement of the sensory innervation to the scalp.

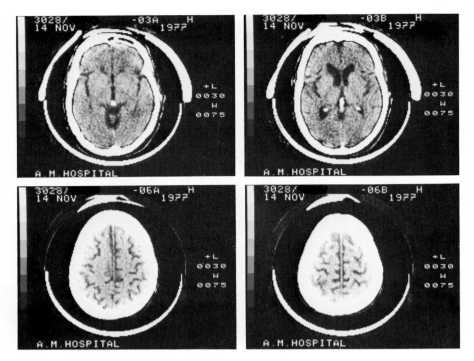

FIG. 18-11. CT scan of cerebral atrophy. Note the enlargement of the lateral ventricles, increase in the subarachnoid space, and widening of the fissures and sulci. (Courtesy of Dr. James Ambrose)

In the limbs, pain is commonly due to nerve root pressure particulary in the lumbosacral plexus, and paraplegia due to spinal cord or cauda equina compression is occasionally seen.

Diagnosis of Paget's disease is made by the patient's bent posture with enlargement of the head circumference, the typical radiologic picture, the raised alkaline phosphatase level in the blood, the often concomitant high-output cardiac failure, and discovery of a murmur over some affected bones.

Until recently there was nothing to offer these patients, except analgesics and encouragement, but the advent of calcitonin treatment has improved the outlook, and some of my deaf patients have regained a substantial amount of hearing on this therapy. Age is no contraindication for treatment with calcitonin if the serum calcium levels are carefully watched.

Even more recently I have used disodium etidronate for this condition and it has the advantage that is can be given by mouth (see Chapter 30).

Osteoporosis

Osteoporosis is very common in the elderly, and it produces neurologic symptoms owing to its effect on the vertebral column. Pain in the back and occasional root pain occur, but vertebral collapse rarely causes cord or cauda equina compression. Diagnosis is by radiography; there is usually little biochemical change in the calcium or phosphorus content of the serum. Differentiation from secondary deposits or myelomatosis is made by the radiographic appearance of the vertebral column (a general smooth loss of calcium in osteoprosis), the presence of a primary growth with localized osteoporosis or osteosclerosis in carcinoma, and the serum protein changes and high sedimentation rate in myelomatosis.

Treatment is by use of anabolic steroids such as androstalone, because positive nitrogen balance is important for the retention of calcium, much of which is protein bound. The possibility of thyrotoxicosis, even in the elderly, and of osteoporosis owing to corticosteroid therapy should be remembered. Bed rest may be necessary if pain is severe, but non-weight-bearing exercises are extremely important in this case. As soon as the pain has eased, the patient may slowly begin to get up and gradually return to normal activities.

If anabolic steroids produce unwanted androgenic effects and therefore preclude their use in women, estrogen seems to be more effective than calcium supplements in preventing bone loss, particularly in postmenopausal patients (see Chapter 30).

Cervical Spondylosis

The radiographic discovery of cervical spondylosis is common in elderly patients, most of whom show no neurologic abnormality as a result. Occasionally, however, osteophytes may distort the vertebral arteries and interfere with the blood supply to the hindbrain. Thus, transient cerebral ischemic attacks can occur, made worse by neck movements, particularly rotation and extension, and a murmur may be heard over the artery in the supraclavicular fossa (Fig. 18-12). In addition, transverse intervertebral bars may interfere with the blood supply to the cervical cord by direct pressure, and an ischemic myelopathy may result. When this occurs, the patient complains of difficulty in walking, weakness of the legs, clumsiness and paresthesias of the hands, and possibly urinary sphincter disturbances. The neck movements may be limited, and some wasting and loss of tendon reflexes may be found in the upper limbs, with sensory loss of peripheral and occasionally segmental distribution. The lower limbs are spastic, with exaggerated tendon reflexes, clonus, and extensor plantar responses. Although walking is difficult, individual muscular weakness is less than might be expected. The posterior columns are the last to be affected by the cord compression, but they may be affected by the normal aging process. Lumbar puncture usually shows a low cerebrospinal fluid pressure, no subarachnoid block, and a cerebrospinal fluid protein content of 40 mg to 100 mg/dl. Treatment aims at the relief of any cord pressure, thereby improving its blood supply. In spite of the dangers of putting the elderly to bed, this procedure combined with prophylactic bed exercises for the lungs and the legs often improves the physical signs. The upper limb pain diminishes, the lower limbs become less stiff, and extensor plantar responses sometimes change to flexor after 3 weeks in bed. Flexor spasms of the legs sometimes occur at night and are relieved by 5 mg of diazepam given orally in most patients. Some authorities favor cervical traction for these patients, but this can increase attacks of hindbrain ischemia and should not be used in the elderly. Before weight bearing is allowed, a collar must be fitted that restricts neck movements. Most patients tolerate this for 3 to 6 months without much difficulty.

If deterioration continues, a myelogram should be done. This may show a well-localized compressing lesion amenable to surgery. However, even in the most skillful hands, cervical laminectomy in the elderly is considerably hazardous and may make the patient much worse. Differential diagnosis in this age-group should include consideration of spinal cord tumor, subacute combined degeneration, and atherosclerotic myelomalacia. The elderly patient with a cervical cord tumor shows a more rapid onset, greater weakness in his legs, and sometimes a segmental level of sensory impairment. The protein content of the cerebrospinal fluid is higher, and some evidence of subarachnoid block may be present. The patient with myelopathy owing to vitamin B_{12} deficiency usually complains of paresthesia of all four extremities. The sensory loss is of the posterior column type, and the cerebrospinal fluid is normal. Diag-

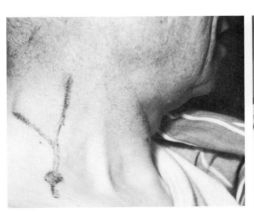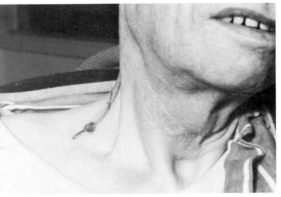

FIG. 18-12. The common site of the systolic murmur heard in some patients with vertebral artery stenosis. (Carter AB: Cerebral Infarction, New York, Pergamon Press, 1964)

nosis is clinched by serum vitamin B_{12} estimations, which are obligatory if there is any doubt. Atherosclerotic softening of the cord may be more difficult, but pain is uncommon, and sphincter disturbances are always present. Occasionally, the onset is very sudden, and the resulting disability is complete.

DISORDERS OF GAIT IN THE ELDERLY

Most elderly people in good health walk as well as they did in youth and middle age, although often with more deliberation. Some tend to walk more slowly, eyeing the ground for unevenness and other pitfalls, and some develop a trifle wayward gait with slight hesitations and deviations from the midline. Many wisely carry a cane for stability and also in these troublesome times for defense. Anything worse than the above is evidence of a disorder of vision, of joints, of the skeletal system, or of the nervous system, and it is this last discipline that concerns us here.

Normal gait depends on the integrity of many parts of the nervous system. There must be sufficient power in the muscles of the trunk and lower limbs, normal sensation in the feet, particularly the sense of position, good coordination, good postural tone, normal righting reflexes in relation to gravity, and a normal desire to walk or run. The more common causes of disorder of gait in the elderly are described below:

In peripheral neuropathy that is either metabolic or infective, *flaccid weakness* is combined with some loss of feeling. The result is a high-stepping gait due to footdrop, a flapping or stamping movement when the foot touches the ground due to loss of feeling for the solidity of the impact, and a general incoordination of movement because weak muscles are always clumsy. The disturbance is usually bilateral and equal on both sides in true peripheral neuropathy but may be unilateral in mononeuritis, in diabetic nerve involvement, or in the early stages of motor neuron disease. Trauma or pressure neuropathy will also frequently produce a unilateral gait problem with a limp and with dorsilumbar scoliosis if the sciatic or femoral nerves are involved. A combination of chronic peripheral neuropathy and loss of position sense that occurs in subacute combined degeneration of the cord (Vitamin B_{12} deficiency) will produce a slow, hesitant, shuffling gait with the eyes turned down toward the ground to compensate for the loss of position.

In the elderly, *spastic weakness,* if unilateral, is almost always due to the effects of a stroke. The problem is stiffness of the affected leg combined with persisting plantar flexion, producing a circumduction of the leg as it is brought forward and a tendency to drag the foot with wearing out of the tip of the shoe or boot. The patient will also lean toward the good side as the foot comes forward and round. Bilateral spastic weakness due to a lesion of both pyramidal tracts produces a shuffling gait with small steps, an inability to lift the feet off the ground, and alternating turning of the body from side to side to obtain forward movement. If the lesion is in the spinal cord there is often spasm of the adductor muscles of the thighs, leading to a scissor gait, with the legs crossing in front of each other, making walking almost impossible.

Parkinsonian gait differs from any other in that the rigidity of muscles combined with their slowness of response produces difficulty in starting any walking movement. Once begun, the gait is shuffling with a forward stooping posture, causing patients to take rapid little steps to avoid falling forward so that they appear in a permanent state of propulsion and find difficulty in stopping. Occasionally a similar problem occurs in a backward direction. When a doorway appears through which they have to pass they tend to freeze into a state of immobility. During the walk the arms do not swing and in the early stages of the disease a unilateral loss of arm swinging may point to the diagnosis.

Ataxic gait may be either sensory or motor. In sensory ataxia the problem is not knowing where the feet are in relation to the ground or to the rest of the body. The gait is slow with the head held down, with the patient hoping that vision may compensate for the sensory deficit as he feels for the ground; walking may be impossible in the dark. Labyrinthine disorders in the elderly are usually vascular in origin and, if acute, produce disorders of equilibrium, making the patient unable to walk at all without clinging to some solid object and progressing from one piece of furniture to another. The ataxia may produce a constant veering to one side or the other, and balance becomes grossly disturbed and made worse by any movement of the head. The slightest push will cause the patient to lose sufficient balance to make a fall almost inevitable. In pure motor ataxia the problem is one of muscular incoordination and the patient walks on a wide base, wandering from side to side and veering in every direction. Balance is also disturbed, and this type of gait is seen commonly in drunkenness. Other causes in the elderly are lesions of the brain stem and cerebellum, either neoplastic or vascular. The earliest signs are loss of arm swinging when walking, some widening of the stance, and poor recovery from tripping or from anything that disturbs the patient's equilibrium. Other gait disturbances, such as the waddling of muscular dystrophy and the spastic-ataxic combination of multiple sclerosis, are unlikely to trouble the elderly since the life expectancy of these conditions is below normal.

NEUROLOGIC INVESTIGATIONS IN THE ELDERLY

Although a more dynamic and less nihilistic approach to the treatment of disease in the elderly is fortunately becoming more accepted by practicing neurologists, it is important to ensure that enthusiastic investigations for this purpose do not cause harm.

Serendipity has brought us many excellent noninvasive techniques and there is little excuse for overdoing the rather more old fashioned exercises.

Lumbar Puncture

My view is that lumbar puncture is mandatory in comatose elderly patients unless gross papilledema or evidence of rapid brain compression is present. It is also necessary in all ill elderly patients with stiffness of the neck or acute recent disorientation and confusion. Only in this way can meningitis and subarachnoid hemorrhage be diagnosed in some patients with minimal or unclear signs. The test is also useful and without harm in those with paraplegia due to injury, vascular catastrophes, infections, or compressing lesions in the spinal column.

In a progressing or straightforward completed stroke, I formerly used this investigation routinely but have mostly given it up with the advent of computed tomography and have not regretted it.

Cerebral Angiography

Cerebral angiography is a particularly invasive investigation with morbidity and mortality rates increasing in the elderly. In one large multicenter trial in the United States, transient complications occurred in 5.4%, permanent deficit in 0.6%, and death in 0.25%. Only those patients who are fit, willing, and suitable for surgery should undergo

this test. My personal indications for surgery have been mentioned earlier in this chapter.

Ultrasound

Ultrasound is a noninvasive investigation that is now capable of showing moderate or severe grades of arterial stenosis and also of demonstrating the direction and volume of the blood flow.

Electroencephalography

Electroencephalography is a harmless investigation that is perhaps a little disappointing in its application to neurologic problems in the elderly. It correlates well with regional reduction in blood flow and clearly demonstrates infarction and can also help to distinguish between transient cerebral ischemic attacks and focal epilepsy but otherwise is probably less useful in the long run than the other tests.

Echoencephalography

Again a noninvasive test, echoencephalography can indicate the presence or absence of midline shift (see Fig. 18-1).

Pneumoencephalography

Pneumoencephalography is a very invasive test with some disastrous results in my experience in the early days (1933), particularly in elderly patients. In my opinion it no longer has any place in the neurologic investigations of patients over 65 years of age.

Computed Tomography (CT Scanning)

Computed tomography represents the greatest advance in noninvasive radiologic investigation for many years. It can locate lesions, differentiate them one from another, define their type, demonstrate edema around them, show up aneurysms, show areas of vasospasm, and show areas of cortical atrophy or the absence of hemispheric cerebrospinal fluid circulation with the greatest of ease. Some invasive techniques have been added to enhance the scans, and these help to pick out smaller lesions and to differentiate even more clearly the pathology of space-occupying lesions. Cerebral hemorrhage of all types can be clearly shown—epidural, subdural, intracerebral, subarachnoid, and even hemorrhagic infarctions—and no one doubts that at present this is the safest, most complete, and most useful investigative technique.

Positron Emission Tomography (PET)

Positron emmission tomography is more recent, noninvasive, but rather more complicated and expensive and perhaps yields less dramatic results than computed tomography. Positrons are positively charged electrons that combine with the tissue electron to produce two high-energy gamma ray protons emitting in opposite directions. Imaging from these can be formed by short-lived isotopes incorporated in metabolites such as glucose and oxygen and thus give some idea of the efficiency of regional brain metabolism in and around areas affected by cerebrovascular disease. Workers in this field consider that the metabolic uptake of radioactive elements is a more sensitive indicator of cerebral dysfunction than computed tomography and can show areas of viable tissue with poor perfusion, not always identified by the CT scan.

The technique is to use radioactive fluorine 18 and oxygen 15, which can be linked to glucose and to oxygen, respectively, and thereby can show areas that may appear to have a normal blood flow but have poor metabolism.

Nuclear Magnetic Resonance

The imaging of nuclear magnetic resonance in the brain is an exciting and fairly recent noninvasive investigation without any known risk. It allows tomographic imaging based on the chemistry and metabolism of thin slices of brain tissue and produces a computerized display scan.

The clinical use is at present mainly in the detection and differentiation of cerebral tumors, and scanning is completely electrical, avoiding the expense of the rotating gantry of the CT scanner.

Modern systems are now designed to eliminate all moving parts so that patient disturbance is minimal and there can be no doubt that this investigation can reveal lesions that cannot be shown on the normal CT scan. It would appear that this investigation would be more useful in the investigation of young and middle-aged patients rather than the elderly.

CONCLUSION

It has been impossible in the confines of a single chapter to give a full account of all the neurologic changes associated with aging. Fortunately an excellent and wider ranging book has been published on this subject with extensive references to the appropriate literature, and this volume can be strongly recommended to those interested in the study of and research into the effects of old age on the nervous system.[23] Emphasis in this present contribution has been placed on the importance of accurate diagnosis in the treatable and reversible conditions, which are more common than most physicians think. In particular, organic dementia is a dangerous diagnosis, leading to a nihilistic therapeutic approach unless particular trouble is taken to exclude such conditions as subdural hematoma; meningitis; and deficiency states including hypothyroidism, hypoglycemia, and drug intoxication. Similarly, neurotic symptoms are uncommon in elderly patients, and unexplained headache may be due to arteritis, Paget's disease, cervical spondylosis, or trigeminal and postherpetic neuralgia. Even degenerative occlusive vascular disease has treatable manifestations, and no one should be denied the benefit of thorough investigation and of appropriate treatment solely because of old age.

The author wishes to thank the editor of the *Practitioner* for permission to reproduce some of the illustrations and excerpts from the previous published writings—especially Figures 18-1, 18-2, 18-5, 18-6, and 18-10.

REFERENCES

1. Adams GF: Cerebrovascular Disability and the Aging Brain. London, Churchill Livingstone, 1974
2. Adams GF, Hurwitz LJ: Mental barriers to recovery from strokes. Lancet 2:533, 1963
3. Alvarez WC: Little Strokes. Philadelphia, JB Lippincott, 1966
4. Barnett HJM, Peerless SJ, McCormick CW: In answer to the question: 'As compared to what?' A progress report on EC/IC bypass study. Stroke 11:137, 1980
5. Bhatia SP, Irvine RE: Electrical recording of the ankle jerk in old age. Gerontol Clin 15:357, 1973
6. Blaschko H: Metabolism and storage of biogenic amines, Experientia 13:9, 1957
7. Brodie BB, Shore PA: A concept for a role of serotonin and norepinephrine as chemical mediators in the brain. Ann NY Acad Sci 66:631, 1957
8. Carter AB: Cerebral Infarction. New York, Pergamon Press, 1964
9. Chamberlain W: Restriction in upward gaze with advancing age. Am J Ophthalmol 71:341, 1971
10. Cotzias GC, van Woert MH, Schiffer LM: Aromatic

amino acids and modification of parkinsonism. N Engl J Med 276:374, 1967

11. Critchley M: The neurology of old age. Lancet 1:1119, 1931

12. De Bakey ME, Crawford ES, Cooley DA, Morris GC, Garrett HE, Fields WS: Cerebral arterial insufficiency: One to eleven year results following arterial reconstruction. Ann Surg 161:921, 1965

13. Fields WS, Maslenikov V, Meyer JS, Hass WK, Remington RD, Macdonald M: Joint study of extracranial arterial occlusion. JAMA 211:1993, 1970

14. Fisher CM: Cerebral Vascular Disease (Second Princeton Conference), p 81. New York, Grune & Stratton, 1958

15. Goldberg AD, Raftery EB, Cashman PMM: Ambulatory electrocardiograph records in patients with transient cerebral attacks. Br Med J 4:569, 1975

16. Harrison MJG: Vascular surgery for ischaemic stroke. Br J Hosp Med 24:108, 1980

17. Hornykiewicz O: Dopamine (3-hydroxytyramine) and brain function. Pharmacol Rev 18:925, 1966

18. Howell TH: Senile deterioration of the central nervous system. Br Med J 56, 1949

19. Impallomeni M, Kenny RA, Flynn MD, Pallis CA: The elderly and their ankle jerks. Lancet 1:670, 1984

20. Irvine WT, Luck RJ, Sutton D, Walpita PR: Intrathoracic occlusion of great vessels causing cerebrovascular insufficiency. Lancet 1:1177, 1963

21. Johnson RT: Viral infections of the Nervous System. New York, Raven Press, 1982

22. Juel-Jensen B: Chemotherapy for varicella-zoster infections. Antimicrob Chemother 2:261, 1976

23. Katzman R, Terry R: The Neurology of Aging. Philadelphia, FA Davis, 1983

24. Lambert HP: Personal communication, 1977

25. Licht S: Stroke and Its Rehabilitation. Baltimore, Waverly Press, 1975

26. Marshall J: Dilemmas in the management of the neurological patient, p 54. London, Churchill Livingstone, 1984

27. McKissock W, Richardson A, Taylor JC: Primary Intracerebral haemorrhage: A controlled trial of surgical and conservative treatment in 180 unselected cases. Lancet 2:221, 1961

28. McKissock W, Richardson A, Walsh L: Spontaneous cerebellar haemorrhage. Brain 83:1, 1960

29. Prakash C, Stern G: Neurological signs in the elderly. Age Ageing 2:24, 1973

30. Ross-Russell RW: Observations on intracerebral aneurysms. Brain 86:425, 1963

31. Ross-Russell RW: Cerebral Arterial Disease, p 221. London, Churchill Livingstone, 1976

32. Ross-Russell RW: Vascular Disease of the Central Nervous System, p 216. London, Churchill Livingstone, 1983

33. Sandok BA, Furlan AJ, Whisnant JP, Sundt TM: Guidelines for the management of transient ischaemic attacks. Mayo Clin Proc 53:665, 1978

34. Sommerville JG: The rehabilitation of the hemiplegic patient. Proceedings of the World Federation of Occupational Therapists, 1967

35. Stanford JR, Lubour M, Vasko JS: Prevention of stroke by carotid endarterectomy. Surgery 83:259, 1978

36. Taverner D, Fearnley ME, Kemble F, Miles DW, Peiris OA: Steroid therapy in Bell's palsy. Br Med J 1:391, 1966

37. Thompson JE: Surgery for Cerebrovascular Insufficiency. Springfield. IL, Charles C Thomas, 1968

38. Timbury C: Acyclovir. Br Med J 285:1223, 1982

19 Genitourinary Disease in the Elderly

Selwyn Z. Freed

Most genitourinary disease is associated with aging. The incidence of urinary tract infections, neuromuscular voiding disabilities, and urinary tract neoplasms increases steeply in the later decades; prostatism in the male and sexual dysfunction in both sexes are predictable. Past the age of 50 a progressive increase in the collagen content of the detrusor muscle of the bladder occurs in both sexes.[59] Increase in collagen is largely responsible for a parallel reduction in detrusor contractility and helps explain urinary retention even in women. In addition, intravesical prostatic obstruction in the male is another cause of detrusor collagenesis. Whether this results in work hypertrophy (trabeculation) or simple passive distention, the consequence is even more collagen deposition and diminished detrusor contractility. Even in men who have had a prostatectomy there is a gradual decrease in the force of the stream with advancing age.

THE PROSTATE

The prostate gland, which is associated with but not essential for reproduction and dispensable for health generally, is unrivaled as the most frequently diseased human organ. It is the site of the most common neoplasm, benign prostatic hyperplasia (BPH), of the most frequent malignancy, and of several inflammatory conditions. The enormous incidence of physician visits (to all physicians, not just urologists) occasioned by it requires accurate knowledge of its diseases and of the imprecision of available examinations. An example is the extensive mythology surrounding the term *prostatism*. Although the etiology of neither BPH nor

carcinoma of the prostate is known, requisites for both are aging and a sufficiency of testicular androgen. Castration before puberty prevents either condition, yet testosterone administration by itself cannot cause them. BPH and carcinoma occur in different portions of the prostate, and neither predisposes to the other. There is some regression of BPH (as well as carcinoma) by castration or antiandrogen medication, but this is inconsistent at best and largely abandoned as a therapy. More than 80% of males past age 60 have BPH, and half of these will suffer from some urinary dysfunction but only about 10% will require surgery to relieve obstruction.

Benign Prostatic Hyperplasia

It cannot be overemphasized that bladder outlet obstruction is the essential issue, but its documentation is often neglected. The actual size of the gland is rarely crucial. Many men have very large prostates without suffering any urinary difficulty. It is indefensible that some are advised to undergo prostatectomy on this basis alone, or even if accompanied by only mild symptoms. Symptoms such as frequency, nocturia, and urgency ("prostatism") may have little or no correlation with the severity of bladder outlet obstruction.[9] One may reflect that these same symptoms are often present in women. They may well be due to irritable contractions of the bladder detrusor, which is common in both sexes. Other conditions that present similarly include cystitis and other bladder diseases, stress, neuropathies such as diabetes, and parkinsonism, while medications such as diuretics and α-adrenergics often alter urinary patterns. The determination must be made as to whether the

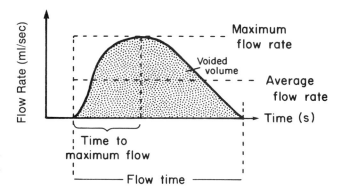

FIG. 19-1. Diagram of urinary flow demonstrating peak flow, voiding time, average flow, voiding curve pattern, and voided volume.

symptoms of detrusor instability are related to prostatic obstruction and, therefore, whether surgery or medical management is to be prescribed.

Traditional urologic workup of patients with prostatism usually includes an appraisal of the symptoms, rectal digital assessment of the size and texture of the prostate, intravenous urography, and cystoscopy. The role of each currently requires reevaluation. Symptoms may not necessarily be related to the degree of prostatic obstruction. Rectal digital examination is only a rough gauge of prostatic size,[40] though essential to discovering carcinoma or abscess. Intravenous urography for determining obstruction is controversial. It may reveal unsuspected disease in the upper tracts or bladder, but the yield is small.[10,53] The post-voiding film for residual urine at best yields only a rough estimate of the prostatic problem. Routine intravenous pyelography has been challenged as not cost effective, and sonography is now an acceptable alternative. When indicated, a retrograde cystogram can be a useful option. The simple passage of a catheter with instillation of radiopaque fluid is quick, easy, and eminently cost effective. It uncovers or rules out a urethral stricture and precisely documents the post-void residual, and a single roentgenogram clearly delineates bladder diverticula and ureteral reflux. Cystoscopy is mandatory for investigating most cases of hematuria or intractable pyuria. There are other specific indications, but its routine value in prostatism is questionable. The urologist cannot ''see'' obstruction; visualizing the configuration and size of prostatic lobes does not determine whether obstruction does in fact exist. However, if the decision for surgery has been made, cystoscopy may be helpful in choosing the most suitable type of prostatectomy.

The deficiencies of traditional investigation have been largely overcome by modern urodynamic studies, which include urinary flow rate, cystometrics, urethral pressure profile, and electromyography. Only the first should be routine. Cystometry is usually helpful, but the latter two are sophisticated tests for more complicated cases.

Assessment of urinary flow rate is the simplest and the most important. It reflects the net result of bladder contractibility and outlet resistance and should therefore be the primary screening procedure (Fig.19-1). Measurements include peak flow rate, average flow, flow-voided curve pattern, and the voiding volume and time. The peak flow rate is the most important single parameter. In males, rates above 15 ml/sec may be considered normal but a flow rate below 10 ml/sec suggests intravesical obstruction. Repeating the test at intervals provides a practical way of following obstruction or detrusor decompensation. Serial tests eventually document the effectiveness of treatment (Fig. 19-2).

Intravesical prostatic obstruction is generally indicated by a diminished flow, but there are caveats. A low-voided volume of less than 125 ml cannot produce a good flow. Dyssynergia (failure of sphincteric muscles to relax at the time of detrusor contraction), urethral stricture, or a weak detrusor (as in the hypotonic bladder of diabetes mellitus) will also result in a low flow. The clinical suspicion of these possibilities should be pursued by cystometry. Although this requires catheterization it is a relatively simple procedure that measures residual urine, bladder pressure, and capacity, and by it irritable (unstable) bladder is diagnosed (Fig. 19-3).

Sometimes, in prostatic obstruction, the flow rate remains normal due to early detrusor compensation. A more sophisticated study, called synchronous pressure flow, can then be invoked; intravesical pressure and flow are thereby measured simultaneously. Many bladders go through such a

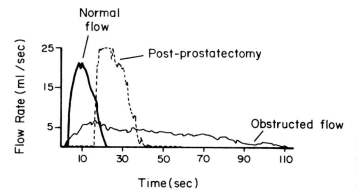

FIG. 19-2. Diagram of urinary flow demonstrating a normal curve, an obstructed flow pattern, and the usual appearance after a prostatectomy.

phase of hypertrophy, so-called silent prostatism, before decompensating in a state of distention. This leads to increased post-void residuals and potential complications such as bladder diverticula, overflow incontinence, vesicoureteral reflux, and eventual renal damage. Generally, patients with increased intravesical pressure will do well after surgery; those with diminished pressure tend to have voiding problems postoperatively. If the bladder is severely and chronically hypotonic, surgery should not be performed at all. Such patients are best managed by intermittent catheterization.

With the affirmation that outlet obstruction is present and due to a prostatic disorder, surgery may be advised with the promise that the flow will be greatly improved. However, the symptoms of an unstable bladder when present in addition to obstruction will resolve in only three fourths of patients; in the remainder the symptoms persist.[60] This approximates the usually incidence for this age-group.

The ability of elderly patients to withstand sur-

gical procedures seems to be based not so much on age itself but on the presence of significant diseases in other organs. Three to 6 months should elapse after a myocardial infarction before elective surgery. Preparations should be made for inhalation therapy postoperatively for patients with pulmonary insufficiency. Depressed renal function due to acute bladder neck obstruction may be greatly improved by an indwelling catheter for a few days preoperatively. In chronic renal failure, sophisticated monitoring of fluid and electrolyte balance is mandatory. Systemic bleeding problems must be anticipated, anticogulants discontinued, and chronic salicylate habit questioned.

There are four main types of prostatectomy: transurethral, suprapubic, retropubic, and perineal (Fig. 19-4). Total removal of all of the intracapsular prostate is the goal of each procedure. Transurethral resection is presently the procedure of choice for about 80% of cases in Western countries. It is usually chosen if the weight of the prostate is estimated to be less than 60 g. This proce-

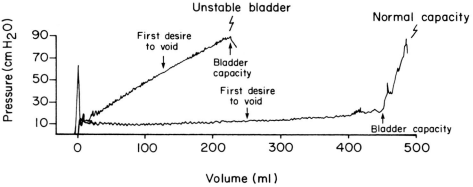

FIG. 19-3. Diagram of a cystometrogram, demonstrating a normal pattern and the pattern of an unstable bladder.

Transurethral

Retropubic   Suprapubic

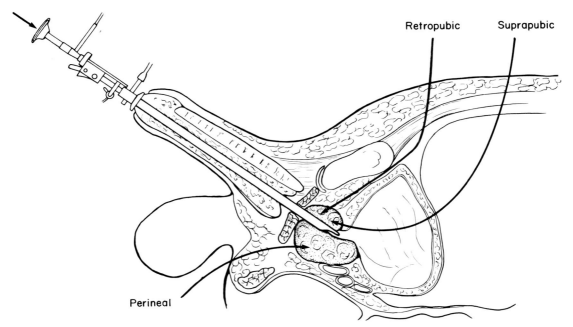

Perineal

FIG. 19-4. Drawing indicating the surgical approach to each of the four types of prostatectomy.

dure is especially attractive since there is no external wound. It is not the procedure of choice if the prostate is very large, if ankylosis of hips prevent the lithotomy position, or if concomitant surgery for bladder diverticulum, large vesical stone, or inguinal hernia is necessary.

Open prostatectomy is better suited for very large prostates, and the suprapubic (transvesical approach) is still the most popular worldwide because of its brevity and technical simplicity. However, the retropubic procedure ensures better hemostasis and functional outcome. The perineal postatectomy is not popular because of probable impotence. It is technically more difficult, but the postoperative course tends to be especially bland. I recommend that it be considered for the elderly, poor-risk patient for whom sexual activity is no longer an issue. For all these procedures, modern surgical technique and anesthesiology, antibiotics, and the like have reduced the mortality to approximately 0.5%, owing in most instances to cardiovascular complications or pulmonary embolism. Ten percent of post-prostatectomy patients continue to be troubled by symptoms of varying kinds. The urinary infection and transient incontinence of the immediate postoperative period are usually managed by the urologist, but he may hear

complaints even at later times. For example, some men with persistent nocturia from habit, insomnia, or reverse diurnal rhythm will have a normal urodynamic evaluation. More commonly, persistent urgency and frequency will be found to be due to detrusor instability. A slow stream, with possible retention of urine, is most often due to a hypotonic bladder. Both of these conditions may have been present preoperatively but were overlooked. Detrusor instability should be treated by restriction of fluids and anticholinergic medication. The severely hypotonic bladder requires intermittent catheterization; cholinergic therapy is rarely of value and an indwelling catheter should be avoided if at all possible. Incontinence (see Chapter 43), when it occurs after prostatectomy is probably due to sphincter injury during surgery, most often transurethral resection, which has an incidence of approximately 0.03%. Other causes of incontinence include drug-unresponsive detrusor instability, overflow from a hypotonic bladder, fundamental sphincter weakness, or a combination of these factors. Stress incontinence, unusual in males, has nevertheless been demonstrated by urethral pressure profiles in post-prostatectomy and even nonoperated patients to be due to low sphincter pressures.[2] Incontinence due to severe sphincter damage may be controlled by prosthetic devices.[8,32]

Prostatitis

Prostatitis is as confused and nonspecific a term as *prostatism*. Clarification has been made possible by the techniques of differential microscopy and cultures for voided urine specimens and rectally expressed prostatic secretions.[37] Prostatic pathogens in the presence of a sterile urine establishes a diagnosis of bacterial prostatitis, which may be acute in febrile episodes but is more often chronic. Nonbacterial prostatitis is diagnosed if the expressed secretion shows 10 or more white blood cells per high-power field but no pathogens; this merges inevitably with the most common condition of all, which is variously called prostatosis, prostatodynia, or prostatic congestion.

All these conditions occur in all age-groups after puberty, are generally suspected and promptly diagnosed in younger men, but are often overlooked in the elderly. The diagnosis is not usually made unless it is first suspected. Symptoms are the same as for the "prostatism" of BPH, unstable bladder, and so on but are apt to include dysuria and an ill-defined perineal discomfort. Relapsing cystitis may be due to an otherwise asymptomatic chronic bacterial prostatitis. Rectal palpation may be helpful if the prostate is tender or boggy but is often not diagnostic. Cystoscopy is not helpful and is usually contraindicated.

Treatment may result in a long history of frustration for both physician and patient. Human prostatic secretions have a bacterial inhibiting factor, probably zinc.[18] Nevertheless, there is no good evidence that zinc administration offers any therapeutic advantage. Antibacterial management over many weeks, based on culture and sensitivity reports, remains the treatment of choice for bacterial prostatitis, but one must be prepared for relapses. A radical transurethral resection of all the infected prostatic tissue is advocated by some[55] but I do not consider it advisable. It is curious that men with chronic bacterial prostatitis seldom develop BPH.

Prostatodynia, or chronic congestion, is by far the most common inflammatory condition of the prostate in men of all ages. The prostate may or may not feel boggy or produce the characteristic penile tip discomfort. Expressed secretions may or may not show white blood cells, and no consistent pathogenic organism is cultured. Sexual dysfunction is often present, although its relationship is not clear. There is usually an obvious psychic com-

ponent, and the patient is often greatly relieved when the association is pointed out. Old-fashioned remedies such as hot baths and bland diet (elimination of alcohol and spicy foods) seem helpful, prostatic massage much less so. Antibacterial medication is worth a try but rarely helps if the diagnosis of abacterial prostatitis is correct.

Carcinoma of the Prostate

The third of the triad of prostatic diseases in the elderly male is carcinoma. It is the most common malignancy, with a substantial morbidity and mortality (25,000 deaths annually in the United States alone). Yet most men with undiagnosed and untreated prostatic carcinoma live without apparent ill effect; probably only one third of all cases are recognized clinically.[21] Since the histology of both clinically active and inactive malignancies is the same, there has been much effort to understand the disease and much controversy regarding management. One hypothesis is that there are two biological types, and one is inactive. A better documented concept is that prostatic cancer is a slow-growing malignancy that may be diagnosed early or late. An octogenarian in whom the disease is detected early, as a small nodule, will probably die of another cause. The same small nodule in a man with a greater life expectancy must be considered for what it is, a lethal cancer. If age-corrected actuarial survival curves are employed and further corrected for histologic differentiation, presence of metastases, and so on, then survival with prostatic cancer is unrelated to age.[26,56] The persistent view that prostatic cancer is more benign in the elderly (and conversely more malignant in younger men) is refuted by studies that show no significant biologic differences in the two age-groups.[30]

Curable cancer of the prostate depends on several factors but none so vital as early detection of localized disease. In this era of sophisticated diagnostic equipment it is nevertheless the time-honored, cost-effective simple digital rectal examination that continues to be the mainstay. This should be done routinely and compulsively in all adult males regardless of the absence of symptoms. Any nodule or firm area in the prostate should be considered suspicious and at any age histologic identification is advantageous. The best procedure for this purpose is transrectal fine needle aspiration. This simple office procedure, which at most occasions minor discomfort, is as reliable as needle biopsy. The aspirate should be read by an experienced cytologist. A serum prostatic acid phosphatase elevation signifies metastatic disease. A normal value does not rule it out; not all metastases release this enzyme. A prostatic carcinoma calls for a judgment regarding management, based not only on age but also on life expectancy, the extent of the malignancy, and its microscopic differentiation. Stage B in prostatic cancer is by definition confined to the prostate and is therefore curable, especially with the "B1" nodule; with intraprostatic spread (stage B2) this is less so. Stage C means invasion of the prostatic capsule; stage D, metastatic disease. Stage A, unsuspected and so-called "occult" carcinoma, is disclosed only by prostatectomy.

Prostatic cancer spreads in three ways: (1) local growth, (2) hematogenously, and (3) via the lymphatics. The rectal finger is the best guide to the size of the tumor. Hematogenous spread is usually primarily to bone, so bone roentgenograms or preferably the more sensitive radioisotope bone scan is the next step.[4] If these are negative, and the acid phosphatase level is not elevated, potential lymphatic spread is next evaluated. Although still controversial, it is largely agreed that the best method is pelvic lymphadenectomy; lymphangiography and computed tomography are unreliable.[44] There are several approaches to lymphadenectomy; my preference for ipsilateral pelvic lymph node dissection is based on the observation that cells from a nodule in the right lobe of the prostate, as an example, spread primarily to the lymph nodes on the right. If they cross to the left pelvic nodes, it is only after involving the nodes on the right. This ipsilateral drainage has also been documented by lymphoscintigraphy.[24]

There are five basic categories of therapy: (1) surgery, (2) irradiation, (3) hormonal therapy, (4) chemotherapy, and (5) "watchful waiting." A B1 nodule in a man over 80 years of age merits only the last "therapy"; close observation should include periodic rectal examinations, determinations of the serum acid phosphatase level, and bone scans. A man in his 60s with the same nodule and normal acid phosphatase, bone scan, and lymph nodes is a candidate for cure. Recent studies support the increasingly prevailing view that radical prostatectomy is more likely to be curative than exogenous megavoltage radiation.[45] Radiation, external or interstitial (iodine 125 or gold 198) offers an acceptable alternative if surgery is inadvisable and effectively sterilizes the prostate of its malignant cells in 30% to 50% of suitable cases.[28] However, radical prostatectomy is increasingly recommended for otherwise healthy elderly men, even well into their 70s.[33]

Most men, unfortunately, present with stage C or D disease. An elevated acid phosphatase level, a positive bone scan, or lymph nodes or a large mass of prostatic tumor makes curative procedures unrealistic. One now turns to hormonal manipulation, which includes any of the androgen suppression modalities, such as bilateral orchiectomy, exogenous estrogens, or antiandrogens such as cyproterone. It should be reaffirmed that such therapy does not prolong survival and is therefore not indicated in asymptomatic patients. Diethylstilbestrol in a dosage of 3 mg/day will decrease serum testosterone levels to the castrate range; lower doses are ineffective, and higher doses have no additional effect. Estrogens increase the risk of cardiovascular disease,[48] so bilateral orchiectomy would seem best for both efficacy and safety. There is no advantage in combining two or more androgen suppressant therapies at one time nor in administering another when one is no longer effective. Bone pain from metastases sometimes responds to direct radiation. Chemotherapy may be employed as a last resort but has thus far been largely ineffective.

URINARY DYSFUNCTION IN THE ELDERLY WOMAN

Consideration of urinary disorders in women shifts the emphasis from bladder outlet obstruction to incontinence (see Chapter 43). Nonetheless, urinary retention is a problem in some elderly women.

Age-related changes prominently influence lower urinary tract function. The postmenopausal decline in estrogen secretion affects the urethra as much as the vagina since their epithelium has a common embryologic heritage. Postmenopausal atrophic urethritis should be suspected in symptomatic elderly women who had minimal or no symptoms in their reproductive years. Urethroscopy is not necessary to confirm the presence of a sore, tender, thin, reddened epithelium because these changes can be deduced from the vaginal appearance. The estrogen deficiency often results in a change in the vaginal bacterial flora so that bacterial cystitis or abacterial "urethral syndrome" can plague these women, sometimes to the extent of causing a urethral obstruction.[35]

Functional changes occur in the bladder and urethra with increasing age even in the absence of dysfunction.[6] Trabeculation and hypertrophy are common and may or may not be related to uninhibited contractions (unstable bladder),[36] readily diagnosed by simple urodynamic studies.

Although lower urinary tract disorders are not geriatric inevitabilities but rather represent pathologic conditions it must be conceded that there are predisposing age-associated factors. Cognitive and sensory impairment, problems in walking, and the like interfere even with simple toilet functions. They are often aggravated by common disease processes such as arthritis, hip fractures, stroke, dementia, and Parkinson's disease. An added factor is the wide use of drugs, many of which are antidepressants, analgesics, and antihistamines, that have a profound anticholinergic effect, thus favoring urinary retention.

Urinary Retention in the Elderly Woman

Urinary retention in elderly women must therefore be reckoned with. Intrapelvic tumors such as fibroids, retroverted uterus,[15] or even vaginal tumors may be culpable.[22] Retention can occur when prolapse pulls the bladder into the vagina.[7] More common are the neurologic impairments of diabetes (hypotonic bladder) or nerve damage from neoplasms or herniated disks. One must rule out fecal impaction for which an enema may be curative. The diagnosis of retention of urine may be as easy as palpating a distended bladder. Simple catheterization discloses the post-voiding retained urine, and further workup may then include cystometry, cystoscopy, or intravenous urography as indicated.

Postmenopausal urethritis, stricture, or meatitis can be successfully managed by urethral dilatation and estrogens, either locally or systemically. Used alone estrogen therapy increases the risk of endometrial carcinoma, and combination with progesterone is desirable. Bacteriuria should be treated with appropriate antibiotics.

When significant urinary retention persists, we are confronted by the issue of catheterization. The catheter is a great convenience for the staff in hospitals and nursing homes when an elderly patient has some urinary dysfunction. However, an indwelling catheter is attended by a high morbidity, and even mortality may result from the inevitable infection. Intermittent catheterization is overwhelmingly preferable; it does not carry nearly as high a risk of infection. The urothelium of the bladder has inherent antibacterial properties effective as long as it is usually empty and in the absence of a foreign body such as a catheter. Elderly persons at home can be taught to catheterize themselves or a family member or nurse can do it for them. In institutions, intermittent catheteriza-

tion should also be the rule. A regular schedule with measurement of residual urine is advisable. When the amount of urine residual drops below 50 ml the catheterization may be discontinued.[23] At home, a clean technique, which includes simple washing of the catheter before use, is acceptable.

Sterility should be observed in hospitals or nursing homes because of the virulence of nosocomial organisms. As with indwelling catheters, systemic antibiotics should not be used routinely, although mild urinary antiseptics (methenamine) and acidifiers (ascorbic acid) may be beneficial.

SEXUAL DYSFUNCTION

Societal mores have traditionally interpreted the normal changes of aging as indications that it is no longer necessary or even appropriate to engage in sexual intercourse. Aging changes and religious proscriptions against sex have even greater impact on the elderly woman than on the elderly man. An aging woman may have difficulty adjusting to the loss of youth and beauty. She may confuse loss of reproductive ability with sexuality and become sensitized to diminution in her partner's interest in sex. A study of 800 perimenopausal women in Sweden found that lower socioeconomic status and good mental health were the two most important determinants of sexual attitudes, in contrast to organic and other factors.[25] There are, of course, organic factors, but the older woman often has difficulty in articulating her concern and may use physical complaints to mask a sexual problem.

Postmenopausal women, although still normally desirous of sexual activity, undergo changes in the labia, vagina, uterus, and breasts caused by estrogen and progesterone deprivation. Vaginal length and width decrease, and elasticity diminishes as the walls become thinner and more rigid. Lubrication may be delayed despite strong sexual stimulation. Penetration then becomes painful, and orgasm results in uterine cramps. "Coital anxiety" replaces pleasure, as the effect on the male creates a self-perpetuating cycle of disinterest.[13] There is a fear of failure and ridicule in both sexes. A significant factor is the limitations our culture and institutions impose by depriving the elderly of opportunity and privacy.[34]

Despite these difficulties, men and women of all ages should have the ability to enjoy sex throughout their lives. There has been a dramatic change in attitudes toward sexual behavior and greatly increased information about its physiology.

Nonetheless it is usually the male partner who continues to be responsible for continuity or cessation of sexual activity.

A man's erectile capacity involves several factors: libido, hormonal sufficiency, normal anatomy of the penis with an adequate blood supply, and neural regulation. Seminal emission and ejaculation are separately regulated, and orgasm is chiefly cerebral. Dysfunction of any of these factors results in erectile problems.

The plasma level of testosterone begins to diminish at about age 60, but its relation to erectile capacity remains unclear. The fall is probably due less to diminished secretion than to increased production of serum hormone binding globulin. During the night, the concentrations vary and peak values occur at the time of rapid eye movement sleep. Lower plasma levels of testosterone were once believed responsible for lessened sexual activity. This view has been modified by the finding that sexual intercourse raises the plasma levels of testosterone.[20]

Penile tumescence is the result of vascular engorgement of the corpora cavernosa, so that insufficiency of the arterial blood supply during sexual stimulation will result in erectile dysfunction. Arteriosclerosis and other diseases of blood vessels, especially diabetes, are more common in aging men and are no doubt culpable.[50] Erectile dysfunction may be the first symptom of intermittent claudication in arteriosclerotic patients and of disordered glucose metabolism in diabetics. There is also a "steal syndrome," in which the erection disappears immediately after initiating coital movements.[39] In such cases, blood flow to the penis is sufficient for a normal erection but fails when activity results in dilatation and flow into the arteries of the legs and gluteal region. This is often misinterpreted as being psychogenic.

Diabetes

If has been known for many years that erectile failure is a more common problem among diabetics than in the general population. Frequency of sexual dysfunction in younger diabetic males is around 50%.[49] It is even higher in older diabetics irrespective of the duration of the disease, no doubt a result of the prevalence of diabetic complications with increasing age.[14] Sexual dysfunction in diabetics can be attributed to one or more neurologic, vascular, psychogenic, and possibly hormonal factors. Peripheral neuropathy has been significantly correlated with sexual dysfunction.[17]

Norepinephrine, the probable neurotransmitter in the corpora cavernosa, has been found to be deficient in diabetic men.[38] Vascular changes affect both large and small vessels in long-term diabetics, resulting in penile arterial insufficiency. Techniques of penile blood pressure measurement have demonstrated such a reduction.[1] Pathologic conditions in the arterial bed supplying the penis have been observed in diabetics.[50] Studies of endocrinologic disorders affecting diabetics have not been conclusive, but a hypogonadotropic hypogonadism with response to chorionic gonadotropin and testosterone has been claimed.[52] Much more convincing has been the psychologic aspects. Some diabetics, with knowledge of the relationship, assume impotence even if it is not truly present. Depression, anxiety, fear of complications, and the daily restrictions of the disease all play a significant role.[47]

Heart Disease

Every man knows that disease not directly affecting the genital area can decrease sexual drive. With advancing age, illnesses occur more frequently and are often multiple. Fatigue is a frequent complaint in the geriatric group and certainly erodes sexual inclination. Men who have survived a coronary occlusion or are coronary prone are often afraid of coitus and "the strain on the heart." Erectile failure may be due to lowering of blood pressure, systemic and penile, by drugs such as β-blockers or digitalis. Well-treated chronic heart disease should not significantly increase sexual risk. In a study of men with coronary disease the mean maximal heart rate during intercourse and orgasm was 117 beats/min while during their usual occupational activity it was 120 beat/min. Electrocardiographic changes and anginal symptoms were comparable in the two situations.[27] Diminished sexual desire and erectile failure in those on long-term digoxin treatment has been ascribed to hormonal derangement, but one study showed no correlation between levels of testosterone or estradiol and sexual functioning.[43]

Chronic Renal Failure

Uremia undoubtedly diminishes libido in both men and women. Loss of libido is often worsened by dialysis but dramatically improves after renal transplantation. The mechanisms involved are not clear, but metabolic derangements and hormonal changes can be significant. Prolactin increase may be an important cause of erectile failure inasmuch as it can depress testosterone secretion. Treatment with bromocriptine, which lowers serum prolactin, has been observed to restore sexual function.[57]

Chronic Lung Disease

Dyspnea is a prominent symptom during sexual intercourse. The physical requirements for coitus in terms of oxygen consumption can be considerable.[3] Although erectile failure in men with chronic bronchitis, asthma, or emphysema is common, a careful study showed that this was due less to the pulmonary disorder than to interpersonal problems created by the disease.[31] Information on sexual techniques such as having male patients adopt the side-by-side position or lying supine with the partner on top can be very helpful.

Neurologic Disease

A host of neurologic disorders interfere with potency. In spinal cord injury, in cases of a high lesion, erectile capacity is maintained; cervical lesions leave almost all patients with an intact reflexogenic pattern.[5] Complete lower neuron lesions incapacitate 90% sexually.[12] Special measures such as prostheses are usually necessary.[11]

Parkinsonism accelerates the attrition of potency in aged males who may be otherwise healthy. Even women with this disease are aware of decreased orgasmic potential. Akinesia and rigidity are associated with fatigue, and a sense of worthlessness is additive.[46] Levodopa was touted as an aphrodisiac a decade ago, but this has proved to be a disappointment. Discussion and reassurance is extremely relevant in this disease.

Stroke patients stabilized after the acute phase are often depressed and demoralized with respect to sexual activity. Paralysis and sensory loss can profoundly impair the patient's body image. However, unless there has been severe cerebral insult, the sexual response is usually preserved through the limbic system and spinal cord. There is little effect on most autonomic functioning so that erection and ejaculation in the male and lubrication in the female can usually occur. Despite aphasia and cognitive loss, obstacles to sexual activity can be overcome with reassurance and education. For patients with motor problems, communication between spouses about comfortable positioning and the use of props such as pillows can be effective.

Arthritis

There is a mechanical barrier to sexual functioning in arthritic patients, especially when there is involvement of the hip joints. The FABER maneuver, an acronym for *f*lexion, *ab*duction, and *e*xternal *r*otation at the hips, performed supine is helpful in identifying mechanical limitations that may interfere with coitus.[16] Pain can be a dominant problem. Nevertheless the patient should be encouraged to try a variety of positions to discover which is most comfortable and requires the least energy expenditure. Many couples have found that side-by-side positions are the most satisfactory (either face to face or back to front) when spine and hip mobility are problems.

Back pain is yet another problem in the elderly. Most back pain is due to muscle weakness and inelasticity, but herniated disks with sciatica may occur. Again, sexual activity is not precluded. Prior to intercourse it may be wise for the patient to take a hot bath or use other heat applications, a counterirritant, and an analgesic. If the female partner has the back problem, the above position may be used by the male without discomfort if she places a pillow under her buttocks. In other cases, the side-by-side position causes least pain. If the male has the back pain, it may be necessary to abandon the male-above, female-below position and encourage the woman to be more active.

Prostatectomy

There have been numerous reports of sexual activity being adversely affected by prostatectomy.[29] However, there is no specific reason why this should be so. Psychological factors are important and may be accentuated by prostatectomy-induced retrograde ejaculation. However, studies indicate that patient's level of anxiety and preoperative patient education are determining factors.[61] Nocturnal penile tumescence monitoring preoperatively and postoperatively in 35 randomly selected patients showed no significant difference between recordings for any given patient.[58] I, too, have found the most important factor to be preoperative reassurance and discussion of the anticipated retrograde ejaculation to explain the absence of an ejaculate.

Drugs

Many classes of medication have been described as possible factors in impotence. Excluding the obvious antiandrogenics, the drugs most often reported include the antihypertensive medications, especially propranolol and clonidine; sedatives; and antidepressants, both the monoamine-oxidase inhibitors and the tricyclics. Controlled studies of their effects on potency are lacking, so in individual cases the physician can only discontinue each drug for several weeks and observe. Alcohol affects both the neural mechanisms and the individual's psychologic status; a trial on disulfiram (Antabuse) would seem to be worthwhile. Methyldopa depletes biogenic amines and also increases the prolactin level, so it is difficult to be precise about its specific antierection effect. More recently, tobacco has been accused of causing erectile problems.[19]

Differential Diagnosis of Psychogenic and Organic Erectile Failure

Failure of erection can have a variety of causes. Of primary importance is the history and the obtaining of a precise description of the dysfunction. If a man has good erections during the night or on awakening, or with masturbation, the essential mechanisms must be considered to be intact and therefore difficulty with intromission is probably psychogenic. These facts are not always easily documented, and some basic tests are generally required. After the physical examination, plasma levels of testosterone and prolactin, penile blood pressure measurements, and nocturnal penile tumescence studies are desirable. When indicated, infusion cavernosonography can be helpful in localizing defects or shunts in the corpora. However, in many cases accurate diagnosis can be made by history and physical examination alone without expensive or invasive laboratory tests.[51]

Therapy

Management of sexual problems in the elderly requires a sensitive and informed physician. It must be appreciated that sexual desire and expression are normal in the elderly and total functional loss is unusual. A sympathetic, nonjudgmental approach may reveal sexual dissatisfactions to be an important basis for vague complaints about health and even for hypochondriasis. There is a great variation in capacities, which are sometimes quite robust, and in realities, which are not.

For the male, morning erections, wet dreams, and masturbation are physical signs of potency. Retarded ejaculation, lengthening of refractory periods, and slower achievement of full erection are normal in advancing years, and I have found the elderly patient to be highly receptive to this affirmation of normality. He must be dissuaded from the rather destructive attitude that normal sexual performance is nothing less than the solid erection and vigorous orgasm of youth.

Women are often relieved to learn that the painful intercourse due to an estrogen-deprived vaginal muscosa is eminently treatable by topical hormonal creams and lubricants. Her partner's noninterest in sex may be misinterpreted as her failure. For these and other reasons, masturbation is common among elderly women, but there is even greater reluctance to discuss this than among men.

Since women statistically outlive men, the proportion of older women increases especially in settings such as the nursing home. Nonjudgmental discussion on finding a sex partner may include advice regarding the male's delay in achieving erection and the verbal and physical assistance required. "Stuffing" the flaccid penis into the vagina is a rewarding technique for both partners, and there is nothing perverse about an orgasm for one while the other enjoys the intimacy. For some, touching, caressing, closeness, companionship, and caring are satisfying alternatives.

More active therapy is demanded by others. Indiscriminate prescription of hormonal therapy in the elderly has been disappointing. Testosterone is clearly helpful in hypogonadal men and to others who otherwise inexplicably have low serum testosterone levels.[54] Bromocriptine is effective in hyperprolactinemia (but testosterone is not).[57] Even in the absence of hypogonadism, testosterone sometimes has a placebo effect, and there are scattered reports of some benefit over and above this effect. A drug called Afrodex may be in this category[41]; it consists of 5 mg nuxvomica extract, 5 mg methyltestosterone, and 5 mg yohimbine hydrochloride. The reclamation of yohimbine, an x-adrenergic antagonist and a traditional aphrodisiac, has led to popular empiric use (6 mg three times a day).[42]

Finally, penile prosthetic implantation is available if desired by both partners. Currently the two better choices are the inflatable and the semi-rigid prostheses. Technical success with both is high, but the former has a higher complication rate and for the older man the semi-rigid prosthetic implantation would be more advisable.

The geriatrician should also be aware of the deviant sexual behavior infrequently seen in the elderly. Long after sexual performance has waned or vanished, delusions of infidelity may appear. Behavioral disturbances include exhibitionism, voyeurism, and pedophilia. These profound disturbances of senile dementia require expert psychotherapy. There are anecdotal instances of aggressive copulation or masturbation behavior in elderly nursing home residents. Control of a sexually oriented wanderer may call for use of tranquilizers.

REFERENCES

1. Abelson D: Diagnostic value of the penile pulse and blood pressure: A Doppler study of impotence in diabetics. J Urol 113:636, 1975
2. Abrams PH: Investigation of postprostatectomy problems. Urology 15:209, 1980
3. Bartlett RG Jr: Physiologic responses during coitus. J Appl Physiol 9:469, 1956
4. Bisson J, Vickers M Jr, Fagan WT Jr: Bone scan: In clinical perspective. J Urol 111:665, 1974
5. Bors E, Comarr AE: Neurological disturbances of sexual function with special reference to 529 patients with spinal cord injury. Urol Survey 10:191, 1960
6. Brocklehurst JC, Dillane JB: Studies of the female bladder in old age. Gerontol Clin 8:285, 1966
7. Brown ADG: Post menopausal urinary problems. Clin Obstet Gynecol 4:181, 1977
8. Brown AG, Turner-Warwick R: A urodynamic evaluation of urinary incontinence in the female and its treatment. Urol Clin North Am 6:31, 1979
9. Castro JE, Griffiths HJL, Scheckman R: Significance of signs and symptoms in benign prostatic hypertrophy. Br Med J 2:598, 1969
10. Christoffersen I, Moller I: Excretory urography: A superflous routine examination in patients with prostatic hypertrophy. Eur Urol 7:65, 1981
11. Cole T: Sexuality and the spinal cord injured. In Green R (ed): Human Sexuality: A Health Practitioner's Text, 2nd ed. Baltimore, Williams & Wilkins, 1979
12. Comarr AE: Sexual function among patients with spinal cord injury. Urology 25:134, 1970
13. Cooper A: Outpatient treatment of impotence. J Nerv Ment Dis 149:360, 1969
14. Deutsch S, Sherman L: Previously unrecognized diabetes mellitus in sexually impotent men. JAMA 244:2430, 1980
15. Doran J, Roberts M: Acute urinary retention in the female. Br J Urol 47:793, 1975
16. Ehrlich GE: Total Management of the Arthritic Patient. Philadelphia, JB Lippincott, 1973
17. Ellenberg M: Impotence in diabetes: The neurologic factor. Ann Intern Med 75:213, 1971
18. Fair WR, Couch J, Wehner N: Prostatic antibacterial factor. Urology 7:139, 1975
19. Forsberg L, Gustavii B, Hojerback T, Olsson AM: Impotence, smoking and β-blocking drug. Fertil Steril 31:589, 1979
20. Fox C, Ismail A, Love D, Kirkham K, Loraine J: Studies on the relationship between plasma testosterone levels in human sexual activity. J Endocrinol 52:51, 1972
21. Franks LM: Latent carcinoma of the prostate. J Pathol Bacteriol 68:603, 1954
22. Freed S, Haleem S, Wiener I, Feldman J: Bladder outlet obstruction caused by vaginal fibromyoma: female prostate. J Urol 13:30, 1974
23. Freed SZ: Urinary incontinence in the elderly. Hosp Pract March 17(3):81, 1982
24. Gardiner RA, Fitzpatrick JM, Constable AR, Cranage RW, O'Donoghue EPN, Wickham JEA: Improved techniques in radionuclide imaging of prostatic lymph nodes. Br J Urol 51:561, 1979
25. Hallstrom T: Sexuality in the climacteric. Clin Obstet Gynecol 4:227, 1977
26. Harrison GSM: The prognosis of prostatic cancer in the younger man. Br J Urol 55:315, 1983
27. Hellerstein HK, Friedman EH: Sexual activity in the post coronary patient. Arch Intern Med 125:987, 1970
28. Herr H, Whitmore WR Jr: Significance of prostatic biopsies after radiation therapy for carcinoma of the prostate. Prostate 3:339, 1982
29. Holtgrewe HL, Valk WL: Late results of transurethral prostatectomy. J Urol 92:51, 1964
30. Huben R, Natarajan N, Pontes E, Mettlin C, Smart CR, Murphy G: Carcinoma of prostate in men less than 55 years old: Data from American College of Surgeons National Survey. Urology 20:585, 1982
31. Kass I, Updegraff K, Muffly RB: Sex in chronic pulmonary disease. Med Aspects Human Sexuality 6:33, 1972
32. Kaufman JJ, Raz S: Symposium on Male Incontinence. Urol Clin North Am 5, 1978
33. Kraus CT, Persky L: Radical perineal prostatectomy in patients over age of seventy. Urology 18:368, 1981
34. Laury GV: Reflections in aging in the United States. Geriatrics 28:178, 1973
35. Lipsky H. Urodynamic assessment of women with urethral syndrome. Eur Urol 3:202, 1977
36. McGuire EJ: Urinary dysfunction in the aged: Neurological consideration. Bull NY Acad Med 56:275, 1980
37. Meares EM, Stamey TA: Bacteriologic localization patterns in bacterial prostatis and urethritis. Invest Urol 19:31, 1981
38. Melman A, Henry D: The possible role of the catecholamines of the corpora in penile erection. J Urol 121:419, 1979
39. Metz P, Mathiesen FR: External iliac "steal syndrome" leading to a defect in penile erection and impotence. Vasc Surg 13:70, 1979
40. Meyhoff HH, Hald T: Are doctors able to assess prostatic size? Scand J Urol Nephrol 12:219, 1978
41. Miller W: Afrodex in the treatment of impotence:

A double-blind crossover study. Curr Ther Res 10: 354, 1968

42. Morales A, Surridge DHC, Marshall PG, Fenemore J: Nonhormonal pharmacological treatment of organic impotence. J Urol 128:45, 1982

43. Neri A, Aigen M, Zukerman Z, Bahary C: Subjective assessment of sexual dysfunction of patients on long-term administration of digoxin. Arch Sex Behavior 9:319, 1980

44. Paulson DF: Assessment of Anatomic Extent and Biologic Hazard of Prostatic Adenocarcinoma. Urology 15:537, 1980

45. Paulson DF, Lin GH, Hinshaw W, Stephani S, and the Urology-Oncology Research Group: Radical surgery versus radiotherapy for adenocarcinoma of the prostate. J Urol 128:502, 1982

46. Paulson GW: The psychological aspects of parkinsonism. Ohio State Med J 77:711, 1981

47. Renshaw D: Impotence and diabetes mellitus. Compr Ther 2:47, 1976

48. Robinson RMG, Thomas BS: Effect of hormonal therapy on plasma testosterone levels in prostatic carcinoma. Br Med J 4:391, 1971

49. Rubin A, Babbott D; Impotence and diabetes mellitus. JAMA 168:498, 1958

50. Ruzbarsky V, Michel V: Morphological changes in the arterial bed of the penis with aging. Invest Urol 15:194, 1977

51. Saypol DC, Peterson AG, Howards SS, Yazel JJ: Impotence: Are the newer diagnostic methods a necessity? J Urol 130:260, 1983

52. Schoffling K, Federlin K, Ditschuneit H, Pfeiffer EF: Disorders of sexual function in male diabetics. J Am Diab Assoc 12:519, 1963

53. Siegelman S, Freed S: Serendipity in the diagnosis of renal carcinoma. J Can Assoc Radiol 23:251, 1972

54. Skakkeback N, Bancroft J, Davidson D, Warner P: Androgen replacement with oral testosterone undecamoate in hypogondal men: A double blind controlled study. Clin Endocrinol 14:96, 1981

55. Smart CJ, Jenkins JD: The role of transurethral prostatectomy in chronic prostatitis. Br J Urol 45:654, 1973

56. Smedly HM, Sinnott M, Freedman LS, Macaskill P, Naylor CPE, Pillers EMK: Age and survival in prostatic carcinoma. Br J Urol 55:529, 1954

57. Spark R, White R, Conally P: Impotence is not always psychogenic. JAMA 243:750, 1980

58. So EP, Ho PC, Bodenstab W, Parsons CL: Erectile impotence associated with transurethral prostatectomy. Urology 19:259, 1982

59. Susset JG, Servot-Viquier D, Lamy F, Madernas P, Black R: Collagen in 155 human bladders. Invest Urol 16:204, 1978

60. Turner-Warwick R: Clinical urodynamics. Urol Clin North Am 6:13, 1979

61. Zohar J, Meiaz D, Maoz B, Durst N: Factors influencing sexual activity after prostatectomy: A prospective study. J Urol 116:332, 1976

20   Geriatric Gynecology

Hugh R. K. Barber

The number of individuals in the United States over the age of 65 is currently estimated at over 25 million. By the year 2000 it is expected that this will rise to 31 million, and by 2020 to over 45 million. In addition, life expectancies have been on the rise during the 20th century. These two trends will create a population of elderly that is large in number and also older in years. Since women are more likely than men to survive into late life, there are 1.3 women for every man over the age of 65. It is obvious that geriatric gynecology will play an increasingly important role in the care of American women as this century draws to a close and a new century starts.

There are hardly any persisting differences of opinion on the concepts of menopause, premenopause, postmenopause, and climacteric. The usefulness of the division into early and late postmenopause is also generally recognized. Because of the increasing life expectancy of women, postmenopause is the part of their life that is becoming longer. Many women will spend one third of their lives in the postmenopause and will be affected by metabolic, cardiovascular, degenerative, and neoplastic disorders that may present as or be complicated by gynecologic symptoms and signs.

There has been much written and much disagreement both here and abroad on the time concepts of aging and of geriatric gynecology. Writing some 30 years ago, Stieglitz considered geriatric medicine to begin with the 40th year of life.[4] He distinguishes a period of later maturity, 40 to 60 years; a period of senescence, 60 to 75 years; and a period of senility after the 75th year of life. Russian aging parameters were suggested by Vojta, in 1965, as follows: elderly people, 60 to 74 years; old people, 75 to 89 years, and very old people, 90 years old and older.[5] The senium is taken to mean the last stage of old age. However, there is still no agreement as to whether all elderly female patients or only especially elderly patients are to be assigned to the senium.

In this chapter, geriatric gynecologic problems will be designated as beginning at the age of 65. However, even in gynecology it is more and more difficult to refer to the senium from the 65th or even from the 60th year of life and to designate all female patients as aged women from this age on. In the view of Kraatz,[2] the first phase of geriatric gynecology might approximate the late menopause, and the senium begins only after the 70th year of life or even later.

EVALUATION OF THE PATIENT

Common Signs and Symptoms of Gynecologic Disease

The most frequent symptom that occasions an inpatient admission is genital bleeding. Its causes in the postmenopausal women will be discussed later in the chapter. The management of genital displacement in elderly women is very common. Urinary incontinence is frequently associated with genital displacements and constitutes not only a medical problem but also social and nursing problems, especially in very old women. Pruritus vulvae is also one of the most frequent symptoms in geriatric gynecologic pathology.

History

The confidence of the patient must be gained, a relaxed and friendly atmosphere must be created, and the practitioner must be prepared to be unhurried when taking a history from an elderly woman.

A significant number of elderly women may be unable to give a useful history of their obstetric and gynecologic experience or the age at which menopause occurred. These patients are often not clear on whether they ever had any hormone therapy. Their past medical and surgical histories are often difficult to obtain. It is useful if a relative or a close friend of the patient is available, but often this is not possible. Some elderly patients may complain of, or be referred for, so-called vaginal bleeding but on close questioning are uncertain whether the bleeding is coming from the urethra, vagina, or the anal area.

Fortunately, many elderly patients are fully alert and possess excellent recall. Thus, usually an accurate obstetric, menstrual, postmenopausal, and gynecologic history can be taken. The patient should be asked about drug ingestion, particularly of hormones. It is also important to explore the patient's eating habits and nutrition.

Epidemiologic data suggest that anxiety disorders are exceedingly common, occurring more frequently in women than men across all age-groups. It is estimated that approximately 5% of all women, at some time in their lives, will have an anxiety disorder of sufficient severity to interfere with function in their usual roles. An estimated 10% to 15% of women over the age of 65 experience anxiety sufficiently severe to warrant medical intervention. Anxiety in the elderly may present as neurologic, gastrointestinal, cardiovascular, or respiratory symptoms. The two most common genitourinary symptoms are pruritus vaginae or ani or dyspareunia.

The Victorian concept that all sexual activity ends at the time of the menopause is totally inaccurate. Many studies have shown that men and particularly women are able to function sexually late in their lives. Therefore, it is very important to ask the patient about sexual function. If the inquiry is approached in an open but discerning manner, it reinforces the patient's regard for the physician.

Sexuality and sexual function in the menopausal and postmenopausal years is now receiving a great deal of attention in the literature. It seems that women who are sexually active during this period of their lives are approximately 22 pounds heavier than those who are not. Thus, in terms of estrogen storage and conversion, as well as sexual activity, some adiposity is probably important. This focuses attention on the importance of diet and nutrition on some of the age-related processes.

Gynecologic Examination

The geriatric patient often is reluctant to have a gynecologic examination and must be educated to the need for periodic examinations. The patient must be impressed with the fact that cancer of the genitalia or breast can occur at any age; for example, cancer of the ovary peaks in incidence at around age 77 to 80. Many older patients recognize that they have atrophic vaginal and vulvar tissue and that an examination may be painful. Therefore, they are inclined to avoid routine examinations. It is important that the patient receive as little discomfort and pain as possible during the examination.

The examining physician should carefully observe the vulva, urethra, and Bartholin's and Skene's glands, and it is important to palpate the texture of the structures. A small speculum or Peterson vaginal speculum should be carefully inserted, holding the blades parallel to the introitus. The instrument is turned slowly so that the posterior blade rests against the posterior wall of the vagina. Gentle downward pressure on the instrument opens the vagina without disturbing the sensitive organs anteriorly. The cervix is identified, any vaginal secretion is removed, and a careful Papanicolaou smear is taken from the cervical canal if possible and also from the posterior fornix. Although it is most important to screen the endometrium, it is better to do this later in the examination or to schedule it as a separate procedure after the patient has established confidence in the physician–patient relationship.

A careful one-finger examination of the entire length and breadth of the vagina including the fornices should be carried out first. Next the uterus should be outlined as to size, shape, and mobility, and then the adnexal area is examined. It is important to explain each step of the examination to the patient and to assure her that if there is any pain the examination will be stopped immediately. Following this, the lubricated middle finger is inserted into the patient's rectum for a rectovaginal examination that explores the rectovaginal septum and the cardinal as well as the uterosacral ligaments. A careful rectal examination should be carried out, including a test for occult blood.

It is often necessary to have one or more attendants to help lift and position a patient for the gynecologic examination. The patient's breasts and abdomen must be routinely palpated. In the presence of neurologic, neuromuscular, or skeletal disorders, the patient's legs may have to be supported by the attendants. If a severely disabled patient is brought on a stretcher for examination, it may be necessary to perform the examination on the stretcher in the left, lateral (Sims) position. In this instance the speculum examination may be difficult, even dangerous, because of the severe, atrophic vulvitis and vaginitis. The physician must decide whether symptoms warrant speculum examination and whether a routine Papanicolaou smear is necessary in view of the low yield of cytologic abnormalities in the asymptomatic patient over 60 years of age. A rectal examination should be performed routinely in all such patients as a separate procedure distinguished from the so-called pelvic examination.

DISEASES OF THE VULVA

The vulvar and vaginal tissues of every woman who is several years postmenopausal and who does not take estrogen are more or less atrophic. Shrinkage, loss of elasticity, and dryness of the vaginal mucosa are due to estrogen withdrawal. Puckering of the vulvar tissue and of the introitus, even in the multipara, may make penile intromission exquisitely painful, and deflection of the penis anteriorly by a rigid perineum may create pressure on the urethral meatus, causing urethritis, local inflammation, and dysuria.

Many vulvar diseases are similar in different age-groups. In the geriatric group there is an increase in the incidence of diabetic vulvitis, hypertrophic dystrophy, hypotrophic dystrophy, and lichen sclerosus. Women with these lesions often present with burning, pruritus, or difficulty in coitus.

Intertrigo, although encountered in patients of all ages, is frequently seen in obese older individuals who have difficulty in bathing and cleansing their perineum and vulva. In consequence, the skin covering their perineum, genital crural folds, labia majora, and thighs is constantly moistened by perspiration and soiled by urine. Those with intertrigo usually complain of perineal itching and burning. Inspection shows the area to be superficially denuded, shiny, hyperemic, and moist; a scanty, malodorous discharge may cover the affected area.

Senile angiomas are small, usually multiple, red, elevated papules that are up to 3 mm in diameter and that bleed freely when scrubbed or scratched. They are quite innocent, but the bleeding frightens patients. Senile angiomas are not excised unless the patient is unduly alarmed.

Sebaceous cysts of the vulva are small yellowish-gray nodules in the skin covering the labia; they are rarely more than 1 cm in diameter. The foul-smelling, purulent material extruded when a sebaceous cyst becomes infected and ruptured or the discovery of the small lump may frighten the patient. Very large sebaceous cysts that become repeatedly infected should be removed.

Clitoral phimosis may cause an inspissated smegma to collect beneath the prepuce, producing discomfort. The area is usually very red and resembles balanitis in men.

For many decades vulvar diseases characterized by pruritus, atrophy, and/or hyperplasia (kraurosis, leukoplakia) were assumed to be precursors of vulvar cancer. However, the term *dystrophia* is now given to this group to obviate the old concept relating them to vulvar neoplasms.

The dystrophies are chronic disorders that persist over many years. Pruritus, often to a marked degree, is their most universal symptom and may make a patient a veritable invalid. Stenosis due to atrophy of the vestibular mucosa may prevent coitus and often interferes with normal urination.

Treatment of vulvar dystrophy depends on the diagnosis that is made. It is axiomatic that any lesion that persists for 3 or 4 weeks should be biopsied. One of the estrogenic vaginal creams applied just to the vulvar area may be tried. However, in some patients this causes a hyperemia of the vulva that may become so uncomfortable that treatment must be stopped. For atrophy of the vulva with persistent burning, application two or three time daily of an ointment of 2% testosterone propionate in white petrolatum seems to have the best effect. It should be continued daily for 6 weeks and then reduced to two or three times weekly and maintained, or the condition will return.

There are certain cases with hypertrophic dystrophy that are best treated with an antipruritic agent such as crotamiton (Eurax) combined with betamethasone (Valisone) ointment (Eurax, 30% and Valisone 70%) applied twice daily. Combined with ice bags to the perineum this medication gives patients marked relief and sometimes breaks the cycle of burning and itching. Combined testosterone-corticosteroid therapy is used in the treatment of mixed dystrophy: testosterone may be applied on alternate days, the corticosteroids on the intervening days. Testosterone must be continued, but corticosteroids can be discontinued after the symptoms resulting from the mixed dystrophy have been relieved.

Primary malignant disease of the vulva represents 5% to 10% of female cancers. The most common lesion is invasive or intraepithelial epidermoid cancer, which is most often seen in women well over 60 years of age. Epithelial dysplasia coexists with about 50% of invasive cancers and is considered by many oncologists to be a premalignant vulvar disease. A second primary malignancy affecting the cervix, breast, or uterus is found in about 15% of the patients, often in association with a primary vulvar neoplasm. It is obvious that these patients should have careful evaluation with biopsy.

Treatment for invasive carcinoma of the vulva is surgical with a radical or modified radical excisional vulvectomy and superficial inguinal node dissection. The decision about excision of the deep nodes is usually left to the responsible surgeon. Radiation therapy is often given to the nodal areas, and the results seem favorable.

DISEASES OF THE VAGINA

Reduction of estrogen support is responsible for most of the common symptoms associated with vaginal disorders. The vaginal epithelium becomes thin and relatively avascular and inelastic; rugae disappear, and the epithelium appears dry and glazed.

The most common symptoms suggestive of vaginal disease are leukorrhea, frequency and urgency of urination, dyspareunia, itching, and bleeding. In elderly women 80% of the patients studied cytologically are estrogen deficiency. Patients who complain of these symptoms may have no findings other than those associated with senile vaginitis. In the absence of a proven pathogen the most common treatment for senile vaginitis is topical estrogen cream. This therapy should be continued for at least 1 month. The patient should be instructed to insert about one fourth of an applicator of estrogen cream into the vagina every fourth night for approximately 2 months. Inserting a full applicator of the cream usually results in some of the cream running out, and having been mixed with vaginal secretion, it may cause a marked irritation around the vulva.

Infections with *Trichomonas vaginalis* and occasionally *Candida* may be superimposed on senile vaginitis. The diagnosis should be confirmed, and in addition to treating the senile vaginitis, infection should be treated with metronidazole for 10 days and the *Candida* infection treated with a topical antifungal agent for approximately the same time.

Primary vaginal carcinoma is uncommon, accounting for less than 1% of cancers of the female reproductive tract, compared with 3% or 4% incidence of vulvar cancer. It is usually epidermoid, presenting as an ulcer high in the posterior vaginal fornix. Any persistent lesion in the vagina must be biopsied and a decision made on the management. Radiation therapy is the usual method of treatment.

DISEASES OF THE CERVIX

The cervix often undergoes atrophic changes that are referred to as atrophic cervicitis. This is usually associated with atrophic vaginitis and is best treated with an estrogenic cream. Chronic inflammation of the cervix in the geriatric patient may occur secondary to an atrophic cervicitis. It may also result from chronic irritation by pessaries or poor hygiene. Frequent offending organisms include streptococci, *E Scherichia coli,* and a wide variety of other organisms. Acute cervicitis was once rare in the postmenopausal patient but with changes in life style involving intercourse with more partners, the postmenopausal patient is experiencing acute cervicitis more frequently. *C. albicans, T. vaginalis, Chlamydia,* and human papilloma virus are occasional causes of acute cervicitis postmenopausally.

Benign tumors of the uterine cervix are uncommon with the exception of cervical polyps. In addition, several proliferative but nonspecific conditions may produce swelling of the cervix such as endocervical glandular hyperplasia. Postmenopausal patients with a lacerated cervix may develop ectropion.

With the increased use of the Papanicolaou smear and greater awareness of the pathology that can occur in the uterus and cervix more cases of cervical intraepithelial neoplasia are being found in patients in the postmenopausal years. These include the whole spectrum from mild through severe dysplasia on to *in situ* carcinoma and microinvasive carcinoma. Because the squamocolumnar junction is high in the canal and is often stenotic, some of these patients need a cone biopsy for a definitive diagnosis. Further treatment will depend on the microscopic pathologic findings.

Sarcomas and melanomas are rare tumors that may arise in the uterine cervix. Also, metastases and spread from other nearby organs to the cervix have been reported.

Carcinoma of the cervix is encountered less often in the postmenopausal patient than in the younger patient. The difference in the incidence is due to no small part to the widespread use of Papanicolaou smears as screening procedures. Even so, elderly patients should be examined for cervical carcinoma just as they were premenopausally.

DISEASES OF THE UTERUS

The uterus undergoes retrogressive changes and becomes small and atrophic. Leiomyomas tend to atrophy, although they may still present problems. There are many causes for postmenopausal genital bleeding, but endometrial carcinoma must always be ruled out. Treatment with estrogens, anticoagulants, or a number of other medications, as well as the presence of blood dyscrasia, should always be considered. Bleeding may be due to estrogen therapy, to a collection of bloody fluid in the endometrial cavity bursting through an occluded cervix, to an estrogen-producing ovarian tumor, to a lesion of the vagina or vulva, or to coital, instrumental, or digital trauma. Whatever its presumed cause, it is mandatory that such procedures as are necessary be performed to exclude endometrial cancer or other genital cancer. Endometrial biopsies and lavages are often ill suited for studying the endometrium of the senescent patient. She should, instead, be hospitalized for a thorough examination, including curettage.

Carcinoma of the uterus ranks as the fifth most common cause of death in women in whom cancer develops and who are 75 years of age or older. Diabetes mellitus, obesity, certain ovarian tumors, and hypertension are among the risk factors for uterine cancer. In patients who are unable to distinguish bleeding from the urethra, the vagina, or the anal canal, it may be necessary to perform cystoscopy and sigmoidoscopy in addition to investigating the reproductive tract.

The management of endometrial carcinoma has evolved from preoperative irradiation followed by hysterectomy to surgery as an initial procedure followed by a decision about the type and extent of the external irradiation. All patients with carcinoma of the endometrium are given a radiation implant into the vagina. This has decreased the number of recurrences of cancer of the vaginal vault. Patients with a normal-sized uterus and a well-differentiated adenocarcinoma confined to stage I can be treated with surgery alone without additional radiation therapy.

DISEASES OF THE OVARY

The ovary is atrophic in the postmenopausal period. Acute oophoritis may occur secondary to diverticulitis of the large bowel.

There are no functional disorders of the ovary in the geriatric female and any enlargement has to be regarded as a neoplasm but not necessarily a malignancy.

Cortical stromal hyperplasia is characterized by moderate to marked nonneoplastic proliferation of the ovarian stroma. The disease is more likely to occur in the postmenopausal patient, in whom a slight degree of hyperplasia of ovarian stroma should not be considered as significantly abnormal. Patients may present with signs of virilization such as hirsutism owing to the overproduction of androgen. If the ovary can be palpated and is equal in size to that in the premenopausal patient, it is abnormal and should be surgically excised.

The palpable postmenopausal ovary may contain fibroma or Brenner cell tumor. Most of these are benign and are clinically suspected at the time of pelvic examination. However, thecomas, if they function, produce signs of estrogenic stimulation in the postmenopausal woman. Thecomas are generally benign tumors. Many gynecologists believe that granulosa cell and thecal cell tumors often occur together and that with appropriate stains the thecal elements can be identified.

The ovary is unique in that it not only gives rise to a great number of tumors but it is also the recipient of metastases from a variety of organs. The breast and colon are the two most commonly encountered cancers that metastasize to the ovary. Thus it is important that patients have a thorough metastatic workup to make sure that the tumor is primary in the ovary. An example of secondary tumors is Krukenberg tumors, which present as kidney shaped, bilateral ovarian tumors with a histology characterized by signet ring cells.

Ovarian carcinoma, the leading cause of death from gynecologic cancer, is the most frustrating problem that the physician faces. The difficulty in making an early diagnosis is evidenced by the fact that 60% or 70% are already in stage III and IV when they present for initial treatment. Overall survival for the truly invasive, common epithelial cancer is seldom better than 25% at 5 years.

The greatest number of patients appear between ages 50 and 70, but the peak incidence is about age 77. It is obvious that the ovary gets too old to function but never gets too old to form a cancer. Although it has been stated that there are no early symptoms of ovarian cancer, reports in the literature contradict this statement. A great number of women with ovarian cancer have vague abdominal complaints for a long time before the diagnosis is made. Many of these women have had a thorough workup, including barium enema and gastrointestinal series before a serious attempt at a pelvic examination was carried out. It is, therefore, important to rule out ovarian cancer in any woman over age 40, particularly if nulliparous or with a history of involuntary sterility or multiple spontaneous abortions who presents with vague abdominal symptoms not identified by the usual workup. These patients must be watched very carefully, and if indeed the suspicion is great enough, the patient should have surgical exploration. It is important to examine patients over age 40 every 6 months. They should be instructed to use an enema before coming in for a pelvic examination. Any woman more than 2 years postmenopausal who presents with a palpable ovary that is normal for the premenopausal years should have a careful workup. If on a repeat examination findings are confirmed, surgical exploration should be carried out. This finding has been designated the postmenopausal palpable ovary (PMPO) syndrome.

The treatment for carcinoma of the ovary is surgical removal of the uterus, fallopian tubes, ovaries, omentum, and appendix. The surgery should be aggressive without creating an inordinate morbidity and mortality. Radiation therapy has value in the management of germ cell tumors and gonadal stromal tumors, but in common epithelial ovarian cancer external radiation therapy should be used to treat supraclavicular and inguinal nodes. If there is an involved area of residual cancer against the pelvic wall, this can be outlined by metal clips and radiation can be directed to that area. The adjuvant treatment of choice is triple chemotherapy. The drugs most often employed are cyclophosphamide, *cis*-platinum, and doxorubicin (Adriamycin). Since these patients are elderly, it is important to make sure that the cardiac ejection fraction and the electrocardiogram are within normal limits before administering doxorubicin and the renal function must be carefully evaluated before *cis*-platinum is given.

DISEASES OF THE FALLOPIAN TUBE

Inflammation of the fallopian tube, a common disorder in the childbearing age, is extremely rare in the postmenopausal patient. Hydrosalpinx, a dilated fallopian tube with accumulation of clear, serous fluid related to an acute process that occurred years before, is rarely found in the postmenopausal patient.

Benign neoplasms of the fallopian tube are uncommon. They are usually asymptomatic and are discovered as incidental findings when the abdomen is explored for other reasons. Adenomatoid tumor, the most common benign tumor of fallopian tube, can also be seen on the surface of the uterus, ovary, and cul-de-sac. Other rare benign tumors include leiomyomas of the fallopian tubes and, very rarely, adenomyomas and papillomas may occur. Clinically, any pathology found in the fallopian tube in the postmenopausal patient must be considered as a neoplasm.

Primary carcinoma of the fallopian tube is rare and constitutes 0.3% of all gynecologic malignancies. The mean age is 55 years, with a range from 18 to 88 years. The disease is seldom diagnosed before laparotomy. Twenty percent of cancers are bilateral. If confined to the fallopian tube, a clinical diagnosis of hydrosalpinx or pyosalpinx may be made. Only half the cases show the classic triad of bleeding, abdominal pain, and pelvic or abdominal mass. The most common presenting symptom is abnormal bleeding or discharge. Spread of this neoplasm is similar to the common epithelial ovarian cancer, and the same treatment is employed for carcinoma of the fallopian tube as for carcinoma of the ovary.

DISEASES OF THE BREAST

The breast may be the site of contusions and lacerations secondary to trauma. Elderly women often fall against objects. It is not uncommon to see a contusion of the breast with or without a hematoma, and fat necrosis may resemble a neoplastic process in the elderly female patient. Inflammatory lesions do occur in the geriatric patient; most are secondary to scratching or to insect bites. Fibrocystic disease, especially in the form of nodules, is occasionally seen in the postmenopausal patient. Nodular fibrosis, an entity distinct from fibrocystic disease, occurs in the patient over 65 years of age. Intraductal papilloma and duct ectasia, which usually occur in the patient under age 55, may occur postmenopausally. A nipple discharge, especially if there is any discoloration or blood, must be suspect for a neoplastic process. Paget's disease of the nipple does not conform to the usual clinical picture of a carcinoma. It usually presents with eczema of the nipple and the patient complains of itching and scaling. The lesions require adequate biopsy to make sure that there is no underlying invasive neoplasm. Approximately 25% of patients presenting with Paget's disease of the nipple have had or will have Paget's disease of the vulva.

Carcinoma of the breast is the second leading cause of death from cancer among women. Each year there are approximately 114,000 new cases, and 36,000 women will die of the disease. It is obviously important that great effort be directed toward reducing breast cancer mortality. The principles that should be followed are as follows:

Breast examinations should be an integral part of the routine gynecologic examination for all patients.

Patients should receive instruction in the technique of life-long periodic breast self-examination.

Proper ambulatory surgical facilities suitable for performing breast biopsies should be developed.

The final diagnosis rests on careful histologic examination of a biopsy specimen (biopsy is necessary for all true, solid, three-dimensional masses).

Research, both basic and clinical, on etiology, diagnosis, and treatment of breast lesions must be encouraged.

Innovative screening programs such as mammography for high-risk patients might be included in this effort. Residency training programs in obstetrics and gynecology should include specific instruction in early detection techniques of breast cancer. The American Cancer Society has information on the step-by-step breast examination for the physician as well as pamphlets for the patient to learn breast self-examination.

CYSTOURETHROCELE AND UTERINE DESCENSUS

It is generally agreed that support of pelvic structures depends on the endopelvic fascia, the uterosacral and cardinal ligaments, and the levator muscle. An intact fascial system with its attachments to the vaginal fornices and upper two thirds of the lateral vagina provides a well-supported vaginal tube, which in turn is the most important supporting structure for the uterus and vaginal vault. Traumatic (obstetric) stretching, occupational and unusual athletic endeavors, heredity, and the postmenopausal attentuation all contribute in varying degrees to the development of pelvic relaxation. Additional contributing factors that promote uterine descensus are obesity, asthma, and other chronic lung diseases.

Descent of a portion of the posterior bladder wall and trigone into the vagina is usually due to the trauma of parturition. Urethrocele (sagging of the urethra) is commonly associated with cystocele and frequently occurs in women who have urinary stress incontinence. However, urethrocele is not a cause of urinary incontinence. It is interesting that in women with large cystoceles there is seldom any stress incontinence, but these patients often have repeated bouts of cystitis: the large cystocele often pulls on the trigone, and the patient has the constant urge to urinate.

The common symptoms and findings include a sensation of vaginal fullness, pressure, or falling out; a feeling of incomplete emptying of the bladder, urinary frequency, and perhaps a need to push the bladder up in order to empty it completely; the presence of a soft, reducible mass bulging into the anterior vagina and distending the vaginal introitus; and with straining or coughing, increased bulging and descent of the anterior vaginal wall as well as the urethra.

The cystocele requires surgical repair if there are repeated bouts of cystitis or trigonitis, if it gets so large than the patient cannot adequately empty her bladder, or if it protrudes to the vaginal introitus and causes an ulceration of the vaginal wall. The various kinds of pessaries usually do not help cystoceles and very often create stress incontinence.

Many older women tolerate large cystourethroceles and some degree of descensus without complaint, but massive procidentia (complete prolapse) is always disabling and occasionally is associated with trophic ulceration of exposed vaginal mucosa or with kidney dysfunction caused by kinking of the ureters. These conditions are best treated surgically, and even the most elderly can tolerate the surgery quite well. However, in women for whom it is advisable not to perform surgery, a vaginal pessary of the Gellhorn disc type or a Smith-Hodge type of pessary may support the uterus and bladder. Although the patient will require repeated visits for removal and cleansing of the pessary, it decreases the need for an operation. The pessary is usually considered a last resort measure. However, when indicated, it can be a great comfort, for example, to a very sick old woman with severe heart disease or emphysema in the presence of procidentia.

RECTOCELE

Bulging of the posterior vaginal wall and underlying rectum through the rectovaginal fascia results in a rectocele. A mild degree of rectocele (rarely causing symptoms) is usually present in all multiparous patients. A large rectocele may produce a sense of pelvic pressure, rectal fullness, or incomplete evacuation of stool. Occasionally a patient may find it necessary to reduce the posterior vaginal wall manually in a backward direction to evacuate stool effectively in the lower rectum. Distinguishing a high rectocele (involving the entire rectovaginal septum) from an enterocele may sometimes be difficult. Generally with the patient straining, a rectovaginal examination will confirm the presence of abdominal contents sliding into the enterocele sac. Pessaries are not helpful for this condition, and if the enterocele is causing a great deal of discomfort, surgical repair is indicated.

ENTEROCELE

An enterocele results when the small bowel pushes into the peritoneum between the rectum and the vagina. Large enteroceles occasionally cause upper abdominal distress because of the pull on the mensentery of the bowel. The diagnosis is made by having the patient stand, by inserting the index finger into the rectum and the thumb into the vagina, and by asking the patient to strain or cough. An impulse of the small bowel is almost certain to be caused by an enterocele. If the enterocele is large and bulges through the introitus, or if there is a great deal of abdominal discomfort, the enterocele should be repaired surgically.

STRESS INCONTINENCE

Urinary incontinence and lower genital tract disorders occur more frequently after the menopause. The lower urinary tract and the lower genital tract are of the same embryologic origin and influence each other in physiologic and pathophysiologic conditions.

Stress incontinence is defined as involuntary loss of urine due to a sudden increase in intra-abdominal pressure, such as occurs with laughing, coughing, or sneezing. It must be distinguished from overflow incontinence, enuresis, and urgency incontinence.

The causes of genuine stress incontinence are urethral sphincter incompetence, an anatomical,

scarred urethra (iatrogenic or traumatic), or urethral denervation. During the stress of coughing, the proximal portion of the urethra drops below the pelvic floor. The increase in intra-abdominal pressure induced by coughing transmits to the bladder but not to the urethra. As the urethral resistance is overcome by the increased bladder pressure, leakage of urine results. On urodynamic evaluation there is a decreased functional length of the urethra, decreased urethral closure pressure, and abnormal response of the sphincteric mechanism in reaction to stress, assumption of the upright position, and bladder filling. Stress incontinence occurs when the urethra sags away from its attachment to the symphysis. It may appear before the menopause, but for many women it becomes increasingly distressing after the age of 60. Loosening of the pelvic supporting tissue, damaged years earlier by vaginal deliveries and aggravated by years of standing, becomes more marked after estrogen secretion decreases following menopause.

Half of the women with stress incontinence can avoid surgery if they have good pubococcygeal tone and faithfully practice pubococcygeal exercises (puckering the vagina and urethral supporting tissues in a manner comparable to stopping a stream of urine.). The patient is advised to carry out this exercise for 2 minutes four times a day. It takes aproximately 2 months before positive results are seen in most cases. Incontinence will recur if the exercises are not continued.

Three fourths of the women with stress incontinence are asymptomatic after surgery to repair a cystourethrocele and return the urethra to its normal position above and behind the symphysis. This procedure is not effective if loss of urine is due to another cause.

EXOGENOUS ESTROGENS AND ENDOMETRIAL CANCER

It has been estimated that approximately 25% of women of menopausal age have symptoms of such severity as to warrant estrogen therapy. Although the evidence is not conclusive, it is suggested that replacement estrogen therapy has long-term metabolic benefits by reducing the incidence of strokes, heart attacks, osteoporosis, and fractures. However, a number of case control studies have indicated that estrogen replacement alone is associated with a 5- to 15-fold increased relative risk of endometrial cancer.

These figures, although alarming, should not

discourage the physician from using estrogen replacement therapy when indicated. The common symptoms of decreased estrogen function include flushes, flashes, sweats, insomnia, and a dry vagina. As the patient gets older, the flushes and sweats and insomnia disappear but the dry atrophic vagina gets worse. Since osteoporosis accelerates in the postmenopausal period, the use of estrogen in a prophylactic manner or to prevent progress of the disorder is repeatedly raised. Although the risk of endometrial cancer is increased, the physician must treat the symptomatic patient. One regimen that will provide relief of symptoms and perhaps some protection against the progress of osteoporosis is to give estrogen 5 days a week and every other month to add a progesterone derivative for 10 days. Occasionally this will cause vaginal bleeding; if the patient is monitored and has endometrial screening this should not be a deterrent.

OSTEOPOROSIS

Although the subject is covered in detail elsewhere (see Chapter 30), it is important to take note of osteoporosis here since many women especially, those in the postmenopausal years, inquire about osteoporosis when visiting their primary physician or obstetrician-gynecologist. Osteoporosis has often been called the silent disease, because it produces absolutely no symptoms until a fracture occurs. The patient predisposed to osteoporosis is a postmenopausal woman who is slender, with very fair skin and small bone structure. There are other contributing factors that may predispose to osteoporosis, namely, a family history of the disease, never bearing a child, lack of physical activity, poor diet, calcium deficiency, vitamin D deficiency, smoking, use of alcohol, change in estrogen balance, and change in calcium metabolism. Therapy for established disease includes calcium supplements, vitamin D, estrogens, androgens, fluoride, and calcitonin. Treatment should be carried out under continued supervision. Osteoporosis cannot be cured but the patient can be made more comfortable by treatment. Progression of osteoporosis may be slowed if not prevented.

SEXUALITY

With better nutrition, more cholesterol in the diet, more rest, and better health, women are maintaining an interest in sexual function well into their postmenopausal years. Continued sexual outlets and functioning are the most important factors in maintaining sexual interest and capacity in the older woman. If for any reason a woman is sexually inactive for some years in the postmenopausal period, there may be difficulty with reinstitution of sexual function.

In 1953 Kinsey reported that the sexual activity of unmarried women remains relatively constant until age 55, whereas that of unmarried men declines progressively after adolescence.[1] Among married couples as well, the frequency of sexual intercourse appears to decline in similar fashion with aging. Kinsey concluded that in women, age has no effect on sexual activity until very late in life, and suggested that reduction in sexual activity may be due primarily to diminution in the sexuality of the male partner.

A study of the sexual activity of single women between 50 and 69 years of age compared previously married subjects with those who had never been married. Both groups reportedly maintain sexual activity, including masturbation (59% of previously married and 44% of never married), coitus (37% and 25%, respectively), and orgasmic dreams (35% and 52%, respectively).

Alterations in sexual response associated with aging are a result of generalized decrease in tone, strength, and elasticity of tissues and lengthening of response time. In older women vaginal lubrication may take 3 to 5 minutes to occur, whereas in a young woman this takes only 15 to 20 seconds. At the same level of arousal, the older woman will have a smaller volume of lubrication. Again, provided that she is in good health and especially if there has been continuing sexual functioning, lubrication for intercourse will be adequate. However, use of commonly available lubricants may be helpful. A recent example is Lubrin, a vaginal lubricating insert that is unscented and colorless and provides long-lasting lubrication for sexual intercourse.

The menopausal woman complaining of sexual inadequacy is often told by her physician that loss of sexual function is to be expected with the change of life and that there is nothing to be done about it. Although sexual behavior is the sum total of the individual make up (including chromosomal sex, gender identification, gonadal adequacy, childhood rearing, environmental influences, a possible hypothalamic sensitization, and hormone factors), there is a role for hormone therapy in modifying sexual responsiveness. Combinations of estrogen and androgen are often beneficial. Equine conjugated estrogen or its equivalent in a dose of 0.625 mg with 5 mg methyltestosterone is recommended. In some women, methyltestosterone, 10 mg three times a day for 2 weeks, will often increase the libido, and if the patient indulges in intercourse, sexual desires will continue without needing any stimulation from hormonal therapy. In women in whom intercourse is difficult because of the shrinkage secondary to estrogen withdrawal, hormonal cream is often beneficial. It should be applied around the inside lips of the small labia, up around the clitoris, and around the fourchette. The treatment should be carried out two to three times a week until the tissue has undergone a period of rejuvenation, and then it can be continued at less frequent intervals. A fourth of an applicator of estogenic cream inserted into the vagina every 2 to 3 weeks usually keeps the upper part of the vagina pink and moist.

Some women seek advice about masturbation. Since they are elderly, they believe that it is a sign of some abnormal psychological condition. The patient must be instructed that it has no harmful physical effects and is within normal limits. However, if the patient raises a moral issue about masturbation it is best to refer her to her clergyman.

Masters and Johnson have shown that all four stages of the response cycle (excitement, plateau, orgasm, and resolution) are somewhat diminished with increased age.[3] In the excitement phase, breasts are less engorged and the sexual flush may be absent. The clitoris enlarges normally, but there is no noticeable change in the labia majora. Vaginal lubrication is reduced. Vaginal ballooning occurs later in the plateau phase and is often less marked. Orgasms continue to occur, but their duration is shorter and muscular contractions may also be less intense. Uterine spasms may render some orgasms painful. The resolution phase is rapid in elderly women and occasionally because of urethral trauma is accompanied by a desire to void. Decrease in the strength of vaginal contractions occurring with orgasm is another change that occurs in elderly women. This decline is recordable and has been documented. However, older women may report no diminution in the experience of pleasure or release gratification.

MAJOR GYNECOLOGIC SURGICAL PROCEDURES IN THE AGED

Disorders of the female genital organs are certainly not among the major causes of death. Yet they give rise to important illness-producing discomfort and disability and therefore warrant treatment.

Most of the gynecologic complaints of elderly women are related to genital prolapse. Contrary to the practice in younger patients, most of the operations in the elderly are carried out by the vaginal route. Vaginal hysterectomy is the preferred procedure in most cases of uterine prolapse.

Medical advances in diagnosis and treatment and the better understanding of physiologic and pathophysiologic processes in the elderly now justify the performance of major operations in this group. Numerous reports have shown that age alone does not contraindicate surgical intervention if due regard is paid to the patient's general condition. It is important for the physician to bear in mind that sexual activity in some women continues into very old age. Therefore, vaginal surgery should be performed with this in mind.

The duration of operation should be kept as short as possible because the prolonged lithotomy position invites even more complications than does prolonged anesthesia. Mini-heparinization should be started the evening before surgery and continued through surgery and for the first few days postoperatively. The regimen I use calls for approximately 3000 units per 24 hours.

As the geriatric population increases and women no longer accept age alone as a barrier to active life, more elective surgery will be demanded by patients and performed by gynecologic surgeons. Contraindications to surgical intervention should not include chronologic age.

REFERENCES

1. Kinsey AC et al: Sexual Behavior in the Human Female. Philadelphia, WB Saunders, 1953
2. Kraatz H: Geriatrische Fragen in der Gynakologie. Dtsch Ges Wes 16:1204, 1961
3. Masters WH, Johnson VE: Human Sexual Response. Boston, Little, Brown & Co, 1966
4. Stieglitz EJ: Foundations of Geriatric Medicine. In Stieglitz EJ (ed): Gereatric Medicine, 3rd ed., pp 3–26. Philadelphia, JB Lippincott, 1954
5. Vojta M: Prevence v peci a zeny ve stari. Cesk Gynekol 30:405, 1965

SUGGESTED READINGS

Hoffman JW: Gynecologic disorders in the geriatric patient: Geriatric gynecology. Postgrad Med 71:38, 1982
Hoffman JW: The diagnosis and treatment of gynecologic disorders in elderly patients. Compr Ther 9:54, 1983
Iosif CS, Bekassy Z: Prevalence of genitourinary symptoms in late menopause. Acta Obstet Gynecol Scand 63:257, 1984

Masters WH: The sexual response cycle of the human female: Vaginal lubrication. Ann NY Acad Sci 83:301, 1959

McKeithen WS: Major gynecologic surgery in the elderly female. Am J Obstet Gynecol 59:63, 1975

Wingate MB: Geriatric gynecology. Primary care 9:53, 1982

Yarnell GW, Voyle GJ: The prevalence and severity of urinary incontinence in women. J Epidemiol Commun Health 35:71, 1981

21 Dermatologic Disorders in the Elderly

Barbara A. Gilchrest

Few statistics are available concerning the burden of dermatologic disorders in the elderly. However, a federally sponsored examination of more than 20,000 noninstitutionalized Americans revealed that 40% of those aged 65 to 74 years suffered from a skin disease sufficiently severe in the opinion of the consulting dermatologist to warrant at least one physician visit, and the average affected individual had 1.5 such disorders. The prevalence of and disability from skin disease in the population greater than 74 years old, the most rapidly enlarging age cohort, can only be larger. Moreover, these figures do not include the omnipresent "normal" changes in aging skin that may have devastating psychological effects and that may predispose the elderly to certain infections and inflammatory diseases. It is the goal of this chapter to outline some of the recent advances in our understanding of old skin and its special problems, as well as to provide guidelines for the treatment of selected common geriatric dermatoses.

IMPORTANCE OF SKIN DISEASES

Because skin is visible, patients are distressed not only by cutaneous discomfort and loss of function but also by changes in appearance. From antiquity the presence of skin lesions has created fear of contagion and/or stigmatization, typified by the biblical classification of patients now known to have had psoriasis or vitiligo as "lepers." The intensity of these now sometimes subconscious attitudes in modern society has been well documented and should not be underestimated. With regard to the elderly in our youth-oriented culture, the visible signs of aging in the skin and its appendages have a measurable negative impact not only on a person's self-image but also on society's perception of him. The more than $10 billion spent annually in this country for cosmetic products, largely in the vain hope of retarding or reversing aging of the skin, is testimony to the horror with which many people regard this process. "Rashes," "growths," and other cutaneous abnormalities add immeasurably to this psychosocial burden.

In addition to disfigurement, skin disease frequently produces itching or pain. Intensity and duration of these symptoms varies widely among diseases and among individuals but especially for the elderly may interfere significantly with normal daily activities and with sleep, creating further disability.

The strictly monetary costs to society and the individual for diagnosis and management of dermatologic disease are also difficult to determine. However, it has been estimated that at least 7% of all physician visits in the United States are prompted primarily or exclusively by disorders of the skin. And although hospitalization is infrequently required for dermatologic disease alone, such disorders as decubitus ulcers and drug rashes may greatly complicate and prolong other hospitalization for the elderly.

GLOSSARY OF TERMS

Proper usage of dermatologic terms facilitates communication between primary care providers and their dermatologic consultants and renders more meaningful textbook and journal accounts of cutaneous pathology. The terms employed in this chapter are defined in Table 21-1.

TABLE 21-1   Glossary of Dermatologic Terms

Term	Definition
Bulla	Fluid-filled lesion greater than 5 mm in diameter
Cream	An oil-in-water preparation, usually "vanishing" and nongreasy
Crust	Dried serum and other material overlying an erosion or ulcer
Dermatitis	Inflammation of the skin (no etiology implied)
Eczema	A pruritic rash characterized by erythema and vesiculation or bulla formation in severe, acute cases and by scaling and lichenification (coarsening of the skin markings) with or without erythema, hyperpigmentation, and vesiculation in chronic cases. Common etiologies include irritant or allergic contact dermatitis and atopic dermatitis (also called "eczema"). Eruption is always at least partially steroid responsive.
Erosion	Absence of part or all of the epidermis; a superficial wound
Macule	Flat lesion of any size in the plane of the normal skin
Neoplasm	New growth
Nodule	Raised solid lesion of any size having most of its mass below the skin surface
Ointment	A water-in-oil preparation, usually somewhat "greasy" and occlusive
Papule	Raised solid superficial lesion less than 5 mm in diameter
Plaque	Raised solid superficial lesion greater than or equal to 5 mm in diameter
Scale	Retained stratum corneum
Scar	Permanent alteration in the skin following trauma or inflammation; associated with increased or decreased cutaneous mass, often "sclerotic"
Ulcer	Absence of epidermis and part or all of the dermis; a deep wound
Vesicle	Fluid-filled lesion less than 5 mm in diameter

AGE-ASSOCIATED CHANGES IN NORMAL SKIN

The skin consists of three distinct compartments: (1) the epidermis, (2) the dermis, and (3) the subcutaneous fat. The epidermis is composed primarily of keratinocytes (80% to 90% of all epidermal cells) that differentiate to make the stratum corneum, the major chemical and mechanical barrier of the body. During embryogenesis, subpopulations of keratinocytes invaginate into the dermis to form the epidermal appendages: hair follicles, sebaceous (oil) glands, and eccrine and apocrine (sweat) glands. Epidermal keratinocytes may be further subdivided into germinative (basilar) and terminally differentiated (suprabasilar) populations, and individual cells traverse the 0.1 mm to 0.2 mm deep epidermis for approximately 1 month before being shed from the skin surface into the environment. The second major cell type of the epidermis (2% to 4% of cells) is the melanocyte, a neural crest derivative that migrates into the skin and functions primarily to make melanin pigment granules, which provide protection against damaging solar radiation. Langerhans cells, the third major cellular constituent of the epidermis (1% to 2% of cells), are derived from bone marrow and are possibly transient, appearing to function primarily in antigen recognition and processing.

The dermis is a complex fibrous matrix, 1 mm to 4 mm thick, set in a mucopolysaccharide gel, through which run blood vessels, lymphatic channels, nerves, glandular ducts, and hair follicles. Cellular constituents of the dermis include fibroblasts, endothelial cells, mast cells, and histiocytes or "fixed tissue macrophages." The fibrous proteins collagen and elastin, produced by fibroblasts, provide tensile strength and elasticity to the skin. The dermal vasculature is the most extensive of any organ system and helps regulate core body temperature through vasoconstriction and vasodilation.

The subcutaneous fat, populated primarily by adipocytes, provides mechanical protection and insulation for underlying structures.

Morphologic Changes

The major aging changes in gross morphology of the skin include "dryness" (by which is meant roughness), wrinkling, laxity, uneven pigmentation, and a variety of proliferative lesions. The most striking and consistent histologic change is flattening of the dermoepidermal junction with reduction in the number of interdigitating papillae and rete pegs per unit skin surface length, resulting in a considerably smaller contiguous surface between the two compartments and presumably less "communication" and nutrient transfer and less resistance to shearing forces. Average epidermal thickness is relatively constant in sun-protected skin with advancing age, although variability in thickness increases.

A decrease of 10% to 20% of the skin's enzymatically active melanocyte population each decade reduces the protective barrier against ultraviolet light. The number of melanocytic nevi (moles) also progressively decreases with age from a peak of 15 to 40 in the third and fourth decades to an average of 4 per person after age 50, with moles rarely observed in persons beyond age 80. A nearly 40% reduction in the number of morphologically identifiable epidermal Langerhans cells occurs between early and late adulthood and may account in part for the age-associated decrease in immune responsiveness observed in the skin.

Loss of dermal thickness approaches 20% in elderly individuals and may account for the paper-thin, sometimes nearly transparent, quality of their skin. The remaining dermis is relatively acellular and avascular. Precise histologic concomitants of wrinkling, if any, are unknown, although age-related loss of normal elastin fibers may be contributory. An approximately 50% reduction in mast cells, with a corresponding reduction in histamine release following a standardized challenge, may be responsible for the reduced rate of immediate hypersensitivity reactions ("prick tests") and acute urticaria in the elderly. The striking age-associated loss of vascular bed is believed to underlie many of the physiologic alterations in old skin, as well as the gradual atrophy and fibrosis of hair follicles and eccrine, apocrine, and sebaceous glands.

Approximately half the population by age 50 years has at least 50% gray (white) body hair with an even higher proportion of depigmented scalp hair, and virtually everyone has some degree of graying, due to progressive and eventually total loss of melanocytes from the hair bulb. Loss of melanocytes is believed to occur more rapidly in hair than in skin because the cells are called on to proliferate and manufacture melanin at maximal rates during the growth phase of the hair cycle (especially long on the scalp), while epidermal melanocytes are comparatively inactive throughout their life span. Advancing age is also accompanied by a gradual decrease in number of hair follicles, and remaining hairs may be smaller in diameter and grow more slowly. The independent process of "balding" on the scalp is actually an androgen-mediated reduction in hair diameter, maximal length, and pigmentation that, at least by certain criteria, increases in prevalence among men from 3% at the end of the third decade to more than 25% by the seventh decade.

Eccrine sweat glands decrease in average number during adulthood in most body sites and grad-

ually accumulate lipofuscin ("age pigment"). Sebaceous gland size and number appear not to change with age, despite decreased function. The cutaneous end organs responsible for pressure perception and light touch progressively decrease to approximately one third of their initial average density between the second and ninth decades of life and display greater variation in size and structure.

Functional Changes

The major cutaneous functions that decline with age and the presumed physiologic consequences are listed in Table 21-2. In many cases, the functional changes can be presumed to result directly from the aforementioned morphologic changes.

Dermatoheliosis (Sun-induced Aging)

Dermatoheliosis is a term describing the chronically sun-exposed skin in middle-aged and elderly adults, widely mislabeled as "aging," "premature aging," or "accelerated aging." Features include atrophy, prominent scaliness or "dryness," irregular pigmentation, coarse wrinkling, "pseudoscars," elastosis (fine nodularity), telangiectasia ("broken blood vessels"), purpura, and actinic keratoses (red-brown, sandpaperlike, premalignant lesions). These changes in appearance are generally accompanied by an exaggeration of age-associated functional losses in affected skin (see Table 21-2).

The importance of differentiating dermatoheliosis from intrinsic aging lies partly in the strong statistical assocation between sun damage and skin cancer (see below), mandating a careful annual examination of the entire exposed skin surface. In addition, patients should be educated regarding the total preventability and even partial reversibility of these unattractive changes by regular use of an effective sunscreen, preferably one with an SPF 15 rating.

COMMON DERMATOSES

Inflammatory Conditions

Xerosis

"Dry skin" can be prevented or improved by daily hydration of the affected areas in the bath or shower or even with a moist cloth, followed immediately by the use of a topical emollient to re-

TABLE 21-2 Age-Associated Losses in Cutaneous Function and Their Consequences

Functional Loss*	Presumed Consequence
Barrier function	More rapid and extensive entry of certain irritants or allergens
Cell replacement	Decreased epidermal turnover rate; prolonged exposure of stratum corneum cells to the environment; slow wound healing
Chemical clearance	Greater accumulation and longer exposure to absorbed irritants or allergens; prolonged ecchymosis following trauma; compromised dispersion of medications administered percutaneously
Dermoepidermal adhesion	Tendency to "torn skin," abrasions, and blisters following trauma
Immune responsiveness	Decreased prevalence of hypersensitivity reactions (positive skin tests, contact dermatitis); increased photocarcinogenesis
Injury response	Poor wound healing; weak scars; reduced inflammatory response
Mechanical protection	Increased frequency and/or severity of injury to subcutaneous structures; increased vulnerability to decubitus ulcer formation over bony prominences
Sebum production	None known
Sensory perception	Increased frequency and/or severity of skin injury
Sweat production	Decreased thermoregulation
Thermoregulation	Tendency to hypothermia and heat stroke during temperature extremes
Vascular responsiveness	Less intense erythema during inflammation (*e.g.*, infections, burns)
Vitamin D production	Increased risk of osteomalacia and bone fractures

* Losses measured for most functions approximate 30% to 50% during adulthood. Conclusions in some instances are based on single and unconfirmed studies.

tard water loss. "Heavy" moisturizers such as Eucerin or Nivea are often more effective than more expensive or cosmetically elegant preparations, especially for the lower extremities. Hydration of the stratum corneum in this way relieves pruritus and prevents fissuring through the barrier layer, with subsequent entry of irritants into the viable epidermis. The etiology of xerosis is poorly understood but probably reflects life-long minor cumulative injuries to the skin, ultimately interfering with normal epidermal maturation. On the lower legs, vascular insufficiency may also contribute. "Dry skin" does not result from loss of water or oil in the viable epidermis, notwithstanding transient improvement in cutaneous appearance with hydration of the abnormal stratum corneum.

Seborrheic Dermatitis

The exceedingly common problem of seborrheic dermatitis is characterized by erythema and usually minimal scaling principally involving the nasolabial folds, eye brows, hairline, and scalp. In severe or neglected cases, involvement may extend to the presternal area or indeed may become generalized. Dramatic improvement of skin lesions usually occurs within a few days of instituting hydrocortisone cream twice daily. Failure to improve should indeed suggest the possibility of an

incorrect diagnosis. Scalp involvement usually responds well to frequent use of tar or zirconium shampoos, although severe cases may also require daily application of a corticosteroid lotion. Treatment of both skin and scalp lesions must continue indefinitely, although good control can be maintained with intermittent medication in some patients. The pathophysiology of seborrheic dermatitis is unknown.

Contact Dermatitis

Either irritants or allergens may produce an eczematous dermatitis at sites of percutaneous penetration. The eruptions are clinically indistinguishable; diagnosis is based on a careful history and (in the case of suspected allergens only) patch testing. Referral to an experienced dermatologist is usually quite worthwhile in all but the most straightforward cases.

In the elderly, recognition of contact dermatitis may be complicated by a muted inflammatory response and a vague or inaccurate history of local exposures. An unusual "geometric" or "outside" configuration of an itchy rash is the best clue. Contact dermatitis usually responds within several days to twice-daily use of a fluorinated corticosteroid (*e.g.*, fluocinonide or fluocinolone) once the precipitating agent is removed. In the absence of corticosteroid contraindications, very severe cases producing extensive bulla formation, facial edema, or incapacity should be treated with oral prednisone, 20 mg to 30 mg twice daily, tapered to nothing over 2 weeks. Without treatment, the eruption slowly improves over 2 to 3 weeks, although even minimal intermittent exposure to the contactant may perpetuate it.

Stasis Dermatitis

Stasis dermatitis is best managed by intermittent elevation of the legs, reduction of dependent edema, and correction of underlying venous insufficiency whenever possible. The inflammatory, often pruritic eruption responds well to twice-daily application of a fluorinated steroid ointment, followed by once-daily application of hydrocortisone or an emollient alone after symptoms improve. In no case, however, should potent corticosteroid preparations be continued beyond a few weeks, especially in patients with past or present stasis ulcers. Slow response or inadequate relief of the itching should suggest an incorrect diagnosis or superimposed allergic contact dermatitis.

Lichen Simplex Chronicus

Older individuals may develop one or more intensely pruritic areas, often near the ankle, that engender habitual scratching over a period of months to years in the absence of any recognized precipitant (Figure 21-1). Established lesions are eczematous plaques with prominent lichenification, excoriations, and often brown-purple discoloration due to repeated self-induced capillary bleeding. Overnight application of a fluorinated corticosteroid ointment under plastic occlusion (*e.g.,* Saran wrap) and behavioral modification, providing an alternative to prolonged strenuous scratching or rubbing, is usually quite helpful. Cordran Tape, a corticosteroid-impregnated adhesive plastic film, is an attractive alternative approach: a length of tape sufficient to cover the lesion is cut from the roll, applied directly over the affected skin, and replaced as necessary every 12 to 24 hours, providing both anti-inflammatory medication and a mechanical barrier to further scratching.

Pruritus

Patients presenting to the physician because of pruritus may in fact have an eruption that is responsible for the symptoms, although its other manifestations may be so subtle that the patient

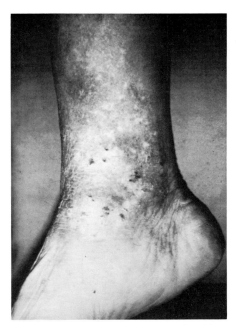

FIG. 21-1. Lichen simplex chronicus. Isolated lesions show classic features of irregular hyperpigmentation and small hemorrhagic erosions where patient has scratched. (Courtesy of Rita Berman, MD)

or even the physician does not notice the rash. Because cutaneous inflammatory responses may be muted in the elderly, a careful history and physical examination are necessary before excluding primary disorders of the skin, such as scabies, atopic dermatitis (eczema), bullous pemphigoid, miliaria (prickly heat), contact dermatitis, urticaria (hives), or pediculosis. Proper identification of a causative dermatosis not only leads to effective treatment in most patients but also avoids the workup for unexplained generalized pruritus.

Among patients seeking medical attention for pruritus without a rash, up to half may have an underlying systemic disease. The most common known cause of persistent generalized pruritus is chronic renal failure, although it is unlikely that mild to moderate renal insufficiency, frequently present in elderly patients, may also be responsible. Hepatic cholestasis, hematopoietic disorders (especially lymphomas), hyperthyroidism, and ingestion of certain drugs are other associations to be considered.

Optimal therapy for generalized pruritus is that for the underlying disease, but unfortunately the responsible disorder is often either uncorrectable or, indeed, undetectable. For those patients whose pruritus is idiopathic, nonspecific therapies must be employed. Often it is worthwhile to prescribe an emollient even in the absence of clinical xerosis, since minimal or intermittent dryness, present in virtually all elderly individuals, may notably exacerbate pruritus of another cause. Topical application of menthol, 0.25% to 0.5%, or the anesthetic phenol, 0.5% to 1.0%, in an appropriate vehicle such as Eucerin lotion also may provide considerable temporary relief; other topical anesthetics can be used only at the risk of allergic sensitization. Topical corticosteroids are ineffective. Oral antihistamines are widely prescribed for pruritus of all causes, although the efficacy is slight in most instances, and these agents may produce paradoxic restlessness or significantly impair psychomotor function in the elderly.

Pruritus Vulvae/Ani

Itchiness restricted to the perineal area deserves separate consideration because of its different etiologic associations and approaches to management. Diabetics and immunocompromised patients sometimes suffer from this distressing problem as a result of low-grade *Candida albicans* infection. Better control of the diabetes or improvement in immune status coupled with good hygiene and frequent applications of nystatin or another effective antifungal agent in a cream base should greatly improve symptoms. In postmenopausal women, pruritus vulvae may result from estrogen deficiency and secondary mucosal atrophy. Daily application of an estrogen-containing cream to the affected skin may be curative; even 1% hydrocortisone ointment may greatly reduce chemical and mechanical irritation.

Patients for whom the above is irrelevant or insufficient represent a major therapeutic challenge. For many, the problem is so longstanding that scratching and rubbing have become reflexive and themselves major exacerbating factors that are no longer under the patient's control. Obesity, even minimal degrees of urinary or fecal incontinence, or difficulty in maintaining personal hygiene are frequent contributing factors in the elderly that are equally difficult to address. The involved area must be kept scrupulously clean. Ideally, the patient should bathe or shower after each bowel movement; a bidet or sitz bath can provide excellent cleansing without the need to totally undress. Simply wiping the skin with toilet paper is likely to leave a residue of irritant material; Tucks are glycerin-soaked pads that are less mechanically irritating than dry paper and perhaps more effective at cleaning the skin. Wipes contain-

ing alcohol or soap frequently aggravate the preexisting dermatitis and should be avoided. Hydrocortisone 1% ointment applied immediately after the bath (or equivalent) provides some barrier to future cutaneous contact with urine and feces, as well as a direct anti-inflammatory effect. Stronger corticosteroid preparations that may produce atrophy in intertriginous areas are inappropriate.

Bullous Pemphigoid

Bullous pemphigoid is an idiopathic, immunoglobulin-mediated disease of the skin, characterized clinically by large, tense bullae arising on either erythematous or normal-appearing skin. The elderly are affected most commonly, and conversely, bullous pemphigoid is almost certainly the most common blistering disease affecting older patients. Untreated, bullous pemphigoid varies in severity from mild to disabling and may be fatal. The disease is self-limited, lasting months to years, with recurrences following disease-free periods in a substantial minority of patients.

Blisters occur most often on the trunk and proximal extremities, often preceded or accompanied by pruritus (Fig. 21-2). Approximately one third of patients have oral lesions. Diagnosis should be confirmed by an experienced dermatopathologist through biopsy of an early lesion for both routine and immunofluorescent histologic studies. Immunofluorescent staining of perilesional skin reveals linear deposition of C_3 in all patients and of immunoglobulin in most patients along the basement membrane zone (BMZ); indirect immunofluorescent studies using patient serum and monkey esophagus or other cutaneous preparation demonstrate anti-BMZ antibodies of the IgG class in approximately two thirds of patients.

Corticosteroids are the mainstay of therapy. In mild or localized cases, topical application of a potent corticosteroid cream once or twice daily may control the lesions, but most patients require prednisone or its equivalent. Dosage and schedule of administration are determined by the extent, severity, and rate of progression of the disease as well as by the age of the patient and the presence or absence of relative contraindications, such as hypertension, diabetes, osteoporosis, or infection. Patients with extensive and/or rapidly progressive, disabling bullous pemphigoid should begin therapy with prednisone 60 mg to 100 mg/d (some authors recommend two to three times this dose). This therapy should be reevaluated at weekly intervals, and the dosage of prednisone reduced rap-

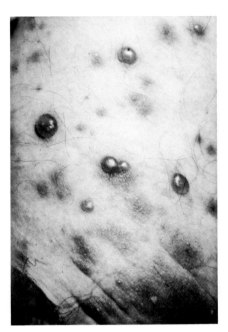

FIG. 21-2. Bullous pemphigoid. Multiple tense blisters arise on either erythematous or normal appearing skin. Individual lesions may enlarge, evolve into crusted erosions, or resolve spontaneously. (Courtesy of Rita Berman, MD)

idly (*e.g.*, 10 mg to 20 mg/week) as new blisters cease forming and clinical remission is achieved. An immunosuppressant such as azothioprine, 150 mg/day, or cyclophosphamide, 100 mg/day, may be added to the regimen initially or at the time of remission in order to reduce the eventual maintenance level of prednisone; 6 to 8 weeks are required for full expression of the steroid-sparing effect. Patients with less severe bullous pemphigoid may initiate therapy with alternate-day prednisone, 40 mg to 60 mg, and/or daily use of an immunosuppressant. Drug dosages are decreased gradually to zero over many months, provided the disease remains in remission. Sulfapyridine or sulfones may be valuable alternative therapies for patients with major contraindications to systemic corticosteroids. Most patients achieve prolonged remission and at least half can ultimately discontinue treatment without recurrence of lesions, although frequent exacerbation of the bullous pemphigoid and potential complications of therapy require close monitoring of all patients throughout the course of their disease.

Concern that bullous pemphigoid might be a marker for concurrent or subsequent development of malignancy has not been substantiated by con-trolled studies. The prevalence of malignant neoplasms appears to be approximately 10% both in patients with bullous pemphigoid and in age-matched controls.

Drug Rashes

Approximately 3% of elderly hospitalized patients experience a drug rash; rates among elderly outpatients are presumed proportional to the number of drug exposures in this population. Exanthematous ("maculopapular") eruptions comprise nearly half of these cases and urticarial eruptions ("hives") nearly one fourth. Bullous drug eruptions, erythema multiforme, fixed drug eruptions, drug-induced toxic epidermal necrolysis, and phototoxic ("exaggerated sunburn") reactions also occur. Statistically, allergic reactions are most likely to occur within the first week after initiating therapy but may begin at any time up to at least 2 weeks after the last drug dose. Eruptions associated with sporadically used medications, self-prescribed over-the-counter medications, or agents such as food additives not regarded by the patient as drugs may be particularly difficult to diagnose.

Treatment consists of discontinuing the causative drug and providing symptomatic relief as needed. If multiple drugs are being used, it is preferable to discontinue all, although practical considerations sometimes dictate beginning with the statistically most likely culprit(s) only and accepting the small but finite risk that a minor annoyance may become life threatening if the responsible agent is mistakenly continued. For most drug rashes, tepid oatmeal (Aveenol) baths *ad libitum*, topical emollients, and (cautiously) oral antihistamines provide adequate relief of pruritus during the initial 1 to 2 weeks and no further therapy is needed. Topical corticosteroids add more to the cost than to the effectiveness of most regimens.

Exceptions to the above approach are erythema multiforme major (Stevens-Johnson syndrome) and toxic epidermal necrolysis (TEN), which warrant immediate hospitalization to maintain hydration, to prevent sepsis, and, in many cases, to administer parenteral corticosteroid therapy. Physicians and families must be aware that TEN especially has a mortality rate exceeding 50% among older adults.

Infectious Conditions

Herpes Zoster

Herpes zoster or "shingles," due to reactivation of latent varicella virus in the dorsal sensory ganglia of a partially immmune host, is most common in older patients, with an age-adjusted annual incidence rate exceeding 10 per 1000 population at age 80 years. The disorder usually begins with dysesthesia or paresthesia of the involved dermatome that persists for days to rarely longer than a week before the appearance of vesicles and may mimic angina, spinal cord compression, renal or biliary colic, muscle sprains, or many other disorders.

The diagnosis is usually made from the appearance of clustered vesicles in a dermatomal distribution (Fig. 21-3) and is confirmed by Tzanck stain of material scraped from the base of an intact vesicle. New lesions continue to appear for several days, often progressing distally along the dermatome. Pain and hyperesthesia are frequently prominent during the first days of the eruption, although their severity is unrelated to either the risk or severity of post-herpetic neuralgia in individual patients. Vesicles usually begin to crust in the second week and resolve within 4 weeks. The course of herpes zoster infection in young and old adults differs primarily in the incidence and severity of post-herpetic neuralgia. This problem occurs in approximately 10% of patients overall, but affects more than half of those above 60 years old. The increase in severity and duration of post-herpetic neuralgia with age is even more marked than the increase in incidence. Persistent pain is especially common in patients with trigeminal involvement or immunosuppression.

During the acute phase of the infection, some patients require narcotic analgesics for adequate relief of pain. Early skin lesions are best treated with local compresses of Burow's solution (1:20 in cool water) or similar hypertonic soaks for 10 minutes three or four times daily followed by gentle washing with Hibiclens or other antibacterial soap, to hasten drying and prevent bacterial superinfection. Topical antibiotic ointment may be applied twice daily to already crusted lesions. The longest-standing and most readily available treatment for the devasting problem of post-herpetic neuralgia is orally administered prednisone or prednisolone, 40 mg/day for 10 days, then tapered over 3 weeks. The drug is most effective if begun during the first 3 to 5 days of the eruption, when it is also helpful in reducing edema and pain. Side-effects seem surprisingly infrequent in the older population at risk, although the relative contraindications must be considered for each patient. Corticosteroids are ineffective in the treatment of established post-herpetic neuralgia. More rapid healing and decreased pain during the acute herpes zoster infection have also been reported for

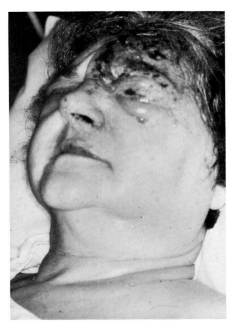

FIG. 21-3. Herpes zoster ophthalmicus. Striking periorbital edema with grouped hemorrhagic vesicles and erosions in the affected dermatome is seen. Lesion at the nasal tip warns of associated corneal involvement.

elderly patients treated with the guanine derivative acyclovir, 5 mg/kg intravenously for 5 days, beginning by the third day of the eruption, but the small experience to date does not suggest a beneficial effect on post-herpetic neuralgia. Treatment of established neuralgia is often frustrating, but the long list of anecdotally helpful procedures and medications deserves exploration for each sufferer.

Tinea (Fungus)

Low-grade tinea infections are very common in the elderly, and treatment is not always indicated. For example, "moccasin foot" with or without nail involvement (onychomycosis) is usually chronic, asymptomatic, harmless, and very difficult to eradicate (Fig. 21-4). However, prominent involvement of the digital web spaces with fissuring warrants local treatment to prevent bacterial superinfection with its attendant risk of cellulitis or sepsis; and tinea involving body locations other than the feet almost always warrants treatment because of pruritus and/or cosmetic concerns. Effective broad-spectrum antifungal agents now available in cream preparation include haloprogin, clotrimazole, and miconazole.

The drug should be applied to the affected area twice daily for at least 3 to 4 weeks and for at least

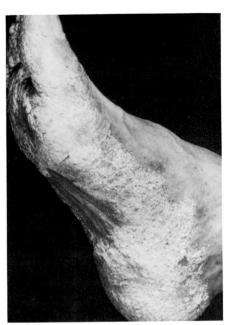

FIG. 21-4. Tinea pedis. Diffuse scaling indicative of chronic fungal infection. If asymptomatic, treatment may not be necessary.

2 weeks after disappearance of the eruption. In sites prone to immediate reinfection, such as the feet or the groin, an antifungal powder should then be applied indefinitely on a daily basis. Only very extensive cutaneous involvement warrants use of oral griseofulvin or ketoconazole.

It should be noted that tinea corporis ("ringworm") is much less common in the elderly than is patchy eczematous dermatitis of a noninfectious etiology. Diagnosis should always be confirmed by a fungal culture or potassium hydroxide stain of lesional scale. Conversely, both eczema and tinea may appear to improve during topical corticosteroid therapy, due to reduced inflammation, but a fungal infection will continue to spread and eventually "rebound."

Candidiasis (Yeast)

Candida infections are also common among the elderly, especially obese individuals confined to warm environments, reflecting the organisms' preference for warmth and moisture. Intertriginous involvement is classically manifested by bright-red, sharply demarcated, tender or pruritic areas with "satellite" papules and pustules along the borders (Fig. 21-5). "Bland" intertrigo, maceration of body folds in the absence of superinfection, is usually (but not always) less symptomatic and lacks pustules. Both conditions respond favorably to improved ventilation of involved areas or frequent application of absorbent, nonmedicated powder. Cornstarch, which is metabolized by yeasts, and occlusive dressings or ointments should be avoided. In cases known to represent candidiasis, treatment may be initiated with nystatin or a broad-spectrum antibiotic such as miconazole or haloprogin in a cream or more drying alcohol-based solution. Specific therapy should be continued until the eruption clears, unless skin irriation occurs: prophylactic daily use of absorbent powder should then be continued indefinitely. Hydrocortisone cream or other corticosteriod-containing preparation predisposes macerated skin to bacterial or fungal superinfection and therefore should be applied sparingly and only in very symptomatic cases not responsive to the above measures.

Perlèche is the name given to candidiasis of the corners of the mouth, an area predisposed to maceration in the elderly by deep skin folds and a

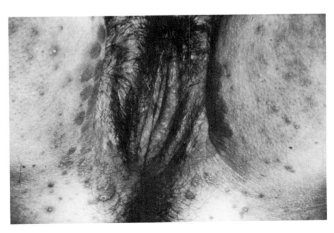

FIG. 21-5. Candidiasis of the groin, showing classic satellite pustules.

tendency toward local pooling of oral secretions. Inflammation and fissuring usually resolve rapidly with twice-daily application of Mycolog cream, a combination corticosteroid-antibiotic product. Intraoral candidiasis or thrush occurs primarily in the debilitated elderly patient, especially during administration of broad-spectrum antibiotics. The diagnosis should be confirmed by potassium hydroxide stain of material scraped from the characteristic tender white mucosal plaques, since bits of adherent food or medication can sometimes be mistaken for yeast infection. Treatment consists of oral nystatin rinses held several minutes in the mouth and then swallowed. In patients unable to cooperate with this regimen or those at risk for aspiration, the oral cavity can be painted twice daily with gentian violet, a fungicidal dye that is effective, if messy and unattractive.

Bacterial Infections

Bacterial infections of old skin are not known to differ substantially from those of young skin, but certain features are noteworthy. First, the age-associated diminution of the inflammatory response may complicate recognition of cellulitis or similar problems. Lack of initial rubor, tumor, calor, and dolor may also render less impressive the patient's response to approriate antibiotic therapy, which is usually quite dramatic in younger individuals. Second, slow healing even in healthy older skin, frequently compounded by diabetes, vascular insufficiency, and other diseases, may result in persistent ulcerations with bacterial superinfection poorly responsive to systemic antibiotics. Such lesions are frequently managed by long-term application of topical antibiotic ointments, but only at the risk of allergic sensitization. Neomycin is perhaps the most frequent offender. Often safer and more effective alternatives include frequent wet-to-dry saline compresses or use of the newer synthetic wound dressings such as Neoderm or Vitaderm if infection can be temporarily eradicated.

Scabies

Although properly speaking an infestation, not an infection, scabies remains an underestimated problem among the elderly, especially those in group residences. Known in Napoleon's time as "the seven-year itch," scabies produces an insidious, progressive, usually extremely pruritic dermatitis that is easily mistaken for eczema or "neurotic" excoriations. The expected concentration of lesions along the flexor wrist and digital web

spaces may be lacking and linear burrows often are. In males, excoriated papules on the glans penis are common and virtually pathognomonic if present (Fig. 21-6). The axillary folds, periumbilical area, and intergluteal cleft are frequent sites of involvement in both sexes. Whenever possible, the diagnosis should be confirmed by microscopic identification of mites or eggs in lesional scrapings. Treatment consists of two 24-hour applications of gammahexabenzene (Kwell) 1 week apart. The entire body surface from the jawline down should be treated, with careful attention to lesion-bearing skin and body folds. In addition, all bed linen, clothes, towels, and other articles in contact with the patient during each 24-hour treatment period should be washed immediately thereafter in hot water. No new lesion should form after the first treatment course, but pruritus often diminishes gradually over 1 to 2 weeks. Topical corticosteroid creams and oral antihistamines during this time may hasten resolution of the secondary eczematous dermatitis. Because infestation with *Sarcoptes scabei* may remain totally asymptomatic for several weeks prior to the patient's developing delayed hypersensitivity to the mites, it is also advisable to treat all close contacts of a documented case, in order to prevent "ping-pong" infestation.

Neoplastic Conditions

Benign Lesions

Neoplasia is associated with aging in virtually all organ systems but is especially characteristic of skin. One or more benign proliferative growths is present in nearly every adult beyond age 65 years, and most individuals have dozens of lesions. Their importance lies in the cosmetic distress they cause many older individuals (whether or not this information is volunteered to the physician) and in the need to differentiate them from various malignant and premalignant lesions, as discussed next. Acrochordons (skin tags) are common on the lateral neck and areas of friction, especially in obese individuals. There are no recognized disease associations. Unsightly lesions can readily be removed by grasping the tip with forceps, by cutting the base with iris scissors, and by applying pressure or a styptic to stop the usually minimal bleeding. Pain from the procedure is minimal in most cases, and local anesthesia is optional.

Seborrheic or "stucco" keratoses are raised, slightly scaly light brown to dark brown plaques, most often on the face and trunk. Curettage under

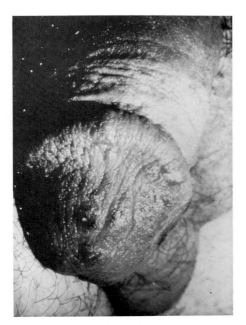

FIG. 21-6. Scabies involving the glans penis. Excoriated papules and diffuse erythema are apparent.

local anesthesia often removes even large lesions without scarring; liquid nitrogen cryotherapy is an alternative approach. The lesions are virtually always without medical significance, although the explosive appearances of *many* keratoses, known as the sign of Leser-Trélat, may indicate occult malignancy.

Cherry angiomas, bright red papules most often on the trunk, are capillary dilatations easily eradicated by electrocautery or argon laser therapy.

Lentigines, evenly pigmented macules also called "age spots," are a completely benign form of melanocytic hyperplasia that can be lightened or removed by liquid nitrogen cryotherapy. Topical hydroquinone (Porcelaina, Artra, Melanex) is much less effective.

Premalignant Lesions

Actinic Keratoses

Actinic keratoses are exceedingly common lesions, present in most fair-skinned elderly individuals, that are best recognized by their sandpaperlike texture; most are red-brown and slightly scaly, more apparent during times of frequent sun exposure with near-total regression after several months of sun avoidance. Management is complicated by the unknown risk of progression to in-

vasive squamous cell carcinoma, variously estimated at less than 1% to more than 20%. Prominent infiltrated (raised) lesions or any of cosmetic concern may be treated individually with liquid nitrogen cryotherapy; scattered inconspicuous lesions can probably be managed with sunscreens only in reliable patients. Extensive involvement is most comprehensively approached by topical use of 5-fluorouracil (5-FU), which destroys abnormal keratinocytes. A 2% to 5% cream preparation is applied twice daily to the entire area at risk, such as the face or upper trunk, until all keratoses "light up" (2 to 3 weeks) then discontinued to allow healing (another 2 to 3 weeks). Patient and physician have the satisfaction of knowing that all keratoses have been treated, but patients must be highly motivated, since 5-FU treatment of severely sun-damaged skin produces widespread tender unslightly erythema often lasting a month or more. There is no advantage to restricting 5-FU application to a selected few keratoses, since treatment is then prolonged and reliant on patient compliance without elimination of clinically inapparent disease. Lesions not eradicated by a course of 5-FU should be biopsied to exclude the possibility of invasive carcinoma.

Leukoplakia

Gradual transition from benign to malignant status for mucous membrane lesions is often accompanied by persistent white discoloration or leukoplakia. The oral cavity is most often involved, but any mucous membrane may behave in this way. Because early invasive carcinoma can be difficult to differentiate from leukoplakia, consultation with an appropriate specialist is usually warranted. Immediate discontinuation of all irritant or carcinogenic exposures, such as tobacco for oral leukoplakia, is imperative. Other measures depend on severity and location of the metaplasia.

Lentigo Maligna

Lentigo maligna is an infrequent precursor to melanoma that is found on sun-exposed skin and differs from the much more common "senile" lentigo by its larger size and greater variation in color. Suspicious lesions deserve biopsy and/or consultation with an experienced dermatologist. Because most lesions progress slowly to malignant melanoma, immediate surgical excision in the elderly is not always warranted, but alternative management approaches should be considered and frequent observation is mandatory.

Malignant Lesions

Virtually all cutaneous malignancies can be attributed to chronic sun damage rather than to aging itself. Regular use of an effective sunscreen beginning early in life will therefore provide great benefit, but anecdotal evidence suggests that avoidance of further exposure beginning even in the seventh or eighth decade may also markedly reduce sun-related morbidity over the ensuing years. In particular, patients with a previous skin cancer have a one-in-three chance of developing a new malignancy each year and therefore should avail themselves of a highly protective (SPF 15) sunscreen during all intentional sun exposures. The role of the primary care physican in management of malignant skin lesions is principally that of early detection, prompt referral, and appropriate follow-up. Basal cell carcinomas and squamous cell carcinomas should be treated by an experienced specialist with one or more of the following: electrosurgery (curettage and electrodesiccation); excision with primary closure, tissue flap rotation, or split-thickness grafting; radiation therapy with external beam or radium implants; and liquid nitrogen cryotherapy or microscopically controlled (Mohs') chemosurgery. Cure rates for primary (nonrecurrent) nonmelanoma skin cancer exceed 90% in all large series and approach 100% for small lesions, regardless of treatment modality. Approach to a specific lesion is therefore based on multiple criteria including cell type, tumor size and location, cosmesis, patient comfort and convenience, and cost, in addition to anticipated success rate. For elderly patients, general health and mental acuity, presence of specific systemic disease, ambulatory status, and home environment are frequently important factors in the physician's choice of therapy. Issues directly related to cutaneous aging have not yet been addressed in the literature but include rate of healing for various types of wounds, character of the resulting scar, intensity of the inflammatory reaction during and after certain procedures, and risk of superinfection. Successful treatment of malignant melanoma depends even more strongly on early diagnosis and definitive surgical treatment.

Basal Cell Carcinoma

Most skin cancers are basal cell carcinomas. Early lesions are asymptomatic, firm, opalescent, or "pearly" papules with fine telangiectases on the surface. More than 90% occur on the habitually

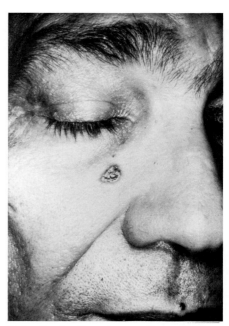

FIG. 21-7. Basal cell carcinoma. Fine rolled border surrounds a crusted central ulcer.

sun-exposed areas of the face and neck (Fig. 21-7). Basal cell carcinomas enlarge very slowly, and 4-mm lesions may have been present for several years. The classic neglected "rodent ulcer" is much less common today but can still be identified by its firm, opalescent telangiectatic rolled border. Differential diagnosis includes dermal nevi, which are flesh-colored but not as firm, and sebaceous hyperplasia, which is also less firm and is characterized by a slightly yellow color and a central punctum, the sebaceous orifice.

Squamous Cell Carcinoma

Squamous cell carcinomas occur in the same fair-skinned patient population as basal cell carcinomas, primarily in habitually sun-exposed areas, but occasionally in sites of chronic ulceration or other skin damage. Early lesions are asymptomatic firm red papules or plaques, usually with scale; more advanced lesions are often ulcerated (Fig. 21-8). Differential diagnosis usually involves various premalignancies that require similar treatment in any case, but verrucous lesions occasionally resemble viral warts, rare among older adults. A cutaneous horn may arise from a well-differentiated squamous cell carcinoma.

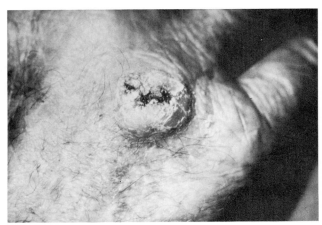

FIG. 21-8. Squamous cell carcinoma. Asymptomatic scaly and crusted firm nodule over the fourth metacarpophalangeal joint arising from sun-damaged skin. Rate of metastasis is lower than for carcinomas arising in sites of chronic ulceration. (Courtesy of Rita Berman, MD)

Melanoma

Malignant melanoma is rare in comparison with nonmelanomatous skin cancer but is increasing in incidence at an alarming 6% annually, approximately sixfold over the past 4 decades. Depending on the subtype, peak incidences occur in the fifth to eighth decades of life. Clinical criteria for the diagnosis of melanoma include diameter greater than 7 mm, irregular border and surface topography, and variation in color ("red, white, and blue"). Loss of skin surface markings, easy bleeding, ulceration, and local discomfort are late findings. Differential diagnosis in the elderly usually involves seborrheic ("stucco") keratoses and lentigines ("age spots"). The former are usually multiple, evenly pigmented with a "regularly irregular" papillated surface and slight scale; and the latter are macular (flat) and evenly pigmented. Nevocellular nevi (moles) rarely arise in the el-

derly. Conversion of lentigo maligna to invasive melanoma is accompanied by the development of raised areas within the otherwise flat lesion.

SUGGESTED READINGS

Balin AK, Kligman AM, Grove GL: Aging and the Skin. New York, Raven Press (In press)

Carter DB, Balin AK: Dermatological aspects of aging. Med Clin North Am 67:531–534, 1983

Gilchrest BA: Age-associated changes in the skin: Overview and clinical relevance. J Am Geriatr Soc 30:129–143, 1982

Gilchrest BA: Skin and Aging Processes. Boca Raton, Fl, CRC Press, 1984

Selmanowitz VJ, Rizer RL, Orentreich N: Aging of the skin and its appendages. In Finch CE, Hayflick L (eds.): Handbook of the Biology of Aging, p 496. New York, Van Nostrand Rheinhold Co, 1977

22 Hematologic Disorders in the Elderly

Mervyn L. Goldstein

Hematologic evaluation of the older patient benefits from the same thorough history and physical examination that form the basis of successful medical care for all age-groups. "Routine" ethnic data may have a profound impact on hematologic differential diagnosis. For example, it has been estimated that up to 25% of New York City residents of black African background have an α-thalassemia variant that can give their red blood cells a benign hypochromia and microcytosis; this could cause the clinician to start testing for many irrelevant diseases. Similarly, recent emigrants from the Indo-Chinese peninsula have a high incidence of hemoglobin E, which can impart target cells and microcytosis to red blood cells. A person named O'Leary, for example, might have had a Sicilian mother and be subject to occult anemia related to β-thalassemia minor. Northern Europeans appear more subject to pernicious anemia. In yet another example there is more Gaucher's disease reported in Eastern European Jews, while their Middle Eastern cousins have glucose-6-phosphate dehydrogenase (G-6-PD) deficiency.

Chronic occupational exposures must be considered in the evaluation of anemia. Disorders caused by occupational and household exposures to organic solvents, insecticides, and other potential toxins also warrant consideration.

The tendency for polypharmacy in the elderly makes the drug history particularly important. It is not enough to ask, "Do you take aspirin?" The patient might deny using aspirin, yet be taking Bufferin, Excedrin, Darvon Compound, Coricidin, Alka Seltzer, or any of the more than 900 medications that contain acetylsalicylic acid. It is better to ask, "If you have an ache or a pain, what do you take for it?" Do you take any medication to help you sleep or calm your nerves?" It's often

worthwhile to have the patient bring all medications including vitamins from his medicine cabinet. A prescription vitamin might have folic acid, masking vitamin B_{12} deficiency; a vitamin with "minerals" might have iron, masking anemia due to blood loss. An antihypertensive agent containing methyldopa (Aldomet) could result in a clinically confusing positive Coombs test. One notable patient was receiving very low dose methotrexate from a dermatologist for psoriasis, phenytoin (Dilantin) from a neurologist, and trimethoprim-sulfamethoxazole from her family physician for recurring urinary tract infections. She became profoundly pancytopenic owing to the combined anti–folic acid effects.

One has to question the patient carefully[33] about possible bleeding in the evaluation of anemia. Any patient, but particularly an elderly person might not look at the stools regularly. In contrast, blood in the urine would be rapidly noticed by most males. It is rare for hematuria *per se* to cause anemia directly; it is much more likely that what is causing the bleeding is also causing the anemia.

The patient must check for low-grade occult fever in the evening, rather than at the time of the office visit. Oral thermometers are often improperly positioned, especially by the elderly. Failing eyesight may preclude accurate readings.

Symptoms in the gastrointestinal tract provide a wealth of clues to hematologic disease, including those related to ulcers, malignancies, hemorrhoids, hiatal hernia, polyps, early gallbladder disease, and others. Chronic constipation and a tendency to bundle up when others feel warm might be considered normal in the elderly but might also be clues to an underactive thyroid gland. An otherwise healthy older patient might complain of problems walking to the bathroom, alleviated by a night light, as the first clue to the proprioceptive difficulty of his pernicious anemia.

In the elderly patient who is unable to give a reliable history, physical findings become even more important. Anemias associated with smooth tongue, small or large thyroid gland, and enlargement of lymph nodes, liver, or spleen are well known. With the patient still in the right lateral decubitus position for examination of the left upper quadrant, the physician might divert briefly to the ankles to test deep tendon reflexes. This posture is generally well tolerted by the elderly, and the examiner can get a good appreciation of the slow return characteristic of the sluggish thyroid. Simultaneously, the physician can test vibration at the malleoli. When testing for position sensation in the toes, the examiner's fingers should be holding the lateral edges of the toe, avoiding contact with adjacent toes, to preclude tactile clues that allow the patient to give the right answer although he lacks proprioceptive skills. Anemia in the elderly demands a rectal examination with testing for blood in the stool.

LABORATORY EVALUATION OF ANEMIA

Although there are conflicting data as to whether there is a minor fall in hematocrit late in life, blood counts remain remarkably stable with age in the otherwise healthy person, despite decreasing marrow cellularity.

In evaluating the patient with anemia, the physican often relies on such basic studies as the hematocrit, red blood cell indices, serum iron level, vitamin B_{12} and folate levels, the Coombs test, and automated chemistries. Unfortunately, laboratory tests can be deceiving, even with these basic parameters. In contrast to red blood cell indices, morphology of cells as discerned on the blood smear is so important that it might well be considered part of the physical examination of the anemic patient.

A patient with rouleaux formation may have significant elevation of his mean corpuscular volume and mean corpuscular hemoglobin. If this is interpreted as macrocytosis, an exhaustive search for vitamin deficiency or a fruitless trial of therapy might be initiated. Since the sedimentation rate, (*i.e.*, rouleaux formation) increases with age, this artifact is more likely in the elderly. Equally important, if the patient really has a microcytic anemia, his indices might be normalized by the rouleau artifact, and early diagnosis of iron deficiency could be missed.

The packed cell volume obtained by centrifugation is not the same as the number calculated by an automated cell counter. For example, the rigid red cells of iron deficiency anemia do not pack as readily as normal red cells. Thus the spun packed cell volume may be several points higher than the automated counter printout. Thus interpretations of blood loss could be significantly distorted.

Another source of erroneous interpretation is in the leukemic patient with a high white cell count and reduced red cells; his buffy coat will make up a significant proportion of the calculated packed cell volume. In contrast, when his blood is spun, the technician will read only to the top of the packed red cell layer to give the hematocrit and then note the size of the buffy coat separately. Were the technician relying solely on the automated count, he could easily wonder why symptoms of anemia were disproportionate to the laboratory value.

The serum iron value and iron binding capacity are frequently used to determine the presence of iron deficiency, despite an estimated error rate of up to 20% with this test.

Serum ferritin is a far more reliable measure of iron stores. It is particularly good in screening otherwise healthy people. However, malignancy, liver disease, and chronic inflammatory disorders raise the ferritin level and may mask the fact that the anemia is due to blood loss. Since in these diseases iron status is most crucial, even this test must be used judiciously.

The Coombs test is commonly used to ascertain if a patient is undergoing hemolysis. However, up to 10% of patients with autoimmune hemolysis have a negative Coombs test and require a more sensitive method of detection, such as the Lalezari-Polybrene test[25]; 20% of patients receiving methyldopa may develop a positive Coombs test, but less than 1% will develop hemolysis. Considering the widespread use of methyldopa among the elderly, the physician must use caution in interpreting the Coombs test for up to 2 years after this medication is discontinued.

A standard commercial radiodilution assay kit was totally ineffective in screening for vitamin B_{12} deficiency.[8] Thus the diagnosis of pernicious anemia may have been incorrectly dismissed in many patients. Failure to diagnose vitamin B_{12} deficiency has potentially tragic consequences while neurologic deterioration, possibly blamed on age, continues. The serum folate level suffers from similar pitfalls, since it measures diet and absorption much more than it reflects folate stores or anemia due to folate deficiency. The red cell folate, a better test for this problem, is not as readily available or used.

Physicians rely on the prothrombin time as a basic tool when treating with coumarin anticoagulants. Yet if one takes citrated blood, splits it into three parts, and runs prothrombin times with three different sources of tissue factor, results that are two, two and one-half, and three times the control value can be obtained. Thus the results from the hospital laboratory, the commercial laboratory, or the hematologist might be different. The implications for managing a given patient are obvious.

For routine screening, the automated platelet counter gives more accurate and reproducible results than manual methods. However, in patients with paraproteins, schistocytes, and sometimes for no apparent clinical reason, there are gross discrepancies between the automated platelet count and the "real platelet count" as documented by blood smear estimates and the tedious and time-consuming manual methods.

We often place great reliance on chemical analyses. Besides the pathologic and physiologic factors that can modify them, a long list of medicines, vitamins, alcohol, and other agents can alter results. Hormones, diuretics, anti-inflammatory agents, antibiotics, psychoactive medications, cardioactive drugs, laxatives, and others can alter one or another standard chemistry determination. Thus despite the seeming logic of starting the evaluation of disorders of the blood with examination of the blood, the physician must be aware of the pitfalls.

Hemolysis Versus Decreased Blood Production

When initial findings suggest a specific disorder, one can go on to very selective confirmatory tests. However, when the diagnosis is not immediately apparent, there is a tendency to use a shotgun approach. The charts in many fine teaching hospitals will show admission orders for barium enema, gastrointestinal series, liver and spleen scans, vitamin B_{12} and folate levels, iron and iron binding capacity, haptoglobin and Coombs test, and routine and not so routine chemistries and serologies, often suggesting lack of thought as to pathogenetic mechanisms. Mechanistically, anemia is due to poor blood production, increased blood destruction, blood loss, or some combination of these disorders.[9,33] Certain tests will rapidly distinguish among them.

An often overlooked test is the reticulocyte count. Reticulocytes decrease with poor blood pro-duction and increase with increased blood destruction. Perhaps the lack of appreciation of this test is related to a frequent misinterpretation of the result. Since a normal marrow can produce seven to ten times the usual number of reticulocytes, failure to do so when challenged by anemia represents poor production. For example, a 4% reticulocytosis in response to profound anemia reflects poor production, even when one has made the required correction in the count for the level of anemia. A better appreciation of the reticulocyte count might be obtained if thought of in absolute numbers rather than percentages. A normal count would be 50,000 per mm^3 and a diagnosis of hemolysis typically would have over 250,000 per mm^3.

Blood Loss

Early recognition of iron deficiency in the elderly patient may well be critical. It can mean the difference between an operable lesion in the colon or death from metastases. A clinician does a disservice by giving iron therapy for anemia if he has not proven lack of iron is the cause. Proving iron deficiency is not enough; bleeding is the most likely cause, and the source of bleeding must be determined.

The blood smear does not correlate well with iron deficiency until the hematocrit falls below 30%. Since it takes perhaps 7 to 10 days to deplete the body of iron stores, the bleeding patient will not produce even one hypochromic microcytic cell until these stores are used up; thus the classic smear might not be apparent for at least several weeks. The stool may become negative a few days after a bleeding episode or may be positive due to unrelated factors. Thus even key parameters may be deceiving.

Commonly, the next laboratory studies obtained are the iron level and iron binding capacity or serum ferritin value, although they are subject to major errors, as discussed earlier. Were there no other reason for doing a bone marrow examination in an anemic patient, the early and accurate diagnosis of iron deficiency would be sufficient. Other information gleaned from the marrow is so critical, definitive, and rapidly obtained that it is a key tool.

MANAGEMENT OF IRON DEFICIENCY ANEMIA

Once the diagnosis and cause of iron deficiency anemia have been evaluated, correcting it in the

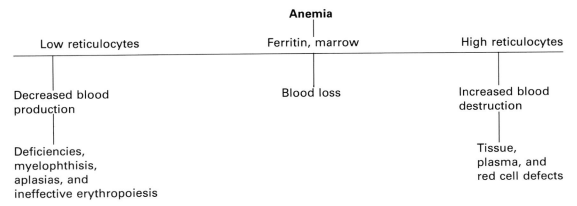

Anemia

Low reticulocytes — Ferritin, marrow — High reticulocytes

Decreased blood production — Blood loss — Increased blood destruction

Deficiencies, myelophthisis, aplasias, and ineffective erythropoiesis — Tissue, plasma, and red cell defects

FIG. 22-1. Algorithm showing conditions in which bone marrow fails to respond to anemia:

Deficiencies: Fe^{++}, B_{12}, folate, "B_6," protein, vitamin C, others

Myelophthisis: carcinoma, leukemia, myeloma, fibrosis, granulomata, lipid storage, other

Aplasias: pure red cell (idiopathic, thymoma, lupus, carcinomata, others), aplastic anemia (idiopathic, drug-related, toxic, other)

Ineffective erythropoiesis: infection, inflammation, malignancy, endocrinopathy, toxic/suppressive state, thalassemia minor, others

Tissue defects: hypersplenism, microangiopathic hemolytic anemias

Plasma defects: antibodies (warm or cold reacting), nonantibody

Red cell defects: membrane (hereditary spherocytosis and elliptocytosis, PNH), enzymes (G-6-PD, P-K, etc.), and hemoglobin (production or structure)

majority of patients is readily accomplished with the least expensive iron tablet. In the elderly, additional factors may change one's approach.

The decrease in gastric acidity with aging may lessen absorption of iron. Adding vitamin C to the regimen occasionally seems to overcome this. A corollary is that the simultaneous use of antacid will greatly inhibit the therapeutic benefit of iron. The two medications should not be taken within several hours of each other.

The older patient may suffer vague abdominal distress or change in bowel habits sometimes attributed to iron therapy. In the patient who has had gastric surgery, the iron tablet may be rapidly delivered distal to the area of optimum absorption. In such patients, an iron suspension, such as Fer-in-Sol Pediatric Suspension, without the high concentrations of alcohol found in an "elixir," can be very effective. The major shortcoming of liquid iron preparations is their propensity to stain teeth or dentures. To avoid this, the medication can be placed on the back of the tongue, swallowed, and rinsed down with water.

Although the young, healthy patient classically shows some hematologic response in as little as 5 days, the older sick patient may not respond for several weeks and may never show a reticulocyte surge. If the patient's blood count does not return to normal after a reasonable period, one has to search for other problems, such as continued bleeding, combined deficiencies, or a second illness.

"FAILURE" OF BLOOD PRODUCTION

Conditions in which the bone marrow cannot mount the usual reticulocyte response to anemia are frequently associated with a mildly shortened red blood cell survival (*i.e.*, an element of hemolysis), but the limiting factor is subnormal marrow response. It is useful to categorize these conditions under four major headings (Fig. 22-1) so one can quickly identify the problem.

DECREASED BLOOD PRODUCTION

Deficiencies

Iron Deficiency

Based on World Health Organization statistics, the most common cause of anemia worldwide is dietary deficiency of iron, without specific mention of associated blood loss. This is based on automated methods of determining hemoglobin, mean corpuscular volume, and mean corpuscular hemoglobin. In view of accumulating data that large populations have α-thalassemia variants and others have myriad diseases causing hypochromia and microcytosis, this conclusion is open to question. Intestinal mechanisms seem geared mainly to keep excess iron out. Before blaming diet for iron deficiency, it behooves the clinician to rule out occult bleeding.

Vitamin B_{12} and Folic Acid Deficiencies

The megaloblastic anemias are the next major nutrient deficiencies causing anemia.[18] A strong suspicion of lack of vitamin B_{12} or folic acid can be obtained from the history and physical examination. Classic features include insidious onset of symptoms, anemia out of proportion to clinical appearance, complaints related to malabsorption, thyroid disease, posterolateral column degeneration, and so on. Mental status changes due to vitamin B_{12} deficiency might be considered even in the absence of anemia, especially if the patient has had sources of folic acid that might have corrected the hematologic picture. When smooth tongue, neurologic changes, chronic alcohol ingestion, or an anti–folic acid medication all point in a particular direction, simple confirmatory tests can be obtained. Macro-ovalocytosis and hypersegmented granulocytes on blood smears provide much more reliable clues than elevated indices from automated blood cell counters. The bone marrow is exquisitely sensitive to these deficiencies. With vitamin B_{12} and folic acid deficiency, marrow changes are usually profound and generally not confused with the less pronounced cytonuclear changes seen with azotemia, malignancies, and other conditions. Determining the mechanism for the vitamin deficiency would include blood levels of the vitamins, determination of the serum thyroxine value, upper gastrointestinal series plus small bowel follow through, the various measures for assessing malabsorption, gastric analysis or endoscopic biopsy as appropriate evaluation for intrinsic factor antibody, and the Schilling test.

Since the Schilling test is critical, it must be remembered that up to 40% of patients with pernicious anemia develop a secondary malabsorption reflected in low vitamin B_{12} excretion for both phase I and phase II of this laboratory examination. Repeat study several weeks later after the malabsorptive problem is corrected by vitamin B_{12} therapy will ensure proper diagnosis. An *in vitro* technique using nucleic acid incorporation into lymphocytes is being used investigationally to diagnose vitamin B_{12} and folic acid deficiency up to 1 month following therapy.

With an inexpensive, nontoxic medication such as vitamin B_{12}, it seems wise to err on the high side in replacing it. One might give 1 mg every other day for seven doses, followed by 1 mg per month thereafter.

Initial therapy in the elderly can pose special problems. The rapid flux of potassium into billions of developing cells poised to synthesize nucleic acids has reportedly caused hypokalemia-induced arrhythmias. Correction of potassium loss should be dictated by serum determinations. Despite a lack of symptoms, the older patient with a very low hematocrit is frequently transfused. Since the heart may be functioning poorly because of the vitamin deficiency, routine transfusion can lead to refractory congestive heart failure. This problem is addressed by reserving transfusion for symptomatic or profound anemia, infusing the blood very slowly, giving the patient a diuretic at the time of transfusion, or even removing equal volumes of anemic blood from one arm while administering the transfusion into the other arm.

The progressive fall in red blood cell 2,3 diphosphoglycerate (2,3 DPG) with storage in the blood bank is a well described phenomenon. Such 2,3 DPG deficient blood does not efficiently release its oxygen to the tissues until the body synthesizes adequate replacement levels. It might even decrease oxygen delivery tissues with the paradoxical potential for harming the tenuous patient. To avoid this possibility, the physician can ensure that the cells for transfusion, collected in citrate-phosphate-dextrose (CPD) solution, were in the blood bank less than 10 days to minimize the effect that reduced 2,3-DPG levels have on oxygen delivery to the tissues.

Folic acid deficiency in the elderly is more commonly dietary in origin than vitamin B_{12} deficiency but may result from anti–folic acid agents such as trimethoprim-sulfamethoxazole, alcohol, or anticonvulsants. Tropical sprue can evolve even years after a patient has left an endemic area. Inflammatory or lymphomatous involvement of the bowel may also be discovered. Despite malabsorption of naturally occurring folic acid, the medicinal form given orally is generally well absorbed. Care must be used when folic acid is given to the person receiving phenytoin since there is some evidence this may lessen anticonvulsant activity. Vitamin B_{12} deficiency should generally be ruled out before prescribing folic acid to preclude masking anemia while neurologic damage progresses.

Miscellaneous Deficiencies

Anemia has been associated with profound protein deficiency, vitamin C deficiency, and lack of various B vitamins. Pyridoxine–responsive anemias are rarely deficiency states in the classic sense but represent a category in which pharmacologic as opposed to physiologic doses of this vitamin can be beneficial. The diagnosis is generally made by observing ring sideroblasts in a marrow obtained from a patient with a hypochromic, microcytic, or two-population anemia. The marrow finding is frequently a surprise that then prompts the physician to look for an underlying hematologic or epithelial malignancy or chronic inflammatory disease. About one third of such patients have a partial response to 300–600 mg of pyridoxine daily, or to pyridoxal-5-phosphate.

These miscellaneous nutritional deficiencies are best diagnosed by careful history and physical examination. For example, one would not obtain leukocyte or platelet ascorbic acid levels unless he has seen perifollicular hemorrhages in the clinical setting of vitamin C deficiency.

Myelophthisic Anemias With Decreased Blood Production

The myelophthisic anemias include widespread marrow replacement by epithelial tumor, hematologic malignancy, fibrosis, lipid-laden macrophages as in Gaucher's disease, and disseminated granulomas. Unexplained nucleated red blood cells in the peripheral blood, so often a marker of extramedullary hematopoiesis, are frequent clues to osseous metastases or primary hematologic malignancy in the elderly.

When metastases to bone are suspected, a bone biopsy is more likely to provide useful material than an aspirate alone. Whether or not the biopsy is performed, a specimen of aspirated marrow can be allowed to clot firmly, placed in appropriate preservative, and delivered to the pathologist for processing without the usual need for decalcification. This additional material aids in diagnosis and is suitable for many special stains that cannot be performed on the standard core of bone. When marrow cannot be aspirated, slides of material obtained by imprinting the bone core or needle edge can be diagnostic of cancer.

When prostatic carcinoma is a consideration, the physician can aspirate additional material for a bone marrow acid phosphatase, which is a more sensitive measure of bone involvement than the regular serum level. Because of the temperature sensitivity of this enzyme, the specimen must be processed rapidly in the chemistry laboratory or an appropriate preservative must be used.

Therapy of the anemia of myelophthisic diseases is generally that of the underlying primary disorder. Hematologic malignancies are discussed later in this chapter.

Red Cell Aplasias

Red cell aplasia may involve purely the red cells or be part of an aplastic anemia. The former is much rarer and is characterized by a virtual lack of red blood cell precursors in the bone marrow. The possibility of a thymoma must be considered and mediastinal computed tomography performed if routine chest films are not diagnostic. Various malignancies and a long list of medications have also been associated; in many cases, no cause is found. Again, therapy is aimed at the underlying disorder (*e.g.,* discontinuing medications, thymectomy). Androgens, corticosteroids, and splenectomy have been used in patients refractory to the removal of the thymic tumor.

Aplastic anemia, unless rapidly reversed by discontinuing an offending agent, is devastating in all age-groups, but particularly in the elderly. Patients with severe cases often present in the throes of life-threatening complications.[15] The elderly are not amenable to bone marrow transplantation. Androgens, although seemingly beneficial in individual patients, do not appear to alter outcome significantly in large studies. Supportive measures related to infection, bleeding, and anemia are generally required but are frequently futile. Investigations with antithymocyte globulin may provide a therapy in the future.

The diagnosis is made by the combination of pancytopenia and hypoplastic bone biopsy (as opposed to just a hypocellular marrow aspirate) to ensure that a lack of cells is not in reality the lack of an adequate specimen. The presence of nucleated red cells in the peripheral blood or of splenomegaly make the diagnosis of classic aplastic anemia virtually untenable, and another cause for pancytopenia should be sought.

Ineffective Erythropoiesis

The combination of anemia with reasonable representation of red cell precursors in the bone marrow yet poor reticulocyte response defines ineffective erythropoiesis. The red cells do not seem to get out into the circulating blood. This is often called the anemia of chronic disease and in the elderly is a "waste basket diagnosis" inappropriately considered an endpoint in itself. A systematic differential diagnosis will often direct one to studies that pinpoint manageable disorders.

Ineffective erythropoiesis is commonly seen with infection, chronic inflammatory disorders, azotemia, liver disease, malignancy, endocrinopathy, toxic or suppressive states, and thalassemia minor. This list should prompt the physician to delve more deeply into these possibilities. Should the patient check his temperature at night? Is there a hidden abscess? Is there a past history of blood transfusion or an exposure to hepatotoxins, including alcohol? Are there signs and symptoms of occult thyroid or other glandular disease? Is the sedimentation rate over 100 ml/h Westergren without good clinical explanation, suggesting malignancy? Has the patient taken medication with the potential for toxic or idiosyncratic damage to the marrow? Is the patient of Mediterranean background? These and similar questions can provide the clinician with meaningful answers.

INCREASED BLOOD DESTRUCTION

A steady or falling hematocrit associated with reticulocytosis generally indicates clinically significant hemolysis. If the hematocrit is rising, reticulocytosis reflects regeneration of blood, as might be seen with treated pernicious anemia. The pathogenesis of red cell destruction generally falls into one of three broad categories: (1) defects of tissues, (2) abnormalities in the plasma, or (3) defects of the red cell itself.[13]

Tissue Defects

The most common "tissue defect" encountered is hypersplenism. When fully evolved, it is characterized by pancytopenia; when a single cell line is decreased, although splenectomy may be curative, the pathogenesis is generally not a large spleen alone but is related to another problem such as a connective tissue disorder or antibody formation. The marrow in hypersplenism shows at least adequate representation of the normal cell lines and is usually hypercellular. A third feature is palpable enlargement of the spleen. Although additional confirmatory data can be obtained with a chromium-51 red cell survival study with splenic uptake, the definitive diagnosis is dependent on relief by splenectomy.

Hypersplenism can complicate any of the long list of diseases that cause enlargement of the spleen, including a wide variety of infections, hemoglobinopathies, granulomatous diseases, liver disease, malignancies, connective tissue disorders, infiltrative diseases, and so on. The majority of such patients will never require splenectomy, especially in the older age-groups. However, when painful splenomegaly, inordinate pressure symptoms, or profound cytopenia occur, splenectomy can be performed with significant benefit and acceptable morbidity and mortality.

The other tissue defects resulting in hemolysis are the macroangiopathic and microangiopathic hemolytic anemias. A tight aortic valve or certain artificial aortic valves can traumatize red cells sufficiently to cause hemoglobinemia, hemoglobinuria, or hemosiderinuria. The microangiopathic disorders often present with the hemorrhagic features of an associated disseminated intravascular coagulation (DIC).

Thrombotic thrombocytopenic purpura presents as fever, neurologic and renal manifestations, bleeding, and hemolytic anemia. Current management includes plasma infusion or exchange and agents that inhibit platelet aggregation. Disseminated intravascular coagulation syndromes in the elderly are generally associated with malignancies, shock, sepsis, and malignant hypertension. Management of disseminated intravascular coagulation is best aimed at the underlying cause, with antibacterials, blood pressure support, antitumor therapy, and similar specific therapies. Heparin has beneficial effects on laboratory parameters more than on clinical outcome, except in rare instances such as hypergranular acute leukemia. The angiopathic syndromes can be strongly suspected when helmet cells and schistocytes are prominent on the blood smear.

Plasma Abnormalities

Although chronic diseases may shorten red cell survival through plasma abnormalities, ordinarily plasma factors causing hemolysis refer to the cold- or the warm-reacting antibodies that may be idiopathic or associated with medications or disease.

Typical anti-I, cold-reacting, IgM antibodies are present in titers up to 64 in normal serum. They are also seen in higher titers in patients with atypical pneumonias, connective tissue disorders, lymphomas, and an idiopathic hemolytic disorder.

When a patient presents with a syndrome suggesting infection caused by *Mycoplasma pneumoniae*, the physician often orders a cold agglutinin test, expecting to find a "diagnostic" elevation. More typically, the patient has a normal titer at the time of respiratory symptoms, with the serum antibody level rising to perhaps 1000 as the pneumonia is resolving. Hemolysis is generally mild and may be missed. Thus, the cold agglutinin titer at the time of presentation should be taken as the baseline by which to gauge the subsequent diagnostic elevation several weeks later. The hemolysis is generally self-limited, requiring no specific management other than ensuring that the patient keeps away from cooling blankets should fever be present or recur.

Connective tissue disorders and lymphomas may be associated with either warm- or cold-reacting antibodies or with both. The cold agglutinin titer often ranges as high as 100,000 and may be associated with significant hemolysis. With these syndromes, therapy is aimed at the underlying disease. Once again, the patient is kept warm, and any infused products are best warmed before they are given.

Idiopathic cold agglutinin disease may be associated with titers in the millions and can be clinically devastating. Exposure to air conditioning or swimming in a lake can cause profound hemolysis. Attempts at management have included corticosteroids, plasmapheresis, immunosuppressives, depolymerizing agents for macroglobulin, and splenectomy. Patients may be forced to move to a warm climate and must wear clothing protecting all parts of the body in cold weather. This disorder, although rare, tends to occur late in life and should be considered in the differential diagnosis of hemolytic disorders of the elderly.

The autoimmune hemolytic anemias associated with warm-reacting antibodies are commonly idiopathic or associated with medications, connective tissue disorders, lymphoproliferative diseases, and other malignancies. Diagnosis is generally made by reticulocytosis and a positive Coombs test. The occurrence of both false positives and false negatives in this basic test for antibodies, or the confusion caused by administration of methyldopa, make the Lalezari-Polybrene test useful.[25]

Transfusion of patients with red cell antibodies can be hazardous[22] because of cross-matching difficulties and because the infused blood is destroyed as rapidly as the patient's own. Thus the patient with the most severe hemolysis, who is most in need of transfusions, is the one least able to tolerate them.

Numerous medications, including methyldopa, penicillins, cephalosporins, quinidine, quinine, and sulfa derivatives, have been associated with hemolysis. Patients are managed by stopping potential offending agents and providing support during the days required for the reaction to subside. In the lymphomas and connective tissue disorders, therapy aimed at the underlying disease is generally beneficial. Corticosteroids are a mainstay of therapy in patients with warm-reacting antibodies that are not drug induced. Other immunosuppressives have been used with mixed results. Controversy exists as to whether splenectomy should be done within the first few weeks before corticosteroids have had their adverse effects on tissues and wound healing or be delayed in the hope that low doses will minimize future life-threatening episodes. Age itself does not appear to preclude a good outcome.

Although rarely encountered in the routine medical practice, malaria, babesiosis, clostridial infection, and other bacterial, viral, and protozoan infections have been associated with hemolysis. Therapy is aimed at the underlying cause when possible, supplemented by transfusion and supportive measures.

Defects in the Red Cell

Red cell abnormalities associated with hemolysis include defects in the membrane, the hemoglobin, and the other cellular contents.

One does not generally think of hereditary spherocytosis as a disease of the elderly. The typical patient is young; is anemic; has splenomegaly and mild icterus; has a family history of anemia, gallbladder disease, or splenectomy; and has the diagnosis readily made by examination of the blood smear. However, the disease can be much more occult when it is mild. Such patients may reach old age without a diagnosis having been made. Anemia may be mild or intermittent. A major clue could be cholecystectomy at a very early age. Some patients have been diagnosed as having recurrent hepatitis because of a history of recurrent jaundice. The blood smear may be contributory only if examined with this diagnosis in mind since the milder cases that reach old age have less morphologic change than the more typical pediatric case. One subtle clue is a mean corpuscular hemoglobin concentration over 36 g/dl of red cells. A patient who has reached old age with hereditary spherocytosis and his spleen might go on without surgery, although this is still the treatment of choice. As in any chronic hemolytic anemia, treatment with folic acid can be beneficial because of increased requirements for this substance.

Hereditary elliptocytosis can be found in the elderly since there are usually no clinical manifestations throughout life. In my experience, significant hemolysis is generally associated with a second major illness, including Gaucher's disease, multiple myeloma, and others. When required, the therapy is similar to that for hereditary spherocytosis. Spherocytosis, when manifest in the elderly, often requires some form of the osmotic fragility test for confirmation. In contrast, the diagnosis of elliptocytosis is readily made from the blood smear.

Congenital hemoglobinopathies with associated hemolysis will generally have been diagnosed before the patient reaches the geriatric age range.[16] Hemoglobin C disease, sickle trait, β-thalassemia minor, and the α-thalassemias, with minimal or no clinical manifestations, are to be excluded as causes of abnormal blood smears. The older patient with sickle trait might present with hematuria and undergo extensive if not dangerous and unnecessary evaluations. In addition, general anesthesia or pulmonary compromise could conceivably precipitate a sickle crisis.

Clinically significant red cell enzyme deficiencies are likely to have been diagnosed before old age. However, unexplained hemolysis in patients of appropriate ethnic background, exposed to agents such as sulfa drugs (including most diuretics and oral hypoglycemics), requires appropriate screening tests to rule out G-6-PD deficiency.

EVALUATION OF THE BLEEDING PATIENT

Bleeding phenomena can range from mild purpura to panic-producing intraoperative hemorrhage. A common reaction is to pour in large volumes of blood products and "hemostasis-promoting" agents. Occasionally, empiric therapy with one or more modalities may be required. Optimally, a patient should be evaluated preoperatively for potential bleeding disorders. If the disorder occurs intraoperatively or postoperatively, the chart must be gleaned for enough data to allow a reasonable diagnosis. No matter what the circumstances, a logical thought process will greatly enhance appropriate clinical management.

The normal elements involved with hemostasis include the blood vessel wall and its supporting structures, the circulating platelets, and the various plasma materials associated with clotting.

Disorders of the Blood Vessel and Supporting Structures

Inordinate bruising and petechiae may be seen with advancing age alone ("senile" purpura). Included in the differential diagnosis are thrombocytopenia, exogenous corticosteroids or Cushing's

disease, the microvascular abnormality of diabetes mellitus, vasculitis, the paraproteinemias (which can also affect the other components of hemostasis), various infectious diseases, autoimmune and drug-related purpuras, scurvy, connective tissue diseases, and milder forms of Marfan's syndrome.

If combined with such data as whether "spontaneous" purpura is in exposed areas, the capillary fragility test may be useful in distinguishing whether ecchymoses are due to a bleeding disorder or to trauma. Other tests for suspected clinical entities might include blood sugars, blood cultures, skin biopsy, or even platelet vitamin C levels.

Platelet Abnormalities

Platelet problems involve their number or their function. High platelet counts appear to be associated with bleeding only when part of a myeloproliferative disorder such as essential thrombocythemia, polycythemia vera, myelofibrosis, and the myeloid leukemias. Besides tests of platelet function, diagnostic studies are aimed at the underlying disorders, and management generally involves cytotoxic agents including radioactive pharmaceuticals. Paradoxically, despite the high platelet counts, bleeding episodes can be treated in such patients with platelet infusions; platelet pheresis has also been used pending the effects of cytotoxic therapy.

Low platelet counts are a far more common cause of bleeding phenomena. In the elderly this commonly presents as petechiae distal to garters, under tight-fitting clothing, or simply on dependent parts of the body. Major bleeding can also be the first overt manifestation.

Identifying causes of thrombocytopenia can follow a logic parallel to, although not identical with, that used in evaluating anemia. There are disorders of platelet production, platelet destruction, and, in cases of massive blood replacement, platelet loss. Decreased platelet production can again be broken down into deficiency states, myelophthisic disorders, megakaryocytic hypoplasias, and "ineffective thrombopoiesis" as noted in a variety of chronic diseases. Although there is no exact counterpart for thalassemia minor involving platelets, there are parallel abnormalities such as the May-Hegglin anomaly in which both number and content of platelets are affected.

The comparison also extends to increased platelet destruction, wherein mechanisms include defects in the tissues (spleen and blood vessels), immune and nonimmune plasma defects, and intrinsic platelet abnormalities.

As in asymptomatic anemia, milder reductions

in platelet counts should be evaluated before bleeding occurs. The list of medical and environmental agents that can cause a low platelet count is so long, virtually any exogenous material is suspect. Careful attention to exposure to such agents is particularly warranted in the elderly.

Although many hemostatic abnormalities follow open heart surgery, the associated decrease in platelet numbers and function proves most important responding to postoperative, posthypothermic platelet infusions.

The ready availability of platelet counts precludes less reliable screening tests; if a bleeding disorder is a strong clinical consideration, a "normal" automated platelet count should be checked manually or on blood smears. When relying on platelet estimates, one must remember that platelets are compared in relative numbers with other cell lines. Thus, if platelets appear normal on smear and the patient's hematocrit is half normal, the corresponding platelet count is half normal.

Although visible manifestations of bleeding start near a count of 100,000/cu mm, one can often perform minor invasive procedures with slightly lower counts; however the likelihood of complications rises. The changes of spontaneous major bleeding go up at perhaps 20,000/cu mm, and "spontaneous," life-threatening bleeding is common below 10,000/cu mm. An underlying myeloproliferative disorder, antiplatelet immune phenomena, or agents causing platelet functional abnormalities greatly enhance the risk of bleeding at a given platelet count. High platelet turnover seems associated with less hemorrhage at a given platelet count than low platelet turnover, perhaps reflecting better platelet function in younger platelets.

Platelet functional defects may be congenital or acquired. In the elderly, the importance of medications in inhibiting thrombus formation is dramatically emphasized by the clinical use of aspirin, dipyridamole (Persantine), and sulfinpyrazone (Anturane), in an attempt to prevent thrombotic phenomena. Antibiotics, antidepressants, anticoagulants, antitussives, antihistamines, analgesics, and alcohol are among the many agents found to impair platelet function. Azotemia, paraproteins, and myeloproliferative disorders can do likewise.

Von Willebrand's disease is an example of a congenital platelet functional defect caused by a deficiency of a circulating clotting factor. When mild, this disorder can escape detection throughout life.

The bleeding time is a reliable screening test for abnormalities of platelet function or thrombocytopenia. A more quantitative measure of platelet function is obtained by aggregometry. Although particularly useful in defining congenital platelet abnormalities and von Willebrand's disease, its correlation with clinical bleeding problems leaves much to be desired.

Management of bleeding problems in patients with platelet abnormalities requires a knowledge of the underlying mechanisms. Conditions with high platelet turnover, such as autoimmune thrombocytopenia, are unlikely to benefit from platelet infusions, since foreign platelets are destroyed at least as rapidly as the patient's own. Depending on the cause, therefore, therapy might consist of corticosteroids, danazol, intravenous γ-globulin, *Vinca* alkaloids, other immunosuppressives, plasma infusions or exchange, and splenectomy.[17] Thrombocytopenia due to an exogenous agent generally responds to avoidance of this substance. Corticosteroids seem to decrease bleeding even without accelerating a rise in platelet counts.

Platelet infusions can give temporary benefit to patients with low platelet production but may require mono-donor, tissue-matched sources if repeated infusions become necessary. Aminocaproic acid (Amicar) has been found useful in preventing rebleeding in patients with hypomegakaryocytic thrombocytopenia. The other major use for this agent is for the prevention and treatment of lower urinary tract bleeding secondary to local causes.

It is particularly important to judge whether the patient with active bleeding has a local bleeding problem compounded by his hemostatic abnormality. Such bleeding, whether from a dental extraction or more extensive surgical procedure, requires local therapy such as pressure or clamping, with systemic measures generally being of secondary importance.

Platelet functional abnormalities due to exogenous materials generally respond to removing the offending agent. When the abnormality is related to uremia, dialysis and cryoprecipitate therapy can be beneficial. Posterior pituitary derivatives are being used investigationally in von Willebrand's disease and mild hemophilia with benefit.

CLOTTING FACTOR ABNORMALITIES

The elderly present many special problems relating to clotting factor abnormalities. They are more likely to have diseases of the liver and gallbladder, consumptive coagulopathies, spontaneous circulating anticoagulants; to be on anticoagulant therapy; or to have vitamin K deficiency. Even congenital disorders such as von Willebrand's disease, Factor XI deficiency, or fibrin-stabilizing factor deficiency can have variable or minimal manifestations until the challenge of some surgical procedure in old age.

In certain instances, the history can be critical. The only clue to mild von Willebrand's disease or even hemophilia might come from a personal or family history of modest bleeding out of proportion to the associated trauma. Factor XIII deficiency can be associated with delayed bleeding and poor wound healing. The recent use of anticoagulants or broad-spectrum antibiotics, significant hepatobiliary disease, or recent surgical procedures are generally evident.

Occasionally laboratory values can be misleading. If blood is drawn through a heparin lock or other heparinized system, a failure to discard 15 ml or more of blood before switching syringes for the clotting studies can give falsely abnormal readings with standard clotting tests. The bedside clotting time performed at ambient temperatures is a poor screen except perhaps for severe hemophilia or circulating antibodies to Factor VIII. The screening tests for clotting factor deficiencies most commonly include the prothrombin time and the activated partial thromboplastin time. The former detects such problems as vitamin K deficiency and liver disease, most patients with consumptive coagulopathies, and patients on anticoagulants. When these screening tests can be supplemented by assays for Factors V and X and for fibrinogen and split products and by a thrombin time and Reptilase time, the distinction among these clotting disorders can be readily made.

In the presence of a normal prothrombin time, the activated partial thromboplastin time serves to screen for deficiencies of Factors VIII, IX, XI, and XII. Except as mentioned previously, such defects do not generally present for the first time in senior citizens. Perhaps, therefore, the most common use of the partial thromboplastin time in the elderly is to monitor heparin therapy.

Management of clotting factor abnormalities in the older patient follows general rules but with certain special considerations. Indiscriminate use of large volumes of plasma can tax the older patient's heart, making specific diagnosis and therapy important when feasible. When vitamin K deficiency is a major consideration, one can give 2 mg of vitamin K_1 oxide slowly intravenously at the time clotting studies are drawn. Some 4 hours later, if the diagnosis is correct, the prothrombin time will be close to normal. When a vitamin K antagonist such as warfarin (Coumadin) is to blame, however, the required dose of vitamin K is in the range of 25 mg to 50 mg. Intravenously,

this should not be given at a rate faster than 5 mg min. Once this dose is given, the patient will not respond to further warfarin for several days, and anticoagulation medication, if required, is switched to heparin. Management of von Willebrand's disease and consumptive coagulopathies is discussed under platelet defects. The other plasma factor deficiencies are generally treated with fresh frozen plasma.

The rare phenomenon of spontaneous antibodies to Factor VIII has a predilection for the elderly. This condition may be exacerbated by infusion of Factor VIII concentrates; attempts at managment may be made using appropriate Factor IX concentrates that have activated clotting factors that bypass the offending antibody.

In summary, bleeding problems in the elderly involve defects in the blood vessel and its surrounding structures, the number and function of platelets, and the clotting-related materials present in the plasma. Screening tests for disorders of hemostasis include the capillary fragility test, platelet estimate on smear or formal platelet count, the bleeding time, the prothrombin time, and the activated partial thromboplastin time. Combining these with a few selected additional tests and the clinical data allow rapid identification of the cause of bleeding and specific appropriate therapy to correct the problem.

ANTITHROMBOTIC AGENTS

Recommendations for the use of anticoagulants have varied markedly over the years; future adjustments are also to be expected. Currently, prophylactic use of mini-heparin, monitored or unmonitored, is advocated for virtually all patients confined to bed, unless they are undergoing procedures such as intracranial or eye surgery or total hip replacement. The large number of widely used medications that interact with warfarin must be kept in mind, especially when they are started, stopped, or used intermittently. The growing popularity of the thrombolytic agents streptokinase and urokinase presents special problems that may be precluded by the less toxic tissue-associated plasminogen activator (investigational).

NEOPLASTIC DISEASES OF THE BONE MARROW, LYMPH NODES, AND SPLEEN

As in epithelial malignancies, neoplasms of blood-related organs tend to increase with advancing age. When the normal cellular elements of the marrow are displaced, the resulting cytopenias give rise to fever and infections, bleeding, and weakness. When the disease involves enlargement of organs, initial presentation may be with lymphadenopathy or splenomegaly. When the cells involved have unique biochemical features, the presentation may be with kidney stones, pruritus, proteinuria, hyperviscosity symptoms, or immune phenomena. Of special importance in the elderly is that some diseases require little or no active therapy and others have a dramatic change in prognosis with relatively benign treatments. Illnesses that are statistically rapidly fatal sometimes seem to smolder in the aged and warrant at least a brief period of observation of progression. Age alone, however, should not preclude therapy.

Because of the relative ease with which affected tissues can be biopsied, hematologic malignancies have been the prototypes for study of therapeutic modalities. For this reason, protocols evolve quickly and their message is then used in the broader range of malignant diseases. In this chapter, emphasis will be on broad principles specific for the older age-group. Reference should be made to active protocols or referrals made to major oncology centers.[7,10,11,14,27,31]

Myeloproliferative Disorders

The basic components of the bone marrow are red cell, white cell, and platelet precursors. Neoplasia can occur involving any one or more of these cell lines and may be chronic or acute.

Polycythemia vera is a profound pancytosis that may present dramatically with thromboembolic or hemorrhagic phenomena or less dramatically with intense pruritus, kidney stones, gout, plethora, or vague neurologic or abdominal symptoms. Physical examination demonstrates modest splenomegaly and plethora. Routine blood cell counts generally show increases in all three cell lines. The bone marrow has reduced iron stores and marked hypercellularity, especially involving megakaryocytes.

Particularly if erythrocytosis rather than pancytosis is present, or if the other previously mentioned clinical features are missing, one must consider hypoxia, renal pathology, Cushing's disease, plasma volume depletion such as from use of diuretics, hepatic malignancies, and even uterine fibroids in the differential diagnosis. In the absence of specific neurologic findingss, a search for the rare posterior fossa tumor, often mentioned in the differential diagnosis, does not seem warranted.

Ancillary tests including arterial oxygen saturation, red blood cell mass, abdominal ultrasonography, erythropoietin assay, leukocyte alkaline phosphatase, and many others may be indicated. Although it is the serum uric acid that is routinely obtained, a study of the urine for crystals or of a 24-hour urine collection for a total uric acid excretion greater than 700 mg/day will determine the need for therapy, such as with allopurinol.

Randomized protocol studies have been the mainstay of progress in management of diseases such as polycythemia vera; however, not all patients will fit neatly into protocol categories; some might not meet all rigid criteria for a diagnosis of the disease although the diagnosis is unequivocal. Similarly, protocol arms indicating one mode of therapy to the exclusion of others might not result in optimum therapy for all patients. Thus one may choose to make phlebotomy the basic mode of treatment with radioactive pharmaceuticals and cytotoxic agents reserved for problem cases. Conversely, an elderly patient may safely obtain prolonged clinical benefit from one injection of radioactive phosphorus without as great a need for frequent monitoring as would be necessary with oral chemotherapy.

When phlebotomy is used in the older patient, smaller volumes of blood may be removed at each visit until a normal hematocrit is obtained. This is particularly required if the patient is volume depleted due to diuretics.

Studies using chlorambucil therapy suggest a resultant higher incidence of leukemia and other malignancies, however, the overall mortality rate approximates those of other treatments.[5] The apparent increased incidence of second malignancies may have been related to the relatively high doses of chlorambucil used. Although it is possible that lower doses would have been associated with fewer second malignancies, the recent trend has been to use hydroxyurea or other agents.

Occasional patients with polycythemia vera develop severe pain in the toes, apparently related to platelet sludging rather than to gout. The pain might not respond to narcotics or acetaminophen but has a dramatic response to as little as one aspirin every 2 or 3 days. Aspirin must be used judiciously in this disease because of a tendency to bleeding as well as to thrombosis.

Essential or hemorrhagic thrombocythemia can almost be considered an offshoot of polycythemia vera in which the platelet count stands out as being profoundly abnormal, the spleen is also often enlarged, and the bone marrow shows marked increase in megakaryocytes, with other clinical and laboratory features being more variable. Platelet aggregometry can generally demonstrate a functional defect. A markedly elevated sedimentation rate should prompt one to look for a nonhematologic cause of a secondary thrombocytosis. Clinical manifestations vary from none, to hemorrhage, to thromboembolic phenomenon. Although statistical benefit has been hard to prove, many clinicians will start cytotoxic therapy with hydroxyurea, radioactive phosphorus, or other agents when the platelet count approaches 1 million/cu mm.

Chronic granulocytic leukemia in the elderly shares the name and the high white cell count of the disease seen in younger patients.[23] Otherwise, it tends to run a different course. Problems associated with anemia and thrombocytopenia occur earlier in the course of the disease. Splenomegaly, although present, is generally not as prominent. The Philadelphia chromosome is less likely to be found. Cytotoxic therapy may lower the white cell count, but often at the expense of the hematocrit and platelet count. The accelerated or blastic phase comes earlier; the overall median survival is shorter. Despite this bleak description, some older patients go on for years with relatively benign therapy and without morbidity, especially with the chronic myelomonocytic picture.

Agnogenic myeloid metaplasia is currently conceived of as a disorder of hematopoietic cells with a secondary fibrotic reaction. Presentation is commonly from pain or pressure symptoms related to the spleen or from hematologic compromise. The diagnosis might also be obtained from fortuitous palpation of the abdomen or from workup of the characteristic leukoerythroblastic blood smear, with its typical teardrop-shaped red blood cells. Diagnosis is confirmed by bone biopsy sections. Other causes of marrow fibrosis such as metastatic carcinoma, lymphoma, or mast cell disease must be excluded.

Many patients require nothing but supportive care; others require splenectomy. Occasionally androgens seem to relieve the need for transfusions temporarily. Corticosteroids, vitamin B$_6$, folic acid low-dose cytotoxic agents, and radiation therapy gingerly administered to the spleen have been tried with at best mixed results. Studies suggesting major clinical benefit from the antifibrosis agent *p*-aminobenzoic acid (PABA) have yet to be confirmed.

Acute leukemia in the elderly is most frequently granulocytic. Occasionally it smolders along with minimal progression for months or even years,[30] and supportive therapy is all that is necessary.[6] For most patients, progressing disease mandates highly toxic intensive chemotherapy.[11] The older patient in particular may benefit from insertion of a Hickman catheter for venous access, to tide him over the chemotherapy and the long period of antibiotic and blood product infusions that characterize induction therapy. With therapy, 60% to 80% of younger patients, but only 20% to 40% of the elderly, attain complete remission. Once having achieved complete remission, prognosis is similar in both age-groups.

Widely used agents include cytarabine, thioguanine, and the anthracycline antibiotics.[12,14] Therapeutic failure may well be related to a lessened marrow reserve in older patients. The cardiotoxic effects of the anthracyclines are especially noted with preexisting heart disease.

Immunoproliferative Disorders

Malignancies of lymph nodes and lymphocyte-derived cells include such diverse disorders as the Hodgkin's and non-Hodgkin's lymphomas, multiple myeloma, and macroglobulinemias. Although Sir Thomas Hodgkin did his work on this family of diseases more than a century ago, they are undergoing rapid evolution with regard to diagnosis and management. Only general principles as they pertain to the elderly can be given.

Multiple Myeloma

Multiple myeloma can be among the most devastating of hematologic malignancies. By destroying bone, it results in pain that can be focal or diffuse and is often excruciating. Displacement of normal marrow elements by myeloma cells gives rise to symptoms of anemia, bleeding, and infection. Inability to produce normal antibodies enhances this propensity to infection, especially fulminant pneumococcal sepsis. Paraproteins, especially if combined with dehydration, can rapidly compromise kidney function.

One can suspect myeloma just by watching the rapidity with which the patient's blood settles, a reflection of the exceedingly high sedimentation rate in relation to the paraprotein. The diagnosis rests on demonstrating the triad of serum or urine protein spike, osteolytic bone disease, and plasmacytosis of the bone marrow.

Management involves cytoreductive and supportive measures. If hydration is not ensured, renal failure will obviate subsequent response to chemotherapy. With signs of infection, appropriate cultures should be rapidly obtained and antibiotic therapy initiated immediately, usually including an antipneumococcal, bactericidal agent. Hypercalcemia must be looked for and addressed. Measures for controlling bone pain are often crucial. Remarkable relief can sometimes be obtained simply by placing the patient on a water mattress, which distributes his weight over a much wider area. Nonsteroidal anti-inflammatory agents, narcotics, local radiation therapy, and prophylactic or therapeutic internal fixation of bones may be required. The large, heavy, metal orthopaedic brace sometimes causes as much pain as it relieves; a simpler lighter cloth support with Velcro closure may be more effective. Early mobilization to prevent further resorption of bone is important. Some authors have suggested that normocalcemic patients with myeloma receive combinations of calcium, fluoride, androgens, and vitamin D to develop stronger bones.[24]

Standard chemotherapy includes an alkylating agent such as melphalan (Alkeran) or cyclophosphamide, often combined with corticosteroids. Melphalan may be used either with intermittent pulse doses or on a regular daily schedule as titrated against blood cell counts.

Corticosteroids are generally administered intermittently, perhaps 1 week of every month. High doses seem beneficial to younger patients but appear to shorten median survival in the elderly, and more modest doses are generally used. Corticosteroids may promote infections, bleeding, and thinning of the bones. Although corticosteroids are associated with a decrease in the protein spike, this could be a nonspecific catabolic effect in addition to any reduction of tumor burden. Their usefulness in hypercalcemia is unequivocal.

Some investigators combine multiple agents, such as cyclophosphamide (Cytoxan), vincristine, prednisone, nitrosoureas, and melphalan in a single chemotherapeutic program. The combination is remarkably well tolerated; whether it should be used initially or following relapse or whether it offers any significant benefit is still controversial. Although additional agents such as the anthracyclines and interferon have antimyeloma activity, they are currently considered second-line therapies.

Hodgkin's Disease

In the early 1950s, if a patient presented with fever, weight loss, and enlargement of lymphoid tissues, the finding of Reed-Sternberg cells on lymph node biopsy was a prelude to palliative therapy and only slightly delayed death. Enor-

mous strides have been made since then. Therapy cures a large number of patients with localized disease, and even in advanced disease there is a reasonable chance for cure.[20,21]

Within this optimistic framework, the elderly do not fare quite as well as younger patients[3]: the morphologic features are more likely to be unfavorable; symptoms are more likely to indicate advanced disease; and tolerance to therapy can be adversely affected by lower marrow reserve and other system failures.

However, the otherwise healthy older person deserves his chance at prolonged survival. Early biopsy of suspicious nodes offers the best chance of making a diagnosis in the early stages of the disease, when therapy is most efficacious. Routine staging,[1] including isotope studies, computed tomography, ultrasonography, and lymphangiography when pulmonary disease is not a problem are generally worthwhile. Diagnostic laparotomy, when it is reasonably likely to define management, can be done in selected patients.

With localized disease, radiation therapy can be used effectively. Mustargen, Oncovin, procarbazine, and prednisone (MOPP) is still the standard of comparison for other chemotherapeutic regimens.[7,10] In the elderly it will generally be initiated at lower doses in anticipation of lower tolerance.

Non-Hodgkin's Lymphomas

The non-Hodgkin's lymphomas are a diverse family of diseases that share a proliferation of lymphoid elements. They range from indolent[28,29] to very aggressive[19,32] and may present with enlargement of affected sites, symptoms referable to displacement of normal elements, or unique features such as the paraprotein spike of macroglobulinemia. One might also include with this group chronic lymphocytic leukemia in which the lymphoid proliferation is manifest primarily in the bone marrow and peripheral blood.

A virtual revolution in identifying specific cell markers[26] is bringing a new understanding to this family of diseases.[4] Current therapies generally involve some combination of vincristine, prednisone, and/or an alkylating agent such as cyclophosphamide or chlorambucil, with the addition of doxorubicin (Adriamycin) for the histiocytic lymphomas.[2,31] Radiation therapy can play an important role in some patients. Methotrexate, asparaginase, and several other agents are also widely used.

In diseases such as chronic lymphocytic leukemia, it is common practice to avoid chemotherapy until the clincial situation pushes one into it.[27] An aggressive lymphoma gives no such option. The principles of management therefore largely parallel those previously outlined for acute leukemia.

REFERENCES

1. Aisenberg AC: The staging and treatment of Hodgkin's disease. N Engl J Med 299:1228, 1978
2. Bagley CM Jr, Devita VT, Berard CW, Cenellos GP: Advanced lymphosarcoma: Intensive cyclical combination chemotherapy with cyclophosphamide, vincristine, and prednisone. Ann Intern Med 76:227, 1972
3. Bearman RM, Pangalis GA, Rappaport H: Hodgkin's disease, lymphocyte depletion type. Cancer 41:293, 1978
4. Berard CW, Greene MH, Jaffe ES, Magrath I, Ziegler J: A Multidisciplinary approach to non-Hodgkin lymphomas. Ann Intern Med 94:218, 1981
5. Berk PD, Goldberg JD, Silverstein MN et al: Increased incidence of acute leukemia in polycythemia vera associated with chlorambucil therapy. N Engl J Med 304:441, 1981
6. Bodey GP, Rodriguez V, Change H, Narvoni G: Fever and infection in leukemic patients. Cancer 41:1610, 1978
7. Canllos GP, Come SE, Skarin AT: Chemotherapy in the treatment of Hodgkin's disease. Semin Hematol 20:1, 1983
8. Cohen KL, Donaldson RM: Unreliability of radio-dilution assays as screening tests for cobalamin (vitamin B-12) deficiency. JAMA 244:1942, 1980
9. Crosby WH: Red cell mass: Its precursors and its perturbations. Hosp Pract 15:81, 1980
10. DeVita VT, Canellos GP, Moxley JH III: A decade of combination chemotherapy of advanced Hodgkin's disease. Cancer 30:1495, 1972
11. Esterhay RJ Jr, Wiernik PH, Grove WR, Markus SD, Wesley MN: Moderate dose methotrexate, vincristine, asparaginase, and dexamethasone for treatment of adult acute lymphocytic leukemia. Blood 59:334, 1982
12. Foon KA, Gale RP: Controversies in the therapy of acute myelogenous leukemia. Am J Med 72:963, 1982
13. Forget BF: Hemolytic anemias: Congenital and acquired. Hosp Prac 15:67, 1980
14. Gale RP, Foon KA, Cline MJ, Zighelboim J, the UCLA Acute Leukemia Study Group: Intensive chemotherapy for acute myelogenous leukemia. Ann Intern Med 84:753, 1981
15. Goldstein ML: The aplastic anemias. Hosp Pract 15:85, 1980
16. Hanash SM, Rucknagel DL: Clinical implications of recent advances in hemoglobin disorders. Med Clin North Am 64:775, 1980
17. Harrington WJ, Ahn YS, Byrnes JJ, So AG, Mylvaganam R, Pall LM: Treatment of idiopathic thrombocytopenic purpura. Hosp Pract 18:205, 1983
18. Herbert V: The nutritional anemias. Hosp Pract 15:65, 1980
19. Horwich A, Peckham M: "Bad Risk" non-Hodgkin lymphomas. Hosp Pract 15:35, 1980
20. Kaplan HS: Hodgkin's disease: Biology, treatment, prognosis. Blood 57:813, 1981
21. Kaplan HS, Rosenberg SA: Hodgkin's disease: Current recommendations for management. Ca 25:306, 1975
22. Katz AJ: Transfusion therapy: Its role in the anemias. Hosp Pract 15:77, 1980
23. Koeffler HP, Golde DW: Chronic myelogenous leukemia—new concepts. N Engl J Med 304:1269, 1981
24. Kyle RA, Jowsey J: Effect of sodium fluoride, calcium carbonate, and vitamin D on the skeleton in multiple myeloma. Cancer 45:1669, 1980
25. Lalezari P, Oberhardt B: Temperature gradient dissociation of red cell antigen-antibody complexes in the Polybrene technique. Br J Haematol 21:131, 1971
26. Li C: Immunocytochemical techniques for identifying leukemia. Mayo Clin Proc 59:185, 1984
27. Liepman M, Votaw ML: The treatment of chronic lymphocytic leukemia with COP chemotherapy. Cancer 41:1664, 1978
28. Portlock CS: "Good risk" non-Hodgkin lymphomas: Approach to management. Cancer 41:25, 1978
29. Portlock CS, Rosenberg SA: No initial therapy for stage III and IV non-Hodgkin's lymphomas of favorable histologic types. Ann Intern Med 90:10, 1979
30. Rheingold JJ, Kaufman R, Adelson E, Lear A: Smoldering acute leukemia. N Engl J Med 268:812, 1963
31. Rodriguez V, Cabanillis F, Burgess MA, McKelvey EM, Valdivieso M, Bodey GP, Freireich EJ: Combination chemotherapy ("CHOP-Bleo") in advanced (non-Hodgkin) malignant lymphoma. Blood 49:325, 1977
32. Rosenberg SA: Non-Hodgkin's lymphoma—selection of treatment on the basis of histologic type. N Engl J Med 301:924, 1979
33. Spaet TH: Anemia is a symptom. Hosp Pract 15:17, 1980

23
The Eye in Old Age

Frank G. Berson

Like many organs of the human body, the eye is capable of quite adequate function well into the extremes of old age. Although accommodation inexorably decreases with age, with little residual focusing power after age 60, many elderly individuals retain adequate, albeit subnormal, vision to age 90 and beyond.[13] Frequently, the elderly patient is able to function quite well with monocular or fair vision owing to limited activities.

Nevertheless, two important factors emerge. First, the increasing frequency of many eye diseases with age coupled with the increasing success of many treatments demands early recognition and diagnosis. Second, the elderly no longer accept poor vision and resultant dependence as a natural consequence of aging. Just as they can expect a prolongation of their life span, with certain limits, so too can they expect a higher quality to their existence. The relationship between vision and quality of life is self-evident.

In this chapter common eye conditions of the elderly will be discussed, with emphasis on diagnosis, indications for referral, and basics of management. Many of these conditions are not unique to the aging eye, but they constitute the major part of eye pathology in the geriatric population and account for most of the visual loss.[12]

EVALUATION OF THE PATIENT

The primary care physician, internist, or geriatrician plays an important role in the eye health of the elderly. Although many older patients receive continuing followup and care from an ophthalmologist, many others do not, especially if they are relatively confined at home or in an extended care facility.

As part of a routine eye examination or evaluation for a specific complaint, two tests are extremely important. First is the testing of visual acuity, which can be accomplished with a portable near-vision chart (Fig. 23-1). This is the single most meaningful test in the examination and yields more information on ocular function than anything else. Each eye must be tested individually, and poor acuity may help confirm the diagnosis, or at a minimum, form the basis for a referral. Good acuity, although not a guarantee of eye health, rules out many significant problems (*e.g.,* advanced cataract, inflammation, vitreous hemorrhage, macular degneration). It is essential to remember that many patients, young or old, can almost totally lose the sight of one eye yet not complain to a physician if the fellow eye sees well. Second is the testing of intraocular pressure, which can easily be accomplished with a portable Schiotz tonometer. This is especially valuable in screening patients for chronic open-angle glaucoma or ruling out acute glaucoma in a painful eye.

CATARACT

Cataract is the most common cause of visual loss in the elderly yet, at the same time, is the most amenable to treatment. Any opacification of the crystalline lens is technically a cataract but is often visually insignificant in its early stages.

Patients often complain of gradual, painless visual loss and may be bothered by the glare from bright lights. With the direct ophthalmoscope, and enhanced with pupillary dilation, the cataract may be manifested by a general dullness in the red reflex (nuclear sclerosis), peripheral "spokes" (cortical), or a central discrete opacity (posterior

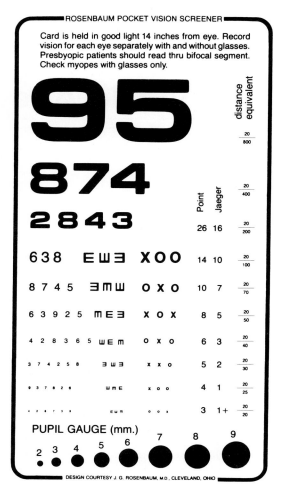

ROSENBAUM POCKET VISION SCREENER

Card is held in good light 14 inches from eye. Record vision for each eye separately with and without glasses. Presbyopic patients should read thru bifocal segment. Check myopes with glasses only.

		Point	Jaeger	distance equivalent
95				20/800
874				20/400
2843		26	16	20/200
638 ЕШЭ ХОО		14	10	20/100
8745 ЭПШ ОХО		10	7	20/70
63925 ПЕЭ ХОХ		8	5	20/50
428365 ШЕП ОХО		6	3	20/40
374258 ЭШЭ ххо		5	2	20/30
937826 ШПЕ хоо		4	1	20/25
427732 Ешп оох		3	1+	20/20

PUPIL GAUGE (mm.)

2 3 4 5 6 7 8 9

DESIGN COURTESY J. G. ROSENBAUM, M.D., CLEVELAND, OHIO

FIG. 23-1. The Rosenbaum Pocket Vision Screener is readily available and quite adequate for measuring acuity in the office or at the bedside.

subcapsular). The latter is usually the most visually disabling.

Indications for cataract extraction center around the extent to which the patient is visually disabled in the context of his daily living pattern. A thoughtful discussion with the patient is as useful as the examination itself. In relatively few patients, cataract extraction is medically indicated when the lens becomes totally opaque (mature cataract). In such patients there is an increased risk of lens-induced inflammation and/or glaucoma.[3]

Modern surgical techniques have had a major impact on the treatment of this condition.[10] The operating microscope, finer sutures, and better instruments have enabled less traumatic surgery and better wound closure. Aspiration devices, used with or without an ultrasonic device (phacoemul-

sification), can remove the lens through a smaller incision. The intraocular lens, implanted once the lens is removed, has rapidly gained popularity over the past decade and is used in the vast majority of operations currently performed in the United States. It is usually superior to the contact lens or spectacles for correction of aphakia. There is, however, a slightly greater complication rate with lens implantation, and certain badly diseased eyes should not have implants. For those patients who originally had a cataract extraction without lens implantation for one reason or another, a secondary implant can be performed with relatively low risk if a contact lens or spectacles prove unsatisfactory.

Although research is progressing in search of medical treatment for the prevention or inhibition of cataract formation,[6,7] surgery is the only viable alternative at present for those patients with visually disabling cataracts. The ability to perform surgery relatively quickly under local anesthesia, often on an outpatient basis, enables most elderly patients, including those with serious medical problems, to withstand the procedure with a minimum of physical stress. Nevertheless, no immature cataract should be removed unless there is a demonstrable visual need. Furthermore, the type of surgery and desire for lens implantation must always be a secondary consideration to whether the patient's own lens needs to be removed.

GLAUCOMA

Glaucoma is an eye disease in which the intraocular pressure is sufficiently elevated to cause characteristic optic disc changes and visual field defects, eventually leading to blindness in some patients. A pressure greater than 22 mg Hg is considered abnormal but not necessarily an absolute indication for treatment. Although there are many different types of glaucoma, the vast majority of affected individuals have so-called chronic open-angle (or "simple") glaucoma. The prevalence of this disease increases with age, rising from a very low level in young adults to as high as 5% to 10% in the eighth decade.[12,13]

Since chronic open-angle glaucoma is essentially asymptomatic until a very advanced stage, and visual loss is essentially permanent, the primary physician plays a key role in early diagnosis. Routine Schiotz tonometry, easily performed in most patients with the aid of topical anesthesia, will yield a reasonably accurate intraocular pressure. Disc examination with a direct ophthalmoscope may reveal pathologic cupping or simple asymmetry of cup size. Visual acuity and confrontation fields, although affected relatively late, will alert the examiner to the problem and potentially save the *fellow* eye, in which vision may be intact.

The ophthalmologist examining a patient suspected of having glaucoma will perform a variety of special tests, in addition to doing a routine comprehensive examination. The latter may reveal other causess of elevated intraocular pressure, such as inflammation, hypermature cataract, neovascularization, or intraocular tumor. Gonioscopy with a contact lens enables visualization of angle structures. Visual fields can be measured with a variety of devices, some now using sophisticated technology, and are important in assessing both the degree of functional visual loss as well as progression of disease. Stereophotography of the disc provides the best documentation for future reference. Tonography measures the facility of outflow, which remains relatively constant despite wide diurnal variation in intraocular pressure. This test is especially useful when the disc and/or field suggest glaucoma but pressure measurements are normal or borderline.[3]

Four types of drugs are often prescribed for glaucoma patients, and they constitute a significant percentage of drugs prescribed by ophthalmologists. All physicians should be aware of the potential systemic side-effects of these medications, even when administered topically.[9] Miotics (*e.g.*, pilocarpine) can commonly cause headaches and rarely excessive sweating, salivation, and diarrhea from parasympathetic stimulation. Cholinesterase inhibitors (*e.g.*, phospholine iodide) are "strong miotics" that contraindicate the use of succinylcholine during general anesthesia, since prolonged apnea may result. β-Adrenergic blockers (*e.g.*, timolol maleate) can exacerbate heart block and cause congestive heart failure and can also result in respiratory decompensation in susceptible patients with asthma or emphysema. Topical administration of epinephrine may further complicate unstable angina or poorly controlled systemic hypertension. Finally, orally administered carbonic anhydrase inhibitors (*e.g.*, acetazolamide and methazolamide) can cause numerous significant systemic side-effects.[2] Among these are a symptom-complex of malaise, fatigue, anorexia, and weight loss, related to the induced metabolic acidosis, and gastrointestinal disturbances, related to local irritation of the mucosa. Nephrolithiasis is a less common side-effect. Carbonic anhydrase inhibitors can also cause severe hypokalemia when administered concomitantly with a thiazide diuretic for systemic hypertension.

Argon laser trabeculoplasty has proven to be an extremely effective treatment for open-angle glaucoma inadequately controlled on maximum-tolerated medical therapy. Originally reported in 1979, this method of laser therapy involved the application of multiple laser burns spread evenly around the circumference of the trabecular meshwork.[25] Although the mechanism of action is still uncertain, it is thought that mechanical tightening or a stretching of the meshwork facilitates the outflow of aqueous. The short-term complication rate is extremely low, with 1% to 2% experiencing significant pressure elevations and/or severe inflammation. Long-term data are still being accumulated. Argon laser trabeculoplasty is probably one of the greatest advances in ophthalmology in this century and has helped countless glaucoma patients avoid traditional surgery. It can be performed on an outpatient basis on anyone who can sit up and place his chin at the slit lamp biomicroscope without excessive tremulousness.

When medical and laser therapy have failed to control intraocular pressure adequately, surgical intervention becomes necessary. There are a variety of operations for glaucoma, the most common being the filtering procedure.[3] The basic principle of this operation, usually performed under local/standby anesthesia, is to create a drainage channel for aqueous humor from the anterior chamber to the subconjunctival space. Although pressure control is achieved in at least 80% of cases, a significant number of patients can develop a cataract as a complication of surgery. Fortunately, such cataracts can be removed subsequently without compromising the filtering site in most cases.

MACULAR DEGENERATION

As a leading cause of legal blindness in the elderly, macular degeneration is probably the least amenable to medical or surgical treatment. Patients usually complain of slow, painless progressive visual loss in one or both eyes. The fundus picture may vary and can include drusen, pigmentary atrophy and clumping, subretinal fluid and hemorrhage, and a large subretinal ("disciform") scar. The latter is a consequence of a breakdown in Bruch's membrane, enabling growth of new vessels from the choriocapillaris underneath the pigment epithelium.[14,15,26]

Decreased acuity and an abnormal appearance to the macula should alert the examining physican to the possibility of this diagnosis. An ophthalmologist who is referred such a patient may obtain a fluorescein angiogram in an effort to locate possible subretinal neovascularization that might be amenable to treatment with the argon laser. If such vessels can be obliterated, fluid can resorb and subsequent hemorrhage and scarring can be averted.

Despite the recent enthusiasm for laser treatment and a national study proving its efficacy,[17] the vast majority of patients are either never amenable to laser therapy (generalized atrophy) or are diagnosed too late (large disciform scar). There are two important considerations for such patients. First, special magnifiers and reading aids may be of tremendous benefit to highly motivated patients. Second, the ophthalmologist must stress that this condition does not progress to "total blindness" but only involves the loss of central or "reading" vision. Thus with the benefit of an intact peripheral field, patients with this condition have good mobility and can function relatively independently.

DIABETIC RETINOPATHY

Although adult-onset diabetes mellitus is usually diagnosed prior to age 65, the ocular sequelae can certainly develop and/or progress in the elderly. In addition to retinopathy, diabetics suffer from a higher incidence of other eye diseases, most notably cataracts and chronic open-angle glaucoma.

The fundus findings in diabetic retinopathy primarily involve the posterior pole of the eye and include microaneurysms, dot and blot hemorrhages, and hard (waxy) and soft (cotton wool) exudates. Proliferative retinopathy is characterized by new vessels on the disc and elsewhere and by preretinal or vitreous hemorrhages. Nonproliferative retinopathy (*i.e.*, without new vessels that can bleed) causes central visual loss due to maculopathy. Hemorrhages, exudates, edema, and capillary dropout can all contribute to macular dysfunction. Proliferative retinopathy, often superimposed on nonproliferative retinopathy, causes more devastating blindness due to vitreous hemorrhage and traction retinal detachment.[16] Once a patient has lost peripheral vision in addition to central vision, mobility becomes a major problem.

Modern technology has facilitated major progress in the treatment of diabetic retinopathy and its complications. Panretinal laser photocoagulation (PRP) has been shown definitively in a national collaborative study to reduce the incidence of blindness in patients with proliferative disease.[23] Vitrectomy has been enormously helpful in clearing the ocular media of persistent hemorrhage resulting from neovascular bleeding.[18] However, the efficacy of laser treatment of nonproliferative disease, specifically maculopathy, has not been proven but is under investigation. Thus, many diabetics who have undergone "successful" treatment (*i.e.*, PRP or vitrectomy) may remain legally blind on the basis of irreparable macular dysfunction.

THE RED EYE

The differential diagnosis of the acute red eye (conjunctivitis, iritis, scleritis, keratitis, acute glaucoma) can be applied to patients of all ages.[20] However, physicians caring for the elderly should be particularly aware of conditions most likely to occur in their patients.

Exposure keratopathy occurs whenever the upper eyelid fails to cover the cornea on a frequent basis, thereby causing drying of the epithelium. This can be seen in patients with decreased blinking, anesthetic corneas, loss of consciousness, and facial nerve palsies. In addition to conjunctival swelling and hyperemia, the cornea will usually stain abnormally with fluorescein, indicating an epithelial defect or deeper corneal ulceration. Treatment initially consists of frequent lubrication with artificial tear solutions or ointment and taping of the eyelids to maintain closure. Patching of the eye is useless if the eye remains open behind the patch. Tarsorrhaphy may be necessary as a temporary or permanent maneuver to protect the cornea.

Acute angle-closure glaucoma will present with similar findings, regardless of age, but treatment may be delayed in the elderly individual who is bedridden or confined to a nursing home. Findings such as decreased vision, perilimbal injection, corneal edema precluding a clear view of the iris and fundus, and a larger, poorly reactive pupil should make the physician suspect this diagnosis. Such patients need emergency treatment with a miotic, a carbonic anhydrase inhibitor, an osmotic agent, and then iridectomy, which is now usually performed with a laser.[1,22] Late diagnosis can lead to permanent angle closure and a difficult management situation.

Entropion and ectropion of the lower eyelid cause inflammation of the conjunctiva that is predominantly inferior. In the former the lower lid lashes rub against the globe and may damage the corneal epithelium. This condition may not be apparent to the examiner unless the patient is asked to squeeze the lids together, thereby revealing an intermittent entropion. In ectropion, the conjunctiva of the lower lid is not adequately apposed to the bulbar conjunctiva and this results in exposure, drying, inflammation, and discomfort. Both entropion and ectropion can be corrected by a variety of surgical procedures that are routinely performed under local anesthesia on an outpatient basis.[21]

Tear deficiencies are quite common in the elderly and cause patients to complain of a burning sensation or sandy feeling. The eye is usually minimally inflamed and may actually reveal excessive tearing, a reflex phenomenon. The diagnosis of a dry eye is confirmed most easily with the Shirmer test by assessing the extent of wetting of a thin strip of litmus paper after 5 minutes. If a presumptive diagnosis is made, frequent use of artificial tear solutions often provides significant relief, whereas application of antibiotic ointment for ''conjunctivitis'' often makes the patient feel worse.

Corneal ulcers can occur not uncommonly in elderly and debilitated patients. Lid malpositions may be a contributing factor. An opaque area of the cornea with fluorescein staining should alert the physician to this potentially dangerous situation. Emergency management, including hospitalization and frequent application of topical antibiotics, is necessary to minimize corneal scarring and prevent perforation.

Dacryocystitis, with swelling and tenderness in the area of the lacrimal sac as well as generalized lid edema, may accompany a conjunctivitis and excessive tearing. Treatment consists of warm compresses along with topical and systemic administration of antibiotics; hospitalization is seldom required. Subsequent permanent obstruction to outflow through the nasolacrimal duct may result in continuous tearing, requiring a dacryocystorhinostomy.[11] Extirpation of the lacrimal sac in elderly patients with serious medical problems is usually well tolerated if repeated abscesses of the sac necessitate surgical intervention.

Herpes zoster ophthalmicus often results in ocular involvement. Patients with a vesicular eruption near the tip of the nose, indicating nasociliary involvement, should have an ophthalmic evaluation. The cornea, uveal tract, and optic nerve may all be involved. There is no specific antiviral agent for dendritic keratitis, but corticosteroids are helpful in the management of intraocular inflammation.

ACUTE VASCULAR OCCLUSIONS

Arterial and venous occlusions of the retinal vasculature must always be considered in the differ-

ential diagnosis of sudden visual loss. These conditions are quite different both in terms of fundus appearance, acute management, and medical evaluation for possible etiologic factors.[4]

With arterial occlusions, abnormalities of blood flow are seen within the affected vessel(s) as well as retinal edema in the distribution of the vessel(s). Typically, a cherry-red spot is seen in the center of the macula when the central retinal artery is occluded. If recognized quickly, this condition is an ocular emergency requiring immediate referral to an ophthalmologist. Therapeutic maneuvers include efforts to lower intraocular pressure (eyeball massage, parenteral carbonic anhydrase inhibitor, paracentesis) and increase arterial blood flow (breathing a mixture of CO_2 and O_2, using a paper bag if necessary). The rationale is to propel a possible embolus distally before irreversible retinal necrosis occurs. Such patients should also undergo a thorough in-hospital medical evaluation, including a search for an embolic source. If an embolus is not seen in the fundus, invasive studies should not be performed automatically since the occlusion may well be thrombotic. This is certainly true in central retinal artery occlusions, whereas branch retinal artery occlusions are more likely to be embolic.[24]

With venous occlusions vascular dilation and tortuosity are accompanied by superficial retinal hemorrhages. In the full-blown picture one is struck by a ''blood and thunder'' appearance of the fundus. From an ophthalmic standpoint, there is no immediate treatment. Once most of the hemorrhaging has resolved, fluorescein angiography is performed to assess the degree of ischemia. Useful vision may return if the retina is not particularly ischemic. Neovascularization of the anterior segment is a serious sequela of retinal ischemia and may superimpose intractable glaucoma on the poor vision caused by the occlusion. Medically, patients can be examined on an outpatient basis to seek possible associated conditions, including hypertension, diabetes, and hyperviscosity syndromes.

ISCHEMIC OPTIC NEUROPATHY

When an elderly patient complains of acute, profound visual loss, ischemic optic neuropathy must be considered.[4] Eye findings usually include decreased acuity, ''altitudinal'' field loss demonstrable by confrontation testing, an afferent pupillary defect, and pale swelling of the optic disc. Immediate sedimentation rate and ophthalmologic referral are indicated in an effort to rule out temporal arteritis as the cause of presumed ischemic optic neuropathy. An elevated sedimentation rate or classic clinical picture is an indication for a temporal artery biopsy. Long-term systemic corticosteroids can protect the vision in the fellow eye and avert a stroke elsewhere, but they should not be used unless one is reasonably secure in the diagnosis of temporal arteritis. The potential complications of such therapy are such that the ophthalmologist and internist must work closely together in the management of these patients. For nonarteritic ischemic optic neuropathy due to presumed thrombosis, there is no effective treatment.

RETINAL DETACHMENT

Separation of the retina secondary to a tear or hole, so-called rhegmatogenous detachment, can be seen in all age-groups but is more common in patients who have undergone cataract extraction. Thus, it is not a rare occurrence in the elderly aphakic population.

Patients experiencing a retinal detachment usually notice a shadow approaching the visual axis from the periphery that was preceded by flashes and/or floaters (a vitreous detachment inducing a retinal break or hemorrhage). It is difficult to make the diagnosis without pupillary dilation and indirect ophthalmoscopy. Thus, the diagnosis should be suspected on the basis of symptoms, visual acuity, and confrontation field, and the patient should be referred immediately for a complete ophthalmic evaluation.

Untreated retinal detachment almost inevitably leads to total blindness in the involved eye. Treatment of most cases consists of a scleral buckling operation, usually performed under general anesthesia. If the detachment involves the macula and is longstanding, central vision may not return despite successful surgery. Thus, in a patient who is in very poor health or is quite elderly, one needs to balance the anesthetic risks against the overall impact of the surgery on visual function. If the fellow eye is in good shape, one may want to forego the stress of surgery.

TUMORS

Lid tumors are a common occurrence in the aged.[19] Solid benign lesions include the papilloma, verruca, keratoacanthoma, seborrheic keratosis, and molluscum contagiosum. Cystic lesions include the chalazion, sudoriferous cyst, and sebaceous cyst. The most common malignant lesions are basal cell carcinoma and squamous cell carcinoma, whereas sebaceous carcinoma and malignant melanoma are much rarer. An excisional biopsy is indicated for any suspicious lesion. Although local excision can usually be accomplished for small tumors, larger or more invasive malignant tumors may require a wide excision, necessitating complex reconstructive surgery to close the lid defect.[21] Cryosurgery is often used for large basal cell carcinomas.

Malignant melanoma of the choroid is the most common intraocular neoplasm in adults. The patient usually does not complain of visual disturbances unless the macula is involved or there is a secondary retinal detachment. These tumors are most often, but not always, pigmented so that the examiner notes a dark reflex when looking at the involved quadrant with a direct ophthalmoscope. Enucleation has long been the standard of treatment to prevent metastases, but proton beam irradiation has been shown to be a promising alternative in eyes with useful vision.[8] The ophthalmologist must be certain the choroidal tumor does not represent a metastasis from another site, in which case the eye is often not treated.

OCULOMOTOR PARALYSES

Sudden onset of diplopia often indicates a palsy of the third, fourth, or sixth cranial nerve.[5] Ptosis of the upper lid will accompany a complete third nerve palsy. Nerve infarction, related to diabetes and/or hypertension, is a common etiology. Other causes include myasthenia gravis, trauma, temporal arteritis, and intracranial tumors. When pupillary dilation accompanies a third nerve palsy, intracranial aneurysm must be considered. A neuro-ophthalmic evaluation is warranted for any patient with acute diplopia.

REFERENCES

1. Abraham RK, Miller GL: Outpatient argon laser iridectomy for angle closure glaucoma: A two-year study. Trans Am Acad Ophthalmol Otolaryngol 79:529, 1975
2. Berson FG: Carbonic anhydrase inhibitors of the eye: A review. J Toxicol 1:169, 1982
3. Chandler PA, Grant WM: Glaucoma. Philadelphia, Lea & Febiger, 1979
4. Cogan DG: Neurology of the Visual System. Springfield, IL., Charles C Thomas, 1966

5. Cogan DG: Neurology of the Ocular Muscles, 2nd ed. Springfield, IL, Charles C Thomas, 1977

6. Cotlier E: Senile cataracts: Evidence for acceleration by diabetes and deceleration by salicylate. Can J Ophthalmol 16:113, 1981

7. Datiles M, Fukui H, Kuwabara T, Kinoshita JH: Galactose cataracts prevention with Sorbinil, an aldose reductase inhibitor: A light microscopic study. Invest Ophthalmol Vis Sci 22:174, 1982

8. Gragoudas ES, Goitein M, Verhey L, Munzenreider J, Urie M, Suit H, Koehler A: Proton beam irradiation of uveal melanomas: Results of 5½ year study. Arch Ophthalmol 100:928, 1982

9. Havener WH: Ocular Pharmacology, 5th ed. St. Louis, CV Mosby, 1983

10. Jaffe NS: Cataract Surgery and Its Complications, 3rd ed. St. Louis, CV Mosby, 1981

11. Jones LT, Wobig JL: Surgery of the Eyelids and Lacrimal System. Birmingham, AL, Aesculapius Publishing Co, 1976

12. Kahn HA et al: Framingham eye study: I. Outline and major prevalence findings. Am J Epidemiol 106:17, 1977

13. Kornzweig AL, Feldstein M, Schneider J: The eye in old age: IV. Ocular surgery of over one thousand aged persons: With special reference to normal and disturbed visual function. Am J Ophthalmol 44:29, 1957

14. Kornzweig AL: The eye in old age: V. Diseases of the macula: A clinicopathologic study. Am J Ophthalmol 60:835, 1965

15. Kornzweig AL: Changes in the choriocapillaris associated with senile macular degeneration. Ann Ophthalmol 9:753, 1977

16. Little HL, Jack RL, Patz A, Forsham PH: Diabetic Retinopathy. New York, Thieme-Stratton, 1983

17. Macular Photocoagulation Study Group: Argon laser photocoagulation for senile macular degeneration: Results of a randomized clinical trial. Arch Ophthalmol 100:912, 1982

18. Michels RG: Vitreous Surgery. St. Louis, CV Mosby, 1981

19. Oculoplastic surgery for the aging eye. Ophthalmic Forum 1(5):00, 1983

20. Ophthalmology Study Guide for Students and Practitioners of Medicine, 4th ed. San Francisco, American Academy of Ophthalmology, 1982

21. Reeh MJ, Beyer CK, Shannon GM: Practical Ophthalmic Plastic and Reconstructive Surgery. Philadelphia, Lea & Febiger, 1976

22. Robin AL, Pollack IP: Argon laser peripheral iridotomies in the treatment of primary angle closure glaucoma: Long term follow up. Arch Ophthalmol 100:919, 1982

23. The Diabetic Retinopathy Study Group: Photocoagulation treatment of proliferative diabetic retinopathy: The second report of Diabetic Retinopathy Study findings. Ophthalmology 85:82, 1978

24. Wilson LA, Warlow CP, Russell RWR: Cardiovascular disease in patients with retinal artery occlusion. Lancet 1:292, 1979

25. Wise JB, Witter SL: Argon laser therapy for open-angle glaucoma. Arch Ophthalmol 97:319, 1979

26. Yannuzzi LA, Gitter KA, Schatz H: The Macula: A Comprehensive Text and Atlas. Baltimore, Williams & Wilkins, 1979

24 Deafness, Tinnitus, and Dizziness in the Aged

Victor Goodhill

Diseases of the external, middle, and inner ears and lesions of the eighth nerve and central nervous system (CNS) auditory and vestibular pathways are common in the aged population. The same otologic problems that affect the young can also affect the old. The term *presbycusis* has been classically applied to the aging process in the auditory system. Tinnitus may or may not accompany presbycusis. Equilibrium disturbances can involve true vertigo, dysequilibrium, or motion sickness.

DEAFNESS

Although the common word "deafness" is used universally to denote hearing loss, it should be reserved for severe hearing impairments that cannot be treated or aided by amplification with hearing aids.

Presbycusis, normal hearing loss attributable to age alone, varies in degree and in auditory patterns and is characterized primarily by degenerative cochlear changes. However, it is now clear that other aging lesions also occur (*i.e.*, in the middle ear, in the auditory nerve, in the cochlear nucleus, and in various levels within the central auditory nervous system).

Differential diagnosis includes consideration of all diseases of the ear that can cause hearing losses occurring in the sixth, seventh, eighth, and ninth decades. Thus, external ear diseases, middle ear diseases, otomastoiditis, otosclerosis, ossicular fixations, temporal bone dystrophies, tumors, direct trauma, barotrauma, acoustic trauma, ototoxic drugs, syphilis, labyrinthine membrane ruptures, viremias, vascular lesions, and other causes must be considered. In addition, differential diagnosis must be concerned with a number of systemic diseases producing hearing losses that can be mistaken for the normal aging patterns of presbycusis.

The senior citizen can have any one of the many otologic diseases with superimposed normal presbycusis. Because of the potential multiple causality inherent in the aged population with hearing losses, it is important to avoid a simplistic stance in considering diagnostic and management aspects of hearing losses in older people. The label "presbycusis" is tenable only when no other specific cause for hearing loss in older adults can be found on careful otologic study.

Ear Examination

Examination of the aged patient with hearing loss includes physical examination of the external ear, and tympanic membrane, audiometric studies, and screening Schuller and Stenver's radiograph views. Simple radiography of the mastoid and internal auditory canal regions is essential to rule out unsuspected or previously undiagnosed diseases of the temporal bone in the mastoid region and possible lesions in the internal auditory canal such as eighth nerve tumors.

External Ear Diseases

Cerumen impactions frequently produce conductive hearing losses. In the aged population, males with hairy external canals, which tend to block normal cerumen extrusion, have predispositions for cerumen impactions. Benign bony growths that narrow the external auditory canal also predispose patients to impacted cerumen. They consist either of benign osteophytes, which may narrow the canal medially, or benign lateral osteomas.

Although otoscopic examination is essential, it is not always possible to remove cerumen safely or adequately with the use of the otoscope. The head mirror or head light is useful in visualization and removal of cerumen.

Cerumen removal is usually performed by curette or syringe irrigation with room temperature water. However, it is inadvisable to remove cerumen with irrigation in a patient whose tympanic membrane has not previously been examined and found to be intact, with no perforation, no evidence of infection, or unusual atrophy.

External otitis may be due to either bacterial or fungus infections. Cultures should precede treatment with appropriate ear drops.

Middle Ear Diseases

Secretory Otitis Media

Secretory otitis media (SOM) produces a painless conductive hearing loss with levels ranging from 10 db to 50 db loss. Bilateral SOM is a sequel of the common cold, allergic rhinitis, or sinus disease. Unilateral secretory otitis media is unusual unless there is evidence of previous middle ear disease, and one must consider the possibility of nasopharyngeal carcinoma in geriatric patients. Treatment usually involves decongestant and antibiotic therapy, but myringostomy, aspiration, and middle ear ventilation (MEV) tubes may be necessary.

Chronic Otitis Media with Perforation

Chronic otorrhea from a central perforation is usually due to previous acute otitis media and eustachian tube disease, trauma, type A (potentially reversible) otomastoiditis, or type B (irreversible cholesteatoma or tympanosclerosis) otomastoiditis. Most type A cases will respond to local therapy. Perforations may close spontaneously following appropriate local therapy or may heal when patched with a cigarette paper or Gelfilm patch.

No attempt should be made to patch any perforation until audiometric, radiographic, and bacteriologic studies have ruled out the possibility of type B otitis and mastoiditis, which usually requires surgical management.

Ossicular Fixation

An intact tympanic membrane can be immobilized by lateral ossicular fixation owing either to malleal fixation, incudal fixation, or combined fixation. Diagnosis requires an audiologic conductive loss test battery and tympanometry to measure impedance of the middle ear and stapedius reflex responses. Management of ossicular fixation is surgical, but amplification by a hearing aid is an alternative.

Otosclerosis

This disease, affecting 10% to 12% of the population, is usually bilateral and most commonly starts in early adult life. However, it may start in middle age, and it may not be recognized until secondary normal presbycusis sets in, adding aging hearing loss to a previously unrecognized borderline conductive loss.

The otosclerotic patient has normal tympanic membranes, a conductive hearing loss varying from 30 db to 90 db, with an air–bone gap varying from 20 db to 55 db. Speech discrimination scores are usually within normal limits, until presbycusis of the cochlear type is added to the problem, when discrimination scores drop.

Otosclerosis is managed by stapedectomy, which can be performed virtually at any age. It should be considered in elderly patients if there is no medical contraindication to a relatively short local anesthetic procedure. Elimination of the conductive component of a combined otosclerosis–presbycusis condition will frequently improve the hearing sufficiently so that the presbycusis component is not handicapping by itself.

Other Middle Ear Diseases

In addition to the more common problems mentioned previously, a number of other middle ear and mastoid conditions, which are less common, are seen in older people. These include temporal bone granulomas and dystrophies and temporal bone tumors. Trauma to the ear and temporal bone can produce a variety of conductive and mixed hearing losses.

Inner Ear Diseases—Presbycusis

The classic normal presbycusis (hearing loss due to age) condition is primarily a cochlear (inner ear hair-cell) lesion. However, degenerative changes of aging can also be produced by lesions in the middle ear, eighth nerve (spiral ganglion), and cochlear nuclei, and higher CNS auditory pathways.

Pathology

In 1937, von Fieandt and Saxen[5] reported temporal bone findings in 33 cases of persons 50 years of age or older. They described senile atrophy of spiral ganglion and angiosclerotic degeneration of cochlear duct epithelial elements.

Suga and Lindsay,[13] in a report of temporal bone histopathology in 17 aged patients, all of whom had bilateral sensorineural hearing losses, pointed out the primary findings of decrease in the population of spiral ganglion cells. In many cases there was also a diffuse senile atrophy of the organ of Corti and stria vascularis (Figs. 24-1 and 24-2).

Johnsson and Hawkins[10] illustrated both sensory and neural degenerations associated with aging in human inner ear microdissections.

Goodhill[6] reported high frequency bone conduction (BC) losses in lateral ossicular fixation. Belal and Stewart[2] described arthritic changes in middle ear ossicular joints with fibrous and calcific changes resulting in ankylosis.

Degenerative changes in the arteries have been demonstrated within the internal auditory meatus. Osseous changes can produce compression of auditory nerve bundles in the internal auditory meatus. Plugging of vascular canals in the otic capsule have been related to the aging process.[7]

Changes in the ventral cochlear nucleus have been reported by Dublin.[3,4] In addition, changes have been seen in the inferior colliculus with cellular degeneration in the medial geniculate body as well as in the auditory cortex.

Audiologic Patterns of Presbycusis

Sensorineural hearing loss patterns in presbycusis fall into several types. The losses rarely show an air–bone gap. One type of decade pattern for normal aging hearing loss is seen in Figure 24-3, but such decade patterns are variable. Pure-tone sensorineural hearing-loss (SNHL) patterns can vary considerably and comprise at least three types— flat, mildly sloping, and severely sloping curves.

Pure tone audiograms and speech discrimination scores are illustrated in Figures 24-4 and 24-5. Occasionally, a moderate flat or mixed pure-tone sloping pattern will be combined with exceedingly poor speech discrimination scores as a result of cochlear degeneration (phonemic regression) possibly related to CNS pathway lesions.

A serious dilemma is the difficulty of evaluating components of the presbycusis pattern relative to (1) true aging phenomena, which are moderately variable; (2) the results of environmental noise or other causes of noise-induced hearing loss; and (3) results of undiagnosed cochlear lesions that may have nothing to do with age. In clinical practice, rather marked variations are found in the so-called normal hearing levels of persons in various age-groups.

Nonpresbycusis Lesions (Pseudopresbycusis)

A number of variants of other sensorineural hearing loss lesions can produce presbycusislike degenerative patterns. These can be considered pseudopresbycusis lesions.

Phonemic regression in some older people (hearing for speech much poorer than the pure-tone audiogram might suggest) might be the result of reduced cerebral function, rather than to cochlear presbycusis. The emergence of more refined central auditory function tests will be useful in diagnosis. Patients with CNS auditory pathway lesions may have greater difficulty with speech in a noisy background.

A one-time audiogram does not necessarily reflect the true diagnosis in every case. Fluctuating

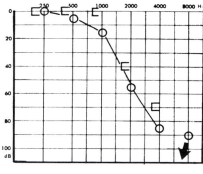

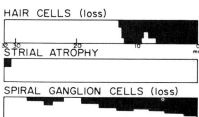

FIG. 24-1. The audiogram and the graphic reconstruction of hair cells of the organ of Corti, the stria vascularis, and the spiral ganglion cells of the right cochlea. (Suga R, Lindsay J: Histopathological observations of presbycusis. Ann Otol Rhinol Laryngol 18:169, 1976)

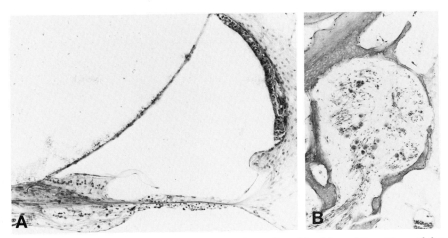

FIG. 24-2. The cochlear duct (*A*) and the spiral ganglion (*B*) of the midbasal turn of the right cochlea. Atrophy of the organ of Corti and the spiral ganglion is severe, while the stria vascularis and the tectorial membrane appear normal. (Hematoxylin & eosin) (Suga F, Lindsay J: Histopathological observations of presbycusis. Ann Otol Rhinol Laryngol 85:169, 1976)

pure-tone and SDS values may be indicative of complicating metabolic, vascular, or CNS problems. Mild presbycusis may appear to be more severe than it really is, as the result of other conditions producing intermittent superimposed cellular hypoxia, which can play a role in fluctuating cochlear hearing levels in patients with thyroid disease, diabetes, arteriosclerosis, hypertension, and other systemic conditions. Thus, periodic reexamination of the patient with presbycusis is advisable.

The label of presbycusis can be incorrectly applied also to a patient who has inner ear hearing loss of ototoxic nature. For example, salicylate and other ototoxicities can be superimposed on a mild subclinical presbycusis to produce handicapping hearing losses.

Last, but not least, is the consideration of hearing loss caused by acoustic trauma and noise in many older patients. In many male patients, the diagnosis of presbycusis is complicated by additional prepresbycusic changes owing to the noise-

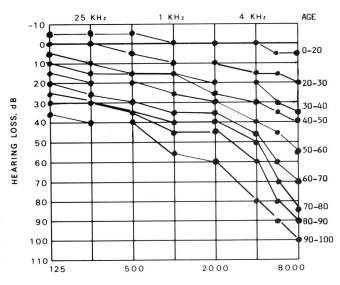

FIG. 24-3. Decade audiogram illustrating normal aging. Audiometric patterns encountered in urban otologic practice. (Goodhill V: Ear Diseases, Deafness and Dizziness. Hagerstown, MD, Harper & Row, 1979)

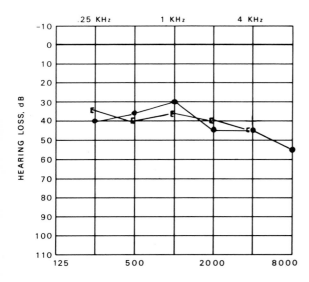

FIG. 24-4. Audiogram representing flat SNHL presbycusis. The SRT (35 db) is consistent with pure-tone average and discrimination ability is good (88% at 65 db +30). ●—●, AC, unmasked RE; [—[, BC, masked RE. (Goodhill V: Ear Diseases, Deafness and Dizziness. Hagerstown, MD, Harper & Row, 1979)

induced hearing losses of industry, military, aircraft, hunting, and other sources of acoustic insults. In the entire older population, sociocusis (hearing loss produced by the noises of society) must be considered as an additional problem to that of normal presbycusis.

Management of Presbycusis

Many drugs, vitamins, and other modalities have been suggested in the treatment of presbycusis and in other SNHL lesions. Nicotinic acid, other vitamins, and numerous esoteric preparations to prevent further presbycusis hearing losses have been

empirically advised. There is no effective medical or surgical treatment for presbycusis.

The patient with presbycusis requires a program of rehabilitation. Many elderly patients with relatively flat audiometric configurations in the 15- to 20-db region, who need no amplification, have been sold hearing aids. Unnecessary hearing aid use not only confuses and upsets a patient, but it can also convince the patient of the existence of a progressively hopeless hearing loss problem. For patients with mild presbycusis, there is usually no need for anything other than lip reading, the use of a telephone buzzer or amplifier, a loud door buzzer instead of a bell, radio and television ear-

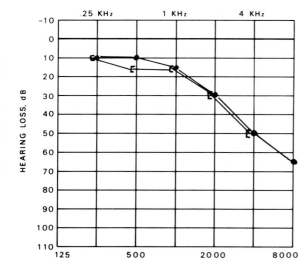

FIG. 24-5. Audiogram representing mild sloping SNHL presbycusis. The SRT (15 db) reflects normal low frequency hearing with mildly decreased discrimination ability (70% at 45 db [+30]; 82% at 55 db [+40]. ●—●, AC, unmasked RE; [—[, BC, masked RE. (Goodhill V: Ear Diseases, Deafness and Dizziness. Hagerstown, MD, Harper & Row, 1979)

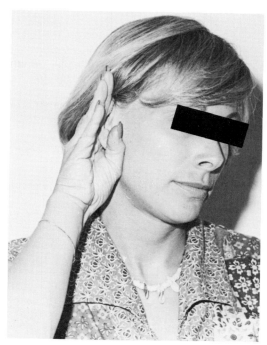

FIG. 24-6. Ideal cupping technique with the auricle cradled in the closed hand and gently pushed forward slightly. Care must be taken not to occlude ear canal. (Goodhill V: Ear Diseases, Deafness and Dizziness. Hagerstown, MD, Harper & Row, 1979)

phone attachments, and above all, an understanding of the social aspects of mild hearing loss on the part of members of the family. Such understanding, the use of ear cupping (Fig. 24-6), and "acoustic strategy" will solve most, if not all, of the communicative problems of many older people with mild sensorineural hearing problems.

When indicated, hearing aid selection by patients with presbycusis should be advised by the otologist in collaboration with an audiologist and a skilled and conscientious hearing aid dispenser. Newer types of amplification devices are successfully being used by patients with presbycusis, even with sloping high frequency SNHL.

Hearing Aids

An amplification system seldom restores normal audition, even in the most satisfactory cases. On the other hand, in virtually all cases of hearing loss that do not yield to medical or surgical management, an appropriate hearing aid can be a significant element in a comprehensive rehabilitation plan if the patient understands the nature of the ear problem and the way in which this loss limits the degree of improvement one may realistically expect.

Once a hearing aid has been selected and fitted, it is necessary that a patient learn to use the instrument and make it a part of his everyday life. Older patients require encouragement and must be taught to insert and remove the earmold, install a fresh battery when required, regulate volume, and manipulate switches and controls to best advantage. Instruction must be provided concerning the care of the instrument and recognition of malfunction. The hearing aid user must learn how to cope with a seemingly hostile environment, filled with noise, unfamiliar sounds, and even familiar sounds that are not heard in a familiar way. Skills required to get the greatest benefit from a hearing aid are not assimilated rapidly but rather slowly over a period of time, and not without informed guidance. A definite program of aural rehabilitation, including hearing aid use, speech reading, auditory training, and counseling is advisable. The necessary skills are mastered through repetition; by patiently guiding fingers crippled by arthritis or rendered insensitive by age, in inserting an earmold or locating a volume control; and by confronting unrealistic expectations and explaining time and time again why the hearing aid cannot eliminate unwanted sounds and transmit only those sounds that the wearer wishes to hear.

TINNITUS

Everyone may have normal tinnitus in special situations. The healthy person with no ear complaints who goes into an audiometric sound-proof booth or into an anechoic chamber and sits quietly in such an acoustically shielded environment will usually hear internal body sounds. This visceral tinnitus is normal and represents an awareness of one's own body at work—of sounds produced by breathing, heart action, blood circulation, and middle ear muscle contractions—by living. We usually ignore such sounds. Tinnitus as a *symptom* occurs when such internal sounds are of higher intensity levels (louder) than the intensity level (loudness) of masking environmental sounds.

Tinnitus can be a troubling human symptom, which may or may not be of ear origin. Tinnitus is not a disease and is not a syndrome. Tinnitus must be considered a *symptom* resulting from any one of a number of lesions.

Subjective Tinnitus

Subjective tinnitus is an auditory sensation of ringing, humming, whistling, roaring, clicking, or any other sensation of tones or noise.

Objective Tinnitus—Bruit

Objective tinnitus refers to a tone or sound that can be heard by an examiner (the physician) as well as by the patient. Objective tinnitus should be described as a bruit.

From the point of view of location, two types of tinnitus must be distinguished: (1) ear tinnitus (tinnitus aurium); and (2) head tinnitus (tinnitus cranii or tinnitus cerebri).

Tinnitus is a common symptom in older people. Since it may represent a component of a number of diseases, it may be the first symptom to bring the patient to the physician for diagnosis and management. Tinnitus may be dismissed as psychogenic when indeed it may be a symptom of a definitive lesion. For example, unilateral tinnitus may very well be the first symptom of a tumor of the internal auditory meatus or of the cerebellopontine angle. Tinnitus, unilateral or bilateral, may be the first symptom of beginning otosclerosis. Tinnitus may herald the presence of a glomus jugulare tumor, and it may be the presenting symptom of a vascular lesion in the temporal bone or skull.

Ear Tinnitus (Tinnitus Aurium)

Ear tinnitus is usually accompanied by hearing loss. Both of the two classic types of hearing loss, conductive and sensorineural, may be accompanied by tinnitus. Tinnitus may precede hearing loss, the two may appear simultaneously, or tinnitus may follow the onset of hearing loss.

Any conductive lesion can be accompanied by tinnitus. Simple cerumen in the external ear canal may cause hearing loss with tinnitus. Tympanic membrane perforation, otitis media, and any ossicular lesion may produce hearing loss and tinnitus. If the middle-ear lesion is bilaterally equal (*e.g.,* in symmetrical bilateral otosclerosis), the bilateral ear tinnitus may resemble a nonlocalizing central tinnitus similar to that of tinnitus cranii.

Cochlear and retrocochlear lesions can produce unilateral tinnitus.

Ménière's disease is frequently accompanied by ipsilateral tinnitus along with hearing loss and vertigo. Acoustic neurinoma and cerebellopontine angle tumors are usually characterized by ipsilateral tinnitus as the first symptom prior to hearing loss and vertigo.

Noise-induced hearing loss, with bilateral 4 kHz audiometric notch, will be accompanied by bilateral tinnitus aurium, which may resemble tinnitus cranii because of bilateral cochlear hearing loss symmetry.

Last, but not least, bilateral cochlear presbycusis may be accompanied by bilateral tinnitus aurium.

Head Tinnitus (Tinnitus Cranii)

True cranial tinnitus is frequently associated with cerebrovascular and other intracranial lesions. However, because any tinnitus, even though non-localizing, may be of ear origin, an otologic examination is always indicated.

Cranial tinnitus is frequently confused with ear tinnitus and may actually coexist with it. Cranial tinnitus is a nonlocalized subjective sensation of sound that is usually diffuse in the head and has a nonspecific quality. It is frequently described as a roaring or rushing sound, not directed to the ear region. It may be accompanied by bruits. Its diffuse character may be confused with somatic sensations of the neck and upper thorax and, indeed, may be due to vascular phenomena in these areas as well as intracranially. Usually tinnitus cranii is due to vascular disease. Both extracranial and intracranial vascular lesions and a number of intracerebral lesions may be accompanied by the symptom of nonlocalizing head tinnitus. Circulatory problems such as anemia, polycythemia, hypertension, and hypotension may also play etiologic roles.

Compensated and Decompensated Tinnitus

Compensated Tinnitus

Compensated tinnitus is present in much of the population and accompanies a number of otologic lesions and some constitutional conditions. In most of these instances the tinnitus is not noticeable to the patient except in an extremely quiet environment, therefore not constituting a clinical problem requiring management. Many conductive and sensorineural hearing losses in lesions of varying etiologies may be accompanied by minimal tinnitus. Such patients may not complain of the tinnitus at all but will acknowledge the presence of the symptom when the history is taken. The complaint of tinnitus is usually not volunteered in patients with compensated tinnitus but can be elicited.

Decompensated Tinnitus

The term *decompensated tinnitus* describes the tinnitus that is the major ear complaint of the patient. There are two types of otologic problems that will produce decompensated tinnitus. The first is the tinnitus of low acoustic intensity in a patient with significant psychosomatic stress factors. The second is the tinnitus of high acoustic intensity in which the complaints are related to the severity of the organic ear lesion and are not related to psychosomatic or stress factors.

Management of Tinnitus

There is no specific treatment for tinnitus aurium.

The goals in the management of the patient with tinnitus aurium are dual. The first goal is specific medical or surgical ear therapy for the underlying condition. If the tinnitus persists despite adequate otologic treatment, the second goal is an attempt to convert decompensated tinnitus into compensated tinnitus.

Regardless of the underlying lesion and the therapy directed to the lesion, the patient whose tinnitus is a major symptom requires special attention, and this should be carried out by the same physician (otologist or generalist) who has treated the underlying organic cause.

For many patients the symptom of tinnitus is very frightening. Anxieties regarding the tinnitus may not be volunteered by the patient. Among such anxieties are those derived from family, friends, folklore, and other sources. Some patients think that tinnitus is the prelude to total deafness. To others, tinnitus implies a sign of a brain tumor. To still others, tinnitus means a prelude to a stroke. For some patients tinnitus may be mistakenly interpreted as the beginning of serious mental disease. Although there are remote realities to some of these concerns, for most patients these worries are inappropriate. Such anxieties may even be concealed by the patient.

Simple reassurance as to the real cause and significance of the tinnitus as a component of an ear condition will go far in helping alleviate such anxieties. Inappropriate concerns should be discussed frankly. Reassurance by the physician who carried out the original otologic diagnostic studies and therapy is infinitely more effective than reassurance by another physician or by a psychotherapist.

It is necessary to explain to the patient what ear tinnitus usually represents—that it is real and not imagined, that it is not an illusion or a hallucination or a delusion. It is an auditory paresthesia. In this regard, it is frequently valuable to give the patient the example of the phantom limb with neuron memory. The amputee with no leg may have "pain" in his absent little toe. The high-pitched tinnitus in a patient with 4 kHz noise-induced hearing loss and a cochlear basal turn lesion may have a phantom neuron memory tinnitus comparable to the phantom limb amputee.

In the vast majority of patients, the tinnitus accompanying a nonprogressive conductive or sensorineural lesion will become less of a problem with the passage of time. In most patients, such tinnitus may disappear completely as a symptom but may return temporarily at times of fatigue, stress, or upper respiratory infections. It is thus appropriate and imperative that an optimistic prognosis be given. Such reassurance *per se* is necessary and will convert decompensated tinnitus in many patients.

Acoustic "sedation" is very helpful in many cases of tinnitus, especially in regard to difficulty in sleep, which is a great problem for many patients. The reason for greater difficulty at that time is the reduction in ambient masking noise levels in the quiet of the night, which increases awareness of the ever-present auditory paresthesia. The use of a bedside radio or tape recorder is frequently helpful in providing an artificial source of ambient noise to mask out the subjective tinnitus.

When there is a lesion for which amplification with a hearing aid is a possibility, even if borderline, such patients should have a hearing-aid consultation. In many cases, a properly fitted hearing aid may be extremely helpful in providing sufficient ambient environmental noise to mask the tinnitus. The hearing aid may also be helpful in reducing the tension that accompanies borderline hearing losses. The hearing aid will be of help as an auditory rehabilitation device as well as a masking device. It is only rarely that a hearing aid accentuates tinnitus rather than masking it.

There is no specific medical therapy for ear tinnitus. Tinnitus is a symptom, not a disease. Sedative therapy, however, is a palliative measure, not only for daytime use but especially for bedtime tinnitus irritability. Drugs such as phenobarbital, various tranquilizers, and other sedatives in small doses will be helpful. There is no one drug with specific tinnitus sedation qualities. No one drug should be used for any long period. It is helpful to alternate the medications so that habituation possibilities are diminished.

There is no effective surgery for tinnitus *per se* at the present time. Obviously surgery is indicated if there is an underlying otologic disease requiring a surgical procedure. However, when the underlying otologic disease is only a marginal indication for surgery, such surgery should not be recommended specifically for the tinnitus component.

There is no clear-cut indication for endolymphatic sac decompressions or shunts, surgical sympathectomy, labyrinth cryosurgery, sacculotomy, labyrinthectomy, eighth nerve section, or other procedures advocated for the treatment of Ménière's and related diseases if the purpose of the operation is primarily the treatment of the accompanying tinnitus. Reports of successes in tinnitus surgery are, of course, entirely subjective, for which no validation is available.

The patient with persistent unexplained tinnitus as an isolated symptom, in whom thorough medical and otologic studies disclose no evidence of disease, requires reexaminations at definite intervals. Tinnitus may be the first symptom in some conditions, long before hearing loss or other findings occur. Reexaminations should include both general medical and otologic studies.

Efforts have been made to relieve troublesome tinnitus, with relaxation training assisted by biofeedback techniques.

Auditory Hallucinations

Many musicians, composers, and music lovers can "hear" entire musical scores as phenomena of normal cerebration. Beethoven "heard" his later compositions when he was totally deaf. Playwrights can "hear" the words of future actors in scenes and acts in conceptual states. These phenomena are certainly not hallucinatory but are related to creative thinking.

Auditory hallucinations are auditory cerebral phenomena unrelated to creative thinking. If they are verbal, they are described as offensive or threatening words or expressions. If they are musical, they are described as uncontrollable musical experiences, unrelated to a desire to recall a tune or to compose a melody.

Auditory hallucinations have not been shown to be related to peripheral ear disease.

The patient with formed auditory hallucinations (words, sentences, singing, or instrumental music) should be examined neurologically. Formed auditory hallucinations occur in ictal states, temporal lobe seizures, and tumors. If no neurologic etiology can be demonstrated, psychiatric referral is indicated.

DIZZINESS

Normal Equilibrium

Normal equilibrium is a state of harmonious symmetry between the right and left vestibular systems as they function to maintain the proper relationships between the person and the environment. The vestibular systems are complex, involving the right and left peripheral vestibular labyrinths, each with three semicircular canals and utriculosaccular organs; the lower CNS vestibular pathways; and the higher integrative CNS vestibular pathways involving cerebellar or cerebral functions.

Dizziness, Vertigo, Dysequilibrium, and Motion Sickness

Dizziness and vertigo are not necessarily synonymous. Terms such as *giddiness, imbalance, wooziness, faintness,* and *passing out* are frequently loosely equated with equilibrium disorders. Thus, the word "dizziness" may be used to describe cortical or visual disorientations, altered states of consciousness, and limb incoordinations in addition to equilibrium disorders.

Two major categories will be used to describe these disorders: vertigo and dysequilibrium.

Vertigo

The term *vertigo* is used specifically to describe symptoms of the vestibular (equilibrium) system. This includes peripheral labyrinthine, retrolabyrinthine, and CNS vestibular system disorders.

Dysequilibrium

The term *dysequilibrium* is used to described symptoms of spatial disorientations not caused by either labyrinthine or CNS vestibular system disorders. It also includes ataxia (CNS-limb incoordinations) as a form of dysequilibrium.

Misunderstandings of the differences between vertigo and dysequilibrium are responsible for confusion in diagnosis and for much inappropriate drug and surgical therapy for the "dizzy patient." The basic differences in symptoms, findings, and causes between vertigo and dysequilibrium are presented in Table 24-1.

True motion sickness is a complex syndrome related to the vestibular, proprioceptive, and visual systems. It is a maladaptation syndrome related to various types of motion. Thus, it includes vertigo,

TABLE 24-1 Dizziness: Differentiation Between Vertigo and Dysequilibrium

	Vertigo	Dysequilibrium
Symptoms	True sensations of disturbed motion	Illusions of spatial disorientation or incoordination
Findings	Nystagmus	No nystagmus
Causes	Peripheral (labyrinthine or retrolabyrinthine) or CNS vestibular system disorders	Systemic disorders or non-vestibular CNS disease

(Goodhill V: Ear Diseases, Deafness and Dizziness. Hagerstown, MD, Harper & Row, 1979)

with superimposed symptoms of pallor, cold sweating, nausea, and vomiting and differs from dysequilibrium in that it does involve peripheral and central vestibular pathways.

Vertigo and Nystagmus

Vertigo—the Symptom

Specific illusions of motion are related either to a sensation of turning or to a sensation of falling and result from an asymmetrical neuronal firing pattern between the right and left vestibular systems. Vertigo may be objective in which the patient feels that the environment is turning or falling, or it may be subjective in which the patient feels that he is turning or falling. Combinations of both may occur.

Nystagmus—the Finding

Nystagmus is an objective finding that accompanies vertigo. It is usually an alternating involuntary movement of both eyes, characterized by slow movement (slow component) to one side with a corrective fast return movement to the other side (quick component). By convention, nystagmus is identified by the direction of the quick component. Thus, a nystagmus to the left means a nystagmus that has a slow movement to the right and a quick corrective component to the left. The quick component actually represents the CNS corrective reflex.

The direction of nystagmus may be horizontal, vertical, diagonal, or rotary. Nystagmus may be manifest or occult. Manifest nystagmus can be observed with the naked eye in ordinary light. Occult nystagmus is that which can be observed either under magnification using +20 Fresnel lenses to abolish fixation or that recorded by electronystagmography in the dark with abolition of ocular fixation.

Causes of Vertigo and Nystagmus

Vertigo and nystagmus can be produced either by peripheral labyrinthine or by central CNS disorders of the vestibular system and by combined lesions.

Peripheral vertigo and nystagmus can originate from the semicircular canals and probably from the utricle and saccule of the labyrinth. They may originate from extralabyrinthine pathways (*i.e.,* the vestibular neurons and ganglia [Scarpa's ganglion]) and from central afferent vestibular nerves in the internal auditory canal and meatus.

Labyrinthitis, Ménière's disease, and labyrinth fistulas are common causes of peripheral vertigo. The symptoms of vertigo may be accompanied by symptoms of nausea, vomiting, and generalized malaise.

Peripheral vestibular or labyrinthine system vertigo is due either to intralabyrinthine or extralabyrinthine causes. Both intralabyrinthine and extralabyrinthine lesions may involve either cochlear and vestibular sense organs (cochleovestibular) or vestibular sense organs alone.

Central vertigo and nystagmus may be caused by a tumor in the temporal lobe (transverse gyrus of Heschl), by cerebral arteriosclerosis, and by lesions of the midbrain, pons, cerebellum, and brain stem. Lesions of the posterior-inferior cerebellar artery will involve vestibular nuclei and their connections to the medial longitudinal fasciculus. Peripheral and central pathways can interact.

Vertigo and Dysequilibrium

Because the aged patient with the complaint of dizziness may or may not have true vertigo, the first task is to differentiate between the possibilities of vertigo and dysequilibrium. In the differential diagnostic approach, the first step is a special dizziness history, followed by a basic medical examination and a basic otologic examination. This preliminary study of the dizzy patient will frequently result in the diagnosis of dysequilibrium, and a detailed vestibular electronystagmographic study will not be necessary.

Dysequilibrium

Dysequilibrium is characterized by subjective symptoms of spatial disorientation. No nystagmus can be detected and no disturbances of vestibular function can be elicited on vestibular examination.

These patients may use the word "dizziness" to convey the feelings of blacking out, fainting, sinking, instability, light-headedness, inability to concentrate, floating in space, or visual confusion.

Dysequilibrium includes a host of nonspecific illusions of orientation characterized by vagueness, lack of directionality, and unclear time-linked relationships and is usually constitutional in etiology. It may be related to cerebral oxygenation, blood pressure changes, or to various metabolic disorders. It may be due to drugs, visual disturbances, or to emotional disturbances.

No significant auditory or vestibular symptoms are associated with dysequilibrium. There is no spontaneous or positional nystagmus, caloric responses are usually normal on electronystagmographic vestibular examination, and auditory tests are usually normal for the age of the patient.

Some Causes of Dysequilibrium

Postural hypotension is a common cause of dysequilibrium. Hyperventilation also produces dysequilibrium. Arteriosclerosis with symmetrical changes involving the carotid and vertebral systems rarely produces true episodic vertigo. In the majority of such patients, dizziness is most commonly due to dysequilibrium. The transient ischemic attack (TIA) is a frequent cause of dysequilibrium, but it can produce vertigo and nystagmus if the lesion is specifically unilateral in relation to lower CNS vestibular pathway lesions.

Vestibular Examination

Examination of the vestibular system involves detection of, first, spontaneous nystagmus and then positional nystagmus. Evoked nystagmus studies following rotation and calorization stimuli complete the vestibular study.

The basic vestibular study does not require elaborate equipment. Electronystagmography is useful, but it is not always essential. It is frequently possible to get adequate diagnostic information by ordinary visual examination for manifest (spontaneous and positional) and evoked nystagmus.

The use of +20 diopter Frenzel lenses will eliminate eye reflex inhibition by gaze fixation.

Spontaneous Nystagmus

The Romberg and past-pointing tests precede a search for spontaneous nystagmus. The patient, sitting erect, may show evidence of spontaneous nystagmus of first, second, or third degree. Gaze nystagmus may be noted on lateral gaze command.

Positional Nystagmus

Positional testing is performed with patient lying on a couch in a number of positions. Spontaneous horizontal nystagmus is usually of peripheral origin (labyrinthine or vestibular disease). Spontaneous vertical, rotary, or diagonal nystagmus is usually of CNS origin. Positional direction-changing nystagmus without apparent vertigo is highly suggestive of a CNS lesion. Extremely active spontaneous nystagmus without vertigo indicates a CNS lesion.

Evoked Caloric Nystagmus

The Hallpike bithermal caloric test is performed by having the patient lie on a couch with head elevated on a pillow at 30°. Comparisons between right and left ear responses and between warm (44°C) and cold (30°C) calorization responses make possible such definitive findings as those of a hyporeactive (canal paresis) labyrinth, a nonreactive (dead) labyrinth, or directional nystagmus preponderance.

Vestibulometry by Means of Electronystagmography

Although valuable and frequently diagnostic vestibular information can be obtained without instrumentation, a number of diagnostic advantages make electronystagmographic examination preferable.

For example, although the Hallpike bithermal caloric test can be performed and give useful information without recording techniques, it is far more valuable to be able to examine and measure an electronystagmographic record and thus quantify test findings. The measurement of nystagmus amplitudes, latencies, and duration can be accomplished by electronystagmographic recording of nystagmus beats and nystagmus patterns. Vestibulometry gives information regarding specific amplitudes of slow and quick components, dysrhythmia, and other graphic aspects of the response pattern. Information from vestibulometry as an analogue to audiometry has expedited otologic differential diagnoses.

The problem of ocular fixation can cause confusion in nonelectronystagmographic studies of nystagmus patterns, although it is possible to reduce ocular fixation by the use of +20 diopter glasses. In electronystagmographic vestibular examinations carried out in a darkened room, abolition of ocular fixation is possible, and responses with both eyes either closed or open can be obtained. Both responses are useful diagnostically.

Peripheral Vestibular Diseases

Peripheral vertigo is due either to intralabyrinthine or extralabyrinthine causes. The prototype intralabyrinthine auditory-vestibular disorder is Ménière's disease. A number of other lesions can mimic Ménière's disease.

The most significant extralabyrinthine lesions causing cochleovestibular disorders are eighth nerve tumors and lesions of the cerebellopontine angle.

Vestibular disorders producing only vertigo and nystagmus consist also of intralabyrinthine lesions (uncommon) and extralabyrinthine lesions such as viral vestibular neuronitis.

Vestibular disorders without hearing loss also involve the consideration of motion sickness, which is a congenital vestibular end organ asymmetry, definitely related to motion. The most common varieties of motion sickness are seasickness, airsickness, and carsickness. In patients who complain of any one or all three of these categories of motion sickness, spontaneous or positional nystagmus may occasionally be elicited. Vestibular asymmetry is frequently found on caloric studies, noted as labyrinthine preponderance. Hearing is usually normal.

No definitive treatment other than the use of vertigo sedatives is of value. Dimenhydrinate and similar drugs, administered orally or intramuscularly, are useful in management. A combination of promethazine hydrochloride, 25 mg, and dextroamphetamine, 10 mg, is useful. Diazepam, 10 mg, may also give symptomatic relief, as well as prophylactic therapy.

Benign paroxysmal positional vertigo is paroxysmal vertigo that occurs only on positional change. The self-limited vertigo is unaccompanied by hearing loss or tinnitus. It has variously been attributed to labyrinthine anomalies or to metabolic or psychogenic problems and is characterized by the following syndrome:

The attack occurs when the patient assumes a supine position with the head turned so that the involved ear is undermost.

There is almost always a latent period, 5 or 6 seconds, before the onset of symptoms.

The nystagmus is chiefly rotatory, the direction being toward the undermost ear.

Central Vestibular Diseases

Central vestibular diseases are most common in the geriatric population. In CNS lesions involving the central vestibular system, true vertigo can occur.

The most common causes of vertigo arising from the brain stem are vascular lesions, such as thrombosis of the posterior-inferior cerebellar artery or basilar artery insufficiency. Localized brain stem encephalitis produces vertigo, but primary tumors of the brain stem or cerebellum less frequently give rise to true vertigo. A type of systemic imbalance—dysequilibrium—is more commonly noticed with such tumors of the brain stem or cerebellum. Metastatic tumors of the brain stem or cerebellum, however, may be accompanied by true vertigo. Although multiple sclerosis does produce vertigo, its most common vestibular symptom is dysequilibrium or systemic imbalance.

Eighth nerve tumors are not always associated with vertigo as a major symptom. Acoustic neurinoma (vestibular schwannoma) or the less common internal auditory meatus or cerebellopontine angle meningiomas or epidermoid cysts rarely give rise to vertigo because of their characteristic slow growth. However, cerebellopontine angle lesions involving arterial or venous malformations may produce severe prolonged and sometimes incapacitating attacks of vertigo, which may very easily be confused with Ménière's disease.

The association of hearing loss and tinnitus with vertigo becomes less common as one deals with lesions in the upper portion of the CNS. In addition to dissociation between vestibular and audiologic symptoms in higher CNS lesions, there are frequent involvements of other cranial nerves. Thus, there may be alterations in facial sensation (fifth nerve), ocular paralyses (third, fourth, and sixth nerves), conjugate ocular deviation, difficulty in swallowing, and hoarseness (tenth nerve).

In cerebellar lesions, arm or leg ataxia, intention tremors, and unsteady gait may be noted.

Vertiginous lesions of the CNS can be divided

into vascular and nonvascular etiologies. A number of "steal" syndromes, vertebrobasilar system lesions, and other vascular phenomena, especially TIA's, characterize vascular etiology. Disseminated sclerosis, cerebellar tumors, and head injuries are included in the nonvascular group.

Extracranial arterial lesions primarily affect the vertebrobasilar system. The two major arteries involved in this system are the anterior-inferior cerebellar artery, which is a branch of the basilar artery, and the posterior-inferior cerebellar artery, which is a branch of the vertebral artery. Symptoms are due either to a TIA or to actual occlusive syndromes. Intermittent vertebrobasilar insufficiency involving the entire system may produce a constellation of syndromes. One of the most common problems is the insufficiency secondary to vertebral artery compression by cervical spondylosis, with vertigo owing to arterial compression on turning of the neck.

In a patient suffering occlusive syndromes, the vertigo is sudden and usually severe. The "drop" attack throws the patient to the ground, is accompanied by nausea, and lasts for hours.

Patients with this syndrome have cochlear hearing loss only if the anterior-inferior cerebellar artery is involved. (This artery supplies the cochlea.) The vestibular findings are usually those of positional nystagmus without vestibular paresis. An evoked positional nystagmus is elicited by neck torsion or sudden change of posture. The normal cochlear findings and absence of contralateral labyrinthine preponderance (canal paresis) point to a vertebrobasilar system lesion.

In vertebrobasilar disease, there are four characteristic symptoms. Barber[1] has suggested a very useful "4D" mnemonic approach. The 4Ds include dizziness, diplopia (transient), dysphasia (speech slurring), and drop attacks.

In some cases, these are potentially prestroke lesions. There may be visual disturbances (*e.g.*, diplopia, blurred vision, or transient blindness). Vertigo is the most common symptom in intermittent vertebral insufficiency, occurring in about 45% of cases and usually provoked by postural changes. Occasionally, there will also be ataxia, seventh nerve paralysis (upper motor neuron), and hemiparesis.

Arteriography is indicated unless there is a specific contraindication. Arteriographic studies may point to the need for definitive surgical treatment, such as endartectomy or arterial bypass, or for orthopedic surgical procedures, such as removal of cervical osteoarthritic spurs.

The most significant finding on neuro-otologic examination is the presence of evoked postural nystagmus with or without caloric abnormality and without cochlear hearing loss.

Treatment is basically medical, neurologic, or orthopedic. No definitive otologic therapy is indicated.

The subclavian steal syndrome is due to occlusion of the proximal subclavian artery, in which the most distal vertebral artery acts as a collateral to the arm. The blood is thus siphoned from the vertebrobasilar system into the distal subclavian bed. The low pressure in the arm and the low peripheral resistance of arterial arborization causes reversal of blood flow in the vertebral system and results in symptoms of vertebrobasilar insufficiency by exercise of the involved arm. In addition, fatigue or claudication of the involved forearm is noted on exercise. A systolic bruit may be heard in the supraclavicular fossa, and there is quite frequently a disparity of arm blood pressures of 30 mm Hg or more. Blood pressure differences and a bruit would call for the consideration of arteriography. There may be indication for subclavian endartectemy or a supraclavicular carotid-subclavian graft.

Vertigo, with or without ataxia, accompanied by systolic cervical bruit points to the possibility of extracranial arterial insufficiency, a possible prestroke lesion.

The occipital steal syndrome, as a variant of the subclavian steal syndrome, may produce unilateral vestibular abnormalities and a concomitant cochlear hearing loss similar to that of Ménière's disease. An abnormal communicating anastomosis between the vertebral and occipital arteries may produce a shunt away from vertebral circulation.

Posterior-inferior cerebellar occlusion will produce a lateral superior medullary infarct, known as the Wallenberg or lateral superior medullary syndrome. This is characterized by a rather abrupt onset. The patient may be thrown to the ground with nausea and vomiting that are exaggerated by movement and may last hours, days, or weeks. The lateral medullary syndrome has associated neurologic symptoms including gait difficulty, Horner syndrome, facial analgesia, and palate weakness.

Internal auditory artery occlusion (vestibular or cochlear branch) is not a common lesion. The entire internal auditory artery, a branch of the anterior-inferior cerebellar artery, may occlude, with sudden hearing loss as well as sudden vertigo. The symptoms and findings resemble peripheral labyrinthine lesions.

The patient with an isolated complaint of sudden dizziness should be carefully questioned for these other symptoms because they may well be prodromas of an impending stroke that might be averted by appropriate anticoagulant therapy in time. The presence of a coarse nystagmus between dizzy spells, excessive imbalance, and the Horner syndrome would also point to basilar ischemia. Nausea, vomiting, diarrhea, sweating, chills, pallor, faintness, a sense of limbs floating in the air, generalized weakness, staggering, ataxia, and blurred or dim vision may be all signs linked to a potential TIA or a true stroke when they accompany dizziness that cannot be explained on any other grounds.

Guide to Differential Diagnosis

In evaluating the entire group of syndromes involving the vertebrobasilar system, a simple guide in differential diagnosis is the question of associated symptoms. A patient with unilateral tinnitus and hearing loss accompanying an acute episode of vertigo should be considered to have a peripheral labyrinthine lesion if there are no signs of brainstem involvement. If such a patient, however, has concomitant ipsilateral Horner's syndrome, facial analgesia, palatal weakness, limb ataxia, and contralateral analgesia of the body and limbs, a definite central lesion exists unless proven otherwise. Differential diagnosis calls for careful cochlear and vestibular studies by quantitative audiologic techniques and by quantitative vestibular studies using electronystagmography, in addition to neurologic examination.

Normal Aging Changes and Dizziness

Aging phenomena in the auditory system, usually termed *presbycusis*, have analogies in the vestibular system, which I suggest should be termed *presbyvertigo* and *presbyataxia*.

Schuknecht[11] has suggested a useful classification of four types of aging phenomenon in the vestibular system—three peripheral and one central.

Cupulolithiasis (Presbyvertigo)

Cupular deposits in the posterior semicircular canal produce a gravity type of response, which causes episodes of sudden, short attacks of falling.

Ampullar Presbyvertigo

This type of vertigo is associated with angular head movements, without falling, which may last for several hours. (It may be difficult to dissociate this from cervical vascular vertigo.)

Macular Presbyvertigo

Vertigo on getting out of bed may be related to saccular macular atrophy described in 1965 by Schuknecht and co-workers.[12] In 1969, Johnsson and Hawkins[9] stated that, as in ampullar vertigo, it is not possible to eliminate cervical circulatory factors from this type of vertigo. An interesting senile saccular change has been reported by Johnsson.[8]

Presbyataxia

This dysequilibrium syndrome is probably of CNS origin and is an ataxia that occurs primarily when walking.

REFERENCES

1. Barber HO: Diagnostic techniques in vertigo. J Vertigo 1:1, 1974
2. Belal A, Stewart T: Pathological changes in the middle ear joints. Ann Otol Rhinol Laryngol 83:159, 1974
3. Dublin WB: The combined correlated audiohistogram. Ann Otol Rhinol Laryngol 85:813, 1976
4. Dublin WB: Fundamentals of Sensorineural Auditory Pathology, pp 173–183. Springfield, IL, Charles C Thomas, 1976
5. Fieandt H von, Saxen A: Pathologic und Klinik der altersschwerhorigkeit. Acta Otolaryngol, Suppl 23, 1937
6. Goodhill V: External conductive hypacusis and the fixed malleus syndrome. Acta Otolaryngol, Suppl 217, 1966
7. Gussen R: Plugging of vascular canals in the otic capsule. Ann Otol Rhinol Laryngol 78:1305, 1969
8. Johnsson L-G: Degenerative changes and anomalies of the vestibular system in man. Laryngoscope 81:1682, 1971
9. Johnsson L-G, Hawkins J Jr: Nerve degeneration and vascular changes in Corti's organ based on surface preparations of the human cochlea. Proceedings of the IX International Congress Oto-Rhino-Laryngology, Mexico, 1969. Amsterdam, Excerpta International Congress Series No. 206.
10. Johnsson LG, Hawkins J Jr: Sensory and neural degenerations with aging, as seen in microdissections of the human inner ear. Ann Otol Rhinol Laryngol 81:179, 1972.
11. Schuknecht HF: Pathology of the Ear. Cambridge, MA, Harvard University Press, 1974
12. Schuknecht HF, Igarashi M, Gacek R: The pathological types of cochleo-saccular degeneration. Acta Otolaryngol 59:154, 1965
13. Suga F, Lindsay J: Histopathological observations of presbycusis. Ann Otol Rhinol Laryngol 85:169, 1976

25   Endocrine Diseases

Paul J. Davis and Faith B. Davis

The recognition of endocrinopathy in elderly patients requires knowledge of the changes in endocrine function to be expected with normal aging, the impact of age on the expression of endocrine disease, and the masking effect that coincident nonendocrine diseases have. Unstable angina pectoris may herald the onset of hyperthyroidism in older patients, but the anginal syndrome itself may be dramatic enough to divert attention from the thyroid disease. The absence of goiter in young patients with suspected thyrotoxicosis makes the latter diagnosis unlikely, whereas 40% of older hyperthyroid subjects lack goiter. Failure to appreciate that the responsiveness of the renin-aldosterone axis to assumption of the upright posture and to salt restriction declines with normal aging can lead to an erroneous diagnostic impression of hyporeninemic hypoaldosteronism in elderly hyperkalemic subjects. Blunted pituitary secretion of thyroid stimulating hormone (thyrotropin, TSH) in response to administration of thyrotropin releasing hormone (TRH) is common in normal elderly men and may erroneously indicate the presence of hyperthyroidism or hypopituitarism. Finally, fatigue, psychomotor retardation, and constipation are all acceptable consequences of "normal aging"; both hypothyroidism and apathetic hyperthyroidism in the elderly can present as this triad of findings and may be overlooked unless one's threshold is low for diagnosing thyroid dysfunction. Treatment of certain endocrinopathies in the elderly should be adjusted on an age-specific basis (*e.g.,* thyroid hormone replacement dosage in elderly myxedematous patients). The purpose of this chapter is to provide information that will facilitate the diagnosis of endocrine disease in older patients and to review its treatment on an age-specific basis.

THYROID DISEASE

Hyperthyroidism

Twenty percent of hyperthyroid patients are over 60 years of age. As we have emphasized elsewhere,[11] the majority present with symptoms and signs indistinguishable from those experienced by young patients with this disorder. The age-specific problems in recognition are the following:

Twenty-five percent of elderly hyperthyroid individuals present with an apathetic or otherwise atypical syndrome frequently affecting a single organ system (particularly the cardiovascular or central nervous system).

Even in the conventionally symptomatic older patient population, goiter is absent in 40%.

The spectrum of cardiac manifestations is distinctive in hyperthyroidism of the aged: sinus tachycardia occurs in a minority. Atrial fibrillation occurs in 40% or more and has a relatively low rate of spontaneous reversion to sinus mechanism; slow ventricular response to atrial fibrillation is relatively common.

The disease is frequently coincident with important systemic illnesses—such as pneumonia or coronary artery disease—that direct the attention of the diagnostician away from the possibility of thyroid disease.

Definitive treatment of the elderly thyrotoxic patient with radioactive iodide carries a substantive risk of thyroid storm, unless adjunctive antithyroid therapy is undertaken or the patient is returned to the euthyroid state by the use of thioamide drugs prior to administration of the radioactive iodide.

A comparison of the frequency of symptoms and signs associated with thyrotoxicosis in old and

TABLE 25-1   Comparison of Clinical Features of Hyperthyroidism in Elderly and Young Patients

	% of Patients	
Clinical Feature	Elderly*	Young†
Nervousness	55	99
Hyperhydrosis	38	91
Heat intolerance	63	89
Palpitation	63	89
Fatigue or weakness	52	88
Weight loss	75	85
Dyspnea	66	75
Polyphagia	11	65
Diarrhea	12	23
Anorexia	36	9
Constipation	26	4
Tachycardia	50	100
Goiter	63	100
Thyroid bruit	27	77
Eye signs	57	71
Atrial fibrillation	39	10

* Taken from a study of 85 patients over age 60 years.[11]
† Taken from a study of 247 patients with thyrotoxicosis.[21]

young patients is shown in Table 25-1. Although weight loss occurs frequently in both patient populations, polyphagia and increased stool frequency are encountered far less often in the older hyperthyroid group. Constipation is noted surprisingly frequently in thyrotoxic elderly subjects, perhaps representing a preexistent symptom unaffected by the supervention of thyroid disease. The cluster of constipation, weight loss, and loss of appetite, suggesting gastrointestinal tract malignancy, occurred in 15% of our thyrotoxic patient population.[11]

Infiltrative ophthalmopathy and thyrotoxic dermopathy ("pretibial myxedema") are both uncommon in older hyperthyroid subjects. Severe eye disease and dermopathy are associated in younger patients with Graves' disease. Graves' disease is defined as diffuse toxic goiter on an autoimmune basis, regardless of the presence or absence of infiltrative cutaneous or eye findings. Diffuse (nonnodular) involvement of the thyroid in the thyrotoxic process occurred in more than half of our own study group of elderly hyperthyroid patients, indicating that, previous impressions to the contrary, Graves' disease is relatively common in the aged.

Thyrotoxic hypertension is readily curable. Widening of the pulse pressure, characteristic of hyperthyroidism in younger subjects, is less frequently seen in older individuals, and we have attributed the finding of relatively normal heart rates in the face of atrial fibrillation and hyperthyroidism to concomitant coronary artery disease with a high degree of intrinsic atrioventricular conduction block. Liver enlargement is relatively common in elderly thyrotoxic patients and in most, but not all, cases is attributable to coincident diseases unrelated to hyperthyroidism (*e.g.*, hepatic cirrhosis). Tremor of various etiologies, increasingly common with age, is a poor discriminant for the presence of thyroid disease in the elderly.

Confirmation of the diagnosis requires the presence of elevated circulating levels of thyroid hormone and a supportive, independent test of thyroid function. Serum thyroxine (T_4) by radioimmunoassay is used to screen for elevated thyroid hormone levels; concomitant measurement of serum triiodothyronine (T_3) resin uptake should also be elevated, indicating that an elevation of thyroxine-binding globulin (TBG) does not account for the high thyroid hormone concentration. Free T_4 index measurements also serve to exclude TBG abnormalities. In as many as 10% of elderly patients subsequently shown to be hyperthyroid, serum T_4 by radioimmunoassay is normal and serum T_3 concentration by radioimmunoassay—not the T_3 resin uptake—is elevated. The latter condition is termed T_3 *toxicosis.* Thus, in patients in whom the suspicion of hyperthyroidism persists in the face of a normal serum T_4 level, measurement of serum T_3 levels should be carried out. We have reported that the thyroidal radioactive iodide uptake test is uniformly elevated in elderly patients with thyrotoxicosis,[11] except in the setting of T_3-toxicosis. The serum free T_4 test lacks specificity in all age-groups; in the presence of systemic, nonthyroidal disease states (infection, cardiovascular catastrophe) the free T_4 may be elevated (up to twice the upper limit of normal). In hyperthyroid patients, however, the serum free T_4 is usually elevated to a level more than twice normal.

Occasionally, the suspicion of hyperthyroidism in older patients is rewarded only by borderline high values for serum T_4, serum T_3, and thyroidal radioactive iodide uptake. In this situation, use of the TRH test should be considered. In the presence of autonomous hyperfunction of the thyroid, administration of exogenous TRH results in no increase in serum concentration of TSH. The TRH test is a reliable index of excessive thyroid hormone action over the life span in women; in normal elderly men with normal thyroid function, however, responsiveness to TRH may be suppressed.[35] A normal TRH test in an elderly man suspected of having thyrotoxicosis indicates that hyperthyroidism is not present. A suppressed TRH response is not diagnostically valuable, since it is consistent with either normal thyroid function or hyperthyroidism. Regardless of a patient's sex or age, failure to respond to TRH administration is also consistent with hypopituitarism or excessive exogenous thyroid hormone administration.

Other laboratory tests that are not specific for thyroid disease should be mentioned. In contrast to thyrotoxicosis in younger patients, hypercalcemia rarely occurs in the older hyperthyroid subject. Serum cholesterol concentration has no discriminant value in the setting of thyroid hyperfunction. Pernicious anemia occurs in as many as 3% of patients with Graves' disease, and undiagnosed anemia (hematocrit value <35%) occurs in about 20% of older hyperthyroid individuals, perhaps reflecting "chronic disease." No elevation of circulating activities of muscle enzymes occurs in thyrotoxic myopathy. Serum liver function test abnormalities are common in older hyperthyroid patients, with the most frequent finding an elevated serum alkaline phosphatase. A large number of other common nonthyroidal diseases are associated with abnormal alkaline phosphatase activity. Elevated alkaline phosphatase values should not be attributed to thyroid disease until biliary tract disease, liver disease, and osteoblastic bone disorders have been ruled out.

Short-term goals and strategies in the management of severe hyperthyroidism include the following:

Control of certain effects of thyroid hormone on peripheral tissues by pharmacologic blockade of β-adrenergic receptors (propranolol administration).
Inhibition of thyroid gland release of thyroid hormone (inorganic iodide administration).
Inhibition of hormonogenesis within the thyroid gland (iodide and thioamide administration).
Specific treatment of nonthyroidal systemic illnesses which, by unknown mechanism(s), may exacerbate hyperthyroidism.

Whether pharmacologic inhibition of the conversion of circulating T_4 to T_3 by peripheral (*i.e.*, extrathyroidal) tissues hastens the return of patients to the euthyroid state is not yet established. Propylthiouracil (PTU), a commonly used thioamide drug, inhibits T_4 to T_3 conversion extrathyroidally and blocks hormonogenesis within the thyroid gland. Pharmacologic doses of corticosteroids, such as prednisone, also inhibit peripheral conversion of T_4 to T_3. Short-term prednisone use (40 mg/day for 7 days) is endorsed for the management of acute, severe hyperthyroidism in the elderly. The clinical setting in which the strategies listed are all used, together with corticosteroid administration, is that of suspected "thyroid storm," in which exaggerated clinical findings of hyperthyroidism are accompanied by fever and, usually, severe tachycardia. The use of propranolol in the elderly hyperthyroid subject with an antecedent or current history of congestive heart failure has material clinical risk. We recommend a cautious trial of propranolol in this setting when ventricular rate is 140 beats/min or greater (heart rate—dependent heart failure). Recommended dosages of the agents cited above are shown in Table 25-2.

In contrast to the presentation in thyroid storm, an elderly patient with mild thyrotoxicosis may require no more than PTU administration for a period sufficient to achieve a euthyroid state. At that time definitive treatment by ablative radioactive iodide administration should be considered. An alternative strategy is administration of an arbitrarily chosen oral dose of propranolol (*e.g.*, 10 mg to 20 mg four times daily) in the mildly thyrotoxic patient and radioactive iodide administration 1 to 2 weeks thereafter. We have not encountered exacerbation of hyperthyroid symptoms by radioactive iodide administration in elderly patients with the latter regimen.

If PTU alone is used to threat hyperthyroidism, therapy should be interrupted at 6 to 12 months to determine if spontaneous remission has occurred. High-dose thioamide therapy (>450 mg PTU daily) should be avoided, since, in patients over the age of 40 years it has an increased risk of bone marrow suppression (granulocytopenia).[9]

Hypothyroidism

Thyroid gland failure and consequent hypometabolism are states encountered more frequently in patients above the age of 50 years than in younger subjects. Thus, the signs and symptoms of hypothyroidism have been well defined in terms of the elderly population. Profound, life-threatening hypothyroidism (myxedema, stupor, or coma) are almost never encountered in younger patients. Worth remembering with regard to hypothyroidism in the elderly are the following:

Many of the symptoms and signs of hypothyroidism (constipation, cold intolerance, psychomo-

TABLE 25-2   Treatment of Hyperthyroidism in Elderly Patients

Medication	Action	Dose	Comments
Short term			
Propranolol	Controls effects of thyroid hormone on peripheral tissues by β-adrenergic blockade	20–40 mg orally q6h	Dose titrated to maintain heart rate at approximately 100/min; may cause exacerbation of congestive heart failure or bronchospasm
Inorganic iodine	Blocks release of hormone from gland; inhibits organification of iodide during hormone synthesis	Lugol's solution 2 drops (16.6 mg) in water daily	Onset of effect in 1–2 days; maximum effect in 3–7 days; escape from effect in 2–6 weeks; may cause rash
Propylthiouracil (PTU) Methimazole (M)	Inhibit organification of iodide; PTU also inhibits conversion of T_4 to T_3 in peripheral tissues	PTU: 100–150 mg q8h orally M: 10–15 mg q8h orally	Onset of effect in 2–4 weeks; maximum effect in 4–8 weeks; drug dose may be titrated downward once disease is controlled; may cause rash, granulocytopenia
Glucocorticoids	Inhibit extrathyroidal conversion of T_4 to T_3	Hydrocortisone 100 mg (or equivalent) orally or intravenously q8h	Use in severe thyrotoxicosis (storm) for 7–10 days; may cause psychosis
Long term			
Radioactive iodide	Radiation damage to thyroid tissue	5–15 mCi; up to 25 mCi for toxic nodules	Definitive therapy; may cause transient release of hormone from gland; give only after hyperthyroidism controlled with propranolol, PTU, or M; may cause transient or permanent hypothyroidism

tor retardation, decreased exercise tolerance) are consistent with normal aging and may be attributed to the latter rather than to thyroid hypofunction.

Hypothyroidism is a cause of hypertension, and the latter may respond to thyroid hormone replacement.

Cognitive changes present at the time of diagnosis infrequently respond to thyroid hormone replacement.

Although pericardial effusion is common in myxedema, it is rarely of hemodynamic consequence.

Hypothyroid myopathy may be associated with extraordinary elevations of circulating creatine phosphokinase (CPK) activity (values up to 5,000 units/liter or more) and such values persist until the initiation of thyroid hormone replacement therapy. The CPK isoenzyme primarily elevated is that of skeletal muscle origin, but

we occasionally see modest elevations of the isoenzyme of myocardial origin in hypothyroid patients who otherwise lack evidence of myocardial disease.

Regardless of patient age, the diagnosis of hypothyroidism rests on the finding of depressed serum levels of T_4 and the hallmark of elevated serum TSH concentration. In fewer than 3% of elderly hypothyroid patients, the serum TSH level is low, signaling the presence of pituitary hypothyroidism. Serum free T_4 concentrations are of no diagnostic value in the setting of suspected hypothyroidism. As is the case in hyperthyroidism, measurement of the serum cholesterol level has low discriminant value in hypothyroidism. A trend upward in serum cholesterol occurs in mild to moderately hypothyroid patients, but severely myxedematous subjects may have normal or even low serum cholesterol levels. As many as 10% of patients with spontaneous hypothyroidism (thyroid hypofunction not attributable to thyroid surgery or radioactive iodide administration) have concomitant pernicious anemia.

Profound myxedema is a medical emergency characterized by altered sensorium, hypothermia, and, usually, hypotension and bradycardia. Care of such patients is to be instituted in a medical intensive care unit and consists of intravenous administration of high doses of L-thyroxine (250 μg to 500 μg) 12 to 24 hours apart, looking for improvement in sensorium, body temperature, or blood pressure within 24 hours. If two such doses of T_4 fail to effect significant clinical improvement, the diagnosis of hypothyroidism should be reconsidered. Support with stress levels of corticosteroid (100 mg to 200 mg of hydrocortisone/24 hours intravenously) is indicated, particularly when hypotension and hyponatremia are present. Hyponatremia in this setting may be due to relative adrenocortical insufficiency (manifested during the period of administration of high-dose T_4 replacement) or to hypothyroidism, itself. When due to the latter, depressed serum sodium concentration is a function of impaired free water clearance, reflecting inappropriate hypersecretion of endogenous antidiuretic hormone (ADH) or altered renal hemodynamics. When a severely hypothyroid patient responds appropriately to high-dose intravenous T_4 management, the patient is then maintained subsequently on low-dose daily oral T_4 therapy (25 μg) for 1 to 2 weeks. Stepwise 25-μg increments are then made at 2- to 4-week intervals until full replacement is achieved with 75 μg to 150 μg/day.

The major issue in treatment of the mildly hypothyroid elderly patient is the initial dose of T_4 to be used. In the setting of any evidence of heart disease (*e.g.*, a history of angina pectoris, myocardial infarction, heart failure, tachyarrhythmia, or tachybradyarrhythmia), low-dose initial replacement therapy is mandatory. Such oral therapy is begun with 25 μg T_4 daily for 1 to 3 weeks, followed by 25-μg increments at similar intervals thereafter until full replacement dosage is obtained. The end point for therapy is that dose of T_4 obtained in 25-μg steps that first lowers the elevated serum TSH level into the normal range.[10] Although more sophisticated measurements may be carried out to confirm the appropriateness of the replacement dose of thyroid hormone, we have found that the regimen recommended is satisfactory in elderly patients. If symptoms or signs of exacerbation of concomitant heart disease are worsened by stepped thyroid hormone replacement, it is judicious to return to a lower level of

replacement dosage for 4 weeks and then institute 12.5 μg increments. Concomitant propranolol therapy may be efficacious in controlling angina pectoris that arises in the course of stepped thyroid hormone therapy.

ADRENAL DISEASE

Hypoadrenocorticism

Primary adrenocortical insufficiency (Addison's disease) is uncommon in the elderly; fewer than 5% of patients with Addison's disease are over the age of 60 years. The issue of Addison's disease is often raised because of the frequency with which the triad of azotemia, hyponatremia, and trivial hyperkalemia is encountered. Although consistent with Addison's disease, this constellation in elderly subjects more commonly represents intravascular volume contraction on a nonadrenal basis superimposed on age-dependent decline in glomerular filtration rate; depressed serum sodium concentration may reflect decreased free water clearance (due to thiazide or other drug administration or to the syndrome of inappropriate secretion of antidiuretic hormone [SIADH]). Despite the relatively common finding of "non-Addison's disease," the prognostic implications of untreated authentic adrenocortical insufficiency are so dire than an evaluation of adrenocortical function must be carried out whenever clinical or laboratory findings suggest that the condition is present.

Authentic Addison's disease in the elderly manifests most of the features encountered in younger patients. Cutaneous hyperpigmentation, however, may be subtle or absent in elderly Addisonian patients, and gingival pigment is lacking in edentulous patients. The clustering of pernicious anemia and Addison's disease persists over the lifespan, whereas other overlap autoimmune syndromes (*e.g.*, the combination of Hashimoto's thyroiditis and Addison's disease [Schmidt's syndrome]) are encountered infrequently in older subjects.

The pathogenesis of adrenocortical insufficiency in the elderly is similar to that in young patients, namely, destruction of the adrenal cortex by autoimmune or granulomatous processes. Failure of the adrenal cortex to recover from suppression by steroid therapy is an important cause of adrenocortical insufficiency in patients of all ages. Bilateral adrenal gland hemorrhage, usually in the setting of bacteremia and azotemia,[37] and adrenal gland destruction due to bilateral mestastases from lung carcinoma, although more common in the older population, remain unusual causes of adrenal gland disease.

Confirmation of the diagnosis of adrenocortical insufficiency, regardless of patient age, depends on measurements of serum cortisol concentration; these are usually measured at 8 AM when, under normal circumstances, endogenous cortisol levels are highest. The stress of systemic, nonadrenal disease and hospitalization may cause patients without adrenocortical disease to lose the normal diurnal variation in serum corticosteroid levels and maintain high concentrations of cortisol throughout the day. It should be remembered that failure to elevate serum cortisol levels in the face of acute systemic disease reflects impaired adrenocortical function ("low adrenocortical reserve"). Thus, a morning serum cortisol level that is in the lower one half of the normal range in a patient with serious systemic infection or myocardial infarction indicates some degree of adrenocortical compromise. Such patients fail to respond to the administration of exogenous synthetic ACTH (cosyntropin) by further increases in serum cortisol levels. Normal aging, *per se,* has no effect on cortisol secretion in response to ACTH.[16] When available and reliable, measurements of serum endogenous ACTH by radioimmunoassay are diagnostically elevated in patients with primary adrenocortical insufficiency. The combination of low serum ACTH and low serum cortisol concentrations signals the presence of hypopituitary adrenal failure.

Corticoid replacement therapy is not age adjusted. Thus, in the elderly a regimen of 20 mg hydrocortisone equivalent orally in the morning and 10 mg in the evening is usually sufficient. Fludrocortisone, 0.05 mg/day or every other day, is required by a minority of patients specifically to support mineralocorticoid deficit. Such a deficit is signaled by persisting asthenia, orthostatic hypotension, hyponatremia, and hyperkalemia.

Hypoaldosteronism

A selective form of adrenocortical insufficiency has been recognized with increased frequency in elderly type II diabetics with mild renal impairment (serum creatinine concentration <2.5 mg/dl). This syndrome of isolated hypoaldosteronism has been attributed to deficient renin production by the kidney ("hyporeninemic hypoaldosteronism") and is characterized clinically by hyperkalemia, sometimes of a marked degree,[13] not explained by the modest fall in glomerular filtration rate. Hyponatremia and evidence of volume depletion are not a part of this syndrome. The validity of the diagnosis is often suspect because of the decline, which occurs in the course of normal aging, of basal and stimulated renin and aldosterone secretion.[36] Thus, an elderly patient with hyperkalemia of any cause may be found to have decreased renin and aldosterone production in response to the conventional stimuli of volume depletion and assumption of the upright posture. The pathogenesis of the authentic syndrome of hyporeninemic hypoaldosteronism may not reside at the level of defective release of renin, since some of these patients with hyperkalemia and hypoaldosteronism have been found to have expanded plasma volume, in which setting the low levels of serum renin and aldosterone reflect functional (*i.e.,* normal) suppression of this axis. Very rarely, deficient aldosterone secretion is an isolated biochemical defect in the adrenal cortex, and circulating levels of renin are expectedly high in this setting. This form of hypoaldosteronism is not seen with increased frequency in the elderly population.

Regardless of pathogenesis, the findings of severe hyperkalemia (serum potassium >6.5 mEq/liter) and hypoaldosteronism are treated similarly in young and elderly patients. Infusions of glucose and insulin and induction of kaliuresis (use of a potassium-wasting loop diuretic) or dialysis are alternative therapies, the choice among which will be dictated by each patient's renal function. Chronic management of hyperkalemia in the elderly, however, poses special problems, unless diuresis is effective. A conventional approach to the hyperkalemia of hypoaldosteronism is the administration of a potassium-losing mineralocorticoid (fludrocortisone). The dosage of this agent required to induce significant kaliuria may be high (0.1 mg to 0.3 mg/day of fludrocortisone) and may promote volume expansion, hypertension, and edema. In patients with, or predisposed to, congestive heart failure, this drug may exacerbate failure.

Adrenocortical Hyperfunction

Spontaneous hyperfunction of the adrenal cortex (due to unilateral adenoma or carcinoma) or bilateral adrenocortical hyperplasia and hyperfunction due to central overproduction of ACTH (Cushing's disease) are uncommon findings in the elderly population. The clinical manifestations of hypercortisolism are similar in old and young patients. The diagnostic evaluation of patients suspected to have adrenocortical hyperfunction is the same in adults of any age.

One form of adrenal gland hyperfunction that occurs with increased frequency as aging progresses is that due to ectopic ACTH secretion.[3] There is an age-dependent facet to this syndrome because of the increasing risk of carcinomas of nearly all types as normal aging proceeds. The syndrome results from the uncontrolled release of ACTH from tumors, usually carcinomas, of non-pituitary origin. Small cell carcinoma of the lung is the most common source of ectopic ACTH production. Although circulating levels of serum cortisol in this condition are very high (usually >100 μg/dl) and substantially above those associated with Cushing's disease, the majority of patients with ectopic ACTH syndrome do not survive long enough to develop classic clinical manifestations of adrenocortical hyperfunction such as obesity, rounded facies, and abdominal striae. A hallmark of this state, however, is hypokalemia, occurring in more than 80% of such patients. Depressed serum potassium concentrations reflect the mineralocorticoid effects of very high levels of endogenous glucocorticoids induced by ectopic ACTH, as well as the stimulation by ACTH of aldosterone secretion by the adrenal cortex.

The hypokalemia associated with ectopic ACTH production is often severe (<2.0 mEq/liter) and life threatening. Measurement of urinary potassium excretion provides an index to the amount of potassium supplementation required to support current levels of serum potassium, but does not index total body potassium deficit. The latter may be extraordinary. The enteral route for potassium replacement is to be preferred, since it allows for the administration of larger quantities of potassium than does the intravenous route. Untreated, significant hypokalemia in the elderly is particularly troublesome because of cardiac arrhythmias, which may be superimposed on preexistent cardiac disease, and induction of digitalis intoxication in patients receiving this drug. In patients in whom survivorship associated with the underlying tumor is relatively long, control of the primary neoplasm with chemotherapy or induction of chemical adrenalectomy are chronic approaches to the management of the ectopic ACTH syndrome. Chemical adrenalectomy may be accomplished with administration of aminoglutethimide,[38] a drug that is preferable to mitotane because of fewer side-effects.

Hyperaldosteronism

The incidence of primary hyperaldosteronism (Conn's syndrome) peaks at the age of 50 years. Hallmarks are volume-dependent hypertension, hypokalemic alkalosis, and normal serum sodium concentration; carbohydrate intolerance and hy-

pomagnesemia may also occur. The presentation in elderly patients is no different from that in younger individuals, and the diagnostic evaluation is similar. Excessive aldosterone secretion originates either from a unilateral adrenocortical adenoma or from bilateral hyperplasia of the glomerulosa layer of the adrenal cortex. Confounding the diagnostic evaluation in older subjects is the increasing frequency over the life span of nonfunctional adrenocortical adenomas.[31] Thus, essential hypertension in an elderly patient and an unrelated (nonfunctional) adrenal adenoma, detected by computed tomographic (CT) scanning, may lead to an initial diagnostic impression of hyperaldosteronism. Diuretic treatment of hypertension may induce hypokalemia in such patients and further mislead the diagnostician. The sensitivity of CT scanning in detecting adrenocortical pathology is exquisite, but the technique of course does not define functional status of the nodules so identified. Chemical hyperaldosteronism, however, is not present in the setting of essential hypertension and nonfunctional adrenal adenomas. The treatment of primary hyperaldosteronism is not altered by patient age.

ADRENOMEDULLARY DISEASE

Pheochromocytoma

The peak incidence of pheochromocytoma occurs in the third and fourth decades and in various series the incidence in patients over 60 years of age has ranged from 0 to 8%. Autopsy data have suggested a substantially higher prevalence of pheochromocytoma in elderly patients,[25] but the majority of such lesions were nonfunctional. The risk of malignant pheochromocytoma is not increased over the life span.[34]

There are no age-specific clinical features of pheochromocytoma that facilitate its diagnosis in the older patient. However, the tumor may exacerbate congestive heart failure in patients with preexistent arteriosclerotic heart disease, and catecholamines, themselves, can induce a primary cardiomyopathy. The possibility of pheochromocytoma should be considered in patients with conventional clinical syndromes of heart disease who manifest excessive sweating, with or without tachycardia, after routine treatment of cardiac symptoms and signs. The diagnosis should also be entertained when routine institution of β-blockade in hypertensive patients accelerates hypertension (due to the state of unopposed α-adrenergic activity).

PITUITARY DISEASE

Hypopituitarism

Tumor registry data indicate a slowly progressive increase with age in clinically apparent pituitary tumors. Autopsy data indicate that the prevalence of clinically inapparent pituitary microadenomas is more than 20%,[7] without age specificity. Regardless of adult patient age, the most common cause of pituitary insufficiency remains pituitary tumor. Occasionally, hypopituitarism in the elderly woman is attributed to partial pituitary necrosis dating to postpartum complications many years earlier. Cranial arteritis is a rare cause of hypopituitarism in the elderly.

The clinical findings of hypopituitarism are unchanged over the life span, except that the sensitive clinical clues in younger patients that relate to loss of gonadal function are lost in postmenopausal women and muted in elderly men in whom decreased sexual function may be attributed to "normal aging." Integumentary changes expected with normal aging, including loss of body hair, may also prevent the physician from considering hypopituitary loss of adrenal androgen production in women and of testicular androgen production in men when hair loss is noted.

The management of patients with hypopituitarism is modified in the elderly to include considerations of age-specific adjustment in thyroid hormone replacement dosage (see Hypothyroidism) and instituting or withholding sex steroid replacement in elderly males according to expressed psychosocial needs. Estrogen replacement therapy in elderly women, regardless of the state of their pituitary function, serves to reduce the risk of clinically significant metabolic bone disease.[32]

The incidence of prolactin-secreting pituitary tumors in the elderly is difficult to estimate because the clinical manifestations of such lesions are primarily reflected in suppressed gonadotropin release (and amenorrhea) and/or galactorrhea. The latter is not likely to be encountered in elderly women. Decreased luteinizing hormone production in elderly men will be associated with decreased sexual function.

Water Metabolism

Abnormalities of free water clearance in older subjects are common because drugs capable of inducing impaired free water clearance (such as diuretics and chlorpropamide) are commonly in use in the elderly patient population and the incidence of certain carcinomas, particularly small cell carcinoma of the lung, capable of synthesizing antidiuretic hormone (ADH; arginine vasopressin [AVP]), is also increased in older subjects. The management of hypo-osmolar syndromes due to both of these factors has been well described elsewhere,[4] but approaches such as high-dose demeclocycline therapy or repetitive intravenous furosemide administration[19] (alternating with parenteral hypertonic saline injection) require extraordinarily close supervision in hospitalized older individuals.

The syndromes of diabetes insipidus and nephrogenic diabetes insipidus are uncommon in elderly subjects, except that transient nephrogenic diabetes insipidus complicates mechanical relief of obstructive uropathy and hydronephrosis; the latter are, of course, encountered more commonly in the elderly male.

PARATHYROID DISEASE

Hypoparathyroidism

The diagnosis of hypoparathyroidism is usually suggested by routine serum chemistries, rather than a syndrome of neuromuscular irritability. The hallmark findings of hypocalcemia and hyperphosphatemia are far more commonly due today to renal failure (and are associated with secondary hyperparathyroidism) rather than to hypofunction of the parathyroid glands. Hypocalcemia without hyperphosphatemia is usually of nonparathyroid origin (*e.g.*, liver disease or other states associated with hypoalbuminemia). In some subjects, particularly the elderly, phosphate depletion may obscure the tendency toward elevated serum phosphate in authentic hypoparathyroidism. Phosphate depletion may be due to decreased dietary intake (calcium and phosphate intake both are decreased over the life span) or to decreased gastrointestinal tract absorption of phosphate. The pathogenesis of decreased parathyroid function in the elderly population includes, as it does in younger patients, autoimmune destruction of the parathyroid glands and surgical sacrifice of the parathyroids in the course of removal of the thyroid gland. Post-thyroidectomy hypoparathyroidism may not express itself for several years after thyroid surgery. Radioactive iodide ablation of the thyroid gland appears to pose an insignificant risk of hypoparathyroidism.

There are other mechanisms by which hypocalcemia may result from abnormalities of the parathyroid axis.[29] For example, we have encountered five patients over 60 years of age whose hypocalcemia was associated with serum levels of immunoreactive parathyroid hormone (PTH) in the mid-normal range. In the parathyroprival patient, such levels should be immeasurably low, and in patients whose hypocalcemia is on a nonparathyroid basis, serum concentrations of PTH should be high. End-organ resistance to PTH also results in high levels of serum PTH and hypocalcemia. Thus, we speculate that these elderly patients with clearly normal PTH levels and hypocalcemia have parathyroid glands that secrete a species of PTH with an abnormal amino acid sequence. The hormone cross-reacts in the PTH immunoassay but is biologically relatively inactive. How common this syndrome is in younger patients is not clear.

The widespread availability of accurate measurements of serum PTH by radioimmunoassay has greatly facilitated the diagnosis of hypoparathyroidism. Assays are available that specifically recognize the intact PTH molecule, the C- (or carboxy-) terminal portion of the molecule, the N- (or amino-) terminal fragments of PTH, or the N-terminal end of the intact hormone. In primary hypoparathyroidism, any of these assays will document low or absent levels of circulating PTH. Measurements of phosphaturia or tubular reabsorption of phosphate are unnecessary and have not been standardized in normal elderly subjects in whom insidious declines in glomerular filtration rates are expected.

It is important to recognize that magnesium depletion is associated with a functionally hypoparathyroid state. Hypomagnesemia results at any age from decreased magnesium intake, gastrointestinal tract malabsorption syndromes, and magnesuria such as that induced by chronic diuretic therapy or aminoglycoside administration. In magnesium depletion, parathyroid gland release of PTH is impaired and serum levels of calcium and PTH are both low. Some degree of end-organ resistance to PTH action may also be present in states of excessive magnesium loss.

The treatment of hypoparathyroidism has relatively few age-specific refinements. When present, hypomagnesemia should be aggressively treated with parenteral administration of magnesium sulfate. Orally administered magnesium is virtually without effect in some patients, particularly those with liver disease, who do not absorb magnesium well. Management of authentic hypoparathyroidism involves optimizing calcium intake and, in the vast majority of patients, administration of vitamin D. Optimizing calcium intake in the elderly hypoparathyroid patient may be difficult. First, the standard dietary source of calcium, dairy products, may not be palatable, particularly

in those patients who have in adulthood developed intestinal disaccharidase deficiency. The therapeutic goal of 1 g of elemental calcium intake daily can be achieved with 1 quart of milk, but few elderly patients comply with this recommendation. Second, the use of calcium carbonate as a dietary calcium source has been widely recommended and is available on a prescription basis or in an over-the-counter antacid (*e.g.,* Tums, 300 mg calcium per tablet). However, in the absence of gastric acid, calcium carbonate is a nonabsorbable form of calcium, so that calcium carbonate therapy in elderly hypocalcemic patients is sometimes singularly unsuccessful. After initiating calcium carbonate in elderly patients, we measure urinary excretion of calcium to document the increase in calcium excretion we expect with normal hydrolysis of calcium carbonate and absorption of calcium ion. Such measurements may need to be carried out only once or twice after dietary intake of calcium has been effectively increased to 1 g/day. Other calcium salts (lactate or gluconate) are widely available in place of calcium carbonate but have the disadvantage of containing relatively little calcium and thus require the intake of a large number of tablets daily. Salts other than calcium carbonate may also be irritating to the upper gastrointestinal tract.

A number of forms of vitamin D are suitable for use in the older hypocalcemic patient. Although widely available and the most biologically active analog of vitamin D, 1,25-dihydroxycholecalciferol is an expensive agent that we have avoided using in patients with fixed incomes. The dosage of this agent is not age specific and 0.25 μg/day may suffice, in the setting of adequate dietary intake of calcium, to normalize serum calcium levels. An alternative, lower-cost agent is dihydrotachysterol (DHT). Careful refinement of the dose of this agent is required in order to avoid hypercalcemia, since the latter state may persist for a week or more after DHT therapy is interrupted; in contrast, hypercalcemia induced by 1,25-dihydroxycholecalciferol remits in 24 to 48 hours after stopping the agent. The least expensive form of vitamin D therapy is ergocalciferol (vitamin D_2); disadvantages of this preparation, however, are slow onset and dissipation of effect (2 to 3 weeks).

Hyperparathyroidism

The near-universal, repeated measurements of serum calcium concentration in outpatients as well as inpatients has resulted in the past decade in the recognition of a large population of patients with asymptomatic, mild hypercalcemia.[8] The majority of these patients have primary hyperparathyroidism of, at least initially, an indolent nature. For 5 years or more after recognition, this hyperparathyroid state is clinically inactive in 80% of patients; follow-up of such patients for a decade, however, reveals an increasing burden of complications of parathyroid hyperfunction.[33] Fifty percent of asymptomatic hyperparathyroid patients are discovered after they reach age 50 years. Our group currently follows a cohort of 10 patients over the age of 70 years with asymptomatic primary hyperparathyroidism. Surgical management of these patients with serum calcium levels of less than 12.5 mg/dl has been proscribed by the concomitant presence of unrelated medical illnesses, such as chronic obstructive pulmonary disease and coronary artery disease.

Thiazide diuretic therapy provokes hypercalcemia in a small number of patients treated with such agents for hypertension or heart failure. Experience elsewhere has suggested that virtually all of these thiazide-treated patients have latent hyperparathyroidism that has been unmasked by drug therapy. (Thiazides decrease renal tubular excretion of calcium.) We classify all patients who develop hypercalcemia on thiazide therapy as primary hyperparathyroidism suspects.

The signs and symptoms of severe hyperparathyroidism and hypercalcemia are unchanged in the course of aging. The bone-resorbing effect of mild or severe hyperparathyroidism is obviously of concern to physicians who manage elderly patients with preexistent metabolic bone disease. The availability of the technique of photon absorptiometry to estimate bone mineral content has allowed us to monitor asymptomatic elderly hyperparathyroid patients for increased rate of bone mass loss. Measurement of bone mineral content that has documented an annual loss rate of 3% or more in an asymptomatic patient causes us to recommend surgical neck exploration for definitive management of hyperparathyroidism.

For asymptomatic hyperparathyroidism in otherwise healthy patients of age 60 years or less, we have endorsed definitive (surgical) treatment of parathyroid disease. Such patients are expected to survive 20 years or more, and we are concerned about the long-term adverse effects of parathyroid disease on the skeleton, kidneys, and other organs.

Nonparathyroid Hypercalcemia

The nonparathyroid causes of hypercalcemia are many and have been well reviewed elsewhere.[22] Several of these states deserve specific mention in a consideration of hypercalcemia in the older patient population. High doses of vitamin A in Europe have been used for putatively chemotherapeutic purposes in patients with cancer. Such therapy is of unproven value but may promote hypercalcemia by increased gastrointestinal tract absorption of calcium. In the United States, anticarcinogenic effects of vitamin A have been suggested in laboratory animals, but results of these studies cannot be extrapolated to humans. The general availability of preparations of vitamin A allow patients to make such applications. Thus, any hypercalcemic patient encountered should be questioned for intake of vitamin A as well as vitamin D. Estrogen management of metastatic breast carcinoma, as well as treatment with tamoxifen, can provoke clinically important, even life-threatening, hypercalcemia.[23]

Pagetic patients are usually over the age of 50 years and normocalcemic. Enforcement of bed rest in patients with Paget's disease can provoke significant hypercalcemia in this state of excessive bone resorption. Other than in pagetic individuals, "immobilization hypercalcemia" is thought to be a state experienced chiefly by young patients placed in total body casts or their equivalent. Occasionally, however, mild hypercalcemia will be seen in elderly patients with nonpagetic demineralizing bone disease (osteoporosis) when they are placed at bed rest. Restoration of physical activity in such patients results in normalization of the serum calcium levels.

Epidemiologically and clinically, the most important nonparathyroid hypercalcemic state is that associated with neoplastic disease.[24] Although it was once thought that various epithelial cancers ectopically secreted authentic parathyroid hormone (PTH), it is now known that this event rarely, if ever, occurs. Tumoral hypercalcemic states result from the secretion by tumor cells of substances that promote bone resorption locally or systemically.[26] Such substances include polypeptides that are PTH-like in bioactivity (but that cross-react only partially with antibody to PTH in most radioimmunoassays), osteoclast-activating factor (OAF), and, perhaps, prostaglandins. Production of OAF is common in patients with multiple myeloma and breast carcinoma, resulting in hypercalcemic states that respond to corticosteroid (prednisone) administration. The vagaries of PTH immunoassay can make the diagnostic distinction between tumoral hypercalcemia and primary hyperparathyroidism quite difficult. We have discussed this diagnostic dilemma elsewhere.[12] Nonparathyroid hypercalcemic tumoral states might be expected to result in suppressed, that is, undetectable, levels of authentic PTH in serum. In some PTH radioimmunoassays, however, high levels of PTH-like polypeptides are measured as "normal" levels of authentic PTH. In patients with well-documented cancer, the finding of high levels (three or more times the upper limit of the normal range) of authentic PTH indicates that primary hyperparathyroidism is present, in addition to the already-diagnosed malignancy.

The management of nonparathyroid hypercalcemia is little affected by patient age. Removal of offending drugs (thiazides, vitamin A or vitamin D) is an obvious step. Steroid therapy is effective in hypercalcemic states due to breast cancer, myeloma, vitamin A or D intoxication, adrenal insufficiency, and sarcoidosis. Sarcoid hypercalcemia, however, is not a problem of the geriatric population. In the management of severe, acute hypercalcemia of tumoral origin in the elderly, we favor the initial use of calcitonin (2 to 8 MRC units/kg daily subcutaneously in four divided doses). The drug is nontoxic, infrequently results in allergic responses, and can be self-administered subcutaneously as maintenance therapy once the acute phase is successfully treated. Maintenance therapy may consist of a single daily dose or several doses weekly of calcitonin. Calcitonin therapy is, however, expensive. Mithramycin is an alternative agent, administered as one or no more than two doses of 25 µg/kg intravenously (the second dose to be given 24 hours after the initial dose). The use of additional doses of mithramycin is frequently associated with gastrointestinal tract and bone marrow toxicity. Outpatient management of hypercalcemia in the elderly can also be accomplished with oral phosphate administration, in the form of flavored phosphate salts (Neutra-Phos) or as a commercial cathartic (Phospho-Soda).

GONADAL DISEASES

Male Hypogonadism

Although modest declines in serum testosterone concentration occur in the normal aging male,[14] most of these alterations occur within the normal range. Decreased testicular Leydig cell number is found in elderly males to account for decreased androgen production. Trivial increases in serum luteinizing hormone (LH) also occur in normal elderly males.[20]

Clinically significant hypogonadism in the elderly male is uncommon. On the other hand, its presence may be unrecognized because the phy-

sician fails to question elderly subjects about sexual dysfunction and concomitant systemic illness (particularly disease of arteriosclerotic origin) may be of sufficient prominence to divert attention from hypogonadism. Serious systemic illness serves to decrease serum testosterone levels, and the diagnosis of hypogonadism due to testicular failure is not established until concomitant systemic illness is stable, serum testosterone concentrations remain low, and serum LH levels are elevated.

There is no mandate for the routine institution of testosterone therapy in elderly asymptomatic men. In elderly males with symptomatic hypogonadism, androgen replacement is available in the form of oral testosterone analogs (such as fluoxymesterone, 10 mg to 20 mg/day) or parenteral testosterone once or twice monthly. Doses of these agents are titrated against libido and/or sexual function.

Measurements of serum testosterone and LH allow endocrine sexual dysfunction to be segregated from disorders of sexual function relating to vascular disease (*e.g.*, Leriche syndrome), neuropathy of various causes, and psychological problems.

Menopause

The programmed decline in ovarian function in middle-aged women may culminate in a variety of symptoms and signs attributable to estrogen withdrawal. The Consensus Conference on the Menopause sponsored by the National Institutes of Health was held to define indications for institution of systemic estrogen replacement in postmenopausal women.[28] It was concluded that women with an early surgical menopause or primary hypogonadism (Turner's syndrome) should receive chronic estrogen therapy to minimize risk of osteoporosis, as should those menopausal women whose symptoms of vasomotor instability ("hot flashes") interfere with activities of daily living. Although the conference did not definitively advocate the use of estrogen replacement in women with spontaneous menopause for the prophylactic management of osteoporosis, evidence published subsequent to the conference has been particularly convincing that estrogen therapy reduces hip and wrist fracture rate in postmenopausal women.[32]

In the woman who is a candidate for estrogen treatment and who has previously undergone hysterectomy, chronic estrogen replacement (such as conjugated estrogens, 0.625 mg/day orally) is endorsed and has a high degree of safety. Cyclic estrogen–progesterone therapy is indicated in the patient with an intact uterus in order to minimize the risk of endometrial cancer associated with chronic estrogen therapy.[17] Such cyclic therapy results in monthly vaginal bleeding, which may be unacceptable to the postmenopausal patient.

We do not endorse routine institution of estrogen replacement in the postmenopausal patient for prophylaxis of osteoporosis. However, we identify by photon absorptiometry those patients who, at the time of the menopause, already have decreased bone mineral content relative to the general female population. Patients so identified are begun on estrogen replacement.

Regardless of bone mineral content, postmenopausal women are urged to maintain an adequate daily dietary calcium intake (1.0 g elemental calcium). Dairy product sources or supplemental calcium carbonate is used. Because hypochlorhydria may develop in the course of normal aging, calcium carbonate is not always an ideal source of calcium supplementation (the compound is hydrolyzed in the presence of gastric acid). Thus, when we institute dietary calcium supplementation we verify by collection of a 24-hour urine specimen for calcium excretion that dietary calcium is being absorbed normally. Exercise has been routinely recommended to elderly patients as a measure that helps to maintain bone integrity, but its efficacy has not been rigorously proved.

DIABETES MELLITUS

In the elderly, diabetes mellitus is generally characterized by overweight and modest degrees of peripheral tissue insensitivity to insulin action.

These patients have nonketosis-prone, type II diabetes mellitus, also called noninsulin-dependent diabetes mellitus (NIDDM). Many do require exogenous insulin therapy for control of blood sugar concentrations, since the small amounts of endogenous insulin that prevent lipolysis and suppress ketone production are insufficient to control hyperglycemia.

Diagnosis is based on the relatively new diagnostic standards developed by the National Diabetes Data Group.[27] As shown in Table 25-3 the diabetic state is established when the fasting venous plasma glucose is greater than 140 mg/dl or the 2-hour postprandial glucose level, plus another glucose level during the 2 hours, are over 200 mg/dl. Normal glucose tolerance is defined by a fasting glucose level below 115 mg/dl and the 2-hour postcibal value below 140 mg/dl. The transitional zone between these two sets of values is currently termed *impaired glucose tolerance* (IGT), recognizing the deterioration in glucose tolerance that occurs in normal subjects as a consequence of aging.[1]

Obesity is an important factor conditioning peripheral tissue insulin resistance.[30] Significant weight loss can normalize carbohydrate tolerance or convert the latter to the IGT state in patients who met diagnostic criteria for type II diabetes mellitus when overweight. Although the precise biochemical mechanism by which such normalization occurs is unknown, the improvement in peripheral tissue sensitivity to insulin action involves repair of a so-called post-receptor defect, perhaps at the membrane glucose transporter level.

Uncontrolled type II diabetes mellitus culminates in a life-threatening state of cellular dehydration termed *hyperglycemic nonketotic stupor* or *coma*. Osmotic diuresis of several days' to several

TABLE 25-3 Criteria for Diagnosis of Diabetes Mellitus

	Venous Plasma Glucose (mg/dl)		
	Fasting	*OGTT *:2 hours*	*30 min–2 hours*
Normal	<115	<140	<200
Impaired glucose tolerance	<140	140–200	>200
Diabetes mellitus	≥140　　*or*	≥200	≥200

* OGTT: 75 g glucose po.
(Data from National Diabetes Data Group: Classification and diagnosis of diabetes mellitus and other categories of glucose intolerance. Diabetes 28:1039–1057, 1979)

weeks' duration results in decreased plasma volume, a fall in glomerular filtration rate, decreased extracellular volume, and, finally, intracellular dehydration. Only when the glomerular filtration rate has declined can the blood glucose concentration achieve levels of 1000 mg to 2000 mg/dl or higher. Because ketosis is minimal in such patients, the serum creatinine concentration (which can be artifactually elevated by ketonemia in standard automated methods for creatinine measurement) remains an accurate insight into renal function in hyperglycemic nonketotic stupor. This hyperosmolar state can be accompanied by focal neurologic deficits, a variety of movement disorders and other aberrations of central nervous system function.[2,18] The acute management of the hyperglycemic nonketotic state requires restoration of body water and solute and low-dosage regular infusion (5–10 U/hr) (see Chapter 37).

Serum potassium levels can plummet dramatically when cellular uptake of glucose is restored by insulin administration in profoundly hyperglycemic patients. Thus, careful monitoring of serum potassium concentration is mandatory. There is no indication for phosphate administration in the hyperglycemic nonketotic setting, or in diabetic ketoacidosis,[15] unless the patient's history includes alcoholism or gastrointestinal tract disease in which absolute phosphate deficiency can be expected.

Several facets of the long-term management of elderly patients with type II diabetes deserve comment. First, the complications of diabetes mellitus encountered in patients with type I (retinopathy, nephropathy, and neuropathy) are also encountered in patients with type II. Death from nondiabetic causes may supervene before the 10 years or more of hyperglycemia required for expression of complications of diabetes mellitus. Hyperkalemia is common in elderly diabetics with minimal renal dysfunction (serum creatinine concentration <2.5 mg/dl). This is usually attributed to the syndrome of "hyporeninemic hypoaldosteronism."[13] The difficulty in defining this syndrome in elderly patients has already been discussed (see section on hypoaldosteronism).

The prescription of carbohydrate-restricted diets for elderly type II diabetic subjects is rarely, if ever, indicated. Restriction of total caloric intake is indicated in overweight diabetic patients to effect weight loss and improve peripheral tissue sensitivity to insulin. However, liberalized carbohydrate intake on an isocaloric basis may be helpful in improving carbohydrate tolerance in patients with mild abnormalities of glucose metabolism.[5]

The long-term effects of normalizing the fasting and postprandial blood sugar concentrations in elderly diabetics have not been studied. We nonetheless recommend that in compliant diabetic patients up to 70 years of age, efforts be made to normalize blood glucose levels. By this we mean maintenance of fasting plasma glucose below 120 mg/dl and postprandial values below 140 mg/dl; the hemoglobin A_{1c} value should also be normal.[6] We believe this effort is indicated because of the expected survival of euglycemic (nondiabetic) subjects to age 80 to 85 years unless other substantive disease states are present. In compliant, intact patients with adequate home support, insulin therapy is introduced by us in subjects up to age 70 years.

The clinical safety of long-term use of oral sulfonylureas is not established, but the majority of elderly new-onset type II diabetic patients over 70 years of age receive oral agents, usually for reasons of convenience and the expressed preferences of the patients. In diabetic patients who are prone to hyponatremia (*e.g.*, patients on thiazide diuretic therapy or those with previously expressed hyponatremia in the setting of acute or chronic illness), an oral agent should be used that does not promote water intoxication. Sulfonylureas that do not promote water intoxication (and, in fact, increase free water clearance) include tolazamide and "second generation" sulfonylureas, such as glyburide and glipizide. It is particularly desirable in elderly diabetics to avoid hypoglycemia (and attendant myocardial or brain ischemia), and oral sulfonylurea therapy should be initially instituted at minimal dosage.

REFERENCES

1. Andres R: Aging and diabetes. Med Clin North Am 55:835–846, 1971
2. Arieff AI, Carroll HJ: Cerebral edema and depression of sensorium in nonketotic hyperosomolar coma. Diabetes 23:525–531, 1974
3. Baylin SB, Mendelsohn G: Ectopic (inappropriate) hormone production by tumors: Mechanisms involved and the biological and clinical implications. Endocrinol Rev 1:45–77, 1980
4. Berl T, Anderson RJ, McDonald KM, Schrier RW: Clinical disorders of water metabolism. Kidney Int 10:117–132, 1976
5. Brunzell JD, Lerner RL, Hazzard WR, Porte D, Jr, Bierman EL: Improved glucose tolerance with high carbohydrate feeding in mild diabetes. N Engl J Med 284:521–524, 1971
6. Bunn HF: Evaluation of glycosylated hemoglobin in diabetic patients. Diabetes 30:613–617, 1981

7. Burrow GN, Wortzman G, Rewcastle NB, Holgate RC, Kovacs K: Microadenomas of the pituitary and abnormal sellar tomograms in an unselected autopsy series. N Engl J Med 304:156–158, 1981
8. Christensson T, Hellstrom K, Wengle B, Alveryd A, Wikland B: Prevalence of hypercalcemia in a health screening in Stockholm. Acta Med Scand 200:131–137, 1976
9. Cooper DS, Goldminz D, Levin AA, Ladenson PW, Daniels GH, Militch ME, Ridgway EC: Agranulocytosis associated with antithyroid drugs. Effects of patient age and drug dose. Ann Intern Med 98:26–29, 1983
10. Davis FB, LaMantia RS, Spaulding SW, Wehmann RE, Davis PJ: Estimation of a physiologic replacement dose of levothyroxine in elderly patients with hypothyroidism. Arch Intern Med 144:1752–1754, 1984
11. Davis PJ, Davis FB: Hyperthyroidism in patients over the age of 60 years. Medicine 53:161–181, 1974
12. Davis PJ, Davis FB: Diagnosis of hyperparathyroidism. Otolaryngol Head Neck Surg 93:62–64, 1985
13. DeFronzo RA: Hyperkalemia and hyporeninemic hypoaldosteronism. Kidney Int 17:118–134, 1980
14. Deslypere JP, Vermeulen A: Leydig cell function in normal man: Effect of age, life style, residence, diet and activity. J Clin Endocrinol Metab 59:955–962, 1984
15. Fisher JN, Kitabchi AE: A randomized study of phosphate therapy in the treatment of diabetic ketoacidosis. J Clin Endocrinol Metab 57:177–180, 1983
16. Gherondache CN, Romanoff LP, Pincus G: Steroid hormones in aging men. In Gitman L (ed): Endocrines and Aging, p 76. Springfield, IL, Charles C Thomas, 1967
17. Greenblatt RB, Gambrell RD Jr, Stoddard LD: The protective role of progesterone in the prevention of endometrial cancer. Path Res Pract 174:297–318, 1982
18. Guisado R, Arieff AI: Neurologic manifestations of diabetic comas: Correlation with biochemical alterations in the brain. Metabolism 24:665–679, 1975
19. Hantman D, Rossier B, Zohlman R, Schrier R: Rapid correction of hyponatremia in the syndrome of inappropriate secretion of antidiuretic hormone. Ann Intern Med 78:870–875, 1973
20. Harman SM, Tsitouras PD: Reproductive hormones in aging men: I. Measurement of sex steroids, basal luteinizing hormone, and Leydig cell response to human chorionic gonadotropin. J Clin Endocrinol Metab 51:35–40, 1980
21. Ingbar SH, Woeber KA: The thyroid gland. In Williams RH (ed): Textbook of Endocrinology, p 187. Philadelphia, WB Saunders, 1981
22. Lee DBN, Zawada ET, Kleeman CR: The pathophysiology and clinical aspects of hypercalcemic disorders. West J Med 129:278–320, 1978
23. Legha SS, Powell K, Buzdar AU, Blumenschein GR: Tamoxifen-induced hypercalcemia in breast cancer. Cancer 47:2803–2806, 1981
24. Mazzaferri EL, O'Dorisio TM, LoBuglio AF: Treatment of hypercalcemia associated with malignancy. Semin Oncol 5:141–153, 1978
25. Melicow MM: One hundred cases of pheochromocytoma (107 tumors) at the Columbia-Presbyterian Medical Center, 1926–1976. Cancer 40:1987–2004, 1977
26. Mundy GR, Ibbotson KJ, D'Souza SM, Simpson EL, Jacobs JW, Martin TJ: The hypercalcemia of cancer: Clinical implications and pathogenic mechanisms. N Engl J Med 310:1718–1727, 1984
27. National Diabetes Data Group: Classification and diagnosis of diabetes mellitus and other categories of glucose intolerance. Diabetes 28:1039–1057, 1979
28. National Institutes of Health Consensus Development Conference: Estrogen use and postmenopausal women. Ann Intern Med 91:921–922, 1979
29. Nusynowitz ML, Frame B, Kolb FO: The spectrum of the hypoparathyroid states: A classification based on physiologic principles. Medicine 55:105–119, 1976
30. Olefsky JM, Kolterman OG: Mechanisms of insulin resistance in obesity and non-insulin-dependent (type II) diabetes. Am J Med 70:151–168, 1981
31. Prinz, RA, Brooks MH, Churchill R, Graner JL, Lawrence AM, Paloyan E, Sparagana M: Incidental adrenal masses detected by computed tomographic scanning. JAMA 248:701–704, 1982
32. Riggs BL, Seeman E, Hodgson SF, Taves DR, O'Fallon WM: Effect of the fluoride/calcium regimen on vertebral fracture occurrence in postmenopausal osteoporosis. N Engl J Med 306:446–450, 1982
33. Scholz DA, Purnell DC: Asymptomatic primary hyperparathyroidism: 10-year prospective study. Mayo Clin Proc 56:473–478, 1981
34. Scott HW Jr, Reynolds V, Green N, Page D, Oates JA, Robertson D, Roberts S: Clinical experience with malignant pheochromocytomas. Surg Gynecol Obstet 154:801–818, 1982
35. Snyder PJ, Utiger RD: Response to thyrotropin-releasing hormone (TRH) in normal man. J Clin Endocrinol Metab 34:380–385, 1972
36. Weidman P, DeMyttenaere-Burzstein S, Maxwell MH, deLima J: Effect of aging on plasma renin and aldosterone in normal man. Kidney Int 8:325–333, 1975
37. Xarli VP, Steele AA, Davis PJ, Buescher ES, Rios CN, Garcia-Bunuel R: Adrenal hemorrhage in the adult. Medicine 57:211–221, 1978
38. Zachmann M, Gizelmann RP, Zagalak M, Prader A: Effect of aminoglutethimide on urinary cortisol and cortisol metabolites in adolescents with Cushing's syndrome. Clin Endocrinol 7:63–71, 1977

26   Infectious Diseases

David W. Bentley

In order to provide detailed, practical information, this chapter is restricted to some major infections in elderly patients. These include two respiratory infections, influenza virus infections and bacterial pneumonia; urinary tract infections; infective endocarditis; and herpes zoster. For a more comprehensive approach, the reader is referred to two recent books on infectious diseases in the elderly.[2,4] Noted here are those age-related and chronic disease–related host factors that cause elderly patients to be more susceptible.[6] Some of these infections may be difficult to diagnose because the onset is insidious and vague or the clinical manifestations may be remote from the actual site of infection. Therefore, aspects of presentation, clinical and laboratory features, and diagnosis that pertain to elderly patients are also emphasized.

Treatment of each infection is discussed in detail; more comprehensive reviews of antibiotics in the elderly are available elsewhere.[1,3,5] Readers are advised to check the instructions for use noted in the package insert for each individual drug. When specific doses are stated, normal renal function is assumed. Renal insufficiency, however, occurs frequently in elderly patients despite minimal elevations in blood urea nitrogen or serum creatinine levels; appropriate dosage adjustments must be made for anti-infectives, especially aminoglycosides, that are excreted primarily by the kidney.

Lastly, preventive therapy, which is the method of choice in approaching the problems of infections in the aged,[7] is discussed, including the three most important vaccines for the elderly patient: (1) tetanus–diphtheria toxoid, (2) influenza vaccine, and (3) pneumococcal vaccine.

INFLUENZA VIRUS INFECTIONS

Influenza virus infections are one of the most important communicable diseases for older persons, especially those with chronic cardiac and respiratory conditions. Persons 65 years of age and older make up about 13% of the total population, and their rates of infection with influenza virus are relatively low, approximately 10%. However, they account for at least 50% of the hospitalizations and 75% to 80% of the deaths attributed to influenza.[23]

In the past several years, the predominant influenza viruses that affected all ages and circulated throughout the world were influenza A (H_3N_2) strains, closely related to A/Bankok/79, and influenza A viruses H_1N_1, including A/Brazil/78. These viruses circulated primarily in children and young adults, although a small outbreak was reported in elderly patients in a chronic disease hospital.[20] In 1979–1980, a new antigenic variant of influenza B virus (B/Singapore)[10] was epidemic in the United States and caused outbreaks in older persons in long-term care facilities[24] and in hospitals.[26]

Sufficient antigen variation or "drift" within the same subtype, such as A/Texas/77 (H_3N_2) and A/Bangkok/79 (H_3N_2), may occur over time so that infection or immunization with one strain may not induce immunity to distantly related strains. Major antigenic shifts, which herald pandemic influenza, produce "new" viruses to which the population has no immunity, such as the shift in 1957 from H_1N_1 to H_2N_2.

Pathogenesis

Pathogenesis in the elderly appears to be the same as in younger persons.[14] Infection is the result of transfer of virus-containing respiratory secretions via small particle ($< 10 \mu m$) aerosols from infected persons who are sneezing, coughing, or talking vigorously to a susceptible person. The earliest response to infection is the production of interferon, which is detectible in the respiratory secretions 1 to 2 days following onset of virus shedding. It reaches a maximum titer by 3 to 6 days and correlates well with the decrease in virus titers and clinical improvement. Secretory antibodies, predominantly IgA, in saliva, nasal secretions, sputum, and tracheal washings reach a peak titer 14 days after infection. Neutralizing, hemagglutination-inhibiting, and complement-fixing antibodies, primarily IgG antibodies, begin to develop in the serum by 14 days and reach peak titers by 4 to 6 weeks following infection.[14]

Presentation

Clinical Findings

The classic syndrome of uncomplicated influenza is similar in younger and older persons. After an incubation period of 1 to 2 days, there is an abrupt onset of systemic symptoms, including feverishness, chilliness or frank chills, headache, myalgias, and malaise.[21] These features last approximately 3 days and parallel the height of the fever, which ranges from 100°F to 104°F (37.8°C to 40°C). Local respiratory signs and symptoms (e.g., cough, nasal obstruction, and nonexudative pharyngitis) become predominant and may be present for several days after the patient is afebrile. Ocular symptoms, including photophobia, tearing, or pain on eye movement are helpful additional clues to distinguish milder cases from rhinovirus common colds.[14] In an outbreak, some elderly patients may have a milder illness indistinguishable from respiratory syncytial virus or influenza B virus infections.[21,26]

Laboratory Findings

During the first 24 to 36 hours of illness, the peripheral white blood cell count is usually slightly elevated (*e.g.,* 10,000 to 12,000/cu mm, with the differential predominantly polymorphonuclear leukocytes), changing within a few days to a normal white blood cell count with predominantly mononuclear cells. In patients with uncomplicated influenza or with bronchitis, the Gram stain of the sputum contains few inflammatory cells, and on chest roentgenography there is no infiltrate but there may be an increase in interstitial markings. The course may be complicated by pneumonia (see laboratory findings in the section on bacterial pneumonia).

Diagnosis

The diagnosis of influenza infection in the elderly is frequently made on clinical-epidemiologic grounds when a community outbreak is in progress. The specific methods of virus diagnosis, however, are often necessary to identify the etiologic agent in the first few cases. This is especially true in long-term care facilities when respiratory syncytial virus can cause concurrent outbreaks of a clinically similar illness.[21]

The virus can be readily isolated from throat swabs or sputum in the majority of specimens within 3 to 5 days of inoculation; final identification may require another week. A fourfold or greater rise (or fall) in complement-fixing antibody titers from acute and convalescent serum specimens obtained 10 to 20 days later is considered diagnostic. Rapid diagnosis using radioimmunoassay, enzyme-linked immunosorbent assay (ELISA), or immunofluorescent techniques are becoming more widely available. These studies provide an etiologic diagnosis within 24 hours of receipt and will allow more effective use of specific chemotherapy.[14]

Treatment

Treatment of influenza A infections include nonspecific symptomatic measures such as bed rest, adequate fluids, aspirin or other analgesics, and the use of nasal sprays or drops and cough syrups as required. Specific treatment consists of amantadine hydrochloride (Symmetrel), which was licensed in 1976 as an oral antiviral compound for respiratory illnesses caused by all strains of influenza A virus. Amantadine has no effect on influenza B viruses.[15] The exact mechanism of action is undefined, but it appears to inhibit an early stage in the virus replication cycle.[16]

In young persons amantadine is rapidly absorbed after ingestion and is not metabolized; 90% is excreted unchanged in the urine. The mean plasma half-life in young subjects is 12 to 17 hours with a wide range.[16] The plasma half-life increases in the elderly and in patients with impaired renal function.[18,22] Adverse reactions are dose-related minor gastrointestinal and central nervous system complaints that often resolve despite continued administration and are completely reversible after discontinuing the drug.[16] Subjective complaints include confusion, drowsiness, nervousness, insomnia, difficulty in concentration, and auditory or visual hallucinations. Objective findings include ataxia, slurred speech, and, rarely, convulsions. Anticholinergic side-effects such as dry mouth, visual disturbances, urinary retention, and constipation are occasionally seen. Adverse reactions occur in approximately 10%, are usually mild, and occur mainly during the first week of administration. Reactions are related to elevated plasma concentrations; toxicity may be more frequent in older persons because of mild to moderate renal dysfunction.

The appropriate dosage of amantadine in older persons is unknown. The usual dosage in young adults is 200 mg initially and 100 mg twice daily thereafter; recent studies indicate that 100 mg/day is as effective as 100 mg twice daily in the treatment of uncomplicated influenza A infections.[28] The duration of treatment is for 3 to 5 days. Young adults demonstrate a decreased shedding of virus and a 50% reduction in the duration of fever and respiratory signs and symptoms versus placebo.[26] Amantadine demonstrates a similar advantage when compared with aspirin.[28] In addition, amantadine prevents progression of pulmonary function abnormalities and accelerates their resolution.[19] Observations in older persons consist of a single study with similar results.[27] No controlled studies have documented that amantadine prevents pneumonic complications of influenza or is useful in patients with established pulmonary complications.[16]

Guidelines for the treatment in this high-risk population, when influenza A viral infections have been documented in the community or strongly suspected, include the following[17]

Use for febrile influenzalike illness, which began less than 48 hours ago, in an elderly person with high-risk or moderate-risk conditions (see section on immunization).
Use for life-threatening suspected primary influenzal pneumonia.
Use dosage of 100 mg to 200 mg/day for 3 to 5 days.
Reduce dosage according to package insert if estimated creatinine clearance is less than 40/ml/min.

Course

The course of uncomplicated influenza infections in the elderly may be prolonged, with dry cough, lassitude, and malaise persisting for 2 to 4 weeks. Pulmonary and nonpulmonary complications of influenza are common in older persons. Pulmonary complications include primarily tracheobronchitis, acute exacerbations of chronic bronchitis, and secondary bacterial pneumonia. These occur with an overall rate of 35% to 75% for persons

over 60 and over 70 years of age, respectively.[15] Primary influenza pneumonia appears to be rare in older persons.

The signs and symptoms of bronchitis are similar to those in younger persons with persistent irritating productive cough with moderate to profuse mucopurulent sputum that is occasionally bloodstreaked. Complications occur generally in the 5th through 10th day of the illness, often following signs of improvement. Recommendations for treatment of postinfluenza bronchitis are the same as the regimens noted in the chapter on pulmonary disease. Empiric treatment of postinfluenza bacterial pneumonia is frequently necessary because of the rapidly progressive and severe nature of the illness; antibiotic regimens appropriate for the most frequent potential pathogens, *Streptococcus pneumoniae, Hemophilus influenzae,* and *Staphylococcus aureus,* are recommended (see section on bacterial pneumonia). Nonpulmonary complications consist primarily of congestive heart failure.

Influenza virus infections cause epidemics of excess hospitalizations and death nearly every year. High-risk conditions include chronic disorders of the cardiovascular or pulmonary systems, chronic metabolic diseases (including diabetes mellitus), renal dysfunction, anemia, immunosuppression, and asthma that are severe enough for patients to have required regular medical follow-ups or hospitalization during the preceding year.[10] Excess hospitalization rates during influenza A epidemics for those individuals 65 years of age and older rise from 150 to 172 per 100,000 population without underlying high-risk conditions to 476 to 636 per 100,000 population with underlying high-risk conditions.[9] In this group mortality rises from 9 per 100,000 with no high-risk conditions to 217 per 100,000 with one high-risk condition to 306 per 100,000 with two or more high-risk conditions. The highest estimated rates are among persons with underlying cardiovascular disease in combination with either diabetes or chronic pulmonary disease.[8]

Chemoprophylaxis

Amantadine, although licensed and effective for the prevention of upper respiratory tract illnesses caused by all strains of influenza A virus, is greatly underused. Numerous studies, primarily in younger persons, indicate that amantadine will prevent about one half of influenza A infections and about two thirds of the illnesses.[11,12,14] The prophylactic effectiveness of amantadine is, therefore, equivalent to the vaccine, can be demonstrated against all subtypes of influenza A virus studied, is not affected by antigenic variations in the type A viruses (unlike the vaccines), and is additive to that of the vaccine. Rimantadine hydrochloride, a structural analogue of amantadine, is associated with a lower frequency of side-effects, especially those of the central nervous system,[13] probably because it is primarily metabolized by the liver. Rimantadine administered prophylactically to institutionalized elderly is as well tolerated as placebo and substantially reduces the incidence of clinical influenza.[14]

In outbreaks of influenza A infection in the community, amantadine (or rimantadine when it is licensed) is recommended in the dose of 100 mg twice daily (or 100 mg/day) for older persons in the following circumstances[10]:

As an adjunct to late immunization of high-risk persons. Because the development of a protective antibody response to vaccination requires approximately 2 weeks, the drug should be used during this interim. There is no interference with the antibody response.

As an adjunct to the vaccination program during a nursing home outbreak. The drug should be given early in the outbreak in an effort to reduce the spread of infection and provide an additional margin of protection for the high-risk patients. The duration of prophylaxis should be for 2 to 4 weeks until the outbreak has subsided.

To supplement protection afforded by vaccination. Because the overall vaccine efficacy may be as low as 65%, amantadine may provide an additional margin of protection for high-risk patients in communities or institutionalized in nursing homes during a community epidemic. The duration of prophylaxis should be for 6 to 12 weeks.

As the only prophylactic measure. This would be an unusual prophylactic use for the few high-risk patients for whom influenza vaccine is contraindicated because of an anaphylactoid hypersensitivity to egg protein or previous severe reactions associated with influenza vaccines (*e.g.,* Guillain-Barré syndrome). The duration of prophylaxis should be for the duration of the expected influenza season or approximately 12 weeks.

BACTERIAL PNEUMONIA

Epidemiology

Bacterial pneumonia is probably the most important infection of older persons because it occurs frequently and with increased morbidity and mortality. The incidence of community-acquired bacterial pneumonia in older persons is 20 to 40 per 1000 per year, depending on the characteristics of the population.[39,46] The rates of institution-acquired pneumonia may be as high as 70 to 115 per 1000 per year for older persons so disabled that they must reside in a nursing home or other long-term care facility.[31] The incidence of a hospital-acquired bacterial pneumonia is 8.6 per 1000 admissions per year; the rate for persons over 65 years of age is two times higher than for persons 18 to 50 years of age.[40] Pneumonia (and influenza) is the fourth leading cause of death in the United States population 65 years of age and over, accounting for 184.8 deaths per 100,000 persons.[34] Mortality rates range from 10% to 40% for pneumonias due to organisms causing minimal lung destruction (*e.g., Streptococcus pneumoniae*[41] to as high as 80% for pneumonias due to *Staphylococcus aureus* or gram-negative bacilli that frequently cause necrosis of the lung.[50]

Pathogenesis

The reasons for the high incidence and high mortality are unclear. Bacterial pneumonia in older persons often follows oropharyngeal colonization with respiratory pathogens, aspiration of these pathogens or normal flora alone, and impaired clearance of these bacteria-laden oropharyngeal secretions by the lung. Possible predisposing age-associated factors include increased oropharyngeal colonization rates by gram-negative bacilli and *Staphylococcus aureus*, increased silent aspiration, decreased effective cough and mucociliary transport mechanisms, possible intrinsic defects in alveolar macrophages and polymorphonuclear leukocytes, and an unknown role of impaired T-cell function. In addition, several disease- or condition-associated factors that predispose to pneumonia are more frequent or affect the elderly more severely, such as chronic bronchitis, congestive heart failure, cerebrovascular accidents, and dementia.[30]

Presentation

Clinical Findings

Pneumonia in older persons usually presents as an insidious or nonspecific deterioration in general health or activities. Confusion, or a change in interest in one's surroundings, is a very common early sign. The confusion is frequently sudden in onset and not correlated with the degree of hypoxia. An unexplained fall is often part of the antecedent history as it is for other serious diseases. Pneumonia may present as a sudden deterioration or a slowed recovery from an existing primary disease. Two frequent settings are a relapse in congestive heart failure despite apparently adequate treatment or a deterioration and/or extension of a previously stable cerebrovascular accident. Fever may be minimal or absent in up to 25% of older persons.[29,38] The sudden onset of rigors, characteristic of pneumococcal pneumonia in younger persons, occurs in only 10% of the elderly with bacteremic pneumococcal pneumonia.[37]

The findings on physical examination are also frequently nonspecific and confusing. Signs of consolidation (*e.g.,* bronchial breath sounds, egophony, and whispered pectoriloquy) are seldom present; although recent studies suggest no age-associated differences in the prevalence of these findings.[37] Rales (especially basilar) are often present in many healthy older persons because of increased airway closure even at normal tidal volumes.[33] Dullness to percussion is always present, but this is nonspecific and does not distinguish between pneumonia and atelectasis. An early clue to the diagnosis may be an elevated respiratory rate (*i.e.,* greater than 26 breaths/min, which may antedate the clinical diagnosis by 24 hours.[44]

Laboratory Findings

There are no specific laboratory findings in older persons with pneumonia. Peripheral blood leukocytosis, a white blood cell count of greater than 10,000/cu mm, is present in approximately 80% of community-acquired and institution-acquired pneumonias and may be an important early clue in the elderly.[29] In cases without leukocytosis, bands and other early forms of the granulocyte series (*i.e.,* a left shift) are often present. Hypoxemia, as documented by peripheral arterial blood gases, is the rule because of the increased regional hypoventilation and inequality of the ventilation–perfusion ratio, which adds to the baseline hypoxia noted in healthy older persons.[49] Elevated blood urea nitrogen and serum creatinine values, reflecting prerenal changes secondary to dehydration are frequently noted.

Roentgenographic Findings

Because of these difficulties, the chest roentgenogram must be obtained whenever pneumonia is suspected in the elderly patient with certain roentgenographic findings unique to this high-risk population. *Incomplete consolidation* is the usual pattern noted in older persons with pneumonia, including patients with bacteremic pneumococcal pneumonia, the prototype for lobar pneumonia.[53] The predominance of incomplete consolidation is probably due to small areas of emphysematous foci scattered throughout the aging lung.[33] A practical implication of this finding may be a delay in appropriate treatment for pneumonias that the physician usually associates with complete consolidation (*e.g.,* those due to *Streptococcus pneumoniae* and *Klebsiella pneumoniae*).

Delay in resolution may occur despite appropriate treatment. Clearing, even of infiltrates due to pneumococcal pneumonia, may require as long as 14 weeks in older patients versus 6 to 8 weeks in those under 50 years of age.[43] Delay in resolution may be further prolonged if alcoholism or chronic obstructive airway disease is present. Important consequences of delayed resolution include prolonged fever and leukocytosis, which may lead to inappropriate changes to more toxic antibiotics. Furthermore, if this delay is not appreciated in older persons it may lead to unnecessary readmissions to rule out bronchial obstruction, lung cancer, and so on.

Other diseases that occur frequently in older persons may be difficult to distinguish roentgenographically from bacterial pneumonia. These disorders include atelectasis, congestive heart failure, pulmonary emboli, and/or infarction, and lung cancer.

Diagnosis

Respiratory Secretions

The etiologic agent(s) causing bacterial pneumonia in the elderly is usually identified by collecting respiratory secretions from the lower respiratory tract. Sputum, the most frequently obtained specimen, is rarely satisfactory because older patients with pneumonia are often dehydrated and have an ineffective cough. This frequently results in specimens composed entirely or primarily of oropharyngeal secretions that are often heavily contaminated with respiratory pathogens. The same holds for nasopharyngeal aspirates.[47,51]

The role of respiratory bacterial pathogens isolated from cultures of sputum or nasopharyngeal aspirates can be assessed by direct microscopy of Gram-stained respiratory secretions to identify the numbers and proportions of squamous epithelial cells and white blood cells per low-power field or $100\times$ magnification (Table 26-1). Respiratory pathogens classified as probable or possible may be considered the putative etiologic agent(s). The role of the pathogen(s) from cultures with more than 25 squamous epithelial cells per $100\times$ magnification, regardless of the number of white blood cells, is unknown. These specimens should not be submitted for culture because they contain an unacceptable amount of oropharyngeal contamination.

Transtracheal, or more accurately infralaryngeal, aspiration (TTA) is an invasive procedure that requires puncture of the cricothyroid membrane. Studies indicate that TTA is a safe and useful procedure in the management of bacterial pneumonia in severely ill elderly patients.[32] If there are no contraindications, and if a skilled and experienced operator is available, a TTA should be performed for an elderly patient with a life-threatening pneumonia that responds poorly to antibiotics selected on the basis of the Gram stain and/or culture of a sputum or NPA or when the possibility of superinfection exists. The role of TTA in managing life-threatening pneumonia prior to starting antibiotics requires more careful study.

Other Specimens

Two blood cultures should be collected prior to treatment, especially if the patient is severely ill and the sputum or nasopharyngeal aspirate demonstrates gram-positive cocci on Gram stain or is not acceptable for culture or not diagnostic or if a TTA cannot or will not be performed. All pleural effusions should be aspirated or drained, immediately examined by Gram stain, and cultured aerobically and anaerobically. Respiratory pathogen(s) isolated from the blood, pleural fluid, or TTA (except from patients with chronic bronchitis) may be considered definite etiologic agent(s). Examining the urine by counterimmunoelectrophoresis or latex agglutination to detect capsular antigen from *Streptococcus pneumoniae* or type B *Hemophilus influenzae* may be very helpful in identifying these etiologic agents, especially when the patient is admitted to the hospital after antibiotics have been started.

Acute and convalescent serology for unusual pathogens should be obtained in patients with an atypical pneumonia syndrome or pneumonia that fails to respond to antibiotic treatment. These studies should include tests for *Legionella pneumophilia*, *Chlamydia trachomatis* and *C. psittaci*, *Coxiella burnetii*, and common respiratory viral agents, including influenza virus and respiratory syncytial virus.

Etiologic Agents

The etiology of bacterial pneumonias in the elderly is poorly understood because of the difficulty in obtaining reliable specimens from the lower respiratory tract for Gram stain interpretation and subsequent culture results and the low yield from blood cultures and other specimens. In addition, as a result of aspiration of oropharyngeal secretions and presumed decreased clearance at the alveolar surfaces, a substantial portion of pneumonias in the elderly are caused by mixed flora (*e.g.*, two or more respiratory pathogens, oropharyngeal commensals, or both). Finally, bacterial pneumonia occurs in several different settings (*e.g.*, community, institution [nursing home or other

TABLE 26-1 Classification of Bacterial Agents Isolated from Sputum of Nasopharyngeal Aspirate based on Gram Stain Findings

| | No. Cells/Low-Power Field ($\times 100$) | |
Classification	Squamous Epithelial Cells	White Blood Cells
Putative		
Probable	<10	>25
Possible	10–25	>25
Unknown	>25	>25

(Adapted from Murray PR, Washington JA II: Microscopic and bacteriologic analysis of expectorated sputum. Mayo Clin Proc 50:339, 1975)

**TABLE 26-2   Estimated Prevalence (%) of Etiologic Agents
Causing Bacterial Pneumonia in the Elderly According to Setting**

	Setting		
Agent	*Community Acquired*	*Institution Acquired*	*Hospital Acquired*
Streptococcus pneumoniae	55	35	20
Hemophilus influenzae and other *Hemophilus* species	10	5	5
Staphylococcus aureus	1	1	5
Gram-negative bacilli	5	15	35
Mixed flora*	25	40	30
Other†	4	4	5

*Two or more respiratory pathogens, normal oropharyngeal commensals, or both
†Other = *Legionella pneumophilia*, anaerobes, fungi, unknown
(Data from Bentley DW, Mamot K et al: Pneumococcal vaccine in the institutionalized
elderly: Design of a nonrandomized trial and preliminary results. Rev Infect Dis 3:S71, 1981;
Ebright JR, Rytel MW: Bacterial pneumonia in the elderly. J Am Geriatr Soc 28:220, 1978; and
Verghese A, Berk SL: Bacterial pneumonia in the elderly. Medicine 62:271, 1983)

long-term care facility] or hospital). It is likely that each setting plus associated host conditions predispose to different etiologic agents.[31,36,52] The estimated prevalence of etiologic agents causing pneumonia in the elderly in these settings is presented in Table 26-2.

The syndrome of atypical pneumonia is characterized by constitutional symptoms (*e.g.*, headache, myalgia, diarrhea, and so on, which are more frequent than the specific respiratory findings); a physical examination that initially demonstrates few, if any, signs of consolidation; pulmonary involvement on the roentgenogram that is more extensive than suspected; and sputum that is frequently mucoid or mucopurulent. *Mycoplasma pneumoniae* is the most frequent cause of this syndrome in young persons but rarely affects persons over 50 years of age; *Legionella pneumophilia* is the most frequent cause in the elderly. Additional pathogens that may be associated with this syndrome are noted in the section on diagnosis.

Treatment

When a reliable interpretation of the Gram stain can be made, the choice of therapy depends on the pathogen(s) suspected, regardless of whether the bacterial pneumonia is community acquired, institution acquired, or hospital acquired. Recommendations for treatment of bacterial pneumonia in the elderly, when initial therapy can be guided by Gram stain, have been discussed[29,42] and are similar to guidelines in textbooks of medicine.

The choice of initial therapy frequently cannot be based on the interpretation of the Gram stain because no predominant organism can be identified. In this case, the antibiotic regimen now must be selected empirically based on clinical and epidemiologic characteristics of similar patients. These characteristics include certain host features and the setting in which the pneumonia occurs. Recommendations for treating suspected bacterial pneumonias acquired in these settings are summarized in Table 26-3.[29,48]

Approximately 80% of community-acquired pneumonias are caused by *Streptococcus pneumoniae* and mixed flora; the latter pneumonias, in general, respond the same as if *S. pneumoniae* had been identified on Gram stain. The drugs recommended assume that the patient is hospitalized and that parenteral therapy is warranted. Patients with pneumonias and minimal signs of toxicity can be managed as outpatients with oral antibiotics; suitable choices in this setting are amoxicillin and erythromycin. The increasing frequency of gram-negative bacillary pneumonias in community-residing older persons and the associated increase in mortality rate, warrants appropriate empiric treatment for life-threatening situations. Future studies may demonstrate the efficacy of the less toxic regimen of third-generation cephalosporins alone in this setting in which a *Pseudomonas* pneumonia is uncommon. Chloramphenicol is an alternative drug for patients with a history of anaphylactic reaction or interstitial nephritis from either a penicillin or a cephalosporin and is the drug of choice when infection with *Hemophilus influenzae* is sus-

TABLE 26-3 Recommended Empiric Antibiotic Regimens for Suspected Bacterial Pneumonia in the Elderly

Setting	Usual Pathogen(s)	Antibiotic Therapy*	
		Not Life-Threatening	*Life-Threatening*
Community	*Streptococcus pneumoniae,* mixed flora, *Hemophilus influenzae,* gram-negative bacilli	Penicillin G or ampicillin, (first- or second-generation cephalosporin), or (clindamycin)	(Third generation cephalosporin) or (chloramphenicol) plus aminoglycoside
Institution	Mixed flora, *Streptococcus pneumoniae,* gram-negative bacilli	As per community setting	Third- or fourth-generation penicillin or (third-generation cephalosporin) or (trimethoprim-sulfamethoxazole) plus aminoglycoside
Hospital			
Not immunocompromised	Gram-negative bacilli, *Straphylococcus aureus, Streptococcus pneumoniae,* mixed flora	(Third generation cephalosporin) plus aminoglycoside	Maximum doses
Immunocompromised	As above plus *Legionella pneumophilia*	Maximum doses: (third generation cephalosporin) plus aminoglycoside plus erythromycin	Same: maximum doses plus trimethoprim-sulfamethoxazole

*The antibiotic regimen(s) listed first are the drug(s) of choice. The first antibiotic regimen listed within the parentheses is an alternate choice for penicillin-allergic patients with a history of a delayed hypersensitivity–type reaction. The second antibiotic regimen listed within the parentheses is an alternate choice for patients with a history of anaphylactic reaction or interstitial nephritis from either penicillin or cephalosporin.

(Data from Bentley DW: Bacterial pneumonia in the elderly: Clinical features, diagnosis, etiology, and treatment. Gerontology 30:297, 1984, and Rozas CJ, Goldman AL: Responses to bacterial pneumonia. Geriatrics 37:61, 1982)

pected in a patient with a life-threatening pneumonia.

Occasionally, empiric antibiotic regimens should be modified for specific pathogens that are frequently associated with a particular syndrome. The syndromes primarily affect older persons residing in the community and include those associated with diseases or conditions that increase the risk of oropharyngeal colonization with certain respiratory pathogens or predispose to aspiration. These syndromes and the usual pathogens associated are previous upper respiratory tract infection: *Streptococcus pneumoniae, Hemophilus influenzae,* and *Staphylococcus aureus;* chronic bronchitis or a history of heavy cigarette smoking: *Streptococcus pneumoniae, Hemophilus influenzae,* and *Legionella pneumophilia;* alcoholism: *Streptococcus pneumoniae, Klebsiella pneumoniae, Staphylococcus aureus,* and *Hemophilus influenzae;* aspiration: anaerobes and mixed flora; and atypical pneumonia: *Legionella pneumophilia.* Antibiotic regimens for

these suspected respiratory pathogens are discussed elsewhere and are not unique for the elderly.[35]

The initial choice of antibiotics for institution-acquired pneumonia should be the least toxic regimen that is effective against pneumonias caused by aspiration of bacteria-laden oropharyngeal secretions. In the absence of prior antibiotics, the most frequent etiologic agents are mixed flora and *Streptococcus pneumoniae.* The antibiotics in these circumstances are the same as those recommended for non-life-threatening community-acquired pneumonias. In life-threatening situations, or in moderately to severely ill patients, the regimen should be directed against aerobic gram-negative bacilli, especially if the patient was receiving antibiotics or was exposed to them in the previous 4 weeks. Although *Klebsiella pneumoniae* is the usual respiratory pathogen involved, other bacilli, including *Pseudomonas aeruginosa,* may cause gram-negative bacillary pneumonias in the institutionalized elderly. For this reason, the regimen selected initially should include a third- or fourth-generation penicillin or a third-generation cephalosporin with good anti-*Pseudomonas* activity plus an aminoglycoside. Depending on the penicillin-allergy history, a third-generation cephalosporin or an investigational intravenous use of trimethoprim-sulfamethoxazole, (TMP-SMX) are suitable alternative drugs, although the latter is not effective against *Pseudomonas aeruginosa*.

The initial choice of antibiotics for hospital-acquired pneumonia must include coverage for aerobic gram-negative bacilli and *Staphylococcus aureus* plus *Streptococcus pneumoniae*. An appropriate regimen for the nonimmunocompromised patient, such as the older person in the intensive care unit with cardiac or respiratory failure or postoperation, is a third-generation cephalosporin plus an aminoglycoside. In a life-threatening situation, maximum doses of each drug are required. In immunocompromised patients, with hospital- or acquired community-acquired pneumonia, the initial choice of antibiotics should include maximum doses of the same regimen plus erythromycin to include coverage for *Legionella pneumophilia*. In life-threatening situations, high intravenous doses of TMP-SMX should be added, especially if a diffuse interstitial pattern is present on chest roentgenogram, to include coverage for *Pneumocystis carinii*.

General supportive measures include adequate oxygen and hydration, antipyretics for patients with persistently high temperature and limited cardiac reserve, and nutrition supplements. Although chest physiotherapy does not decrease the duration of pneumonia, fever, or hospital stay or the mortality rate in younger patients with uncomplicated pneumonia, it should probably be instituted routinely in elderly patients.

Course

Within 48 to 72 hours of starting the antibiotic regimen, additional laboratory and clinical information will become available. Treatment should be directed at any respiratory pathogen(s) isolated from the blood, pleural fluid, or TTA or evidence of *Streptococcus pneumoniae* or *Hemophilus influenzae* capsular antigen in the urine. When possible, drug regimens should be adjusted specifically for the pathogen involved. If broad-spectrum coverage was started with antibiotics active for staphylococci and gram-negative bacilli and if the patient improves dramatically by 48 to 72 hours of treatment, it is unlikely that the pneumonia was due to these organisms. Simpler low-dose and less ex-

pensive regimens, such as those used for pneumococcal pneumonia or aspiration pneumonia, should be considered.

The optimum duration of treatment of bacterial pneumonia in the elderly is unknown. In general, patients with pneumonias that are not life threatening are treated through 3 to 5 days of baseline conditions or for a minimum of 7 to 10 days, whichever is shorter. For pneumonias of unknown etiology complicated by necrosis, treatment should be for a minimum of 14 days.

Prevention

Specific measures to prevent bacterial pneumonia in older persons include influenza and pneumococcal vaccines. Appropriate measures to decontaminate respiratory treatment equipment and control delivery of respiratory care are important. Nonspecific preventive measures have not been adequately studied to see if they can help reduce the incidence of pneumonia in this high-risk population. These measures probably depend on increased attention to positioning, feeding, suctioning, and so on, to reduce the risk of aspiration in elderly patients who have had recent thoracoabdominal surgical operations, depressed levels of consciousness, dysphagia due to neurologic or esophageal disorders, and nasogastric tubes in place.

URINARY TRACT INFECTIONS

Epidemiology

The urinary tract is the most frequent site of bacterial infection in older persons. The prevalence of bacteriuria increases with age, level of care, and decreasing functional capacity (Table 26-4). The vast majority of urinary tract infections (UTIs) in the elderly are asymptomatic, but much controversy exists regarding the natural history of the bacteriuria. In women, the rate of loss may be as high as 70% but the overall prevalence remains elevated as new persons become bacteriuric.[82] Bacteriuria tends to persist in men, especially in chronic disease hospitals.[77] Some reports demonstrate an increased association of renal dysfunction and hypertension with bacteriuria,[73,74] whereas others do not.[54,77] Some reports indicate a higher mortality in older persons with bacteriuria,[61,82] whereas others do not.[77] All agree that bacteriuria, especially in association with obstructive uropathies and instrumentation, can be a serious problem for older persons. Approximately 55% of com-

TABLE 26-4 Estimated Prevalence (%) of Bacteriuria According to Age and Level of Care

Age	Women	Men
<65 Home	5	<1
65–79	20	10
Over 80	40	20
Over 65		
Nursing home	25	20
Acute hospital	30	30
Chronic disease hospital	40	35

(Modified from Kaye D:Urinary tract infections in the elderly. Bull NY Acad Med 56:209, 1980)

munity-acquired and nosocomial gram-negative bacteremias occur in persons over 65 years of age, and UTIs, with or without genitourinary manipulation, are the source for 33% of these cases.[68]

Pathogenesis

The reasons for these high rates for UTIs are unknown, but several factors may be responsible. In men, they include increased residual urine and obstructive uropathy with subsequent instrumentation and surgery, chronic prostatitis caused by age-associated prostatic microcalculi, and possible alterations in normal bactericidal characteristics of the prostatic secretions. In women, they include residual urine secondary to loss of pelvic support; contamination of the perineum, which is increased with fecal incontinence; and possible loss of local bladder mucosal defense mechanisms secondary to decreased local antibody and/or epithelialization of portions of the bladder mucosa associated with menopause.[57a,67]

Presentation

Clinical Features

The clinical features of UTIs in older persons differ from those in younger persons in several ways. Symptomatic lower UTIs, (*e.g.*, cystitis) may present as urinary frequency, nocturia, urgency, and dysuria, features that are difficult to interpret because they occur in older persons in the absence of infection as the result of underlying bladder abnormalities, especially neurogenic bladder dysfunction.[54,59] Confusion and incontinence are presenting features of UTIs more frequently noted in older persons, but both are confounded by other variables and are not significantly associated.[60]

Symptomatic upper UTIs (*e.g.*, acute pyelonephritis) are rare in older persons in the absence of major upper or lower tract outflow obstruction and/or instrumentation. Fever and flank pain, cardinal features of this syndrome, may be absent. Signs and symptoms, especially gasatrointestinal, respiratory, or nonspecific signs of toxicity, frequently direct attention away from the urinary tract. Features more frequent in older persons include a markedly confused state and rapidly increasing blood urea nitrogen value, which is usually associated with severe dyhydration.[63]

Acute bacterial prostatitis is a diffuse inflammatory process that may present as fever, chills, back pain, and symptoms of UTI, including urgency and dysuria. The prostate is warm, swollen, and tender on examination per rectum. Chronic bacterial prostatitis, however, is a focal nonacute inflammatory process and is the most common cause of recurring UTI in older men. It is very difficult to diagnose because there may be few or no symptoms related to the infection. The main clinical clues are perineal pain, low back pain, and difficulty in urinating. Fever is low grade, unless a septic local process (*e.g.*, pyelonephritis) or a contagious process (*e.g.*, vertebral osteomyelitis) is present. Symptoms of UTI may appear periodically.[75]

Laboratory Features

Pyuria, the presence of at least 5 to 10 white blood cells per high-power field of a resuspended centrifuged urine, is absent in 35% to 80% of older persons with significant bacteriuria (*i.e.*, urine with bacterial counts of greater than 10^5/ml).[67] The lack of correlation between pyuria and bacteriuria is due to the increased frequency in the elderly of bladder colonization and asymptomatic UTIs. In the majority of symptomatic UTIs, pyuria is usually present and serves as a helpful screening test. Other causes of pyuria in older persons include vaginitis, severe hypertension, renal ischemia, tuberculosis and regular consumption of analgesics.[72] Proteinuria or albuminuria is poorly correlated with UTIs except in end-stage renal disease.[70] Leukocytosis, however, is not as helpful and may be absent in 33% of older persons with acute bacteremic pyelonephritis.[63]

Diagnosis

Although a single midstream urine specimen with more than 10^5 bacteria/ml has an 80% probability of identifying infection in younger persons, the same specimen in an elderly woman will identify "true" bacteriuria with a 45% to 80% probability, depending on the degree of compliance and mental and physical disabilities.[76] Thus contamination of midstream specimens is a major problem for elderly women, and a second confirmatory specimen is necessary. Obtaining a valid sample of urine to document bacteriuria poses no special problems in elderly men.[65]

When it is important to diagnose the etiologic agent without delay, a single catheterization with the smallest catheter available and careful technique should be employed, especially in frail or bedridden elderly women. In urine thus collected, true bacteriuria is usually identified by counts greater than or equal to 10^5/ml, although counts as low as 10^3 to 10^4/ml may signify true bacteriuria.

When acute pyelonephritis is suspected, two blood cultures over a 30- to 60-minute period should be obtained. The multiple blood cultures are necessary because the bacteremia associated with pyelonephritis is not persistent. A positive blood culture for the same pathogen noted in the urine identifies the urinary tract as the site of infection in a febrile elderly patient. Bacteriuria is so frequent in older persons that it alone cannot be accepted as sufficient evidence for acute pyelonephritis.[64]

In acute bacterial prostatitis, prostatic secretions can be expressed to demonstrate polymorphonuclear leukocytes and the infecting organism on Gram stain, but this may precipitate bacteremia and should be discouraged. Because acute cystitis frequently accompanies acute prostatitis, the causative agent can generally be identified by culturing the midstream urine specimen. In chronic bacterial prostatitis, pyuria is frequently absent and polymorphonuclear leukocytes in expressed prostatic secretions are not helpful. Diagnosis can be made only by quantitative localization techniques, which evaluate concomitant cultures of urethral urine, midstream urine, prostatic secretions expressed by massage or by ejaculation, and urine voided after massage. These studies must be performed at a time when bacteriuria is absent.[75]

For short-term use of indwelling urethral catheters (IDUCs), the criteria for bacteriuria have not yet been defined but generally range from 10^3 to 10^5 bacteria/ml.[78] For long-term or chronic use of IDUCs (*i.e.,* catheters in place more than 30 days), the bacterial counts are usually more than 10^5/ml. Cultures obtained by aspirating the catheter yield additional organisms and in higher counts than the bladder bacteriuria.[83] In both settings, pyuria may be absent.

The frequent practice in institutions of attaching a sterile condom catheter collecting system to obtain urine for culture in men has not been evaluated as a culture technique. If used, the collection bag must be monitored at 15-minute intervals and the specimen must be cultured within 90 minutes of collection or held in the refrigerator for a maximum of 48 hours prior to plating. This collection system has also been identified as an increased risk for new UTIs, especially when used for long-term drainage in the uncooperative patient.[66]

A number of diagnostic tests are used to differentiate between lower and upper track infections because patients with the latter require long-term antibiotic treatment and follow-up in hopes of preventing renal damage. These tests, which are generally helpful in younger persons, probably will be less useful in older persons. The bladder washout (Fairley) test is not reliable in patients with neurogenic bladders.[69] A false-positive antibody-coated bacteria test can be seen when infection is confined to the bladder or surrounding structures (*e.g.,* vaginitis, prostatitis, or severe cases of cystitis with bladder calculi). In addition, both false-negative and false-positive tests occur frequently in patients with neurogenic bladders.[80] The single-dose antibiotic test, which will eradicate uncomplicated cystitis in more than 90% of young women, has not been studied in elderly women but will probably be less satisfactory because of the frequent finding of residual urine secondary to decreased pelvic support and neurogenic bladder. This test is not appropriate for elderly men who rarely have uncomplicated cystitis and frequently have chronic prostatitis.[77]

The frequently benign course of asymptomatic bacteriuria in the elderly argues against vigorous urologic workups, including intravenous pyelograms. The genitourinary tract should be evaluated in all men with UTIs, including initial asymptomatic UTIs, and in elderly women with two or more symptomatic relapses of bacteriuria during a 12-month period or with signs suggesting renal infection. The workup should include an intravenous pyelogram with post-voiding films of the bladder to identify any neurologic dysfunction, structural anomalies, or calculi. Elderly patients who are at increased risk for radiocontrast-induced renal failure (*e.g.,* patients with diabetes mellitus or preexisting renal failure) should not be dehydrated or receive high doses of contrast material. Nucleotide scans and sonography may be especially helpful in ruling out anatomical abnormalities and detecting calculi in these patients.

Urinary retention should be considered in any elderly patient with a UTI, especially if the infection is symptomatic. Causes include fecal impaction, prostatic hypertrophy, atonic neuropathic bladder, and the use of certain drugs, especially antidepressants, antiparkinsonism drugs, and anticholinergics.

Etiologic Agents

The etiologic agents causing UTIs in the elderly depend on the setting and associated factors, including disease, disability, and other conditions such as antibiotic usage and the presence of indwelling bladder catheters (IDUCs) (Table 26-5). In community populations of women, *Escherichia coli* accounts for up to 75% of UTIs, whereas the predominant uropathogens in men are polymicrobial infections such as those caused by *Klebsiella* species and *Staphylococcus epidermidis* and *S. saprophyticus*.[77,82] Similar polymicrobial infections are frequently present in institutionalized residents and patients exposed to multiple courses of antibiotics or who have chronic IDUCs.[81] In addition, anaerobic bacteria (*e.g.,* anaerobic streptococci, *Bacteroides* species, *Clostridium* species) may be present.[55,83]

In hospitalized elderly patients *Escherichia coli, Pseudomonas aeruginosa,* and enterococcus are frequently noted because of an increased length of stay, frequent instrumentation and use of short-term IDUCs, and more exposure to antibiotics.[81]

Multiple-resistant bacteria are often noted in institutionalized and hospitalized older persons with UTIs because of repeated courses of antibiotics, frequent use of IDUCs, and prolonged rectal carriage of multiple-resistant strains.[56,81]

In acute bacterial prostatitis, aerobic gram-negative bacilli and enterococci are the most frequent etiologic agents and are usually isolated from midstream urine cultures in counts of greater than or equal to 10^5 bacteria/ml. In chronic bacterial prostatitis, *Escherichia coli* is the most frequent pathogen, but *Proteus* species, enterococcus, and other gram-negative bacilli may be present.[75]

Treatment

Asymptomatic Bacteriuria

Although controversial, aggressive treatment of asymptomatic bacteriuria in elderly women is probably not warranted because most persons are reinfected with different organisms within 2 weeks or more of stopping the initial treatment and there is no convincing evidence that asymptomatic chronically bacteriuric older women who have no obstructive uropathy are at risk for progressive renal impairment or hypertension. In addition, a large number of patients who would require multiple courses of antibiotics would face an increased number and severity of adverse reactions.

TABLE 26-5 Estimated Prevalence (%) of Etiologic Agents Causing UTIs in the Elderly According to the Setting

	Setting		
Agent	*Community Acquired*	*Institution Acquired*	*Hospital Acquired*
Escherichia coli	21–72*	20–38	34
Klebsiella species	24–5	6–28	10
Proteus species	12–17	29–18	11
Pseudomonas aeruginosa	7–0	13–8	31
Other gram-negative bacilli	4–3	12–8	0
Enterococci	9–3	10–0	14
Other gram-positive organisms	23–0	8–0	0
Polymicrobial	30–10	30–30	NI+

*Hyphenated percentages indicate prevalence for men-women.
+NI = no information.
(Data from Aktar AJ, Andrews GR, Caird FL et al: Urinary tract infection in the elderly: A population study. Age Ageing 1:48, 1972; Cape RDT, Ehtisham M, Zirk MH: Management of bacteriuria in the elderly female: Urinary tract infection. Proceedings of the 2nd National Symposium, March 1972. Oxford, Oxford University Press, 1973; Platt R: Quantitative definition of bacteriuria. Am J Med 75:44, 1983; Sherman FT, Tucci V, Libow LS et al: Nosocomial urinary tract infections in a skilled nursing facility. J Am Geriatr Soc 28:456, 1980; and Wolfson SA, Kalmanson GM, Rubini ME et al: Epidemiology of bacteriuria in a predominantly geriatric male population. Am J Med Sci 250:168, 1965)

TABLE 26-6 Recommendations for Treatment of Urinary Tract Infections in the Elderly

Severity of Illness	Setting	Antibiotic Regimens	Duration
Asymptomatic, uncomplicated	Community, institution, hospital	Avoid in the absence of obstructive uropathy	
Uncomplicated cystitis	Community	Sulfonamides, amoxicillin, first-generation cephalosporin, trimethoprim-sulfamethoxazole	7 days
	Institution or hospital	Oral carbenicillin, third-generation cephalosporin, aminoglycosides	7–10 days
Suspected pyelonephritis, septicemia, complicated UTIs	Community, institution, hospital	Ampicillin plus aminoglycosides followed by oral antibiotics as above	14 days
Chronic relapses or reinfection	Community, institution, hospital	As per uncomplicated cystitis, trimethoprim-sulfamethoxazole, nitrofurantoin, urinary antiseptics	6 weeks to 6 months
Bacterial prostatitis			
Acute	Community, institution, hospital	As per uncomplicated cystitis	14 days
Chronic	Community, institution, hospital	Trimethoprim-sulfamethoxazole, carbenicillin, fourth-generation penicillins	6 weeks to 6 months
Indwelling urethral catheter (IDUC) associated	Community, institution, hospital	Avoid unless septicemic	2–10 days of baseline condition

(Data from Gleckman R, Blagg N, Hibert D et al: Community-acquired bacteremic urosepsis in the elderly patients: A prospective study of 34 consecutive episodes. J Urol 128:79, 1982; Kaye D: Urinary tract infections in the elderly. Bull NY Acad Med 56:209, 1980; and Sherman FT, Tucci V, Libow LS et al: Nosocomial urinary tract infections in a skilled nursing facility. J Am Geriatr Soc 28:456, 1980)

Asymptomatic bacteriuria in elderly men is usually associated with obstructive uropathy, calculi, or chronic prostatitis. If the former is identified, intensive therapeutic efforts are warranted in an effort to prevent renal damage. If chronic prostatitis can be diagnosed, or cannot be ruled out, continued medical treatment of symptomatic episodes is warranted.

Symptomatic Bacteriuria

Initial symptomatic UTIs should be treated in young and old persons but usually it will be necessary to begin treatment before the culture and sensitivity results are available. The antibiotic regimen selected depends on the severity of the infection, the patient's location, and any prior history of instrumentation or treatment. Recommendations for specific antibiotics for initial empiric therapy for community-, institution-, and hospital-acquired UTIs in the elderly have been discussed and are summarized in Table 26-6.[63,67,81]

Uncomplicated community-acquired infections can be treated effectively with oral agents that provide adequate antibacterial levels in the urine. If the patient has no IDUC and is in a long-term care facility or hospital where antibiotic-resistant *Escherichia coli*, *Klebsiella* species, *Proteus* species, and *Pseudomonas aeruginosa* are prevalent, it may be best to wait for the identification and sensitivity results. If symptoms are severe and this delay is not appropriate, treatment should be started with an antibiotic effective against *Pseudomonas aeruginosa* for the reasons that follow. When sensitivity results are available, the most appropriate antibiotic (i.e., the least toxic and the least expensive drug) should be selected and adequate doses given for 7 to 10 days. Management of less severe UTIs in the elderly with urinary antiseptics (e.g., methenamine mandalate, hippuric acid, oxalinic acid) plus an initial course of antibiotics may be more successful than antibiotics alone.[58] The results of single-dose regimens in this high-risk group to date are not encouraging.[71,77]

Pyelonephritis, Septicemia, or Complicated UTIs

Suspected pyelonephritis or septicemia in the elderly (*e.g.*, rigors, high fever, shock) generally occurs in patients with complicated UTIs with obstructive uropathies or recent instrumentation. Older persons in the community should be hospitalized because they develop bacteremia and septic shock more frequently than younger persons.[63] Regardless of the setting (*e.g.*, community, institution, or hospital), initial empiric antibiotic treatment should be with a parenteral broad-spectrum antibiotic regimen with bactericidal activity for *Pseudomonas aeruginosa* because, unlike in younger persons, *Escherichia coli* accounts for less than or equal to 50% of UTIs in the elderly, even for community-acquired episodes; the Gram stain assessment of the urine cannot distinguish between members of the Enterobacteriaceae family (*e.g.*, *Proteus* species, *Klebsiella* species, and *Pseudomonas aeruginosa*; and *P. aeruginosa* must be considered with the predisposing conditions frequently present.[64]

The regimen most frequently recommended is an aminoglycoside effective against *Pseudomonas* plus parenteral ampicillin.[79] This is appropriate for UTIs due to gram-negative bacilli and enterococci; vancomycin should be substituted for ampicillin in the penicillin-allergic patient when the Gram stain of the urine suggests enterococcal or staphylococcal UTI. Newer wide-spectrum antibiotic agents (*e.g.*, the third-generation cephalosporins or the fourth-generation penicillins) may be as effective when used as single agents in the initial treatment of complicated UTI.[62,79]

After 2 to 3 days of the initial regimen, if an appropriate antibiotic has been selected, there will be no bacteria noted on the Gram stain or in the urine sediment and the culture will be negative. This evaluation is imperative if the patient is not responding clinically or, as is the usual case with older persons, there is a question of resistant organisms or the UTI is complicated by mechanical or neurologic obstruction. If no bacteriuria is detected and the patient is afebrile for at least 2 days, the initial parenterally administered antibiotic can be discontinued; then the most appropriate orally administered antibiotic is selected based on sensitivity results and continued for a total of 14 days. If no bacteriuria is present but the patient remains clinically ill, an urgent workup with nuclide scans or sonography is required to assess the likely site of obstruction.

Chronic Recurrent Bacteriuria

If the patient relapses with the same pathogen within 2 weeks of discontinuing an appropriate antibiotic, a predisposing condition is usually present (*e.g.*, renal involvement, a structural or neurologic abnormality of the urinary tract, or chronic bacterial prostatitis.[67] Urologic evaluation and, if an abnormality is found, corrective action should be considered. Older patients with relapse in the absence of structural abnormalities or patients with obstructive uropathies that cannot be corrected should be treated for 6 weeks with the same agents as recommended for the initial treatment course. If relapse occurs despite a 6-week course of treatment, more prolonged treatment for approximately 6 months or chronic suppressive therapy should be considered. The preferred oral antibiotics in this setting are TMP-SMX and urinary antiseptics.[79]

Reinfection is the recurrence of symptoms with a new organism(s). It is usually associated with bladder bacteriuria without renal infection and is caused by the entry of new organisms into the bladder from the fecal-perineal reservoir. Each reinfection is managed as noted for symptomatic infection; asymptomatic infection should not be treated. Prolonged prophylaxis with TMP-SMX or urinary antiseptics should be considered in elderly patients who are symptomatically incapacitated or asymptomatic but with the likelihood of renal damage secondary to concomitant obstructive uropathy.[67,79]

Bacterial Prostatitis

In acute bacterial prostatitis many antibiotics diffuse well into the acutely inflamed prostate. Therefore, appropriate systemic antibiotics, similar to the oral agents recommended in the treatment of symptomatic UTIs, are recommended and will provide adequate blood levels. During the acute stages, urethral manipulation and indwelling catheters are contraindicated. Chronic bacterial prostatitis is very difficult to cure because few antimicrobials penetrate adequately into the noninflamed prostate. TMP-SMX is presently the most effective therapy, but only approximately one third of cases can be cured. If failure occurs either the acute exacerbations of UTI are treated or chronic suppressive treatment with low-dose

TMP-SMX is attempted. If enterococcus is present, oral administration of erythromycin is the treatment of choice. If *Pseudomonas aeruginosa* is present, carbenicillin is given via the oral route; prior parenteral injection of ticarcillin or a fourth-generation penicillin may prove helpful in some cases.[75]

UTIs Associated with IDUCs

Acute symptomatic UTIs associated with short-term or long-term catheter use require prompt attention to avoid serious consequences, especially gram-negative bacteremia. Recent instrumentation, manipulation, and obstruction of the catheter are the usual predisposing events. For the latter, percussion of the bladder is performed to detect retained urine and search for leakage around the catheter, which would indicate catheter dysfunction. If either is noted, the catheter is removed promptly and a new one carefully reinserted to promote effective drainage. If there is no evidence of obstruction, the catheter can be removed after the first dose of the selected antibiotic .

If a recent urine culture is available (*i.e.,* within 2 weeks of the event) an appropriate antibiotic can be chosen. If no culture is available, or was obtained more than 2 weeks previously, or a septicemic syndrome is present, an aminoglycoside effective against *Pseudomonas aeruginosa* plus ampicillin is selected. The antibiotic regimen should not be continued for the usual 14 days because the infection cannot be eliminated as long as the IDUC is in place and resistant organisms will rapidly emerge. Instead, treatment is continued for 2 days after the patient's vital signs have returned to baseline values. If bacteremia is documented, the regimen should be continued for 7 to 10 days.

Repeated symptomatic episodes, especially in the absence of catheter obstruction, suggests the presence of infected bladder or renal calculi and warrants further investigation. Asymptomatic reinfection should be expected and should not be treated. There is no value in monitoring urine cultures at 1-month intervals to allow a better selection of antibiotic regimens because of rapid changes of uropathogens.[57] Asymptomatic bacteriuria associated with short-term catheterization past 10 to 12 days is difficult to prevent and UTIs associated with chronic IDUCs are impossible to prevent. Daily care of the urethral catheter junction with soap and water and careful positioning of the urine collection bag are helpful measures. Neither systemic antibiotics nor antibacterial rinses of the bladder or the collecting system are effective in reducing the presence or risk of the associated bacteriuria.

INFECTIVE ENDOCARDITIS

Infective endocarditis is the current term to denote infection of the endocardial surface of the heart (*e.g.,* natural valves, mural thrombi) and is preferable to the term *bacterial endocarditis*. Prosthetic valvular endocarditis (PVE) is a syndrome that occurs following infection of artificial or homograft valves at cardiac surgery. There is little information on how this syndrome is unique for older persons, and this section will include information only on treatment and prevention of PVE.

Epidemiology

Infective endocarditis has become a disease of the elderly. In the preantibiotic periods the mean age of patients with this disorder was 31; less than 5% were 60 years of age and older.[89] At the present time, the mean age is approximately 55 and 55% of patients are 60 years of age and older.[105,120] The increased number of cases in the elderly appears to be due to an absolute increase in the number of cases of infective endocarditis and a shift in the percentage of cases in older persons.[103] This changing prevalence is due to a number of factors, including an increased percentage of elderly in the general population, increased survival of the very old, an unexplained decline in new cases of and increased survival of patients with rheumatic heart disease, and an increased frequency of older persons with hospital-acquired bacteremia secondary to multiple and prolonged procedures and operations.[97] The male to female ratio is approximately 2:1 to 5:1, depending on the location and etiologies noted.[111]

Pathogenesis

The pathogenesis of infective endocarditis is best understood from information obtained in experimental studies.[96] Any structural alteration of endothelial surfaces apparently leads to deposition of aggregates of platelets and fibrin to form a nidus of vegetation termed *nonbacterial thrombotic endocarditis* (NBTE). The vegetations tend to localize where blood turbulence is generated by jetty from high pressure sources to low pressure sites. Transient bacteremia as from multiple minor and major insults allows bacteria to colonize the NBTE. Factors enhancing bacterial adherence provide an advantage to certain organisms (*e.g.*, streptococci and staphlycocci) for local attachment.[114] The fibrin mesh tends to shield the bacteria from phagocytic white blood cells and allows multiplication, invasion, and subsequent valvular damage. Age influences on these pathophysiologic and pathogenic factors have not been defined.[90]

Previous studies noted that 40% to 50% of elderly patients with infective endocarditis had no valvular disease or undetermined heart disease.[87] Multiple cardiac abnormalities, however, are present in the elderly that cause irregularities in the endothelial surface, including mitral ring degeneration, aortic cusp disease without stenosis, calcified congenital bicuspid valve, and degenerative calcified aortic stenotic changes.[107] Atherosclerotic disease, previously considered a rare predisposing factor, is now thought to be an important cause of atheromatous deposits that can cause turbulent flow and thrombus formation.[120] Mural thrombi secondary to myocardial infarction are probably a more frequent site for turbulence in older persons.[111]

The portals of entry or sources of transient bacteremia in the elderly are unknown in 28% to 63% of cases. Known sources include oral-dental conditions, including edentulousness (5% to 14%), genitourinary instrumentation (5% to 17%), skin, including decubitus ulcer (0 to 17%), intravenous catheters (0 to 18%), and status post surgery with wound infection (0 to 17%).[87,112] Gastrointestinal lesions, especially cancer of the colon, are the usual source for *Streptococcus bovis* endocarditis, which occurs primarily in the elderly.[104,106] Diagnostic and other therapeutic procedures, noted in the prevention section, are also becoming an increasingly important source of bacteremia for the elderly.

Presentation

The pathologic findings in patients with infective endocarditis are the same regardless of age.[94] The site of the disorder in the elderly is equally distributed among the major valves: mitral valve alone (25% to 35%), aortic valve alone (20% to 30%), and both valves (25%).[111]

Gastrointestinal lesions, especially cancer of the colon, are the usual source for *Streptococcus bovis* endocarditis, which occurs primarily in the elderly.[104,106] Diagnostic and other therapeutic procedures, noted in the prevention section, are also becoming an increasingly important source of bacteremia for the elderly.

The pathologic findings in patients with infec-

tive endocarditis are the same regardless of age.[94] The site of the disorder in the elderly is equally distributed among the major valves: mitral valve alone (25% to 35%), aortic valve alone (20% to 30%), and both valves (25%).[111]

Clinical Findings

Several studies have emphasized the atypical noninfectious disease and nonspecific features of infective endocarditis in the elderly.[87,93,98,103,111,112,116] The onset is frequently insidious, and clues that might suggest the diagnosis are frequently overlooked, ignored, or attributed to "old age" or other concurrent or suspected diseases frequently present in the elderly. Some of the presenting features and possible misdiagnoses are listed in Table 26-7.[111] Furthermore, it may be exceedingly difficult to date the onset of infective endocarditis because approximately 40% of older persons with viridans streptococcal endocarditis have had symptoms for more than 8 weeks.[115]

The classic clinical syndrome of infective endocarditis with fever, changing murmurs, splenomegaly, mucocutaneous petechiae, and embolic manifestations is seldom noted in older persons, although the individual findings frequently occur (Table 26-8).

Fever may be absent in as many as 25% of cases. Conditions that predispose to afebrileness include prior treatment with antibiotics or antipruritics, congestive heart failure, and azotemia. Afebrile bacteremia in older persons with other types of infections has been noted.[99] If temperatures are taken rectally four times a day during the first week of evaluation, however, fever will be documented in nearly 100% of elderly patients with infective endocarditis. The fever is usually low grade and, unfortunately, is frequently assigned to a suspected respiratory or genitourinary infection.[111]

Absence of heart murmurs has been reported in approximately 15% of elderly patients with this disorder, although this may be fictitiously high. Systolic murmurs occur frequently, are considered "benign" despite evidence to the contrary, and are often overlooked in older persons.[103] Congestive heart failure is more frequently noted in elderly patients than in a series representing the general population with infective endocarditis.[97] The failure is related to valve destruction, cardiac arrhythmias, or heart block frequently associated with myocardial abscesses.

TABLE 26-7   Presenting Features of Infective Endocarditis in the Elderly and Possible Misdiagnoses

Signs or Symptoms	Misdiagnoses
Nonspecific	"Old age"
Weight loss	Carcinoma
Anorexia	
Fatigue	
Depression	
Anemia	
Neurologic	Arteriosclerotic cerebrovascular disease
Aphasia	
Hemiplegia	
Confusion	
Delirium	
Psychosis	
Transient ischemic attacks	
Headache	Brain tumor
Cardiac	Arteriosclerotic cardiovascular disease
Congestive heart failure, ar-rhythmias, and heart block	
Musculoskeletal backache	"Old age"
	Degenerative spine disease
Renal	
Uremia	Arteriosclerotic renal-vascular disease
Hematuria	Genitourinary neoplasm
Pyelonephritis	Urinary tract infection

(Adapted from Ries K: Endocarditis in the elderly. In Kaye D (ed): Infective Endocarditis. Baltimore, University Park Press, 1976)

Neurologic signs and symptoms occur in approximately 25% of cases. These findings, in addition to those noted in Table 26-7, include toxic encephalopathies, cranial nerve paralysis, and a large number of neuropsychiatric disorders ranging from impaired consciousness to severe neurosis and psychosis.[111]

Cutaneous signs (*e.g.*, petechiae, splinter hemorrhages, Osler's nodes and Janeway's lesions) occur in elderly patients with infective endocarditis in a similar frequency (40%) as noted in the general population with the disease.[97] Splenomegaly occurs in approximately 25% of elderly patients but may be as high as 40% in more indolent chronic forms (*e.g.*, viridans streptococcal endocarditis).[115]

Laboratory Findings

Several laboratory findings are frequently noted in infective endocarditis (Table 26-9). The prevalence of these findings, however, is similar in both elderly patients and younger patients and has limited value because they may be normal or negative when the disease is present. The erythrocyte sed-imentation rate (ESR) rises normally with age and may be as high as 30 mm to 40mm/hr in healthy aged individuals.[102] A positive latex agglutination test for rheumatoid factor is present in approxi-

TABLE 26-8   Clinical Findings of Infective Endocarditis in the Elderly

Findings	Frequency (range [mean])
Fever	50–100 (74%)
Murmurs	78–93 (87%)
Congestive heart failure	11–64 (30%)
Neurologic signs	8–36 (23%)
Cutaneous signs	20–58 (40%)
Splenomegaly	16–43 (26%)

(Data from Anderson HJ, Staffurth JS: Subacute bacterial endocarditis in the elderly. Lancet 2:1055, 1955; Applefeld MM, Hornick RB: Infective endocarditis in patients over 60. Am Heart J 88:90, 1974; Cummings V, Furman S, Dunst M et al: Subacute bacterial endocarditis in the older age group. JAMA 172:137, 1960; and Robbins N, DeMaria A, Miller MH: Infective endocarditis in the elderly. South Med J 73:1335, 1980)

TABLE 26-9 Laboratory Findings of Infective Endocarditis in the Elderly

Findings	Frequency (range [mean])
Elevated erythrocyte sedimentation rate	89–100 (94%)
Hematocrit <35%	40–86 (64%)
White blood cell count ≤12,000/cu mm	15–62 (58%)
Positive latex agglutination test	31 (31%)
Hematuria	24–27 (25%)

(Data from Anderson HJ, Staffurth JS: Subacute bacterial endocarditis in the elderly. Lancet 2:1055, 1955; Applefeld MM, Hornick RB: Infective endocarditis in patients over 60. Am Heart J 88:90, 1974; Hebte-Gabr E, January LE, Smith IM: Bacterial endocarditis: The need for early diagnosis. Geriatrics 28:164, 1973; and Robbins N, DeMaria A, Miller MH: Infective endocarditis in the elderly. South Med J 73:1335, 1980)

mately 40% to 50% of all patients with infective endocarditis, especially when the duration is more than 6 weeks. This test is frequently positive in normal older persons but usually at a titer of less than 1:80. The concentration of serum C3 complement component is reduced in approximately one half of the patients with infective endocarditis, especially those with renal involvement.[121] Microscopic hematuria is noted in approximately 25% of elderly patients with the disease; additional findings of associated renal disease include proteinuria, pyuria casts, elevated blood urea nitrogen and serum creatinine values, and the clinical features of pyelonephritis or uremia.[93]

Diagnosis

Strict case definitions for diagnosing infective endocarditis have been defined[117]:

1. Definite case: histologic or microbiologic evidence of valvular infection
2. Probable case when one of the following conditions exist:
   a. Persistently positive blood cultures in a patient with a new regurgitant murmur or a predisposing heart lesion and peripheral manifestations of infective endocarditis
   b. Negative or intermittent positive cultures in a patient with fever, new regurgitant murmur, and peripheral manifestations of infective endocarditis

Unfortunately, the clinical features of the disease in elderly patients, at least initially, are often vague and nonspecific; new regurgitant murmurs are infrequently noted; and peripheral manifestations do not occur in 40% or more of patients. The majority of elderly patients, however, have fever and murmurs. If the rule of obtaining blood cultures in all patients with fever and murmurs is faithfully followed, the diagnosis will be made in a majority of elderly patients with infective endocarditis.[111]

Because the bacteremia associated with this intracardiac focus is usually continuous, it is not necessary to wait for the presence of fever or rigors. The first two blood cultures will yield the etiologic agent in more than 90% of the cases. However, if antibiotic treatment occurred in the previous 2 to 4 weeks, the rate of positive blood cultures can be as low as 65%.[108] Therefore, three venipunctures for three separate blood culture sets should be obtained over a 24-hour period; additional blood cultures will be necessary if the patient previously received antibiotics. Details concerning the workup and interpretation of the blood cultures have been summarized elsewhere.[118]

Other studies ancillary to blood cultures may be helpful in elderly patients who have received prior antibiotics or have culture-negative infective endocarditis. In the absence of renal failure, congestive heart failure, or intravascular coagulation, a normal ESR (<40 mm/hr, Wintrobe method) is against the diagnosis.[113] Circulating immune complexes, with levels less than 100 μg of aggregated human γ-globulin equivalent per milliliter, are specific for infective endocarditis but are noted in only 35% of cases.[88] The sensitivity of detecting vegetations by myocardial imaging with gallium 67 and other radiolabeled compounds needs improvement, but these techniques may be potentially useful diagnostic tools.[123] Two-dimensional echocardiography has variable sensitivity (from <50% to >90%) for detecting vegetations and is, therefore, useless in excluding infective endocarditis. It is valuable, however, in evaluating the need for surgical intervention by assessing local complications of the disease, especially around the aortic valve, and by identifying vegetations that can give rise to systemic embolization.[109]

Etiologic Agents

The blood culture results from two retrospective series of infective endocarditis in elderly patients that used appropriate case definitions are summarized in Table 26-10.[87,112] Viridans streptococci ac-

TABLE 26-10 Etiologic Agents of Infective Endocarditis in the Elderly

Agent	% of Cases
Streptococci	41–57
Viridans streptococci	24–34
Enterococci	10–16
Other	7
Staphylococci	24–36
Coagulase-positive	21
Coagulase-negative	3–5
Gram-negative aerobic bacilli	2–3
Fungi	0–5
Miscellaneous bacteria	0–3
Mixed infection	0
"Culture negative"	0–9

(Data from Applefeld MM, Hornick RB: Infective endocarditis in patients over 60. Am Heart J 88:90, 1974, and Robbins N, DeMaria A, Miller MN: Infective endocarditis in the elderly. South Med J 73:1335, 1980)

count for approximately 70% of cases in persons under 35 years of age but only 40% of cases in persons over 55 years of age.[90] This decrease in prevalence is partly due to fewer predisposing events (*e.g.,* dental manipulations and edentulousness) but also to an increase in the prevalence of other streptococci, especially enterococci and *S. bovis*. Group D streptococci are commensals in the gastrointestinal and genitourinary tact. Enterococci (*S. faecalis*) can account for as high as 25% of infective endocarditis cases occurring in persons over 70 years of age.[92] *S. bovis,* a nonenterococcal group D streptococcus, is the cause of infective endocarditis in less than 5% of young adults but accounts for as high as 25% of cases in persons over 55 years of age.[91]

Staphylococcus aureus (coagulase positive) causes approximately 20% of infective endocarditis. The clinical syndrome usually has an abrupt onset, a fulminating course, and a mortality rate as high as 85%.[119] In 15% of elderly patients, the diagnosis is made *post mortem*. *S. epidermidis* (coagulase negative) accounts for less than 5% of infective endocarditis but is the most frequent cause of PVE.[122]

"Culture-negative" endocarditis occurs in 10% to 20% of elderly patients with a clinical syndrome compatible with infective endocarditis. The usual cause is prior antibiotic therapy, which may be prescribed more commonly to older patients for bacterial pneumonia or other intercurrent infections, especially genitourinary tract.[111] Other causes are a chronic course of more than 3

months, especially if uremia intervenes; mural endocarditis associated with postmyocardial infarction thrombus or pacemaker wires; subacute right-sided process; slow growth of fastidious bacterium, and an obligate intracellular parasite (*e.g.,* rickettsiae).[113] Avoidance of indiscriminate use of antibiotics, attention to proper collection of blood cultures, and newer diagnostic techniques may reduce the frequency of "culture-negative" cases.

Treatment

General Principles

The pathology of infected vegetations determines the unique response to antibiotic treatment of infective endocarditis. Despite often exquisite sensitivity of the organism, complete eradication takes weeks and relapses are frequent. The high counts (*e.g.,* 10^8 to 10^{10} colony forming units per gram) of relatively inert bacteria and the ineffective phagocytosis by white blood cells demands the following general principles of treatment[113]:

Use high doses of parental drugs for prolonged treatment courses.

Determine the etiologic agent's minimum inhibitory concentration (MIC) and minimum bactericidal concentration (MBC) for the usual antibiotics selected.

Select a regimen based on bactericidal activity and predictable toxicity; avoid bacteriostatic drugs.

Know that combination therapy should demonstrate synergistic killing as tested by standard techniques.

Obtain blood cultures early in the course of treatment to ensure eradication of bacteria.

Monitor serum bactericidal titers periodically; peak titers of more than 1:8, although not well correlated with therapeutic success, are reasonable guidelines.

Specific Regimens

The current recommended antibiotic regimens for the treatment of elderly patients with infective endocarditis are summarized in Table 26-11.[113] The choice of penicillin alone for "penicillin-sensitive" streptococci (*e.g.,* *S. viridans* or *S. bovis*) avoids the risk of streptomycin-induced irreversible ototoxicity, which frequently occurs with the combination of penicillin and streptomycin (0.5 g IM q12H for first 2 weeks). This combination should be used, however, in elderly patients with a compli-

TABLE 26-11   Antibiotic Treatment for Elderly Patients with Infective Endocarditis

Organism	Regimen*	Duration of Therapy (wk)	Regimen in Penicillin-allergic Patients
Susceptible streptococci (MIC < 0.2 µg/ml penicillin G) (*e.g.*, viridans strepto-cocci, *S. bovis*)	Aqueous penicillin G 2 Mu IV q4h	4	Cephalothin, 2.0 g IV q4h or Vancomycin, 0.5 g IV q4h
Resistant streptococci (MIC ≥ 0.2 µg/ml penicillin G) (*e.g.*, enterococcus)	Aqueous penicillin G, 2 Mu IV q4h plus Gentamicin, 1.7 mg/kg IV q8h	4–6	Vancomycin, 0.5 g IV q4h
Staphylococcus aureus (MIC ≥ 0.2 µg/ml)	Oxacillin or nafcillin, 2.0 g IV q4h	6	Vancomycin, 0.5 g IV q4h
Methicillin-resistant *S. aureus*	Vancomycin, 0.5 g IV q4h	6	Same
Staphylococcus epidermidis (MIC ≥ 12µg/ml)	Vancomycin, 0.5 g IV q4h plus Rifampin, 300 mg po q12h	6	Same
Empiric regimen, bacteria not yet identified	Aqueous penicillin G, 3.5 Mu IV q4h plus Gentamicin, 1.7 mg/kg IV q8h	4–6	Vancomycin, 0.5 g IV q4h

*All doses are for patients with normal renal function.
(Data from Scheld WM, Sande MA: Endocarditis and intravascular infections. In Mandell GL, Douglas RG Jr, Bennett JE [eds]: Principles and Practice of Infectious Diseases, p 504. New York, John Wiley & Sons, 1985)

cated course, in those with a history of disease of more than 3 months' duration, or when PVE is due to susceptible strains.

Successful treatment of "penicillin-resistant" streptococcal endocarditis (*e.g.*, enterococcus) requires an aminoglycoside in combination with the penicillin to achieve a synergistic bactericidal effect. Gentamicin is the preferred aminoglycoside because it is effective against "high-level" streptomycin-resistant strains (MIC >2000 µg/ml) noted in 20% to 50% of enterococcal strains and it avoids irreversible ototoxicity due to streptomycin. Reversible gentamicin-associated nephrotoxicity, defined as a twofold increase in the serum creatinine, occurs regularly with this regime, however, and careful monitoring of serum levels for toxicity and avoidance of intravenously administered diuretics are recommended. In elderly penicillin-allergic patients, careful monitoring of serum at the vancomycin levels is required to avoid ototoxicity.

For fulminant cases of staphylococcal endocarditis due to *Staphylococcus aureus*, the initial recommended regimen is oxacillin or nafcillin plus gentamicin (1.7 mg/kg IV q8h) for the first 3 to 5 days. Methicillin-resistant *S. aureus* strains require vancomycin alone. *S. epidermidis* causes less

than 5% of cases of infective endocarditis but approximately 30% of cases of early and late PVE. These strains are usually resistant to methicillin and require a combination of vancomycin and rifampin. The remaining causes of PVE are several different pathogens; the management of these infections and the indications for surgical treatment for valve replacement have been summarized elsewhere.[100]

Empiric therapy should be started if infective endocarditis is suspected in an elderly patient with clinical evidence of extreme toxicity, shock due to sepsis, rapidly progressive heart failure, new regurgitant murmur, or evidence of embolization to a major organ (*e.g.*, brain, lung, kidneys).[90] The regimen for suspected natural valve infection, including cases of culture-negative endocarditis, should be adequate for the entercoccus. If blood cultures are negative, treatment is continued for 6 weeks; if clinical improvement is noted in the first week, some recommend discontinuing the aminoglyocoside after 2 weeks.[113] In patients with suspected PVE, the treatment regimen should include vancomycin and gentamicin (1.0 mg/kg IV q8h). The drug regimen is appropriately adjusted following recovery of the etiologic agent and appropriate susceptibility test.

Course

One measure of a satisfactory response to treatment in an elderly patient is improved feeling of well-being and evidence of improved mental state, appetite, and weight. An elevated temperature may take 10 to 14 days or longer to return to normal despite effective treatment.[94]

Complications of infective endocarditis occur more commonly in elderly patients. These complications can involve the heart (*e.g.*, perforation of the valve leaflet, myocardial abscess, myocardial infarction); systemic emboli; infarction or glomerulonephritis of the kidney; mycotic aneurysms; central nervous system (*e.g.*, emboli infarction or abscesses); and infarction or abscesses of the spleen.

Mortality rates remain high (30% to 60%) for elderly patients with infective endocarditis despite effective antibiotics, although the rates may be as low as 0% in patients with viridans streptococcal endocarditis.[115] Factors that increase the mortality rates include unsuspected or delayed diagnosis, severe disease unrelated to endocarditis, severe cardiovascular or neurologic complications, resistant organisms, and age 70 years or older. The major causes of death are congestive heart failure, annular or myocardial abscesses, heart block, coronary emboli, or neurologic complications.[94]

Prevention

Most authorities recommend prophylaxis during certain procedures associated with transient bacteremia and a substantial risk of endocarditis.[95] Underlying cardiac conditions frequently noted in elderly patients include *high risk*: prosthetic heart valves, atrial and mitral valve disease, mitral stenosis or insufficiency, and previous infective endocarditis; *intermediate risk*: mitral valve prolapse, calcific degenerative changes; *lower negligible risks*: atherosclerotic plaques, coronary artery disease, and cardiac pacemakers.

The procedures associated with bacteremia and a risk for developing infective endocarditis on natural heart valves include *high-risk procedures*: dental and oral surgical procedures that cause gingival bleeding, urologic and gynecologic operations and procedures especially in the presence of urinary or pelvic infection, drainage of abscesses or operations on affected soft tissues, and open heart surgery, and *lower negligible risk*: dilatation and curettage in the absence of pelvic infection, diagnostic cardiac catheterizations, insertions of pacemakers and coronary artery surgery, and other diagnostic

procedures (*e.g.*, endoscopy of upper and lower gastrointestinal tract, barium enema, liver biopsy, bronchoscopy). Current recommendations are that elderly patients with natural valves and high- and intermediate-risk cardiac conditions should receive prophylaxis prior to all high-risk procedures. Patients with prosthetic heart valves should receive prophylaxis for either high- or low-risk procedures.[95]

Widely known and respected recommendations for antibiotic prophylaxis of infective endocarditis are rather lengthy, complex, and often ignored.[85,110] Simplified regimens are being developed in an attempt to improve compliance. An example of these recommendations is noted in Table 26-12. These regimens are empiric suggestions for patients with normal renal function and are not meant to cover all clinical situations. Practitioners should use their own judgment on safety and cost-effective issues in each individual case.[95]

HERPES ZOSTER

Herpes zoster is the second most important viral infection afflicting older persons because it occurs frequently in older persons and with substantial morbidity. The epidemiologic, immunologic, virologic, biochemical, and biophysical evidence to date confirms that the virus causing varicella and zoster is the same.[129]

Epidemiology

Unlike varicella, which usually occurs in young children, zoster is seen in all ages, but especially in the elderly. The overall incidence is 3.4 per 1000 per year in a busy medical practice, rising to approximately 6.5 per 1000 per year in persons 60 to 79 years of age and approximately 10 per 1000 per year in persons 80 years of age and older.[137] The overall frequency of zoster in this same population is 5.4% and reaches a high of 16.2% in persons 80 years of age and older. In the general population, the incidence is closer to 1.3 per 1000 per year.[146] Zoster affects males and females equally, has no racial predilection, and, unlike varicella, has no seasonal variation.

The varicella-zoster virus is very labile so that inanimate objects play a minor role in transmission. It is shed from the site of the localized eruption for up to 8 days,[125] but the infection is considerably less contagious. Chickenpox can be acquired by susceptible individuals after exposure to zoster, although not as frequently as after ex-

TABLE 26-12 Recommendations for Prophylaxis of Endocarditis in the Elderly

Standard Regime	For dental procedures and oral or upper respiratory tract surgery	Penicillin V, 2.0 g orally 1 hr before, then 1.0 g 6 hr later
Special Regimens	Parenteral regimen for high-risk patients; also for gastrointestinal or genitourinary tract procedures	Ampicillin, 2.0 g IM or IV plus 1.5 mg/kg gentamicin IM or IV, ½ hr before
	Parenteral regimen for penicillin-allergic patients	Vancomycin, 1.0 g IV slowly over 1 hr, starting 1 hr before; add gentamicin, 1.5 mg/kg IM or IV if gastrointestinal or genitourinary tract is involved
	Oral regimen for penicillin-allergic patients (oral and respiratory tract only)	Erythromycin, 1.0 g orally 1 hr before, then 0.5 g 6 hr later
	Oral regimen for minor gastrointestinal or genitourinary tract procedures	Amoxicillin, 3.0 g orally 1 hr before, then 1.5 g 6 hr later
	Cardiac surgery, including implantation of prosthetic valves	Cefazolin, 2.0 g IV with induction of anesthesia, repeated 8 and 16 hr later, or vancomycin, 1.0 g IV slowly over 1 hr starting at induction, then 0.5 g IV 8 and 16 hr later

(Adapted from Durack DT: Prophylaxis of infective endocarditis. In Mandell GL, Douglas RH Jr, Bennett JE (eds): Principles and Practice of Infectious Diseases, p. 539. New York, John Wiley & Sons, 1985)

posure to chickenpox.[133] Although reports have suggested that zoster may behave as a transmissible disease,[145,150] careful study indicates that the initial dermatome eruption was zosterformlike, that an incubation period of 11 to 25 days between cases was apparent, and that these cases probably represented varicella in patients already immunocomprised by disease or treatment.[143] There is no evidence that zoster occurs following exposure to varicella-zoster virus in persons already infected with this virus, that is, in those with a past history of clinical or subclinical chickenpox.

Pathogenesis

Varicella infection with varicella-zoster virus occurs primarily in childhood and conveys life-long immunity against exogenous reinfection due to the development and persistence of serum antibody against the virus.[140] Following varicella infection, the virus remains in a latent form in the sensory nerve root ganglia; the state of the virus during latency and the factors maintaining latency are unknown.[129] Zoster occurs primarily in healthy older persons and in immunocompromised persons with underlying malignancy and those re-

ceiving cancer chemotherapy, immunosuppressive therapy, including corticosteroids, or both. A decrease in cell-mediated immune functions is characteristic of patients with malignancy and immunosuppressive treatment. Studies of the immune response of varicella-zoster virus in older persons demonstrate a waning cell-mediated immunity, as documented by decreased skin test and lymphocyte stimulation responses to varicella-zoster antigen, and intact humoral immunity with persistent antibody levels, as measured by fluorescent antibody against varicella-zoster membrane antigen, into the ninth and tenth decades of life.[131]

As a result of the decrease in cell-mediated immunity, the latent infection in the sensory ganglia is no longer maintained, and once reactivated, varicella-zoster virus moves along the nerve axons to the skin and produces the characteristic eruption. Additional predisposing factors associated with reactivation include local areas of tumor, lymph node disease, local irradiation, trauma, surgery, lead, arsenic, and syphilis.[133,137] Recurrences of zoster in older persons occur at about the same rate, approximately 6%, and usually in the same dermatomal site as initial attacks.[137] These recurrences are associated with consistently high antibody titers but with minimal reactivity of cell-mediated immunity, and older persons remain predisposed throughout life to recurrent zoster.[131]

Presentation

Clinical Findings

Pain in a dermatomal distribution is usually the first complaint and may occur 1 to 10 days before the eruption.[142] There is no apparent relationship of pain to the severity of the skin involvement.[130] Occasionally the pain is the only manifestation (zoster sine herpete), although usually regional lymph nodes and often a faint maculopapular eruption in the same dermatomal distribution provide a clue to the diagnosis. As many as one third of patients have no pain.[130]

The typical eruption or rash is a bandlike pattern of grouped vesicles on erythematous bases, morphologically resembling varicella. The eruption involves one or more adjacent dermatomes, with the following distribution in older persons: thoracic, 50% to 60%; trigeminal, 10% to 20%; cervical, 10% to 20%; lumbar, 5% to 10%; and sacral, less than 5%.[130,137,146,149] Although there is frequently a typical progression from vesicles to pustules (2 to 5 days) to dry crusted areas (10 to 12 days) to clearing of the skin (2 to 3 weeks), careful observations during antiviral treatment trials indicate that as many as one third of patients 60 years of age or older present with 50% of the skin lesions in the papule stage and that about 50% of these papules never evolve to vesicles or pustules but simply disappear.[128] The duration to clearing is prolonged in older persons and is related to the severity of the skin infection.[130] Constitutional features are usually absent, although fever, (<101°F [38.3°C]), malaise, and regional lymph nodes are occasionally noted; approximately 5% of patients have a headache and a stiff neck if cranial nerves are involved.[130,142]

Laboratory Findings

There is little information on laboratory studies in older persons with zoster. A mild peripheral leukocytosis (10,000 to 12,000/cu mm) may be present. Because zoster involves the spinal root ganglia, as many as 40% of patients with uncomplicated cases may have mild pleocytosis, slightly increased protein concentration, or both in the cerebrospinal fluid. These patients, however, have few if any signs or symptoms suggestive of meningitis or encephalitis.[148]

Diagnosis

The diagnosis is usually apparent once the eruption appears. The varicella-zoster virus can readily be isolated from vesicular fluid using a 25-gauge needle and syringe during the first 3 days following the onset of localized zoster and as long as 10 days after onset in patients with disseminated zoster. The virus can also be isolated from the cerebrospinal fluid in patients with cervical or trigeminal dermatome distribution. Laboratory confirmation is rarely necessary in clinical practice except when eruptions resembling zoster are present in patients suspected of herpes simplex. Zoster infection can be confirmed by demonstrating a fourfold rise in the complement fixation antibody titer in serum specimens obtained within the first week and 4 weeks later.[129]

Course

Approximately 70% of older persons with zoster diagnosed or treated at a medical center will return to baseline by 8 weeks after the onset versus approximately 90% resolution in persons under 60 years of age.[149] In this population, moderate to severe pain or complications were noted in 44% and 10%, respectively, versus 25% and 6%, respectively, for persons under 60 years of age. Mortality rates, on the other hand, are less than 2% in normal as well as immunosuppressed older persons.

The most common cause of morbidity is postherpetic neuralgia (PHN), frequently defined as pain in the involved dermatome lasting for more than 1 month following the acute episode. It occurs with a frequency of 10% to 50% depending on whether older persons with zoster are seen in the community or admitted to the hospital.[126] The dermatomal distribution does not appear to be well correlated with the frequency of PHN except for the trigeminal nerve, which has a worse prognosis.[142] The cause of PHN is obscure but may be related to postinflammation fibrosis in the dorsal root ganglia, which is perpetuated by a central mechanism.[138]

Cutaneous disseminated zoster, defined as the appearance of vesicles outside the initial dermatome may occur in healthy older persons and especially in the immunosuppressed. A benign type of dissemination occurs in approximately 15% of healthy older persons in whom the scattered vesicles begin to occur about 1 week after the onset of the localized eruption and continue over the next 3 to 5 days. The distribution is generally sparse with a maximum of 15 to 30 new lesions. In this limited type of dissemination, there is no increase in morbidity or mortality. In immunosuppressed patients more extensive and prolonged skin lesions and visceral dissemination can occur. Even this generalized type of dissemination, however, is rarely life threatening.[133] It generally occurs in patients with lymphoma or other malignancies who are receiving immunosuppressive treatment and represents prolonged blood-borne spread of varicella-zoster virus early during the reactivation period when absent or low levels of circulating antibody and vesicular fluid interferon titers are present.[141,151]

Herpes zoster ophthalmicus occurs in 2% of the general population,[146] with ocular involvement reported in approximately 20% of older persons in the general population and in 75% of those referred to an opthalmology service.[146,155] Early zoster lesions on the top or side of the nose, sensory areas served by the nasociliary nerve, may prewarn of infection in the eye.[142] Late central nervous system complications, presenting as contralateral hemiplegia or segmental cerebral arteritis, can occur several months after zoster ophthalmicus, causing the association to be overlooked.[155]

Neurologic complications such as encephalitis, meningitis, myelitis, or peripheral neuropathies occur in less than 0.5% of the general population.[146] In cases of encephalitis, the symptoms usually occur near the end of the first week of the rash and, rarely, before the rash. One third of these patients have ophthalmic zoster and contralateral hemiplegia that are ascribed to a granulomatous angiitis.[148] Motor neuropathies are the most common neurologic complication, accounting for up to 30% of cases.[148] In 90% of these cases, the muscle paralysis occurs within the dermatome affected by the rash.

Lumbosacral involvement is frequently associated with constipation, urinary retention, polyuria, and impotence. Other rare complications include Bell's palsy, Ramsay Hunt syndrome, and Guillain-Barré syndrome. Approximately 75% of zoster-associated paralyses recover completely. Zoster neurologic complications contribute great morbidity, but mortality is rare even in cases of meningoencephalitis.[148]

There is no increase in risk for subsequent cancer in normal healthy elderly patients with zoster or in those with serious complications such as gangrenous zoster, PHN, dissemination, or ophthalmic zoster. Therefore, there is no support for investigations for occult cancer at the time zoster is diagnosed or enhanced surveillance afterward.[147]

Treatment

Uncomplicated Zoster

Uncomplicated zoster is treated symptomatically with wet compresses and mild analgesics. Orally administered narcotics may be required. Levodopa, 100 mg, and benserazide, 25 mg, orally three times a day for 10 days significantly shortens the time for skin healing, disappearance of pain, and sleep problems but does not reduce the chances for PHN.[139] No specific antiviral treatment is required.

Complicated Zoster

Systemic corticosteriods given in the first week of zoster significantly decrease PHN,[134,138] and many recommend that this treatment be used in all but the mildest cases.[149] The most frequently used regimen is a rapidly tapering dose of prednisone, 40 mg to 60 mg/day for the first week, then 20 mg to 30 mg/day for the second week, and 10 mg to 15 mg/day during the third week, discontinuing treatment in the fourth week. Using this regimen, or an equivalent dose of prednisolone or triamcinolone, PHN is decreased to 15% to 30% versus 65% to 75% in patients treated with analgesics or placebo. Dissemination or other complications of zoster or corticosteroid use have not been noted.[134,138] The effect of steroids is not usually apparent until the second or third week of treatment. If the pain dramatically decreases within several days of starting steroids, this response most likely represents the natural course of the disease, and the steroids should be discontinued.[126]

Once PHN is present, treatment results are much less satisfactory. A randomized placebo-control trial with amitriptyline, a tricyclic antidepressant, provided good to excellent relief of pain in two thirds of patients with PHN for at least 3 months.[153] An initial dose of 25 mg was increased to a maximum dose of approximately 125 mg (median dosage in older persons approximately 65 mg) as tolerated once at bedtime. In most patients, no antidepressant effect could be demonstrated. Other regimens that have demonstrated some success in relieving the pain include intralesional injection of triamcinolone,[135] carbamazepine,[134] and chlorprothixene.[136]

Varicella-zoster virus is a herpesvirus that, like other members of this group, contains DNA and can be treated by a variety of DNA inhibitors such as idoxuridine, vidarabine, and acyclovir.[129] Idoxuridine must be dissolved in dimethyl sulfoxide (5% to 40% IDU and 100% DMSO) and applied frequently to the skin infection. Experimental studies demonstrate a decreased time to healing with decreased duration of pain, but the Food and Drug Administration (FDA) has approved idoxuridine only for topical treatment of herpes simplex.

Vidarabine, 15 mg/kg/day for 5 days, in immunosuppressed patients reduces the time to healing, the total duration of PHN, the frequency of cutaneous dissemination, and the frequency of visceral dissemination.[154] Vidarabine is approved by the FDA for normal hosts, but the intravenous infusions require 1.5 to 2.5 liters of fluids per day, the primary route of clearance is renal, and dose-related gastrointestinal toxicities and neural toxicities, including pain syndromes of the extremities, occur.[16]

Acyclovir, a purine nucleoside analogue, is given by intravenous infusion in a dose of 5 mg to 10 mg/kg every 8 hours for 5 days. As of 1985, it has not been approved for vericetta-zoster virus infections, although several studies have demonstrated significant reductions in the time to healing of skin lesions, duration of pain, and duration of viral shedding.[125,144] Acyclovir has no effect on the incidence of severity of PHN. In immunocompromised patients, acyclovir significantly reduces cutaneous dissemination and visceral complications.[124] Acyclovir is excreted primarily by the kidney, and elevated serum creatinine levels, which are reversible, are frequently noted in older persons.[125] An oral preparation of acyclovir is under investigation.

Varicella-zoster immune globulin (VZIG) prepared from sera of patients who have recently recovered from zoster contains high titers of anti-varicella-zoster antibody. Observations that patients can be protected against varicella by passive immunization with VZIG has stimulated interest in its use in the management of patients with zoster. The clinical course of zoster, however, is not related to decreased levels of serum antibody to varicella-zoster virus, and administration of VZIG to older patients with zoster would be of no benefit.[152]

Prevention

Prevention of zoster for the healthy elderly person requires a return of the normal cell-mediated immune functions that have been slowly but steadily declining since early adulthood. Replacement therapy (*e.g.*, thymic hormones) are not available for this use. Live-attenuated varicella-zoster virus vaccine can improve reduced *in vitro* lymphopro-

liferative responses of older persons to the varicella-zoster virus.[127] Further trials are necessary to determine if improvement in this measure of cell-mediated immune response will protect against reactivation of zoster infection. Although most older persons are not susceptible to varicella because of previous chickenpox infection, contact with persons with varicella or zoster should be avoided if the older person has a malignancy such as a lymphoma or is immunosuppressed.

IMMUNIZATION

Tetanus–Diphtheria Toxoid

Although the total number of cases, approximately 100 per year, is low in the United States compared with other countries, tetanus is a serious health problem for the elderly. In the United States in 1979, persons 60 years of age and older accounted for more than 50% of the reported cases, with a case-fatality rate of 75%. In one series from the United States, less than 20% of cases were associated with injuries that occurred on farms and more than 50% with injuries that occurred in the home. Nine cases with 6 deaths, almost exclusively in older persons, occurred following surgery, especially amputation of gangrenous extremities or abdominal surgery. Twenty cases, including 19 deaths, were related to chronic skin ulcerations, infected pressure ulcers, and varicose veins.[174] There is no natural immunity to the toxin of *Clostridium tetani*; tetanus occurs almost exclusively in persons who are unimmunized, who are inadequately immunized, or whose history of immunization is unknown.

Although recent studies demonstrate a low prevalence of diphtheria-protective antitoxin antibody levels in older persons, diphtheria does not appear to be as serious a problem for the elderly as is tetanus. In this section we will not comment further on diphtheria but recommendations for tetanus-diphtheria toxoid will provide protection against it as well.

Immunizing Agent

Tetanus and diphtheria (Td) toxoids—adsorbed for adult use is a combined preparation recommended for all persons over 7 years of age.[165] The toxoids are prepared by formaldehyde treatment of the respective toxins and standardized for potency. The dose and administration of Td follow the recommendations in the package insert, and the preparation is administered intramuscularly.

Adverse Reactions

Information on the risk of adverse reactions following Td toxoid in older persons is scant; observations are mainly based on studies in young adults and children. Local reactions, generally erythema and induration, occur in up to 40% but are usually self-limited, lasting only 1 to 2 days. Major local reactions (*e.g.,* Arthus-type hypersensitivity reactions starting 2 to 8 hours after the injection) occur primarily in persons with elevated antibody levels following multiple boosters. Severe systemic reactions are rare. The only contraindication to Td is a history of a neurologic or severe hypersensitivity reaction associated with a previous dose. Passive immunization with human tetanus immune globulin should be considered in those persons whenever an injury other than a clean wound is sustained.[165]

Immunogenicity and Efficacy

Protective serum antibody levels (*i.e.,* 0.01 unit/ml in persons over age 60) are present in only 40% of men and 30% of women.[168] Other studies from Great Britain and Australia also document the high proportions of nonimmune older persons.[156,167] The prevalence of protective titers in nursing home residents is approximately 50%.[179]

There is little information on the effectiveness of tetanus toxoid as an immunizing agent for older persons. Protective antitoxin antibody levels following immunization occur in 85% to 100% of older persons following a second booster dose of Td.[179a,181] Approximately 25% of older persons, who were immunized 8 years previously, have antitoxin serum levels of less than 0.01 units/ml, but 93% of these persons respond to a booster immunization with protective antibody levels.[182]

Current Recommendations

Immunization is recommended for all older persons who are unimmunized, who are inadequately immunized, or whose history of immunization is unknown. The routine immunizing schedule for older persons requires a series of three doses called primary immunization and is identical to that recommended for all adults.[165] The booster immunization, also Td, is administered every 10 years after the last dose, provided the primary series has been completed. The recommendations for tetanus pro-

phylaxis or the use of passive immunization with human tetanus immune globulin in the management of wounds will not be reviewed here; these details have been published elsewhere.[165]

Strategies for Implementing Current Recommendations

There is substantial indirect evidence that the low incidence of tetanus is a result of widespread immunization and that tetanus immunization is the only means of eliminating the disease. Despite repeated urgings emphasizing the need for tetanus immunization in adults, there has been no real decrease in the number of cases reported per year in older persons in the United States.[165] If the number and severity cases of tetanus are to be reduced in older persons, current recommendations must be implemented and new strategies developed to deliver tetanus toxoid to this high-risk population. To do this, the following points should be emphasized:

Consider routine immunization with the full primary series for those likely to be inadequately immunized or not immunized at all. Today, this is primarily the elderly and, especially, elderly women.

Give single booster doses, after the initial series, every 10 years regardless of the patient's age. *Do not overlook the elderly.*

After an injury, do not give a single booster to an older person with an unknown immunization history. More than 15% of tetanus cases occur in this setting. If the history is doubtful the elderly patient should receive Td and passive immunization if the trauma is more than a clean minor wound. The primary immunization series should then be completed.

Promptly immunize or give boosters as indicated for debilitated patients, especially those prone to cutaneous ulceration or vascular complications.

Determine the immunity status of older persons prior to elective surgery, especially surgery including the gastrointestinal tract, and provide adequate immunization.

Know that although it may not be cost-effective in the usual sense, the increased frequency and severity of tetanus in older persons, the likelihood of high-risk conditions afflicting the institutionalized elderly (*e.g.,* cutaneous ulcers and peripheral gangrene), and the fact that tetanus toxoid is inexpensive, safe, and highly effective support the concern that nursing home residents should receive immunization.

Inactivated Influenza Virus Vaccines

Immunizing Agent

In general these vaccines contain both A and B type virus, usually the types isolated in the previous winter's influenza season. The formulation contains 15 µg of hemagglutinin from each antigen in a 0.5-ml dose administered intramuscularly. Only one dose is required for older persons.[10]

Adverse Reactions

Vaccine-associated reactions include local reactions with mild discomfort in 25% to 50% and moderate discomfort in 5%, generally lasting less than 2 days post vaccination. Fever, with or without a flulike illness, occurs in less than 1% and begins 6 to 12 hours post vaccination, persisting for 1 to 2 days. Guillain-Barré syndrome, which was noted in approximately one per 100,000 persons who received A/New Jersey/76 swine influenza vaccine in 1976–1977, is not significantly associated with the more recent vaccine preparations.[173] Systemic reactions appear to be less severe in the elderly.[12] Contraindications to vaccination include a previous history of Guillain-Barré syndrome post vaccination or anaphylactic hypersensitivity to eggs.[10]

Immunogenicity

Antibody responses following immunization are similar to that of natural infection, including the presence of detectable secretory antibody and respiratory secretion. Protection against infection is generally noted with serum hemagglutination-inhibiting titers of greater than 1:40, serum neutralizing titers greater than 1:8 and nasal neutralizing antibody titers greater than 1:4. Optimal protection probably occurs when both types of antibodies are present.[12] Antibody responses to vaccination in older persons are comparable to those in young, healthy adults.[12]

Efficacy

The best assessment of the effectiveness of influenza vaccines in high-risk older persons is protection against disease. In young, healthy adults, the overall efficacy rate for reducing influenza infection is approximately 65%. Although fewer studies have been performed in older persons, similar efficacy rates have been noted when the vaccine more closely matches the epidemic strain.[160] A retrospective study demonstrated that influenza vaccine reduced pneumonia- and influenza-associ-

ated hospitalizations and deaths among older persons residing in communities by 72% and 81%, respectively.[159] Recent uncontrolled prospective and retrospective studies indicate that influenza vaccine can reduce illness, hospitalization, pneumonia, and death in influenza A outbreaks in nursing homes.[162,177]

Current Recommendations

Current recommendations include a reclassification of the previously broadly defined high-risk group. The elderly for whom active targeted vaccination efforts are most necessary include persons with chronic disorders of the cardiovascular or pulmonary systems that are severe enough to have required regular medical follow-ups or hospitalization during the preceding year and residents of nursing homes and other long-term care facilities. In addition, physicians, nurses, and others with extensive contact with these high-risk patients should also receive influenza vaccination annually.[10]

With a slightly lower priority, the vaccine should also be readily available to persons at moderately increased risk of serious illness compared with the general population. These include persons 65 years of age and older who have chronic metabolic disease (including diabetes mellitus), renal dysfunction, anemia, and immunosuppression or asthma that is severe enough to have required regular medical follow-ups or hospitalization during the previous year and those otherwise healthy persons.[10]

Strategies for Implementing Recommendations

Prevention of influenza virus infections, however, is a formidable task. In most past years only 20% of the group, defined at high risk on the basis of medical condition or age, received influenza vaccine. Efforts to implement the recommendations will require dramatic new strategies to identify persons with high-risk conditions, improve acceptance of older persons, and improve the delivery of the vaccine. This will require a renewed interest and effort by older persons, their physicians, and other members of the health care team.

Pneumococcal Vaccine

Immunizing Agent

The current recommended immunizing agent is pneumococcal vaccine, polyvalent. The original vaccine contained purified capsular polysaccharides from 14 of the 83 different types of *Streptococcus pneumoniae*. In July 1983, an expanded 23-serotype vaccine was licensed. Pneumococcal vaccine and influenza vaccine can be given at the same time, if different sites are used, without decreasing the antibody response of either vaccine or substantially increasing side-effects.[166]

Adverse Reactions

Vaccine-associated reactions occur within 24 hours of injection in 10% to 15% of elderly vaccinees and consist primarily of discomfort, erythema, and induration that lasts approximately 2 to 5 days. Fever of 100°F (37.8°C) or greater occurs in approximately 2% and generally lasts less than 24 hours.[161] Severe local and systemic reactions with fever (>103°F [39.4°C]) headache, myalgias, and chills have been reported.[169] These reactions occur 2 to 8 hours following the injection and probably represent an Arthus-type hypersensitivity reaction. Acute anaphylactoid reactions are rare, occurring in approximately five per million doses administered.[166] The only contraindication to the vaccine is a history of allergy to one of the vaccine components, usually the diluent.

Immunogenicity

Antibody responses to the pneumococcal vaccine are type specific, that is, antibodies are produced only against the 23 serotypes represented in the vaccine. The mechanism of protection is similar to natural infection and depends on the production of opsonizing antibodies that promote phagocytosis of the homologous types. Although adequate levels of serum antibody to the pneumococcal type-specific capsule following infection are considered the basis for immunity to pneumococcal disease, the opsonizing function may not be well correlated with the serum anticapsular antibody concentration.[170] The level of the antibody, which is protective against each type, has not been determined but appears to be greater than 300 ng Ab N/ml.[175] Most adults respond to the vaccine in 2 weeks, with a maximum response in 4 to 6 weeks.

Limited available studies suggest that the immune response to the vaccine in older persons is satisfactory.[157,172] Preliminary findings, however, indicate that the total antibody responses in a small group of ambulatory institutionalized elderly differ significantly from the responses in young, healthy adults in terms of lower levels of preimmunization titers, a decrease in frequency of two-fold increases following immunizations, and decrease in the frequency of "protective" antibody levels 1 month post immunization.[160]

The duration of protective levels of antibody in the elderly following vaccination is unknown, although antibody to serotypes of *Streptococcus pneumoniae* represented in the vaccine persist at 30% to 50% of peak levels among healthy, middle-aged persons for at least 5 to 6 years.[176] Because there is an increase in adverse reactions among adults that appears to correlate with elevated antibody,[163] and because additional doses of pneumococcal vaccine provide a poor "booster" response, the vaccine should be given only once to adults.[166] Preliminary studies, already noted, however, demonstrate a rapid decline in postimmunization antibody titers that result in 12-month postimmunization "protective" levels markedly reduced from levels 1 month post immunization. As a group, persons 80 years of age and older have the most impaired response.[160] Studies with larger numbers of volunteers are in progress to examine this important issue.

Efficacy

In randomized controlled trials, the vaccine is approximately 80% effective in decreasing pneumococcal disease in young, healthy adults.[158] Preliminary reports of efficacy studies in older persons, however, indicate no notable differences in the frequency of pneumonia (total), pneumococcal pneumonia (nonvaccine-type or vaccine-type), or mortality (total or pneumococcal) in persons residing in communities or in the institutionalized elderly.[180] An alternate method for evaluating the efficacy of pneumococcal vaccine, one that compares the distribution of serotypes of pneumococci isolated from the blood of vaccinated and unvaccinated persons, reports an estimated efficacy of 60% to 80% for persons over 60 years of age with no underlying illness or no chronic pulmonary disease, chronic heart disease, or diabetes mellitus.[164]

Current Recommendations

The recommendations of the Immunization Practices Advisory Committee, an advisory group to the US Public Health Service and the Centers for Disease Control, for older persons are as follows:[166]

Those with chronic illnesses, especially cardiovascular disease and chronic pulmonary disease, who sustain increased morbidity with respiratory infections

Those with chronic illnesses specifically associated with an increased risk of pneumococcal disease or its complications (*e.g.*, those with splenic dysfunction or anatomical asplenia, Hodgkin's disease, multiple myeloma, cirrhosis, alcoholism, renal failure, cerebrospinal fluid leaks, and conditions associated with immunosuppression

Persons aged 65 and older who are otherwise healthy

Persons undergoing elective splenectomy or immunosuppressive treatment, as in patients who are candidates for organ transplants, should be vaccinated at least 2 weeks, or as long as possible, prior to the treatment.

Strategies for Implementing Recommendations

For older persons residing in communities, the frequency (75% to 85%) of vaccine-type pneumococcal pneumonia and the potential for healthy life-years gained,[183] warrants use of the pneumococcal vaccine. The acceptance of the vaccine by this group, however, is poor; one study noted only 4% had received pneumococcal vaccine versus 28% who had received influenza vaccine.[178] Efforts to improve vaccine delivery in this group include the following[166]:

Identify older persons who have already received, or are candidates for, influenza vaccine. Although pneumococcal vaccine can be given at any time of year, it is convenient for physicians to give the vaccine in the autumn during the same visit when influenza immunization is given, provided the vaccines are given at different sites.

Promote hospital-based programs to vaccinate the patients prior to discharge. Studies demonstrate that two thirds of persons with serious pneumococcal disease have been hospitalized within 5 years before the onset of the pneumococcal illness.[171]

Promote office-based and clinic-based programs to identify and immunize the frequent user of medical care. Older persons who visit physicians frequently and have chronic conditions are likely to be at higher risk of pneumococcal infection than those who require infrequent visits.

It is recommended that more effective programs are needed for giving pneumococcal vaccine in nursing homes and other chronic care facilities.[166] There are several concerns, however, with recommending the vaccine for general use in the institutionalized elderly. Although the incidence of

pneumococcal pneumonia in this population is very impressive (approximately 15 per 1000 per year), nonvaccine serotypes are effectively selected by widespread use of the vaccine and account for as high as 70% of pneumococcal pneumonia cases in those vaccinated during the first postvaccination year.[31] Pneumococcal vaccine should be promoted in nursing homes for those individual residents with cardiopulmonary conditions requiring active treatment. These individuals are the same highest-risk residents and patients who are already receiving, or are candidates for, influenza vaccine. Pneumococcal vaccine should also be used in the presence of an epidemic or a high endemic rate of vaccine-type pneumococcal pneumonia.

REFERENCES

1. DeTorres OH, Marr FN Jr: Antimocrobial agents. In Gleckman RA, Gantz NM (eds): Infections in the Elderly, p 13. Boston, Little Brown Co, 1983
2. Fox RA: Immunology and Infection in the Elderly, p 379. Edinburgh, Churchill Livingstone, 1984
3. Gleckman RA, Esposito AL: Antibiotics in the elderly: Skating on therapeutic thin ice. Geriatrics 35:26–28, 33–37, 1980
4. Gleckman RA, Gantz NM: Infections in the Elderly, p 360. Boston, Little Brown Co. 1983
5. Grieco, MH: Use of antibiotics in the elderly. Bull NY Acad Med 56:197, 1980
6. Schneider EL: Infectious diseases in the elderly. Ann Intern Med 98:395, 1983
7. Yoshikawa TT: Geriatric infectious diseases: An emerging problem. J Am Geriatr Soc 31:34, 1983
8. Barker WH, Mullooly JP: Pneumonia and influenza deaths during epidemics: Implications for prevention. Arch Intern Med 142:85, 1982
9. Barker WH, Mullooly JP: Impact of epidemic type A influenza in a defined adult population. Am J Epidemiol 112:798, 1980
10. Centers for Disease Control: Prevention and Control of Influenza. Recommendation of the Immunization Practices Advisory Committee. Ann Intern Med 101:218, 1984
11. Consensus Development Conference Panel: Amantadine: Does it have a role in the prevention and treatment of influenza? A National Institutes of Health Consensus Development Conference. Ann Intern Med 92:256, 1980
12. Couch, RB, Jackson GG: Antiviral agents in influenza—summary of influenza workshop VIII. J Infect Dis 134:516, 1976
13. Dolin R, Reichman RC, Madore HP et al: A controlled trial of amantadine and rimantadine in the prophylaxis of influenza A infection. N Engl J Med 298:516, 1978
14. Douglas RG Jr, Betts RF: Influenza virus. In Mandell GL, Douglas RG Jr, Bennett JE (eds): Principles

and Practice of Infectious Diseases, p 846. New York, John Wiley & Son, 1985

15. Fry J: Influenza, 1959: The story of an epidemic. Br Med J 2:135, 1959

16. Hayden FG, Douglas RG Jr: Antiviral agents. In Mandell GL, Douglas RG Jr, Bennett JE (eds): Principles and Practice of Infectious Diseases, p 270. New York, John Wiley & Sons, 1985

17. Horadam VW, Sharp JG, Smilack JD et al: Pharmacokinetics of amantadine hydrochloride in subjects with normal and impaired renal function. Ann Intern Med 94:454, 1981

18. Ing TS, Daugirdas JT, Soung LS et al: Toxic effects of amantadine in patients with renal failure. Can Med Assoc J 120:1695, 1979

19. Little JW, Hall WJ, Douglas RG Jr et al: Amantadine effect on peripheral airways abnormalities in influenza. Ann Intern Med 85:177, 1976

20. Mathur U, Bentley DW, Hall CB et al: Influenza A/Brazil/78(H1N1) infection in the elderly. Am Rev Respir Dis 123:633, 1981

21. Mathur U, Bentley DW, Hall CB: Concurrent respiratory syncytial virus and influenza A infections in the institutionalized elderly and chronically ill. Ann Intern Med 93:49, 1980

22. Montanari C, Ferrari P, Bavazzano A: Urinary excretion of amantadine by the elderly. Eur J Clin Pharmacol 8:349, 1975

23. Schoenbaum SC: A perspective on the benefits, costs, and risks of immunization. In Weinstein L, Fields BN (eds): Seminars in Infectious Disease, p 294. New York, Thieme-Stratton, 1980

24. Silverstone FA, Libow LS, Duthie E et al: Outbreak of influenza B, 1980, in a geriatric long-term care facility. Gerontologist 20:200, 1980

25. Van Voris LP, Belshe RB, Shaffer JL: Nosocomial influenza B virus infection in the elderly. Ann Intern Med 96:153, 1982

26. Van Voris LP, Betts RF, Hayden FG et al: Successful treatment of naturally occurring influenza A/USSR/77 H1N1. JAMA 245:1128, 1981

27. Walter HE, Paulshock M: Therapeutic efficacy of amantadine HC1. MO Med 67:176, 1970

28. Younkin SW, Betts RF, Roth FK et al: Reduction in fever and symptoms in young adults with influenza A/Brazil/78 H1N1 infection after treatment with aspirin or amantadine. Antimicrob Agents Chemother 23:577,1983

29. Bentley DW: Bacterial pneumonia in the elderly: Clinical features, diagnosis, etiology, and treatment. Gerontology 30:297, 1984

30. Bentley DW: Pathogenesis of bacterial pneumonia in the elderly: The effects of normal aging processes. In Steel K (ed): Geriatric Education, p 161. Lexington, MA, The Collamore Press, 1982

31. Bentley DW, Ha K, Mamot K et al: Pneumococcal vaccine in the institutionalized elderly: Design of a nonrandomized trial and preliminary results. Rev Infect Dis 3:S71, 1981

32. Berk SL, Wiener SL, Eisner LB et al: Mixed *Strep-tococcus pneumoniae* and gram-negative bacillary pneumonia in the elderly. South Med J 74:144, 1981

33. Campbell EJ, Lefrak SS: How aging affects the structure and function of the respiratory system. Geriatrics 33:68, 1978

34. Kovar MG: Health of the elderly and use of health services. United States—1977. Hyattsville, MD, Division of Vital Statistics, National Center for Health Statistics. Public Health Report 92:9, 1977

35. Donowitz GR, Mandell GL: Empiric therapy for pneumonia. Rev Infect Dis 5:S40, 1983

36. Ebright JR, Rytel MW: Bacterial pneumonia in the elderly. J Am Geriatr Soc 28:220, 1978

37. Esposito AL: Community-acquired bacteremic pneumococcal pneumonia. Arch Intern Med 144:945, 1984

38. Finkelstein MS, Petkun WM, Freedman ML et al: Pneumococcal bacteremia in adults: Age-dependent differences in presentation and in outcome. J Am Geriatr Soc 2:19, 1983

39. Fried MA: An analysis of the controlled field trial of docecavalent pneumococcal vaccine. San Francisco, Kaiser Permanente Medical Center, 1978

40. Haley RW, Hooton TM, Culver DH et al: Nosocomial infections in US hospitals, 1975–1976: Estimated frequency by selected characteristics of patients. Am J Med 70:947, 1981

41. Hook EW, Horton CA, Schaberg DR: Failure of intensive care unit support to influence mortality from pneumococcal bacteremia. JAMA 249:1055, 1983

42. Horton JM, Pankey GA: Pneumonia in the elderly. Postgrad Med 71:114, 1982

43. Jay S, Johanson WG, Pierce AK: The radiographic resolution of *Streptococcus pneumoniae* pneumonia. N Engl J Med 293:798, 1975

44. McFadden JP, Price RC, Eastwood HD et al: Raised respiratory rate in elderly patients: A valuable physical sign. Br Med J 284:626, 1982

45. Murray PR, Washington JA: Microscopic and bacteriologic analysis of expectorated sputum. May Clin Proc 50:339, 1975

46. Oseasohn R, Skipper BE, Tempest B: Pneumonia in a Navajo community. Am Rev Respir Dis 117:1003, 1978

47. Phair JP, Kauffman CA, Bjornson A: Investigation of host defense mechanisms in the aged as determinants of nosocomial colonization and pneumonia. J Retic Soc 23:397, 1978

48. Rozas CJ, Goldman AL: Responses to bacterial pneumonia. Geriatrics 37:61, 1982

49. Sorbini CA, Grassi V, Solinas E, Muiesan G: Arterial oxygen tension in relation to age in healthy subjects. Respiration 25:3, 1968

50. Sullivan RJ, Dowdle WR, Marine WM et al: Adult pneumonia in a general hospital. Arch Intern Med 129:935, 1972

51. Valenti WM, Trudell RG, Bentley DW: Factors predisposing to oropharyngeal colonization with

gram-negative bacilli in the aged. N Engl J Med 298:1108, 1978

52. Verghese A, Berk SL: Bacterial pneumonia in the elderly. Medicine 62:271, 1983

53. Ziskind MM, Schwarz MI, George RB et al: Incomplete consolidation in pneumococcal lobar pneumonia complicating pulmonary emphysema. Ann Intern Med 72:835, 1970

54. Aktar AJ, Andrews GR, Caird FL et al: Urinary tract infection in the elderly: A population study. Age Ageing 1:48, 1972

55. Alling B, Brandberg A, Seeberg S et al: Aerobic and anaerobic microbial flora in the urinary tract of geriatric patients during long-term care. J Infect Dis 127:34, 1973

56. Bendall MJ, Gruneberg RN: An outbreak of infection caused by trimethoprim-resistant coliform bacilli in a geriatric unit. Age Ageing 8:231, 1979

57. Breitenbucher RB: Bacterial changes in the urine samples of patients with long-term indwellng catheters. Arch Intern Med 144:1585, 1984

57a. Brocklehurst JC: The urinary tract. In Rossman I (ed): Clinical Geriatrics, 2nd ed., pp 317–328. Philadelphia, JB Lippincott, 1979

58. Brocklehurst JC, Bee P, Jones D et al: Bacteriuria in geriatric hospital patients: Its correlates and management. Age Ageing 6:240, 1977

59. Brocklehurst JC, Dillane JB, Griffiths L et al: The prevalence and symptomatology of urinary infection in an aged population. Gerontol Clin 10:242, 1968

60. Cape RDT, Ehtisham M, Zirk MH: Management of bacteriuria in the elderly female: Urinary tract infection. Proceedings of the 2nd National Symposium, March 1972. New York, Oxford University Press, 1973

61. Dontas AS, Kasviki-Charvati P, Panayiotis CL et al: Bacteriuria and survival in old age. N Engl J Med 304:939, 1981

62. Gillenwater JY: Use of Beta-lactam antibiotics in urinary tract infections. J Urol 129:457, 1983

63. Gleckman R, Blagg N, Hibert D et al: Community-acquired bacteremic urosepsis in the elderly patient: A prospective study of 34 consecutive episodes. J Urol 128:79, 1982

64. Gleckman R, Blagg N, Hibert D et al: Symptomatic pyelonephritis in elderly men. J Am Geriatr Soc 30:690, 1982

65. Gleckman R, Esposito A, Crowley M et al: Reliability of a single urine culture in establishing diagnosis of asymptomatic bacteriuria in adult males. J Clin Microbiol 9:596, 1979

66. Hirsh DD, Fainstein V, Musher DM: Do condom catheter collecting systems cause urinary tract infections? JAMA 242:340, 1979

67. Kaye D: Urinary tract infections in the elderly. Bull NY Acad Med 56:209, 1980

68. Kreger BE, Craven DE, Carling PC et al: Gram-negative bacteremia: III. Reassessment of etiology, epidemiology and ecology in 612 patients. Am J Med 68:332, 1980

69. Kuhlemeier KV, Lloyd LK, Stover SL: Failure of antibody-coated bacteria and bladder washout tests to localize infection in spinal cord injury patients. J Urol 130:729, 1983

70. Kunin CM: Detection, Prevention and Management of Urinary Tract Infections, 3rd ed., p 32. Philadelphia, Lea & Febiger, 1979

71. Lacey RW, Simpson MHC, Lord VL et al: Comparison of single-dose trimethoprim with a five-day course for the treatment of urinary tract infections in the elderly. Age Aging 10:179, 1981

72. Lye M: Defining and treating urinary infections. Geriatrics 33:71, 1978

73. Marketos SG, Dontas AS, Papanayiotou P et al: Bacteriuria and arterial hypertension in old age. Geriatrics 25:136, 1970

74. Marketos SG, Papanayiotou PC, Dontas AS: Bacteriuria and non-obstructive renovascular disease in old age. J Gerontol 23:33, 1969

75. Meares EM Jr: Prostatitis and related diseases. DM 26(8):40, 1980

76. Moore-Smith B: Suprapubic aspiration in the diagnosis of urinary infection in the elderly. Mod Geriatr 1:124, 1971

77. Nicolle LE, Bjornson J, Harding GKM et al: Bacteriuria in elderly institutionalized men. N Engl J Med 309:1420, 1983

78. Platt R: Quantitative definition of bacteriuria. Am J Med 75:44, 1983

79. Ronald AR: Current concepts in the management of urinary tract infections in adults. Med Clin North Am 68:335, 1984

80. Sheldon CA, Gonzalez R: Differentiation of upper and lower urinary tract infections: How and when? Med Clin North Am 68:321, 1984

81. Sherman FT, Tucci V, Libow LS et al: Nosocomial urinary tract infections in a skilled nursing facility. J Am Geriatr Soc 28:456, 1980

82. Sourander LB, Kasanen A: A 5 year follow-up of bacteriuria in the aged. Gerontol Clin 14:274, 1972

83. Warren JW, Tenney JH, Hoopes JM et al: A prospective microbiologic study in bacteriuria in patients with chronic indwellilng urethral catheters. J Infect Dis 146:719, 1982

84. Wolfson SA, Kalmanson GM, Rubini ME et al: Epidemiology of bacteriuria in a predominantly geriatric male population. Am J Med Sci 250:168, 1965

85. American Heart Association Committee on Prevention of Bacterial Endocarditis: Prevention of bacterial endocarditis. Circulation 56:139A, 1977

86. Anderson HJ, Staffurth JS: Subacute bacterial endocarditis in the elderly. Lancet 2:1055, 1955

87. Applefeld MM, Hornick RB: Infective endocarditis in patients over 60. Am Heart J 88:90, 1974

88. Bayer AS, Theofilopoulos AN, Eisenberg R et al: Circulating immune complexes in infective endocarditis. N Engl J Med 295:1500, 1976

89. Blumer G: Subacute bacterial endocarditis. Medicine 2:105, 1923

90. Cantrell M, Yoshikawa TT: Infective endocarditis in the aging patient. Gerontology 30:316, 1984

91. Cantrell M, Yoshikawa TT: Aging and infective endocarditis. J Am Geriatr Soc 31:216, 1983

92. Cherubin CE, Neu HC: Infective endocarditis at the Presbyterian hospital in New York City from 1938–1967. Am J Med 51:83, 1971

93. Cummings V, Furman S, Dunst M et al: Subacute bacterial endocarditis in the older age group. JAMA 172:137, 1960

94. Denham MF: Septicaemia and infective endocarditis. In Fox RA (ed): Immunology and Infection in the Elderly, p 137. New York, Churchill Livingstone, 1984

95. Durack DT: Prophylaxis of infective endocarditis. In Mandell GL, Douglas RG Jr, Bennett JE (eds): Principles and Practice of Infectious Diseases, p 539. New York, John Wiley & Sons, 1985

96. Durack DT, Beeson, PB: Pathogenesis of infective endocarditis. In Rahimtoola SH (ed): Infective Endocarditis. New York, Grune & Stratton, 1978

97. Gantz NM: Infective endocarditis. In Gleckman RA, Gantz NM (eds): Infections in the Elderly, p 217. Boston, Little, Brown & Co, 1983

98. Glecker WJ: Diagnostic aspects of subacute bacterial endocarditis in the elderly. Arch Intern Med 102:761, 1958

99. Gleckman R, Hibert D: Afebrile bacteremia: A phenomenon in geriatric patients. JAMA 248:1478, 1982

100. Gnann JW Jr, Cobbs CG: Infections of prosthetic valves and intravascular devices. In Mandell GL, Douglas RG Jr, Bennett JE (eds): Principles and Practice of Infectious Diseases, p 530. New York, John Wiley & Sons, 1985

101. Griffiths RA, Sheldon MG: The clinical significance of systolic murmurs in the elderly. Age Ageing 4:99, 1975

102. Hayes GS, Stinson IN: Erythrocyte sedimentation rate and age. Arch Ophthalmol 94:939, 1976

103. Hebte-Gabr E, January LE, Smith IM: Bacterial endocarditis: The need for early diagnosis. Geriatrics 28:164, 1973

104. Klein RS, Recco RA, Catalan MT et al: Association of *Streptococcus bovis* with carcinoma of the colon. N Engl J Med 297:80, 1977

105. Lowes JA, Williams G, Tabaqchali S et al: Ten years of infective endocarditis at St. Bartholomew's Hospital: Analysis of clinical features and treatment in relation to prognosis and mortality. Lancet 1:133, 1980

106. Murray HW, Robert RB: *Streptococcus bovis* bacteremia and underlying gastrointestinal disease. Arch Intern Med 138:1097, 1978

107. Pomerance A: Pathogenesis of aortic stenosis and its relation to age. Br Heart J 34:569, 1972

108. Pazin GJ, Saul S, Thompson ME: Blood culture positivity: Suppression by outpatient antibiotic therapy in patients with bacterial endocarditis. Arch Intern Med 142:263, 1982

109. Popp RL: Echocardiography and infectious endocarditis. In Remington JS, Swartz MN (eds): Current Clinical Topics in Infectious Diseases, p 98. New York, McGraw-Hill, 1983

110. Prevention of bacterial endocarditis. Med Let 26:3, 1984

111. Ries K: Endocarditis in the elderly. In Kaye D (ed): Infective Endocarditis, p 143. Baltimore, University Park Press, 1976

112. Robbins N, DeMaria A, Miller MH: Infective endocarditis in the elderly. South Med J 73:1335, 1980

113. Scheld WM, Sande MA: Endocarditis and intravascular infections. In Mandell GL, Douglas RG Jr, Bennett JE (eds): Principles and Practice of Infectious Diseases, p 504. New York, John Wiley & Sons, 1985

114. Scheld M, Valone JA, Sande MA: Bacterial adherence in the pathogenesis of endocarditis. J Clin Invest 58:1394, 1977

115. Tan JS, Watanakunakorn C, Terhune CA Jr: *Streptococcus viridans* endocarditis: Favorable prognosis in geriatric patients: Prognosis depends on correct identification of the organism and appropriate antibiotic therapy. Geriatrics 28:68, 1973

116. Thell R, Martin FH, Edwards JE: Bacterial endocarditis in subjects 60 years of age and older. Circulation 51:174, 1975

117. Von Reyn K, Levy BS, Arbeit RD et al: Infective endocarditis: I. An analysis based on strict case definitions. Ann Intern Med 94:505, 1981

118. Washington JA II: The role of the microbiology laboratory in the diagnosis and antimicrobial treatment of infective endocarditis. Mayo Clin Proc 57:22, 1982

119. Watanakunakorn C, Tan JC, Phair JP: Some salient features of *Staphylococcus aureus* endocarditis. Am J Med 54:473, 1973

120. Weinstein L, Rubin RH: Infective endocarditis—1973. Prog Cardiovasc Dis 16:239, 1973

121. Williams RC, Kunkel HG: Rheumatoid factors and their disappearance following therapy in patients with SBE. Arthritis Rheum 5:126, 1962

122. Wilson WR, Jaumin PM, Danielson GK et al: Prosthetic valve endocarditis. Ann Intern Med 82:751, 1975

123. Wiseman J, Rouleau J, Rigo P et al: Gallium-67 myocardial imaging for the detection of bacterial endocarditis. Radiology 120:135, 1976

124. Balfour HH, Bean B, Laskin O et al: Acyclovir halts progression of herpes zoster in immunocompromised patients. N Engl J Med 308:1448, 1983

125. Bean B, Braun C, Balfour HH: Acyclovir therapy for acute herpes zoster. Lancet 2:118, 1982

126. Bentley DW: Management of infection in the elderly. In Cape RDT, Coe RM, Rossman I (eds): Fundamentals of Geriatric Medicine, p 197. New York, Raven Press, 1983

127. Berger R, Luescher D, Just M: Enhancement of varicella-zoster-specific immune responses in the elderly by boosting with varicella vaccine. J Infect Dis 149:647, 1984

128. Betts RF, Dawlat AZ, Douglas RG et al: Ineffectiveness of subcutaneous cytosine arabinoside in localized herpes zoster. Ann Intern Med 82:778, 1976

129. Brunell PA: Varicella-zoster virus. In Mandell GL, Douglas RG Jr, Bennett JE (eds): Principles and Practice of Infectious Diseases, 2nd ed, p 952. New York, John Wiley & Sons, 1985

130. Burgoon CF, Burgoon JS, Baldridge GD: The natural history of herpes zoster. JAMA 164:265, 1957

131. Burke BL, Steele RW, Beard OW et al: Immune responses to varicella-zoster in the aged. Arch Intern Med 142:291, 1982

132. Crill WE: Carbamazepine. Ann Intern Med 79:844, 1973

133. Dolin R: Varicella-zoster virus infections. In Dolin R (moderator): Herpes zoster-varicella infections in immunosuppressed patients. Ann Intern Med 89:375, 1978

134. Eaglstein WH, Katz R, Brown JA: The effects of early corticosteroid therapy on the skin eruption and pain of herpes zoster. JAMA 211:1681, 1970

135. Epstein E: Treatment of herpes zoster and post-zoster neuralgia by sublesional injection of triamcinolone and procaine. Acta Derm Venereol 50:69, 1970

136. Farber GA, Burks JW: Chlorprothixene therapy for herpes zoster neuralgia. South Med J 67:808, 1974

137. Hope-Simpson RE: The nature of herpes zoster: A long-term study and a new hypothesis. Proc R Soc Med 58:9, 1965

138. Keczkes K, Basheer AM: Do corticosteroids prevent post-herpetic neuralgia? Br J Dermatol 102:551, 1980

139. Kernbaum S, Hauchecorne J: Administration of levodopa for relief of herpes zoster pain. JAMA 246:132, 1981

140. Mazur MH: Immunodiagnosis and immunoprophylaxis. In Dolin R (moderator): Herpes zoster-varicella infections in immunosuppressed patients. Ann Intern Med 89:375, 1978

141. Mazur MH, Whitley RJ, Dolin R: Serum antibody levels as risk factors in the dissemination of herpes zoster. Arch Intern Med 139:1341, 1979

142. Miller LH: Herpes zoster in the elderly. Cutis 18:427, 1976

143. Morens DM, Bregman DJ, West CM et al: An outbreak of varicella-zoster virus infection among cancer patients. Ann Intern Med 93:414, 1980

144. Peterslund NA, Ipsen J, Schonheyder H et al: Acyclovir in herpes zoster. Lancet 2:827, 1981

145. Rado JP, Tako J, Geder L et al: Herpes zoster house epidemic in steroid-treated patients. Arch Intern Med 116:329, 1965

146. Ragozzino MW, Melton LJ, Kurland LT et al: Population-based study of herpes zoster and its sequelae. Medicine 61:310, 1982

147. Ragozzino MW, Melton LJ, Kurland LT et al: Risk of cancer after herpes zoster: A population-based study. N Engl J Med 307:314, 1982

148. Reichman RC: Neurologic complications of varicella-zoster infections. In Dolin R (moderator): Herpes zoster-varicella infections in immunosuppressed patients. Ann Intern Med 89:375, 1978

149. Rogers RS, Tindall JP: Geriatric herpes zoster. J Am Geriatr Soc 19:495, 1971

150. Schimpff S, Serpick R, Stoler B et al: Varicella-zoster infection in patients with cancer. Ann Intern Med 76:241, 1972

151. Stevens DA, Ferrington RA, Jordan GW et al: Cellular events in zoster vesicles: Relation to clinical course and immune parameters. J Infect Dis 131:509, 1975

152. Uduman SA, Gershon AA, Brunell PA: Should patients with zoster receive zoster immune globulin? JAMA 234:1049, 1975

153. Watson CP, Evans RJ, Reed K et al: Amitriptyline versus placebo in postherpetic neuralgia. Neurology 32:671, 1982

154. Whitley RJ, Soong S-J, Dolin R et al: Early vidarabine therapy to control the complications of herpes zoster in immunosuppressed patients. N Engl J Med 307:971, 1982

155. Womack LW, Liesegang TJ: Complications of herpes zoster ophthalmicus. Arch Ophthalmol 101:42, 1983

156. Ad-hoc Working Group: Susceptibility of diphtheria. Lancet 1:428, 1978

157. Ammann AJ, Schiffman G, Austrian R: The antibody responses to pneumococcal capsular polysaccharides in aged individuals. Proc Soc Biol Med 164:312, 1980

158. Austrian R, Douglas RM, Schiffman G et al: Prevention of pneumococcal pneumonia by vaccination. Trans Assoc Am Phys 89:184, 1976

159. Barker WH, Mullooly JP: Influenza vaccination of elderly persons. JAMA 244:2547, 1980

160. Bentley DW: Immunisation. In Fox RA (ed): Immunology and Infection in the Elderly, p 333. Edinburgh, Churchill Livingstone, 1984

161. Bentley DW: Pneumococcal vaccine in the institutionalized elderly: Review of past and recent studies. Rev Infect Dis 3 (suppl):S61, 1981

162. Betts RF: Inactivated influenza vaccine reduces frequency and severity of illness in the elderly (abstr). Program and Abstracts of the 24th Interscience Conference on Antimicrobial Agents and Chemotherapy. Washington, DC, American Society for Microbiology, 1984

163. Borgono JM, McLean AA, Vella PP et al: Vaccination and revaccination with polyvalent pneumococcal polysaccharide vaccines in adults and infants. Proc Soc Exp Biol Med 157:148, 1978

164. Broome CV, Facklam RR, Fraser DW: Pneumococcal disease after pneumococcal vaccination: An alternative method to estimate the efficacy of pneumococcal vaccine. N Engl J Med 303:549, 1980

165. Centers for Disease Control: Diphtheria, tetanus, and pertussis: Guidelines for vaccine prophylaxis and other preventive measures. MMWR 30:393–396, 401–407, 1981

166. Centers for Disease Control: Update: Pneumococcal polysaccharide vaccine usage—United States. Ann Intern Med 101:348, 1984

167. Chapman WG, Davey MG: Tetanus immunity in Busselton, Western Australia, 1969. Med J Aust 2:316, 1973

168. Crossley K, Irvine P, Warren JB et al: Tetanus and diphtheria immunity in urban Minnesota adults. JAMA 242:2298, 1979

169. Gabor EP, Seeman M: Acute febrile systemic reaction to polyvalent pneumococcal vaccine. JAMA 242:2208, 1979

170. Giebink GS, Foker JE, Kim Y et al: Serum antibody and opsonic responses to vaccination with pneumococcal capsular polysaccharide in normal and splenectomized children. J Infect Dis 141:404, 1980

171. Fedson DS, Chiarello LA: Previous hospital care and pneumococcal bacteremia: Importance for pneumococcal immunization. Arch Intern Med 143:885, 1983

172. Hilleman MR, Carlson AJ Jr, McLean AA et al: *Streptococcus pneumoniae* polysaccharide vaccine: Age and dose responses, safety, persistence of antibody, revaccination, and simultaneous administration of pneumococcal and influenza vaccines. Rev Infect Dis 3(suppl):531, 1981

173. Kaplan JE, Katona P, Hurwitz ES et al: Guillain–Barré Syndrome in the United States, 1979–1980 and 1980–1981: Lack of an association with influenza vaccination. JAMA 13:248, 1982

174. LaForce FM, Young LS, Bennett JV: Tetanus in the United States 1965–1966. N Engl J Med 280:479, 1969

175. Landesman SH, Schiffman G: Assessment of the antibody response to pneumococcal vaccine in high-risk populations. Rev Infect Dis 3(suppl):S184, 1981

176. Mufson MA, Krause HE, Schiffman G: Long-term persistence of antibody following immunization with pneumococcal polysaccharide vaccine. Proc Soc Exp Biol Med 173:270, 1983

177. Patriarca PA, Weber JA, Parker RA et al: Efficacy of influenza vaccine in nursing homes: Reduction in illnesses, hospitalizations, pneumonia, and deaths during an influenza A (H3N2) epidemic in Genesee County, Michigan (abstr). Program and Abstracts of the 24th Interscience Conference on Antimicrobial Agents and Chemotherapy. Washington, DC, American Society for Microbiology, 1984

178. Pianko L, Sherman F, Rehr H et al: Acceptance of pneumococcal vaccination by the community residing elderly (abstr). Gerontologist 21(special issue):43, 1981

179. Ruben FL, Johnston F, Streiff EJ: Influenza in a partially immunized aged population. JAMA 230:863, 1974

179a. Ruben FL, Nagle J, Fireman P: Antitoxin responses in the elderly to tetanus-diptheria (td) immunization. Am J Epidemiol 108(2):145, 1978

180. Schwartz JS: Pneumococcal vaccine: Clinical efficacy and effectiveness. Ann Intern Med 96:208, 1982

181. Solomanova K, Vizev S: Secondary response to boostering by purified aluminium-hydroxide-adsorbed tetanus anatoxin in aging and in aged adults. Immunobiology 158:312, 1981

182. Solomonova K, Vizev S: Immunological reactivity of senescent and old people actively immunized with tetanus toxoid. Z Immun Exp Klin Immunol 146:81, 1973

183. Willems JS, Sanders CR, Riddiough MA et al: Cost effectiveness of pneumococcal vaccine. N Engl J Med 304:116, 1981

27 Surgical Problems in the Aged

Kevin Morrissey and Clarence J. Schein*

Although a formalized subspecialty of geriatric surgery does not presently exist, specialized knowledge as well as a broad perspective are required to deal skillfully with surgery in this age-group. A realistic knowledge of the surgical risk in relation to the symptoms and progress of the untreated disease is a prerequisite. The surgeon should also be sensitive to the dignity and right to self-determination that many elderly or infirm patients hold on to tenaciously. Information gleaned from relatives or friends, if the patients is unable to communicate adequately, may profoundly influence the indications for surgery, the timing of operative intervention, and the magnitude of excisional procedures. The surgical procedure itself should be oriented toward maximal preservation of functional integrity. It is an exercise in futility to convert a functioning patient into a surgically cured unhappy invalid. The surgeon has to balance the realistic operative risk for that person in terms of invalidism, morbidity, and mortality, not against the estimated salvage time alone but also against the quality and degree of restored or retained independent functioning.

One must also learn to recognize that the surgical problem may be the final episode in a series of events from which the patient could not survive. For example, 2 decades ago it may have been acceptable and even heroic surgical practice to attempt proximal gastrectomy in a patient with cancer of the cardia and severe pulmonary insufficiency with cor pulmonale, but today it would be considered foolhardy. Fortunately, a host of endoscopic and other less traumatic alternatives to major surgery are rapidly evolving to assist in care and palliation of disorders of the elderly.

It is no longer necessary for individual surgeons to rediscover the risks of standard procedures in the geriatric age-group since there is now a substantial published experience detailing risk factors, preventive measures, complications, operative mortality, and survival rates.[34,41,42,52,53,66,75,92,93,99]

Despite the enormous interest in analyzing the surgical problems associated with aging, an impediment exists in the variable manner of reporting geriatric surgical studies.[59,80] Many interesting or provocative small studies cannot easily be incorporated into statistical analysis. In a review of 108 such studies over the past 40 years, Linn and co-workers[59] were unable to find a clear answer to the crucial question of relative risk of surgery with advancing age. Sources of confusing variance among such studies include dissimilar age criteria for the term *elderly*; uneven and incomplete classification of mortality data (*e.g.*, immediate or late postoperative, caused by or unrelated to surgery; classification as a death whether occurring during hospitalization or after discharge); and poor distinction between emergency and elective surgical procedures. Nevertheless, much has been learned about risk factors and perioperative maneuvers to correct or minimize them.

RISK FACTORS FOR SURGERY

Age

Depending on how one views it, chronologic age is or is not a risk factor for predicting mortality and morbidity figures in the elderly.[13,27,48,59,66] Many cumulative reports provide age-related data such as comparatively increased mortality figures for the geriatric population by specific surgical procedure.[99] However, emergency as well as elective procedures are grouped together with other risk

* Deceased.

factors that may be associated with but not necessarily due to advancing age. It is best when evaluating an individual patient to view age as a contributing but not a global depressing factor affecting all other parameters.

Goldman and associates[38,39] have delineated the role of age *per se* as a very important predictor of cardiac complications. In their series, the risk of perioperative cardiac death was increased by a factor of 10 for patients older than 70 years. Hirsch and Schwartz[48] documented an increased mortality among elderly patients undergoing cataract extraction. Adult-onset diabetes commonly associated with cataract did not account for the excess mortality. The conclusion of their study was that the development of clinically important senile cataracts was not a local disorder but a result of systemic processes associated with aging and poorer survival from an otherwise minimally traumatic operation.

Cardiac Risks

Ischemic heart disease (in particular, a recent myocardial infarction) is the most serious risk factor in elderly patients. A myocardial infarction, either subendocardial or transmural, within 3 months preceding surgery, is associated with either another myocardial infarction or cardiac death in 30% of patients. This figure decreases to 15% if surgery occurs 3 to 6 months following a heart attack and decreases further to a constant 5% risk after the 6-month interval.[38,86,92] More recent data indicate that myocardial infarction risk rates within 0 to 6 months of surgery may have been reduced further owing to advances in anesthesia, preoperative assessment, and perioperative monitoring and treatment of arrhythmias and hemodynamic problems.[7,26,45,96]

Congestive heart failure from all causes, but especially a prior myocardial infarction, valvular heart disease, and fluid overload, is another major risk factor in elderly patients. The ability to correct or control preoperative congestive heart failure substantially reduces the risk of surgery.[39] Cardiac arrhythmias such as frequent ventricular premature contractions or a rhythm other than normal sinus rhythm may be a sign of serious coronary artery disease and ventricular dysfunction that will predispose to cardiac complications. Some cardiac related factors, such as hypertension, hyperlipidemia, stable angina, and cigarette smoking, surprisingly do not correlate with increased risk of cardiac complications following general anesthesia and surgery.[38]

Pulmonary Risks

The usual age-related changes in arterial Po_2 and other tests of lung function (see Chapter 14) without coincident cardiac or pulmonary disease do not appear to be severe enough to increase significantly the risk of pulmonary complications in elderly patients.[53] However, the common pulmonary complications (respiratory insufficiency, pneumonia, and atelectasis) certainly do occur more often in patients with preexisting chronic lung disease.

Nutritional and Immunologic Status

Many elderly patients, particularly those with cancer or facing emergency surgery, have evidence of significant nutritional deficits.[8,72] The general assumption has long been that starved patients tolerate surgery or any stress less well. There is now considerable interest in documenting less obvious nutritional depletion and relating nutritional replacement or maintenance to improved morbidity and mortality. With regard to important aspects of immunologic status, healthy older patients appear similar to younger ones preoperatively.[58] Although some aspects of the immune responses are more depressed by surgery in healthy older patients, these are not significant enough to affect adversely the outcome of surgery, and in fact the clinical outcome of an elective surgical procedure is no different between healthy young and old patients. The effects of nutritional deficiency on immunologic function are only beginning to be appreciated,[3] and efficacious ways of correcting or compensating for nutritional deficits in elderly patients facing surgery need to be developed.

Emergency Surgery

Elderly patients undergo more emergency operations than the young or middle-aged, and this is unequivocally a major predictor of increased complications and fatal outcome.[9,37,39,41] On average, an emergency operation carries about three times increased risk of major morbidity and mortality than the same elective procedure. Cardiac complications alone are up to four times more common following emergency procedures. When the magnitude of an emergency operation can be lessened or staged to a second more elective procedure (*e.g.*, colostomy instead of obstructive resection or endoscopic decompression of sigmoid volvulus rather than emergency colostomy), there are significant reductions in surgical mortality.

Other Factors

Demented patients do far less well than those in command of their mental faculties. Chronic renal disease and diabetes are generally associated with poorer patient response to stress, which is not necessarily peculiar to the aged population. The type of general anesthesia administered is not a risk factor. Local anesthesia avoids some of the cardiopulmonary risks of general anesthesia and is preferable when possible. Spinal anesthesia does not diminish risks to the cardiovascular system except perhaps in patients with congestive heart failure and should not be chosen solely on this basis. Often careful balanced general anesthesia in good hands avoids other problems with muscular relaxation, pain, and patient anxiety that might adversely affect the duration or difficulty of the same procedure under local anesthesia.[39,64] The mental health of the patient (*e.g.*, depression) affects the ability to cooperate with medical personnel in combating the stresses of illness in general and surgery in particular, and dementia is a major impairment in this regard.

RISK REDUCTION AND PERIOPERATIVE MANAGEMENT

Identification of pertinent risk factors leads naturally to measures to monitor and correct or compensate for them.[33,38,53,95] An interested consulting physician is often the cornerstone of the global care of the elderly patient. He fills in the important gaps in nonsurgical care. Care must be taken in evaluating the cardiopulmonary status of the patient, in particular, in adjusting or discontinuing some chronic medications (*e.g.*, analgesics, anticoagulants, bronchodilators, and cardiovascular and diuretic drugs).

Only if historical data warrant it are special pulmonary function tests, arterial blood gases, cardiac exercise tests, or angiographic studies indicated preoperatively. Their routine use, as well as the practice of routine pulmonary artery catheterization and hemodynamic measurements that have been advocated by some clinicians, are associated with low rates of surgical complications in the elderly, but it appears that the same results can be achieved by risk assessment and management relying on more conventional noninvasive measures.[26]

It is well to remember that even with apparently uncomplicated surgery the elderly patient with underlying ischemic heart disease remains at risk for significant cardiovascular problems for up to 6 days postoperatively; too early relaxation of attention can be catastrophic.

Many elderly patients have known persons who have died after an operation. Their anxieties, feelings of hopelessness, and isolation are understandable. It should be the definitive responsibility of at least one senior member of the surgical team to be the patient's doctor and help by explaining, in advance, what will happen. The use of tubes, catheters, intravenous feedings, and respirators should be anticipated by explanations in the patient's own language. The postoperative procedures should be explained in advance, so that respiratory care and the management of pain, drains, and dressings do not come as unanticipated assaults that have dire implications.

First-night care is particularly critical. If a member of the surgical team is present on the evening of the operation to assist in the problems of voiding, ventilation, and pain, the patient is more likely to be cooperative and to develop an optimistic attitude toward survival.

At the extremes of age there is less latitude for error in equivocal decisions. The best results can be anticipated when the surgery does only what is required and avoids or manages in advance events that contribute to the morbidity of a particular procedure.

Sometimes it is best not to intervene surgically. Thus the surgeon cannot disregard the social implications of advanced organic mental syndrome. The patient's motivation and future prospects play an important role in decision making.

HERNIAS

The indications for hernioplasty in the elderly are not as absolute as in the pediatric age-group or in young adults. Also, the appearance of the bulge in the abdominal wall may herald an occult neoplasm within the peritoneal cavity, benign prostatic hypertrophy, or progressive respiratory disease. Thus, supportive laboratory and radiologic studies are indicated prior to elective hernia repair.

Surgery for intra-abdominal tumors often permits concomitant hernioplasty, particularly in the case of ventral incisional hernia from a previous abdominal operation. For a small congenital inguinal hernia defect, simple plication of the peritoneum and adjacent fascial margins suffices. In some instances, the celiotomy incision may be planned so that simultaneous repair of a groin hernia could be done by a properitoneal approach.

In the majority of such cases, however, longstanding groin hernias that are easily reducible, either direct or indirect but with a wide neck to the hernia sac, should be left alone, and attention should be directed to the expeditious surgical handling of the major intra-abdominal problem.

Progressive pulmonary insufficiency in an elderly patient with a symptomatic inguinal hernia is a surgical trap. Every effort should be made to improve the pulmonary status of the patient, thereby relieving both respiratory and hernia symptoms. Hernia repair is indicated only in the event of incarceration and should be done under local anesthesia, with maximum medical support to avoid postoperative endotracheal intubation and further respiratory failure.

In the elderly man, the coexistence of inguinal hernia and prostatism is so common that the relationship must not be overlooked. Urologic consultation, with tests of urine flow, residual volume, and urodynamics, should be obtained preoperatively; if the enlarged prostate requires resection, this should precede the hernioplasty.[22]

In the elective repair of inguinal and femoral hernias, local anesthesia is preferred. General or spinal anesthesia is not necessary and may predispose to significant cardiopulmonary and urologic complications.[71]

The repair of groin hernias under local anesthesia has several advantages, not the least of which is the opportunity for intraoperative testing of the repair with the patient voluntarily straining.[21,57] Prompt ambulation often avoids postoperative urinary retention in the male; there is an early restoration of well-being and a sense of not having been through an extensive ordeal.

Indirect Hernia

Indirect inguinal hernias are particularly apt to become incarcerated. Acutely incarcerated bowel, with or without strangulation, demands emergency surgery. Resection of the small bowel is frequently indicated and often can be carried out through the inguinal incision. The surgeon should not hesitate to extend the inguinal incision or make a separate laparotomy incision if necessary to reduce the hernia or resect the bowel. The risk of entering or resecting the bowel is high in any patient with an incarcerated hernia, and the administration of broad-spectrum antibiotics preoperatively and intraoperatively is advisable. Such perioperative antibiotic coverage, as well as the technique of leaving the skin and subcutaneous fatty layers of the wound packed lightly open, in the event the bowel has been entered, will substantially decrease the incidence of sepsis, wound infection, and subsequent hernia recurrence. If there is any concern by the surgeon about the viability of incarcerated bowel after it has been reduced by manipulation, it is better to resect the intestine than risk subsequent bowel infarction and emergent re-laparotomy with its substantially higher mortality and morbidity.

When an indirect hernia becomes progressively larger or symptomatic, early surgical intervention is advised by most groups experienced in the care of elderly patients. On the other hand, a hernia may be carefully followed in poor-risk, elderly patients. Either the patient or a responsible member of the family is thoroughly briefed on the complications and danger signals of incarceration. Surgery is delayed until significant symptoms appear. However, when considering a course of expectant treatment rather than immediate surgery, it is well to keep in mind that the reported mortality for emergency inguinal hernia repair in the aged ranges between 7% and 22%, while elective hernia repair carries only a 1.2% to 2% operative mortality in the properly prepared elderly patient.[71]

Large neglected scrotal hernias often of the indirect type are not unusual in the aged. Their repair cannot be considered routine. The abdominal wall defect may be so large as to preclude a primary repair without tension. The available fascial margins may be of poor quality or the right of domain may have been lost and the scrotum may contain a large portion of the abdominal viscera. Elective resection of such viscera is not indicated in an attempt to achieve intra-abdominal restoration. Pulmonary insufficiency secondary to elevation of the diaphragmatic leaflets or focal atelectasis owing to retained secretions, bilateral testicular compromise, and higher rates of recurrence and wound infections dissuade many surgeons from undertaking such repairs.

Huge scrotal hernias can be repaired in intact and physiologically sound geriatric patients. It is very gratifying to observe the personality alterations after removal of what has been virtually an accessory appendage that is repugnant, difficult to clean, and often a hindrance to daily activities.

Special measures helpful in the successful operative management of scrotal hernias are as follows: Mechanical bowel preparation to reduce the volume of large bowel that may need to be reduced in size to accommodate intraperitoneal replacement of the hernia contents; a 2- to 3-day preoperative skin care regimen with mild detergent soaps that along with perioperative antibiotics may reduce the incidence of postoperative wound infection; and preoperative and postoperative blood gas determinations and, if indicated, a period of postoperative endotracheal intubation and positive-pressure ventilatory support.

Synthetic abdominal wall replacements by plastic meshes as well as autogenous fascia are important adjuncts to the management of such large hernias.[61] Repair may be facilitated by orchiectomy and excision of the spermatic cord or by division of the spermatic cord at the level of the internal spermatic ring without testicular mobilization. Preservation of extraspermatic blood supply to the testis avoids tecticular atrophy and the major problem of infarction with abscess formation. Such complications contribute to recurrence of the original problem.

Direct Hernia

Because direct inguinal hernias rarely strangulate, expectant rather than surgical treatment is often quite satisfactory, and use of a truss may be successful. In contrast, with an indirect inguinal hernia, the obliquity of the inquinal canal makes the truss virtually useless and perhaps even dangerous. Complications such as superficial and deep decubiti, infections, and desmoplasia may occur when a truss is improperly used. Although trusses are readily available and easily applied, it is best to restrict their use to direct inguinal hernias for which surgery is otherwise contraindicated. The clinical distinction between a direct and an indirect hernia is not always correct, and direct hernias may become incarcerated. Thus, one should not preclude surgery for a presumed safe, longstanding direct hernia.

Femoral Hernia

A high index of awareness increases the diagnosis of uncompromised femoral hernia, especially in the elderly female. Elective surgery is almost always advised because incarceration is so frequent and carries a high mortality.[91] Occasionally, femoral hernias are mistaken for inguinal hernias. The repair from above, in which the medial portion of the femoral canal is obliterated after entering the inguinal canal through the external oblique aponeurosis, is the procedure of choice. The alternative procedure is the repair from below, in which the inguinal ligament is sutured to the pectineus fascia after ligation and reduction of the femoral sac. The latter approach is particularly innocuous in the geriatric patient who requires urgent repair with minimal manipulation and anesthesia time.

Umbilical Hernia

All symptomatic umbilical hernias should be repaired, preferably under elective circumstances. Umbilical hernia is a common defect in the aged and has a high incidence of incarceration. If strangulation is suspected, surgical reduction and repair should be done promptly.

Ventral Incision Hernia

Incisional hernias are very common in elderly, obese patients. Local factors to be evaluated include location, size, quality of fascial margins, and condition of skin. Ventral hernias in the upper abdominal quadrants are less prone to incarceration than those in the lower quadrants, because small bowel is not ordinarily present in the supracolic compartment of the peritoneal cavity. Hernias in this area usually contain omentum, liver, transverse colon, and stomach. If surgical repair is inadvisable, a fitted elastic girdle sometimes provides both physical and psychological relief. However, when the hernia cannot be reduced because of adhesions and interstitial compartmentalization, an external support may be contraindicated. Many obese patients with longstanding incarcerated small bowel in a ventral incisional hernia have this apparently unchanged region quickly passed over when they finally develop symptoms and often have gangrenous bowel before the correct diagnosis and surgical treatment is undertaken.

Hiatal Hernia

The vast majority of sliding hiatal hernias are asymptomatic, and their radiographic demonstration does not require further investigation or treatment. Hiatal hernias in the aged are usually silent, but complications such as bleeding may be life threatening. This is caused by acid reflux esophagitis. Its management is similar to that employed in peptic ulcer. Small intermittent bleeding episodes can be well tolerated; infrequently, massive hemorrhage necessitates surgical intervention. Endoscopic evaluation is mandatory.

Paraesophageal hiatal hernia is uncommon but more apt to be troublesome in the elderly. Incarceration and volvulus of the stomach may occur, requiring emergency treatment. Occasionally, the stomach may be acutely decompressed endoscopically before strangulation or perforation occurs. When strangulation occurs, mortality rises steeply. Elective transabdominal repair of these hernias is simple, dramatically improves symptoms, and carries a very low mortality rate.[77]

MALIGANT NEOPLASMS

Breast Cancer

Carcinoma of the breast is the most common and most lethal form of cancer among women. The specific management of the geriatric patient in the group that is usually 20 or more years post menopause is no better defined than for any other age-group. The standard therapeutic approach had been the radical mastectomy. Simple mastectomy with radiation therapy or each of these alone, modified radical mastectomy, and extended radical mastectomy have all been advocated by those dissatisfied with the unaltered survival rates achieved by the classic operation. Voluminous statistical analyses have been forwarded in the past as arguments in favor of one or the other procedure, but it is doubtful that significant improvement of survival and cure rates will occur until more is known of the biologic predeterminism of breast cancer and its specific growth characteristics. Mammography and newer techniques may ultimately prove to be valuable in leading to earlier diagnosis and treatment, with improved results.[43]

Despite opinions to the contrary, there is good evidence now that breast cancer in elderly patients is every bit as aggressive, grows at an equal rate, and kills as surely as breast cancers in younger women.[1,44,70] Advanced age alone should not be the excuse for doing a less aggressive operation. The hope for long-term survival in the elderly is equivalent to that for the young when treatment methods most likely to effect a cure for a given stage of the disease are used.[21,44,55]

These operations can often be done under local anesthesia by direct infiltration and nerve block techniques. If the surgeon is patient and waits for the full anesthetic effect, 100 ml to 150 ml of 0.5% lidocaine (Xylocaine) is adequate for total mastectomy and axillary dissection. Operative mortality rates for elderly patients undergoing cancer surgery are reported at 4.8% versus 3.4% for all ages.[44]

There is great advantage to doing a preoperative needle aspiration, incisional, or excisional biopsy on an ambulatory basis. One can then specifically plan the optimum operative procedure. It is important to regard all outpatient biopsies as though the patient has a potentially malignant lesion and to submit the tissue for hormonal receptor assay in addition to the usual histologic examination.

The size of the lesion, the condition of the skin, an estimation of survival time in terms of other systems and the expressed wishes of the patient influence the choice of procedure. In general the preference now is for modified radical mastectomy. Simple mastectomy without axillary lymph node dissection may be done in patients less able to tolerate the more extensive procedure. About 50% of women with breast cancer at age 75 will die of the disease before their otherwise approximately 10-year life expectancy has been attained. There is a recent wave of enthusiasm and promising early data for local excision of breast neoplasms, combined with axillary lymph node dissection and supervoltage external beam irradiation. Postoperative radiation therapy does not improve the cure rate but may deter or delay local recurrence of already extensive lesions.

Because cosmetic and sexual factors are not importantly involved in the geriatric patient, the trend toward mastectomy procedures is related to the desire for primary healing, diminished risk of local recurrence, and the opportunity to avoid the problems in transportation and the small but significant morbidity of 4 to 6 weeks of daily radiation treatment. Often, elderly patients' neoplasms are estrogen receptor positive;[62] and such adjuvant treatment, without cytotoxic chemotherapy will prolong disease-free intervals if not survival.[60] There is evidence that tamoxifen alone may induce complete radiologic remissions in elderly women with small neoplasms less than 4.2 cc and who refuse any form of surgical treatment.[43]

Lymph node positivity in elderly patients is a very bad prognostic sign, and many such patients will be dead from their disease within 5 years, regardless of the type of treatment.[1] Reported relative 5-year survival data for patients age 65 and over are 85% for localized disease and 58.2% for regional disease (lymph nodes positive).[44] Such data underline the assertion that elderly breast cancer patients may enjoy the same survival rate as younger patients, if treated by comparable surgical techniques.

Colon and Rectal Cancer

Cancer of the colon and rectum is the leading cancer cause of death among men and women over 50 years of age in the United States. It is a threat to life in the elderly as in the young, and generally the same surgical principles should be applied to its treatment. Age as an isolated factor appears to have little effect on the operative mortality of colon resections for cancer; rather, it is the preexisting diseases that increase with age (*e.g.,* cardiovascular, pulmonary, metabolic, and nutritional problems).[13] When more than one significant preexisting condition occurs in the same elderly patient, and when emergency rather than elective colon surgery is necessary, the operative mortality increases steeply to 16% to 18%, as compared with 5% to 8% for better risk patients over 70 years of age.[18,19] The high risk of emergency colon operation in the aged and its septic complications are particularly aggravated by nutritional or pulmonary deficiencies that could not be corrected preoperatively.

Prevention

Elderly patients who receive good medical care are an ideal group for the prevention of far advanced, chronically bleeding, or acutely obstructing colon cancers. During routine medical visits, care should be taken to inquire about rectal bleeding, change in bowel habit, or symptoms such as syncope, angina or weakness, or abdominal cramps.

A past or family history of colonic neoplasia should be a clear indication to carry out periodic tests for anemia, occult blood in the stool, and radiographic or endoscopic surveillance studies of the colon at 1- to 3-year intervals according to the estimated degree of risk.[98] Timely colonoscopic polypectomy should prove within the next decade capable of dramatically reducing the incidence of colon cancers, as has already been demonstrated in the case of rectal cancers.[32]

Early Cancer

The development of colonoscopy and polypectomy over the past 15 years in the United States has already produced a significant decline in the number, mortality, and morbidity of operations for benign or focally malignant colonic neoplasms.

The decision whether or not to advise colon resection for an elderly patient with invasive cancer in a polyp is controversial. In the younger, good-risk patient, bowel resection is preferable. The presence or absence of significant preexisting diseases rather than advanced age should be a guideline to advising surgery or settling for local control by colonoscopic resection and accepting the small subsequent risk of lymph node and distant spread of disease.[17]

Advanced Cancer

Surgical resection is indicated for all patients young or old in whom colon cancer has thoroughly invaded the wall of the colon and chronic hemorrhage or luminal obstruction is inevitable. An exception to this dictum might be the hopelessly ill patient with widespread metastatic disease

and no hope for cure. Transfusion of blood and low residue diet with stool softeners may suffice to forestall an emergency operation in the brief time remaining. The presence of lymph node or hepatic metastases alone is not a contraindication to surgery even in the aged. Carcinoma of the colon may progress very slowly, even in an advanced stage. If there is no evidence for severe impairment of liver function, and the symptomatic mass of the tumor is resected or can be bypassed, the patient may derive from 3 months to 1 or more years of restored quality of life prior to the eventual death. The computed tomographic (CT) scan has added an extra dimension to the assessment of patients with advanced colon cancer. Thus, at operation when there is no apparent regional or hepatic extension the foreknowledge of intrahepatic or high para-aortic metastatic disease gained by CT scanning is extremely useful in deciding on the extent of surgery for cure or palliation.

Obstructing or partially obstructing neoplasms of the right or left colon pose different problems in optimum surgical management. As a group, half of these patients already have metastatic pericolic lymph nodes and at least 20% have hepatic metastases. Nevertheless, palliative or staged operations can be very beneficial.

Primary resection is usually possible for acutely obstructed right-sided colon tumors. If the patient is severely ill or has multiple risk factors predisposing to septic complications, a proximal ileostomy and distal mucus fistula is preferable to risking the time and problems inherent in a primary anastomosis in unprepared bowel. Partially obstructing tumors can almost always be operated on after a period of mechanical and antibiotic bowel preparation, and if necessary, a 10- to 12-day delay for parenteral hyperalimentation or restoration of other decompensated conditions. If the tumor is found to be unresectable, it can nevertheless be bypassed internally by a side-to-side enterocolostomy, thus avoiding the depressing and debilitating effects of permanent intestinal stomas on elderly patients.

Acute obstruction of the left side of the colon requires a diverting colostomy. Usually this is best done as a loop colostomy in the right transverse colon. Occasionally a sigmoid neoplasm will lend itself to rapid mobilization and resection without anastomosis, bringing out the proximal descending colon as an end colostomy and either closing the distal rectosigmoid segment or tacking it open to the abdominal wall as a mucus fistula. The advantage of this latter alternative is twofold: (1) the more distal colostomy emits less liquid stool, is smaller, and is easier for the patient to manage and (2) as such, it is a preferable long-term colostomy in the event the patient's spread of disease or associated medical problems militate against a subsequent surgical procedure. A proximal right-transverse loop colostomy, on the other hand, relieves the obstructive symptoms, and often the bleeding from a distal colonic neoplasm, but local and distant signs and symptoms from progression of the tumor remain a problem. A subsequent attempt at curative or palliative resection is almost always indicated.

Rectosigmoid and Rectal Cancer

These neoplasms are less often completely obstructing, but frequently present at a far-advanced stage. Even with satisfactory bowel preparation, and time for preoperative preparation, the magnitude of either a low-anterior resection or an abdominoperineal resection adds considerably to the operative surface area traumatized, the duration of operation, and the intraoperative and postoperative blood and fluid requirements. Once again the crucial medical-surgical decision will be the appropriate procedure commensurate with the risk status of the elderly patient.

Rectal cancers confined below the peritoneal reflection in extremely high-risk patients present the possibility of electrocoagulation, laser ablation, or supervoltage x-radiation in lieu of surgical resection. Often these techniques will suffice to avoid or put off a diverting colostomy. When a colostomy does become necessary for control of symptoms of obstruction, pain, bleeding, or incontinence, it may be done with the benefit of preliminary mechanical bowel preparation and local anesthesia. In the better risk patient, an abdominoperineal resection can often be done with less time expenditure or risk of septic complications than a low-anterior resection for a high rectal or rectosigmoid tumor. Both procedures carry a high risk of permanently decompensating marginally symptomatic prostatism in the male, and often need to be followed by a transurethral resection or cystostomy.

A low-anterior resection of the rectum or rectosigmoid is usually a long and difficult operation, particularly in male patients. The use of anastomotic stapling devices has not made the operation appreciably easier or shorter, nor does it necessarily avoid a temporary diverting colostomy or decrease the risk of anastomotic recurrence of tumor. Often in the elderly high-risk patient it is wiser to consider only resection of the tumor, with forma-

tion of a proximal permanent end-sigmoid colostomy and simple closure or drainage of the rectal stump.

There are some patients with impaired vision, poor motor coordination, or senility for whom a colostomy will always be just barely manageable even with constant assistance. On the other hand, a colostomy in a senile patient often facilitates nursing care and avoids the frustration and labors involved in trying to maintain a clean perineum and avoid decubitus ulcers.

Gastric Cancer

The incidence and death rate for gastric cancer in the United States continue to fall. For 1985, the estimated incidence of new cases is 24,700 and of deaths is 14,300,[15] which is a death rate of approximately 8 per 100,000, one-fourth of the death rate 50 years ago. Although early diagnosis and gastric resection improve the overall cure rates slightly, it is seldom possible to detect these tumors at an early stage in elderly patients. Cachexia, considerable weight loss, anemia, and hypoalbuminemia are common presenting signs. Very extensive tumors may also produce disturbances in swallowing or gastric emptying as well.

The diagnosis is usually evident on the gastrointestinal series. Often, endoscopy alone is diagnostic or will be helpful in differentiating the tumor from a large or benign gastric ulcer. If the diagnosis is certain and the tumor is clearly not resectable, nothing more need be done if the patient is asymptomatic. However, if the tumor appears resectable and the patient is a potential candidate for surgery, then an abdominal CT scan is helpful. Many gastric cancers will thus be proven far more widespread than clinical, radiographic, or endoscopic examinations would indicate. Surgery may then be decided against in the very high risk or minimally symptomatic patient, or the nature or extent of the intended operation better ascertained.

Chronically bleeding or partially obstructing tumors are often well palliated by a subtotal gastrectomy. If at all possible, particularly in the incurable patient, one should try to preserve a small cuff of gastric wall in performing a proximal gastrectomy for a high lesion. Preoperative parenteral hyperalimentation and a stapled anastomosis is preferred if esophagogastrectomy is anticipated. Both contribute to a diminished anastomotic leak rate and operative mortality in debilitated patients.

Total gastrectomy is best avoided and is practically never indicated as a palliative procedure.

Gastrostomy or jejunostomy alone, for nutritional purposes, is not advised since it does not relieve symptoms related to obstruction, compression, or blood loss. These problems may be adequately palliated by endoscopic laser therapy or passage of an endoprosthesis, with restitution of ability to take oral feeding.

Pancreatic and Peripancreatic Cancer

The role of surgery in the diagnosis and management of pancreatic and peripancreatic neoplasms has become very limited, especially in the geriatric group. Pancreatic cancer, now the fourth leading cause of cancer death in the United States, can usually be diagnosed and its extent determined by less invasive modalities such as CT scan and sonography with guided percutaneous needle biopsy or by endoscopic retrograde cholangiopancreatography (ERCP), angiography, and laparoscopy. Surgery is rarely curative. In the 40-year experience at the New York Hospital-Cornell Medical Center, long-term survival data of pancreaticoduodenectomy were related to final pathologic diagnosis as follows: adenocarcinoma of the pancreas, 0%; duodenal carcinoma, 38%; ampullary carcinoma, 30%; common bile duct carcinoma, 24%, and benign diseases, usually inflammatory, 100%.[16] Cumulative surgical series continue to report high mortality rates and warn against this operation in patients over 65 years of age.

Operative bypass of the obstructed biliary tree is still an effective palliative procedure.[81] Because of advanced disease in many patients, bypass procedures such as cholecystojejunostomy or choledochojejunostomy carry a high operative mortality in the range of 8% to 33% and yield an average patient survival of only 5 to 6 months. In some cases good palliation can extend well beyond 1 year. If obstruction of the gastric outlet is a result of advanced pancreatic cancer, or appears imminent, then dual bypass of the biliary tree and stomach is to be considered.

During the past 10 years, transhepatic percutaneous biliary stents, and more recently, endoscopically placed biliary stents have revolutionized the management of obstructing tumors of the bile duct system and the head of the pancreas.[83] Survival is not prolonged, but the procedure-related mortality is negligible and the morbidity is very acceptable. Endoscopically placed internal stents are preferable to the percutaneous drains. They avoid one more draining tube with which the debilitated patient has to cope. Cholangitis from stent-catheter sepsis can be a major and recurring problem. It is one reason to consider operative bypass in the better risk patient regardless of age, when the disease appears still limited. A better quality of remaining time might thus be enjoyed without need for repetitive catheter manipulations and courses of antibiotics.

ESOPHAGEAL CANCER

Esophageal neoplasms may be treated in a variety of ways, depending primarily on their anatomical location, gross extent, and histologic type. Elderly people tolerate palliative radiation or laser therapy with a tolerance equal to those in younger age-groups.

With regard to attempts to cure by surgical resection, there is little reported literature specific for the aged.[88] Major resectional and reconstructive procedures have generally been avoided in the elderly because of the very high morbidity and mortality associated with pulmonary and anastomotic complications. Interestingly, the 5-year survival rate of 25% for carefully selected patients operated on for cure is roughly equal for age-groups under 60, 60 to 69, and over 70 years of age. Important considerations are very careful preoperative selection and readiness to continue with mechanical assisted ventilation, frequent endotracheal suction, and attention to cough dynamics during the postoperative period.

ACUTE AND CHRONIC GASTROINTESTINAL DISEASES

Biliary Tract Disease

The septagenarian who, when younger, had a cholecystectomy may be very fortunate, since "benign" extrahepatic bilary tract disease is the bane of the geriatric patient. Operations on the biliary tract account for the majority of abdominal operations and of the surgical mortality in the aged person. The great percentage of operations are for complications of calculous disease, with a lesser percentage for acalculous inflammation and for malignant obstructions of the bile ducts.

Calculous Disease

Cholesterol calculous formation accounts for the prevalence of biliary tract surgery in women between the early and middle years of life. For not fully known reasons, men begin to form pigment or mixed composition gallstones at a greater rate than women after 60 years of age, and so the prevalence of symptomatic biliary tract disease begins to even out for both sexes after the seventh decade. Autopsy studies show a 50% incidence of gallbladder stones in persons over age 70.[24] In many instances such calculus disease was either asymptomatic or tolerably symptomatic, whereas in approximately 8% of cadavers with gallstones, inflammatory biliary tract disease is thought to have been the cause of death.[14] Gallstone disease can be categorized by the severity of signs and symptoms, as follows.

Asymptomatic Patients. Cholecystectomy is generally not advised for patients with silent gallstones. Studies of the natural history of asymptomatic gallstone disease indicate little advantage to prophylactic cholecystectomy, especially in the elderly age-group.[40] Fear of gallbladder cancer as a reason for prophylactic cholecystectomy is not justified, except in the case of a patient with calcifications in the wall of the gallbladder. Twenty-five percent of such ''porcelain'' gallbladders harbor a carcinoma.

Moderately Symptomatic Patients. Symptoms may range from indigestion and fatty food intolerance to periodic attacks of severe colic or even transient bouts of acute cholecystitis or common bile duct obstruction. It should be recalled that at least 20% to 30% of patients over age 70 with symptomatic biliary tract disease will have associated choledocholithiasis.[33,50,89] It has been repeatedly noted that it is difficult to diagnose an acute exacerbation of moderately symptomatic disease in elderly individuals, and therefore a much higher percentage will have acute cholecystitis when finally operated on, often as an emergency.

Current medical practice is to consider an elective cholecystectomy in an elderly patient, depending on the degree of functional disability of the patient and his surgical risk profile, as well as anticipated life expectancy. This equation does not often take into account the unpredictability of disease progression in the aged, nor the tremendous difference in operative risk once the clinical situation becomes acute.

The risk of death following elective cholecystectomy in elderly patients is reported between 2% and 4%, with the increasing incidence proportional to age.[14,50,89] Pulmonary and cardiovascular complications, as expected, are the major causes of mortality and morbidity. Emergency cholecystectomy in the same age-group carries a 10% to

16% mortality and a correspondingly higher morbidity. Confronted with these statistics, the physician must be vigilant in observing symptomatic patients and aggressive in his recommendations for early elective surgical or endoscopic procedures.

Patients with a large solitary gallstone are statistically more likely to develop an acute cholecystitis than patients with smaller stones.[14] However, the latter group has more common duct stones in association with gallbladder lithiasis. Thus elective cholecystectomy may be more readily recommended with a large solitary calculus, with the expectation of probably not finding any reason to explore the common duct as well. Surgery in a moderately symptomatic patient with multiple small stones includes the higher probability of a common duct exploration. A preoperative ERCP or at least an intraoperative cystic duct cholangiogram should be done in such patients.

The extremely high-risk patient with moderately severe symptoms from a large solitary calculus might be considered for a cholecystostomy rather than a cholecystectomy. The probability of recurrent stone formation and inflammation or obstruction during the expected remaining life span will usually be very low. The extremely high-risk patient with moderate symptoms related to multiple stones might be considered for an endoscopic sphincterotomy prior to cholecystectomy. This may often relieve symptoms and allow the physician to reconsider the indications for interval cholecystectomy.[14,79] If surgery still has to be done after an interval, it could be limited to a cholecystectomy or to a cholecystostomy, without need for common duct exploration.

Seriously Ill Patients. Included in this group are patients with life-threatening obstruction and infection of the gallbladder (acute cholecystitis), common bile duct (choledocholithiasis), or intestinal tract (gallstone ileus).

Acute Cholecystitis. Acute cholecystitis should be treated by emergent cholecystectomy or, in rare situations by cholecystostomy. The practice of acute conservative treatment followed by interval elective cholecystectomy is not advisable in the elderly age-group.[34,39] It is less cost efficient, as well as less time efficient; and older persons, particularly men, are prone to free perforation of the acutely inflamed gallbladder. This complication carries a 15% to 25% mortality rate.

As has been noted, the operative mortality for cholecystectomy in elderly patients with acute cholecystitis ranges between 10% and 16%. The

operative mortality for patients undergoing cholecystostomy in the same situation is reported between 10% and 30%. However, patients selected
for cholecystostomy are generally those individuals at increased risk. In approximately 20% of patients treated by cholecystostomy, there is an associated cholangitis secondary to an element of
life-threatening common duct obstruction. The
life-threatening inflammatory process may not
subside with placement of a cholecystostomy tube
alone. If cystic duct patency cannot be reestab-
lished by disimpaction of an obstructed stone, or
if trying to do so risks injury to the common duct
or hilar vessels, then a complementary choledochotomy and drainage of the common duct should
be performed with a No. 16 or No. 20 T-tube.
During the postoperative period, when the patient
is out of danger, any common duct stones may be
percutaneously extracted or a noncalculous obstruction can be either dilated or stented. If the
common bile duct as well as the gallbladder has
been cleared of calculi or an obstructive process,
the cholecystostomy or T-tubes may be removed
with little fear of recurrent illness.

Choledocholithiasis.   Calculous obstruction
of the common duct will produce intermittent or,
more commonly, progressive jaundice and debility,
usually in association with symptomatic infection
of the bile ducts. The gallbladder, if not removed
surgically years before, may be unobstructed and
uninvolved in the inflammatory process, even
though gallbladder lithiasis is usually present. The
primary goal should be relief of common duct
obstruction. In the post-cholecystectomy patient
or in the extremely high-risk patient with an intact
uninvolved gallbladder, open surgery may often
be avoided by endoscopic sphincterotomy and a
stone extraction. Current data indicate that approximately 10% of patients undergoing primary
endoscopic sphincterotomy and stone extraction
will have residual symptoms from their gallbladder
significant enough to warrant its surgical removal
at a later date.[78,83] Mortality figures as low as
0.18% have been reported for large series of elderly patients undergoing endoscopic sphincterotomy for choledocholithiasis.[83] A better risk patient with cholelithiasis and choledocholithiasis is
still advised to have cholecystectomy with common duct exploration, the latter either done preoperatively by the endoscopic technique or as part
of the surgical procedure.

In particular, choledochoduodenostomy is a
rapid, effective way to decompress permanently
the extrahepatic biliary tract in the elderly high-

risk patient. At the Montefiore Medical Center in
New York City, choledochoduodenostomy performed in over 200 patients, mostly over 70 years
of age, had a 3.5% mortality rate.[79] Indications for
its use include multiple or recurrent common duct
calculi, calculi in the secondary hepatic radicles,
and a greatly dilated (>1.2 cm) common duct.
However, unless all common duct stones have
been cleared from the bile ducts, partial obstruction with serious signs and symptoms of cholangitis may persist even after an internal bypass procedure.[63]

Cholangitis.   Occasionally, severe common
duct infection, either a suppurative or an ascending cholangitis, may be present without evident
choledocholithiasis. This may present as sudden
and rapid progression of jaundice and signs of
sepsis (fever, chills, confusion, hypotension) in an
elderly patient without marked abdominal complaints or physical findings. However, the presentation is variable and jaundice may not be present.
Thus a high index of suspicion is helpful in making
the diagnosis, and immediate antibiotic therapy as
well as drainage of the common duct is often necessary by either endoscopic or surgical means.[14]

**Gallbladder Perforation with Biliary-En-
teric Fistulae.**   As has been mentioned, free perforation of the obstructed infected gallbladder is
not uncommon in the aged male. In females, localized perforation of the gallbladder into an adjacent viscus is more common and results in the
formation of a biliary-enteric fistula, usually between the fundus of the gallbladder and the second
part of the duodenum but occasionally to the colon, first part of the duodenum, stomach, or jejunum.[68] Often this event occurs in the absence of
major clinical illness and goes unnoticed by the
patient or physician for months or even years. If
there is no residual common duct obstruction or
infection, such a natural biliary bypass can remain
patent and functional for years or for the life span
of the individual. However, a high percentage of
such patients do have common duct disease that
predisposes to intermittent biliary symptoms, particularly of cholangitis. Such patients may require
operative or endoscopic relief of their common
duct obstruction and often takedown of the fistula.

Two variants of cholecystoenteric fistula invariably require surgery: A cholecystocolonic fistula
is most often associated with life-threatening episodes of ascending cholangitis and as well may
present severe symptoms of intractable diarrhea
and, if not promptly operated on, of a short bowel

malabsorption syndrome. Gallstone ileus is a surgical emergency. This uncommon cause of intestinal obstruction is due to a cholecystoenteric fistula. Depending on the size of the stone, the site of perforation and the variable compliance of the intestinal lumen, the stone may become lodged in the duodenum, distal ileum, jejunum, or sigmoid. Emergency surgery is indicated, with the prime goal to overcome the intestinal obstruction. Ileotomy, gastrotomy, and occasionally a colostomy is needed. No attempt should be made to remove the gallbladder or take down the fistula in the acute situation.

Acalculous Disease

Acute cholecystitis may occur in the absence of gallstones and is often insidious and lethal. This entity is increasingly being diagnosed in elderly male patients, often occurring in the early days following a previous operation or in relation to major trauma, burns, or other septic processes.[35,49] A high index of suspicion and a radionuclide scan are essential to the diagnosis of cystic duct obstruction, although the presence or absence of calculi may not be known for certain until after operation. Early surgery, usually cholecystectomy, is indicated for acute acalculous cholecystitis.

Colonic Diverticulosis and Diverticulitis

Most diverticula of the colon are presumed to represent a degenerative phenomenon related to aging. They are found in about 40% of patients by age 70. However, some patients inherit the tendency for diverticulum formation, without obvious associated smooth muscle dysfunction of the colon or progressive disturbance of bowel habit. Limited left-sided diverticula, or even pan-diverticulosis can be found in many perfectly healthy septagenarians. The complications of diverticulosis occasionally requiring surgery are usually associated with constipation and are the direct result of ulceration and inflammation distal to the diverticular neck obturated by fecal material. The pathogenic sequence is similar to that associated with a fecolith of the appendix, but the prognosis for spontaneous resolution is much greater because of disimpaction of the fecolith into the bowel lumen rather than into the peritoneal cavity.

Hemorrhage

Diverticular hemorrhage occurs in less than 10% of patients with diverticulosis, often in the absence of any signs of inflammation or a history of chronic bowel disturbance. Acute constipation or some other mechanism contributes to the local ulceration and erosion into an arteriole at the neck of usually a single diverticulum. These patients, who often have systolic hypertension and evidence of diffuse atherosclerotic disease, may have a regular or somewhat explosive, formed bowel movement, followed shortly thereafter by a succession of brightly bloody movements, often of life-threatening amount.[11,20] Stroke and myocardial infarction are major possibilities in the wake of such hemorrhages.

Immediate hospitalization, with intravenous resuscitation by Ringer's lactate solution and blood products, as well as a program of complete bowel rest and careful monitoring are indicated. Intermittent or moderate continued bleeding can be assessed by a technetium pertechnetate red cell–labeled or technetium sulfocolloid scan. Alternately, colonoscopy usually to the sigmoid or descending colon reveals an interface of formed normally appearing stool and colonic mucosa proximally, and the relatively feces-free, blood-stained lumen distally. Such endoscopic information, or the angiographic demonstration of the bleeding point that is unresponsive to vasopressin infusion in the event colonic hemorrhage has been continuous and massive,[4] will give the surgeon a map necessary for carrying out a segmental rather than a subtotal colectomy.

More often than not, diverticular hemorrhage will cease before either nuclear scanning or angiography can define the bleeding site. Colonoscopy on the unprepared bowel may still delineate the feces/blood interface mentioned previously. If not, repeat colonoscopy after bowel preparation may rule out other causes of massive colonic bleeding such as vascular ectasias of the cecum and, less commonly, colonic polyps or cancers, a segment of ischemic bowel, or stercoral ulcer. The barium enema is almost never helpful in localizing major colonic bleeding, and if performed during or immediately following a bleeding episode will render subsequent angiography or colonoscopy useless.

Inflammation

The vast majority of patients with nonperforative acute diverticulitis and perisigmoiditis respond to medical management. Contrast enema study in the acute stage is usually not necessary, and, if it is too ardently pursued, it may convert a local process to a free perforation and generalized peritonitis. Barium studies sometimes show obstruction to the flow of barium, suggesting complete sigmoidal obstruction. The patient may, however, have no impediment to the normal flow of stool. Management should be influenced by this consideration. The appearance of extraluminal air or barium confirms the diagnosis of intramural fistulization or perforation with localized abscess.

Surgery is necessary if there are complications such as abscess formation, free perforation, fistulization, or obstructive compromise of the small bowel. Staged procedures with preliminary colostomy and subsequent resection are perhaps the safest, but this involves two and possibly three operations.[20] Sometimes a patient develops a significant medical complication after the colostomy phase of a planned staged procedure. It is proper to leave the poor-risk patient with a colostomy. Resection of the chronically inflamed or perforated segment may be warranted.[29] This will usually prove to be a difficult and tedious procedure by itself.

In a few instances, walled-off perforative disease that has been allowed to subside under medical treatment and is adequately prepared can be safely managed by one-stage resection and anastomosis or by obstructive resection that eliminates the need for subsequent major intra-abdominal surgery.[29,65]

It is occasionally impossible to differentiate radiographically between obstructing diverticular disease and cancer of the colon. Colonoscopic study of the colon with biopsy and washings for cytology can often make this differential diagnosis. If the problem cannot be resolved after 3 weeks of medical management, the indication for surgery exists. Resection is required because intra-abdominal gross examination of the colon may still leave the diagnosis in doubt.

Small Bowel Obstruction

Intestinal obstruction is the most common surgical problem of the small bowel. Its pathophysiology, diagnostic features, and management are amply discussed in standard surgical texts.[81] Differential diagnostic features and treatment strategies pertinent to the aged are discussed here.

Differential Diagnosis

In the aged individual, the hallmark signs and symptoms (vomiting, abdominal distention, colicky pain, and obstipation) may be identical to those in the young or middle-aged person. More often they are muted and accompanied by other unrelated but confusing complaints arising from chronic degenerative diseases. For example, the elderly often have diminished intestinal peristaltic contractile waves. Not only may their chronic constipation be hard to distinguish from true cessation of flatus and feces but also the waves of colicky pain they complain of may be far less severe than those encountered in a healthy young person with small bowel obstruction.

Partial small bowel obstruction can be difficult to distinguish from either a slowly resolving ileus or localized inflammation with altered intestinal motility and a secretory diarrhea in the aged. A nontender left groin nodule that the patient thinks may have been long present may be a partially entrapped loop of small bowel (Richter's hernia) emerging from the femoral ring. The constant danger of postoperative cholecystitis further adds to the trying diagnostic dilemmas.

Adhesions and hernias are the most common cause of small bowel obstruction in the elderly, but overlooking other causes such as primary or recurrent intra-abdominal neoplasm or carcinomatosis may be disastrous. A perforated, walled-off diverticulosis or appendicitis may also be the focus of adhesions obstructing the small bowel. Occasionally, patients never operated on but with congenital bands or adhesions from a long-resolved intra-abdominal inflammatory process may also present with obstruction. Now and then a patient with intra-abdominal adhesions from prior operations may have an attack of obstruction of the small bowel precipitated by severe constipation or any condition or medication leading to colonic hypomotility. Fortunately, sometimes all that is needed to abort the attack is one or two tap water enemas. Cathartics are not advised.

Treatment Strategies

Two principles are most useful when confronted with obstruction of the small bowel in the elderly: (1) do not delay in operating for complete obstruction and (2) give careful attention to maintenance of fluid and electrolyte balance when promptly performing diagnostic studies (sonogram, decida scan of the biliary tree, barium enema, CT scan), which often yield a diagnosis that avoids surgery or facilitates it in a well-prepared patient who has partial rather than complete obstruction.

It is the patient with the completely obstructed bowel who is at most risk from the disastrous consequences of watchful waiting and conservative therapies. The myocardium, kidneys, and intestine of elderly patients do not tolerate hypovolemia and hypoperfusion for long without major multisystem complications. Mesenteric venous thrombosis and arterial inflow arrest occur very rapidly and necessitate bowel resection more often than is otherwise necessary. Prolonged nasogastric decompression of an obstructed individual is an invitation to atelectasis and aspiration pneumonia. The stakes are so high in small intestinal obstruction that it is best to involve the surgeon from the time the diagnosis is first considered.

With regard to operative strategy, certain points are noteworthy. Perioperative antibiotics are recommended because of the high possibility that the intestine may be entered or need to be resected at operation. Often, dense and convoluted adhesions matting many loops of bowel are found; an extensive dissection is often necessary with one or more areas of bowel needing repair or resection. Passage of a Baker tube through a jejunostomy enables the entire small bowel to be stented, thus avoiding recurrent small bowel obstruction or prolonged ileus. Elderly patients will rarely survive a second major operation on the same organ system within a short time interval. The jejunostomy tract may be used to pass a small catheter for enteral feeding supplements after the Baker tube has been removed. In certain instances (*e.g.*, obstructing adhesions in an irradiated pelvis or recurrent carcinoma invading the small bowel), it is often wiser to carry out a limited lysis of adhesions and bypass loops of hopelessly compromised bowel by means of side-to-side enteroenterostomy.

Peptic Ulcer

The past 15 years have seen a definite decrease in the incidence of chronic duodenal ulcer disease in general and of the need for surgery of its complications.[85] In any group, the classic surgical indications for peptic ulcer are hemorrhage, perforation, obstruction, and intractability. Because peptic ulceration is primarily found in the young adult and in middle age, it is not surprising that intractability, as an indication for operation in the elderly, is seldom encountered. In a series of 85 consecutive patients aged 65 or older with complications of peptic ulcer operated on at New York's Montefiore Hospital and Medical Center, the overall mortality rate of 17.6% was linearly related to the interval between onset of bleeding or perforation and the surgery. Other related factors were number and rate of transfusions, extent of peritonitis, and associated cerebral, cardiovascular, and pulmonary disability. In the presence of an organic men-

tal syndrome, the outcome was poor. Chronologic age as such did not directly correlate with complications or death.

Immediate Care and Diagnostic Assessment

The surgical mortality rates for hemorrhage and perforation were 21.3% and 17.9%, respectively. The major advance in lowering the mortality has been a policy of aggressive and early surgery. Initial, rapid resuscitative measures are paramount; central venous pressure should be routinely monitored as a guide to correction of fluid and blood loss. All patients should have upper pan-endoscopy to identify the nature and location of the bleeding lesion preoperatively (see Chap. 15). The unexpected finding of bleeding esophageal varices, a Mallory-Weiss laceration at the esophagogastric junction, a diffuse superficial gastritis, or, as expected, a duodenal bulbar ulcer with or without a visible vessel at its base represents a triumph of present-day endoscopic practice.

Surgical Strategies

The indications for surgery with either perforation or obstruction are clear. This is also true for continuous massive bleeding. When bleeding is intermittent, or ceases spontaneously after each of several major episodes, the issue of surgery often becomes clouded. Further bleeding can produce hypotension and precipitate myocardial infarction, cerebral ischemia, or renal insufficiency. In the otherwise good-risk elderly patient, it is wiser to be aggressive regarding indications for surgery and conservative in choice of procedure. Recurrence of peptic ulcer, increasingly observed in long-term follow-up studies, after vagotomy and drainage procedures, is of less significance with advancing age.[19]

Many surgeons with an interest in gastric physiology are reverting to the direct Billroth I type of gastroduodenal anastomosis whenever the duodenal cuff permits it to be done safely. This avoids some of the postgastrectomy syndromes associated with the Billroth II anastomosis. When gastrectomy is performed using a Billroth II type of reconstruction, a lateral tube duodenostomy is performed for decompression and drainage whenever the duodenal stump is closed, but concern exists regarding the adequacy of the suture line. Another complementary procedure is the passage of a small rubber catheter retrograde into the afferent loop via a jejunostomy; this ensures the patency of the anastomosis and can subsequently serve for enteral feeding supplements. Thus, the immediate and delayed morbid factors in gastric resectional surgery, related to duodenal stump blowout, stomal obstruction, and gastric atony can be eliminated.

Bleeding Ulcer.   A spectrum of procedures is available for the surgical care of bleeding peptic ulcers.[85] The procedure of choice in the good-risk patient is vagectomy and antrectomy. When control of hemorrhage by surgery is a life-saving measure and the patient is very elderly or a poor risk, operating and anesthesia time should be minimal. Ligation of the bleeding vessel and conversion of the pyloric outlet to a pyloroplasty can give gratifying results. Even vagectomy may be omitted if the patient's condition does not warrant the extra time required. In most instances, suture plication of the bleeding ulcer, vagotomy, and pyloroplasty can be readily and safely performed.

Perforated Ulcer.   Simple plication of the perforated peptic ulcer has proven its merit by its simplicity as well as its effectiveness. Studies confirming the high incidence of ulcer recurrence following plication suggest that a definitive procedure such as proximal gastric vagotomy be used when surgery can be performed within 6 to 8 hours of perforation and after appropriate metabolic repletion.[54] We believe that this approach is better limited to the younger age-group. Similarly, proximal gastric vagotomy with oversewing of a bleeding ulcer is not advisable in the elderly high-risk patient. Proximal gastric vagotomy, without opening the stomach is a much lower risk procedure that perhaps might at present be reserved for the unusual instance of an elderly patient with an intractably painful ulcer, without a bleeding or obstructive component.

Pyloric Obstruction.   Chronic obstruction necessitating surgery is infrequent in the aged. Acute obstruction is usually reversible using intubation and subsequent dietary management. Admittedly, dietary management may be difficult in the aged individual who either cannot or will not follow instructions. Because severe distortion of the pyloric region can occur in chronic obstruction, the preferred procedure is vagotomy and gastroenterostomy.

Marginal Ulcer.   Marginal ulcer is a complication of previous surgery. It may not become manifest until the patient reaches old age. If surgery is required, the cause must be identified and corrected. A previous inadequate resection may require further resection, vagectomy, or a combination of procedures. A retained antrum is highly ulcerogenic and must be removed. Prior to the widespread use of histamine H_2-receptor antagonists, the probability of spontaneous or therapeutic healing of marginal ulcers was considerably less than for the primary duodenal ulcer and a more aggressive surgical attitude was usually required. At present, the best approach is to manage the ulcers medically if there is no evidence of a hypersecretory condition but to do prompt corrective surgery if the ulcer persists or after partial healing becomes symptomatic again on chronic cimetidine or ranitidine therapy. There is little geriatric tolerance to the delayed treatment of hemorrhage, sepsis, or obstruction.

Gastric Ulcer

The incidence of gastric ulcer increases with advancing age. The primary problem is to differentiate between benign ulceration and gastric cancer. The policy of observation on strict dietary control with radiographic follow-up belongs to the past. The diagnosis can now be established in over 90% of instances by competent gastroscopic biopsy. When the radiographic features conflict with the tissue report, repeat biopsy is required.

Some of these ulcers get to be very large and quickly extend outside the stomach. Anteriorly they penetrate into the liver and posteriorly into the pancreas. The lesion that is histologically identified as benign can be managed medically unless it becomes complicated by perforation, significant or recurrent hemorrhage, or intractable obstruction.

Gastrectomy is the procedure of choice and frequently can incorporate the ulcer. When the ulcer is in the juxtacardiac region and wedge excision in addition to distal gastrectomy appears difficult or potentially dangerous, healing can nevertheless be anticipated as long as the antral segment of the stomach is excised. Four-quadrant biopsy of the ulcer should be performed whenever it is left *in situ.*[10]

Bleeding gastric ulcers are best managed by gastric resection. However, in poor-risk patients, suture plication with vagotomy and pyloroplasty may decrease operative risk.

Stress ulcers appear as a complication of an extragastric problem, often sepsis. The presentation is with upper gastrointestinal hemorrhage owing to sepsis and low-flow states of varying cause. These ulcers are multiple, superficial, above the muscularis mucosae, and more common in the fundus, although the entire stomach may be involved. The best approach in patients liable to develop stress ulcer is prophylactic alkalinization of the stomach.

In a bleeding patient, the diagnosis can be confirmed only by gastroscopy. Moderate bleeding sites may respond to selective pitressin infusion into the left gastric artery, gastric lavage, and photocoagulation or electrocoagulation. Persistent bleeding requires surgery. In most instances a truncal vagotomy and oversewing of the deep gastric erosions will control the bleeding, but occasionally extensive gastric devascularization or subtotal gastrectomy is necessary.[51] With improved care of hypotensive and septic conditions in an intensive care unit, prophylactic intragastric neutralization, and the use of H_2 blocking drugs, the need for major gastric resectional surgery has greatly decreased.[100]

Peritonitis

There is a group of geriatric patients who present directly from nursing homes. They share a common presentation: virtually no past history, few or no relatives as a source of information, and an acute illness, often tardily recognized as an established moderate to advanced peritonitis. All such patients require surgical intervention.

The differential diagnosis here is less important than recognition that the person requires prompt surgery. The preoperative management includes a chest film, electrocardiogram, blood gas analysis, flat films of the abdomen, complete blood cell count, and a chemical profile. This is directed less at the diagnosis than it is at defining the general status in relation to total management. Because the prior cardiac status is not known, it is wise to establish a central venous pressure line. During the 4 to 6 hours required to complete this workup, an attempt is made to stabilize the patient. Intravenous antibiotics are administered.

The patient is taken to the operating room with the diagnosis of acute surgical abdomen. It is interesting that in the majority of instances the lesions encountered have been correctable. Perforated sigmoid diverticulitis, infarcted bowel, and acute cholecystitis have been the most frequent disorders. Hence the patient with the acute abdomen should be viewed as having a favorable immediate prognosis with surgery.

Appendicitis

In the aged person appendicitis often presents a diagnostic problem because it is unexpected and the symptomatic events may vary as widely and be as ambiguous in the octogenarian as in the 8-year old. During the past 25 years the incidence of appendicitis in the aged has increased considerably to about 7%.[90] Whereas in the very young, males far outnumber females in incidence, the aged population have a more even sex ratio.

Formerly much was made of the different presentation of appendicitis in the elderly, but current assessment does not support this traditional belief.[74] In fact, many elderly patients who prove to have appendicitis do present with right lower quadrant abdominal pain and fairly well-localized tenderness, as well as fever and leukocytosis.

The major problem influencing the outcome is delay in seeking medical care. This results in a greatly increased incidence of rupture and septic complications. The reported incidence of appendiceal rupture in the aged ranges between 37% and 71%, and the mortality rates range from 7% to 9%.[74] There is little to be gained by observation for suspected acute appendicitis in the aged. As in the younger age-groups, a higher index of suspicion, early surgery, and willingness to accept the findings of a normal appendix will result in optimum benefit to all concerned.

Volvulus

Sigmoid volvulus is a common complication in the chronically constipated aged individual. Volvulus is more frequently seen in those with Parkinson's disease and with neuropsychiatric disorders requiring institutional or nursing home care. A routine for making cathartic rounds in bed-ridden patients and a program of once- or twice-weekly enemas may prevent some episodes of obstipation and torsion of the colon.

Volvulus can be suggested in a massively distended, obstipated patient, who is often in abdominal and respiratory distress. The plain film of the abdomen may be almost diagnostic but is often also compatible with nonobstructive colonic distention or a diffuse ileus. An immediate contrast enema (Hypaque is preferred to barium) will confirm or rule out the diagnosis. Volvulus can be decompressed with an 85% success rate by the sigmoidoscope or colonoscope.[5,97]

Decompression of air and feces is the goal in the emergent treatment of sigmoid volvulus. Detorsion of the twisted loop is often not possible, nor is it necessary. Tap water enemas and, if necessary, a repeat endoscopic decompression will control the problem while the patient is prepared for elective surgery.

It is often tempting to discharge the patient to his home or be dissuaded from surgery by an anxious patient or family. In the major clinical series the following data appear again and again: Emergently operated volvulus carries an average 25% to 40% mortality rate, as opposed to a 6% operative mortality in the elective situation; and volvulus that has been endoscopically reduced but not operated on carries a greater than 50% chance of recurrence, with a heightened mortality, regardless of how the recurrence is treated.[5,47,97]

Nonobstructive colonic distention will occasionally be demonstrated in a patient who appears to have an obstruction. Colonoscopic decompression is an effective, temporary treatment for this poorly understood condition. Colonoscopic decompression does not treat the cause of the problem, which is often a systemic response to massive trauma, sepsis, major fractures, or recent surgery. One third of such patients will die of their underlying problem, whether or not the colon is decompressed surgically or endoscopically.

Cecal volvulus also may occur in the aged individual but no more so than in a younger person. Nevertheless it may be lethal if not operated on promptly.[67] Nonresectional procedures such as cecopexy and cecostomy are preferred, unless the viability of the bowel is in question. If a right colectomy is necessary, careful consideration should be given to a temporary ileostomy and mucus fistula rather than risking a primary ileotransverse colon anastomosis in the emergent situation.

Intestinal Ischemia

Acute Mesenteric Ischemia

Acute mesenteric vascular occlusion by thrombosis or embolism is a surgical emergency. The difficulty is in establishing the diagnosis because abnormal physical findings may be minimal during the early stage when the condition is most amenable to vascular correction. An awareness of the possibility of acute visceral occlusion in the patient with fibrillation or with hypotension superimposed on preexistent stenosing lesions can lead to an increased salvage rate.

Both the occlusive and nonocclusive types of mesenteric ischemia may occur seemingly suddenly, but there is always a prodromal stage before there is total intestinal ischemia, peritonitis, and frank perforation. Mortality rates as high as 90% were related to late diagnosis (made at the time of diffuse peritonitis with bowel infarction involving most of the small bowel and right colon), as well as to the primary role of the initially collapsed

circulating system. Earlier diagnosis and treatment are now possible and effective and are discussed in detail in Chapter 15. This aggressive diagnostic and therapeutic approach, championed by Boley, Brandt, and Veith, should be done, if possible, in all suspected instances, including the patient in the intensive care or cardiac care unit, and may be expected to yield a 54% survival rate with preservation of good gastrointestinal function in 85% of the survivors.[12,14]

Chronic Ischemic Syndromes

Chronic ischemic syndromes are discussed in Chapter 16, in which the variable types of injury that result from syndromes of chronic mesenteric ischemia are noted in detail. The definitive treatment of these injuries ranges from emergency surgery for patients with peritoneal signs to conservative management or subsequent elective surgery, depending on the presentation and clinical response of the patient to attentive medical care.

Focal ischemia of the colon has become increasingly common in the older age-group, particularly as a consequence of abdominal aneurysmectomy and sigmoid colectomy and interference with the inferior mesenteric artery circulation. The natural history of this entity is as variable as ischemia involving the small bowel. Most episodes of ischemia involve all or part of the left colon, particularly the splenic flexure, and are usually transient and completely reversible. Some may go on to gangrene and perforation; others may persist as a form of colitis or progress to a late stricture. As with focal ischemia of the small intestine, the treatment of colonic ischemia may vary from a very conservative program of surveillance to one of surgical resection.

Intestinal Angina

Intestinal angina is a syndrome of chronic mesenteric ischemia characterized by postprandial abdominal pain or discomfort, altered intestinal motility, and often malabsorption sufficient to produce marked weight loss. Indeed, before the routine use of the CT scan, many of these patients were suspected of harboring a malignancy in the pancreas. Diffuse atherosclerotic disease often with significant stenosis or occlusion of one or more major mesenteric vessels is present in many cases, although there is no consistent correlation with the degree of atherosclerosis and symptomatology or progression of the condition. The presence of multisystem atherosclerotic disease and the difficulty of ascertaining whether vascular reconstruction will functionally benefit the patient have limited surgical enthusiasm to very carefully selected individuals. Surgeons performing abdominal surgery should note that enlarged peripheral mesenteric vasculature in fact represents compensation for chronic mesenteric ischemia and that all efforts must be made not to injure this collateral circulation.

CARDIOVASCULAR OPERATIONS

In 1981, diseases of the cardiovascular system accounted for nearly 960,000 deaths or 48.5% of all men and women who died in the United States. Diseases of the heart primarily accounted for 38.1%, cerebrovascular disease, 8.3%; diffuse arteriosclerosis, 1.4%; and aortic aneurysm, 0.7%. Of the 753,800 persons dying of heart diseases, about 404,000 were aged 75 years or older. Interestingly, at this age level, 58% of the deaths were in females, whereas in the 55- to 74-year age-group 64% of the deaths were in men. In general, women had more cerebrovascular disease and men had more aneurysmal disease of the aorta.

Cardiac Surgery

Coronary bypass surgery grafting (CABG) is increasingly reported in patients over 65 years of age with a very acceptable operative mortality of 3% to 6%.[56] Hibler and associates[46] analyzed 115 such patients. Early mortality was 6% with a total mortality of 8.7% at the end of 1 year; however, both early and late mortality was increased in patients over age 74 years versus those in the 65- to 74-year range. In addition, to an age factor of 74 years or more, patients with left ventricular ejection fraction less than 35%, in the New York Heart Association (NYHA) class IV, or with diffuse disease requiring more than four bypass grafts, were at increased risk. On the other hand, elderly patients in NYHA classes II or III with good left ventricular function and four or fewer grafted vessels had excellent survival in the hospital and at the end of 1 year post surgery. Long-term functional survival is confirmed by other recent reports of post-CABG patients with somewhat lower median age but who were all capable of undergoing subsequent major general surgical operations without operative mortality.[23,76]

Peripheral Vascular Surgery

The results of elective peripheral vascular reconstructive procedures are encouraging for the elderly patient. Edward and co-workers[28] have re-ported a 5.5% hospital mortality and an acceptable 13.8% complication rate in 144 patients over 80 years of age undergoing vascular operations: Cerebrovascular reconstructions (45 patients), aortic aneurysmectomy (21 patients), grafts of upper and lower extremity vessels (65 patients), and enbolectomy for acute arterial occlusion (14 patients). Similarly, O'Donnell and colleagues reported a 4.7% mortality rate in octogenarians undergoing elective aortic aneurysmectomy[73] and that 86% of the operated patients enjoyed a quality of life equal to or better than their preoperative status. Darling and Brewster have achieved an overall 1.7% operative mortality in their last 500 elective aortic aneurysm resections and have pointed out that the majority of octogenarians in whom surgery was not done died of aneurysm rupture.[73] That, together with the good current survival data, the fact that 25% of abdominal aortic aneurysms 4 cm to 7 cm in diameter do rupture, and the 40% operative mortality rate for ruptured aneurysm hovers about 40%, is a strong argument for elective vascular surgery in carefully screened and prepared elderly patients (see Chap. 12).

TRAUMA

The surgical care of the trauma patient is an expanding, complex subject, beyond the scope of this chapter. For a detailed treatment, the reader is referred to Shires' *Principles of Trauma Care.*[82] Certain aspects of the phenomena of trauma, as they apply to the aged patient, are noted here. The acute nature of most trauma presents increased risk to the elderly patient who may be forced to undergo emergency surgery. The other major risk factors that cannot be satisfactorily compensated for are the age-related cardiopulmonary complications that beset traumatized patients in their 70s or 80s. Thus, the physician consulting with the relatives or friends of a patient about to undergo an emergency surgical effort to remedy the effects of trauma must be very guarded in optimism or prognostic attempts.

Accidents are the fourth leading cause of death in the United States, accounting for 5.1% of the total deaths;[94] and patients at the extremes of age represent a significantly higher percentage than the mean. In men and women over 75 years of age, accidents are the seventh leading cause of death. Patients over age 65 sustaining multiple injuries in a motor vehicle accident were subject to a 50% expected mortality (LD_{50}) despite a graded injury severity score one half that of patients under age 44 years with the same LD_{50}.

Falls, burns, and motor vehicle accidents account for the great majority of accidents in the elderly. Hip fractures alone, usually secondary to falls, have been estimated to yield 2% of the annual deaths in the elderly; and despite much improved specific and supportive care of hip fractures and increased hospital survival, it is hard to show any improvement in the 3-month mortality rates from this injury. Burns in patients over age 65, like multiple injuries, carry a disproportionately increased mortality, with an LD_{50} for a 17% body surface area burn. In contrast, patients aged 15 to 44 tolerated up to a 56% surface area burn before reaching a 50% mortality rate.

Initial Care

It is the elderly more than any age-group who are prone to and will suffer from a delay in medical attention. Fractures and insidious hemodynamic alterations due to occult blood loss may not be recognized for days in nursing home or other mostly bed-ridden patients. Burns may be considered insignificant or not requiring hospitalization and more vigilant monitoring for adequate care. Undesired, self-imposed immobilization of the patient, pulmonary embolus, infection, and often sepsis will supervene in situations of such ''benign neglect.'' The reduced life expectancy of the patient may lead to an erroneously diminished sense of urgency in mobilizing appropriate team members for the patient with multiple injuries or to arrange appropriate transfer to a tertiary care facility.

Initial maneuvers in the care of the traumatized patient of any age deserve emphasis: establish an adequate airway; assess for and control any degree of shock; assess and treat chest injuries; evaluate degree of consciousness/neurologic status; and rapidly achieve surgical preparation. This last item includes completing any further history and physical examination, alerting the blood bank and operating room of an imminent surgical emergency, and placing monitoring devices (*e.g.*, nasogastric tube, urinary catheter, and intravascular hemodynamic recording lines). If the injured patient has become or remains stable, then any fractures may be splinted and, necessary or desirable diagnostic procedures (*e.g.*, angiography, sonography) may be carried out.

Definitive Surgical Treatment

Once the victim of a traumatic injury has been brought through the initial resuscitative phase, specific surgical procedures are often indicated. Good judgment in the timing of such procedures,

their extent, and the goals desired are crucial to the very survival of the elderly patient. One cannot quibble about immediately exploring a limb with ischemia secondary to a vascular laceration or compression associated with fractures. Absence of vascular compromise may permit a beneficial delay in the timing of fracture exploration. Alternatively, a high-risk patient with vascular compromise secondary to bone fractures might just be able to tolerate release or repair of the injured vessel and muscle compartment fasciotomies, leaving further operative care of the fractures for another time. A younger hip fracture victim might do better long term with simple insertion of Knowles' pins and a period of non-weight-bearing in the hope of preserving the head of the femur and the hip joint. A septagenarian with limited ability to comply with ambulation instructions, not to mention a much shorter functional life expectancy, would benefit from a well-timed more extensive operation with stable fixation of the existing joint or primary hip replacement with a prosthesis.

In no area is the application of practiced, well-researched clinical decisions and timely, well-defined and carefully monitored operative procedures more promising than in the care of the trauma patient. This is illustrated by recent reports of increased survival and diminished hospital stay in older burn patients subjected to an early aggressive program of burn wound incision and grafting.[25] The former truism that major burn wounds are lethal in the elderly is being replaced by the realization that the solution to many emergency problems in the elderly lies in altering the physicians' tactical response as much as the patients' metabolic response to the injury.

REFERENCES

1. Adkins RB, Whiteneck JM, Woltering E: Carcinoma of the breast in the extremes of age. South Med J 77:554, 1984
2. Alexander W, Macmillan BG, Stinnett JD et al: Beneficial effects of aggressive protein feeding in severely burned children. Ann Surg 192:505, 1980
3. Antonacci A, Reaves LE, Lowry SE et al: The role of nutrition in immunologic function. Infect Surg 3:590, 1984
4. Athanasoulis CA, Baum S et al: Mesenteric arterial infusions of vasopressin for hemorrhage from colonic diverticulosis. Am J Surg 129:212, 1975
5. Bak MP, Boley SJ: Sigmoid volvulus in the elderly. (in press)
6. Baum S et al: Selective mesenteric arterial infusions in the management of massive diverticular hemorrhage. N Engl J Med 288:1269, 1973

7. Bille-Brahe NE, Eickhoff JH: Measurement of central haemodynamic parameters during preoperative exercise testing in patients suspected of arteriosclerotic heart disease: Value in predicting postoperative cardiac complications. Acta Chir Scand 502:38, 1980

8. Bistrian BR, Blackburn GL, Hallowell E et al: Protein status of general surgery patients. JAMA 230:858, 1974

9. Blake R, Lynn J: Emergency abdominal surgery in the aged. Br J Surg 63:956, 1976

10. Bode WE, Beart RW Jr, Spencer RJ et al: Colonoscopic decompression for acute pseudo-obstruction of the colon: Report of 22 cases and review of the literature. Am J Surg 147:243, 1984

11. Boley SJ, DiBiase A, Brandt LJ et al: Lower intestinal bleeding in the elderly. Am J Surg 137:57, 1979

12. Boley SJ, Sprayregen S, Siegelman SS et al: Initial results from an aggressive roentgenologic and surgical approach to acute mesenteric ischemia. Surgery 82:848, 1977

13. Boyd JB, Bradford B Jr, Watne AL: Operative risk factors of colon resection in the elderly. Ann Surg 192:743, 1980

14. Brandt LJ: Gastrointestinal Disorders of the Elderly. New York, Raven Press, 1984

15. Cancer Rates and Risks. US Public Health Service publication No. 1148. Washington, DC, US Government Printing Office

16. Cohen JR, Kuchta N, Geller N et al: Pancreaticoduodenectomy, a forty year experience. Ann Surg 195:608, 1982

17. Colacchio TA, Forde KA, Scantlebury V: Endoscopic polypectomy: Inadequate treatment for invasive colorectal carcinoma. Ann Surg 194:704, 1981

18. Cole WH: Operability in the young and aged. Ann Surg 138:145, 1953

19. Cole WH: Medical differences between the young and the aged. Am Geriatr Soc 18:589, 1970

20. Colcock BP: Diverticular disease of the colon. In Major Problems in Clinical Surgery. Philadelphia, WB Saunders, 1971

21. Cortese AF, Cornell GN: Radical mastectomy in the aged female. J Am Geriatr Soc 23:337, 1975

22. Cramer SO, Malangoni MA, Schulte WJ et al: Inguinal hernia repair before and after prostatic resection. Surgery 94:627, 1983

23. Crawford ES, Morris GC, Howell JF et al: Operative risk in patients with previous coronary artery bypass. Ann Thorac Surg 26:215, 1978

24. Crump C: The incidence of gallstones and gallbladder disease. Surg Gynecol Obstet 53:447, 1931

25. Deitch EA, Clothier J: Burns in the elderly: An early surgical approach. J Trauma 23:891, 1983

26. DelGuercio LRM, Cohn JD: Monitoring operative risk in the elderly. JAMA 243:1350, 1980

27. Djokovic JL, Hedley-Whyte J: Prediction of outcome of surgery and anesthesia in patients over 80. JAMA 242:2301, 1979

28. Edwards WH, Mulherin JL, Rogers DM: Vascular reconstruction in the octogenarian. South Med J 75:648, 1982

29. Eng K, Ranson JHC, Localio SA: Resection of the perforated segment: A significant advance in treatment of diverticulitis with free perforation or abscess. Am J Surg 133:67, 1977

30. Fisher B: Cooperative clinical trials in primary breast cancer: A critical appraisal. Cancer 31:127, 1973

31. Flanagan L Jr, Bascom JU: Herniorrhaphies performed upon outpatients under local anesthesia. Surg Gynecol Obstet 153:557, 1981

32. Gilbertson VA: Proctosigmoidoscopy and polypectomy in reducing the incidence of rectal cancer. Cancer 34:936, 1974

33. Glenn F: Pre- and postoperative management of elderly surgical patients. J Am Geriatr Soc 21:385, 1973

34. Glenn F: Surgical management of acute cholecystitis in patients 65 years of age or older. Ann Surg 193:56, 1981

35. Glenn F, Becker CG: Acute acalculous cholecystitis: An increasing entity. Ann Surg 195:131, 1982

36. Glenn F, Reed C, Grafe WR: Biliary enteric fistula. Surg Gynecol Obstet 153:527, 1981

37. Goldman L, Caldera DL, Nussbaum SR et al: Multifactorial index of cardiac risk in noncardiac surgical procedures. N Engl J Med 297:845, 1977

38. Goldman L: Cardiac risks and complications of noncardiac surgery. Ann Surg 198:780, 1983

39. Goldman L, Caldera DL, Southwick FS et al: Cardiac risk factors and complications in non-cardiac surgery. Medicine 57:357, 1978

40. Gracie WA, Ransohoff DF: The natural history of silent gallstones: The innocent gallstone is not a myth. N Engl J Med 307:798, 1982

41. Greenburg AG, Saik RP, Coyle JJ et al: Mortality and gastrointestinal surgery in the aged: Elective vs emergency procedures. Arch Surg 116:788, 1981

42. Greenberg AG, Salk RP, Coyle JJ et al: Mortality and gastrointestinal surgery in the aged. Arch Surg 116:788, 1981

43. Helleberg A, Lundgren B, Norin T et al: Treatment of early localized breast cancer in elderly patients by tamoxifen. Br J Rad 55:511, 1982

44. Herbsman H, Feldman J, Seldera J et al: Survival following breast cancer surgery in the elderly. Cancer 47:2358, 1981

45. Hertzer NR, Young JR, Kramer JR et al: Routine coronary angiography prior to elective aortic reconstruction: Results of selective myocardial revascularization in patients with peripheral vascular disease. Arch Surg 114:1336, 1979

46. Hibler BA, Wright JO, Wright CB et al: Coronary artery bypass surgery in the elderly. Arch Surg 118:402, 1983

47. Hines JR, Guerkonk RE, Bass RT: Recurrence and mortality rates in sigmoid volvulus. Surg Gynecol Obstet 124:567, 1967

48. Hirsch RP, Schwartz B: Increased mortality among elderly patients undergoing cataract extraction. Arch Ophthalmol 101:1034, 1983

49. Howard RJ: Acute acalculous cholecystitis. Am J Surg 141:194, 1981

50. Huber DF, Martin EW Jr, Cooperman M: Cholecystectomy in elderly patients. Am J Surg 146:719, 1983

51. Hubert JP Jr et al: The surgical management of bleeding stress ulcers. Ann Surg 191:672, 1980

52. Johnson JC: Surgery in the elderly. In Goldman DR, Brown FH, Levy WK et al (eds): Medical Care of the Surgical Patient. Philadelphia, JB Lippincott, 1982

53. Johnson JC: The medical evaluation and management of the elderly surgical patient. J Am Geriatr Soc 31:621, 1983

54. Jordan PH Jr: Proximal gastric vagotomy without drainage for treatment of perforated duodenal ulcer. Gastroenterology 83:179, 1982

55. Kessler HJ, Seton JZ: The treatment of operable breast cancer in the elderly female. Am J Surg 135:664, 1978

56. Knapp WS, Douglas JS, Carver JM et al: Efficacy of coronary artery bypass grafting in elderly patients with coronary artery disease. Am J Cardiol 47:923, 1981

57. Lichtenstein IL et al: Exploding the myths of hernia repair. Am J Surg 132:307, 1976

58. Linn BS, Jensen J: Age and immune response to a surgical stress. Arch Surg 118:405, 1983

59. Linn BS, Linn MW, Wallen N: Evaluation of results of surgical procedures in the elderly. Ann Surg 195:90, 1982

60. Ludwig Breast Cancer Study Group, Berne, Switzerland: Randomised trial of chemo-endocrine therapy, endocrine therapy, and mastectomy alone in postmenopausal patients with operable breast cancer and axillary node metastasis. Lancet 1:1256, 1984

61. McCarthy JD, Twiest MW: Intraperitoneal polypropylene mesh support of incisional herniorraphy. 142:707, 1981

62. McCarty KS Jr, Silva JS, Cox EB et al: Relationship of age and menopausal status to estrogen receptor content in primary carcinoma of the breast. Ann Surg 197:123, 1983

63. McSherry CK, Fischer MG: Common bile duct stones and biliary-intestinal anastomoses. Surg Gynecol Obstet 153:669, 1981

64. Mann RAM, Bisset WIK: Anaesthesia for lower limb amputation. Anaesthesia 38:1185, 1983

65. Miller DW Jr. Wichern WA Jr: Perforated sigmoid diverticulitis: Appraisal of primary versus delayed resection. Am J Surg 121:536, 1971

66. Mohr DN: Estimation of surgical risk in the elderly: A correlative review. J Am Geriatr Soc 31:99, 1983

67. Morris DM, Eisenstat T, Hall GM: Management of cecal volvulus in debilitated patients. South Med J 75:1069, 1982

68. Morrissey KP, McSherry CK: Internal biliary fistula and gallstone ileus. In Blumgart LH (ed): Surgery of the Liver and Biliary Tract. London, Churchill Livingstone (in press)

69. Morrow DJ, Thompson J, Wilson SE: Acute cholecystitis in the elderly. Arch Surg 113:1199, 1978

70. Mueller CB, Ames F, Anderson GD: Breast cancer in 3,558 women: Age as a significant determinant in the rate of dying and causes of death. Surgery 83:123, 1978

71. Nehme AE: Groin hernias in elderly patients. Am J Surg 146:257, 1983

72. Nixon DW, Heymsfield SB, Cohen AE et al: Protein calorie undernutrition in hospitalized cancer patients. Am J Med 68:683, 1980

73. O'Donnell TF Jr, Darling C, Linton RR: Is 80 years too old for aneurysmectomy? Arch Surg 111:1250, 1976

74. Owens BJ, Hamit JF: Appendicitis in the elderly. Ann Surg 187:392, 1978

75. Palmberg S, Hirsjarvi E: Mortality in geriatric surgery: With special reference to the type of surgery, anaesthesia, complicating diseases, and prophylaxis of thrombosis. Gerontology 25:103, 1979

76. Prorock JJ, Trostle D: Operative risk of general surgical procedures in patients with previous myocardial revascularization. Surg Gynecol Obst 159:214, 1984

77. Reed WP Jr, Steinert H, Badder E: Paraesophageal hernias: Early operation provides the key to safe, simple repair. South Med J 76:27, 1983

78. Safrany L, Cotton PB: Endoscopic management of choledocholithiasis. Surg Clin North Am 62:825, 1982

79. Schein CJ, Gliedman ML: Choledochoduodenostomy as an adjunct to choledocholithotomy. Surg Gynecol Obstet 152:797, 1981

80. Seymour DG, Pringle R: A new method of auditing surgical mortality rates: Application to a group of elderly general surgical patients. Br Med J 284:1539, 1982

81. Shapiro TM: Adenocarcinomas of the pancreas: A statistical analysis of biliary bypass vs Whipple resection in good risk patients. Ann Surg 182:715, 1975

82. Shires GT: Principles of Trauma Care, 3rd ed. New York, McGraw-Hill, 1985

83. Siegel JH: Interventional endoscopy in diseases of the biliary tree and pancreas. Mt Sinai J Med 51:535, 1984

84. Slater H, Gaisford JC: Burns in older patients. J Am Geriatr Soc 29:74, 1981

85. Stabile BE, Passaro E Jr: Duodenal ulcer: A disease in evolution. Curr Prob Surg 21:48, 1984

86. Steen PA, Tinker JH, Tarhan S: Myocardial reinfarction after anesthesia and surgery. JAMA 239:2566, 1978

87. Storer E: Manifestations of gastrointestinal disease: Intestinal obstruction. In Schwartz S, Shires GT, Spencer F et al (eds): The Principles of Surgery. New York, McGraw-Hill, 1979

88. Sugimachi K, Inokuchi K, Ueo H: Surgical treatment for carcinoma of the esophagus in the elderly patient. Surg Gynecol Obstet 160:317, 1985

89. Sullivan DM, Hood TR, Griffen WO: Biliary tract surgery in the elderly. Am J Surg 143:218, 1982

90. Thorbjarnarson B, Loehr WJ: Acute appendicitis in patients over the age of sixty. Surg Gynecol Obstet 125:1277, 1967

91. Tingwald GR, Cooperman M: Inguinal and femoral hernia repair in geriatric patients. Surg Gynecol Obstet 154:704, 1982

92. Topkins MJ, Artusio JF: Myocardial infarction and surgery: A five-year study. Anesth Analg 43:716, 1964

93. Turnbull AD, Gundy E, Howland WS et al: Surgical mortality among the elderly: An analysis of 4,050 operations (1970–1974). Clin Bull 8:139, 1978

94. Vital Statistics of the United States. CA Jan/Feb 1985

95. Wachtel TJ: How to limit the risks of elective surgery. Geriatrics 36:95, 1981

96. Wells PH, Kaplan JA: Optimal management of patients with ischemic heart disease for noncardiac surgery by complementary anesthesiologist and cardiologist interaction. Am Heart J 102:1029, 1981

97. Wertkin MG, Aufses AH Jr: Management of volvulus of the colon. Dis Colon Rectum 21:40, 1978

98. Winawer SJ, Sherlock P, Schottenfeld D et al: Screening for colon cancer. Gastroenterology 70:783, 1976

99. Ziffren SE: Comparison of mortality rates for various surgical operations according to age groups, 1951–1977. J Am Geriatr Soc 27:433, 1979

100. Zinner MJ et al: The prevention of gastrointestinal tract bleeding in patients in an intensive care unit. Surg Gynecol Obstet 153:214, 1981

28 Geriatric Anesthesia

Deryck Duncalf and Edith R. Kepes

Anesthesiology is far from an exact science. Nevertheless, several significant advances in recent years have enhanced our ability to deal with the problems accentuated by frailty and aging. Even minor forms of surgery with local anesthesia in the elderly should not be regarded too casually, as shown in a study demonstrating significant mortality in association with eye operations.[14]

Consider the elderly, brittle diabetic patient with arteriosclerotic heart disease about to undergo minor or major surgery. He needs careful, planned management by surgeon, anesthesiologist, and internist to reduce the risks to an acceptable minimum and to regain well-being in the shortest possible time. At its best, the team approach can be a most effective system for the optimal care of patients undergoing surgery. Division of labor, however, may lead to problems of communication among the specialists concerned. As a result of specialization, we become unfamiliar with the detailed aspects of each other's field. In this chapter, we discuss the scope and limitations of the anesthesiologist's contributions to the medical care of the aged.

AIM OF ANESTHESIA

In order of importance, anesthesia should be safe, provide adequate operating conditions, and prevent pain or discomfort. Achievement of these goals requires careful evaluation and preparation of patients, as well as appropriate selection and management of anesthesia. Frequently, it is necessary to institute supportive measures. Whenever time permits, patients should be brought into optimal physical status preoperatively. In emergency situations, such as ruptured aortic aneurysm, this ideal may have to be compromised.

RESPONSE TO STRESS

Anesthesia and surgery impose stresses that have more marked effects in the elderly patient, whose ability to compensate or adapt is less than that of a younger counterpart. All anesthetic agents depress cellular function to a greater or lesser extent. Suitable combinations of agents and techniques should be chosen to limit unwanted depression of cellular function, particularly in the brain, heart, liver, and kidneys. These considerations assume special importance when the surgery is stressful or associated with significant blood loss or tissue trauma. Cardiovascular homeostatic mechanisms may then approach the limit of their abilities to provide necessary tissue perfusion. In one respect—the adrenocortical response to the stress of surgical trauma and anesthesia—the elderly patient is not at a disadvantage. Adequate stimulation reveals no impairment of capacity by the adrenal cortex to secrete 11,17-hydroxysteroids in the elderly.[43]

PREOPERATIVE EVALUATION

Today, no patient is too old to tolerate anesthesia. If contemplated surgery prolongs life and alleviates suffering, no one should be denied anesthesia and surgery because of age or physical status. Often, well-conducted anesthesia may even support life. The anesthesiologist has the advantage of being in almost full control of physiologic functions during the brief but stressful phase of surgery.

Anesthesia Risk

Operative and postoperative mortality in the aged depends on various factors. The Commission on

494

Professional and Hospital Activities examined hospital mortality for the years 1974–1975.[27] It was found that the risk of a given anesthesia and surgical procedure in an older patient is greater than in a younger one. The hospital death rate was 4.88% for patients 65 years or older, whereas it was 0.75% for those under 65 years of age. According to another study in 148 patients over 65, in which invasive monitoring was used preoperatively,[11] it was found that chronologic age is a poor predictor of the successful or adverse outcome of surgery and anesthesia compared with the physiologic profile of these elderly patients. When the risk of surgery and anesthesia was examined in 500 patients over 80, the 1-month mortality was 6.2%.[13] Myocardial infarction was the leading cause of death. ASA physical status was very useful in predicting the outcome. In patients over age 90 the mortality rose to 29%,[12] but in those without associated preoperative disease, the mortality was only 4.9%.

Age was also studied as one of nine risk factors in patients with cardiac disease in noncardiac surgical procedures.[22] Although age did relate to the outcome, it had only one half the risk value of that of a history of myocardial infarction within 6 months of a surgical procedure.

In general, lower mortality results when surgery is performed as an elective procedure, whereas prohibitively high mortality figures are encountered in emergency surgery on patients with concomitant acute diseases. Therefore, every effort should be made to convert an emergency procedure into an elective operation and to treat the concomitant acute condition first. The only true emergencies that do not allow time for preoperative preparation are uncontrollable hemorrhage and emboli in major vessels. Other acute conditions, such as perforations, intestinal obstruction, and fractures, have a better prognosis if a few hours are taken to correct heart failure, dehydration, or severe anemia.

If time permits, administration of vitamins, correction of hypoproteinemia, augmentation of tissue oxygenation by improving lung function, or treatment of anemia all contribute to better healing.

PREOPERATIVE PREPARATION

The anesthesiologist is at a disadvantage in his efforts to prepare the patient for surgery compared with the internist. Usually, he knows the patient only from a brief preoperative visit the evening before. Early communication between internist, surgeon, and anesthesiologist prevents the exasperation of the last-minute discovery of an essential investigation that has been overlooked.

Just as an infant is not a miniature adult, the geriatric patient is not a feeble version of an adult. The aging process varies from patient to patient, and the chronologic age is a poor guide for therapeutic measures. It is of the utmost importance to approach the anesthetic management on an individual basis, after a careful assessment of the patient's biologic age. In addition, the presence of acute or chronic diseases will influence the evaluation and preparation of the geriatric patient for surgery.

Mental Status

An important aspect of preoperative evaluation is the mental status of geriatric patients. The history may reveal recent personality changes, disorientation, forgetfulness, and related changes owing to arteriosclerotic brain damage. The patient's attitude toward surgery has an important bearing on its ultimate outcome. The will to live may ultimately determine survival from surgical intervention. Many elderly persons are more afraid of going to sleep and not waking up than they are of surgery itself. At the time of the anesthesiologist's preoperative visit, he can do much to alleviate fear by intelligent explanation and reassurance. Even in the alert elderly individual, transient postoperative mental disturbances are frequent. In almost 30% changes occurring after general anesthesia usually consist of confusion, loss of memory, and cognitive ability. These abnormalities usually last 4 to 5 days, but they may even be present 6 weeks after surgery.[4]

Many depressed elderly patients are treated with antidepressant drugs, which may affect the management of anesthesia. These include tricyclic antidepressants, monoamine oxidase (MAO) inhibitors, lithium, and haloperidol. Preoperative management of patients taking tricyclic antidepressants does not require discontinuation of ordinary therapeutic dosages. However these patients need special attention. Because of their anticholinergic effect, the tricyclic drugs may cause tachycardia and minor electrocardiographic changes. In the elderly patient who is taking antihypertensive medication plus a tricyclic antidepressant, the drug interaction may be similar to that in the patient receiving MAO inhibitors, namely cardiac failure or exaggerated response to vasopressors.

The MAO inhibitors such as phenelzine, pargyline, and tranylcypromine, unless discontinued for at least 1 week, may cause serious anesthetic complications. For example, potentiation of central nervous system depressants, such as anesthetics, barbiturates, alcohol, and narcotic analgesics may occur. Before this danger was recognized, several patients receiving meperidine died. The mechanisms of this potentiation are not known. Another problem, hypertensive crisis, is better understood. MAO inhibitors inactivate monoamine oxidase, an enzyme concerned with the destruction of catecholamines. In the absence of this enzyme, epinephrine, norepinephrine, and serotonin stores increase. If, during the course of anesthesia, certain vasopressors such as ephedrine or amphetamine are administered, the excessive catecholamine stores are mobilized and serious hypertension develops. If not treated promptly with phentolamine, cerebrovascular accident, heart failure, pulmonary edema, and death may ensue.

With lithium, the anesthesiologist must be aware of two problems. First, lithium produces a slight neuromuscular blockade and both prolongs and intensifies the neuromuscular blockade produced by succinylcholine chloride, gallamine, and pancuronium bromide. Lithium also prolongs the time required for neostigmine to reverse neuromuscular blockage produced by pancuronium.[26] In addition, it has been demonstrated that the intracellular potassium level is decreased with lithium.[46] Because of these lithium effects, muscle relaxants should be used with caution, and succinylcholine chloride should be avoided unless pretreatment with a nondepolarizing muscle relaxant is carried out. Patients receiving haloperidol may need smaller doses of induction agents if hypotension is to be avoided.

Parkinson's Disease

Levodopa, which is used to treat Parkinson's disease, has been of concern to anesthesiologists. Patients receiving levodopa exhibit a decreased rigidity, akinesia, and tremor, and often the dysphagia, aspiration potential, and ventilation disorder return toward normal. For these reasons, levodopa medication must be continued close to the time of the induction of anesthesia and should be restarted when surgery is completed. However, levodopa is converted to dopamine not only in the brain but also in the rest of the body, resulting in high dopamine blood levels. Dopamine effects are primarily cardiovascular. Myocardial contraction and heart rate are increased as a result of norepinephrine release from catecholamine storage areas in the heart. Dysrhythmias are not uncommon, and peripheral vasoconstriction is present. With lower dopamine levels, vasodilation occurs. This is a dopamine effect not antagonized by α- or β-adrenergic blockers.[21] Dopaminergic receptors may, however, be antagonized by butyrophenones, such as haloperidol and droperidol, and phenothiazines, including chlorpromazine and phenergan. The vasodilation seen with dopamine increases the potential for hypotension during anesthesia. Despite many other side-effects of levodopa medication, such as nausea, psychic abnormalities, and dyskinetic movements, serious complications during anesthesia are rare. Drugs that antagonize dopaminergic effects, such as chlorpromazine and droperidol, should be avoided because they can precipitate parkinsonianlike syndromes. It is also advisable in hypertensive patients on levodopa therapy to reduce the antihypertensive medication in order to prevent severe drops in blood pressure during anesthesia. The peripheral dopamine effects can be avoided if patients with Parkinson's disease are given a combination of levodopa with carbidopa. The latter substance inhibits decarboxylation of peripheral levodopa. It does not cross the blood–brain barrier and, consequently, does not affect the metabolism of levodopa within the central nervous system. Carbidopa, however, does not decrease adverse reactions owing to central effects of levodopa, and the combination of levodopa with carbidopa may on occasion even increase them.

Cardiovascular Status

Heart disease is common among people aged 65 or older, accounting for more than 40% of the deaths in this age-group,[34] and is an important factor affecting postoperative survival.[23] There is an increased incidence of cardiac dysrhythmias[14] and congestive heart failure. As the elastic tissue decreases, vessel walls become more rigid, peripheral vascular resistance tends to rise, and blood pressure is higher than in the young.[19] In managing hypertension in the elderly, the goal should be a reduction in the pressure to 140/90 mm Hg. In the elderly the systolic level is just as important as the diastolic.[8,30] The elderly heart responds poorly to stress, and there is less increase in rate with hypoxia and hypercarbia.[35] The sensitivity of the heart to anticholinergic drugs decreases with age.[41] Electrical activity of pacemaker cells is decreased, and this may account for the increased incidence of cardiac dysrhythmias and altered response to quinidine and lidocaine.[34] Digitalis toxicity is common in the elderly owing to decreased renal excretion of this drug and possibly a reduction in cardiac receptors for digitalis. Both cardiac output and cardiac index are decreased in the aged. All these changes lead to decreased tissue perfusion, a crucial factor in the pharmacodynamics of drug effects. Absorption of drugs from the gastrointestinal tract is diminished, and this route of drug administration is rarely advised in the preoperative period. The rate of absorption from subcutaneous and intramuscular tissues is also delayed.[3] Orders for medication by these routes must be prescribed early enough to allow adequate time for maximal drug effect before the induction of anesthesia. This consideration is especially important in the case of a sedative agent. Should the maximal effect occur after induction of anesthesia, this may cause excessive cardiovascular depression.

Patients with artificial pacemakers usually present no major problems in anesthetic management. Temporary pacing is indicated prior to surgery in patients with various forms of heart block, including second-degree Mobitz type II and third-degree and complete heart block. It may also be indicated when drug therapy results in severe bradycardia.[47]

Antihypertensives, coronary dilators, and other medications that patients with impaired cardiovascular status take should not be discontinued preoperatively, but their pharmacology must be understood if intraoperative complications are to be avoided.

Many antihypertensive agents affect sympathetic neuronal storage, metabolism, or release of neurotransmitters. Reserpine and guanethidine deplete storage of norepinephrine, epinephrine, and dopamine both in the brain stem and in the periphery. The absence of transmitters in sympathetic nerve endings renders drugs such as ephedrine and metaraminol ineffective since such drugs act by releasing catecholamine. Should hypotensive, hypertensive, or bradycardic problems arise, titrating doses of direct-acting vasoconstrictors (phenylephrine), vasodilators (nitroprusside), chronotropes (isoproterenol or dopamine), or vagolytics (atropine, glycopyrrolate) have to be used.

α-Methyldopa is a false neurotransmitter. It replaces norepinephrine in the granules at the nerve ending. The false neurotransmitter is less potent than norepinephrine or dopamine and is one means by which antihypertensive action is produced. It also stimulates the brain stem sympa-

thetic nervous system, which antagonizes the peripheral sympathetic nervous system. When peripheral sympathetic nervous activity decreases, blood pressure is reduced. Other medications used in hypertension are α-adrenergic blockers (*e.g.,* regitine, phenoxybenzamines, and prazosin) and β-adrenergic blockers (propranolol and metoprolol). Abrupt withdrawal of propranolol in the preoperative period may precipitate angina or even myodardial infarction.

Clonidine is an α-adrenergic stimulant in the brain stem. It lowers blood pressure by antagonizing the peripheral sympathetic nervous system. Complications with sudden withdrawal are similar to those seen after discontinuing propranolol abruptly.

Other medications that should be continued are nitroglycerine, which reduces the "preload" and "afterload," and calcium (slow) channel blocking drugs such as verapamil, nifedipine, and diltiazem, which act by slowing the influx of calcium into the muscle cell membrane and repolarization. This results in coronary vasodilation and a myocardial depression. It is believed that the negative inotropic effect of halothane may be related to slow channel blockade, and cardiodepressant interactions have been demonstrated between verapamil and halothane in dogs.[31] Consequently, potent inhaled anesthetics should be carefully titrated in patients being treated with slow channel blockers.

With diuretics such as chlorothiazide, there may be a depletion of extracellular fluids and a loss of potassium. During anesthesia, severe hypotension resistant to vasopressor therapy may develop. If time permits, this drug should be discontinued 2 to 3 days before surgery. In any case, fluid and electrolyte balance, if abnormal, must be corrected preoperatively.

Patients who have had symptoms of cardiac failure, an enlarged heart, and certain electrocardiographic abnormalities must be put on digitalis therapy preoperatively. Oral administration of digitalis should be changed to use of an intramuscular preparation on the day of surgery.

Prophylactic use of digitalis is controversial. There is evidence that in the patient on digitalis therapy, cardiac reserve is increased and the heart is better able to withstand the insult of hemorrhagic shock and trauma.[44] On the other hand, digitalis has a limited margin of safety, with increasing toxicity caused by hypokalemia. Since potassium concentrations can fluctuate widely during anesthesia owing to fluid shifts and ventilatory acid–base changes and since intraoperative arrhythmias caused by digitalis toxicity may be difficult to differentiate from other causes, we avoid prophylactic use of digitalis.

Because a history of recent myocardial infarction increases the risk of postoperative mortality,[23] only the most essential surgery should be carried out in the immediate postinfarction period, and elective procedures should be postponed for at least 3, and preferably 6, months. If sufficient time for healing has elapsed and the patient is asymptomatic, anesthesia and surgery are usually well tolerated. A recent study suggests that preoperative optimization of the patient's status, aggressive invasive monitoring of the hemodynamic status, and prompt treatment of any hemodynamic aberration may be associated with a substantial decrease in perioperative morbidity and mortality in patients with previous myocardial infarction.[40] Cardiac patients on anticoagulant therapy, including mini-heparinization, need special attention if hematomas are to be prevented. Anticoagulants must be discontinued preoperatively and surgery delayed until prothrombin time becomes normal, but only after carefully weighing the increased circulatory risks, including those of pulmonary emboli. Regional anesthesia, such as ankle blocks, that may damage blood vessels should be excluded, unless general anesthesia is absolutely contraindicated.

Choice of anesthesia in the hypertensive elderly patient is often a controversial problem. These patients may suffer serious hypotension once the vascular bed is dilated by preoperative or anesthetic drugs.

Dopamine is useful to restore the blood pressure during surgery, especially cardiac surgery, and septicemia. In addition to its inotropic effect on the myocardium, it dilates the renal vasculature and increases renal blood flow, glomerular filtration rate, and sodium excretion. However, restoration of blood volume should always be instituted prior to or together with dopamine administration. The drug should be administered intravenously with a suitable metering device. Arterial and central venous pressure and, in some cases, pulmonary wedge pressure must be monitored.

Anemia

Anemia is common in the elderly. It should not be accepted as a physiologic process of aging but as a pathologic finding to be corrected before surgery. Its treatment is discussed in Chapter 22.

Respiratory Status

Age-associated changes in the respiratory system decrease functional reserve. After the age of 40 there is a loss of strength of the muscles of respiration and the chest wall compliance decreases. There is also a loss of elastic recoil.[33] The net effect of these changes is an increase in small airway closure,[36] producing a fall in vital capacity and an increase in functional residual capacity and residual volume.[38] The histologic changes with aging are dilatation of alveolar ducts, loss of intra-alveolar septa, and decreased number of alveoli, and the total lung surface area is reduced.[42] There is an increased incidence of postoperative pulmonary complications. Decreased ability to cough, increased secretions, and progressive loss of protective reflexes in the airway[39] increase the risk of postoperative atelectasis. Ventilatory response to hypoxia and hypercapnia is decreased.[35]

Assessment of pulmonary function preoperatively is helpful in predicting the need for ventilatory support postoperatively. The increase in closing volume in elderly patients makes it more difficult to wean them from mechanical ventilation.[25] Arterial oxygen tension declines linearly with age, and oxygen supply to vital organs may be borderline. Consequently, it is especially important to maintain inspired oxygen concentration at a level sufficient to meet tissue organ requirements.

During anesthesia, the efficiency of alveolar-capillary gas exchange is decreased owing to increased shunting, inequality of ventilation–perfusion ratios, and increased physiologic dead space. Alveolar hypoventilation or inadequate inspiratory oxygen concentration in anesthetized patients further reduces oxygen uptake. In the elderly, this train of events may have particularly undesirable consequences because respiratory function is already impaired at the outset. Anesthesia, coupled perhaps with decreased tissue perfusion, may seriously reduce the supply of oxygen to tissues, causing altered function and even tissue death. At the same time, should carbon dioxide retention also occur, cardiac dysthythmias hypertension, and coma may occur. If impaired pulmonary function can be improved by appropriate therapeutic measures, surgery should be postponed until optimal results have been achieved. Respiratory function should, of course, be taken into account in planning a suitable anesthetic technique.

Special Considerations

Secretions may often accumulate in the tracheobronchial tree, owing to increased production and impaired elimination. Retained secretions, aside from interfering with blood gas exchange, predispose to atelectasis and bronchopneumonia. Secretions increase in chronic bronchitis, which is often a feature of old age, and with smoking. Therefore, smoking should be cut down and preferably stopped for at least 1 week before operation. This also decreases the irritability of the tracheobronchial tract and postoperative coughing, making recovery from abdominal procedures more comfortable and decreasing the need for respiratory-depressant analgesics. Coughing postoperatively is particularly undesirable after intraocular operations. A suitable antibiotic may reduce secretions if a bacterial etiology is demonstrated.

The ability to eliminate secretions can be impaired in several ways. Dehydration tends to increase the viscosity of secretions and retards their elimination. Hydration corrects this. When pooling of secretions occurs in bronchiectasis, postural drainage is indicated. Destruction of ciliated epithelium in chronic bronchitis or its impaired function after smoking can impede the removal of secretions.

Weakness of respiratory muscles and narrowing of the airways reduce the peak expiratory velocity and hence the effectiveness of coughing. The cough reflex may itself be depressed. Anesthesia, splinting owing to postoperative pain, and the limitation of respiratory movements owing to surgical factors also tend to reduce the effectiveness of coughing. Occasionally, nebulized bronchodilators, such as metaproterenol or terbutaline, increase the effectiveness of coughing. Ideally, they should be used only after it has been demonstrated that there is a bronchoconstrictive element and that they increase expiratory velocity.

The possibility that asthmatics may have received corticosteroids should not be overlooked. Previous administration of these agents may adversely affect the patient's response to anesthesia and surgery, owing to suppression of the normal adrenocortical response to stress.

Acute upper respiratory infections are contraindications to elective surgical operations because they predispose to pulmonary complications such as pneumonia. These infections should be cleared up, if possible, before surgery is undertaken.

For the most part, changes in the chest wall, respiratory muscles, lungs, and airways that occur in old age are irreversible. In some instances, a bronchodilator may be helpful in increasing the diameter of the airways. Assessment of those changes in pulmonary function that may not be amenable to preoperative correction is still important in the overall management. Chief among them are the following:

Increased functional residual capacity and uneven ventilation and perfusion slow induction and emergence from anesthesia when inhalation agents are used and decrease the efficiency of the alveolar-capillary exchange of oxygen and carbon dioxide.

Decreased compliance increases the mechanical work and oxygen consumption required for breathing, particularly when ventilatory requirements increase. During anesthesia, if assisted or controlled ventilation is used, especially when a positive end-expiratory pressure is added, somewhat higher inflation pressures may be required in the presence of decreased compliance. This may interfere with venous return to the heart, cardiac output, and pulmonary capillary filling.

An increase in the physiologic dead space increases the ventilatory requirements necessary to achieve adequate alveolar ventilation.

Genitourinary Status

Careful evaluation of the genitourinary system helps prevent complications, which are frequent in the geriatric surgical patient. In senescence, the kidney mass decreases and glomerular and tubular function diminishes.[37] Latent renal insufficiency may become manifest in the presence of blood loss, hypotension, dehydration, or urinary retention. In addition, all anesthetics produce a transient depression of renal function. If laboratory tests show significant abnormality of renal function, surgery should be performed, when possible, under regional anesthesia. Many elderly men have an enlarged prostate that is asymptomatic but may cause urinary obstruction postoperatively. If examination reveals this, the opinion of a urologist should be requested. Preoperative indwelling catheter drainage or a limited resection, depending on the urgency of the contemplated surgery, should be considered. Patients in severe renal failure have a poor prognosis unless dialysis is performed preoperatively. Anesthesia is poorly tolerated in patients with electrolyte imbalance, especially hyperkalemia.

Dentition

Peridontal disease is common in old age with varying degrees of mobility of the teeth. There may be complete or partial loss of teeth, with removable or fixed dental prostheses. Loose teeth may become dislodged during and after surgery, so preoperative removal should be strongly considered.

Removable dental prostheses should be taken out before induction of anesthesia.

Metabolic Status

Aging is associated with a significant reduction in basal oxygen consumption. Up to about age 70, many elderly patients are overweight and the adipose tissue is increased in relation to the total body mass. The muscle mass is decreased, and osteoporosis is frequent. Over the age of 70, the body weight is usually decreased. Markedly adipose patients have a lower life expectancy, and most of them do not live to be octogenarians. Diabetes should be carefully controlled during all phases of surgical management (see Chap. 37).

Corticosteroids

Some elderly surgical patients are on corticosteroid medication or have a history of previous cortisone therapy. If necessary, details should be obtained from family members (because some elderly persons are forgetful). In this circumstance, unless hydrocortisone or an equivalent drug is administered to substitute for endogenously produced adrenocortical hormones, cardiovascular collapse may occur during surgery.

With systemic corticosteriods, duration of administration rather than the dose level used seems to be more important in suppressing adrenocortical function. However, after corticosteroids have been administered, ability to respond adequately to surgical stress without supplemental corticosteroid therapy is unpredictable because of individual variations in the degree of adrenocortical depression. Therefore, in the preoperative preparation of patients in whom hypofunction of the adrenal cortex cannot be excluded, arbitrary rules to ensure adequate corticosteroid coverage must be followed. Any patient who has received cortisone or an equivalent for 4 days or longer within the past 6 months should receive hydrocortisone. At least 100 mg of hydrocortisone should be administered intramuscularly, in divided doses, on the day before operation. On the day of surgery, 100 mg should be administered intravenously every 8 hours. Longer-acting corticosteroids, such as methylprednisolone and dexamethasone, can be used in equivalent doses. Requirements may be high and should be at least twice the amount taken for daily maintenance. In some instances, this may have been 500 mg of hydrocortisone or more. Thereafter these drugs should be administered in gradually reduced amounts and finally discontinued over the next 2 to 3 days. In patients receiving a maintenance dose of a corticosteroid, dosage should be gradually decreased to the original level postoperatively. Corticosteroids in very large doses have been advocated in the management of septic shock during surgery.

Alcohol

Alcohol is taken in moderation by many elderly persons as a mood elevator and stimulant or soporific. This comfort should not be denied the patient in the preoperative period. It should be prescribed for patients accustomed to large quantities of alcohol. Alcohol, as a 5% solution intravenously, facilitates induction and maintenance of anesthesia and helps to prevent postoperative restlessness and psychosis (delirium tremens) in alcoholics.

Drug Habituation

Patients who take narcotic analgesics for prolonged periods may become tolerant and drug dependent. Such patients should continue to receive their accustomed amounts of narcotics or an equivalent alternative narcotic if difficulties are to be avoided during and after anesthesia. A similar approach is also recommended for such habituating drugs as barbiturates and tranquilizers. One must remember also that there is considerable cross-tolerance between such drugs and general anesthetics. The large amount of anesthetics these patients can tolerate without ill effect is often surprising in spite of the fact that in aging there is a reduction in the functional state of the microsomal enzyme systems.[24]

Fluid and Electrolyte Disturbances

Fluid and electrolyte disturbances are common in the elderly patient, owing to apathy, lack of appetite, or an unbalanced diet. Blood count and hematocrit determination should be performed on all surgical patients, but, in addition, electrolyte levels should be determined in the acutely sick and in elderly patients who are to undergo major surgery. If time permits, corrections should be carried out until normal values are obtained.

CHOICE OF ANESTHESIA

The choice of anesthesia follows the general principles of management dictated by the patient's state of health and the requirements of the surgical procedure. The duration and location of the operation, the amount of relaxation required, and the need for special techniques such as hypothermia or cardiopulmonary bypass are all determining factors in the ultimate choice of anesthetic management.

The patient's desires should be taken into consideration, provided they do not compromise optimal care. Some anxious elderly patients, like small children, dread the hospital, medical personnel, and operating rooms. Others are too incoherent and senile to cooperate. Such patients, if operated on under regional analgesia, need such heavy sedation that cardiorespiratory depression becomes a real hazard. In these aged patients, general anesthesia is preferable. The anesthesiologist is always in full control of ventilatory function, a parameter that is difficult to control during heavy sedation; thus hypoxia and hypercarbia can be prevented.

The majority of geriatric patients are cooperative and have a strong desire to get well and live longer. As a rule, these patients are best managed with regional methods. All surgical procedures in the lower parts of the abdomen and on extremities can be performed with regional techniques, using local anesthetic agents. Operations frequently performed on the elderly and most suitable for regional techniques include herniorrhaphies, prostatectomies, nailing of hip fractures, embolectomies, arterial bypass grafts, and amputations. Subarachnoid, peridural, or other nerve blocks interfere less with homeostatic mechanisms than presently available inhalation and intravenous drugs. Although skin infection, septicemia, bleeding tendencies, and neurologic diseases are contraindications to regional anesthesia, patients with poor myocardial reserve or liver and kidney failure usually do better with this approach.

PREOPERATIVE MEDICATION

The purpose of preoperative medication is to alleviate apprehension, to reduce secretion of mucus in the upper respiratory tract, and to facilitate the induction and maintenance of general anesthesia.

Age-related functional and pathologic change may interfere with absorption, binding, distribution, metabolism, and excretion of drugs. These factors together with a reduction in number and altered sensitivity of certain receptors, notably in the central nervous system, may result in quantitative and, at times, qualitative differences in the

effects of anesthetic agents, including premedications, in the elderly. The intensity and duration of the therapeutic effects are usually increased. For example the half life of diazepam is increased fourfold to fivefold with increasing age.[32] Moreover, adverse side-effects of drugs are common in elderly patients.

Premedications that cause minimal respiratory and circulatory depression should be selected. If the patient is in the habit of taking a certain tranquilizer, barbiturate, or narcotic analgesic, it is usually safest to continue with the same medication. The central nervous system is probably the organ most sensitive to changes in drug activity in advanced age. These pronounced changes are believed due to a decrease in the number of nerve cells. This results in enhanced activity of depressants,[29] whereas the sensitivity to stimulants is reduced.[16] With narcotics, an increased depressant effect on the central nervous system is particularly marked on the respiratory center. Because respiratory reserve decreases with age, the elderly compensate by increasing the minute volume, primarily through an elevation of the respiratory rate. Because narcotics tend to depress an elevated respiratory rate more than a normal one,[15,33] their greater effect on the respiratory exchange of the elderly is understandable. In elderly persons the cough reflex is depressed, and further depression by narcotics may lead to atelectasis. Narcotics, therefore, should only be used preoperatively if the patient has pain and then should be reduced to one third or two thirds of the usual adult dose.[18] Morphine depresses cardiac output less than fentanyl or meperidine,[45] which is a consideration of special significance in the selection of a narcotic in the elderly. Newer narcotics are becoming available but have yet to find their place in our therapeutic armamentarium. Sufentanyl is five to ten times more potent than fentanyl and has a better analgesic to convulsant ratio. Alfentanyl is not as potent as fentanyl but is shorter acting.

Aged persons often exhibit increased sensitivity to the depressant effects of barbiturates. Furthermore, these compounds may cause excitement and various psychotomimetic symptoms. The sedative effects of diphenhydramine are more predictable than those of barbiturates. Based on clinical experience, paraldehyde, chloral hydrate, and glutethamide are also considered safer than barbiturates in aged patients[2] and are very suitable for preoperative preparation. Flurazepam is currently the most popular hypnotic, and usually 15 mg is a sufficient dose to ensure an adequate night's sleep before operation. Diazepam is a centrally acting sedative, which appears to affect the limbic system, thalamus, and hypothalamus, inducing a calming effect. It is effective for preoperative medication. The recommended dose in the elderly is 2.5 mg to 5 mg by intramuscular injection. It is useful to prevent the recall of many short diagnostic or therapeutic procedures such as colonoscopy, cystoscopy, dental procedures, cardioversion, or electroshock therapy. Lorazepam is a related drug with a longer half-life, but it is less suitable.

Anticholinergic drugs (atropine and scopolamine), which were used almost routinely in the young adult in the past, should always be omitted in the aged. The elderly are more sensitive to the central nervous system and ophthalmic effects of atropine and scopolamine.[2] Glycopyrrolate, an atropinelike drug that does not cross the blood–brain barrier, conceivably might have special application in the elderly because of its absence of central effects. Atropine or glycopyrrolate may be given intravenously in the operating room if drugs such as halothane and succinylcholine, which caused increased vagal stimulation, are to be used. However, the sensitivity of the heart to anticholinergic drugs diminishes with old age,[20] and the dose of atropine may have to be repeated during the course of anesthesia, if bradycardia develops.

ANESTHETIC MANAGEMENT

Position

Careful attention must be paid to the position of the patient on the operating table and stretcher in the immediate perioperative period to avoid cardiorespiratory embarrassment and trauma.

Cardiorespiratory Aspects

Position influences circulation and respiration profoundly, and extremes of posture may cause severe complications. The elderly who suffer from orthopnea should not be transported flat on the stretcher or operated on in the supine position without support in order to prevent cardiovascular complications such as pulmonary edema.

Trendelenburg position or elevation of the legs increases venous return to the heart, which may be dangerous in patients in heart failure. It also causes venous congestion of the head, which can lead to cerebrovascular hemorrhage. The sitting position may cause hypotension, owing to pooling of the blood in the dependent parts of the body. It may decrease pressure in the cerebral arteries, which may lead to cerebral thrombosis, cerebral hypoxia, and permanent brain damage.

The vital capacity is also impaired in some of the positions assumed during surgery. This is important, especially in patients with regional anesthesia, when ventilation is not supported by anesthesiologist.

Trauma

Damage may be done to bones, joints, nerves, and blood vessels by careless positioning of the anesthetized patient. The elderly often suffer from osteoarthritis, wasted flaccid muscles, loss of adipose tissue, and hemiplegia. Unless the spine and limbs are carefully padded and supported in a natural position, fractures, muscle tears, pressure paralysis of the nerves, and damage to blood vessels causing postoperative venous thrombosis may result.

Because of these difficulties, the surgeon must often compromise with the position that would otherwise be optimal for surgical exposure.

GENERAL ANESTHESIA

The response of the geriatric patient to general anesthesia is altered in many ways. Concentrations and amounts of anesthetic agents that are hardly analgesic in the young may cause severe respiratory and cardiovascular depression. Because of the anatomical and functional changes of the lungs, the rate of absorption of drugs administered by inhalation is reduced and the onset of anesthesia is delayed. For the same reason, the elimination of inhalation agents is slowed, and elderly patients remain anesthetized longer at the conclusion of surgery. Altered distribution of inhaled or intravenously administered drugs is another factor in their slow onset and elimination. Lower cardiac output and decreased tissue perfusion slow the onset of drug action and decrease the rate of elimination. Preferential distribution of drugs into areas with the best circulation, such as brain, heart, and muscles,[1] may cause drugs to accumulate in these organs. Decreased hepatic and renal blood flow, on the other hand, hinders the elimination of drugs that depend on metabolic transformation and urinary excretion.

INDUCTION OF ANESTHESIA

Barbiturates

To ensure smooth and rapid induction, a short-acting barbiturate is frequently administered intravenously. Thiopental, methohexital, or thiamylal are injected slowly intravenously; careful individual titration minimizes undesirable side-effects. Neither age nor body weight is a suitable basis for the calculation of the dose to be administered, and only if these drugs are used with caution can cardiorespiratory depression be avoided.

Tranquilizers

Droperidol is quite suitable for the induction of general anesthesia. It has hardly any undesirable effects on the cardiovascular and respiratory systems. The combination of this agent with a narcotic analgesic such as fentanyl has been frequently used in geriatric patients for induction and maintenance of nitrous oxide–oxygen anesthesia. This form of balanced anesthesia has been referred to as neuroleptic anesthesia. With this technique, induction is smooth, depth of anesthesia is easily controllable, and homeostasis is well preserved. During recovery, the patient remains pain free for many hours, owing to persisting narcotic action. The rather prolonged recovery is a disadvantage in elderly patients. The antiemetic property of droperidol almost completely prevents nausea and vomiting.

Instead of droperidol, diazepam may be used to induce anesthesia. Because of its shorter duration of action, it is particularly suitable for operations lasting less than 1 hour. There is some evidence that diazepam may increase myocardial blood flow,[28] a desirable feature in patients with coronary insufficiency. Midazolam, a water-soluble benzodiazepine, has similar pharmacologic properties to diazepam and does not cause pain or irritation at the site of intravenous injection.

Ketamine is a fast-acting drug, whether given intravenously or intramuscularly, which produces a dissociative anesthesia. It appears to interrupt selectively the association pathways of the brain. The anesthesia is characterized by profound analgesia, normal pharyngeal-laryngeal reflexes, enhanced skeletal muscle tone, cardiovascular stimulation, and, occasionally, respiratory depression. The greatest disadvantage is that in a relatively large percentage of patients emergence reactions occur, including vivid hallucinations, delirium, and confusion, which may be accompanied by excitement and irrational behavior. Fortunately, in the geriatric population these complications are somewhat reduced. This anesthetic has a limited application in the elderly patient. It may be useful as the sole anesthetic in short painful procedures such as debridement of wounds, painful dressings, skin grafting in burn patients, and the induction of anesthesia in emergency procedures for poor-risk patients with depression of vital functions.

Maintenance

Maintenance is usually accomplished with one of the inhalation agents.

Nitrous Oxide

Because nitrous oxide is a nonpotent inhalation anesthetic agent, in the presence of adequate oxygen (at least 30%) it barely achieves unconsciousness. Deeper anesthesia requires supplementation with small, intermittent, intravenous doses of a narcotic analgesic, such as fentanyl, meperidine, or morphine, or vaporization of more potent inhalation anesthetics such as halothane, enflurane, or isoflurane. If muscular relaxation is needed for the surgery, homeostasis is maintained better by muscle relaxants than by deepening the plane of anesthesia. Nitrous oxide is highly soluble in tissues; it is able to depress the circulation, it limits the inspired oxygen concentration, it has some neurotoxicity and perhaps carcinogenicity. All these findings have posed some questions whether its advantages over other drugs are as great as once believed.

Halothane

Halothane is not the agent of choice in adults. Its low blood solubility has desirable and undesirable features. Although it produces rapid induction, swift recovery, and easy controllability, the potential hazard of a sudden overdose is especially dangerous in the geriatric patient. Hypotension and bradycardia (conditions to be avoided in the elderly) may appear suddenly. Both myocardial depression and vasodilation are implicated in hypotension, and absence of sympathetic stimulation explains the bradycardia. Cardiac irregularities may also appear. Its hepatoxicity has not been definitely established. Until its effect on liver cells has been clarified, it should be used with caution. Accordingly, it might be prudent not to repeat the administration of this halogenated inhalation agent until at least 1 year has elapsed.

Enflurane

Enflurane, a volatile nonflammable agent, is capable of inducing anesthesia rapidly and smoothly in a similar manner to halothane. It is less soluble in fat than halothane so that emergence from anesthesia is more rapid. It is a fluorinated ether and is metabolized to inorganic fluoride. The rapid clearance of enflurane and its metabolites reduces its potential for acute renal toxicity.

Isoflurane

Isoflurane is an isomer of enflurane. It is similar to enflurane with respect to dose-related depression of respiration and electroencephalographic changes. Isoflurane, however, does not produce electroencephalographic seizure activities. It decreases cerebrovascular resistance and thereby increases cerebral blood flow, but less so than halothane and enflurances. It is more stable than other inhalation agents, and recovery of metabolites in the human is small; therefore organ toxicity is also less. It is probably the inhalation agent of choice in geriatric patients.

MUSCLE RELAXANTS

Neuromuscular blocking agents should always be used in conjunction with general anesthesia if surgery requires muscle relaxation. This is preferable to obtaining similar operating conditions by deep planes of anesthesia with potent inhalation agents. Because of the elderly patient's decreased muscle tone, good relaxation can usually be obtained with smaller doses of muscle relaxants than in young subjects. Moreover, the onset of action of relaxants is delayed and their duration of action is prolonged. Consequently, the patient's requirements should be met by the cautious administration of small fractional doses.

Succinylcholine

Succincylcholine has a rapid onset and brief duration of action. Therefore, it is a useful relaxant to facilitate the introduction of an endotracheal tube or for brief surgical procedures. Succinylcholine depends for its detoxification on plasma cholinesterase, which is synthesized in the liver. In old age, the production of this enzyme is reduced. Liver disease and debility may markedly increase this reduction. Approximately 1 in 3000 patients have atypical plasma cholinesterase levels and hydrolyze succinylcholine very slowly. The usual clinical dose of succinylcholine may produce apnea for several hours.

One of the most frequently used nondepolarizing muscle relaxants is pancuronium, which is five times as potent as *d*-tubocurarine. It has an advantage over the latter drug in that histamine release is insignificant. Pancuronium has little effect on the circulatory system, although transient tachycardia and hypertension occur after its administration. If the plasma protein levels are lowered, the binding of these relaxants is reduced. This results in an increase of the free active drug in the plasma and causes an overdose. Other conditions that alter the patient's sensitivity to these drugs are myasthenia gravis, carcinomatous neuropathy, and potassium deficiency. Atracurium has a duration of action longer than succinylocholine but shorter than pancuronium or *d*-tubocurarine. It has fewer cardiovascular effects than the previously introduced nondepolarizing muscle relaxants. Vecuronium, probably an even more suitable muscle relaxant for the elderly, is now available.

Reversal of Neuromuscular Block

One of the great advantages of the nondepolarizing muscle relaxants over the depolarizing drugs is the ease with which the neuromuscular block can be reversed. Neostigmine or pyridostigmine bromide, together with or preceded by atropine or glycopyrrolate, are effective antagonists. Reversal should usually be carried out if residual curarization exists. Neostigmine and pyridostigmine are cholinesterase inhibitors. Pyridostigmine has advantages over neostigmine in that it has fewer side-effects, such as bradycardia, salivation, and gastrointestinal stimulation. It also has a longer duration of action than neostigmine, and recurarization after reversal is less likely to occur. The clinical impression of persisting neuromuscular block can be confirmed by observing the response to electrical stimulation of the ulnar nerve. Reversal is not an innocuous procedure because both atropine and neostigmine, used for this purpose, have profound effects on cardiac rate and rhythm. Small initial and incremental doses, administered slowly, are recommended in the elderly until muscle tone is normal.

REGIONAL ANESTHESIA

Whenever the surgical requirements are suitable, we prefer regional anesthesia in the elderly. No general anesthetic technique is without unwanted systemic effects, and most of the undesirable side-effects can be avoided by regional anesthesia. Skillfully performed nerve blocks or local infiltration can avoid most systemic side-effects.

No attempt is made here to describe the various

drugs and techniques available, but the general principles on which safe and effective techniques are based are outlined.

Overdose

Overdose of the local analgesic used for the anesthesia of the mucous membrane or skin and underlying tissues is the most frequent complication. To avoid toxic blood levels recommended maximum doses must never be exceeded. Fortunately, conduction of the sensory and motor nerves in the aged can usually be interrupted with lower concentrations and often with smaller volumes of local anesthetic agents than in young adults.

Epinephrine

Systemic toxicity can be reduced further by the admixture of minimum doses of epinephrine. The old patient is usually hypersensitive to the pressor effect of adrenergic drugs, and the possibility of cardiac dysrhythmias is also increased unless dilute solutions are used. If instead of the customary 1:200,000 concentration of epinephrine, 1:400,000 concentrations are employed, systemic effects will be no more frequent than in young adults.

With these general principles, infiltration and nerve blocks should be used in most eye surgery, superficial operations of the head, neck, chest, and abdomen, and operations on the extremities.

Major surgery of limited duration in the chest and abdomen can also be safely performed with the combination of intercostal nerve blocks and very light general anesthesia.

For surgery in the lower abdomen, perineum and on lower extremities, subarachnoid and peridural anesthesia is an excellent choice.

Intravenous Regional Anesthesia

An old method of local anesthesia has been reintroduced in surgery on the extremities. This consists of the administration of a dilute local anesthetic agent intravenously with an occluding cuff around the limb proximal to the injection. This provides excellent local analgesia in the extremity. Systemic reactions can be avoided by slow, intermittent, gradual release of the occluding cuff at the end of surgery.

SUBARACHNOID ANALGESIA

When used correctly, spinal anesthesia is one of the safest techniques for the geriatric patient. The hypotension so much feared in this age-group results from the preganglionic blockade of sympathetic vasoconstrictor fibers. The extent of vasodilatation is in direct ratio to the number of sympathetic segments paralyzed. Provided the subarachnoid block is limited to spinal segments below the T8 level, the resulting vasodilatation is easily controlled with vasopressor drugs, thus avoiding hypotension. Spinal analgesia below the L1 level usually does not lower blood pressure. We therefore recommend limiting spinal anesthesia to operations below the umbilicus (T10). There are fortunately few contraindications to this technique. These include abnormal clotting mechanism, skin infections at the site of lumbar puncture, septicemia, and diseases of the central nervous system. Headache as a complication of spinal anesthesia, for reasons unknown, is rarely seen in the aged person.

Peridural Anesthesia

Peridural anesthesia has several advantages over subarachnoid anesthesia. It involves the introduction of a needle or catheter into the peridural space, into which local anesthetic agents are injected. The catheter may be left in the epidural space for prolonged periods, thus making anesthesia possible for the longest operation. It may also be used in the postoperative period for pain relief and sympathetic blockade. Because the dura is not pierced, postpuncture spinal headache is avoided. The incidence of hypotension is almost the same as in spinal anesthesia and depends primarily on the level of sympathetic blockade.

A disadvantage is that greater skill is needed to avoid failures. Injection into venous plexuses or inadvertent subarachnoid injection of large amounts of local anesthetics must be avoided. In the elderly, only about half the amount of local anesthetic agents used in the young achieves the same anesthesia.[6] The extent of spread of the local anesthetic and, hence, the height of the block becomes less predictable with increasing age.[5] Failure to recognize this will almost certainly result in widespread block. The contraindications and management of complications are similar to those of spinal anesthesia.

MONITORING

The response to the continuing anesthetic and surgical trespasses must be carefully observed and corrective measures instituted when appropriate.

The effects of deep anesthesia, blood loss, fluid and electrolyte derangements, surgical manipulations, trauma, and changes in position and temperature on vital organs must be taken into account. The respiratory and circulatory systems and their interactions on other vital systems are especially important. For example, inadequate blood flow to the brain, liver, and kidneys interferes with their functions and threatens the integrity of these organs at a cellular level, and hypercarbia owing to hypoventilation may increase catecholamine production, causing hypertension and cardiac dysrhythmias.

A complete discussion of the multitude of pathophysiologic changes that can occur during anesthesia can be found in standard texts. At all stages of life, the integrity of the respiratory and circulatory systems is fundamental for tissue perfusion and oxygen supply to cells. With advancing age, degenerative cardiovascular and pulmonary changes reduce the oxygen supply available to tissues. Careful assessment of the adequacy of tissue oxygenation is essential during anesthesia so that potentially harmful changes can be detected and quickly corrected.

Cardiovascular System

Arterial Blood Pressure

Arterial blood pressure is usually measured indirectly by sphygmomanometry. Direct intra-arterial pressure monitoring is desirable during extensive surgery, in cardiac surgery, or when excessive bleeding is anticipated.

Electrocardiography

In elderly patients, one of the most useful monitoring devices is the electrocardioscope. This instrument, although it does not indicate the adequacy of circulation, is valuable in the analysis of dysrhythmias and as a warning of myocardial ischemia and hypercarbia. Atherosclerosis is widespread in three of every five patients over age 60, and it increases the chance of fatal complications to three times that of the nonsclerotic patient.[9]

Central Venous Pressure

Central venous pressure can be measured by inserting a catheter into the internal jugular or subclavian vein and advancing it into the superior vena cava. The basilic and cephalic veins are other routes of access. The catheter is then connected to a suitable manometer. A decrease in central venous pressure below 6 cm H_2O and significant hypotension may be caused by inadequate venous return, owing to hypovolemia or vasodilatation. In this case, blood, plasma, other fluid replacement, or elevation of the legs is indicated.

A high venous pressure (more than 16 cm H_2O) with hypotension may indicate the need for digitalization or the administration of a vasodilator. A rising central venous pressure may indicate overtransfusion. The intraoperative monitoring of the pulmonary artery wedge pressure using a Swan-Ganz catheter is indicated in patients with marginal cardiovascular reserve. This type of monitoring is especially useful in cardiovascular surgery; in patients in whom massive blood loss or extensive fluid shifts are anticipated as may occur during aortic bifurcation graft; and in induced hypotensive anesthesia used during extensive surgery on the head and neck for removal of brain tumors and neoplasms of the eye, tongue, and maxilla.

Pulmonary artery pressure monitoring allows the anesthesiologist to make a differential diagnosis between hypotension owing to myocardial depression, decreased peripheral resistance, and decreased blood volume. This knowledge facilitates the judicious administration of drugs, blood, and crystalloid solutions to correct a drop in blood pressure and to maintain optimal cardiac output.

The Doppler ultrasonic flowmeter permits the detection of air emboli. Patients of any age who undergo neurologic surgery in the sitting position are exposed to the danger of air emboli. Unless this complication is immediately recognized and therapeutic measures are taken at once, cardiovascular collapse results.

Respiratory System

Blood Gas Transport

The adequacy of blood gas transport depends on the efficient exchange of oxygen and carbon dioxide between the pulmonary capillaries and alveoli. If the function of either or both the circulatory and respiratory systems is impaired, oxygen transport is significantly reduced and cyanosis may appear. This should be regarded as a late sign of hypoxia, and the absence of cyanosis does not necessarily imply that tissues are being adequately oxygenated. When accurate assessment of oxygen transport is necessary, arterial blood gas analysis can be used.

Ventilatory Parameters

Respiratory rate is counted at frequent intervals during anesthesia. Tidal volume can be assessed by observation of the amplitude of respiratory movements. For greater accuracy, a ventilation meter should be incorporated into the anesthetic circuit. The information derived from these observations and measurements enables one to estimate the adequacy of alveolar ventilation. If necessary, ventilation should be augmented by manual or mechanical means.

Temperature

Temperature can be monitored by an electronic device with a sensing probe. The probe is usually introduced into the esophagus. Temperature monitoring is mandatory in hypothermic techniques such as surgery for intracranial aneurysm, and it is useful in prolonged surgery, especially when accompanied by multiple transfusions, and in septic shock.

The foregoing examples illustrate the type of observations used frequently during anesthesia to assess the adequacy of vital systems in the geriatric patient. The patient's safety depends on continuous vigilance and appropriate action when deleterious changes develop. In the elderly patient, the ability to compensate for the stresses of anesthesia and surgery is impaired. It is essential to be aware of any undesirable change and the additional information provided by instruments now available should be fully exploited.

SUPPORT OF HOMEOSTASIS

With advancing age, the function of essential organs declines and the mechanisms that preserve function in the face of stress gradually become exhausted. Therefore, supportive measures are more critical in the elderly anesthetized patient than in a younger counterpart. The elderly patient does not tolerate deep anesthesia, principally because of its depressant effects on the circulatory center and myocardium. Consequently, the depth of anesthesia should never exceed the requirements of the surgical procedure. Position during surgery has an important bearing on circulatory homeostasis.

Cardiorespiratory Aspects

Assisted or controlled ventilation affects circulatory dynamics. The inspiratory phase should be kept relatively short, and there should be an adequate expiratory pause. The incorporation of a positive end-expiratory pressure during the expiratory pause is frequently useful to reduce pulmonary shunting, thus facilitating oxygen transport.

Blood Volume and Electrolyte and Fluid Balance

Dehydration and hypovolemia are common in elderly patients. These and other forms of fluid and electrolyte imbalance should be corrected by appropriate parenteral infusion before induction of anesthesia whenever possible. Correction should be continued while the operation is in progress to compensate for additional losses and fluid shifts taking place. Care must be taken to avoid sodium overload. Correction of dehydration is best guided by central venous pressure, pulmonary arterial wedge pressures, and urinary output. In major procedures, a catheter in the bladder enables the output of urine to be measured hourly. This also avoids overdistention of the bladder. The intravascular space may require expansion with blood or a suitable substitute. During surgery in which renal blood flow is impaired, such as that requiring extracorporeal circulation, furosemide may be administered intravenously to improve urinary output.

For adequate cardiac output and tissue perfusion, hypovolemia owing to continuing blood loss or fluid shifts must be corrected. The use of balanced salt solutions (*e.g.*, Ringer's lactate) reduces the need for correction of blood loss, with its attendant risks. However, correction of blood loss is indicated to maintain a satisfactory blood oxygen-carrying capacity. In the estimation of actual blood loss, central venous pressure is a valuable guide.

Because vasopressors constrict the vascular bed and may impair tissue perfusion, they should be used only as a temporary expedient or after spinal or epidural anesthesia. Even in these circumstances, careful technique with the extent of anesthesia limited to the required segments, expansion of the vascular bed by the administration of fluids intravenously, and careful attention to posture reduce the need for vasopressors.

In metabolic acidosis, such as that seen after massive correction of blood loss, quantitation of the severity of the loss in terms of base deficit or plasma bicarbonate enables suitable correction with sodium bicarbonate. For this purpose, analysis of venous blood samples is adequate.

POSTOPERATIVE CARE

The immediate postoperative period is a critical phase of the patient's overall surgical experience. Some residual anesthetic depression of metabolic functions remains. Protective reflexes, such as coughing, have not yet fully returned. Blood gas exchange may be compromised by anesthetic and surgical factors. These include hypoventilation owing to residual curarization, respiratory center depression, diaphragmatic splinting owing to pain, and tight dressing. Early in the postoperative period, new problems may require treatment, such as restlessness owing to pain, nausea, and vomiting.

During this initial period of recovery, the elderly patient is vulnerable to the effects of these stresses. For optimal recovery, careful observation by skilled nurses and appropriate supportive therapy are essential. The recovery room provides the necessary facilities for these measures, including suitable monitoring equipment, as well as immediate emergency treatment should this be needed. Even after relatively minor surgery under local anesthesia, it is usually desirable to admit the elderly patient to a recovery room for observation.

Transport

Postoperative care begins in the operating room. Surgical patients should remain in the operating room until it is safe to transport them to a recovery room. Then they should be gently moved onto recovery room stretchers, which should be equipped with side rails and should be adjustable, so that the lower extremities or upper part of the body can be elevated if necessary.

During general anesthesia, and frequently in association with local anesthesia, patients inspire an oxygen-enriched mixture. It is desirable to continue the administration of oxygen postoperatively by means of a nasal catheter to prevent hypoxemia. In some instances, ventilatory support is also indicated. When necessary, these measures should be instituted during transfer of patients from the operating room and should be continued in the recovery room. When an endotracheal tube is used during anesthesia, it should be left in place to facilitate the transport of patients who require ventilatory assistance. Endotracheal tubes are generally best left in until the reflexes fully return. This is especially important if the possibility of vomiting or regurgitation is present because it prevents aspiration of gastric contents.

Oxygen

Hypoxemia is common, if not universal, in elderly postoperative patients. Arterial oxygen tension tends to decline with age.[10] This is mainly due to increasing mismatching of alveolar ventilation and perfusion. This derangement may be increased during the administration of, and recovery from, anesthesia. Its effect on lowering oxygen tension is enhanced by alveolar hypoventilation. The resulting cerebral hypoxia may cause restlessness, and it is important to distinguish this from the restlessness owing to postoperative pain. The administration of narcotics at this time would cause further respiratory depression and possible fatal consequences if unrecognized.

Fortunately, mild hypoxemia can be corrected simply by administering 4 to 6 liters/min of humidified oxygen through a nasal cannula. This provides an inspired oxygen concentration of 35% to 40%. We recommend its routine use in all elderly patients to prevent hypoxemia for at least the first hour of recovery.

Narcotics

Respiratory depression may be due to the residual effects of narcotic analgesics used to supplement anesthesia, such as morphine, meperidine, or fentanyl. The respiratory rate under these circumstances is typically slow. Naloxone is recommended to reverse this.

Narcotic analgesics should be used sparingly for postoperative pain because of their respiratory depressant effects. In large amounts, they depress the cough reflex and interfere with the sighing mechanism.

Mechanical Ventilation

Mechanical ventilation with oxygen-enriched mixtures may be indicated when hypoxemia is severe. Usually carbon dioxide retention is also a feature, and hypercarbia is itself an indication for mechanical ventilation. Severe respiratory insufficiency can be recognized easily, by observing the patient's respiratory efforts. In less obvious situations, blood gas analysis is helpful in assessing the need for ventilatory therapy. After mechanical ventilation is instituted, blood gas analysis should be repeated at suitable intervals to evaluate treatment.

The oxygen cost of increased ventilatory effort may, under certain circumstances, approach 50% of total oxygen uptake.[7] This is associated with an increase in cardiac output. In the elderly, the demands of heightened ventilatory activity on a circulation that already has little reserve may lead to cardiac decompensation and circulatory failure. Mechanically assisted or controlled ventilation reduces or abolishes the work and oxygen cost of spontaneous respiration. For these reasons, mechanical ventilation may be indicated in elderly subjects with increases in ventilatory effort, that might be safely tolerated by younger persons. If a positive end-expiratory pressure is used during mechanical ventilation, it should be remembered that cardiac output may be decreased as a consequence; this is more likely to happen in elderly persons with impaired circulatory homeostasis.

When continuous mechanical ventilation is required for several hours or days, a cuffed oral endotracheal tube usually provides a satisfactory airway. Endotracheal tubes with soft cuffs are less likely to damage the tracheal mucosa. Tracheostomy is rarely necessary. Secretions must be carefully removed by suctioning with a sterile catheter, at hourly intervals or more frequently if necessary. Mechanical hyperventilation of the lungs every hour helps prevent atelectasis. Frequent turning is also important in this regard. Weaning should be accomplished as soon as feasible, by permitting brief periods of spontaneous ventilation and gradually increasing their duration. Intermittent mandatory ventilation during which spontaneous ventilation is periodically interrupted by mechanical insufflations is often useful during weaning. Blood gas analysis; measurement of vital capacity, tidal volume, and inspiratory force; and calculation of dead space to tidal volume ratios are helpful in determining the time at which weaning can be initiated.

Chest Physiotherapy

Chest physiotherapy consists of breathing and coughing exercises, postdural drainage, and percussion of the chest wall. The patient should be introduced to these exercises preoperatively. Chest physiotherapy is a valuable measure in elderly patients, whether or not they require mechanical ventilation. It reduces the incidence of respiratory complications. The physiotherapist can also play an important role in maintaining muscular power and optimal range of joint movement, thereby facilitating early return to ambulation. This in turn reduces the incidence of pulmonary complications.

CONCLUSION

Life expectancy continues to increase in all segments of the population in the United States. As a consequence, the incidence of geriatric surgical conditions has increased. Improvement of all phases of surgical management, including anesthesia, has made it possible to carry out surgery successfully, in terms of immediate survival, on ever-increasing segments of the geriatric population.

Operations that would not have been deemed feasible a decade ago are being performed today on patients advanced in age. This has been made possible by greater understanding of their reactions to stresses of surgery and anesthesia and of the supportive measures that counteract potentially harmful situations. These measures must be fully exploited for a successful outcome.

However, our increasing successes should not interfere with a realistic appraisal of a given surgical procedure. The gain should be considered soberly from both short- and long-term standpoints. Some of the gross impairments of senescence, such as an advanced organic mental syndrome, are persistent contraindications, even when heroic surgery supported by brilliant anesthesia is instantly available.

REFERENCES

1. Bender AD: The effect of increasing age on the distribution of peripheral blood flow in man. J Am Geriatr Soc 13:192, 1965
2. Bender AD: Pharmacologic aspects of aging: A survey of the effect of increasing age on drug activity in adults. J Am Geriatr Soc 12:114, 1964
3. Bender AD: Pharmacodynamic consequences of aging and their implications in the treatment of the elderly patient. Med Ann DC 36:267, 1967
4. Blundell E: A psychological study of the effects of surgery on eighty-six elderly patients. Br J Soc Clin Psychol 6:297, 1967
5. Bromage PR: Ageing and epidural dose requirements. Br J Anaesth 41:1016, 1969
6. Bromage PR: Speed and site of action of epidural analgesia. Int Anesthesiol Clin 1:545, 1963
7. Campbell EJM: The Respiratory Muscles and the Mechanics of Breathing, p 84. London, Lloyd-Luke (Medical Books), 1958
8. Castelli WP: CHD risk factors in the elderly. Hosp Pract 11:113, 1976
9. Clowes GHA: Special Problems in the aged patient. In Randall HT, Hardy JD, Moore FD (eds): Manual of Pre-Operative and Post-Operative Care, p 243. Philadelphia, WB Saunders, 1967
10. Conway CM, Payne JP, Tomlin PJ: Arterial oxygen tensions of patients awaiting surgery. Br J Anaesth 37:405, 1965
11. Del Guercio LRM, Cohn JD: Monitoring operative risk in the elderly. JAMA 243:1350, 1980

12. Denney JL, Denson JS: Risk of surgery in patients over 90. Geriatrics 27:115, 1972

13. Djokovic JL, Hedley-Whyte J: Prediction of outcome of surgery and anesthesia in patients over 80. JAMA 242:2301, 1979

14. Duncalf D, Gartner S, Carol B: Mortality in association with ophthalmic surgery. Am J Ophthalmol 69:610, 1970

15. Eckenhoff JE, Oech SR: The effect of narcotics and antagonists upon respiration and circulation in man. Clin Pharmacol Ther 1:483, 1960

16. Farner D, Verzár F: The age parameter of pharmacological activity. Experientia 17:421, 1961

17. Fisch C: Electrocardiogram in the aged: An independent marker of heart disease? Am J Med 70:4, 1981

18. Foldes FF, Swerdlow M, Siker ES: Narcotics and Narcotic Antagonists, p. 232. Springfield, IL, Charles C Thomas, 1964

19. Fraser JG, Ramachandran PR, Davis HS: Anesthesia and recent myocardial infarction. JAMA 199:318, 1967

20. Freeman IT (ed): Clinical Principles and Drugs in the Aging, p 122. Springfield, IL, Charles C Thomas, 1963

21. Goldberg LI: D'opamine: Clinical uses of an endogenous catecholamine. N Engl J Med 291:707, 1974

22. Goldman L, Caldera DL: Risk of general anesthesia and elective operation in the hypertensive patient. Anesthesiology 50:285, 1979

23. Goldman L, Caldera DL, Nussbaum SR et al: Multifactorial index of cardiac risk in noncardiac surgical procedures. N Engl J Med 207:845, 1977

24. Greenblatt DJ, Sellers EM, Shader RI: Drug disposition in old age. N Engl Med 306:1081, 1982

25. Hedley-Whyte J, Burgess GE, Feeley TW, Miller MG: Applied Physiology of Respiratory Care, p 299 Boston, Little, Brown & Co, 1976

26. Hill GE, Wong KC, Hodges MR: Lithium carbonate and neuromuscular blocking agents. Anesthesiology 46:122, 1977

27. Hospital Mortality: PAS Hospitals United States 1974–1975, Ann Arbor, Michigan. Commission on Professional and Hospital Activities, 1977

28. Ikram H, Rubin AP, Jewkes RF: Effect of diazepam on myocardial blood flow of patients with and without coronary artery disease. Br Heart J 35:626, 1973

29. Kaiko RF, Wallenstein SL, Rogers AG et al: Narcotics in the elderly. Med Clin North Am 66:1079, 1982

30. Kannel WB, Dawber TR, McGee DL: Perspectives on systolic hypertension. The Framingham Study. Circulation 61:1179, 1980

31. Kapur PA, Flacke WE: Epinephrine-induced arrhythmias and cardiovascular function after verapamil during halothane anesthesia in the day. Anesthesiology 55:218, 1981

32. Klotz V, Avant GR, Hoyumpa A et al: The effects of age and liver disease on the disposition and elimination of diazepam in adult man. J Clin Invest 55:347, 1975

33. Knudson RJ, Clark DF, Kennedy TC et al: Effect of aging alone on mechanical properties of the normal adult lung. J Appl Physiol 43:1054, 1977

34. Kolata GB: The aging heart: Changes in function and response to drugs. Science 195:166, 1977

35. Kronenberg RS, Drage CW: Attenuation of the ventilatory and heart rate responses to hypoxia and hypercapnia with aging in normal men. J Clin Invest 52:1812, 1973

36. Leith DE, Mead J: Mechanism determining residual volume of the lungs in normal subjects. J Appl Physiol 23:221, 1967

37. McLaughlan MSF: The aging kidney. Lancet 2:143, 1978

38. Muisan G, Sorbini CA, Grassi V: Respiratory function in the aged. Bull Physiopathol Respir 7:973, 1971

39. Pontoppidan H, Beecher HK: Progressive loss of protective reflexes in the airway with advancing age. JAMA 174:2209, 1960

40. Rao TLK, Jacobs KH, El-Etr AA: Reinfarction following anesthesia in patients with myocardial infarction. Anesthesiology 59:499, 1983

41. Rusy BF: Cholinergic drugs in the age. In Freeman JT (ed): Clinical Principles and Drugs in the Aging, p 100. Springfield, IL, Charles C Thomas, 1963

42. Ryan SF, Vincent TN, Mitchell RS et al: Ductasia: An asymptomatic pulmonary change related to age. Med Thorac 22:181, 1965

43. Solomon DH, Shock NW: Studies of adrenal cortical and anterior pituitary function in elderly men. J Geriatr 5:302, 1950

44. Strandell T: Circulatory studies on healthy old men. Acta Med Scand [Suppl] 414:1, 1964

45. Strauer BE: Contractile response to morphine, piritramide, meperidine, and fentanyl: A comparative study of the effects on the isolated ventricular myocardium. Anesthesiology 37:304, 1972

46. Wespi H: Active transport and passive fluxes of K, Na and Li in mammalian non-myelinated nerve fibers. Pfluegers Arch 306:262, 1969

47. Zaidu YR: Pacemakers. Anesthesiology 60:319, 1984

IV

Musculoskeletal Problems in the Aged Patient

29 Rheumatic Disorders

David Hamerman

The number of adults who present to primary physicians with arthritic complaints ranges from 20% to 30% of the population, exceeded only by those with cardiovascular diseases and perhaps respiratory diseases.[6,46,55] A National Commission on Arthritis in the United States reported to Congress in 1971 that at least 22 million Americans suffer from arthritis, and this figure did not include approximately 6 million more with related musculoskeletal conditions. These figures are based on those reporting to physicians; estimates of those with arthritic complaints who do not seek medical advice run as high as 75%.[55] Another way to look at the extent of the problem is to assess disability in the home. Defined as a condition in which existence at home without help is impossible, disability increases with age, rising from 12% at ages 65 to 69 to 80% at age over 85, according to one study.[21] Although not all such disability is related to arthritic complaints, almost half may be.[61] In one study musculoskeletal diseases exceeded all other classes of disability except cardiovascular,[46] with a prevalence of 14.2 per 1000 and 17 per 1000, respectively.

All this means that the subject of arthritis in older persons is a highly relevant concern to primary physicians and one in which education in this field for these health care providers has been stressed.[46,50] Special features that relate to arthritis and rheumatologic complaints in the elderly include the following: a high prevalence of certain specific conditions, such as osteoarthritis (OA) and polymyalgia rheumatica (PMR); the greater impact on the elderly that results from immobility; the superimposition of arthritic disorders on other medical problems prevalent in the elderly, such as cardiovascular diseases, anemia, and emphysema;[60] the use of multiple medications by the

elderly for multiple medical conditions, creating the potential for adverse effects from drug interactions;[35] atypical presentations of arthritis that may lead to inappropriate diagnoses, as, for example, casually designating joint complaints as OA, thereby masking or delaying detection of more serious underlying conditions, such as malignancy

A number of excellent books and reviews focus on arthritis in the elderly and divide the discussion of the various arthritic disorders into traditional categories.[3,23,62] In this chapter I will discuss the presentations that might be observed by primary physicians, reviewing in some detail a limited number of conditions rather than discussing the subject exhaustively. Naturally, it should be understood that overlap exists between polyarticular and monoarticular types of presentation, and the format used here should be regarded as a means for a working discussion rather than a rigid classification.

POLYARTICULAR PRESENTATIONS

Rheumatoid Arthritis

Symmetrical polyarthritis with joint swelling, particularly of the metacarpophalangeal (MP) joints, morning stiffness, and a female preponderance are among the typical clinical features of rheumatoid arthritis (RA) in an adult population. The diagnosis is often confirmed by remissions and exacerbations, the presence of subcutaneous nodules, and a positive serologic test for rheumatoid factor ("seropositive RA" as contrasted to "seronegative RA").[11] In patients 60 years of age and over, the incidence of apparent first onset of RA is variously estimated to be between 2% to 15%,[3] and the usual female predominance may revert to equivalence between the sexes. Grahame[28] has commented on the greater tendency of RA in the elderly to commence "in an abrupt and even explosive form," and Corrigan and co-workers[13] have reported on a small subgroup of "aged" patients who show an acute onset with many systemic features (fever, weakness, anemia) who subsequently appear to recover completely. The nonarticular manifestations often associated with vasculitis appear less common in the older age-group. In establishing the diagnosis of RA the following should be considered: the erythrocyte sedimentation rate (ESR) is usually elevated; typical joint erosions on roentgenography are helpful if present and can be distinguished from changes in OA and crystal deposition disease; a positive test for rheumatoid factor is also helpful but must be interpreted with caution due to higher incidence of positive tests in subjects as they age; and long-term observation may be essential to document remissions and exacerbations. The necessity to observe over a long period of time is an obligation for physicians who provide primary care for patients with arthritic disorders. This ensures the establishment of rapport and confidence between patient and physician; sets the appropriate tone for management of a chronic illness especially in the aged where multiple time-consuming, expensive, and physically demanding referrals may be avoided; diminishes unrealistic expectations on the patient's part of a quick "cure" often based on gossip by other patients; reduces the temptation of the pressed physician to start "major league" therapy, particularly corticosteroids, when more conservative medications will be better tolerated in the long run; and provides for clarification of the diagnosis with time.

There are a few special considerations. After the diagnosis of RA is established, the physician must still be aware of certain pitfalls. Presentation of an acute arthritis in one large joint (*e.g.,* the knee) or even multiple joints should not simply be accepted as an "acute flare" of RA, leading the physician to increase anti-inflammatory medication, particularly corticosteroids. Fever and especially mental status changes, with or without an elevated blood leukocyte count, are clues to make the physician think rather of septic arthritis.[47] Areas of skin breakdown or urinary tract infection may form foci for hematogenous dissemination; other predisposing factors include chronic debilitating disease, long-term corticosteroid therapy, ulcerating subcutaneous nodules, and diabetes

mellitus. If unrecognized, septic arthritis can be a highly lethal complication. The diagnosis can only be made or excluded by aspirating the joint and subjecting the fluid to culture and analysis. *Staphylococcus aureus* is the organism involved in most cases.[56] Even when the diagnosis of RA appears likely in a patient with polyarthritis, fever, anemia, elevated ESR, and a positive test for rheumatoid factor, further workup including blood cultures may be needed to exclude subacute bacterial endocarditis. The differential diagnosis between RA and polymyalgia rheumatica (PMR) requires consideration, especially when patients with apparent PMR have synovitis. Healey[32] points out that none of the patients with PMR and synovitis had positive tests for rheumatoid factor, joint damage, or radiographic evidence of erosion during a follow-up period. Therapeutic considerations concerning corticosteroid use as well as the possibilities of temporal arteritis are at stake here.

Malignancy

The primary physician must be alert to older patients presenting with polyarticular complaints in which the underlying problem is a malignancy not readily apparent unless appropriate workup is instituted.

The following are examples of malignancy with arthritis;[5,10,24] discussion will be limited to hypertrophic osteoarthropathy:

Metastatic disease to joints
Primary malignancy of joint components
Hypertrophic (pulmonary) osteoarthropathy
Multiple myeloma with or without amyloid disease of joints
"Carcinoma polyarthritis"
Dermatomyositis
Gout secondary to myeloproliferative disorders

Hypertrophic osteoarthropathy is usually designated as hypertrophic pulmonary osteoarthropathy because most cases are associated with lung cancer. The points to emphasize here are based on a recent review:[52] the symptoms of joint complaints affecting the knees and ankles, and at times small joints of the hands, usually precede by months clinical manifestations of intrathoracic disease; morning stiffness and relief with nonsteroidal anti-inflammatory drugs (NSAIDs) may occur and raise the possibility of RA; clues may be characteristic facial changes with accentuated forehead creases and prominent nasolabial folds; roentgenograms of the lower extremities reveal periostitis, and bone scans show peripheral uptake along the periosteum of all distal long bones; clubbing of the fingers and toes is observed in all cases but at times is a later manifestation. The major point is that if a chest roentgenogram is included in the diagnostic workup, the true nature of the arthritic condition may be apparent. When the tumor is excised (almost always an adenocarcinoma or squamous cell carcinoma), joint manifestations disappear.

Seronegative Spondyloarthropathies

It has become popular among rheumatologists to designate a group of rheumatic disorders as the "seronegative spondyloarthropathies." These conditions are marked by negative serologic tests for rheumatoid factor, strong clinical and familial interrelations, which includes high frequency of positive tests for the genetic marker HLA-B27 (particularly in ankylosing spondylitis), and the high prevalence of coexisting spinal, sacroiliac, and peripheral joint disease, particularly hips and shoulders, in association with involvement of the eye, skin, and bowel:

Ankylosing spondylitis
Psoriatic arthritis
Reiter's disease
Crohn's disease
Ulcerative colitis
Whipple's disease

With the exception of psoriatic arthritis these disorders are not a particularly frequent accom-

paniment of older age and will not be further discussed here.

Polyarticular Osteoarthritis

Osteoarthritis is generally regarded as a rather slowly progressive and noninflammatory condition confined to one or two large weight-bearing joints (hip and/or knee) where it may be variably symptomatic over the years. Polyarticular OA has received more attention recently and is important to recognize because the painful, symmetric involvement of the hands and other joints may lead to confusion with RA. Huskisson and co-workers[33] have specifically addressed this differential in patients observed in a medical (rheumatology) clinic and a summary of their findings is presented in Table 29-1. The clinical picture of polyarticular inflammatory OA is generally clear,[59] although there are nuances in the clinical descriptions and radiographic findings in terms of "primary generalized OA,"[34] "erosive OA,"[42] and "inflammatory OA."[19] Generalized OA with Heberden's nodes is said to be highly familial,[43] while nonnodal OA with proximal interphalangeal (PIP) involvement is less so and more influenced by and associated with climate, obesity, hypertension, and hyperuricemia. The onset of the nodal form is usually abrupt, and almost all patients affected are women in their early 50s or 60s. The distal interphalangeal (DIP) joints are symmetrically involved, swollen, warm, and tender, producing the typical features of Heberden's nodes. The PIP joints are also in-

TABLE 29-1   Comparisons Between Patients with Rheumatoid Arthritis and Osteoarthritis Seen in a Rheumatology Clinic

Criteria	Rheumatoid Arthritis	Osteoarthritis
Age at onset	Younger	Older
Morning stiffness	Prolonged—diffuse	Brief—often 1 site
Pain	Mostly morning	Mostly night
Number of joints	Many	Few
Joints involved	Hands—proximal interphalangeal joints	Hands—distal interphalangeal joints
	Feet	
	Knees	Knees
	Shoulders	
Roentgenographic findings of crystals	Rare	Common
Erythrocyte sedimentation rate	Often elevated	Rarely elevated
Rheumatoid factor	Often present	

(Data from Huskisson EC, Dieppe PA, Tucker AK et al: Another look at osteoarthritis. Ann Rheum Dis 38:423, 1979)

volved in at least half of the patients, with swelling and deformity referred to as Bouchard's nodes. In a smaller proportion of patients the thumb base (carpometacarpal joint) is involved. In Kellgren and Moore's cases,[34] additional involvement was described of the great toes, the first tarsometatarsal joints, and even interfacetal joints of the spine. The hip is occasionally included. Patients may complain of morning stiffness of short duration (less than 30 minutes). The ESR is normal in at least half of the patients and slightly to moderately elevated in the remainder. Tests for rheumatoid factor are generally negative. The condition runs a course measured in a few years and usually subsides, leaving the osteophyte as the typical residue, both clinically and radiographically.

MONOARTICULAR PRESENTATIONS

Indeterminant Diagnosis

A good way to look at establishing the diagnosis of monoarthritis in the elderly is to analyze acute presentations in a population over 70 years of age. Such a study by Gibson and Grahame[25] was carried out "prompted by the suggestion that there exists a senile [sic] monoarticular arthritis peculiar to the aged." Of 59 patients, all but 15 could be diagnosed in conventional terms, including RA, gout, OA, septic arthritis, and so forth. These diagnoses were established by clinical observation, physical examination, tests for serum uric acid, rheumatoid factor, and ESR. In special instances, a joint tap proved diagnostic, as with crystal-induced arthritis or septic arthritis, and perhaps to exclude these conditions in what ultimately was said to be OA confined to one joint (knee) where an effusion was present.

In 11 of the 15 patients with indeterminate monoarthritis potential *multiple* causes existed, such as OA, hyperuricemia secondary to diuretic therapy, and chondrocalcinosis. In 4 others "no evident cause" existed. Two of these patients with knee involvement had benign synovial fluid findings. The follow-up over 13 months generally showed subsidence of symptoms. Thus, a diagnosis could be established in the majority of patients presenting with monoarticular arthritis.

Certain conclusions can be drawn from this assessment. The physician should avoid casually labeling monoarthritis in the aged as "OA," especially when an effusion is present; search for a definite diagnosis, but at least exclude the more serious one (septic joint); and institute appropriate

and conservative forms of therapy while observing the patient for an extended time. The concept of "senile" monoarthritis gains no support: indeed it smacks of ageism.[9]

Osteoarthritis

In this section, OA is considered in its more limited form of knee or hip involvement. The obvious association with weight-bearing joints comes to mind, but we are then confronted by the observations that the ankles rarely have changes compatible with OA, and the non-weight-bearing fingers demonstrate roentgenographic changes in 80% to 100% of the older population.

It is very easy to appreciate that even among experts,[36] OA cannot be organized within the framework of a single encompassing definition. There are obviously multiple predisposing factors as well as types, or subsets. What we lack most are longitudinal data relating to OA over time, but it would be hard to envision the conduct of such a study, extending at least over 30 years.[1] We do not know if OA of the hip or knee is necessarily progressive and in whom it will progress. Forman and co-workers[20] claimed no increased incidence of OA in subjects at a senior center studied at ages of 60 to over 80, but certain pitfalls exist: the study was not longitudinal; criteria for the diagnosis are not necessarily universally accepted; patients with the most severe cases may not have survived; and in some instances advanced disease can become painless.[1]

What can be said of OA of the hip or knee is that there are a host of associated conditions that seem to predispose to joint deformity, such as RA, known trauma, meniscectomy,[18] and, particularly in the hip, congenital deformities such as slipped capital femoral epiphysis, Legg–Calvé-Perthes disease, and congenital dysplasia.[30] All these conform to a category of so-called secondary OA; presumably primary OA exists where there are no known predisposing conditions. However, such a classification does not seem particularly useful and may be misleading.

In the hip, subchondral sclerosis and osteophyte formation occur with other anatomical abnormalities and pain and restriction of movement are major effects. The prevalence of OA of the knee is much greater than OA of the hip, and joint instability is also an associated finding. The condition termed *chondromalacia patellae* applies to gross softening of the articular cartilage of the patella, but this occurs at an earlier age and is said not to progress.[53]

Crystal Deposition Arthritis

The relationship between crystals in the joint fluid and acute arthritis is a fascinating story elucidated in the past 25 years and described by McCarty in his 1982 Heberden oration.[38] It is a subject that concerns us because of its prevalence in the elderly.

Gout is associated with the deposition of monosodium urate crystals. The most frequent nonurate crystal associated with arthritis is calcium pyrophosphate dihydrate (CPPD). These are seen on joint radiographs in a linear array within the menisci or cartilage itself.[44] Radiologic studies suggest a rapidly rising prevalence of chondrocalcinosis with age, so that 30% to 50% of nonagenarians are affected. Radiographic findings may be noted in asymptomatic patients. The clinical presentations are variable:

Acute (pseudogout) attacks with asymptomatic intervals, predominantly in men (20% of cases).
Cases with subacute inflammation of multiple joints, especially wrist and MP, that may mimic RA (5%)
Acute attacks with joint degeneration, usually symmetrical and resembling OA, but involving wrist, carpal, MP, elbow, and shoulder joints more commonly. Isolated patellar-femoral or radiocarpal joint involvement is a radiologic clue to CPPD (50%).

About 10% of the patients with either gout or pseudogout show an acute attack after surgery or an acute medical illness.

Dieppe and colleagues[16] studied 105 patients with pyrophosphate arthropathy, 29 men (mean age 62) and 76 women (mean age 73). There was usually a long history of joint complaints, predominantly in the knee. About half the men and one third of women had acute attacks. All patients showed linear punctate calcification of hyaline and fibrocartilage, associated with typical degenerative changes. In a few cases rapidly progressive joint destruction was observed, resembling Charcot joints; this may require joint replacement or prosthesis of the hip or knee. Hydroxyapatite is another form of crystal deposition associated with acute arthritis[51] and with destructive changes in the shoulder ("Milwaukee shoulder").

It is not entirely clear whether preexisting joint damage predisposes to crystal deposition or whether crystal deposition is a primary event. Such associated joint conditions as OA, hypermobility, prior joint surgery, RA, and chronic steroid therapy seem to predispose to cartilage damage and crystal deposition.

Two nonprimary articular diseases that appear to have an association with crystal deposition are hyperparathyroidism and hemochromatosis.

Septic Arthritis

Septic arthritis for the purpose of this discussion includes nongonococcal arthritis arising as a consequence of joint invasion by bacteria directly from the bloodstream during bacteremia.[26] Aside from patients with preexisting joint involvement due to RA, the classic presentation occurs in a single joint, usually the knee, although at times in multiple joints, with warmth and swelling, with or without fever and chills; although pain is characteristic, it may not be present. Substantial limitation of the range of motion of the joint is the most consistent finding. Joints not usually involved by arthritis may be involved, such as the shoulder, and in particular the sternoclavicular joint. Bacteria associated with septic arthritis in an older age-group are predominantly *Staphylococcus aureus* and streptococci, with a fairly high incidence of gram-negative bacilli other than *Hemophilus influenzae,* which is seen almost always in infants.

In an adult, particularly of an older age-group, there are some potential predisposing conditions that should be kept in mind: RA, immunosuppressive therapy, malignancy, diabetes mellitus, and presence of a joint prosthesis (most of these are recognized within 1 month after surgery). Very important for the older-age group is the presence of an extra-articular focus of infection. Such a primary focus should be sought since its discovery could provide an important clue to bacterial etiology. Thus septic arthritis may be associated with urinary infections due to *Escherichia coli* or *Proteus mirabilis,* skin and soft tissue infections or acute endocarditis with *staphyloccus aureus,* intra-abdominal foci with polymicrobial isolates, including Enterobacteriaceae and anaerobes, and pneumonia with pneumococci or streptococci.

If the primary physician is inexperienced in performing joint aspiration, especially of joints less accessible than the knee, immediate liaison should be established with a physician trained to do so or with the appropriate health facility (clinic or emergency department). Gram stain and culture, white cell count and differential on fluid collected in a tube with heparin, and polarizing microscopy for crystals are essential. Occasionally crystal-induced acute arthritis may coexist with septic arthritis. It must be recognized that negative cultures may be related to prior antibiotic therapy for an extra-articular focus. Antibiotic therapy for the older patient with septic arthritis may require coordinated efforts by the primary physician and consultants in infectious diseases, rheumatology, orthopedic surgery, and rehabilitation medicine. A very good summary has been prepared by Steigbigel.[56] Repeated aspiration of the joint (daily at first) will be needed to remove debris and monitor the outcome of antibiotic therapy. Since a period of non-weight-bearing is advised early, passive range of motion exercises become important in the older patient in whom immobilization has adverse physical and psychological consequences.

PRIMARY MUSCULAR COMPLAINTS

Polymyalgia Rheumatica and Temporal Arteritis

The onset of PMR may be abrupt or occur over a period of 1 or 2 weeks associated with a state resembling a mild viral illness. The patient experiences pain and stiffness in the shoulders and thighs, and these symptoms in an older patient should arouse suspicion of PMR. The stage at which the patient seeks medical advice affects the ease of diagnosis. If mild aching exists, this may tend to be dismissed. When pain and stiffness are paralyzing, simulating "frozen shoulder," or impairing rising from a chair or sitting, the diagnosis may be more apparent.

At this point investigation may reveal a mild anemia and a strikingly elevated ESR, findings which increase probability of PMR. There is no specific way to confirm the diagnosis. The clinical approach often involves excluding other possibilities and instituting a therapeutic trial of low doses of a corticosteroid. The former category would include such medical problems as occult infection,[17] myeloma or carcinoma,[27] polymyositis, and RA. In rare cases the ESR is not highly elevated. A trial of low doses of a steroid (somewhere between 10 mg and 20 mg of prednisone a day) is often so rapidly effective as to constitute a diagnostic test. It should also be pointed out that aspirin and other nonsteroidal drugs have been used when disease seems to be "milder." In any case, over the course of months or years the symptoms gradually subside and the corticosteroid dose or other drug therapy is tapered very slowly.

Of major concern in any discussion of PMR is its relationship to temporal arteritis. Their coexistence converts a benign although painful condition into a potential medical emergency in which blindness may ensue and be nonreversible. The features that strongly indicate the presence of temporal arteritis include headache, tenderness of the scalp and the temples, and intermittent claudication of the jaw muscles. Visual symptoms may precede blindness and include diplopia, spots of light, blurred vision, and ptosis. All these complaints may be superimposed on systemic symptoms that, in addition to PMR, include sweats, anorexia, malaise, low grade fever, and ill-defined depression. In typical cases when the constellation of findings makes the diagnosis apparent, immediate ophthalmologic consultation is advised, and high-dose steroid therapy is begun at once.

Rarely arteritis may be widespread in the cranial arteries, producing a global dementia that may also respond to corticosteroid therapy.[40]

Some comment is needed concerning the question of obtaining a temporal artery biopsy. Dixon[17] has stated that if you suspect temporal arteritis, give corticosteroid therapy, and then arrange for a temporal artery biopsy. However, temporal artery biopsy is not generally done when the diagnosis is obvious because of the recognition of its limitations, including failure to obtain an involved segment and difficulty in determining an acute from a chronic lesion. A floridly positive biopsy showing giant cell arteritis can confirm the diagnosis, but a negative or questionable biopsy cannot exclude it. Biopsy on the contralateral side may be necessary, and thin, consecutive serial sections must be made.[27,29]

To cite one study of 96 patients with the diagnosis of PMR,[12] 40 had a temporal artery biopsy. The results were positive in 14, and 13 of these patients had typical symptoms. The results were negative in 26, and 19 of these patients also had typical symptoms.

NONARTICULAR RHEUMATISM

This section includes fibrositis "striving for recognition and acceptance" (among clinicians and patients alike) and brief mention of two conditions that become important because they are well recognized and remediable: dissection of a popliteal (Baker's) cyst into the posterior calf and carpal tunnel syndrome.[54]

Nonspecific musculoskeletal aching, known as fibrositis or more recently as fibromyalgia syndrome, has certain accepted features, shown below.[63] These are well reviewed in recent articles.[54,57,63]

Terms: *fibrositis, fibromyalgia syndrome*
Aching pains and stiffness, particularly at "trig-

ger" or "pressure points" over the neck, shoulder, elbow, upper and lower back, anterior sternum, and the fat pad medial to the knees

Worse in cold weather, emotional strain

Temporary relief with aspirin, local heat

Sleep disturbance in non–rapid eye movement (REM) sleep with morning stiffness

Symptoms may occur as a "primary disorder" or in association with known articular disease. It is important to exclude PMR by demonstrating a normal ESR. Approaches to therapy include reassurance, conditioning exercises, moist heat, and massage. NSAIDs may be used intermittently.

Fluid in the knee with penetration into a popliteal cyst may lead to a presentation with calf tenderness and swelling suggesting thrombophlebitis. A mass should be sought in the popliteal fossa. A knee arthrogram is the most effective way to demonstrate this, and bed rest with intra-articular administration of corticosteroids will prove helpful.

Entrapment of the median nerve beneath the transverse carpal ligament at the wrist may be idiopathic, or associated with RA, hypothyroidism, amyloid infiltration, and other conditions. The initial symptoms are pain, numbness, and tingling along the palmar surface of the thumb, index, and middle finger, which is often worse at night. If unattended, motor weakness and atrophy develop.

The symptoms can be reproduced by wrist flexion (Phalen maneuver) or percussion of the median nerve at the wrist (Tinel's sign), and the diagnosis is confirmed by electromyographic and nerve conduction studies. A good response usually occurs with a wrist splint and corticosteroid injection. Surgical decompression may be indicated if motor symptoms progress, and the nerve condition remains abnormal.

DIFFUSE IDIOPATHIC SKELETAL HYPEROSTOSIS (DISH)

A great deal of interest has arisen in a condition of diffuse idiopathic skeletal hyperostosis, a new name for a skeletal disorder described for over 35 years in the literature.[45] This subject is important here since it is a disorder of middle-aged and elderly patients,* and radiographic criteria, as described by Resnick and colleagues[45] should distinguish DISH from intervertebral disk degeneration.

---

* Forestier and Rotes-Querol in 1950 described senile (sic) ankylosing hyperostosis of the spine.[22]

DISH shows ossification of the anterolateral ligaments of several contiguous vertebral bodies, absence of "degenerative" disk disease, and absence of apophyseal joint bony ankylosis and sacroiliac joint erosion. Extraspinal radiographic findings may be present, such as irregular excrescences arising from the pelvis, calcaneus, or elbow.

The prevalence of DISH is not clear but may be of "high frequency."[22] It is observed mostly in men, and up to now it has been primarily a radiographic diagnosis. Symptoms referred to the spine such as backache and stiffness are common, but there is not the rigidity of ankylosing spondylitis. Tendinitis may be a complaint in the heel or elbow. Dysphagia may be related to prominent cervical osteophytes. Associated rheumatic diseases (*e.g.,* RA, gout, chondrocalcinosis) may also be present.

THERAPEUTIC CONSIDERATIONS

The primary physician clearly has the initial responsibility to assess the nature of the arthritic complaints that the patient presents, to set in motion necessary diagnostic tests, and to formulate a treatment plan. Depending on the outcome of this first appraisal that may take place over the course of days, weeks, or months, treatment may be modified and consultation with a specialist in rheumatology and/or orthopedic surgery may be desirable. Patient education in the process, with very specific instructions and easy-open containers,[4,31] become particularly important for the elderly patient with arthritis who is likely to be taking multiple other medications. Agate[2] has emphasized an important aspect of geriatric practice that the primary physician is in the best position to follow: knowledge of the patient as a whole in terms of various states of physical disease, mental status, emotional outlook, social environment, and support systems.

In this section a few general principles rather than details of therapy will be discussed. The approach to PMR and temporal arteritis has already been described.

Therapy of a specific nature exists for septic arthritis (antibiotics) and for crystal deposition arthritis. For gout, colchicine (0.65 mg every 2 hours until symptoms subside or diarrhea occurs) has been used as a therapeutic trial, but current practice probably warrants use of the less specific but highly effective NSAIDs, particularly indomethacin, for treatment of any form of crystal-induced acute synovitis. Rodnan[49] prepared an outstanding review of therapy, including indications for the long-term management of tophaceous gout. Some

TABLE 29-2 Partial List of Nonsteroidal Anti-inflammatory Drugs

Class	Generic Name	Trade Name
Salicylates	Acetylsalicylic acid and other salicylates	ASA, aspirin
	Diflunisal	Dolobid
Pyrazoline derivatives	Phenylbutazone*	Butazolidin
	Oxyphenbutazone*	Tandearil
Indoleacetic acid derivatives	Indomethacin	Indocin
	Sulindac	Clinoril
Structural resemblance to indomethacin	Tolmetin	Tolectin
Propionic acid derivatives	Ibuprofen	Motrin
	Naproxen	Naprosyn
	Fenoprofen	Nalfon
Anthranilic acid derivatives	Mefenamic acid	Ponstel
	Meclofenamate	Meclomen
Oxicams	Piroxicam	Feldene

* Cases of marrow dyscrasia, especially aplastic anemia, have been reported in older patients on long-term use.

of the NSAIDs currently available for clinical use in the United States are listed in Table 29-2.[14,41,48,58] Aspirin is included but is not used in crystal deposition disease. Elucidation of the mode of action of the NSAIDs is one of the most exciting recent achievements in biochemical pharmacology. The interested reader may consult recent reviews.[41,48] Some of the biochemical aspects of NSAIDs are shown in Figure 29-1. From cell membrane phospholipid precursors, an enzyme (phospholipase) produces arachidonic acid. Another enzyme (cyclo-oxygenase) converts arachidonic acid to a variety of prostaglandins active in promoting inflammation, with vasodilation, vascular permeability, and so on. The NSAIDs inhibit the enzyme cyclo-oxygenase and thereby arrest synthesis of all prostaglandins nonselectively.

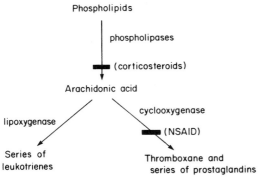

FIG. 29-1. Outline of pathways of arachidonic acid metabolism, showing sites of inhibition of drugs used in the treatment of rheumatic disorders.

There is another pathway of arachidonic acid metabolism not involving cyclo-oxygenase by way of the enzyme lipoxygenase and the series of products called leukotrienes. These are chemotactic for neutrophils and have other inflammatory effects, some in synergy with prostaglandins. The NSAIDs appear not to have major effects on the leukotriene pathway.

Glucocorticoids in contrast to NSAIDs work "earlier" in the biochemical pathway by inhibiting the phospholipase-induced release of arachidonic acid from membrane phospholipids and so appear to have a broader anti-inflammatory role than the NSAIDs.

In crystal deposition–induced acute arthritis, an NSAID is most often used. The toxic or side-effects of the NSAIDs should also be emphasized. These include effects on the upper gastrointestinal tract (erosive gastritis, peptic ulceration) and impaired platelet aggregation (through inhibition of cyclo-oxygenase-induced synthesis of thromboxane A_2), a combination that may produce gastrointestinal bleeding, especially if the patient is also on coumarin derivatives that can be displaced from plasma protein binding sites.[4] Other side-effects include sodium retention (with edema formation), and when renal function is already impaired, a tendency for further compromise with azotemia and hyperkalemia.[7] Abuse of aspirin, phenacetin, and certain other NSAIDs may produce "analgesic nephropathy."[15] Hepatotoxicity, central nervous system changes (headache, confusion), and exacerbation of asthma are additional side-effects.

When the diagnosis of early RA and OA is

made, some debate exists over instituting aspirin or another NSAID in view of the necessity for long-term therapy. High-dose aspirin (up to 3.6 g/day) may be needed to achieve anti-inflammatory effects[31] that then merge into potential hazards (*e.g.,* gastric, tinnitus,* metabolic acidosis).[41] Therefore, some physicians favor another NSAID, but others continue to prefer aspirin as the initial drug of choice. Buffered aspirin has the drawback of adding an alkaline load that may not be well tolerated by the kidney.[31] RA starting in an older subject may remit, and hence "conservative therapy" at the start is always indicated. In the presence of exacerbations, short-term low-dose corticosteroid therapy may be indicated. In the unusual event of serious extra-articular complications with vasculitis or progressively erosive joint disease, gold compounds may be the treatment of choice, and ultimately more potent agents such as penicillamine and immunosuppressive drugs.[37,58] With them the primary physician may well wish to maintain patient care in conjunction with a colleague in rheumatology.

The situation in OA is different. It is likely that the primary physician will see the patient at some point in its evolution. Counseling and judicious use of NSAIDs may provide substantial benefit to patient and family.[39] The role of physiotherapy has been discussed by Agate[2] in a positive encouraging way. Such treatment can also attempt to build up specific muscle groups and provide splintage, footwear, and suitable walking aids. Some specific indications for seeking orthopedic consultation include increasing pain, immobility, instability, and deformity of the affected joint.

* Bluestone[8] points out that elderly patients with a high threshold hearing loss may fail to detect tinnitus as a manifestation of salicylate toxicity.

REFERENCES

1. Acheson RM: Osteoarthritis—the mystery crippler. J Rheumatol 10:174, 1983
2. Agate JN: Physiotherapy problems and practices in the elderly: A critical evaluation. In Wright V (ed): Bone and Joint Disease in the Elderly, pp 237–255. New York, Churchill Livingstone, 1983
3. Baum J: Arthritis in the aged. Current Concepts, Upjohn Co., 1981
4. Beeley L: Prescribing antirheumatic drugs for special groups of patients. Rep Rheum Dis 88: 1984
5. Benedek TG: Associations of rheumatic diseases and rheumatic symptoms with cancer. In Wright V (ed): Bone and Joint Disease in the Elderly, pp 121–149. New York, Churchill Livingstone, 1983
6. Bjelle A: Rheumatic disorders in primary care. Scand J Rheumatol 10:331, 1981
7. Blackshear JL, Davidman M, Stillman MT: Identification of risk for renal insufficiency from nonsteroidal anti-inflammatory drugs. Arch Intern Med 143:1130, 1983
8. Bluestone R: The diagnosis and management of rheumatic disease in the elderly—a special challenge. In Kay MMB, Galpin J, Makinodan T (eds): Aging, Immunity, and Arthritis, vol 11, pp 183–194. New York, Raven Press, 1980
9. Butler RN: Ageism: Another form of bigotry. Gerontologist 9:243, 1969
10. Caldwell DS: Musculoskeletal syndromes associated with malignancy. Semin Arthritis Rheum 10:198, 1981
11. Calin A, Marks SH: The case against seronegative rheumatoid arthritis. Am J Med 70:992, 1981
12. Chuang T-Y, Hunder GG, Ilstrup DM et al: Polymyalgia rheumatica. Ann Intern Med 97:672, 1982
13. Corrigan AB, Robinson RG, Tereny TR et al: Benign rheumatoid arthritis of the aged. Br Med J 1:44, 1974
14. Craig GL, Buchanan WW: Antirheumatic drugs: Clinical pharmacology and therapeutic use. Drugs 20:453, 1980
15. Crowshaw K: Role of inhibition of prostaglandin biosynthesis by antiinflammatory drugs in the pathogenesis of renal damage. In Rainsford KD, Velo GP (eds): Side-effects of Anti-inflammatory Analgesic Drugs, pp 149–158. New York, Raven Press, 1984
16. Dieppe PA, Alexander GLM, Jones HE et al: Pyrophosphate arthropathy: A clinical and radiological study of 105 cases. Ann Rheum Dis 41:371, 1982
17. Dixon AStJ: Polymyalgia rheumatica. Rep Rheum Dis 86: 1983
18. Doherty M, Watt I, Dieppe P: Influence of primary generalized osteoarthritis on development of secondary osteoarthritis. Lancet 2:8, 1983
19. Ehrlich GE: Inflammatory osteoarthritis: I. The clinical syndrome. J Chronic Dis 25:317, 1972
20. Forman MD, Malamet R, Kaplan D: A survey of osteoarthritis of the knee in the elderly. J Rheumatol 10:282, 1983
21. Fox RA: Arthritis in the elderly. Eur J Rheum Inflam 5:285, 1982
22. Francois RJ: Editorial: Vertebral ankylosing hyperostosis: What new bone, where and why. J Rheumatol 10:837, 1983
23. Giansiracusa DF, Kantrowitz FG: Rheumatic and Metabolic Bone Diseases in the Elderly. Lexington, MA, DC Heath & Co, 1982
24. Giansiracusa DF, Kantrowitz FG: Malignancies and rheumatic diseases. In Giansiracusa DF, Kantrowitz FG (eds): Rheumatic and Metabolic Bone Diseases in the Elderly, pp 59–68. Lexington, MA, DC Heath & Co, 1982
25. Gibson T, Grahame R: Acute arthritis in the elderly. Age Ageing 2:3, 1973

26. Goldenberg DL, Cohen AS: Acute infectious arthritis. Am J Med 60:369, 1976
27. Goodman BW Jr: Temporal arteritis. Am J Med 67:839, 1979
28. Grahame R: The problems of diagnosis of arthritis in the elderly. Proc R Soc Med 69:926, 1976
29. Hall S, Lie JT, Kurland LT et al: The therapeutic impact of temporal artery biopsy. Lancet 2:1217, 1983
30. Harris WA: Primary osteoarthritis of the hip: A vanishing diagnosis. J Rheumatol 10 (suppl 9):64, 1983
31. Haslock I: Arthritis in old age: Drug treatment. In Wright V (ed): Bone and Joint Disease in the Elderly. pp 181–196. New York, Churchill Livingstone, 1983
32. Healey LA: Polymyalgia rheumatica and the American Rheumatism Association criteria for rheumatoid arthritis. Arthritis Rheum 26:1417, 1983
33. Huskisson EC, Dieppe PA, Tucker AK et al: Another look at osteoarthritis. Ann Rheum Dis 38:423, 1979
34. Kellgren JH, Moore R: Generalized osteoarthritis and Heberden's nodes. Br Med J 1:181, 1952
35. Klein LE, German PS, Levine DM: Adverse drug reactions among the elderly: A reassessment. J Am Geriatr Soc 29:525, 1981
36. Lequesne M: Clinical features, diagnostic criteria, functional assessments and radiological classifications of osteoarthritis (excluding the spine). Rheumatology 1:1, 1982
37. Lipsky PE: Remission-inducing therapy in rheumatoid arthritis. Am J Med 75:40, 1983
38. McCarty D: Crystals, joints, and consternation. Ann Rheum Dis 42:243, 1983
39. Moskowitz RW: Management of osteoarthritis. Bull Rheum Dis 31:31, 1981
40. Nightingale S, Venables GS, Bates D: Polymyalgia rheumatica with diffuse cerebral disease responding rapidly to steroid therapy. J Neurol Neurosurg Psychiatry 45:841, 1982
41. O'Brien WM: Pharmacology of nonsteroidal antiinflammatory drugs: Practical review for clinicians. Am J Med 75:32, 1983
42. Peter JB, Pearson CM, Marmor L: Erosive osteoarthritis of the hands. Arthritis Rheum 9:365, 1966
43. Peyron JG: Discussion: General and local aspects of osteoarthritis. J Rheumatol 10 (suppl 9):17, 1983
44. Resnick CS, Resnick D: Crystal deposition disease. Semin Arthritis Rheum 12:390, 1983
45. Resnick DR, Shapiro RF, Wiesner KB et al: Diffuse idiopathic skeletal hyperostosis (DISH) (Ankylosing hyperostosis of Forestier and Rotes-Querol). Semin Arthritis Rheum 7:153, 1978
46. Reynolds MD: Prevalence of rheumatic diseases as causes of disability and complaints by ambulatory patients. Arthritis Rheum 21:377, 1978
47. Rimoin DL, Wennberg JE: Acute septic arthritis complicating chronic rheumatoid arthritis. JAMA 196:109, 1966
48. Robinson DR: Prostaglandins and the mechanism of action of antiinflammatory drugs. Am J Med 75:26, 1983
49. Rodnan GP: Treatment of the gout and other forms of crystal-induced arthritis. Bull Rheum Dis 28:43, 1982
50. Rudd E, Lockshin M: Education in rheumatology for the primary care physician. J Rheumatol 5:99, 1978
51. Schumacher HR, Somlyo AP, Tse RL et al: Arthritis associated with apatite crystals. Ann Intern Med 87:411, 1977
52. Segal AM, Mackenzie AH: Hypertrophic osteoarthropathy: A 10-year retrospective analysis. Semin Arthritis Rheum 12:220, 1982
53. Sissons HA: Osteoarthritis of the knee. A review. J Rheumatol 10 (suppl 9):76, 1983
54. Smythe HA, Moldofsky H: Two contributions to understanding of the "fibrositis" syndrome. Bull Rheum Dis 28:928, 1978
55. Spitzer WO, Harth M, Goldsmith CH et al:" The arthritic complaint in primary care: Prevalence, related disability, and costs. J Rheumatol 3:88, 1976
56. Steigbigel NH: Diagnosis and management of septic arthritis. In Remington JS, Swartz MN (eds): Current Clinical Topics in Infectious Diseases, vol 4, pp 1–29. New York, McGraw-Hill, 1983
57. Swezey RL, Spiegal TM: Evaluation and treatment of local musculoskeletal disorders in elderly patients. Geriatrics 34:56, 1979
58. Turner R: Medical management of rheumatoid arthritis. In Yetiv JZ, Bianchine JR (eds): Recent advances in Clinical Therapeutics, Antivirals and Antimicrobials, Anticancer Agents, and Cardiovascular Therapy, vol 3, pp 279–294. New York, Grune & Stratton, 1983
59. Utsinger PD, Resnick D, Shapiro RF et al: Roentgenologic, immunologic, and therapeutic study of erosive (inflammatory) osteoarthritis. Arch Intern Med 138:694, 1978
60. Williamson J, Stokoe IH, Gray S et al: Old people at home: Their unreported needs. Lancet 1:1117, 1964
61. Wood PHN, Badley EM: An epidemiological appraisal of bone and joint disease in the elderly. In Wright V (ed): Bone and Joint Disease in the Elderly, pp 1–22. New York, Churchill Livingstone, 1983
62. Wright V (ed): Bone and Joint Disease in the Elderly. New York, Churchill Livingstone, 1983
63. Yunis MB:a Editorial: Fibromyalgia syndrome: A need for uniform classification. J Rheumatol 10:841, 1983

30

Disorders of the Skeletal System

Herta Spencer, Stephen J. Sontag, and Lois Kramer

OSTEOPOROSIS

Etiology

Many factors have been considered in the etiology of postmenopausal or senile osteoporosis (See Possible Causes of Postmenopausal or Senile Osteoporosis).

POSSIBLE CAUSES OF POSTMENOPAUSAL OR SENILE OSTEOPOROSIS

Calcium loss
Calcium deficiency
    Insufficient calcium intake
    Lactase deficiency
    Impaired calcium absorption
Hormonal deficiency
    Decrease of estrogens or androgens
    Imbalance of sex hormones and of adrenal hormones
    Excess parathyroid hormone
Changes in protein nutrition
Decreased physical activity

Calcium Loss

Loss of calcium may occur via the kidney or intestine (*i.e.*, urinary and endogenous fecal calcium loss). Increased loss of calcium from bone by either route for a sufficiently long period of time could lead to osteoporosis. An example of the renal loss of calcium is idiopathic hypercalciuria; an example of intestinal loss is seen with abnormalities of intestinal structure and function such as nontropical sprue. The demineralization in this condition results from a mixture of osteomalacia and osteoporosis since vitamin D as well as bile salts are malabsorbed. It has also been claimed that patients with osteoporosis continue to excrete increased amounts of calcium in urine even when the calcium intake is reduced. This implies an inability to adapt to the low calcium intake by decreasing the urinary excretion of calcium; this may then lead to a decrease in skeletal mass and osteoporosis. In our experience, adaptation, namely, a decrease of the urinary calcium during a low calcium intake, has been observed in the majority of patients with osteoporosis.

Calcium Deficiency

Insufficient Calcium Intake. In recent years, it has been proposed that a deficient intake of calcium for prolonged periods may lead to loss of calcium from bone and osteoporosis. This concept was mainly based on retrospective histories of dietary intake obtained from patients with osteoporosis. The difficulty in evaluating the accuracy of such histories must be considered since it is frequently difficult, if not impossible, to recall food consumption accurately, particularly by older persons who may have impairment of memory. The average calcium intake of these patients was below the recommended 800 mg/day for adults and lower than the calcium intake of persons without osteoporosis. However, the exact amount of dietary calcium needed to prevent osteoporosis is not known, and great individual variations may exist.

Lactase Deficiency or "Lactose Intolerance." One reason for decreased calcium intake may be the abdominal discomfort, cramps, and diarrhea after ingestion of milk experienced by persons with decreased or absent levels of the intestinal enzyme lactase. Milk is the major source of both calcium and lactose in most Western diets, with 1 liter of milk containing about 50 g of lactose. Persons with lactose intolerance may, consciously or subconsciously, restrict calcium intake by avoiding milk. Over many years this might result in osteoporosis. The incidence of lactase deficiency in patients with osteoporosis is not known; despite a recently reported association, it is unlikely that lactase deficiency is a major factor. Populations with the highest frequency of lactase deficiency have also been reported to have a low incidence of osteoporosis.

Impairment of Intestinal Absorption of Calcium.   Elderly patients with osteoporosis may have a defect in the absorption of calcium. Over a prolonged time the decreased efficiency of calcium absorption could lead to decreased calcium stores in bone and osteoporosis. A less than normal absorption of calcium in the presence of a high calcium intake has been demonstrated. The duration of this defect prior to the diagnosis of osteoporosis is not known. The efficiency of calcium absorption as well as the dietary intake of vitamin D have both been shown to decrease with age. The plasma level of the vitamin D metabolite 1,25-dihydroxy-D_3, active in the transport of calcium across the intestine, has been shown to be decreased in elderly patients with osteoporosis.

Hormonal Changes

Decrease of Estrogens and Androgens. The concept of hormonal deficiency as a cause of osteoporosis was advanced in 1941 by Albright and Reifenstein. Since gonadal hormones decrease with advancing age, a causal relationship between estrogen deficiency in older females and androgen deficiency in older males and osteoporosis has been assumed to exist. The high incidence of demineralization of the skeleton in males with hypogonadism and in females with gonadal dysgenesis supports the hormonal deficiency hypothesis. Estrogens have been shown to block bone resorption induced by parathyroid hormone *in vitro* and to suppress bone turnover *in vivo*. It is thus possible that the decrease in sex hormones in the elderly leaves the activity of parathyroid hormone unopposed, thereby leading to the gradual development of osteoporosis.

Imbalance Between Sex Hormones and Adrenal Hormones.   An imbalance of sex and adrenal hormones may play a role in the development of osteoporosis. A deficiency of estrogen in elderly females or of androgens in elderly males can be considered to lessen an anabolic stimulus for new bone formation. Since the level of adrenocortical hormones remains normal in the older age-group and the levels of estrogens or androgens decrease, the antianabolic effect of adrenal corticoids is unopposed by the anabolic effect of sex hormones. This imbalance would favor catabolism, with decreased bone formation and increased bone resorption and loss of bone mass.

Parathyroid Hormone and Vitamin D. Normally, a low calcium status, resulting from a low intake of calcium, decreased intestinal absorption of calcium, or calcium loss, leads to an increase in parathyroid hormone (PTH) secretion. PTH causes bone resorption and calcium loss, but its role in osteoporosis is not clear. Plasma levels of PTH have been reported to be normal, increased, as well as decreased. Some investigators believe that lower levels of PTH play an important part in osteoporosis, as explained by the following: Patients with osteoporosis shown to have a lower than normal absorption of calcium have no increase in PTH secretion because increased amounts of calcium are released from bone; these calcium levels in the plasma suppress PTH secretion. Lower levels of PTH are of relevance because of their relation to vitamin D metabolism: PTH is necessary for the conversion of 25-hydroxy vitamin D to its active metabolite 1,25-dihydroxy vitamin D_3. Impairment of this conversion would lead to decreased intestinal absorption of calcium. However, some investigators believe that patients who have low levels of PTH have less bone resorption than those who have high levels of PTH. The reported low intakes of calcium and the age-related decrease in intestinal absorption of calcium, owing to low levels of the active vitamin D metabolite, puts elderly persons at risk of a negative calcium balance and bone loss.

Decreased Serum Calcitonin.   The plasma levels of calcitonin, a hormone that decreases bone resorption and serum levels of calcium and phosphorus, have been reported to decrease with age. Infusions of calcium increase the serum calcium level, which normally leads to increased release of calcitonin. In older persons, release of calcitonin in response to calcium infusions lessened. Although calcitonin decreases bone resorption and may thereby stabilize or even increase the bone mass, the significance of lower plasma levels of calcitonin in aging is not known. Also, so far there is no evidence that calcitonin increases bone mass.

Changes in Protein Intake

An increase in dietary protein intake has been reported to result in increased calcium loss via the kidney; however, in most of these studies, purified proteins such as amino acids were used. Studies in our research unit have shown that a high protein intake, given as meat, does not increase the urinary calcium level. The failure of this type of protein to increase the urinary calcium level is probably due to its high phosphorus content since phosphorus has been shown to decrease urinary calcium. High protein intake as meat had no effect on the intestinal absorption of calcium, and the calcium balance remained unchanged. It can therefore be concluded that a high meat intake does not induce calcium loss. In rare instances increased urinary calcium may be observed in the initial phase of the high protein intake, given as meat; if this occurs it is only temporary. The urinary calcium value decreases to control levels within 50 to 60 days during the continued high protein intake, apparently due to compensatory retention of calcium, and decreases even further if the high protein intake is continued. Inadequate intake of dietary protein and also of vitamins such as vitamin C affects all tissues of the body, including bone, and leads to osteoporosis. The "atrophy" of skin, of subcutaneous tissue, and of muscle in malnutrition as well as in aging is well known. Osteoporosis due to protein–calorie malnutrition has been observed during wartime famine. Lack of protein, of vitamins in general, and of vitamin C in particular may play an important role in insufficient or faulty bone matrix formation since vitamin C is essential in the formation of collagen.

Decreased Physical Activity

Muscular stress on bone is an important stimulus for bone formation. A decrease or lack of physical activity in any age-group results in urinary calcium loss and is probably a contributory or even a causative factor in osteoporosis. It has been shown that urinary calcium loss may be decreased by placing patients who are on bed rest in an oscillating bed. It has also been shown that the urinary calcium loss of bed rest patients can be decreased by standing quietly for 3 hours a day, but not by supine ergometer exercise even when continued for up to 4 hours a day. More recent studies have shown a 25% to 45% bone mineral loss in healthy adults restricted to bed rest for 30 to 36 weeks. This mineral loss was reversible during reambulation. An extreme effect of inactivity is the severe osteoporosis produced by complete immobilization in paraplegia or the application of whole body plaster casts for prolonged periods. Indeed, one wonders whether lack of exercise and physical inactivity of the American population may not be a significant contributory factor to the high incidence of osteoporosis.

Pathogenesis

The skeletal structure and the bone mass is maintained by a balance of bone formation and bone resorption. A loss of bone mass (*i.e.*, osteoporosis) could be due either to a decrease in bone formation or to an increase in bone resorption.

Decrease in Bone Formation

About 40 years ago, Albright and Reifenstein proposed that the basic defect in osteoporosis is decreased osteoblastic activity resulting in decreased bone matrix formation. Low levels of sex steroid hormones in elderly women and men were thought responsible for this. The majority of kinetic studies, however, using radioactive calcium, and bone biopsies, using quantitative microradiography, have failed to show a decrease in bone formation. Apparently, bone formation remains unchanged in osteoporosis.

Increase in Bone Resorption

An increase in bone resorption is believed to be the major pathophysiologic change in osteoporosis. Bone resorption may be stimulated by any condition that tends to decrease the plasma level of calcium. This stimulates secretion of parathyroid hormone, which in turn increases bone resorption. Maintenance of a normal plasma calcium level is readily achieved by release of calcium from bone despite great variations in intake and output of calcium. Factors that lower plasma calcium levels (*i.e.*, calcium deficiency and calcium loss) have been discussed in the section on etiology. Bone resorption without compensatory increase in bone formation eventually results in a decreased bone mass, as seen in osteoporosis. The smaller bone mass is normally calcified and of normal chemical composition.

Changes in Acid–Base Balance

It has been suggested that osteoporosis results from continuous removal of small amounts of calcium from bone throughout life in response to a "chronic acidosis," which leads to increased urinary calcium levels. Removal of calcium from bone would occur to maintain a normal plasma *p*H. Chronic low-grade subclinical acidosis has been attributed to the long-term intake of a diet high in meat considered to be an acid-ash diet. However, carefully controlled studies have shown that a loss of calcium does not occur due to the high phosphate content of meat. In the very rare case, increase is only a temporary phenomenon followed by increased retention of calcium.

An example of the effect of acute metabolic acidosis is the severe skeletal demineralization induced in animals by ammonium chloride. In our studies in humans, metabolic acidosis induced by ammonium chloride led to a marked increase in urinary calcium and phosphorus excretion, indicating that both calcium and phosphorus are removed from bone in acidosis.

Diagnosis

The diagnosis of postmenopausal or senile osteoporosis is usually made when the condition is well advanced and perhaps already associated with bone pain and skeletal fractures. The insidious onset and the absence of clinical signs and symptoms result in delayed diagnosis. No clinical indicators or laboratory tests are useful for early detection other than the calcium tolerance test, the retention of calcium in response to an intravenous calcium load. This test is helpful in establishing the diagnosis of osteoporosis in the absence of roentgenographic evidence. It requires hospitalization of the patient. For details of the calcium tolerance test, see the section on laboratory findings. The use and limitations of conventional and specialized roentgenographic procedures will be discussed in the sections on roentgenographic findings and bone densitometry. Early detection and therapy are mandatory if the rate of bone loss is to be slowed and complications avoided. In contrast, the prognosis and alleviation of secondary osteoporosis associated with well-defined causes, such as the use of corticosteroids, thyrotoxicosis, or Cushing's syndrome, depend on the recognition and treatment of the underlying disease.

Clinical Features

Osteoporosis is often asymptomatic and frequently discovered incidentally. Even the collapse of vertebrae may occur insidiously until persons with osteoporosis realize that their stature has become shortened. The most frequent symptom is back pain, localized usually to the midthoracic spine or to the "low back." The lumbar and thoracic vertebrae are involved to a far greater extent than the long bones or skull. The pain is mainly due to associated spasm of paravertebral muscles. The absence of back pain or its severity does not correlate with the extent of osteoporosis. Jarring of the involved area by percussion, flexion, or extension of the spine may elicit or aggravate the pain. In some patients, sudden severe back pain due to vertebral fractures or severe pain due to fracture of the neck of the femur following trauma may be the presenting complaint. Occasionally, compression of nerve roots from collapsed dorsal vertebrae may give rise to substernal pain mimicking angina pectoris or an acute abdomen.

Physical Signs

Localized bone tenderness is usually not a prominent feature. With progression of the disease, recurrent fractures of the vertebral bodies result in spinal deformities, kyphosis of the dorsal spine, reduction of the lumbar lordosis, limitation of motion of the spine, and a decrease in body height. The loss in body height can be demonstrated by a decrease in the crown-pubic distance as compared with the pubic-heel measurement, the appearance of a transverse thoracoabdominal skin fold, decrease of the distance between the anterior ribs, and narrowing of the distance between the costal arches and the iliac crest to an extent that overriding of the two structures increases discomfort. With deformity of the thorax and pain in the spine and ribs, inefficient respiratory motion of the thoracic cage may result in recurrent pulmonary infections and possibly also in changes in cardiopulmonary dynamics.

Roentgenographic Findings

The diagnosis is usually made by roentgenographic findings. The predominant areas of demineralization are the vertebrae of the dorsal and lumbar spine and the pelvis, with the long bones and skull seemingly unaffected for a long time. Routine radiologic methods have limitations in detecting the early decrease in bone density and in diagnosing the early stages. At least 25% of the calcium content of bone has to be lost before demineralization becomes recognizable on roentgenograms. With increasing loss of bone mineral from trabecular bone, the vertebral plates appear accentuated on roentgenograms so that the vertebral bodies can be likened to "empty shells." The vertebral bodies become biconcave; the intervertebral disks expand and become biconvex, producing the "fish-mouth" appearance of adjacent vertebrae. Herniation of the nucleus pulposus into the weakened vertebral bodies produces the "Schmorl's nodes." Vertebral collapse is seen on the roentgenogram as anterior wedging of the vertebra or as complete compression. In addition to evaluating the bone density of the vertebrae on roentgenograms, measurement of the cortical thickness of long bones has been reported to be useful for early detection. Fractures of other skeletal sites occur with relative frequency, particularly of the neck of the femur and of the ribs. The diagnosis of postmenopausal or senile osteoporosis should never be made on roentgenographic findings alone, since these may be indistinguishable from the roentgenographic findings of other bone disorders such as osteomalacia, hyperparathyroidism, multiple myeloma, and osseous metastases.

Bone Densitometry

The drawbacks of routine skeletal roentgenograms have stimulated the development of quantitative radiography. Early, bone density was determined by comparison with a stepwedge made of metal alloy or of ivory. A source of error in this arises from the variable amount of soft tissues surrounding the bone. Extensive studies of bone density have used photon absorptiometry and the cortical index. Photon absorptiometry, which measures the mineral content of long bones, especially of the radius, is available only in certain centers. This technique is most useful for determining the density of certain bones, such as the distal ends of the radius or ulna, the fifth finger and the os calcis, bones not usually involved by osteoporosis to any great extent. The bone density of the vertebral bodies predominantly involved by osteoporosis, cannot be determined with accuracy by present methods. Also, the mineral measurement of the radius does not always accurately reflect the overall skeletal mass. The cortical index can be determined in a roentgenogram of the hands, by measuring the precise cortical thickness and relating it to the total width of the metacarpal bone. Another method is radiographic absorptiometry using

roentgenograms of the hand, and a computer scanner using the density of an aluminum wedge for comparison with the bone density of the hand.

Laboratory Findings

Blood Chemistries

No specific changes in the blood chemistries are indicative of osteoporosis. In fact, the absence of abnormal findings is an aid in the differential diagnosis. The serum calcium level is usually normal. An exception is rapid demineralization, as in immobilization of younger persons in whom rapid release of calcium from bone can elevate the serum calcium. The serum phosphorus level and the serum alkaline phosphatase levels are usually normal. The blood chemistries in osteoporosis and in other bone conditions are listed in Table 30-1.

Urinary Calcium and Phosphorus Excretion

Generally, the urinary calcium excretion is in the normal range or low. Hypercalciuria is rare in osteoporosis. It does occur with immobilization or in cortisone-induced osteoporosis and may be associated with hypercalcemia. The urinary phosphorus excretion is usually in the normal range in uncomplicated osteoporosis. The urinary phosphorus value is increased in immobilization osteoporosis owing to rapid and increased skeletal demineralization with removal of both calcium and phosphorus from bone.

Fecal Calcium Excretion

A high excretion of calcium in stool is observed in patients with almost any type of osteoporosis who are on a high intake of calcium. It is due to the decreased ability to absorb calcium. The increase in fecal calcium is primarily unabsorbed calcium, not increased reexcretion of absorbed calcium into the intestine, the so-called endogenous fecal calcium.

Radioisotope Tracer Studies

Radioactive tracer techniques have been used to measure rates of bone formation and bone resorption. Radioactive calcium tracers are used to determine the intestinal absorption of calcium as well as the endogenous fecal calcium excretion in osteoporosis. This requires a specialized setup and is not a practical aid in diagnosis but is useful in investigations of metabolic bone disease.

TABLE 30-1 Serum Levels of Calcium, Phosphorus, and Alkaline Phosphatase in Skeletal Diseases

Condition or Disease	Serum Levels		
	Calcium	*Phosphorus*	*Alkaline Phosphatase*
Osteoporosis			
Postmenopausal or senile	Normal	Normal	Normal or low
Immobilization	Normal or high	Normal or high*	Normal or low
Cushing's syndrome	Normal or increased	Normal	Normal
Diabetes mellitus	Normal	Normal	Normal
Cortisone-induced	Normal or slightly increased	Normal or decreased	Normal or low
Chronic alcoholism	Normal or low	Normal or low	Normal
Liver disease	Normal	Normal	Normal or increased†
Osteomalacia	Low, normal, or high‡	Low or normal	Increased
Metastatic bone disease	Normal or high	Normal or high*	Normal or increased
Multiple myeloma	Normal or high	Normal or high*	Normal, low, or slightly increased
Hyperparathyroidism	Increased or normal§	Decreased or normal§	Normal‖ or increased
Hyperthyroidism	Normal or increased	Normal or decreased	Increased or normal
Vitamin D intoxication	Increased	Normal or increased	Normal or increased
Paget's disease of bone	Normal, decreased, or increased#	Normal	Increased

  * Usually secondary to renal failure
  † In the presence of jaundice or in cases of osteoporosis and osteomalacia
  ‡ Owing to secondary hyperparathyroidism
  § Serum calcium and phosphorus levels may be normal in hyperparathyroidism
  ‖ Normal in majority of cases with hyperparathyroidism
  # Serum calcium decreased in the predominantly blastic stage, serum calcium increased in the predominantly lytic phase and in immobilization

Calcium Balance Studies

The metabolic balance study technique can determine whether the patient is losing calcium, is retaining calcium, or is in equilibrium during a given calcium intake. These studies do not reflect the functional or structural condition of the skeleton and require a constant strictly controlled diet analyzed for its mineral content. A specially trained team of nurses, dietitians, and physicians is needed. The problem of collecting excreta is not inconsiderable, and special care must be taken to ensure completeness of collections. The metabolic balance technique is especially useful in evaluating the efficacy of any given therapy.

Calcium Tolerance Test

The calcium tolerance test measures the ability of the skeleton to retain a standard amount of intravenously infused calcium. A standard dose of 500 mg calcium as the gluconate is infused in 500 ml 5% glucose in water over 4 hours, while the patient is maintained on a constant low calcium intake of approximately 250 mg/day. Retention of the infused calcium was significantly lower in patients with osteoporosis than in patients without osteoporosis, with the decreased calcium retention reflecting the inability of the decreased bone mass to deposit calcium in the skeleton. This test is useful in diagnosing osteoporosis in the absence of roentgenographic evidence but cannot be performed as an office procedure and requires hospitalization for a minimum of 3 days.

Ancillary Diagnostic Aids

Bone biopsy (needle biopsies) is desirable for establishing the diagnosis of osteoporosis objectively, but this invasive technique is not acceptable to many patients. *Tetracycline* labeling of bone has been used for the estimation of new bone formation and of bone resorption. This is a research procedure and not routine.

There is no specific characteristic anatomical finding in osteoporosis other than the diminished amount of normally calcified bone. The number and width of the bone trabeculae are decreased, but they are fully calcified. The cortex of bone is diminished. Histologic quantitation of bone on iliac crest biopsies has been suggested, using an arbitrary nine-point scale, with a score of less than five regarded as osteoporosis. In evaluating bone biopsies, one has to consider that they may not be representative of the entire skeleton since osteoporosis does not develop in all skeletal sites at the same time.

Differential Diagnosis

The roentgenologic appearance of the skeleton is the same in both primary and secondary osteoporosis; therefore, all causes must be considered in the differential diagnosis.

Osteomalacia

Osteomalacia is infrequent in the United States because of the rarity of vitamin D deficiency. It is most frequently encountered in cases of malabsorption, and thus may be secondary to hepatobiliary disease, nontropical sprue, or chronic pancreatitis. Osteomalacia does occur in elderly persons who have no exposure to sunlight and do not drink vitamin D–fortified milk or take vitamin D supplements. The skeletal changes in osteomalacia are similar to those of osteoporosis, with marked generalized demineralization and vertebral compression fractures. Linear infractions (*i.e.*, greenstick fractures [milkman's pseudofractures]) and bowing of the lower extremities present in osteomalacia are not seen in osteoporosis. The serum calcium level in osteomalacia is usually low, but compensatory overactivity of the parathyroid glands results in secondary hyperparathyroidism so that the serum calcium level may be restored to normal. The serum phosphorus level is usually low and the alkaline phosphatase level is elevated in osteomalacia, values that are normal in osteoporosis. The 24-hour urinary calcium excretion is usually very low. Retention of infused calcium in the calcium tolerance test is very high, in contrast to the low calcium retention of osteoporosis. Also, the intestinal absorption of calcium is low in osteomalacia and can be increased by the use of vitamin D. This is in contrast to the usual lack of effect of vitamin D in osteoporosis, unless there is a coexisting vitamin D deficiency. In osteomalacia secondary to malabsorption, the fecal fat excretion is high; in osteoporosis, the fecal fat excretion is usually normal but has also been reported to be slightly higher than normal.

Multiple Myeloma

Although the typical "punched-out" radiolucent skeletal lesions, visible on roentgenography of the skeleton, are considered characteristic of multiple myeloma, osteoporosis may be the only radiologic manifestation. Punched-out radiolucent areas are found in only 13% of cases of multiple myeloma, most frequently on roentgenography of the skull. Several clinical and biochemical features are more characteristic of multiple myeloma than of osteoporosis. Severe persistent bone pain occurs in about 90% of cases of multiple myeloma, while bone pain in osteoporosis is usually inconstant, less severe, or even totally absent. In advanced osteoporosis, however, the bone pain may be very severe, especially when fractures are present. The serum calcium level may be normal or high in multiple myeloma, while it is normal in osteoporosis. The serum phosphorus and alkaline phosphatase levels are usually normal in both multiple myeloma and in osteoporosis. Occasionally, the serum alkaline phosphatase is slightly to moderately elevated in multiple myeloma, but not to the extent seen in metastatic neoplastic bone disease. The 24-hour urinary calcium excretion may be normal in multiple myeloma, it may be low if the disease is progressing slowly, or it may be very high if the disease is progressing rapidly or in the presence of hypercalcemia. In contrast to manifestations of rapid bone breakdown in multiple myeloma, hypercalcemia and hypercalciuria are not present in osteoporosis, except in immobilization osteoporosis. Multiple myeloma can be differentiated from osteoporosis by characteristic changes in serum and urinary proteins (*i.e.*, by a reversal of the albumin–globulin ratio, hyperglobulinemia, an abnormal electrophoretic pattern of the plasma and/or urine, and the presence of Bence-Jones protein). Also, bone marrow aspirates usually show the presence of abnormal plasma cells. In view of the similarity of the roentgenographic appearances, the diagnosis of multiple myeloma must be ruled out in every case of osteoporosis.

Neoplastic Bone Disease

Metastatic osteolytic bone diseases may present with roentgenographic evidence of what appears to be osteoporosis. A search for a primary neo-plastic lesion, such as a carcinoma of the breast, kidney, lung, thyroid, female genitalia, and intestinal tract, should be made. Even if there is no evidence for a primary neoplastic lesion on physical or roentgenographic examination, elevation of the serum alkaline phosphatase value, hypercalciuria, and hypercalcemia may be indicative of a neoplastic process. These abnormal biochemical findings are not encountered in uncomplicated postmenopausal or senile osteoporosis; for instance, hypercalcemia occurs in cases of osteoporosis only during prolonged immobilization. An increase in the level of the serum alkaline phosphatase may be encountered in cases of osteoporosis if there are complications such as skeletal fractures or in cases of coexisting osteoporosis and osteomalacia. Demonstration of tumor cells on bone marrow aspirates or a bone biopsy may reveal the correct diagnosis of neoplastic bone disease.

Hyperparathyroidism

Excess PTH production due to parathyroid adenoma or hyperplasia causes bone resorption and changes in calcium and phosphorus metabolism. The typical cystic bone changes in primary hyperparathyroidism are rarely seen in this country, probably owing to the relatively high calcium intake and the efficient absorption of calcium from the intestine in hyperparathyroidism. The roentgenographic findings in hyperparathyroidism may frequently be diffuse demineralization indistinguishable from generalized osteoporosis. Other roentgenographic findings that may differentiate hyperparathyroidism from osteoporosis are subperiosteal bone resorption, motheaten appearance of the cortical surface of the phalanges or of the lateral ends of the clavicles, and incomplete outline of the lamina dura. Roentgenograms of the skull in hyperparathyroidism may show osteoporosis and stippled "salt and pepper" appearance not seen in postmenopausal or senile osteoporosis. Recurrent renal lithiasis frequently associated with hyperparathyroidism is not a feature of osteoporosis. The principal diagnostic findings in hyperparathyroidism are hypercalcemia and hypophosphatemia. Several cases of hyperparathyroidism with normal serum calcium levels have been reported. Clinical symptoms of hypercalcemia, such as fatigue, muscle weakness, constipation, anorexia, and at times cardiac arrhythmia are encountered in patients with hyperparathyroidism. The 24-hour urinary calcium excretion is high in hy-

perparathyroidism unless there is impairment of renal function, while in patients with osteoporosis the urinary calcium excretion is usually normal or low. The level of the serum alkaline phosphatase may be normal or high in hyperparathyroidism. Calcium tolerance tests are helpful in the differentiation of osteoporosis and hyperparathyroidism, the calcium retention being low in osteoporosis and normal in the majority of cases of hyperparathyroidism. Also, the decrease in urinary phosphorus excretion on the day of infusion of calcium (*i.e.*, on the day of the calcium tolerance test) is less marked in hyperparathyroidism than in patients with osteoporosis. Studies in our research unit show that the intestinal absorption of calcium is very high in hyperparathyroidism. Numerous tests, including that of the tubular reabsorption of phosphorus (TRP), have been used for the differentiation of hyperparathyroidism from other metabolic bone diseases. PTH assay of plasma to demonstrate excess PTH activity is a reliable indicator of hyperparathyroidism, if positive. Normal or low PTH levels do not exclude the diagnosis, particularly in the presence of hypercalcemia. This test is now available in most institutions.

Hyperthyroidism

Diffuse skeletal demineralization may be seen in hyperthyroidism. The roentgenographic appearance of the skeleton in hyperthyroidism may resemble osteoporosis, osteomalacia, or hyperparathyroidism. Usually the serum calcium and phosphorus levels are normal, but hypercalcemia and hypercalciuria may be present as well as an increase of the serum alkaline phosphatase level. These changes are not encountered in postmenopausal or senile osteoporosis. The diagnosis can be made by determining the serum levels of thyroxine and triiodothyronine.

Excess Vitamin D Intake

The long-term intake of relatively large doses of vitamin D, such as 25,000 to 50,000 IU/day, may lead to bone resorption resembling osteoporosis or osteitis fibrosa cystica as seen in hyperparathyroidism. The differential diagnosis from hyperparathyroidism may be difficult because the excess intake of vitamin D is associated with hypercalciuria, hypercalcemia, and elevation of the alkaline phosphatase, changes observed in hyperparathyroidism. However, in excess vitamin D intake, there is hyperphosphatemia, which is not encountered in hyperparathyroidism. The biochemical changes in excess vitamin D intake may persist for a prolonged period of time after discontinuation of the vitamin. Calcifications of soft tissues, renal calcinosis with or without associated impairment of renal function, and involvement of the cardiovascular system, such as development of supravalvular aortic stenosis, may occur, which are complications not encountered in osteoporosis. Whenever skeletal demineralization is seen on the roentgenogram, a history should be obtained regarding the intake of vitamin D.

Chronic Alcoholism

Generalized demineralization has been observed in patients with a history of prolonged excess alcohol intake. The fractures frequently encountered in patients with alcoholism may be traumatic but also due to bone fragility secondary to demineralization. The mechanism of the bone changes is not clear, but several contributory factors should be considered, such as decrease in protein, calcium, and vitamin D intake as well as possible impairment of hydroxylation of vitamin D, with decreased formation of the 1,25-dihydroxy vitamin D_3 essential for the intestinal absorption of calcium. Other causes may be increased loss of fecal calcium due to steatorrhea and malabsorption secondary to chronic pancreatitis or pancreatic insufficiency. Hormonal changes may also play a role as increased levels of plasma cortisol have been reported in chronic alcoholism and alcohol intake has produced adrenal hyperplasia in animals. Skeletal demineralization in chronic alcoholism may also be a result of increased urinary excretion of calcium and of magnesium for a prolonged period of time. Osteoporosis associated with chronic alcoholism can usually be differentiated from primary osteoporosis by history. This type of osteoporosis is usually encountered in male patients of the younger or middle age-group in whom osteoporosis ordinarily does not occur. The serum levels of calcium and phosphorus are usually normal while the serum alkaline phosphatase is usually elevated and is of hepatic origin. The source of the increased alkaline phosphatase (liver or bone) can be distinguished by special laboratory tests.

Osteomalacia and osteoporosis may be present singly or combined in patients with chronic liver disease. Osteomalacia has been reported to occur in obstructive liver disease associated with jaundice and may be due to impairment of the absorption of vitamin D, while osteoporosis is present more often in patients with hepatocellular damage or in patients with cirrhosis of the liver.

Renal Osteodystrophy

Osteoporosis observed with increasing frequency in patients undergoing hemodialysis is associated with osteitis fibrosa cystica and osteomalacia. The osteomalacia is due to aluminum deposits in bone. It has been suggested that the osteoporosis associated with renal osteodystrophy in chronic hemodialysis may in part be due to the aging process in these patients.

Treatment

The primary goals of treating osteoporosis are to retard its progression, prevent complications, and reverse the demineralization. Inasmuch as a single specific cause for postmenopausal and for senile osteoporosis has yet to be identified, therapy is still in the trial-and-error stage and often limited to symptomatic management. Treatment regimens are based on the various hypotheses regarding causation. They fall into two main sectors: specific therapy and nonspecific therapy. Symptomatic relief and clinical improvement can be achieved in osteoporosis by available therapeutic modalities. The following therapeutic objectives should be considered:

Correction of the process that is presumably the cause of osteoporosis
Symptomatic relief of pain
Treatment of complications, such as fractures
Rehabilitation, which includes correction of inadequate dietary habits, such as poor intake of calcium, protein, and vitamins; the use of physiotherapy or of physical devices; correction of physical inactivity; and psychologic support to encourage motivation and change the hopeless and apathetic outlook frequently encountered in the elderly.

Specific Therapy

Specific therapeutic measures are designed to correct the assumed defects involved in the pathogenesis. Present programs have two main purposes: (1) to inhibit increased bone resorption and (2) to stimulate new bone formation. Estrogens, calcitonin, and, most likely, phosphate relate to the first, while calcium and fluoride supplements probably play a dual role.

Calcium Supplementation. The officially recommended calcium intake is 800 mg/day. Studies in our research unit show this is insufficient for many adults, and particularly for patients with osteoporosis who require a higher calcium intake. For them an intake of approximately 1.5 g/day is recommended. A calcium intake higher than 800 mg/day, approximately 1200 mg, can be achieved by adding three glasses of milk to a general diet. The intake of other dairy products and of other foods relatively high in calcium, such as broccoli, green leafy vegetables, kidney beans, sardines, and almonds, can increase the calcium intake further. One glass of milk provides about 300 mg calcium, and one serving of the foods mentioned above provides about 200 mg calcium. Additional foods that are good sources of calcium are kale, mustard greens, turnip greens, and eggs. One serving of these provides approximately 100 mg calcium, with two eggs being considered as a serving.

Elderly persons may consume insufficient quantities of food, and recommended food items, so supplementation by calcium carbonate, gluconate, or lactate tablets may be necessary. Fewer tablets of calcium carbonate, which contains 40% elemental calcium, are needed than of calcium gluconate or lactate, which contain only 10% calcium. The intake of a large number of tablets can be facilitated by dissolving them in water. Supplements should be given in two or three divided doses per day. Large amounts of calcium may cause constipation, which can be counteracted by use of a high fiber diet. However, foods high in fiber may interfere with the intestinal absorption of calcium.

Calcium balances change from negative to positive values in most patients with osteoporosis receiving a high calcium intake. However, recalcification of the skeleton on the roentgenogram has not been demonstrated but should not be interpreted negatively. Stabilization of the skeleton in the absence of recalcification should be considered a positive result. Inasmuch as bone in osteoporosis is already fully calcified, ''recalcification'' cannot be expected to occur unless there is new bone matrix that can then calcify.

Sex Hormones. Almost 45 years ago, estrogen replacement was introduced to treat osteoporosis in postmenopausal women to improve the quality of the bone structure. Androgens were introduced to promote protein retention and increase formation of the organic bone matrix.

Estrogen produces symptomatic relief in the majority of patients. It slows progression of the disease as evidenced by arrest of the decline in vertebral and body heights and by a decrease in fractures. Metabolic studies show that estrogen decreases the urinary calcium excretion and improves the calcium balance, most likely as a result of decreased bone resorption. Estrogen has also been reported to improve the calcium balance by decreasing the fecal calcium excretion, but no improvement in intestinal absorption of radioisotopic calcium has been demonstrated.

In a 1984 National Institutes of Health Consensus Conference on Osteoporosis, estrogens were recommended for postmenopausal women to prevent the development of osteoporosis. In addition, adequate nutrition, with a calcium intake of 1000 mg to 1500 mg/day, and modest weight-bearing exercise were recommended.

In a 10-year prospective study, postmenopausal women treated with estrogen had either an increase in bone mass or minimal bone loss, while an untreated control group continued to have significant bone loss.

The main effect of androgens is increased retention of protein, while the effect on urinary and fecal calcium excretion is variable.

The following hormonal compounds are generally used:

Estrogens: diethylstilbestrol, conjugated estrogens, ethinyl estradiol
Androgens: testosterone propionate

Dosages. The usually recommended dosage of diethylstilbestrol is 1 mg/day given orally. The dosage of other estrogenic compounds, such as conjugated estrogens, is up to 1.25 mg/day and of ethinyl estradiol, 0.05 mg to 0.1 mg/day. Cyclic therapy, given daily for 3 of 4 weeks, is recommended to diminish breakthrough bleeding and lessen the remote risk of genital or breast neoplasia. The dose of testosterone propionate for male patients with osteoporosis is usually 25 mg to 50 mg intramuscularly one to three times per week.

Side-effects. Estrogens may cause nausea and abdominal discomfort. At the dose levels indicated, diethylstilbestrol should rarely, if ever, result in any untoward effect. It is believed that conjugated estrogens and ethinyl estradiol are tolerated better than diethylstilbestrol.

Methyltestosterone can cause jaundice and is therefore not recommended. Virilization precludes the prolonged use of androgens in females. Both with estrogens and androgens, sodium retention may lead to edema formation and congestive heart failure. Therefore a low sodium intake is recommended during hormone replacement therapy.

Because of the calcium-anabolic effect of estrogens and the protein-anabolic effect of androgens, combinations of both have been advocated. Most investigators question the effectiveness of androgens in females with osteoporosis, but combination therapy is recommended in male patients with osteoporosis to counteract the feminizing effect of estrogens. It is customary to give various combinations of therapeutic agents rather than one modality at a time (*e.g.,* the combination of a high calcium intake and estrogens for the treatment of female patients).

Anabolic Agents. Since the basic aim of androgen therapy is to increase protein anabolism, longer-acting, less virilizing agents are preferable to testosterone propionate. An example is nandrolone phenpropionate, at doses of up to 400 mg intramuscularly once a month. Although some anabolic agents have been reported to be hepatotoxic, this is rarely, if ever, encountered when they are given by the intramuscular rather than the oral route.

Exercise. A growing body of literature strongly indicates that physical exercise results in increased skeletal mass. An adequate bone mass formed in early years may be sufficient to delay or prevent osteoporosis in later life, especially if the physical activity is continued. Physical activity has been shown to retard or prevent bone loss in both postmenopausal and elderly women.

Other Treatment Modalities. Fluoride Therapy. Incorporation of fluoride into bone results in a fluorapatite that is less soluble than the bone crystal hydroxyapatite from which it is formed. The increased hardness of fluorapatite and its greater resistance to dissolution suggested the possible benefit of fluoride for osteoporosis. Varying doses of fluoride, given as sodium fluoride, have been used. Initially, the dosage ranged from 60 mg to 150 mg/day of elemental fluoride, given orally, but smaller dosages, on the order of 20 mg to 50 mg/day of fluoride, have also been used, and the question of whether smaller doses are as effective is unanswered. Some investigators prefer to use 0.5 mg/kg of fluoride. Symptomatic relief of bone pain has been observed with fluoride therapy. Increase in the density of the skeleton on roentgenograms has been described by some investigators. The significance of this is not clear; it may well

indicate deposition of fluoride in bone rather than recalcification of the skeleton. An increase in fluoride content does not necessarily imply increased strength of bones; in fact, excessive fluoride in bone, fluorosis, may increase the brittleness of bone. Metabolic studies show that urinary calcium excretion decreases during the intake of fluoride. This may be due to decreased bone resorption. In our research unit, 45 mg/day of fluoride as sodium fluoride was used; this produced a decrease in the urinary calcium excretion, and the intestinal absorption of calcium did not improve. The change in calcium balance thus depended on the decrease in urinary calcium. This decrease is an important change and may well reflect a decrease in bone resorption. Treatment was given for 3 months and was highly effective in alleviating bone pain. Triple therapy with fluoride, vitamin D, and calcium has been suggested by others, namely, a daily dose of 25 mg fluoride, given as sodium fluoride, together with 900 mg calcium as well as twice weekly doses of 50,000 IU of vitamin D. This regimen has been reported to produce new bone formation without roentgenographic or microscopic evidence of fluorosis.

The investigators who originally suggested the large dose of 50,000 IU of vitamin D subsequently stated that this dose should not be used since it may increase urinary calcium excretion. To our knowledge, data have not been reported on the effect of vitamin D on the intestinal absorption of calcium during fluoride therapy. Our experience is that 50,000 IU vitamin D does not improve the intestinal absorption of calcium in patients with osteoporosis, and increases the urinary calcium, an undesirable effect. Our recommendation is to use 45 mg fluoride, as sodium fluoride, per day for 3 months with a calcium intake of 2 g/day achieved by addition of calcium supplements. A standard diet usually contains between 800 mg to 1000 mg/day of calcium. The dosage of vitamin D should be 400 IU/day, the recommended intake. In the majority of patients this course of treatment alleviated bone pain and no further fluoride therapy was necessary.

Fluoride therapy may cause adverse reactions: gastric discomfort can be effectively counteracted by putting fluoride tablets into gelatin capsules and giving them in three doses with meals. Aluminum-containing antacids inhibit the intestinal absorption of fluoride and should not be given for gastric distress. In our research unit, five sodium fluoride tablets, each containing 1 mg of fluoride ion, are placed into one gelatin capsule and three capsules, each containing a total of 15 mg fluoride, are given with meals. No untoward effects were observed over a 10-year period with fluoride administered in this fashion.

Inorganic Phosphate. Phosphate, intravenously or orally, decreases the serum calcium level in hypercalcemia associated with neoplastic bone disease. In our studies, phosphate, given as glycerophosphate or inorganic phosphate, decreased the urinary calcium excretion, irrespective of the calcium intake. Phosphate supplements were given daily for several weeks in three divided doses.

In view of this effect of phosphate, its use may be beneficial, particularly for patients who have skeletal fractures and a high urinary calcium excretion. However, when a high phosphorus and a high calcium intake was prescribed for prolonged periods, an increase of the mineral content of the radius could not be demonstrated. This may not be a negative result since phosphate may have decreased bone resorption and may have stabilized the bone structure. This desirable effect would not be reflected by increased bone density. Large single doses of oral phosphates have been reported to increase bone resorption in patients with osteoporosis, although the plasma PTH levels were not abnormally elevated. The effect of single large doses of phosphate may differ from the effect of smaller doses given intermittently during the day. Adverse side-effects, such as soft tissue calcifications, should be kept in mind when phosphates are administered for prolonged periods.

The dosage of the oral phosphate supplements are as follows:

Sodium phosphate or potassium phosphate: 600 mg to 1200 mg/day, given in divided doses
Neutral potassium or sodium phosphate (Neutra-Phos K): 1 g to 2 g/day, given in divided doses

The sodium salt of the phosphates should be avoided in patients with hypertension and/or congestive heart failure.

Calcitonin. Thyrocalcitonin has been shown to reduce bone resorption. However, studies in patients with osteoporosis could not demonstrate this despite indications that there may be an increase in bone formation and in bone mass. At present, the use of calcitonin for the treatment of osteoporosis is still investigational.

Infusions of Calcium. Intravenous infusions of relatively large amounts of calcium (15 mg/kg) in patients with osteoporosis originally indicated this treatment to be beneficial. However, data obtained in two subsequent studies could not confirm this.

Infusions of Calcium and Phosphorus. Alternating daily infusions of calcium and phosphorus for several weeks and thereafter twice or three times per week for 10 months has been reported to produce positive calcium and phosphorus balances. Patients experienced relief of bone pain and bone biopsies obtained 1 year after the start of this treatment demonstrated an increased thickness of cortical bone. The rationale is the dual effect of the infusions, namely, osteoblastic stimulation by phosphorus and the inhibitory action of calcium on PTH secretion. Intravenous administration of calcium and phosphorus over prolonged periods may not only be unacceptable to the patient but may possibly induce soft tissue calcifications. Since phosphorus is readily absorbed from the intestine, it appears reasonable that oral phosphate and calcium supplements be used.

Vitamin D. Circulating vitamin D has been reported to be decreased in patients with osteoporosis and the intestinal absorption of calcium in these patients to be slow during a high calcium intake. Vitamin D therapy may therefore be assumed to be beneficial in order to improve the intestinal absorption of calcium. However, it has not been proven that vitamin D increases the absorption of calcium in patients with osteoporosis. In our own studies relatively large doses of vitamin D (10,000 to 50,000 IU/day) had no effect on calcium absorption in these patients, possibly because these patients were not deficient in vitamin D. Vitamin D is therefore not indicated unless there is vitamin D deficiency (*i.e.,* coexisting osteomalacia or intestinal malabsorption), in which case the absorption of both calcium and vitamin D is impaired. However, vitamin D in a dosage not to exceed 5000 IU/day has been given to patients with osteoporosis. A dosage of 1000 IU vitamin D is probably as effective as 5000 IU and there is less likelihood that the smaller dose would cause vitamin D toxicity and an increase in the urinary calcium level.

Studies of two vitamin D metabolites, 1,25-dihydroxycholecalciferol and 1α-hydroxycholecalciferol, have not demonstrated that they are of greater benefit.

Thiazides. In one study of men receiving thiazides for hypertension, bone density was significantly increased as compared with controls. This beneficial effect was apparently due to the ability of thiazides to decrease calcium loss in the urine.

Because thiazide diuretics may also result in potassium loss and other electrolyte abnormalities, they must be used with caution. It is still too early to recommend them for osteoporosis.

Nonspecific Therapy

For the relief of bone pain, whether or not associated with fractures, analgesics or heat application along with appropriate stretching exercises should be tried first to decrease the associated muscle spasm. If these measures fail, more potent means of pain relief should be employed. In the presence of vertebral fractures, the period of immobilization should be as short as possible or even avoided. Early ambulation, physiotherapy, and exercise should be instituted. Braces may relieve pain by providing support and relaxation of muscle spasm shortly after a vertebral fracture is sustained but are not recommended for long-term use.

Malnutrition may be present in patients with osteoporosis. In undernourished persons, the protein and calorie intake should be increased. Although a high protein, high calorie intake may change a negative nitrogen balance to a positive balance, a concomitant increase in calcium retention does not necessarily occur.

Finally, encouragement and moral support by the physician is important since the chronic course of osteoporosis may lead to a sense of hopelessness.

Secondary Osteoporosis

Secondary osteoporosis is either a consequence of another disease or of administration of drugs.

Osteoporosis Due to Immobilization

The disuse of the skeleton and the lack of muscle pull on bone in immobilization results in severe and generalized osteoporosis. Release of calcium and phosphorus from bone leads to increased urinary calcium excretion and frequently to kidney stone formation. When immobilization is partial, the osteoporosis may be localized and affect only the part of the skeleton immobilized. Examples of conditions in which immobilization may be complete are skeletal trauma, paraplegia due to spinal cord injury, bed rest for prolonged periods in patients with severe arthritis, and application of plaster casts for orthopedic disorders.

It has been generally accepted that immobilization osteoporosis is due to an imbalance of bone formation and bone resorption and that the latter predominates. The absence of normal stress (*i.e.,* muscle pull on the skeleton) removes stimuli for bone formation, while normal bone resorption continues unaffected.

Osteoporosis Associated with Endocrine Disturbances

Osteoporosis in Cushing's Syndrome. A cardinal feature of Cushing's syndrome is osteoporosis usually characterized by back pain and roentgenographic evidence of generalized demineralization and vertebral fractures. In contrast to primary osteoporosis, the osteoporosis of Cushing's syndrome usually shows skull involvement.

The excess production of glucocorticoids by the adrenal gland results in osteoporosis, probably by inhibiting bone matrix formation as well as increasing calcium loss. The serum calcium level is usually normal but may be increased in some instances. The urinary calcium excretion may be in the high normal or distinctly elevated range; retention of infused calcium is lower than normal.

Osteoporosis in Hyperthyroidism. Generalized osteoporosis may be present in hyperthyroidism. The serum calcium level may be normal or elevated; the serum phosphorus level may be normal, low, or high; and the serum alkaline phosphatase value is usually elevated. The urinary calcium excretion may be high and may reach levels similar to those observed in hyperparathyroidism.

The cause of the osteoporosis is accelerated bone turnover; both bone resorption and bone formation are increased, with the rate of resorption being greater than the rate of bone formation.

Osteoporosis in Diabetes Mellitus. The cause of osteoporosis observed in diabetes mellitus is not known but has been linked to poor control of the diabetes, to diabetic acidosis, and to a decrease of the intestinal absorption of calcium.

Osteoporosis Induced by the Use of Drugs

Corticosteroid-induced Osteoporosis. The antianabolic properties of glucorticoids were described by Albright and Reifenstein many years ago. Direct skeletal and extraskeletal effects of corticosteroids or a combination of the two may result in osteoporosis. In cortisone-induced osteoporosis there is increased bone resorption as well as decreased bone formation. An increase in urinary calcium excretion may in part be due to decreased tubular reabsorption of calcium. There may also be a decrease in intestinal absorption of calcium. The decrease is believed due to interference of corticoids with the normal vitamin D metabolism in transport of calcium across the intestine. It is tempting to suggest that the calcium loss induced by corticosteroids may be compensated by overactivity of the parathyroid glands in order to maintain normal serum calcium levels. In fact, it has been suggested that this consequence of secondary hyperparathyroidism might be overcome by the intravenous administration of calcium.

Heparin Osteoporosis. The possibility has been raised that osteoporosis may be induced or accelerated by heparin, which is used for prolonged anticoagulant therapy. Heparin has been shown to inhibit new bone formation as well as increase bone resorption. The latter is believed to be dose related, and anabolic agents may offer some protection against heparin-induced osteoporosis. The levels of the serum calcium, phosphorus, and alkaline phosphatase are normal in heparin osteoporosis. Heparin is produced by mast cells, and the number of mast cells in the bone marrow of patients with osteoporosis has been reported to be increased. Excess heparin produced endogenously by increased mast cells in the marrow or administered as a therapeutic agent may contribute to osteoporosis.

Prolonged Intake of Aluminum-containing Antacids. The intake of large amounts of aluminum-containing antacids results in phosphorus depletion and calcium loss. Our studies show that even a dosage of 30 ml three times per day readily leads to phosphorus depletion and secondary loss of calcium via the kidney. This calcium loss is most likely a result of increased bone resorption. If this process continues for many years, skeletal demineralization and even vertebral fractures may develop.

Other Associations in Osteoporosis

Postmenopausal women who are cigarette smokers are reported to have more bone loss than nonsmokers. The bone loss is also greater in nonobese women than in obese women.

PAGET'S DISEASE

Another bone disease in the older age-group is Paget's disease. It is encountered in persons past 40 and is rare before age 30. Men are more frequently affected than women, the incidence ratio being 4:3. Excess bone resorption and excess bone deposition characterize the disease. In some cases, bone deposition predominates, resulting in sclerosis. Severe deformities of the skeleton may occur, hence the name osteitis deformans. The polyostotic form involves multiple areas of the skeleton, but the bone involvement is not generalized and the parathyroid glands are normal in the majority of cases. In 10% of cases, Paget's disease is monostotic and limited to a single bone or to a single area. Comprehensive reviews on the subject have been published.

The etiology is unknown and has been variously ascribed to chronic inflammation caused by several organisms or bacterial toxins, to developmental defects of the skeleton secondary to hereditary factors, and to wear and tear due to the aging process since the common sites are the sacrum and spine. However, the latter could not account for the common involvement of the skull. Ultrastructure studies have revealed nuclear inclusions remarkably similar to those in viral diseases and, therefore, a viral etiology has been considered.

Clinical Features

It is estimated that at least 20% of patients with Paget's disease are asymptomatic and the diagnosis is frequently an incidental finding on roentgenograms. Bone pain is the most common symptom, with its location depending on sites of bone involvement. The most common sites are the lumbar vertebrae, sacrum, the pelvis, long bones, particularly of the lower extremities, and the skull. The ossicles of the ear are apparently not affected. There may be shortening of the stature, bowing of the extremities, enlargement of the skull, and gross deformity.

Complications

In progressive disease, skeletal deformities are common and fractures may lead to severe pain due to nerve root compression or paraplegia due to compression of the spinal cord. Similarly, involvement of the skull may lead to invagination of the base of the brain, to cranial nerve compression, and to deafness.

In extensive disease, high-output failure may occur caused by the multiple small arteriovenous fistulas in the affected bone. Other associated conditions are calcific periarthritis, rheumatoid arthritis, or its variants as well as hyperuricemia.

The incidence of osteogenic sarcoma has been reported to be 5% to 14%. It occurs twice as often in males as females, more commonly in the humerus or femur; vertebrae are rarely involved. Pain, localized swelling, and very high levels of serum alkaline phosphatase are indicators of this complication. The prognosis of sarcoma in Paget's disease is poor.

Laboratory Findings

The serum calcium and phosphorus levels are usually normal. The elevation of the serum alkaline phosphatase level may be striking, occasionally 10 to 20 times higher than normal. The extent of the disease and the elevation of the serum alkaline phosphatase have been reported to be roughly proportional. However, in the early stages in which bone breakdown rather than bone deposition predominates, the serum alkaline phosphatase may be in the high normal or only slightly elevated range. Development of osteogenic sarcoma may be associated with a marked increase in the serum alkaline phosphatase. The urinary excretion of hydroxyproline is increased. The urinary calcium level may be normal or very high depending on the state of activity of the disease.

The roentgenographic appearance depends on the stage of the disease. In the early or porotic phase, lesions appear as sharply demarcated radiolucent areas, "osteoporosis circumscripta." As bone repair sets in, the areas around the porotic lesions become sclerotic. The skull usually presents a "cotton ball" appearance, but there may be large areas of demineralization surrounded by areas of sclerosis. Progression may result in complete diffuse sclerosis of the skull. In the long bones, the early destructive phase of porosis is followed by overgrowth of bone. Successive layering of new bone in the periosteum results in sclerosis and marked thickening of the cortex, the "wide" bone cortex is characteristic of the disease.

Treatment

Different types of treatment have been used for Paget's disease. Large dosages of aspirin, ranging from 4.0 g to 5.0 g/day, have been suggested, with monitoring of serum salicylate levels. Treatment with mithramycin has been reported to have beneficial effects. This drug relieves bone pain, decreases the serum level of alkaline phosphatase and calcium, and also decreases the urinary excretion of both calcium and of hydroxyproline. Small dosages have been used (*e.g.*, 15 μg to 20 μg/kg/day for 10 days). Dosages as high as 20 to 25 μg/

kg/day, given on alternate days for several weeks, may be required to relieve bone pain or improve objective findings. As maintenance therapy the drug can be given once a week for prolonged periods of time, for instance, 1 to 3 years. The drug can cause thrombocytopenia, hemorrhage, renal failure, and impairment of liver function. The smaller dosage of 15 μg/kg/day may result in fewer adverse reactions. Another therapeutic agent is sodium fluoride, which is reported to relieve bone pain in some cases, starting 4 to 6 weeks after its initiation. The serum alkaline phosphatase and the urinary calcium levels decreased, and the retention of calcium increased in some patients. The retention of fluoride was considerably higher in these patients than in patients with osteoporosis treated with fluoride. However, there was no objective evidence of slowing down of this disease process. Fluoride has been studied in only a small number of patients for relatively short periods of time, so valid conclusions of its efficacy cannot be drawn at this time.

The drug of choice in long-term therapy seems to be calcitonin. Usually salmon calcitonin is used, but human calcitonin may also be used, if available. Maximal clinical benefits are achieved during the first 6 to 12 months of treatment. Relief of bone pain has been observed along with decreases of the serum alkaline phosphatase level and of the urinary hydroxyproline excretion. Salmon calcitonin may result in a higher incidence of binding antibodies than porcine calcitonin. However, patients may be completely asymptomatic and this laboratory finding is not an indication for discontinuing calcitonin therapy. Mild nausea and rarely dermal reactions may occur. The initial dosage of calcitonin is 100 Medical Research Council (MRC) units, given daily for 3 to 5 weeks. Subsequently, the dosage can be decreased to 50 MRC units three times per week, intramuscularly or subcutaneously, with the latter route being used more frequently. The patient can be taught to self-administer this medication. The duration of calcitonin therapy has been reported to be 2 to 3 years, and it appears that it may be given indefinitely.

The diphosphonates are a class of compounds that inhibit bone resorption and bone mineralization. Disodium etidronate has been reported to produce relief of bone pain and favorable biochemical changes. Doses of 15 mg to 20 mg/kg, given orally per day up to 7 months, decreased the serum alkaline phosphatase level and the plasma level of hydroxyproline as well as the urinary hydroxyproline excretion. This treatment has not been reported to be associated with significant adverse reactions.

31 Orthopaedic Aspects of the Lower Extremities

Edward T. Habermann

Loss of the capacity for ambulation is a major transition in the lives of the elderly, and a major challenge to the concerned orthopaedist. The orthopaedic surgeon is increasingly confronted with the management of acute and chronic orthopaedic disabilities in the aged. The importance of individualizing the care of elderly patients should be emphasized. Chronologic age may not accurately reflect a patient's health; his capacity for work and self-care are more significant. Patients should be given every opportunity to return to their former self-sufficient status after disability. Certain risks must be appreciated in deciding on appropriate therapy. The mortality and morbidity rates of the elderly, following surgery, are higher than in younger persons, but these rates are on the decline.

The risks of surgery in the elderly are increased by a multiplicity of preexisting medical problems, especially those of the cardiorespiratory and genitourinary systems. Urinary retention, oversedation, overhydration, and poor digitalization are not infrequent. Preoperative and postoperative programs should guard against pulmonary complications. The use of anticoagulant therapy should be considered in patients requiring long periods of bed rest, as with skeletal traction for long-bone fractures or after surgery of the hip joint[74,75,77] necessitating immobilization. Active exercises to reduce the incidence of venous complications should be encouraged and taught preoperatively, if possible. Early return of the patient to his previous environment may also speed recovery.

FRACTURES IN THE LOWER EXTREMITY

In fractures of the lower extremities, the surgeon must critically evaluate the conditions of the pa-

tient at the time of injury, as well as his prior health and activity. Was the patient ambulatory prior to injury, or was he confined to bed or chair? Was the patient institutionalized because of a chronic brain syndrome or other chronic disease requiring long-term nursing care? Are the bones too osteoporotic to hold internal fixation devices? Does the patient's general condition allow for prolonged traction in bed? Is the nursing care skilled enough to prevent complications of prolonged bed rest, such as decubiti and clotting? Does the patient have some preexisting disease in which prolonged bed rest is not tolerated, such as Paget's disease? All these factors alter treatment from one patient to the next, despite the similarity of location and type of the fracture. Heavy plaster casts and heavy braces are often not tolerated, and stabilization must be provided in some other manner.

The healing of fractures in the aged generally occurs predictably, with the length of time for union depending on the site of fracture. In areas such as the middle and distal thirds of the tibia, a longer period for union is required, primarily because of the critical bone blood supply to these areas.

The concept of electrical stimulation for fracture healing and for treatment of nonunions has shown significant promise.[7–9,12,13,29,67] Its role to date has been primarily in the area of nonunion and delayed union of fractures. There are presently three methods of electrical stimulation: (1) via an external source applied directly over a plaster cast at the fracture site, (2) by application via wires placed percutaneously at the fracture site and linked to an external power source, and (3) by surgical placement at the fracture site of a coil attached to an internal power source implanted simultaneously. The three methods range from noninvasive to invasive with obvious advantages and disadvantages to each. The end results of all three methods for fracture healing are comparable.

Fractures About the Knee

Fractures about the knee are primarily patellar, tibial condylar, and femoral supracondylar fractures.

The best treatment for comminuted or markedly displaced fractures of the patella in the aged is patellectomy. It shortens the length of disability. Regaining extension is the key to success. Loss of terminal extension is a frequent finding that does not negate a relatively good end result. Flexion to 90° is expected with adequate motivation and rehabilitation. Tibial condylar fractures often do moderately well with nonoperative treatment—either traction or plaster-cast immobilization. As soon as possible after injury, traction (balanced suspension) should be started so that early motion may be achieved. Following this, the patient is kept non-weight-bearing until the fracture is sufficiently united (usually 8 to 12 weeks). A cast-brace may be helpful to allow flexion and extension of the knee while maintaining the necessary immobilization for fracture healing.

If there is significant depression of one or both of the condyles or inability to obtain a satisfactory

reduction of a split fracture of the condyles, then open surgical reduction with internal fixation is usually required if the patient is medically stable. Depressions of the condyles greater than 1 cm frequently require fixation and bone grafting. Tomography is often very helpful in determining the true status of depressed condylar fractures. One must always be cognizant of associated ligamentous injuries, which may not be readily diagnosed. Failure to provide for stability, either bony or ligamentous, leads to long-term poorer results.

Early mobilization is an important feature of treatment. Both clinical and experimental observations show that intra-articular adhesions form after knee-joint fractures if the extremity is immobilized longer than 1 month. Quadriceps setting exercises are started at the beginning of treatment and are critical to obtaining a good clinical result. The use of internal fixation in selected cases, especially in a noncomminuted displaced fracture of a condyle, may offer early stability and rapid return of motion (Fig. 31-1).

Supracondylar fractures present clinical problems similar to those of the femoral shaft and hip, requiring prolonged bed rest in traction. Many of them can be managed by skeletal traction through the tibial tubercle if the patient is able to tolerate bed status for the necessary period.

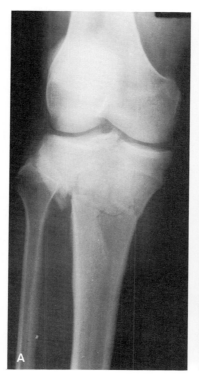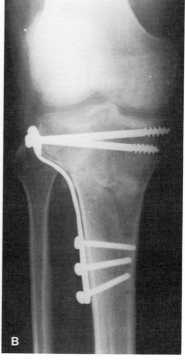

FIG. 31-1. (*A*) Bicondylar tibial plateau fracture in a 67-year-old man. (*B*) Internal fixation with lateral buttress plate restored congruity to the articular surface.

The cast-brace technique[18,19,64] has proved to be of great value in the treatment of supracondylar fractures, allowing for relatively early ambulation and for motion of the knee and ankle while the patient is ambulatory. By this method the time in traction can be decreased, the hospital stay shortened, and ambulatory outpatient care provided. By allowing early knee motion one escapes the prolonged disability of a stiff knee following healing. This has been especially effective in the treatment of comminuted supracondylar fractures, which are not very amenable to internal fixation. The binding down of the quadriceps mechanism had been a significant problem prior to the advent of early knee motion with this technique.

Alternative procedures may be necessary when bed rest and traction cannot be tolerated or are not indicated (Fig. 31-2). Internal fixation may then become a necessity.[14] Osteoporotic bone is the usual finding, and the holding of internal fix-ation devices may be difficult. After healing, flexion and extension about the knee joint are frequently compromised by this fracture, so that secure fixation and early motion of the joint is most important.

The use of methylmethacrylate (bone cement) in selected cases of very difficult fractures along with internal fixation has provided immediate stability to an already compromised geriatric patient. This technique has allowed immediate ambulation under the proper conditions.[42]

Fractures of the tibial and fibular shafts are not common in the aged. Closed reduction and plaster immobilization usually suffice. However, internal fixation or external fixators may be necessary to gain reduction and stability and care for any other associated soft tissue or vascular injury.

Short-leg functional cast braces for most tibial fractures have been successful and allow for both knee and ankle motion and early ambulation.[23,76]

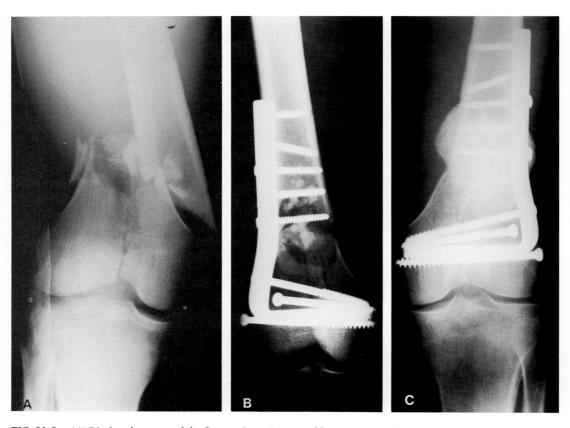

FIG. 31-2. (*A*) Displaced supracondylar fracture in an 81-year-old woman. (*B* and *C*) Internal fixation with 90° angle plate and compression screws. Bone grafting was required. The patient left the hospital in 3 weeks with a functional range of motion of her knee.

Most elderly patients can tolerate this technique after an appropriate period of time in a long-leg cast if the latter is necessary.

Fractures of the Hip

Most hip fractures occur in women over 60. It is well established that operative management decreases morbidity and mortality. There is extensive literature on the treatment of fractures about the hip joint, especially the intracapsular type.[27] An unanswered question with intracapsular fractures is whether one should primarily replace a displaced neck fracture with a prosthesis or attempt a reduction followed by internal fixation. The proponents of both methods are numerous, and treatment is a matter of the surgeon's philosophy. Because of the high success rate in total hip replacement for the arthritides in the geriatric population, total hip replacement in selected cases of intracapsular fractures has also been advocated, especially when there is advanced osteoporosis or any other associated degenerative changes within the acetabulum. The use of bone cement to secure hemiarthroplasty prosthetic components in place, especially in the presence of osteoporosis, has enhanced the end results of prosthetic replacement after hip fractures. Trochanteric fractures are best treated by operation,[35] thereby avoiding prolonged traction and bed rest (Fig. 31-3). These fractures usually unite, and aseptic necrosis and nonunion

are uncommon. In over 1000 cases of intertrochanteric fractures reviewed at my institution a 98% union rate occurred after fixation with a sliding nail and plate device.[36] There are numerous appliances with different types of materials, and each surgeon decides on the special apparatus he prefers. Medial displacement osteotomy[24] for unstable intertrochanteric fractures has been effective in adding stability and reducing the tendency toward varus deformity. Crawford[22] has had good results with nonoperative treatment of impacted fractures of the neck of the femur, but possible displacement at a later date remains a hazard.

The treatment of subtrochanteric fractures in the elderly population is often very difficult. With the advent of the Zickel intramedullary nail,[87,88] secure fixation of most subtrochanteric fractures can be provided and earlier ambulation is possible than with other previous methods of surgery (Fig. 31-4).

Avascular Necrosis

The extent of nonunion and avascular necrosis of the femoral head following displaced neck fractures varies, but an incidence of 20% to 40% is reported in the literature.[6,27,63] The resultant question then is, "Why not perform a primary prosthetic replacement in such fractures if the chances of failure following nailing are so high?" There is no final answer to our question, except that the

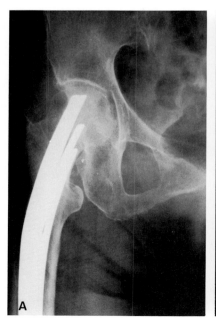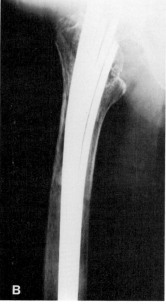

FIG. 31-3. (*A* and *B*) Nondisplaced intertrochanteric fracture fixed with multiple Enders rods in an 82-year-old woman. The patient was allowed to bear weight immediately.

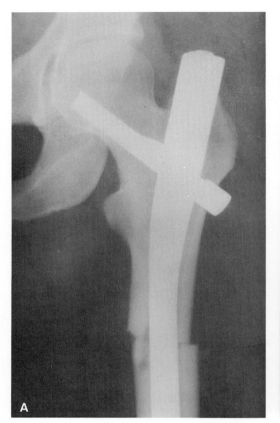

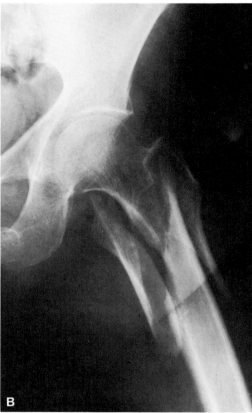

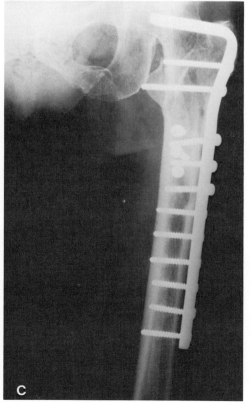

FIG. 31-4. (*A*) Zickel intramedullary nailing transfixing subtrochanteric fracture of the femur. (*B* and *C*) Comminuted subtrochanteric fracture in an 80-year-old woman. Plate and screw fixation was used with anatomical restoration.

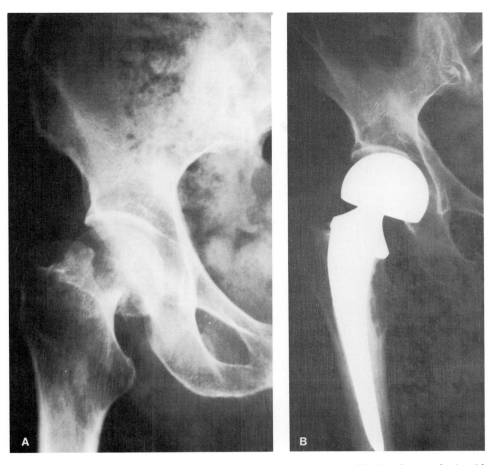

FIG. 31-5. High subcapital hip fracture in a 70-year-old woman treated by bipolar prosthesis with immediate weight bearing. She was discharged ambulating with a walker in 1 week.

patient's healed femoral head is better than any prosthesis. A study of neck fractures using a variable-angle/sliding nail demonstrated a decrease in the incidence of nonunion and a suspected decrease in the rate of avascular necrosis.[38]

Although generally apparent earlier, avascular necrosis may not be detected either radiographically or clinically for several years following injury.[63] Thus, the incidence of avascular necrosis is higher if a long follow-up is maintained. Primary prosthetic replacement of the femoral head or bipolar type of arthroplasty (Fig. 31-5) or total hip replacement is indicated in the following situations: (1) an intracapsular fracture that cannot be adequately reduced, (2) a fracture extending into the femoral head, (3) a displaced high subcapital fracture, (4) a displaced subcapital fracture that is greater than 3 weeks old, and (5) a pathologic fracture. In these instances, primary prosthetic replacement seems to offer better end results than

other methods of treatment. Various methods for predicting viability of the femoral head have been performed, and others are under study. A simple, accurate method for determining the viability of the femoral head may ultimately be the surgeon's best guide in determining the procedure of choice. The use of bone-scanning techniques has been useful in the evaluation of avascular necrosis.[57,78]

In the elderly debilitated senile patient who has been an ambulator and who presents with a displaced subcapital fracture that cannot be reduced, simple resection of the femoral head has provided pain relief and wheelchair status in a rapid fashion. This procedure should be reserved for carefully selected patients. The final solution to intracapsular fractures has not yet been found.

The United States leads the world in the incidence of hip fractures. The estimated costs in 1980 were well over one billion dollars. Although the orthopaedic surgeon has attempted to facilitate the patient's return to preoperative status and his own environment, reality is often unkind. Delays are usually built into the system: (1) There is often no coordinated policy for postfracture rehabilitation in the hospital and commonly no efforts are made to equip patients for return to their own homes. (2) Continuing hospital stay often adds to the patient's mental confusion and deterioration. Confusion is not uncommonly seen in the postoperative period and may be related to the sudden change in environment, overprescription of sedatives or change in metabolic state. (3) Planning for home early in the course of the patient's admission is vital and must include a careful study of the home situation by social workers and professionals trained in this area (See Chapter 44). Home assistance is often needed, especially if the patient lives alone or has a spouse who is unable to help. Can the patient dress and take care of himself? Who will prepare meals and do the shopping? These factors must be worked out prior to discharge and often require weeks to plan. Returning a patient to his own environment in dignity, to become an active member of society, is everyone's goal. Inability of a team effort to achieve this places the patient on an ever-growing waiting list for nursing homes or long ward stays where deterioration becomes more complete.

Patients with hip fractures can be placed in high- and low-risk categories (Table 31-1), and their outcome can often be related to these categories. In a classic study of high-risk patients by Niemann and Mankin,[65] the mortality at 6 weeks was 40% and only 33% survived 1 year. The lower risk group fares better, but the figures are still awesome.

Fractures of the femoral shaft may be treated either by traction or by internal fixation (intramedullary nailing). By nailing, one escapes prolonged bed rest and all its complications. The extent of available nursing care may alter the type of treatment advised for these fractures. When surgery is not advisable owing either to the type of fracture or to the medical status of the patient, fractures of the femoral shaft may be treated by a period of traction followed by cast-brace immobilization and early weight bearing.[18,19,64] The use of a long-leg cast-brace or minispica cast-brace has allowed early ambulation during the course of fracture healing.

INJURIES AROUND THE KNEE

Ligamentous injuries occur much less frequently in the elderly than in a younger, more vigorous population. They must be recognized and appropriately managed to avoid later instability and disability. Lesions of the menisci in the elderly are primarily degenerative rather than the acute traumatic episodes seen in younger patients. In selected patients with persistent findings of meniscal disease, an arthrogram may be helpful in determining the status of the meniscus. Limited procedures through the arthroscope have been reported to give short-term beneficial results. Whether there will be any long-term good results has yet to be determined.

Avulsion of the quadriceps muscle requiring surgical repair is a not infrequent injury. It is usually cause by forcible flexion of the knee while the quadriceps is strongly contracted (*e.g.*, in falling down stairs). Loss of active knee extension with tenderness and swelling of the upper margin of the patella is a clue to the diagnosis. A palpable defect may be present. Primary repair produces the best results if performed early. Knee flexion beyond 90° is usually achieved, and extension may lack the last few degrees, but an early repair provides the best chance for a stable well-functioning knee.

TABLE 31-1   Risk Factors for Patients With Hip Fractures

	High Risk	Low Risk
Age	> 65	< 65
Living at Home	No	Yes
Living with Someone	No	Yes
Mobility	Improved	Unimproved
In a Chronic Institution	Yes	No
Mental Status	Impaired	Unimpaired
Associated Medical Conditions	Many, especially cardiovascular	Few

OSTEONECROSIS OF THE KNEE

Osteonecrosis of the knee in the elderly, now a well-recognized entity, received minimal attention in the past. Since the initial description by Ahlback and Bauer[1] in 1968, it has become clear that it is more common than previously appreciated.[2,70] Spontaneous osteonecrosis may now be considered a not uncommon source of knee pain in patients over the age of 50. It presents with a symptom complex that may often seem confusing to the unwary and hence go unrecognized, especially in the absence of the classic radiographic findings. Initially it had been thought to occur only in the medial femoral condyle. However, it is now described about the tibia and also on the lateral side of the joint. In reviewing 52 patients with osteonecrosis, two thirds had previously been treated for an incorrect diagnosis.[39] Norman and Baker[66] have reported an association of spontaneous osteonecrosis and medial meniscal tears. Physical examination may vary significantly from patient to patient, and findings include local tenderness over the appropriate condyle, some loss of extension and/or flexion, effusion, synovial thickening, and symptoms of an osteoarthritic nature depending on the stage that the diagnosis is made. The patient's complaints may also vary from acute symptomatology, which persists even at rest to symptoms compatible with an arthritic knee. Results of laboratory studies and study of the synovial fluid are consistently unremarkable. Many of the patients present with a normal radiographic examination initially, but a technetium-99-labeled pyrophosphate bone scan that consistently reveals intense focal uptake over the affected condyle can establish a proper diagnosis. The earliest radiographic finding may consist of flattening of the weight-bearing surface of the medial femoral condyle often accompanied by a variable degree of subchondral sclerosis (Fig. 31-6). Many but not all patients will demonstrate a progression from this earlier minimal lesion to the so-called typical lesion of osteonecrosis. However, Lotke and coworkers[61] have described a group of patients treated supportively who go on to complete resolution without the typical progressive lesion. The lesion may progress to severe medial compartment osteoarthrosis with subsequent varus deformity.

Early treatment is supportive when there are minimal roentgenographic findings and includes quadriceps exercises, protected weight bearing, and observation; the course may vary from improvement in symptoms to progressive osteoarthritic changes, which determine further therapy. I have found that arthrotomy and drilling of the lesion in the hope of promoting vascular ingrowth was disappointing. The best results came with high tibial osteotomy,[58] if only a single compartment were involved, to total knee replacement when there was multicompartmental involvement. A clear understanding of the etiology of spontaneous osteonecrosis of the knee remains elusive. It has been attributed to microtrauma with associated microfracture and vascular insufficiency (*i.e.,* bone infarction). Errors in diagnosis may lead to un-

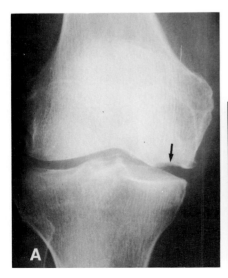
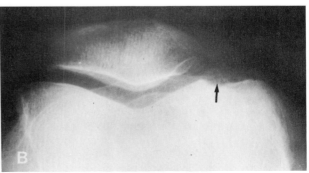

FIG. 31-6. (*A* and *B*) Osteonecrosis of medial femoral condyle as seen on anteroposterior and patella view in a 73-year-old woman who experienced sudden onset of pain without a history of trauma.

necessary surgical procedures. The clinical course is extremely variable, and radionuclide bone scanning remains crucial in establishing diagnosis in the absence of typical radiographic findings. This condition should be suspected in elderly patients presenting with knee pain often in the absence of another cause. Osteonecrosis is known to occur in patients receiving corticosteroids;[49] however, in the patients I have seen corticosteroid therapy was not considered as a factor.

OSTEOARTHRITIS

It is generally believed that osteoarthritis results from the wear and tear of increasing age and repeated trauma and is thus a concomitant of the aging process. Stecher[83] has shown that osteoarthritis is a collection of individual diseases, differing from each other according to the joints involved, sex ratio, age at onset, relation to the menopause, and hereditary factors. Osteoarthritis is not necessarily a disease of old age, and it has been complicated by confusion with aging changes. The aging process begins in joints, as it does in other organs, at an early age, and proceeds at varying rates in different tissues and in different parts of the same tissue. The pathologic changes in osteoarthritis are nonspecific and are seen also in aging. First, changes occur in the cartilage, followed by erosion of the joint surfaces and desquamation, leading finally to a wearing away and loss of cartilage and resultant denuded bone. This process is most marked and most frequently seen in pressure areas, whereas in other areas the cartilage proliferates and builds up. In this connection one should remember that the stress across the hip approximates three times the body weight and that significant stress is applied even with non-weight-bearing.

Studies of the comparative pathology of osteoarthritis seriously question conventional views of the prime responsibility of abnormal mechanical stresses; thus, the weight-bearing human ankle is rarely affected, but the distal joints of the fingers are frequently involved. In contrast, ankles are prone to degenerative arthritis in horses, cattle, and certain breeds of swine.

Osteoarthritis in all joints has features that distinguish it from other types of arthritis. Degenerative arthritis is not associated with demineralization or bone atrophy as in rheumatoid arthritis, nor with constitutional symptoms. The patient is well and vigorous, except for the affected joints. There are no blood or serologic changes.

Salter and Field[71] have shown that compression

of opposing living articular cartilage surfaces in rabbits interferes with the nutrition of the cartilage and results in compression necrosis. If an animal in which this lesion has been produced is allowed to run free, the joint becomes the site of typical degenerative arthritis. Changes that occur in the cartilage as age advances include thinning and even total disappearance of cartilage. Other changes present are congestion of the synovial membrane and capsular fibrosis. There seem to be two different processes working together. One is aging and the other is osteoarthritis. These have in the past been grouped together.

Trueta and Harrison[85] showed that osteoarthritis of the hip is associated with proliferation of blood vessels and an increased blood supply and is not a disease of ischemia as suspected in the past. Alterations in vascularity do not seem to initiate degenerative joint disease but are involved later in the development of some of the characteristic features. In weight-bearing areas, bone sclerosis results from thickening of trabeculae when new lamellae are laid down as the result of proliferation of newly formed vessels. In non-weight-bearing areas, vessel proliferation and resultant stimulation of endochondral ossification may lead to osteophyte formation. Observations in degenerative hip disease suggest that increased vascularity may be responsible for pain and that relief of pain after salicylate therapy or osteotomy may be related to vascular changes.

There are many potential contributing factors that may place an individual at risk, such as congenital deformities, trauma and/or surgery about a joint, obesity, crystal deposition, systemic disease, and family history. However, the specific reasons for progression to osteoarthritis in this group are not known.

It is known that aging produces changes in the composition of glycosaminoglycans, chondroitin sulfate, and keratan sulfate, but there seems to be a complex set of new developments associated with matrix breakdown and major separation and remodeling processes that alter the osteoarthritic joint that differ from the aging process alone.

Structural and biochemical changes alter the geometry of joints, and stimuli for repair appear to be cartilage loss and fibrillations that penetrate the tide mark into the subchondral bone. How to influence and direct cartilage repair is still being studied experimentally.

Osteoarthritis of the Hip

Osteoarthritis of the hip occurs after a variety of disturbances in the joint. Some cases are the result of fracture, dislocation, or avascular bone necrosis unrelated to genetic factors. Others follow congenital dysplasia of the hip, coxa plana, slipped capital femoral epiphysis, or Legg–Calvé–Perthes disease, which are conditions in which the role of heredity has been suspected or demonstrated. Graber-Duvernay[33] stated that osteoarthritis develops only in preexisting deformities of the hip and that 50% of his patients had had previous congenital deformity. Although many believe that most cases could be accounted for on some secondary basis, others hold that primary osteoarthritis of the hip is still an entity. Secondary osteoarthritis is distinguished with difficulty, if at all, from other forms of the disease.

Osteoarthritis of the hip is a unilateral disease in about 50% of patients. It often develops in early adult life but may first become apparent in advanced old age. Its onset is often insidious, and it may develop to a fully recognizable degree unknown to the patient. Clinically, the first sign is a decrease in range of motion that can progress to a nearly complete loss of rotation of the upper leg. As the disease advances, pain becomes troublesome and flexion becomes greatly restricted.

Osteoarthritis of the hip is unpredictable; it may progress rapidly or be dormant for many years. Radiographic changes may not relate accurately to the patient's symptomatology, and the chief consideration for treatment is the severity of the complaint.

The most common clinical manifestations are pain and loss of mobility. Loss of mobility is ascribed to destruction of the articular cartilage, causing joint-surface incongruity; muscle spasm and contracture; mechanical block due to osteophytes and loose bodies; and incongruity of articular surfaces. The origin of the pain in osteoarthritis of the hip remains obscure. Some recognized causes include synovitis, inflammation in the articular capsule, contracture and spasm of the muscles crossing the hip, and cystic changes in the subchondral bone.

Bilateral hip disease is far more restricting and disabling than the unilateral form and more often necessitates surgical intervention. As is true for osteoarthritis of other joints, physiotherapy, weight loss, external support, anti-inflammatory agents, rest, and analgesics may provide significant relief and maintenance of an ambulatory status. Intra-articular corticosteroids are a last resort for patients not amenable to other types of therapy. Degenerative osteoarthritis of the hip joint may progress without response to the medical treatment outlined, and surgery may then be indicated. The most frequent reasons for surgery are to re-lieve pain, to restore motion and function, to correct deformity, to establish stability, and to relieve secondary changes in other joints. In the aged, psychologic blocks are often present, causing reluctance to accept any surgical procedure.

Total hip replacement arthroplasty is the most effective therapy now available for the treatment of arthritic conditions of the hip (Fig. 31-7).[15,16,26,37] The ideal objectives of treatment—relief of pain, restoration of range of motion, and return to a more normal level of function—can be satisfied in the majority of patients. Even in patients with less than perfect results, marked improvement in at least one and usually in all three of these parameters is obtained. Refinement of surgical technique and improvement in design are responsible for extension of the indications for operation to include almost any age-group. Long-term data are now available that reveal the good results as well as the complications of total hip arthroplasty.

Although total hip replacement has virtually supplanted all other methods of treatment for the arthritic hip in the aged,[37] it is important to recall the other procedures used:

1. The girdlestone procedure, an excision arthroplasty of the upper end of the femur, left the patient with shortening and instability requiring external support and far less than optimal results. It is now primarily reserved for failed total hip replacements when a salvage procedure, such as revision, cannot be performed.
2. The mold arthroplasty, used extensively in the past, necessitated long-term rehabilitation and was relatively unpredictable. Cooperation of the patient was of the utmost importance in achieving a good end result.
3. Osteotomy of the hip continues to be of importance in the relief of hip pain secondary to arthritis. Pain is relieved in a significant percentage, although not in all cases.
4. Hemiarthroplasty is not advocated in the present era because of the unpredictable end results when arthritic changes are present on both sides of the joint. It is primarily used in the treatment of fractures of the neck of the femur.
5. Arthrodesis of the hip joint continues to be regarded as an operative possibility for hip disease in a young patient with a unilateral process. Arthrodesis necessitates prolonged immobilization, which is not well tolerated by the aged.

Most of the previous procedures performed for arthritis of the hip are now historical, and, except

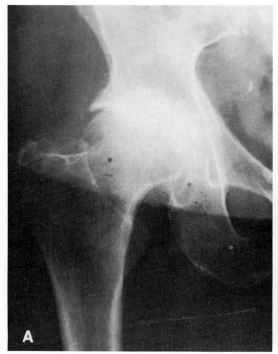
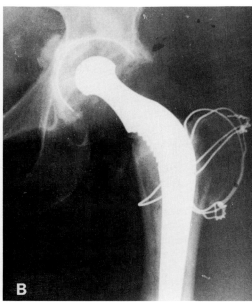

FIG. 31-7. (*A*) Painful osteoarthritis of the hip in a 75-year-old patient. (*B*) Conversion to total hip replacement.

for isolated cases, total hip arthroplasty has supplanted them all.[37] A bewildering array of total hip replacement designs is available. Each of them continues to be refined as experience accumulates. Selection of a specific design is related to the surgeon's experience and preference.

Total hip replacement has also provided an excellent salvage procedure for a variety of failed procedures in the geriatric population. These include failures of surgery in the five procedures noted previously (Figs. 31-8 and 31-9). In my initial series of 377 patients,[38] 21% in the geriatric age-group had total hip replacement as a salvage for failure of other procedures. The outstanding characteristics of total hip replacement are the predictable absence of pain and maintenance of improvement in mobility in a relatively short period of time, with minimal physical therapy. Postoperative ambulation is usually started within the first week. These factors are obviously of great advantage to the aged. Long-term follow-up and analysis of complications has stimulated interest in new designs, better cementing techniques, and other advances. It has been my routine, except where contraindicated, to use some form of anticoagulation,[55,73] as well as prophylactic short-term antibiotic therapy (48 hours) following total joint replacement surgery.

Total hip replacement must be considered one of the most successful procedures in the orthopaedic surgeon's armamentarium,[10,21] but a variety of complications are now well recognized. The most frequent significant complication is that of aseptic loosening (Figs. 31-10 and 31-11). Radiographic loosening may or may not be symptomatic or progressive. However, it must be critically analyzed and defined in each patient so that appropriate treatment can be planned.[3,52] It is important to have adequate roentgenograms taken to determine whether progressive changes are suggestive of loosening or existed on the immediate postoperative films. Loosening may manifest itself symptomatically by pain and radiographically by demonstration of radiolucent zones of increasing size between the bone–cement interface or between the cement–prosthesis interface on the acetabular or femoral side or both.[72] Migration or subsidence of the cement mass into the medullary canal of the femur or shift in the femoral component are relatively easily observed radiographically, as are deformations of the stem or late, incomplete or complete fracture (Fig. 31-12).[17,86] Fragmentation or cracking of the cement column is usually well appreciated, especially when comparing prior roentgenograms. Calcar absorption, which is not an uncommon event, is not specifically related to

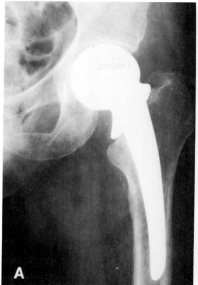
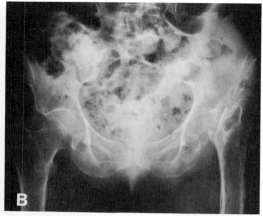
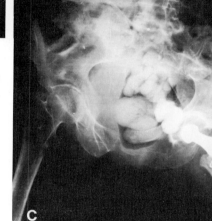

FIG. 31-8. (*A*) Thompson prosthesis in a 78-year-old woman with subcapital hip fracture. Patient has persistent pain in hip. (*B*) The prosthesis was removed and the hip joint converted to pseudoarthrosis because patient could not tolerate the pain, but after this surgery the pain continued and instability followed. (*C*) Conversion from pseudoarthrosis to Charnley-type total hip replacement gave the patient relief from pain and a return to ambulatory status in 4 weeks.

progressive loosening or clinical symptomatology. Cystic changes about the medullary canal and massive osteolysis are ominous signs of failure.[47] On the acetabular side changes of radiolucency may be incomplete but altered position of the acetabular component or erosive changes about the cement–bone interface are obvious signs of failure. A demarcation line about the acetabulum is extremely common radiographically and not necessarily evidence of loosening or failure.[68] The incidence of loosening has had a broad range from less than 5% to greater than 50%. The rate of loosening of the femoral component is higher during earlier follow-up periods and seems to decrease in incidence over time.[82] Conversely, the rate of loosening of the acetabular component is found to increase with time.

Osteolysis about total hip replacements has been encountered with increasing frequency (Fig. 31-13),[47] and it is believed that acrylic cement

plays a significant role. On microscopy, one sees histiocytes, macrophages, and giant cells along with significant amounts of methylmethacrylate debris, without evidence of an inflammatory process or infection. Changes at the bone–cement interface in loose prostheses have been further defined, and Goldring[31] has suggested there is a synoviallike membrane as a biological response to the acrylic cement. Whether motion at this cement–bone interface provides the stimulus for differentiation and organization of cells into synovial tissue is not fully understood, but methylmethacrylate itself may promote formation of a synoviallike membrane. Collagenase and prostaglandin E2, which are both implicated in bone resorption, have been found at this synovial tissue interface. I have had several cases of revision surgery for osteolysis in which the same pathologic process recurred after revision.

It is critical to rule out loosening secondary to

(*Text continues on p. 552*)

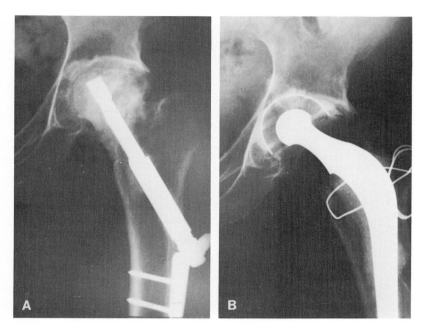

FIG. 31-9. (*A*) Fracture of neck of femur in an 83-year-old woman who developed painful avascular necrosis following hip nailing. (*B*) Conversion to total hip replacement.

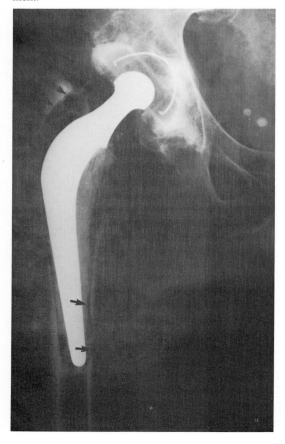

FIG. 31-10. Loosening of femoral component in a 75-year-old woman. Note radiolucency at arrows.

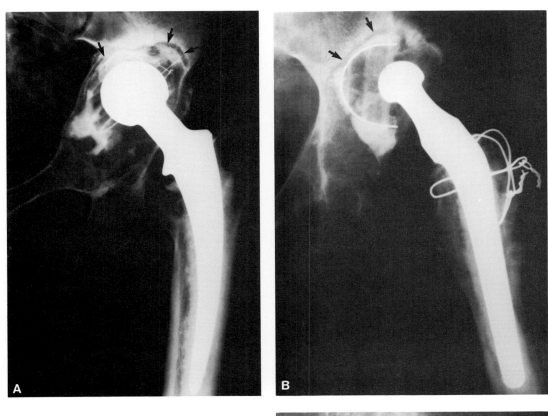

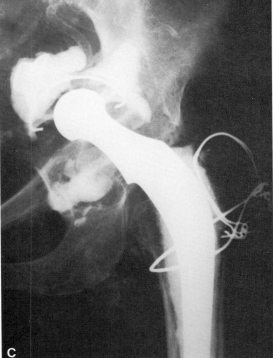

FIG. 31-11. Loose acetabular components of various types. (*A*) Circumferential radiolucency around socket in a 78-year-old woman. (*B*) Loose acetabulum that has shifted to a vertical position with associated radiolucency. (*C*) Acetabulum has migrated into the pelvis of an 80-year-old patient.

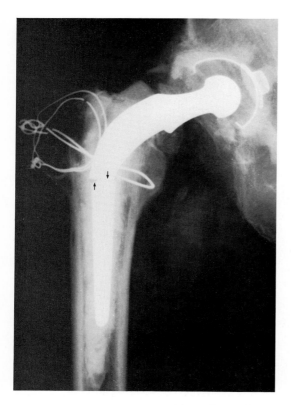

FIG. 31-12. Fracture (*arrows*) of femoral stem due to metal fatigue in this 200-pound, active, 73-year-old patient with loosening at the proximal portion of the prosthesis.

sepsis. Patients with septic loosening often present only with pain and without signs of systemic illness or localizing infection. Basic studies include erythrocyte sedimentation rate, white blood cell count, and radiography of the total hip replacement. Roentgenographic criteria alone are often not definitive enough to differentiate between septic and aseptic loosening (Fig. 31-14). There has been no absolute differentiation between the two on technetium and gallium scanning. However, it has been suggested that a positive gallium scan is more frequently seen in patients with septic loosening. To prove the diagnosis, aspiration of the infected joint should be performed. In addition, biopsy at the time of surgical exploration is very helpful. One of the most common offending organisms is *Staphylococcus epidermidis,* which previously was not regarded as a pathogen. In total joint arthroplasty it is certainly one of the most frequent organisms seen in septic processes. In loosening secondary to sepsis, antibiotic therapy, with removal of the cement and component parts,

followed by either a primary or two-stage revision has given the best results. Conversion to a pseudoarthrosis of the hip, although not ideal, has often eradicated the infection; some patients can manage with external support and without significant pain following this procedure. Gram-negative organisms have a poorer prognosis for exchange arthroplasty than gram-positive ones. It has been my usual policy when the patient's medical condition permits to perform a two-stage procedure rather than a direct exchange arthroplasty.

Hematogenous seeding from transient bacteremias following dental manipulation, urologic procedures, or infections of the urinary tract and other areas are potential sources for infection about a joint arthroplasty. All of my patients have been advised to take appropriate prophylactic antibiotics prior to dental or urologic manipulation.

Heterotopic bone formation is not an uncommon problem following total hip arthroplasty. One can usually identify to some degree high-risk patients such as those with ankylosing spondylitis who have had massive osteophyte formation or heterotopic bone. These high-risk patients are usually placed on low-dose radiation therapy immediately following the total hip replacement. Use of diphosphonates has also been successful in decreasing the incidence of heterotopic bone formation.

Because of increasing problems especially with loosening of prosthetic components in total joint arthroplasty, there have been significant experimental trials in the area of biologic fixation. These trials show that trabecular bone is able to grow into various types of porous-coated prostheses and provide a mechanically effective biologic bond, thereby eliminating the cement interface. With this in mind, clinical studies have been undertaken about the hip and knee to see if biologic fixation can achieve long-term stability and prevention of loosening (Fig. 31-15).[48,52]

Osteoarthritis of the Knee

Osteoarthritis of the knee is a frequent and often disabling condition leading to deformities of flexion, valgus, or varus, of varying degrees. The patellofemoral articulation may be the site of maximum damage. Crepitus of the knee is common in patients without complaints. Its incidence increases as age advances. The cause of crepitus has not been well identified but is believed to result from irregularities of the surface or fibrillation of the cartilage. Crepitus is produced on motion in almost all painful knees. The diagnosis of osteoar-

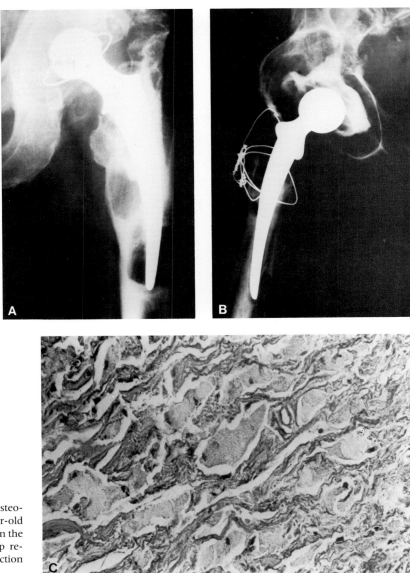

FIG. 31-13. (*A*) Marked osteolysis of the femur in a 72-year-old man. (*B*) Massive osteolysis on the acetabular side of a total hip replacement. (*C*) Histiocytic reaction on pathology section.

thritis should be reserved for knees, with or without crepitus, in which there is pain and limitation of motion. Early, there is a lack of normal hyperextension, then a lack of complete extension, and finally limitation of flexion. Such knees are often slightly tender and enlarged by thickened synovial tissues; they may contain a moderate increase in synovial fluid.

Treatment is instituted in the aged primarily for pain relief and maintenance of an ambulatory status. Severe radiographic changes and gross deformity may be compatible with a painless and stable situation. The quadriceps mechanism is a

key factor in providing this stability, and its continued function should always be encouraged.

The following conservative treatments yield varying degrees of success: active physiotherapy, weight reduction, intra-articular injections of corticosteroids, and bracing, or other forms of splinting and immobilization. If conservative therapy fails to provide relief, surgery must be considered.

Osteotomy of the tibia[20,53] is a well-recognized surgical procedure for osteoarthritis of the knee. Some good results have been achieved, and it should be considered when there is unicompartmental disease but not when both compartments

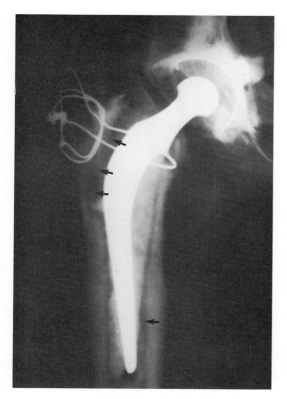

FIG. 31-14. Septic prosthesis in a 69-year-old patient. Note changes at arrows.

are involved in the arthritic process. The osteotomy can correct the deformity as well as relieve pain (Fig. 31-16). Better results can be anticipated when correcting a varus deformity with a high tibial osteotomy. When significant valgus deformity exists a femoral osteotomy may be necessaary.[11]

After the successes of total hip replacement, great enthusiasm for total knee replacement was not long in coming.[34,54,60,69,80,81] With the same type of biomaterials, there were hundreds of different knee replacements being used throughout the world. The primary indications for total knee replacement are to relieve pain, provide stability, and allow motion. The design of the total knee prosthesis will depend on the degree of destruction of the bone, ligamentous stability, other associated joint problems, and the experience and preference of the individual surgeon. Because of the complexity of the knee joint, design considerations and specific criteria for the various prosthesis must be critically analyzed. Follow-up results are now available that indicate that complications are not infrequent. Loosening, instability, wear of the tibial component, malalignment, sepsis, patella prob-

lems, and the necessity for revision surgery are some of the problems encountered. Salvage procedures using other types of knee prostheses are available when earlier designs have failed. Arthrodesis of the knee is sometimes necessary, especially as a salvage procedure. It is rarely used at the present time as a primary procedure for osteoarthritis of the knee in the aged. The Charnley-type compression arthrodesis has been successful. It is also used for salvage of the failed total knee replacement, as in cases of infection. Total knee arthroplasty (Fig. 31-17), has been a great advance in the treatment of arthritis of the knee, providing relief of pain, stability, and motion in a significant percentage of cases. No one knee implant in use at this point satisfies the needs of all types of knee dysfunction. Complications of loosening primarily of the tibial component have been of concern, and the use of porous-coated knee prostheses (Fig. 31-18) along with appropriate design modifications has attractive possibilities.[50,51]

Failure rates with earlier knee designs were not insignificant, necessitating more anatomical designs, better instrumentation so as to achieve alignment, and more precise surgical techniques. Not unlike the hip joint, complications following total knee replacement need careful and critical analysis to determine the etiology of the failure (Fig. 31-19).

The use of a continuous passive motion exerciser following knee reconstruction has been helpful.

Osteoarthritis of the Ankle

Osteoarthritis of the ankle is not nearly as frequent as it is in the other major joints of the lower extremity (*i.e.,* the hip and knee). Osteoarthritis of the ankle can often be managed by conservative means, and, in contrast to the knee and hip, surgical procedures are infrequent. If relief of pain and maintenance of stability cannot be provided by conservative management, then arthrodesis of the joint or total ankle arthroplasty may be necessary. Arthrodesis will give good end results with relief of pain and stability in about 80% of cases.[56,59] Total ankle joint arthroplasty has shown promising results in very carefully selected cases (Fig. 31-20).[25]

THE NEUROPATHIC JOINT

The neuropathic joint was most frequently seen in the past in *tabes dorsalis* and was long regarded as

(Text continues on p. 558)

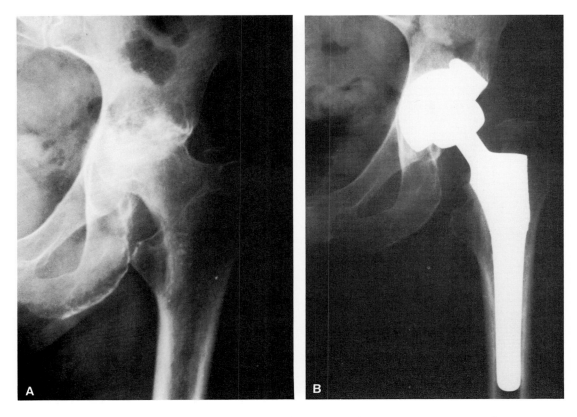

FIG. 31-15. Preoperative view of patient with osteoarthritis (*A*) and postoperative (*B*) views of porous-coated total hip replacement without cement.

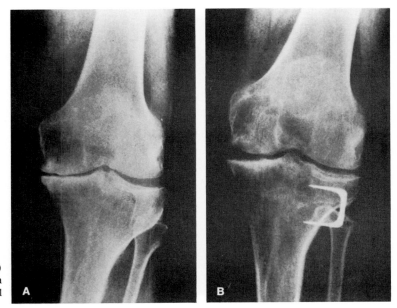

FIG. 31-16. Preoperative (*A*) and postoperative (*B*) views of a high tibial osteotomy for medial compartment osteoarthritis.

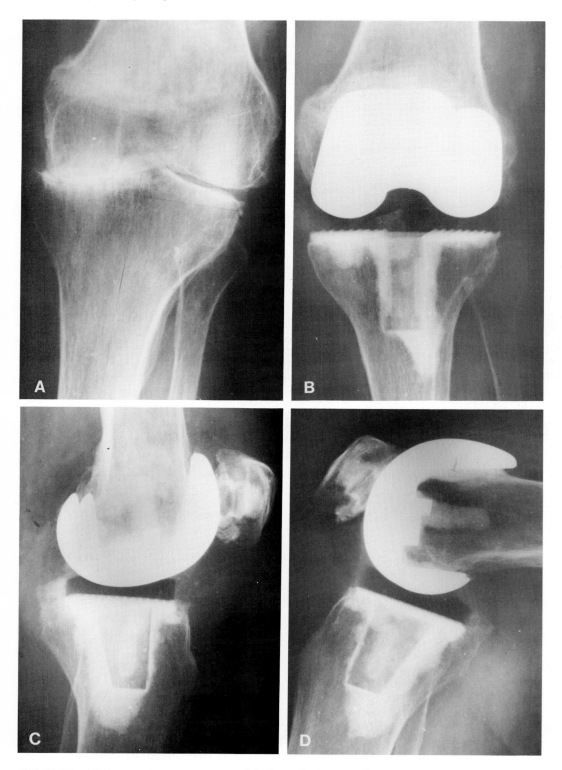

FIG. 31-17.   (*A*) Preoperative roentgenogram of the knee of a 67-year-old woman with loss of medial joint space and severe knee pain secondary to arthritis. (*B, C,* and *D*) Postoperative views of total condylar knee replacement. Resurfacing of the patella was also performed.

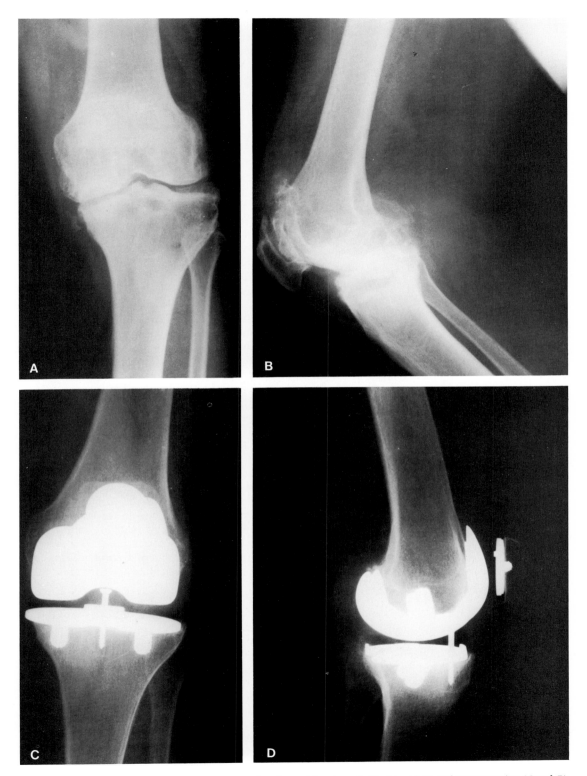

FIG. 31-18.   Preoperative x-rays of patient with osteoarthritis (*A* and *B*) and postoperative (*C* and *D*) views of a porous-coated noncemented total knee arthroplasty in a 62-year-old active woman.

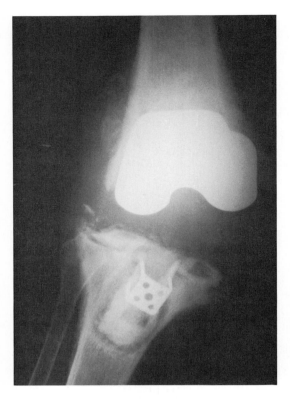

FIG. 31-19. Loose septic total knee replacement (note radiolucency about tibial component) requiring revision surgery. Also note gross instability.

syphilitic. However, it is now known to occur in other conditions as well. Syringomyelia, paraplegia, myelitis, various peripheral nerve lesions, diabetes, leprosy, congenital indifference to pain, and corticosteroid medications have all been incriminated. In *tabes dorsalis*, the joints most frequently affected are the knee, foot and ankle, hip, and spine (Fig. 31-21). In diabetes, the foot and ankle are the primary sites involved (Fig. 31-22). In syringomyelia, involvement is most commonly seen in the upper extremity. Confusion still exists regarding the pathogenesis and treatment of neuropathic disease. It may present a varied clinical picture of rapid or insidious onset.

The introduction of injectable and systemic corticosteroid preparations now being used widely and frequently in the elderly has produced Charcotlike lesions. The mode of action of corticosteroids locally is still not known, but they appear to produce anti-inflammatory effects after absorption into the cells of the synovial lining. This is manifested by a decrease in swelling and by tenderness and local pain. The degree of response varies

greatly, as does the duration of effect. Mankin and Conger[62] have shown experimentally that intra-articular cortisone affects glycine utilization by the articular cartilage cell, and its duration depends on the dose. Repeated intra-articular injection of hydrocortisone in a given joint over a long period may have a deleterious effect on the articular cartilage, not only in the rabbit but also in humans. A neuropathic joint may develop because the lack of pain results in increased trauma to an already damaged articular cartilage. The incidence of neuropathic articular cartilage destruction remains small when the large amount of corticosteroid medication given both systemically and intra-articularly is considered.

Obviously, the best treatment is prevention. Early recognition is of major importance. The early signs of mild swelling, local heat, and early instability or deformity must be critically evaluated. Treatment in this stage often enables repair to take place. Adequate protection should be used until all inflammatory and reactive signs have subsided. This may require prolonged periods of rest and immobilization. Because the patient does not experience normal pain, the clinical findings must be carefully evaluated before the patient resumes activities.

If the joint is seen when destruction is total, arthrodesis may be the procedure of choice. The knee is far more amenable to arthrodesing procedures than is the hip. It is extremely difficult to obtain an arthrodesis of the hip, but with better fixation devices and techniques, limited success has been reported. Also, the elderly do not tolerate the prolonged immobilizaiton so often necessary. In most cases, surgery should be performed after the acute phase of the neuropathic joint has subsided; local findings should be at a minimum. Bracing may be an adjunct to surgery or an alternative that provides stability and protection to the joint.

The complication rate following surgery is higher than in similar procedures carried out on nonneuropathic lesions. Infections are very serious, often necessitating amputation. Failure of arthrodesis is frequently encountered. Surprisingly, neuropathic hips may be relatively stable, even when grossly dislocated; and patients are often able to ambulate without significant difficulty, especially if other joints in the lower extremity are not involved. Total joint replacement in patients with neuropathic joints have been performed in small numbers with uncertain long-term results. There is a significantly higher percentage of complications with any surgery of a neuropathic joint.

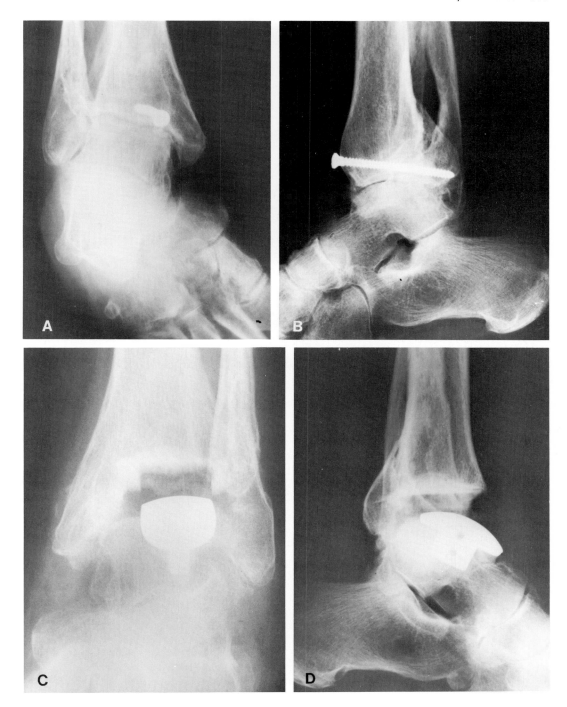

FIG. 31-20. (*A* and *B*) Roentgenograms of the knee of a 66-year-old woman with painful posttraumatic arthritis following open reduction of a fracture. (*C* and *D*) Postoperative views showing conversion to total ankle replacement.

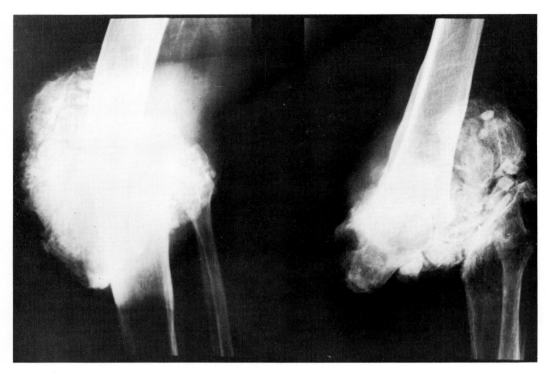

FIG. 31-21. Anteroposterior and lateral roentgenograms of a full-blown neuropathic joint secondary to luetic disease in a 61-year-old man. He had marked swelling and instability without pain. Note marked fragmentation and osseous metaplasia.

Some good results have been reported, but one should weigh the risks of any joint replacement very carefully in this group of patients.

The neuropathic joint associated with diabetes mellitus is now a well-recognized entity and is being seen more frequently. The tarsal and metatarsal joints are most frequently involved; next in decreasing frequency are the ankle joint, knee, hip, and spine. Treatment in a diabetic must be undertaken with considerable caution. On occasion, the neuropathic status of a foot first brings the patient to the physician's attention, and evaluation discloses the diabetic status. Increased infection follows surgical procedures on neuropathic joints, and prolonged drainage may ensue. In some diabetic patients, nonsurgical treatment is feasible, especially when the foot and ankle are in good alignment. Prevention of trophic ulcers of the skin and secondary osteomyelitis is vital.

METASTATIC CARCINOMA TO THE SKELETON

In the lower extremity, the femur is the most frequent bone involved in metastatic disease. Metas-

tases distal to the knee joint are rare. Pain may be present for some time before roentgenographic changes are visible. Pathologic fractures through metastatic lesions are not infrequent. It is unusual for metastatic disease in a weight-bearing bone to be symptomless. In many instances, vague, aching pain, frequently attributed to arthritis, has been present for weeks or months before roentgenographic changes reveal the metastatic disease. A bone scan may be very helpful in a suspected metastatic lesion when roentgenograms are interpreted as negative or inconclusive.

When pathologic fractures occur through metastatic lesions, internal fixation of the fracture has the following advantages: to decrease prolonged confinement to bed with all its subsequent complications, to reduce pain, to enable earlier and easier definitive care, such as radiation therapy, to ease nursing care, to make the patient ambulatory earlier, to avoid external immobilization, and to give the patient greater mobility in his remaining life span. In addition, at the time of internal fixation, tissue may be obtained for histologic interpretation, especially if a positive diagnosis has not been made as to the primary site.

Internal fixation for impending fractures about

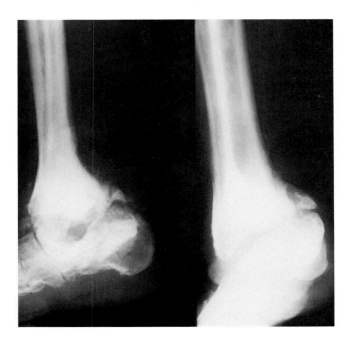

FIG. 31-22. Severe bony changes at the ankle of a 71-year-old woman with diabetic neuropathy.

the femur offers a satisfactory treatment for the patient with metastatic disease (Fig. 31-23). Prophylactic surgery, especially about the hip, has enabled the patient to remain ambulatory when fracture seemed imminent. Postirradiation fractures of the femoral neck are not uncommon.[32]

Primary prosthetic replacement is advocated for gross metastatic disease involving the femoral neck or head. Methylmethacrylate (bone cement) has

added a new dimension in treating pathologic fractures in metastatic disease. In over 500 patients with surgically treated pathologic fractures at my institution, those in whom methylmethacrylate was used as an adjunct to internal fixation had a higher incidence of pain relief, ambulation, and survival when compared with a comparable group in whom internal fixation was used without bone cement.[41] With the adjuvant use of methylme-

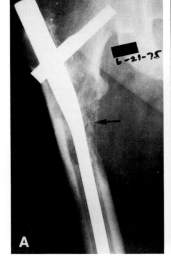
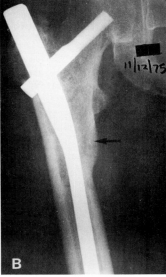

FIG. 31-23. (*A*) A large destructive pathologic lesion from breast metastases with impending fracture in subtrochanteric region in a 68-year-old woman stabilized with a Zickel intramedullary nail (6/21/75). (*B*) Appearance 4½ months post nailing and irradiation. Note healing; patient had been ambulatory without pain and received radiation as an outpatient.

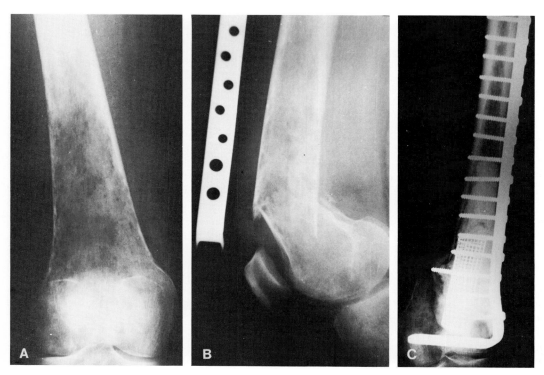

FIG. 31-24. (*A*) A large destructive lytic lesion secondary to breast metastases to distal femur. (*B*) A pathologic fracture as seen on lateral roentgenogram. (*C*) Internal fixation with condylar plate and the adjuvant use of methylmethacrylate (bone cement) and wire mesh to reinforce area of destroyed bone. Patient remained ambulatory.

thacrylate, one can reconstruct the severely destroyed skeleton, maintain ambulation, and gain relief of pain until the terminal event (Fig. 31-24).[40,41,43–45,79]

EMBOLIC PHENOMENA FOLLOWING INJURY OR SURGERY

Pulmonary embolism is of major importance in both management and diagnosis in the aging patient following a fracture of a long bone or surgery involving the lower extremity. Careful postmortem examination reveals pulmonary embolism in more than 25% of these patients.[28]

Anticoagulant therapy has been advocated in the elderly orthopaedic patient, especially after hip fractures or trauma of the lower extremity. Salzman and associates,[75] in 1966, demonstrated a definite decrease in pulmonary embolism in elderly patients with hip fractures following anticoagulant therapy. Investigators have emphasized that in most instances in which pulmonary embolization occurred patients did not manifest phle-

bitis clinically. Harris and co-workers,[46] in a controlled study of elective hip surgery, showed there was a decrease in venous thrombosis and pulmonary embolization following anticoagulation. A study by Fitts and colleagues[28] of 161 patients with fractures of the hip on whom autopsies were performed revealed death due to pulmonary embolization in 38% of these cases.

At my institution some form of anticoagulation has routinely been used in patients with hip fractures, with total hip or knee replacements, and in traction for fractures. This has ranged from aspirin to full heparinization.

Fat embolism is an important cause of morbidity and mortality in patients with fractures. How frequently it occurs is uncertain. Fat embolism may go unrecognized and may be attributed to other causes, especially in the elderly. Fuchsig and co-workers[30] found that fat embolism was the principal cause of death in more than 5% of patients dying as a result of trauma, and in more than 10% it was a secondary cause.

There are many controversies regarding the pathogenesis of fat embolization and the relationship between shock and fat embolism. Pulmonary arterioles and capillaries are plugged, with a subsequent increase in pulmonary resistance and impairment of the gaseous exchange. Severe involvement may cause the patient to die in a short time from left-sided heart failure and hypoxia. However, the body usually copes with this situation and survival is more common.

The diagnosis of fat embolism rests on the degree of suspicion the clinician has in the presence of a history of trauma, dyspnea, tachycardia, fever, and mental and pulmonary deterioration. Petechiae, rapidly dropping hematocrit, urinary and sputum fat, elevated lipid level, and radiographic changes in the chest film substantiate the diagnosis. Symptoms and findings usually appear 24 to 72 hours following injury. The effectiveness of a given treatment is difficult to assess because of the variability of the clinical course. Treatment has included corticosteroids, heparin, alcohol, and low molecular weight dextran. It has been difficult to evaluate these methods of treatment.

The effect of corticosteroids in the treatment of respiratory failure associated with massive fat embolism was ascribed by Ashbaugh and Petty[4] to protection of the endothelium from the free fatty acids and inhibition of local edema and hemorrhage. The effect of heparin has been ascribed to its lipolytic action. Low molecular weight dextran has been thought to act as a dislodging agent and a plasma expander. Alcohol decreases the rate of hydrolysis of neutral fat by lipase, thereby delaying the release of toxic fatty acids. General supportive measures are used in addition to the agents described.

SUDECK'S ATROPHY

Sudeck's atrophy[84] in the lower extremity chiefly involves the ankle and foot. It may follow minimal trauma to the lower extremity and is not infrequently seen following a fracture, incomplete nerve injury, or ligamentous injuries, especially in the region of the ankle. Changes are the result of vasospasm of the terminal arterioles. The picture usually includes swelling, edema, tenderness, glossy and cyanotic skin, and limitation of motion of the affected part.

Pain may be a prominent and persistent feature with complaints of burning and paresthesia. Pain on movement produces a foot or ankle with significantly restricted motion. Radiographically, spotty osteoporosis is seen distal to the site of injury, and the remaining portion of the bone appears relatively uninvolved. Treatment of Sudeck's atrophy includes encouragement of active exercises of the extremity and symptomatic treatment. If pain is severe and persistent and the patient cannot tolerate active exercise, sympathectomy may offer rapid relief.

REHABILITATION OF THE ORTHOPAEDIC PATIENT

Rehabilitating the aged orthopaedic patient presents numerous problems. Treatment often depends on the patient's ability to cooperate in a rehabilitation program within his tolerance. Prolonged immobilization and bed rest present additional problems such as contractures, muscle weakness, decubiti, and concurrent problems arising in the respiratory, urogenital, and gastrointestinal systems. The prevention of complications is of major concern to the physician. Positioning and adequate nursing care can often prevent contractures and decubiti. Muscle-strengthening programs should be instituted prior to surgery, if possible, so that the patient knows what to expect in his postsurgical course. The maintenance of muscle action and joint function is mandatory, not only to achieve a good end result, but also to correct deformities owing to immobilization and faulty positioning.

Return to an ambulatory status with preservation of function is the goal of orthopaedic treatment. In the past, criteria used in gait training of the handicapped patient were based primarily on cosmetic patterns, and there was a tendency to avoid the use of external devices. Recent studies underline the need for using devices that are economical regarding energy expenditure, even at some sacrifice of the cosmetic aspect of the gait pattern. Considerations of energy expenditure are also critically important in determining the physical therapy and occupational therapy techniques to be used in rehabilitation.

Bard and Ralston[5] have studied energy expenditure and have shown that crutch walking is very costly compared with walking with other assistive devices, such as a walker. Crutches may be hazardous because of the excessive work burdens imposed on the patient. Forearm crutches increase the energy expenditure compared with that needed to use other assistive devices. Careful evaluation of each patient before prescribing a form of external support is necessary. The walker has been very effective in rehabilitating patients with hip fractures. In addition, simply giving the patient a cane may often reduce the amount of energy expended in ambulation to a level within his tolerance, when without it, dyspnea may occur.

The importance of an early and adequate rehabilitation program cannot be overemphasized. Without it, the aged patient may be unable to return to the status that existed before his orthopaedic disability.

REFERENCES

1. Ahlback S, Bauer GCH, Bohne WH: Spontaneous osteonecrosis of the knee. Arthritis Rheum 11:705, 1968
2. Ahuja SC, Bullough PG: Osteonecrosis of the knee: A clinicopathological study in twenty-eight patients. J Bone Joint Surg 60A:191, 1978
3. Amstutz HC, Markolf KL, McNeice GM, Gruen TA: Loosening of total hip components: Cause and prevention. In: The Hip: Proceedings of the Fourth Open Scientific Meeting of The Hip Society, pp 102–116. St. Louis, CV Mosby, 1976
4. Ashbaugh DG, Petty TL: The use of corticosteroids in the treatment of respiratory failure associated with massive fat embolism. Surg Gynecol Obstet 123:493, 1966
5. Bard G, Ralston JH: Measurement of energy expenditure during ambulation with special reference to evaluation of assistive devices. Arch Phys Med Rehabil 40:415, 1959
6. Barnes R, Brown JT, Garden RS, Nicoll EA: Subcapital fractures of the femur: A prospective review. J Bone Joint Surg [Br] 58:1, 1976
7. Bassett CAC, Pawluk RJ, Pilla AA: Acceleration of fracture repair by electromagnetic fields. Ann NY Acad Sci 238:242, 1975
8. Bassett CAL: Pulsing electromagnetic fields: a new approach to surgical problems. In Buchwald H, Varco RL (eds): Metabolic Surgery, pp 255–306. New York, Grune & Stratton, 1978
9. Bassett CAL, Valdes HG, Hernandez E: Modification of fracture repair with selected pulsing electromagnetic fields. J Bone Joint Surg 64A:888–895, 1982
10. Breckenbaugh RD, Ilstrup DM: Total hip arthroplasty: A review of three hundred and thirty three cases with long follow-up. J Bone Joint Surg [Am] 60:306, 1978
11. Benjamin A: Double osteotomy of the knee. J Bone Joint Surg [Br] 49:795, 1967
12. Black J, Brighton CT: Mechanisms of stimulation of osteogenesis by direct current. In Brighton CT, Black J, Pollack SR (eds): Electrical Properties of Bone and Cartilage, p 215. New York, Grune & Stratton, 1979
13. Brighton CT, Friedenberg ZB, Black J: Evaluation of the use of constant direct current in the treatment of nonunion. In Brighton CT, Black J, Pollack SR (eds): Electrical Properties of Bone and Cartilage, p 519. New York, Grune & Stratton, 1979
14. Brown A, D'Arcy JC: Internal fixation for supracondylar fractures of the femur in the elderly patient. J Bone Joint Surg [Br] 53:420, 1976
15. Charnley J: The long-term results of low friction arthroplasty of the hip performed as a primary intervention. J Bone Joint Surg 54B:61, 1972
16. Charnley J: Low Friction Arthroplasty of the Hip: Theory and Practice. New York, Springer-Verlag, 1979
17. Charnley J: Fracture of femoral prostheses in total hip replacement: A clinical study. Clin Orthop 111:105, 1975
18. Connolly JF, Dehne E, Lafollette B: Closed reduction and early cast brace ambulation in the treatment of femoral fractures: II. Results in one hundred and forty-three fractures. J Bone Joint Surg [Am] 55:1518, 1973
19. Connolly JF, King P: Closed reduction and early cast brace ambulation in the treatment of femoral fractures: I. An *in vivo* quantitative analysis of immobilization in skeletal traction and a cast brace. J Bone Joint Surg [Am] 55:1559, 1973
20. Coventry MB: Osteotomy about the knee for degenerative and rheumatoid arthritis. J Bone Joint Surg [Am] 55:23, 1973
21. Coventry MB, Beckenbaugh RD, Nolan DR, Ilstrup DM: 2,012 total hip arthroplasties: A study of postoperative course and early complications. J Bone Joint Surg [Am] 56:273, 1974
22. Crawford HB: Conservative treatment of impacted fractures of the femoral neck: A report of fifty cases. J Bone Joint Surg [Am] 42:471, 1960
23. Dehne E: Ambulatory treatment of the fractured tibia. Clin Orthop 105:192, 1974
24. Dimon JH III, Hughston JC: Unstable intertrochanteric fractures of the hip. J Bone Joint Surg [Am] 49:440, 1967
25. Evanski PM, Waugh TR: Management of arthritis of the ankle. An alternative to arthrodesis. Clin Orthop 122:110, 1977
26. Feinstein PA, Habermann ET: Selecting and preparing patients for total hip replacement. Geriatrics 32(7):91, 1977
27. Fielding JW, Wilson SA, Ratzan S: A continuing end-result study of displaced intracapsular fractures of the neck of the femur treated with the Pugh nail. J Bone Joint Surg [Am] 56:1464, 1974
28. Fitts WJ, Lehr HB, Bitner RL, Spelman JW: Analysis of nine hundred and fifty fatal injuries. Surgery 56:663, 1964
29. Friedenberg ZB, Andrews ET, Smolenski BI, Pearl BW, Brighton CT: Bone reaction to varying amounts of direct current. Surg Gynecol Obstet 113:894, 1970
30. Fuchsig P, Briick P, Bliimel G, Gottlob R: A new clinical and experimental concept on fat embolism. N Engl J Med 276:1192, 1967
31. Goldring SR, Schiller AL, Roelke M et al: The synovial-like membrane at the bone-cement interface in loose total hip replacements and its proposed role in bone lysis. J Bone Joint Surg [Am] 65:575, 1983

32. Goodman AH, Sherman MS: Post-irradiation fractures of the femoral neck. J Bone Joint Surg [Am] 45:723, 1963

33. Graber-Duvernay J: L'Aspect clinique des arthritis chroniques de la tranche d'origine consenitale. Rev Rhum Mal Osteoartic 5:304, 1938

34. Gunston FH: Polycentric knee arthroplasty: Prosthetic simulation of normal knee movement. J Bone Joint Surg [Br] 53:272, 1971

35. Habermann ET: Management of intertrochanteric fractures. Contemp Surg 7:35, 1975

36. Habermann ET, Anderson RL Jr, Greenberg BB: Unpublished data

37. Habermann ET, Feinstein PA: Total hip replacement arthroplasty in arthritic conditions of the hip joint. Semin Arthritis Rheum 7:189, 1978

38. Habermann ET, Greenberg BB, Anderson RL Jr: Treatment of 1,000 consecutive hip fractures by the use of the sliding nail-variable angle plate method. J Bone Joint Surg [Am] 57:1022, 1975

39. Habermann ET, Hartzband MA: Spontaneous Osteonecrosis of the knee. In Arlet J, Ficat P, Hungerford D (eds): Bone Circulation, pp 274–285. Baltimore, Williams & Wilkins, 1984

40. Habermann ET, Sachs R, Stern R, Hirsch D, Anderson W: A comparative review of the treatment of pathological fractures of long bones with and without the use of methylmethacrylate. Read at the annual meeting of the American Academy of Orthopaedic Surgeons, Dallas, 1978

41. Habermann ET, Sachs R, Stern R, Hirsh D, Anderson W: The pathology and treatment of metastatic disease of the femur. Clin Orthop Rel Res 169:70, 1982

42. Harrington KD: The use of methylmethacrylate as an adjunct in the internal fixation of unstable comminuted intertrochanteric fractures in osteoporotic patients. J Bone Joint Surg [Am] 57:744, 1975

43. Harrington KD: New trends in the management of lower extremity metastasis. Clin Orthop Rel Res 169:53, 1982

44. Harrington KD et al: Methylmethacrylate as an adjunct in internal fixation of pathological fractures: Experience with three hundred and seventy-five cases. J Bone Joint Surg [Am] 58:1047, 1976

45. Harrington KD, Johnston JO, Turner RH: The use of methylmethacrylate as an adjunct in the internal fixation of malignant neoplastic fractures. J Bone Joint Surg [Am] 54:1665, 1972

46. Harris WH, Salzman EW, DeSanctis RW: The prevention of thromboembolic disease by prophylactic anticoagulation: A controlled study in elective hip surgery. J Bone Joint Surg [Am] 47:81, 1967

47. Harris WH, Schiller Al, Schöller JM et al: Extensive localized bone resorption in the femur following total hip replacement. J Bone Joint Surg [Am] 58:612, 1976

48. Hedley AK, Clarke IC, Kozinn SC et al: Porous ingrowth fixation of the femoral component in a canine surface replacement of the hip. Clin Orthop 163:82, 300, 1900

49. Helfet AJ: Osteochondral fractures of the articular surfaces of the knee. In Milgran JE (ed): The Management of Internal Derangements of the Knee. Philadephia, JB Lippincott, 1963

50. Hungerford DS, Krackow KA, Kenna RV: Preliminary experience with the porous coated anatomic total knee replacement with and without cement. Orthop Clin North Am 13:103, 1982

51. Hungerford DS, Kenna RV, Krackow KA: The porous-coated anatomic total knee. Orthop Clin North Am 13:103, 1982

52. Hungerford D, Hedley A, Habermann E, Borden L, Kenna R: Total Hip Arthroplasty: A New Approach. Baltimore, University Park Press, 1984

53. Insall J, Shoji H, Mayer V: High tibial osteotomy: A five year evaluation. J Bone Joint Surg [Am] 56:1397, 1974

54. Insall JN, Ranawat CS, Aglietti P, Shine J: A comparison of four models of total knee replacement prostheses. J Bone Joint Surg [Am] 58:754, 1976

55. Jennings JJ, Harris WH, Sarmiento A: A clinical evaluation of aspirin prophylaxis of thromboembolic disease after total hip arthroplasty. J Bone Joint Surg [Am] 58:926, 1976

56. Johnson EW, Boseker EH: Arthrodesis of the ankle. Arth Surg 97:766, 1968

57. Korvald E et al: Examination of the vascular disturbance of the femoral head following intracapsular fracture of the hip: A preliminary report using a new isotope complex. Acta Orthop Scand 45:572, 1974

58. Koshino T: The treatment of spontaneous osteonecrosis of the knee by high tibial osteotomy with and without bone grafting or drilling of the lesion. J Bone Joint Surg [Am] 64:47, 1982

59. Lance EM, Pavel A, Patterson RL Jr, Fries L, Larsen IJ: Arthrodesis of the ankle: A follow-up study. J Bone Joint Surg [Am] 53:1030, 1971

60. Laskin RS: Modular total knee replacement arthroplasty: A review of eighty-nine patients. J Bone Joint Surg [Am] 58:766, 1976

61. Lotke PA, Ecker ML, Alavi A: Painful knees in older patients: Radionucleotide diagnosis of possible osteonecrosis with spontaneous resolution. J Bone Joint Surg [Am] 59:617, 1977

62. Mankin HJ, Conger KA: The acute effects of intra-articular hydrocortisone on articular cartilage in rabbits. J Bone Joint Surg [Am] 48:1383, 1966

63. Massie WK: Treatment of femoral neck fractures emphasizing long term follow-up observation on aseptic necrosis. Clin Orthop 92:16, 1973

64. Mooney V, Nickel VL, Harvey JP Jr, Snelson R: Cast-brace treatment for fractures of the distal part of the femur. J Bone Joint Surg [Am] 52:1563, 1970

65. Neimann K, Mankin H: Fractures about the hip in an institutionalized patient population. J Bone Joint Surg [Am] 50:1073, 1968

66. Norman A, Baker N: Spontaneous osteonecrosis of the knee and medial meniscus tears. Radiology 3:653, 1978

67. Paterson D, Lewis GN, Cass CA: Treatment of delayed union and nonunion with an implanted di-

rect current stimulator. Clin Orthop 148:117, 1980

68. Reckling FW, Asher MA, Dillon WL: A longitudinal study of the radiolucent line at the bone–cement interface following total joint replacement procedures. J Bone Joint Surg [Am] 59:355, 1977

69. Riley LH: The evolution of total knee arthroplasty. Clin Orthop 120:7, 1976

70. Rozing PM, Insall J, Bohne WH: Spontaneous osteonecrosis of the knee. J Bone Joint Surg [Am] 62:2, 1980

71. Salter RB, Field P: The effects of continuous compression on living articular cartilage. J Bone Joint Surg [Am] 42:31, 1969

72. Salvati EA, Im VC, Aglietti P, Wilson PD Jr: Radiology of total hip replacements. Clin Orthop 121:74, 1976

73. Salvati EA, Lachiewicz P: Thromboembolism following total hip replacement arthroplasty: The efficacy of Dextran-Aspirin and Dextran-Warfarin prophylaxis. J Bone Joint Surg [Am] 58:921, 1976

74. Salzman EW, Harris WH: Prevention of venous thromboembolism in orthopaedic patients. J Bone Joint Surg [Am] 58:903, 1976

75. Salzman EW, Harris WH, DeSanctis RW: Anticoagulation for prevention of thrombo-embolism following fractures of the hip. N Engl J Med 275:122, 1966

76. Sarmiento A: A functional below the knee cast for tibial fractures. J Bone Joint Surg [Am] 49:855, 1967

77. Sharnoff JG, Rosen RL, Sadler AH, Ibarra-Isunza GC: Prevention of fatal pulmonary thromboembolism by heparin prophylaxis after surgery for hip fractures. J Bone Joint Surg [Am] 58:913, 1976

78. Shoji H, Koshino T, Doherty JH: 85 Sr scintimetry of intracapsular fracture of the hip: A preliminary report. Clin Orthop Rel Res 86:85, 1972

79. Sim FH, Daugherty TW, Ivins JC: The adjunctive use of methylmethacrylate in fixation of pathological fractures. J Bone Joint Surg [Am] 56:40, 1974.

80. Skolnick MD, Bryan RS, Peterson LF, Combs JJ, Ilstrup DM: Polycentric total knee arthroplasty: A two year follow-up study. J Bone Joint Surg, [Am] 58:743, 1976

81. Skolnick MD, Coventry MB, Ilstrup DM: Geometric total knee arthroplasty: A two year follow-up study. J Bone Joint Surg, [Am] 58:749, 1976

82. Stauffer RN: Ten year follow-up study of total hip replacement. J Bone Joint Surg [Am] 64:983, 1982

83. Stecher RM: Osteoarthritis and old age. Geriatrics 16:167, 1961

84. Sudeck P: Ueber die akute (reflektorische) Knockenatrophie nach Entzundungen und Verletzungen an den Extremitäten und ihre klinischen Erscheinungen. Fortschr Geb Röntgenstrahl 5:277, 1901–1902

85. Trueta J, Harrison MHM: Normal vascular anatomy of the femoral head in adult man. J Bone Joint Surg [Br] 35:442, 1953

86. Wroblewski BM: Fractured stem in total hip replacement. Acta Orthop Scand 53:279, 1982

87. Zickel RE: A new fixation device for subtrochanteric fractures of the femur. Clin Orthop 54:115, 1967

88. Zickel RE: An intramedullary fixation device for the proximal part of the femur: Nine years' experience. J Bone Joint Surg [Am] 58:866, 1976

32 Geriatric Aspects of the Foot and Ankle

Melvin Howard Jahss

Of the entire musculoskeletal system the foot is perhaps foremost in showing the ravages of time, abetted by the static stresses imposed by weight bearing and shoes. Longstanding deformities, whether congenital (clubfoot, splayfeet) or acquired (poliomyelitis, trauma), are often at first flexible and asymptomatic but gradually become fixed and rigid. Painful exostoses, calluses, and degenerative changes ultimately develop. After the patient passes middle age, prophylaxis and nonsurgical attempts at correction are no longer indicated because the deformities are already fixed. With further aging and the superimposition of arterial or arteriolar insufficiency, even simple surgical correction may be contraindicated. Treatment becomes palliative, falling into the realm of mechanotherapy: special shoes, shoe corrections, protective paddings, or arch supports.

Some of the most common causes of late foot pain and deformity are due to seemingly innocuous normal variants. A typical example is splayfoot, which basically is a wide forefoot in relation to the heel. Often it is made even wider by an abnormal deviation of the first metatarsal from the second, known as metatarsus primus varus. In childhood, splayfoot goes unnoticed because childrens' shoes normally allow plenty of room for the forefoot. Later, however, especially in women, the commercial shoe is much too narrow and pointed about the forefoot. High heels further jam the forefoot into the narrow toebox. The result is that the toes are forced together. Bunions develop over the medial aspect of the first metatarsal head and over the lateral aspects of the fifth metatarsal head (bunionette, tailor's bunion). Continued pressure against the hallux forces it laterally, thereby creating a hallux valgus deformity. As this deformity increases, the base of the proximal phalanx of the hallux no longer normally articulates

with the head of the first metatarsal, and secondary osteoarthritic changes develop in this joint. The hallux ultimately pushes under and crowds out the second toe, which is displaced dorsally. Hammertoe deformity develops, with a tender dorsal callus from shoe pressure.

THE BLOOD SUPPLY

One of the most serious effects of senescence on the foot is its loss of blood supply. At best, the blood supply to the skin of the foot is not overabundant. Any extensive surgical undermining of skin is prone to slough. Prolonged pressure from an ill-fitting cast, leg traction, or a mattress rapidly results in a chronic ulcer that heals poorly or with painful scar formation. The senile, postoperative, comatose, or bedridden patient is especially prone to develop pressure sores in the avascular skin over the posterior aspect of the heel. Prophylactic treatment consists of the use of massive padding of both feet with sheet wadding or thick sponge rubber.

It must be presumed that there is significant vascular impairment of the foot from arteriosclerosis in patients over 65 years of age and from small vessel disease in younger diabetics. Small vessel disease is present in diabetics even in the presence of palpable dorsalis pedis and posterior tibial arteries. A slight skin crack or infection in such patients is to be considered a medical emergency often requiring immediate hospitalization. Not infrequently an unusually painful plantar callus in a diabetic overlies a deep, necrotic underlying ulcer. Conversely, a perforating foot ulcer in a relatively young person is to be considered diabetic or neurotrophic until proven otherwise.

It must be stressed that with advanced arterial

567

insufficiency, minor trauma, a surgical procedure, or even the application of a relatively strong keratolytic agent such as salicylic acid may precipitate local edema, slough, infection, and gangrene.

In the elderly foot, the skin becomes more atrophic and delicate and it does not readily tolerate adhesive tape. Pressure ulcers develop easily over or under calluses. Not uncommonly, one finds a painful soft corn between two rigid toes that are abnormally pressed together. When the vascular supply of the foot is impaired, the calluses may break down, forming ulcers with incipient gangrene of the adjacent toes.

The subcutaneous tissue of the foot is normally sparse, except for the plantar fat pad. This pad acts as a resilient buffer against the constant pounding of the metatarsal heads and the os calcis against the ground. The fat pad atrophies in the elderly and at earlier ages in those patients with rheumatoid arthritis of the foot. Painful calluses then develop under the metatarsal heads, which become palpable superficially. Atrophy of the heel pad may cause pain under the os calcis.

THE JOINTS

In comparison to the hip and knee, the joints of the foot and ankle develop little evidence of painful osteoarthritis with advancing age. The ankle, especially in obese women, develops general synovial thickening, differentiated from ankle edema by its lack of pitting. The symptoms are relatively mild. Painful osteoarthritis of the ankle does develop following old intra-articular fractures about the ankle. The subtalar joint gradually stiffens with age, and narrowing of the components of the subtalar complex may be seen radiographically. Joint limitation is usually unnoticed by the patient and is not particularly symptomatic. More frequently, the midtarsal joints develop osteoarthritic changes that may be palpated as multiple small bony dorsal exostoses over the midtarsus. Symptoms are frequently mild.

The bones of the foot are not particularly affected by senescence from a clinical viewpoint. Symptomatic osteoporosis, as it occurs in the spine, is not a clinical entity.

SYSTEMIC DISEASES

Systemic disease often attacks the foot, the most frequent (besides diabetes) being gout and rheumatoid arthritis. Frequently the foot is the only area involved. In the aged, especially men, the presence of hallux rigidus is highly indicative of gout, even without a history of acute attacks. Rheumatoid arthritis, as seen in the elderly, is usually burned out. It may present itself as pain under the plantar aspect of the heels or metatarsals, painful spastic subtalar joints, or by multiple toe deformities. Radiographs and laboratory tests are not always diagnostic.

CONSERVATIVE THERAPY VERSUS SURGERY

Many chronic disabilities are readily remediable by simple surgical procedures, thereby eliminating the need for special footwear and chronic podiatric therapy. On the other hand, many patients do not desire surgery, or surgery is contraindicated for various reasons in the aged. Most foot surgery is elective, and alternatives are invariably available. Local vascular insufficiency is a surgical contraindication. Inadvisable surgery resulting in delayed healing, slough, infection, scar formation, secondary contractures, and joint stiffness often causes irremediable permanent painful disability. There are patients in whom major surgery is necessary despite a questionable blood supply. A vascular surgeon should then determine if preliminary sympathectomy or vascular surgery would decrease the hazards of the anticipated foot surgery.

Difficult problems of evaluation and surgical judgment are posed by chronic toe or foot ulcers associated with vascular insufficiency. The decision often involves judgment as to whether to institute chronic conservative care with prolonged bed rest or to do simple definitive amputations—for example, of an ulcerated toe. Unfortunately even this relatively minor surgical procedure may lead to progressive gangrene with amputation at a much higher level.

Plastic surgery may be even more vexing, especially in the aged. Many tender scars and areas of skin loss may be adequately managed by means of special shoes and soft rubber innersoles, but repeated skin breakdown is one indication for plastic surgery. However, in areas of weight bearing or shoe friction, simple split grafts readily break down. Also, rotation flaps about the foot slough, and cross-leg pedicle flaps are usually contraindicated in patients over age 45 because of joint stiffness secondary to the immobilization. Such problems are often insurmountable but should be given the benefit of combined orthopaedic, vascular, and plastic surgical experience.

CONSERVATIVE OFFICE FOOT CARE

The most frequently seen minor foot conditions consist of fungal infections of the skin and nails, hypertrophied and ingrown toenails, hard and soft corns, and minor sprains and fractures. Overtreatment should be avoided, especially for minor trauma. A fractured toe at most needs a simple strapping with tape for 2 weeks plus a wide or cut-out toe box. A fractured metatarsal usually requires only midtarsal strapping for 2 to 3 weeks. Prolonged plaster immobilization may lead to a stiff, painful, or edematous foot and ankle, and even Sudeck's atrophy or a causalgialike state. When the local circulation is poor as in diabetes, use of adhesive tape and plaster should be avoided to prevent skin breakdown. An Unna boot is preferable, especially in ankle sprains. Unless one takes immediate roentgenograms for ankle "sprains," unsuspected fractures and fracture dislocations may be overlooked. Swelling from the "sprain" and the "heavy" ankles found in the elderly owing to pitting edema or synovitis often makes palpation difficult, obscuring bony deformity.

Even though temporary relief may be obtained by removing soft corns and calluses, concomitant paddings or shoe corrections prevent rapid recurrence. In certain cases, permanent relief may be obtained by simple surgical procedures.

The physician must advise his patients in great detail regarding foot care, especially if there is vascular impairment. A mimeographed set of orders is preferable. It should include items on foot hygiene, avoidance of extremes of temperature (such as hot Epsom salt soaks), avoidance of constricting garters, proper stocking and shoe wear, proper trimming of calluses and toenails, and the need for immediate medical attention with the earliest signs of infection, bleb formation, ulceration, or necrosis.

Local anesthetic agents or intra-articular injection of cortisone is often of temporary and even permanent value. Injection into a small area such as a small joint (toe, tarsal joint), tendon sheath, or bursa requires only 0.25 ml of local anesthetic combined with 0.25 ml of injectable cortisone. Patients should be forewarned that there may be a temporary increase in pain for 24 hours. The most commonly involved small joint is the metatarsophalangeal joint of the second toe, which developes a painful synovitis secondary to pressure from a hallux valgus deformity. Larger joints such as the subtalar and ankle joints require double the dosage mentioned previously. Painful tenosyno-

vitis is very common, occurring in order of frequency in the tibialis posterior, flexor hallucis longus, and Achilles tendon. Injection into a deep bursa such as the retrocalcaneal bursa is occasionally indicated. Injection should not be made into superficial or inflamed bursas, because an infection or a draining sinus may result. Aspiration of superficial bursas is contraindicated for the same reasons. Cutting out the shoe over an inflamed or acutely tender superficial bursa for 6 to 8 weeks is much safer and is usually curative.

The most common type of office therapy is mechanotherapy, which encompasses the prescription of appropriate shoes, shoe corrections, arch supports, and, rarely, braces. Specific protective padding (shields) may be applied in the office and also may be ordered commercially. This padding consists of moleskin and adhesive backed piano felt or sponge rubber ranging from $\frac{1}{16}$ to $\frac{3}{16}$ of an inch in thickness. Plain felt or sponge rubber may also be used up to 1 inch in thickness. The felt or sponge rubber is cut out to form a protective shield just proximal to, or encircling, a painful exostosis or callus. A hammertoe or bunion is thus protected from abnormal shoe friction (Figs. 32-1 and 32-2). Thicker padding is used on the plantar aspect of the foot to relieve painful metatarsal calluses from excess weight bearing. The pad is positioned just proximal to the tender area. More permanent forms of relief consist of corrections permanently glued into the shoe or ordered as removable innersoles (arch supports), which can be changed from one shoe to another. Modern supports are lightweight, made of soft rubber, cork-rubber, or closed celled polyethylene foam and provide comfort by cushioning and by redistributing weight away from pathologic areas. This contrasts to older rigid steel arch supports, which were fruitlessly used to correct uncorrectable fixed deformities.

In severe foot deformities, custom-made shoes must be ordered. The shoe should incorporate removable arch supports. Arch supports must not be ordered after a shoe is obtained because their bulk invariably necessitates use of larger (wider) shoes. The shoe and arch support should, therefore, be ordered together. Similarly, shoes should not be ordered immediately postoperatively, when there is still residual edema. It must be remembered that a shoe one size wider is only $\frac{1}{4}$ inch greater in girth. In ordering an elastic stocking for leg or foot edema, the fitting should be done in the morning before the edema increases. Otherwise the stocking will be too loose.

The difference between success and failure in treatment comes from practical experience and

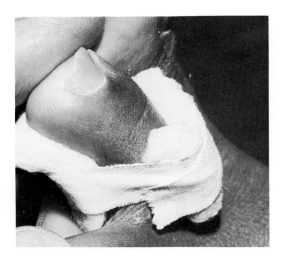

FIG. 32-1. Shield for flexible hammertoe deformity.

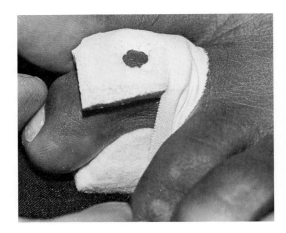

FIG. 32-2. Shield for rigid hammertoe deformity.

scholastic knowledge. Thus, hypersensitive patients are often unable to tolerate a simple metatarsal pad, whereas they benefit by an equivalent outside sole correction such as a Denver bar (heel). However, no type of shoe correction affords relief to a patient suffering from a plantar neuroma misdiagnosed as a metatarsalgia.

COMMON FOOT PROBLEMS

The two most common skin lesions in the aged are painful calluses due to underlying deformities coupled with static stresses and ulcers due to impaired vascular supply (especially in diabetics) or to underlying neurologic disease. Fungal infections, so prevalent in the young, are relatively infrequent in the aged. On the other hand, maceration of a fungal infection (especially interdigital) may lead to secondary infection and cellulitis, and it is of particular danger with impaired blood supply. Similarly, plantar warts are seen mainly in children or relatively young adults. However, warts that have been poorly treated with resultant painful scar formation are seen in the elderly. Rubber arch supports to relieve weight bearing may not be satisfactory; thus, excision of an underlying metatarsal head or excision with a rotation flap may be indicated, depending on the severity and location of the lesion. In general, plantar warts should not be excised because a painful plantar scar may be produced, often with recurrence of the wart in the scar. Irradiation of warts or other lesions is often followed years later by chronic disabling radiodermatitis. The primary

treatment of plantar warts consists of repeated applications of either salicylic acid ointment (50%), salicylic acid plaster, or trichloroacetic acid. If no response is obtained in 6 to 8 weeks, curettement is done. Recurrence is not uncommon.

The elderly are often unable to bend over to cut their toenails. The nails may be too hard and thick to cut, or failing eyesight may cause difficulty. The most common nail deformities are hypertrophy owing often to chronic fungus infection, onychogryposis (ram's-horn deformity), and ingrown toenails with or without secondary infection. In hypertrophy and deformity owing to fungus, detritus lifts the nail up, often as far as its matrix. The nail and underlying detritus should be clipped back as far as possible with heavy nail clippers. The thickened nail may also be ground down with a sanding disk, using a small electric drill. The same type of therapy is used for onychogryposis. Total removal of hypertrophied deformed nails usually results in recurrence of the deformity, owing to permanent damage of the nail bed. Destruction (excision) of the entire nail matrix along with removal of the nail is therefore the surgical method of choice.

For ingrown toenails, treatment depends on whether there is associated chronic nail matrix damage or secondary lateral nail-fold infection. Some may be treated by gently lifting the edge of the nail with a small piece of cotton. Nail packing may have to be continued for several months to effect a permanent cure. Packing along with antiseptic soaks may be used for infected ingrown toenails. If the nail edge is digging into the underlying nail fold, the edge should be removed with the use of local anesthesia. A wide, square toe box, open-toed shoes, or cutting out the shoe over the hallux relieves painful pressure from the shoe. If the condition becomes chronic or recurrent and is associated with permanent nail deformity, removal of the edge of the nail and its underlying matrix is necessary. If both sides of the nail fold are involved, the entire nail and nail matrix should be excised.

Hallux Valgus, Bunions, and Splayfeet

Hallux valgus, bunions, and splayfeet may all be surgically corrected in patients under 65 years of age with no local or systemic contraindications. Over the past year the upper age limit for surgery has been gradually extended and ankle blocks are replacing general anesthesia. In older patients and in diabetic patients, conservative treatment is the method of choice. In severe splaying and deformities, commercial shoes or even a bunion-last oxford is not satisfactory, and a custom-made shoe is necessary. If the foot spreads significantly on standing, the casts for the custom shoes should be made when the foot bears weight. Such shoes should be ordered with removable innersoles in order to make necessary plantar corrections. If there are tender anterior metatarsal calluses, the innersoles should be made of rubber, cork-rubber composition or polyethylene foam with wells (depressions) under the tender calluses and extra anterior metatarsal support proximal to the painful metatarsal heads.

In milder cases of hallux valgus and bunions, bunion-last orthopaedic oxfords may be ordered along with metatarsal pads if there are associated plantar metatarsal calluses. If hammertoe is present, a high toe box should also be ordered. If the patient is unable to tolerate the metatarsal pads, then Denver heels (metatarsal bars) may be substituted. Occasionally, for extra anterior metatarsal support, the metatarsal pads are combined with the Denver heels.

Removable protective bunion and hammertoe shields are available commercially, or a custom-made latex shield may be made.

Hallux Rigidus

Hallux rigidus results in limitation of motion of the metatarsophalangeal joint of the hallux. It may be associated with osteoarthritis and is also seen with gout. It may occur without a history of gouty attacks. If there is no pain, treatment is not necessary. In many cases, motion, especially walking, causes pain. By limiting motion at this joint, pain is relieved. This may be accomplished in women

by the use of rigid sole (*e.g.,* platform shoes). The simplest shoe correction is a ¼-inch sole rocker, which consists of a convex piece of leather tacked across the entire width of the outer sole with its maximum thickness under the metatarsophalangeal joints. This piece of leather prevents motion of the sole at the metatarsophalangeal joint level and, owing to the rocker shape, permits a smooth forward rolling of the foot during ambulation (Fig. 32-3).

Hammertoes

Hammertoes may be congenital or the result of any of several acquired disorders, including rheumatoid arthritis. Perhaps most common is the hammering of the second toe associated with hallux valgus.

As the toe becomes hammered, a painful dorsal callus develops over the dorsum of the proximal interphalangeal joint and occasionally under the pulp of the toe just below the end of the nail (end corn). At first the hammering is flexible and passively correctable, but it ultimately becomes rigid. Gradual dislocation at the metatarsophalangeal joint is frequent but not particularly painful.

Treatment may be conservative or surgical. In severe cases of hammering, a custom-made shoe is necessary; in others a high toe box will suffice. Hammertoe shields (protective pads) are constructed according to whether the hammering is flexible or rigid. The flexible pad consists of a thick half-moon piece of piano felt or sponge rubber placed just proximal to the dorsal corn. On the plantar surface, a plug of felt is placed under the middle phalanx with its proximal portion tapered to a thin edge (see Fig. 32–1). The shield is secured to the toe with thin circular strips of adhesive tape. The dorsal pad tends to push down on the proximal phalanx, and the plantar pad pushes up on the distal portion of the middle phalanx.

In rigid hammertoes, a full oval protective shield of felt or foam rubber with a central aperture is placed over the dorsal corn. On the plantar surface, a plug of felt is cut to fit snugly into the hollow, its distal portion being tapered (see Fig. 32-2). A strip of moleskin with a central aperture may be placed transversely across an end corn. Minimal bulk is essential with these paddings; otherwise the toes will be further cramped in the toe box. As an alternative protection of end corn or hammertoe, a foam plastic toe cap or sleeve may be used (Fig. 32-4). The Budin splint is a

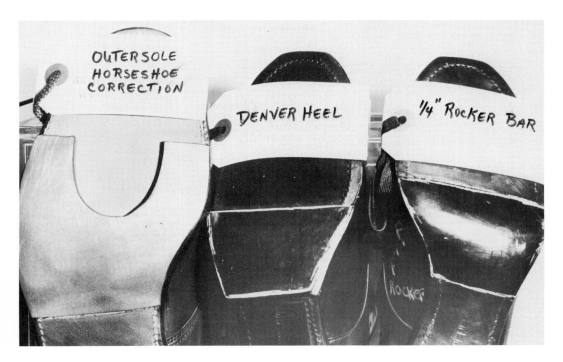

FIG. 32-3.   (*Left*) Outersole horseshoe correction. (*Center*) Denver heel. (*Right*) One-quarter-inch rocker bar.

commercially available rubber appliance that passively holds down a flexible hammertoe. It may also be used postoperatively where there is a tendency for recurrence of a hammertoe deformity.

Corns

The lateral aspect of the fifth toe is the most common site of a toe corn that is caused by pressure from narrow pointed shoes. This area may be protected with a thin shield having a central aperture. A wider, more rounded toe box also relieves the local pressure, or the shoe may be stretched over the fifth toe area. In acute discomfort, the shoe should be cut out or open sandals worn for about 6 weeks. Surgical correction consists of excision of the underlying thickened bone that is invariably present.

The soft corn is seen most often in the depths of the web space between the fourth and fifth toes and usually in association with a wide forefoot. The wide square-shaped toes are cramped together in the usual commercial shoe. Hence, there is often also a hard corn on the lateral aspect of the fifth toe. Treatment consists of a shield or lamb's wool placed between the fourth and fifth toes combined with a wide, square toe box or completely open-

toed shoes. Excision of the bony thickening beneath the soft corn is often indicated. The soft corn, especially when macerated, may be misdiagnosed as an interdigital fungal infection. However, its localization deep within a single web space associated with acute tenderness over the underlying palpable small "bump" is diagnostic.

Tailor's Bunion (Bunionette)

Tailor's bunion is a lateral bony thickening of the head and neck of the fifth metatarsal. It is seen mainly in people with splayfeet. Conservative treatment consists of wide shoes, stretching the shoe over the area of abnormal prominence, or the use of a moon-shaped shield placed proximal to the lesion. The exostosis is readily removed surgically under local anesthesia.

Painful calluses and corns may be pared down, but never down to normal skin, which results in undue local sensitivity or danger of bleeding and secondary infection. If the pared calluses are tender, they may be temporarily protected with moleskin. Shielding and padding should be used as a temporary means of obtaining relief until the permanent shoe and shoe corrections are obtained. In multiple foot or toe deformities, it is much sim-

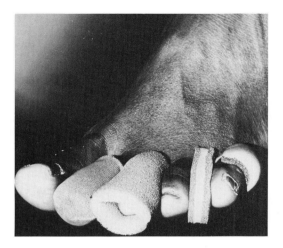

FIG. 32-4. Commercial removable shields. From left to right, foam (polyurethane) toe cap, foam toe sleeve, soft corn shield, fifth toe (hard corn) shield.

pler to order custom-made shoes with soft-rubber removable molded innersoles than to apply repeatedly bulky complicated multiple shields and pads.

Anterior Metatarsalgia

Anterior metatarsal pain accompanying disturbances of the toes is a common disability in women. Because men wear lower-heeled shoes, they are less likely to develop such symptoms. Half the body weight is borne by the metatarsal arch, the other half by the heel. Normally each metatarsal head carries equal amounts of weight except for the first, which carries twice the load. The more severe the relative equinus of the forefoot, the more the weight is borne by the metatarsal heads. In midtarsal or forefoot cavus, the metatarsals point more acutely plantarward. In order to clear the forefoot off the ground in walking, the patient overexerts the dorsiflexors of the toes, ultimately resulting in hammertoe deformities. If the ankle can compensate by excessively dorsiflexing, significant anterior metatarsal calluses do not develop. Anterior metatarsalgia becomes more painful when there is pressure atrophy of the fat pads and development of heavy calluses. Paring offers temporary relief, but rapid recurrence is the rule without shoe corrections, arch supports, or surgery.

Anterior metatarsal pain is typically "burning" in nature. An occult peripheral neuropathy owing to diabetes or peripheral arteriosclerosis obliterans may simulate anterior metatarsalgia. However, in such cases there are usually no anterior metatarsal calluses and, more significantly, no local tenderness under the metatarsal heads.

Plantar Interdigital Neuroma

Metatarsal pain may result from a plantar interdigital neuroma, which is found especially in middle-aged women but also occasionally in the elderly. In such cases the history is diagnostic. The pain occurs only with walking, and it is felt about the plantar aspect of the third and fourth metatarsal heads with occasional radiation into the toes. It often forces the patient to stop walking and even to remove her shoe and rub her foot for relief. The tenderness has pinpoint localization, occurring deeply between two adjacent metatarsal heads, usually the third and fourth. The typical pain is duplicated by compressing the metatarsal heads with one hand while pressing deeply between them with the finger tip of the opposite hand. Conservative treatment with metatarsal pads is relatively ineffective. Removal of the plantar neuroma is the treatment of choice.

Sesamoiditis

Localized pain under the first metatarsal head may be due to sesamoiditis. The tenderness is under the proximal portion of the first metatarsal head, either laterally (lateral sesamoid) or medially (medial sesamoid). Roentgenograms are noncontributory. Treatment consists of the use of a "bat" metatarsal pad, also known as a dancer's pad or a sesamoid pad. This is a rubber metatarsal pad with an extension behind the first metatarsal head (Fig. 32-5). Excision of a sesamoid is rarely necessary although commonly practiced.

Atrophy of Metatarsal Fat Pad

Atrophy of the fat pad under the metatarsal heads may occur in old age and cause anterior metatarsalgia. Severe atrophy with painful calluses, rigidity of the forefoot, and hammertoes are found in rheumatoid arthritis. The metatarsalgia is much more disabling than the toe deformities, but it is often helped by custom-made shoes with removable molded rubber or polyethylene innersoles.

Conservative and Surgical Treatment of Anterior Metatarsalgia

The conservative treatment of anterior metatarsalgia consists of combinations of mechanical means of relieving pressure. Each patient and each foot

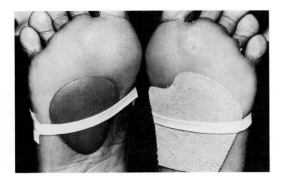

FIG. 32-5. (*Left*) Standard metatarsal pad. (*Right*) "Bat" metatarsal (sesamoid) pad. Pads should be glued onto innersole and covered with thin innersole leather lining.

must be considered individually. Mild cases may be relieved with a ⅛-inch sponge-rubber or polyethyelene innersole. Rubber outersoles, especially resilient ripple soles, relieve pressure. The standard metatarsal pad fits just proximal to the second, third, and fourth metatarsal heads, and it relieves weight bearing on these heads (see Fig. 32-5). If a decided hollow proximal to these heads is noted on deep palpation, a high metatarsal pad should be ordered. These pads are made of firm rubber, and they may also be incorporated into full-length innersoles. When the calluses are severe, "wells" should also be ordered in the innersoles under the involved metatarsal heads.

Often, there is too little weight bearing on the first and fifth metatarsal heads with baby-soft skin noted in these areas. In such cases, in addition to the metatarsal pads, the innersoles are raised about ⅛ inch under the first and fifth metatarsal heads to distribute weight more evenly. The area under the fifth metatarsal head should be raised slightly less than that under the first. The horseshoe outersole correction is an alternative. It is made from a thick piece of leather attached across the proximal half of the outersole proximal to the second, third, and fourth metatarsal heads, and it has extensions past the first and fifth metatarsal heads (Fig. 32-3). A Denver heel (metatarsal bar) provides support for all the metatarsal heads, while the standard metatarsal pad supports mainly the second, third, and fourth metatarsal heads. A combination of both may be useful. In severe anterior metatarsalgia of the second, third, and fourth metatarsal heads with rigid reversal of the transverse anterior metatarsal arch, a horseshoe-type rubber innersole may be combined with an outersole

horseshoe correction. Heel height should be the minimum the patient can tolerate, usually about 1½ inches. If the heel cord is short, lower heels are not tolerated by the patient.

Major procedures such as tarsometatarsal wedge resection or midtarsal wedge resection should be reserved for young adults. Total resection of a metatarsal head is reserved for a persistent painful callus with secondary scar formation, seen with poorly treated plantar warts. Metatarsal shaft shortening and simple osteotomy of a metatarsal shaft with dorsal displacement of the distal fragment are alternative procedures. In rheumatoid arthritis with severe involvement of the metatarsal heads, usually associated with dorsally displaced rigid hammertoes, radical resection of all metatarsal heads and necks is a satisfactory procedure. Injudicious resection of a single metatarsal head throws excessive weight onto the adjacent metatarsal heads, resulting in ultimate painful callus formation.

Perforating Plantar Ulcers

Perforating ulcers are most common under localized plantar bony prominences bearing excess weight, such as the interphalangeal joint of the hallux and under the metatarsal heads. The most common cause is vascular insufficiency, most often due to arteriolar disease. Diabetic or alcoholic neuritis or spinal cord lesions, such as spina bifida and cord tumors, are also causes. Where there is sensory loss, skin breakdown may occur. Repeated skin breakdown may also develop secondary to old trauma, skin loss, scar formation, burns, bed sores, and ill-advised surgical incisions. Perforating ulcers associated with vascular insufficiency are difficult and frustrating. Bed rest, tepid betadine soaks, antibiotic therapy, and sympathectomy may all be of use. The hyperkeratotic ulcer margins may be gently debrided to allow better drainage. Any underlying bone or joint destruction seen radiographically should be disregarded. The bone simply absorbs under the ulcer area and does not sequestrate or form sinuses as it does in other parts of the body. Any removal of bone or incisions for drainage may lead to disaster. Beyond conservative therapy, the surgical approach is ray resection or amputation at the proper level.

With bed rest for weeks or months and no weight bearing, most of the ulcers will granulate in and epithelialize. Before ambulation is allowed, soft, thick (¾-inch minimum) custom-made sponge-rubber arch supports should be made with wells under all calluses. Calluses should be cautiously trimmed and limited weight bearing instituted. Strong keratolytics including salicylic acid ointment should be avoided because they may produce edema and inflammation. Excessive standing or walking may result in rapid breakdown of the avascular, poorly epithelialized scar. Both vascular and neurotrophic types of ulcer tend to recur. Chronic ulcers not associated with neurologic defect or poor blood supply, such as those owing to scar formation following trauma or burns, are more amenable to surgical repair.

More recently, radical surgical prophylactic treatment has been advocated for diabetics with impending ulers under metatarsal heads. This consists of excision of all of the metatarsal heads to prevent such ulceration.

The conservative care of plantar ulcerations calls for bed rest, debridement, antibiotics, and betadine whirlpool. This is followed by early ambulation with total contact casts, which are changed at intervals depending on the amount of drainage.

The Midtarsus

The midtarsus, normally an asymptomatic area of the foot, is frequently the source of mild chronic discomfort in the aged because of osteoarthritic changes. Examination reveals slight irregular bony thickening about the bones of the midtarsus dorsally and roentgenography may reveal osteophytosis. If a specific joint is tender, local anesthetic or corticosteroid injection may offer relief. Antirheumatic medication and analgesics along with well-fitted oxford shoes are also effective. Whenever there are dorsal exostoses, Blucher-style oxfords should be ordered. Such shoes have no transverse dorsal seams, with more room in the uppers; hence, pressure is not exerted on a dorsal exostosis. They are also used for pes cavus deformities, in which the midtarsus is prominently convex dorsally. When a dorsal exostosis is persistently bothersome or unusually large, surgical excision is the simple procedure of choice.

The dorsal ganglion is the most common tumor of the foot, but it is infrequently seen in the aged. At times, it is firm enough to be mistaken for a dorsal exostosis. A ganglion typically grows larger and becomes smaller and is often soft and multiloculated. Surgical extirpation is rarely necessary. The ganglion is needled in multiple directions with a heavy-gauge needle. Then by firm digital pressure, the contents are completely dispersed within the soft tissues of the foot. Permanent cure is often effected in this manner.

The Subtalar Joint

The subtalar joint is the major joint of the foot. It permits the side-to-side motion known as inversion and eversion. It is a complex of joints involving the talus, os calcis, navicular, and cuboid. There is slight side-to-side motion of the subtalar joint in normal walking; this is accentuated on uneven ground. In disease of the subtalar complex, considerable pain occurs on weight bearing and the foot assumes a spastic valgus (flatfoot) position. This is caused by the peroneal tendons becoming spastic and pulling the foot into a valgus deformity. Side-to-side motion becomes limited, and passive motion in these directions (especially inversion) is painful. There is tenderness to deep palpation over the sinus tarsus, which is just anterior (distal) to the lateral malleolus. The syndrome may be caused by any inflammatory, mechanical, or degenerative lesion of the subtalar complex such as traumatic degeneration following fractures of the os calcis, congenital tarsal bars, and longstanding hypermobile flatfeet. Rheumatoid arthritis frequently (almost typically) attacks the subtalar joint before any other peripheral joint is involved. Thus, a diagnostic workup is necessary to determine the etiology of a spastic flatfoot syndrome. Along with routine roentgenography of the foot, an oblique view rules out the presence of a calcaneonavicular bar and a tangential os calcis view rules out talocalcaneal bar. In the elderly, flexibility of the subtalar joint is diminished. However, little or no tenderness is found over the sinus tarsus and passive subtalar motion is not painful.

Treatment of the painful subtalar joint in the adult is difficult. Complete limitation of weight bearing relieves symptoms, but they usually recur when weight bearing is resumed. Palliative therapy consists of limitation of weight bearing, antirheumatic medication such as phenylbutazone and indomethacin, and shoe support. Subtalar rocking may be minimized by using an Ashley heel, which consists of forward placement of the heel (similar to that of a Western-style riding boot) with the addition of inner and outer heel flanges. In normal walking, the foot strikes the ground with the unstable back edge of the heel and rocks. Use of the Ashley heel eliminates this posterior edge, as with the walking heel of a cast. Occasionally, a high-top shoe provides additional support, especially when there is severe valgus deformity of the foot. Injection of 0.5 ml of local anesthetic combined with 0.5 ml of intra-articular cortisone into the sinus tarsus often provides considerable relief, but this usually lasts for only 1 or 2 weeks. The most stubborn cases of painful subtalar joint are those associated with rheumatoid arthritis. Relief usually can be obtained only by using systemic (oral) prednisone often for a prolonged period. The usual dosage is 5 mg three times a day for 3 to 4 weeks. If symptoms and swelling subside and subtalar motion improves, the dosage is gradually reduced.

Ultimately, in most degenerative diseases of the subtalar joint, the symptoms abate with conservative management, and significant pain recurs only years later, or perhaps not at all. When symptoms are persistent, a subtalar or a triple arthrodesis is the surgical method of choice. Painless loss of subtalar motion is not disabling, but such surgery is not usually indicated in patients over 60.

One other relatively common condition in the subtalar area is tenosynovitis of the tibialis posterior tendon just before it inserts in the medial tuberosity of the navicular. Quite often, the medial tuberosity is hypertrophied or a large accessory navicular is present. The collar of the shoe may rub against this medially protruding bump. The shoe upper should extend either above or below this prominence for comfort. Old-style steel arch supports often painfully press on this area. In general, local instillation of corticosteroids into a tendon should be avoided because of increasing awareness of tendon ruptures following such injections. The prominence may also be excised.

The Plantar Heel-Spur Syndrome

In men the most common type of hindfoot pain is the plantar heel-spur syndrome. Marked by pain and tenderness, it is found less frequently in women, especially those who wear high heels with weight bearing thrust against the metatarsal heads. Rheumatoid arthritis and spondylitis frequently cause a periostitis or spurring of the undersurface of the os calcis. The pain is often bilateral and most severe on initiating weight bearing, especially on arising. Most patients have tenderness to deep pressure over the anterior extremity of the medial tubercle of the os calcis; others have tenderness in the middle of the plantar aspect of the heel. In rheumatoid arthritis, the pain and tenderness are often more diffuse and may include the sides of the heel. In the very elderly, in whom the syndrome may be due to heel pad atrophy (not a common cause), the tenderness is usually in the

center of the heel, and there is palpable absence of the fat pad. Roentgenograms may or may not reveal a heel spur, and conversely, many patients with asymptomatic heels have large spurs.

Successful treatment may invariably be accomplished by conservative therapy. Excision of the heel spur, although widely practiced, is not necessary. The wearing of high heels by women or the use of a piece of sponge rubber inside the heel of the shoe give only partial relief. Similarly, plastic heel cups give inadequate relief. A Steindler heel-spur correction should be used. In this technique a well is cut out from the inside of the shoe heel under the painful area. It is then filled with sponge rubber, and the entire heel area is covered with about ⅜ inch of firm foam rubber. This produces a soft and yet resilient, shallow cup into which the heel sinks. For further correction, a ³⁄₁₆-inch (maximum) tapered heel elevation may be added to pitch weight bearing forward off the heel.

If no relief is obtained within 2 or 3 weeks with such corrections and if the pain is somewhat atypical, rheumatoid arthritis should be suspected. The latex fixation test is usually negative, although the erythrocyte sedimentation rate is frequently elevated. Prednisone is given for about 2 weeks, or longer if necessary, until the shoe corrections alone provide the necessary relief. Local injection of Novocain combined with cortisone deep into the heel over the tender area is often effective for about 2 weeks, but it is very painful. Weight reduction in obesity is also imperative.

Tenosynovitis of the flexor hallucis longus is frequently confused with the plantar heel-spur syndrome. Pain occurs on the bottom of the heel, especially with walking, but not on initiating weight bearing. The tenderness is more superficial along the course of the flexor hallucis longus tendon, usually about ½ to 1 inch distal to the usual medial tenderness of the heel spur. Treatment consists of using rubber innersoles, limiting walking, and injecting cortisone into the area of tenderness.

Disabilities of the Posterior Heel

Achilles tendinitis and Achilles bursitis are occasionally encountered in the middle-aged or older patients. The tenderness in Achilles tendinitis is usually in the distal portion of the tendon. Achilles bursitis usually involves the retrocalcaneal bursa, which is small and lies between the Achilles tendon and the posterior superior surface of the os calcis. Treatment consists of use of analgesics, the wearing of high heels, cutting out the heel counter, shielding the tender areas, and local injection of

Novocain and cortisone. In my experience posterior heel pain is not associated with gout or gonorrhea.

Spontaneous rupture of the Achilles tendon may occur in the elderly, but it is most often precipitated by sudden tension on the heel cord, such as in running for a bus. The rupture may be complete or incomplete, and healing may occur with or without elongation or with a considerable defect (palpable gap). The disability in the elderly may not be particularly incapacitating. If diagnosed early, treatment in plaster with the foot in equinus may be elected for milder cases. When the rupture is complete with a wide palpable gap, surgical repair is indicated.

One occasionally encounters annoying heel skin fissures seen radially about the posterior and lateral edges of the heel, especially in obese middle-aged women. Treatment consists of paring the hypertrophic skin and the application of emollients. Chronicity is the rule.

Ankle Trauma

Ankle fractures in the elderly are managed by standard methods except that immediate reduction is more imperative to prevent edema and secondary vascular impairment. Open surgery may be contraindicated with evidence of impaired circulation. Perfect anatomical reduction is less important than a painless, functional, viable foot and ankle. Postoperative care includes rehabilitation of the stiffened ankle and subtalar joints secondary to immobilization. Walking with crutches is not advisable in the elderly. They usually do not have strength or agility and may fall and break a hip.

Small avulsion fractures are often overlooked, especially with inadequate roentgenography. Whenever there is associated tenderness of the foot near the ankle, roentgenograms of the foot as well as the ankle should be taken. Persistent foot and ankle edema often follows sprains and sprain avulsion fractures. Many of these basically innocuous fractures tend to be overtreated. Relatively minor sprains and sprain fractures including fractures of the lower end of the fibula, if not accompanied by ankle mortise distraction or ankle instability, are preferably treated using an Unna boot rather than a cumbersome cast. Elastic anklets tend to cut off local circulation, and Ace bandages are usually improperly applied by the patient.

Synovitis of the Ankle

Synovitis of the ankle is common, especially in obese middle-aged and older women. There is thickening about the ankle and mild limitation of motion. There is no crepitus on motion, and roentgenograms are not remarkable. Discomfort is relatively mild but may be persistent. Treatment consists of weight reduction, salicylates, indomethacin, and, if necessary, local injection of Novocain and intra-articular cortisone. More painful destructive synovitis and arthritis occur in rheumatoid arthritis and are treated systemically. Therapeutic forms of heat may make rheumatoid joints feel worse.

Osteoarthritis of the ankle is surprisingly infrequent in the elderly, except when associated with old fractures or old infections. Conservative therapy includes antirheumatic medication and physiotherapy. A stable shoe with a long sole rocker is helpful when painful loss of motion is significant. The ankle may also be immobilized by a high-top shoe incorporating a steel upright within the upper. Occasionally, an ankle brace is necessary.

Inversion Ankle Instability

Some patients, especially women, complain of inversion instability of the ankle. Cases that follow severe ankle sprains with permanent disruption of the lateral collateral ligament of the ankle may require surgical reconstruction. In milder cases, the patient should be fitted with a relatively low (1.5 inches) broad heel. An outer heel flange or an Ashley heel may further prevent the tendency for the ankle to turn inward.

Tendon Ruptures

Spontaneous tendon ruptures about the ankle usually occur in persons over 44 years of age. The most frequent rupture involves the tibialis posterior, causes a unilateral flat foot, and is often overlooked. It is amenable only to surgical repair. Rupture of the heel cord may also be overlooked. In this case the patient cannot walk tip-toe. This disability, however, is not severe in the elderly. Less common is rupture of the tibialis anterior, which causes a mild dropfoot. Surgical repair may be indicated.

SUMMARY

Foot problems of the elderly are often the residua of diseases, trauma, and deformities of childhood and adult life, and superimposed degenerative and static changes and deformities may also develop. Treatment becomes more difficult because of systemic and local infirmities, the most limiting being the poor vascular status of the foot. Conservative, supportive, and palliative therapy thus replaces definitive reconstructive surgical therapy. Also, co-operation in the elderly may be limited because of organic mental syndromes with forgetfulness and inability to follow orders. Even transportation problems may interfere with the patient seeing the physician at necessary intervals. Consultation with members of the family is advisable to make sure the patient is following medical orders.

SUGGESTED READINGS

Atlas of Orthotics: Biomechanical Principles and Application. St. Louis, CV Mosby, 1975

Bauman JH, Girling JP, Branch PW: Plantar pressure and trophic ulceration: An evaluation of footwear. J Bone Joint Surg [Br] 45:652, 1963

Dickson FD, Dively RL: Functional Disorders of the Foot, 3rd ed, p 345. Philadelphia, JB Lippincott, 1953

DuVries HL: Surgery of the Foot, 2nd ed, p 586. St. Louis, CV Mosby, 1965

Evanski PM: The geriatric foot. In Jahss MH (ed): Disorders of the Foot, vol 1, pp 964–978. Philadelphia, WB Saunders, 1982

Giannestras NJ: Foot Disorders: Medical and Surgical Management, 2nd ed, p 699. Philadelphia, Lea & Febiger, 1973

Gibbard LC (ed): Charlesworth's Chiropodical Orthopaedics, 2nd ed. London, Baillère Tindall, 1968

Gould N: Shoes and shoe modifications. In Jahss MH (ed): Disorders of the Foot, vol 2, pp 1745–1782. Philadelphia, WB Saunders, 1982

Gross RH: Modern Foot Therapy, p 710. U.S.A., Modern Foot Therapy Publishing Co., 1948

Hauser EDW: Diseases of the Foot, 2nd ed, p 415. Philadelphia, WB Saunders, 1950

Jahss MH: Arch supports and miscellaneous devices. In Jahss MH (ed): Disorders of the Foot, vol 2, pp 1733–1744. Philadelphia, WB Saunders, 1982

Jones FW: Structure and Function as Seen in the Foot, 2nd ed. London, Baillère Tindall, 1949

Kelikian H: Hallux Valgus, Allied Deformities of the Forefoot and Metatarsalgia. Philadelphia, WB Saunders, 1965

Klenerman L (ed): The Foot and Its Disorders. Oxford, Blackwell Scientific Publications, 1976

Lake NC: The Foot. London, Baillère Tindall, 1952

LeLièvre J: Pathologie du Pied, 3rd ed. Paris, Masson, 1967

Lewin P: The Foot and Ankle, 4th ed. Philadelphia, Lea & Febiger, 1959

Mercer W, Duthie RB, Ferguson AB: Orthopaedic Surgery, 7th ed, p 1236. London, Arnold, 1973

Milgram JE: Padding and devices to relieve the painful foot. In Jahss MH (ed): Disorders of the Foot, vol 2, pp 1703–1732. Philadelphia, WB Saunders, 1982

Morton DJ: The Human Foot, Its Evolution, Physiology and Functional Disorders, p 244. New York, Columbia University Press, 1935

Orthopaedic Appliances Atlas, vol 1, Braces, Splints, Shoe Alterations. Ann Arbor, MI, JW Edwards, 1952

Regenspurger G: Orthopädische Einlagen und Schuhversorgung, p 307. Leipzig, Barth, 1975

Wickstrom J, Williams RA: Shoe corrections and orthopaedic foot supports. Clin Orthop 73:30, 1970

33 Rehabilitation of the Geriatric Patient

Jerome S. Tobis

Chronic disease with disability is a frequent concomitant of old age. According to data from the 1976 National Health Survey, 43% of the elderly (over age 65) suffered limitations of activity owing to chronic disability. Not only do the elderly show the highest incidence of chronic disease of all age-groups, but multiple impairments are also frequently observed. The concurrence of degenerative disease of many systems is common and may lead to limitations of function. Thus, 12% of those over age 65 are unable to perform three or more activities of daily living.[20] With advanced age these functional losses increase.

MULTIPLE DISABILITIES OF THE AGED

The elderly diabetic may show extensive ischemic vascular changes with symptoms of peripheral vascular disease, heart disease, retinopathy, renal impairment, and cerebrovascular disease. Even when not multicentric, pathologic processes pyramid. The changes resulting from one disorder may have dire consequences on other systems. Thus, osteoporosis leads to fragility of bone, which predisposes the elderly to the risk of fracture (of the hip) or collapse of vertebrae. Diminution of vision may predispose to accident. Psychologic concomitants, such as depression and loss of motivation, further amplify the disability. In addition to interrelated disorders, many of the elderly experience several unrelated diseases. In a study by Wilson[21] of 200 patients serially admitted to a geriatric unit, each had an average of four apparently unrelated diseases, and the mean number of diseases per patient was nearly six.

The multiplicity of disorders in the elderly person not only reduces his capacity to perform the necessary tasks of daily life but also frequently requires the participation of many professional disciplines in the evaluation and management of these disorders, thus causing a need for a variety of ancillary services. In addition to one or more medical specialists, the elderly patient may require the aid of nursing, psychology, physical therapy, audiology, social work, speech therapy, and occupational therapy. These may need to be supplemented by other services such as transportation, housekeeping, home food service, and recreation.

GOALS OF REHABILITATION

Rehabilitation medicine (physical medicine and rehabilitation) seeks to improve the motor performance of the disabled elderly so that they can attain or maintain their premorbid functional status. The techniques that are employed are essentially symptomatic because the chronic diseases of old age are usually degenerative and incurable. The goals of rehabilitation are to reduce the limitations imposed by these impairments and to prevent the sequelae of disease.

For example, a patient with peripheral vascular disease may finally require amputation of the lower extremity. The amputation may prevent his walking again, perhaps further complicated if the patient is kept in bed or in a wheelchair. Resultant contractures of the hip and knee might prevent walking with an artificial limb. The rehabilitative aspects of caring for such a patient might include prevention of contractures; teaching self-care activities; evaluation of cardiovascular and neuromuscular status to meet requirements for walking; prescription and check-out of a prosthesis, if indicated; conditioning exercises to increase motor power; gait training to improve motor skill and cardiovascular performance; evaluation of the patient's psychologic status in terms of his judgment, capacity to learn, and his motivation; and management of the patient and modification of his environment to help the patient attain feasible and safe performance. Carrying out these tasks requires a thorough physical examination with the major emphasis on function. The amputee's vision, his cardiovascular status, his loss of kinesthesis, or ischemic changes in the remaining foot may each be a potential or absolute contraindication to teaching ambulation. Any of them may significantly reduce the capacity of the patient to perform the task safely.

RISKS OF REHABILITATION

Rehabilitation is essentially a learning process. The physician in rehabilitation medicine, often in collaboration with other health disciplines such as nursing, physical therapy, and occupational therapy, teaches the patient to perform a new or renewed task. Such activities often subject a patient to the risk of trauma or significant stress, so the elderly patient must be closely supervised to avoid undue risk. On the other hand, few physicians would prefer the safety of prolonged bed rest for the patient with the consequent deleterious effects of immobilization—in order to avoid the risks of activity and rehabilitation. Nonetheless, the danger of a fall for an elderly, unstable patient who is learning to walk again is ever present. The elderly active patient is more prone to accident than is an inactive counterpart.

INSTITUTIONAL VERSUS HOME SERVICES

Rehabilitation techniques may be carried out in a hospital, home, or nursing home. For the severely involved, the elaborate facilities of a hospital rehabilitation medicine service may be required lest the patient remain completely dependent. In a study[12] of patients with stroke admitted in 1 year to an acute 1000-bed general hospital with an active rehabilitation service, only 3% remained in a severely dependent state at their time of discharge. In another hospital of approximately the same size without formal rehabilitation services, 18% remained severely dependent. These findings suggest that rehabilitation services in a hospital tend to lessen disability in the presence of severe

impairment. On the other hand, hospitalization may not be necessary in some severely disabled, because many therapeutic activities can be carried out at home. In a report describing physical medicine and rehabilitation services in the home care program at New York's Montefiore Hospital, Lowenthal[11] indicates that the patient load in the home setting can be comparable to any inpatient rehabilitation service. Most patients start their rehabilitation while in the hospital. Sometimes, the patient makes more significant progress at home. The following case exemplifies this.

A 66-year-old male truck driver transferred to the inpatient rehabilitation service at Montefiore Hospital in February after being involved in a motor vehicle accident. Roentgenography at the time showed no evidence of a fracture, but advanced spondylosis of the bodies of C6 and C7 was noted.

On admission, the patient was found to have a complete areflexic tetraplegia at the C7 level. The strength in his upper extremities ranged from zero at the fingers to fair at the shoulders. The patient was incontinent of bowel and bladder. There were sacral and left heel decubiti. He was treated for his decubiti with frequent turning to avoid prolonged pressure on any body part, débridement, cleansing, and ultraviolet radiation of the involved areas. Two months later, the sacral decubitus was closed with a rotation flap. Genitourinary evaluation revealed benign prostatic hypertrophy, and in June of the same year, the patient had a transurethral resection, following which he became continent of urine. While hospitalized, the patient was placed on a rehabilitation therapy program, including range-of-motion exercises, training in activities of daily living, and gradual tilting to the erect posture to avoid hypotensive syncopal attacks until he was able to stand erect, fully supported. An appropriate wheelchair was prescribed.

By the time of discharge, the patient had regained some motor and sensory function so that he was independent in the wheelchair, but he was dependent on transfer from bed to chair. He was sent home on the home care service in December of the same year with a hydraulic lift, a wheelchair, a hi-lo bed, and a trapeze for lifting himself in bed. He was unable to stand except for pivoting in transfers. Since being home, the patient has made significant additional improvement in his motor performance with the emotional and physical support of his wife. In part this represents further neurologic return, but the functional improvement exceeds the expectations based on his changing neurologic findings. He now no longer requires a hydraulic lift. He transfers without assistance, and ambulates with a walker and a short leg brace on the right leg.

The second case highlights other advantages to the patient of the familiar surroundings and attention of relatives at home. In this instance, the motor impairment persisted at home, but total function as a human being was greatly improved.

A 73-year-old white male retired minister suffered an attack of left hemiplegia in mid-February. The patient was confused as to time and sometimes to place. He spoke in an extremely low voice, which made conversation extremely difficult, and at times his conversation was unintelligible. He had no spontaneous or voluntary movement of the left upper extremity. He had a spastic left lower extremity with poor hip and knee movers. Sensory examination was completely unreliable.

This man was evaluated on the rehabilitation ward over a 3-week period. During this time, it was evident that he was a severely brain-damaged patient who had no significant neurologic return following the stroke. The patient was incontinent of urine. Attempts at involving him in occupational therapy or physical therapy programs during this time showed very little progress. The results of his rehabilitation program were nil, and therefore he was discharged in May of the same year to live with his family and to return to the care of his family physician.

In November of the following year, the patient was seen in the follow-up clinic. The report includes the following: "Today the patient's family claims the patient has shown marked improvement in mentation. He is now able to read, write, and keep his correspondence. He is able to communicate and converse with relatives. As for motor activities, the patient is dependent in activities of daily living and transfer. With moderate assistance and holding himself on the hand rails he can go to the bathroom." The patient became continent of bladder and bowel at home.

In nursing homes, rehabilitation services are generally indicated for only a small minority of the patient population.[16] In a 3-year study[14] of approximately 400 public assistance recipients in nursing homes in New York City, the efficacy of complete medical rehabilitation services was evaluated. It was hoped that with such services some patients might improve their self-care or possibly return to community living. Unfortunately, this study tended to support earlier work showing the low rehabilitation potential of physically impaired nursing-home residents. The population whose modal age was in the 70s was chronically ill with a poor prognosis for survival. Realistically, increased independence in self-care was probably an irrelevant goal for such a group because their significant medical problems, and dependence on

public agencies for financial, medical, and social services, considerably antedated their entry to the nursing home. Such patients, by and large, need social stimulation such as recreational and group-work services rather than an elaborate medical rehabilitation program. On the other hand, with proper selection as shown in a study by Gordon and co-workers,[8] a minority of elderly patients in nursing homes can achieve significant improvement in functional status.

Economical use should be made of rehabilitation facilities and services for the chronically ill generally, but especially for the elderly. Each patient should obtain all the rehabilitation services he can profitably use when increased performance is a realistic goal—no less, but also no more.

MODALITIES OF PHYSICAL MEDICINE

Physical medicine techniques are symptomatic therapies prescribed for the following indications: relief of pain, increase in range of motion, increase in motor power, increase in skill, and increase in endurance. The approach to management depends on the etiology underlying the symptom. This has been summarized in Figures 33-1, 33-3, 33-5, 33-7, and 33-8.

Because disturbances in one or more of these areas are common in the elderly, physical agents are frequently prescribed by the family physician. Provided there are no contraindications, physical modalities often give effective symptomatic relief. They include heat, cold, massage, electrotherapy, hydrotherapy, and ultraviolet radiation. Occupational therapy and braces, splints, and prostheses may then be used to enhance function, will be better tolerated, and will be of maximal use to the patients.

Relief of Pain

Heat is a valuable agent in providing pain relief in musculoskeletal disorders of the aged such as those due to rheumatic diseases. It may be given to superficial structures by a hot-water bag, paraffin bath, or an infrared lamp and to deep structures by a diathermy, microwave, or ultrasound machine. Heat is contraindicated locally in the presence of occlusive vascular disease, in which increased tissue metabolism cannot be met by increased blood flow. It is also contraindicated in the presence of cancer. When there is acute inflammation involving a nonexpansible area such as bursitis, heat may exacerbate the pain. Intermit-

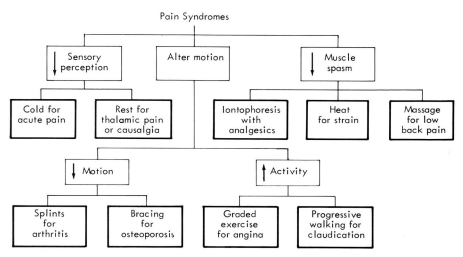

FIG. 33-1. Modalities of physical therapy applicable to pain syndromes. (Charts 1 to 5. Light boxes—symptom or affected function; heavy boxes—specific therapy; ↑ , increase; ↓ , decrease.)

tent cold packs (ice) or fluoromethane spray may then be useful as an analgesic. In some patients with exquisitely painful musculoskeletal disorders such as acute low back pain or even pain of radicular distribution, cold may provide symptomatic relief.

The application of heat and cold to elderly patients should be carried out with awareness of pathophysiologic considerations, which are of less consequence when younger persons are treated. The elderly often have diminished perception of heat and cold. Without the protection of normal sensation, they may be subjected to the risk of trauma from these modalities. Occlusive vascular disease may compound the injury. It is often present without a history of intermittent claudication, because the inactive elderly person may not walk long enough to develop typical symptoms. Thus, the near-basal condition in which the oldster has lived may lead the physician to overlook a potentially ischemic extremity. For example, if an older person soaks his feet in very hot water, irreparable skin damage may result. Furthermore, a hot bath for musculoskeletal complaints may place undue stress on an already embarrassed cardiovascular system. It can produce a sudden marked increase in the functional vascular bed with major shifts of blood from one region to another and concomitant increase in circulating blood volume. If the compensatory mechanisms governing this reaction are deficient, hemodynamic changes may lead to hypotensive and even syncopal episodes.

Thermoregulatory mechanisms may be im-

paired in the elderly. Prolonged exposure to body heating may result in hyperpyrexia, and exposure to cold may result in hypothermia. One of my elderly patients, who was placed on a water mattress because of a sacral decubitus, developed an unrecognized and significant drop in body temperature. The water, at room temperature beneath the rubber sheet, conducted heat away from the patient's body.

Increase in Range of Motion

The elderly tend to develop contractures relatively quickly if they are bedridden for a time or in a wheelchair most of the day or if a body part is immobilized by a cast. A young person may have an extended knee maintained in a cast for 6 weeks with return of full range of flexion after a few weeks of exercise and passive stretching. If the same procedures are done with the elderly, significant flexion may never be regained. Thus, immobilization of a body part should be as short as possible in the elderly. At best, the range of motion of the major synovial joints of the elderly is generally restricted at the extremes of extension and flexion. Thus, there is a tendency to walk without full extension of the knees and hips.

Range of motion of a joint may be increased by the use of passive exercises or stretching. Stretching should be accomplished only by a physical therapist or other trained person to avoid trauma and aggravation of underlying disease. For example, a 10° to 15° flexion contracture of a knee joint might be overcome by the therapist applying firm pressure over the anterior surface of the thigh and calf. Stretching may also be attempted mechanically by use of a brace or cast with a turnbuckle or ratchet device that can lock in progressively greater angles until full extension is obtained. Such an appliance may be applied for minutes to hours. Preferably, if feasible, as in rheumatoid arthritis, the extremity should be removed from a cast or splint and put through range of motion passively every day.

As in stretching, passive motion must be done cautiously to avoid trauma or bleeding in or around a joint. In the hemiplegic or paraplegic, passive exercise may occasionally be associated with heterotopic ossification. The following report highlights such a case.

A 70-year-old woman has had a longstanding history of hypertension and heart disease with atrial fibrillation and congestive failure.

In September, she had the onset of a right hemiplegia with a dense global aphasia. She was admitted to another hospital, where some return of function in the right leg was noted. The arm was essentially flail. A brace was ordered, and she ambulated with maximum assistance in the parallel bars. One month later she was transferred to my service. Bilateral Babinski signs were elicited. This apparently represented a change over the earlier findings. Her nurse reported a deterioration in functioning. Because of the possibility that her new condition might have resulted from cerebral embolism, anticoagulation was begun.

In early December of the same year, she began crying and exhibited discomfort when manipulations of her right hip were carried out or in walking with her long leg brace. Roentgenograms revealed considerable bony density between the right ilium and right upper femoral shaft on both sides of the shaft. This represented a form of heterotopic ossification (Fig. 33-2).

Although trauma is not the only cause of this phenomenon, it must be kept in mind as a risk of passive motion of a joint that has impaired sensation.

Stretching in the form of traction is occasionally used for radicular pain of the cervical region, often the consequence of cervical spondylosis in the elderly. Such stretching may be applied with the use of an electrical traction instrument that pulls on the head through the attachment of a halter (Sayre's suspension). The force may be applied continuously or intermittently with graduated forces used, starting with 15 lb. Inexpensive, non-

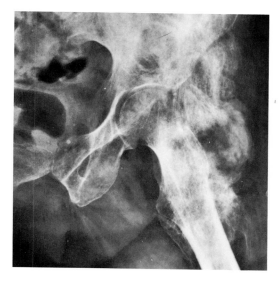

FIG. 33-2. Heterotopic ossification of the left femur and pelvis in a patient with hemiplegia.

electrical traction devices for home use are available (Fig. 33-3).

Increase in Motor Power

Aging is associated with a decrease in strength, speed, and coordination. The decrease in strength may be related primarily to the decrease in size of motor units as found by Gutmann and Hanzlekova.[9] There is also a decrease in the diameter of muscle fibers according to Rowe[18] which may lead to reduced strength. Campbell and co-workers[6] have shown that there is, in old age, a loss of the number of functioning motor units. Furthermore, the speed of mobilization of motor units decreases owing to slowing of impulse conduction. However, in addition to these peripheral mechanisms, the changes in motor performance in old age must also include central mechanisms as well.

Weakness is a frequent complaint in the elderly. It may represent the aging process itself, for the strength of a young adult diminishes as he ages. It may result from acute or chronic systemic illness. Or weakness may result from a pathologic process in the nervous system—the brain (mild hemiparesis), spinal cord (amyotrophic lateral sclerosis), peripheral nerve (polyneuropathy), myoneural junction (myasthenia gravis), or the muscle (myopathy). Electrodiagnostic techniques including low-voltage currents, chronaxy, and electromyography, which are employed by the physiatrist, may help identify the cause. Several systemic neurologic sequelae of cancer (lung and

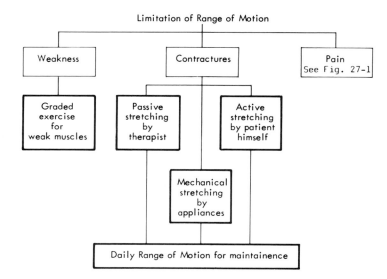

FIG. 33-3. Modalities of physical therapy applicable when there is limited range of motion. (Light boxes—symptom or affected function; heavy boxes—specific therapy; ↑, increase; ↓, decrease.)

pancreas) have been identified by Brain and Norris.[5] Conditions like the (pseudo) myasthenic syndrome of Lambert,[17] which is occasionally found in patients with intrathoracic cancer, may be definitively identified by an electrodiagnostic technique.

Increase in motor power is obtained by active exercise. Passive exercise, no matter how prolonged, does not effect strength. Active exercises produce increased strength by bringing about hypertrophy of muscle fibers with an associated increase in the glycogen and myoglobin storage in the individual cell. Exercise thus produces a change in the contractile elements of the muscle fiber. Active exercise may be graduated from assistive to resistive. Such exercises may be performed either as calisthenics or by the use of occupational therapy procedures (Fig. 33-4).

Much has been written in lay and scientific literature concerning isometric versus isotonic exercises. Isometric contraction is one in which the length of the muscle remains essentially unchanged and, therefore, is occasionally referred to as static exercise. Isotonic exercise, on the other hand, refers to a changing length of muscle with changes in joint motion and, therefore, is referred to as phasic, or dynamic, exercise.

Regarding elderly persons, isometric exercises should be avoided. Isometric exercise may produce the effect of a Valsalva maneuver that, in turn, places an undue pressure load on the heart. This is observed if one attempts to lift an immovable object from the floor. Even if the breath is not held, Donald and colleagues[7] have shown that an isometric sustained contraction of a muscle group

of the arm that is as little as 15% of the maximum voluntary contraction results in a significant rise in blood pressure. This may be an inappropriate stress for the cardiovascular system of an elderly person, who all too often suffers from arteriosclerosis of the vascular tree and ischemic heart disease.

In addition to these considerations, isotonic exercises are preferred for other reasons. They encourage full range of motion of joints and counteract the restrictive effects of immobilization. Thus, the isotonic exercise associated with walking or climbing stairs tends to extend the hips and knees maximally and helps overcome any mild contractures of these joints (Fig. 33-5).

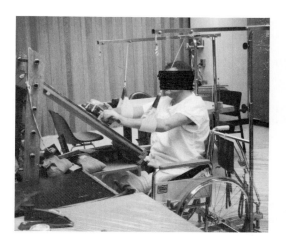

FIG. 33-4. Active exercise with the use of occupational therapy techniques.

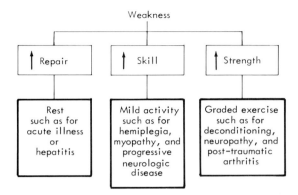

Weakness

↑ Repair	↑ Skill	↑ Strength
Rest such as for acute illness or hepatitis	Mild activity such as for hemiplegia, myopathy, and progressive neurologic disease	Graded exercise such as for deconditioning, neuropathy, and post-traumatic arthritis

FIG. 33-5. Modalities of physical therapy applicable to weakness. (Light boxes—symptom or affected function; heavy boxes—specific therapy; ↑, increase; ↓, decrease.)

Increase in Skill

Repetitive exercises tend to improve motor skill by improving the efficiency with which a given task is performed. This applies to any motor task, whether it be walking or wielding a heavy hammer to hit a nail.

When a person limps, the energy cost of walking is much higher than the cost of normal gait. Molbech[13] has estimated that even a moderate limp provides an additional energy requirement that corresponds to what a normal person would experience carrying a heavy weight. In a group of 24 patients with various types of musculoskeletal and neuromuscular disabilities, Molbech determined the cost of walking to be almost double that of the normal person. Thus, if skill in walking can be improved and made more efficient, this in turn reduces the energy expenditure in the elderly person. In disabled elderly people, the modest difference in caloric expenditure between skilled and unskilled performance may determine the level at which the patient may function—ambulating versus wheelchair-bound. Even a minor modification of a shoe—for example, a lift—on the uninvolved leg of a hemiplegic may permit the involved leg with a foot drop to clear the floor more easily (Fig. 33-6).

Improvement in skill may also be obtained by the use of assistive devices, braces, and canes. For example, Bard and Ralston[4] have shown that the energy requirements for walking in an elderly hemiplegic with the use of a brace and cane may be significantly less than with the cane alone. Furthermore, they found that walking with a crutch in the above-knee amputee was very costly met-

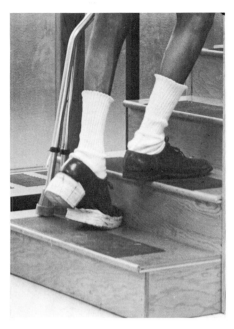

FIG. 33-6. A temporary lift of the left shoe, which may be used to assist a right hemiplegic to clear the floor.

abolically, compared with the use of an artificial limb (Fig. 33-7).

Increase in Endurance

Isotonic exercises have a training effect on the cardiovascular system and the heart itself. Such exercises may lead to an increase in endurance— that is, the length of time or the number of times that an activity can be carried out. Isotonic exercises train both skeletal and heart muscle and may produce changes in the oxygen transport system. Intracellular muscle enzymes increase, which thereby causes economy in the use of oxygen. Other changes may include a greater arteriovenous oxygen difference and a marked increase in the number of capillaries supplying a given area of muscle tissue. In addition, there is evidence of a training effect on the myocardium itself, so that the resting pulse rate may diminish and stroke volume may increase.

Exercise programs for the elderly have been organized both in this country and abroad, for example, in the Soviet Union and Holland.[19] They consist of calisthenic, rhythmical tasks, some of which may be performed in a chair. It might be feasible to organize such group programs in nursing homes, where the patients often show the ravages of deconditioning and disuse.

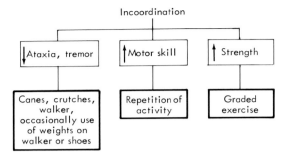

FIG. 33-7. Modalities of physical therapy applicable to incoordination. (Light boxes—symptom or affected function; heavy boxes—specific therapy; ↑, increase; ↓, decrease.)

Obviously, any exercise that the elderly carry out should be aerobic, with a steady state easily attained, and, therefore, submaximal, with avoidance of any oxygen debt.[22]

One simple technique for monitoring the elderly during any exercise activity is the pulse rate. Because there is a direct relationship between the pulse rate and oxygen consumption, beyond a minimum level, the severity of an exercise or activity for an elderly person and the oxygen consumed are directly related to his pulse, providing there is a regular sinus rhythm.

Anderson[1] monitored the pulse of 52 inpatients whose average age was in the mid-60s. All were severely disabled. He found that particular attention should be paid to the elderly patient whose resting pulse is above 100 or whose immediate postambulation pulse exceeded 120. A pulse rate over 130 often was indicative of excessive stress and could lead to dire consequences. Consequently, exercise producing a pulse above 130 was interdicted for the elderly convalescent inpatient.

That no elderly patient was allowed to exercise to a pulse level above 130 is of special interest in light of physiologic data. The maximum pulse rate with exercise for healthy persons of 65 is around 165.[2] It has been estimated that for a cardiovascular training effect, a pulse rate 60% to 80% of the maximum must be obtained (99 to 132 beats/min). The upper range (120 to 132 beats/min) includes values the elderly disabled patient seldom achieves and certainly does not sustain in a rehabilitation program. It appears that the exercises performed by the elderly in a typical rehabilitation program improve motor skill and efficiency of performance but may not significantly influence cardiovascular fitness (Fig. 33-8).

Despite those considerations of the limitations of the elderly and the elderly disabled, there is

evidence that the later years of life for many older individuals living in the community is "characterized by substantial physical ability." According to Jette and associates,[10] although advancing age is associated with a consistent increase in physical disability, the magnitude of the risk is less than is generally presumed.

A THERAPEUTIC PROGRAM FOR REHABILITATION

The first step in the rehabilitation management of an elderly patient is to evaluate his functional status. This would encompass the factors reviewed—namely range of motion, motor power, neuromuscular performance, and cardiopulmonary capacity. To this should be added the psychological and social status of the patient.

Evaluation

Because hemiplegia is so common among the elderly, let us use it as a prototype. In addition to the routine neurologic assessment of the patient, his psychologic status should be evaluated. Is the patient obtunded? Is he aphasic? Can he completely comprehend the simple and more complex directions that may be given? The patient's capacity for communication must be assessed. Obviously, with a dense aphasia, many tests that require his cooperation might be invalid. Rehabilitation is essentially a learning process and requires the patient to retain for tomorrow the skill acquired today. Sometimes the experienced clinician may use supplementary techniques for evaluation such as the double simultaneous stimulation test, in which the patient is touched simultaneously on the face and dorsum of the hand. The patient may err repeatedly by only perceiving the more cephalad stimulus. Another helpful test is to request the patient to keep his eyelids closed or his tongue protruded for as long as 20 seconds. In the presence of an organic mental syndrome, the patient may not be able to carry out these tasks appropriately.

Testing for sensory and sensorial loss is of major importance. Hemianopia is often associated with a hemisensory loss. These perceptual factors may create a far greater loss in motor skill than muscular weakness.

Management

Incontinence of bladder and bowel is seen early in the more severely involved. Urethral catheteriza-

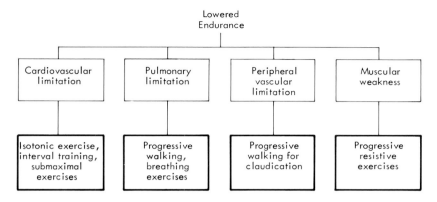

FIG. 33-8. Modalities of physical therapy applicable to lowered endurance. (Light boxes—symptom or affected function; heavy boxes—specific therapy; ↑, increase; ↓, decrease.)

tion may be required for the elderly male, although a condom sheath with a collecting bag is preferable in order to avoid urinary tract infections. Often with ambulation, incontinence improves, and the drainage devices can be discontinued.

At the Bedside

An activity program to prevent the sequelae of deconditioning can be started even during the acute stage of an illness. Such activity should, of course, be within the tolerance of the patient. Thus, initially for the patient with hemiplegia from a stroke the following schedule of activities might be provided. The paralyzed extremities are passively moved through their range of motion to prevent contractures. Proper positioning of the patient's limbs in bed might include a pillow under his arm and hand to prevent swelling of the hand from dependency and contractures, sandbags lateral to the leg to prevent prolonged external rotation of the hip, and a footboard to prevent a dropfoot from being maintained in plantarflexion.

Exercise Program

As soon as the patient's neurologic status is stabilized, and even within the first 1 or 2 days, mild activity or active assistive exercises may be initiated for the uninvolved side. Within a few days, self-care techniques may be taught so that the patient may learn to perform bimanual activities unimanually. The patient may also be assisted in transferring from bed to chair or wheelchair. An arm sling may be given if there is subluxation of the paralyzed shoulder (Fig. 33-9). Later the patient may be started on an ambulation program,

first standing between parallel bars, then walking in parallel bars, and finally progressing to the use of a cane outside the bars. Obviously, the rate of progress depends on the severity of the case. For the patient treated at home, substitutions may be developed with ingenuity. For example, straight-back chairs may substitute for the bars.

Skilled evaluation is needed regarding the use of a brace. Most hemiplegics can learn to walk either without any brace or with a below-knee brace, which provides stability at the ankle. Occasionally, a T-strap is attached at the ankle to correct medial or lateral deviations of the joint. For the knee that buckles on weight bearing, a full length leg brace may be required. Such a brace is heavy, difficult to put on independently, and tends to produce a clumsy gait pattern. It usually precludes significant walking, except for transfer purposes or taking several steps within the home. Occasionally, a long leg brace may be prescribed as an intermediate step to early ambulation with the hope that it may be cut down to a below-knee brace as the patient's functional status improves. If a long leg brace is prescribed, it should have a knee lock on the inner longitudinal bar so that the uninvolved hand can more easily lock or unlock it (Fig. 33-10).

Such a patient is also likely to need a wheelchair, which should be thoughtfully prescribed to meet the patient's size and type of use. It should have foot supports and brakes.

Speech Therapy

Speech therapy is provided for the aphasic patient through formal training by a qualified speech clinician. The family should be advised of techniques

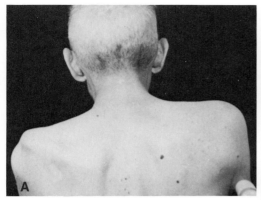

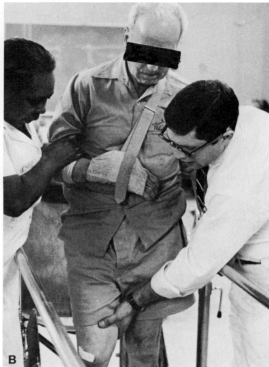

FIG. 33-9. (*A*) Subluxation of the left shoulder in a left hemiplegic. (*B*) Right hemiplegic wears an arm sling that may be used for subluxation of the paralyzed shoulder.

for helping the patient to improve his ability to communicate. These techniques used by the family may include repetition, speaking slowly and simply, using gestures, and maintaining a well structured and nondistractive environment.

Psychological Factors

Emotional support may be invaluable in overcoming the depression that results from the realization of the severity of the disability. In fact, depression as a temporary state is part of the process of readjustment. The patient who does not experience a "period of mourning" in recognition of his loss often reflects severe intellectual deficit due to brain injury.

Motivation plays a very important role in the ability of a patient to regain the lost or impaired skills of daily living. For the severely disabled patient, all who provide care should be sensitive to creating the optimal conditions for learning required tasks. One invaluable method is to demonstrate success to the patient with small tasks of progressive complexity that he can perform. Short-

term goals that are too ambitious may be demoralizing.

PROGNOSIS FOR REHABILITATION

There are some guidelines to help in predicting recovery from chronic disability such as that produced by stroke. In general, as with many neurologic disorders of brain, spinal cord, or peripheral nerve, the earlier that return of function appears, the greater the return that takes place. For example, if there has been no significant return of function in a flail arm and hand 1 month after a stroke, they are likely to remain nonfunctional.[3]

Incontinence of bladder and bowel that persists in a stroke patient for more than several days is a poor prognostic sign. Bowel incontinence of central origin usually signifies severe organic mental syndrome. Although depression as a transitional state is almost a necessary process in the patient's early rehabilitation, the converse is also true. The stroke patient who is euphoric—for example, one with an organic mental syndrome or with a per-

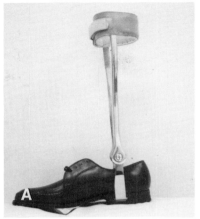

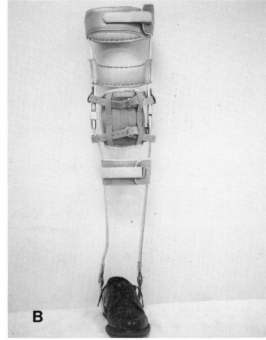

FIG. 33-10. (*A*) Below-the-knee brace with 90-degree stop. (*B*) Full-length leg brace with medial lock.

sistent dense aphasia—has a poorer prognosis for rehabilitation.

Left hemiplegia is often associated with a poorer outcome than right hemiplegia. The left hemiplegic, even though he usually has no language disorder, often shows poor judgment, disturbance in abstract thought, and perceptual motor disorders such as constructional apraxia (an inability to reproduce geometric designs). These characteristics interfere with carrying out the tasks of daily life, and they may subject the patient to undue risks of trauma.

Chronologic age *per se* is not closely correlated with successful outcome in rehabilitation. Physiologic age is often the more significant determinant. For example, a man of 75 with the same amputation as a 55-year-old man may suffer less severe disability if he is thinner, if he had been athletic as an adult in contrast to sedentary habits in the younger man, and if he has no other significant health problem such as cardiac disease or arthritis, which could be found in the 55-year-old man.

Concomitant disabilities may influence the outcome. For example, if the amputee needs to use one or two canes but has rheumatoid arthritis in his wrists, his capacity to walk would be seriously

compromised because he would need his arms for assisting in his ambulation.

Finally, the *sine qua non* for success is either the patient's motivation or an environment that influences him to attain feasible goals.

REHABILITATION SERVICES FOR THE ELDERLY

For the institutionalized aged, the resources of physical medicine and rehabilitation should be made available through the consultation services of a physiatrist. Under his supervision, a meaningful program of physical activity might be devised to counteract the consequences of deconditioning. This might prevent deformities such as contractures and weakness owing to disease. It might improve motor skill and possibly cardiovascular performance. The objective should be maintaining or regaining the maximum capacity at which the elderly person can safely perform. But most elderly people live in the community with families rather than in institutions. For them, the capacity to perform independently is often determined by the environment. Thus, architectural barriers, such as flights of steps or bathroom thresholds that do not permit a wheelchair to cross, may limit performance. Other limitations may be imposed by inappropriate furniture such as a chair that is so low that an arthritic cannot stand up because of weakness and pain of the hip extensors. A bed that is too high for the stroke patient may make independent transfer to a chair impossible.

Simple modifications in the home ensure greater safety and function for the disabled elderly. They may include a grab bar in the bathtub or beside the toilet seat, or modifications in the kitchen that enable the disabled housewife to perform her daily work. An extensive list of self-help devices has been made[15] that may enhance the performance of disabled hands. Examples include increasing the size of a handle for a toothbrush and modifications in clothing—large buttons, elastic shoelaces, and a long-handled shoehorn.

When the resources of the physiatrist and other members of the rehabilitation group are available (physical therapist, occupational therapist, speech therapist, recreation worker), their skills may be very valuable for attaining higher levels of physical performance by the elderly. Many areas lack such services, but with ingenuity on the part of physician and family much can be devised to help the disabled elderly to live with dignity and usefulness.

REFERENCES

1. Anderson AD: The use of the heart rate as a monitoring device in an ambulation program—a progress report. Arch Phys Med Rehabil 45:140, 1964
2. Astrand I: Aerobic work capacity—its relation to age, sex and other factors. In Physiology of Muscular Exercise, American Heart Association Monograph No. 15. New York, American Heart Association, 1967
3. Bard G, Hirschberg G: Recovery of voluntary motion in upper extremity following hemiplegia. Arch Phys Med Rehabil 46:567, 1965
4. Bard G, Ralston HJ: Measurement of energy expenditures during ambulation with special reference to evaluation of assistive devices. Arch Phys Med Rehabil 40:415, 1969
5. Brain L, Norris F Jr: The remote effects of cancer on the nervous system. In Contemporary Neurology Symposia, vol I. New York, Grune & Stratton, 1964
6. Campbell MJ, McComas AJ, Petito F: Physiological changes in aging muscles. Neurol Neurosurg Psychiatry 36:174, 1973
7. Donald KW et al: Cardiovascular response to sustained (static) contractions. Circ Res [Suppl] 20:1, 1967
8. Gordon EE et al: A study of rehabilitation potential in nursing home patients over 65 years. J Chronic Dis 15:311, 1962
9. Gutmann E, Hanzlekova V: The motor unit in old age. Nature 209:921, 1966
10. Jette AM, Branch LG: The Framingham Disability Study: II. Physical Disability among the Aging. Am J Public Health 71:1211, 1981
11. Lowenthal M: Experience in physical medicine and rehabilitation on a home care program. J Chronic Dis 6:153, 1957
12. Lowenthal M, Tobis JS, Howard IR: An analysis of the rehabilitation needs and prognoses of 232 cases of cerebral vascular accident. Arch Phys Med Rehabil 40:183, 1959
13. Molbech S: Energy cost in level walking in subjects with an abnormal gait. Communications from The Danish National Association for Infantile Paralysis, 1966, No. 22
14. Muller JM, Tobis JS, Kelman HR: The rehabilitation potential of nursing home residents. Am J Public Health 53:243, 1963
15. National Foundation for Infantile Paralysis: Self-Help Devices for Rehabilitation. Dubuque, IA, William C. Brown, 1958
16. Reynolds FW, Abramson M, Young A: Rehabilitation potentials of patients in chronic disease institutions. J Chronic Dis 10:152, 1959
17. Rooke ED, Lambert EH, Hodgson CH: Myasthenia and malignant intrathoracic tumors. Trans Am Neurol Assoc 84:24, 1958
18. Rowe RWD: The effect of senility on skeletal muscles in the mouse. Exp Gerontol 4:119, 1969
19. Schreuder JTR: Maintaining physical fitness as a therapeutic measure in old age. Sandoz J Med Sci 8:8, 1968
20. Shanas E: Self assessment of physical function: White and black elderly in the United States. Second Conference on the Epidemiology of Aging. NIH. publication No. 80-969. Washington, DC, US Government Printing Office, 1980
21. Wilson LA, Lawson IR, Brass W: Multiple disorders in the elderly—a clinical and statistical study. Lancet 2:841, 1962
22. Zohman L, Tobis J: Cardiac Rehabilitation. New York, Grune & Stratton, 1970

V

Psychiatric and Behavioral Considerations in the Aged Patient

34 Psychiatric Disorders

Dan Blazer

Although true psychiatric disorders (except for the dementias) are less common in late life than at other stages of the life cycle, the combination of these disorders with physical illness and the inevitable involvement of the family with health care professionals render an understanding of these disorders essential for geriatricians and primary care physicians. Unfortunately, a traditional pessimism about the physical and mental capacities of older persons continues to pervade the conceptualization and practice of medicine, nursing, social work, and other health professions. Studies at Duke University's Center for the Study of Aging and Human Development and other centers around the country have demonstrated that the many ingrained beliefs regarding older persons are ill founded, because not only do the elderly demonstrate considerable malleability in their functioning, but they also are much happier and healthier than was originally believed.[21,22] In this chapter, four of the more common psychiatric disorders in late life will be discussed: (1) primary degenerative dementia, (2) affective disorders, (3) hypochondriasis, and (4) paranoid disorders. For each of these disorders, information will be presented regarding the epidemiology, etiology, diagnosis, and treatment. Each disorder will be used to illustrate how myth and fact must be separated if effective care is to be provided for older adults.

PRIMARY DEGENERATIVE DEMENTIA

According to the third edition of the *Diagnostic and Statistical Manual of Mental Disorders (DSM–III)*, the essential feature of the primary degenerative dementias is a loss of intellectual abilities of sufficient severity to interfere with social or occupational functioning.[10] The deficit found in the dementias is multifaceted and involves memory, judgment, abstract thought, and a variety of other higher cortical functions, including changes in personality and behavior.

Epidemiology

Most older persons complain that they have more difficulty remembering than at earlier stages of their lives. Unfortunately, this has created the illusion that older persons will "lose their minds" and become hopelessly senile if they survive to advanced old age. Nothing could be farther from the truth. Much recent attention has been directed to the primary degenerative dementias, specifically Alzheimer's disease and/or senile dementia of the Alzheimer's type. Although Alzheimer's disease is the most common experienced in late life, at no stage of the life cycle is the prevalence of dementia greater than 30% to 40%. Of all persons over the age of 65, less than 4% suffer from Alzheimer's disease. Although the risk of developing Alzheimer's disease certainly increases with age, the likelihood of an older adult contracting the disease between the ages of 65 and 70 is less than 5%.[1]

The clinical course of Alzheimer's disease varies in duration with age, since younger patients have a more malignant course and a shorter life expectancy. Nevertheless, the typical stages of the condition are generally predictable regardless of age and are presented in Table 34-1. Stage I is unnoticed by the family until the patient moves, is hospitalized for a physical illness, or is stressed with sudden increased responsibilities. This stage usually lasts 1 or 2 years. Stage II is by far the longest, lasting from 3 to 7 or 8 years and presents significant problems to family members. Patients are

TABLE 34-1 The Evolution of Dementia

Stage	Characteristics
I	Forgetfulness, concern (especially among the well educated and professionals), avoidance of groups, symptoms often unnoticed by the family
II	Confusion, denial of memory problems, rambling conversations or poverty of speech, disorientation, flattening of affect, impairment in social functioning and usual business or household tasks, suspiciousness
III	Wandering, impaired activities of daily living, "lives in the past," angry outbursts, frank delusional thoughts, incontinence

difficult to manage but generally can be maintained at home and are usually aware enough to protest institutionalization. Stage III is often the transition period between community and institutional care and usually lasts 1 to 2 years.

Etiology

Etiology of the dementias varies with the type of primary degenerative dementia being considered. A number of hypotheses have been suggested for Alzheimer's disease, senile dementia of the Alzheimer's type, multi-infarct dementia, and Pick's disease. Genetic factors undoubtedly contribute to some of these conditions, especially the presenile forms of Alzheimer's disease. Most relatives of a person with senile dementia of the Alzheimer's type can simply ignore their own risk for developing a dementia. However, there are families with appreciably greater risks, among whom relatives exhibit more severe disease and more members are affected. Early onset also suggests both an increased severity of the disease and a larger proportion of affected relatives.[14]

Much attention has been directed to the neurotransmitter deficits associated with Alzheimer's disease. A decline in the amount of the neurotransmitter acetylcholine has been implicated as causal in the decreased memory of dementia patients. Evidence for this has been primarily indirect—notably the recognition of decreased levels of choline acetyltransferase and acetylcholine esterase in the autopsied brains of the deceased demented.[6] This pathophysiologic change, however,

has not been totally explained. Coyle and his colleagues at Johns Hopkins University have suggested that the decline occurs secondary to a degeneration of nerve cell bodies in the nucleus basalis of Meynert.[8] The axons that project from this nucleus transmit information via the neurotransmitter acetylcholine.

Some "slow" viruses are known to affect the brain, and dementia of Alzheimer's type may be similar in etiology to the degenerative viral-related dementias such as scrapie (the disease of sheep and goats), kuru (a dementing illness limited to certain groups of natives in New Guinea), and Creutzfeldt-Jakob disease, which is characterized by a relatively rapid downhill course (months rather than years). Others have implicated heavy metals poisoning, especially that of aluminum, since the brains of victims of Alzheimer's disease contain high concentrations of aluminum in the characteristic neurofibrillary tangles. Epidemiologic studies have not confirmed a relationship between dietary intake of aluminum and the prevalence of this dementia. Finally, the immune system has been implicated—one of the components of another neuropathologic feature, the senile plaque, contains amyloid, which is present in many immune system disturbances. Despite ignorance regarding etiology, there is no question that Alzheimer's disease is a true disease, although many of the pathologic findings can be seen to a lesser degree in the normal aging brain.

The etiology may be more obvious in other dementias. For example, multi-infarct dementia is almost always associated with hypertension and is secondary to multiple small infarcts. Both Parkinson's disease, which is secondary to decreased levels of dopamine primarily in the substantia nigra, and Huntington's disease, a genetic disorder, are marked by variable degrees of dementia. The etiology of substance-induced dementia, specifically alcoholic amnestic disorder, has been known for many years to result from dietary deficiencies in thiamine following long-term excessive alcohol intake.

Diagnosis

The history and mental status examinations are the essential components of the diagnostic workup. Although it is frequently difficult to elicit a history from the patient, a family interview usually generates information needed for a reasonably correct diagnosis. This information should include a history of the onset, symptoms at various points through the course of the illness, a family history of dementia, concurrent physical and psychiatric illness (especially a history of depressive disorder and alcohol abuse), and a history of medication intake.

The mental status examination can be systematized by using an instrument such as the *Mini-Mental Status Exam.*[11] Basically, the mental status examination should include assessment of orientation and memory, judgment, and affectivity. Short-term memory can be tested by asking the patient the time of day, the date, the location, and so forth. Although near-miss answers are of less concern, gross inaccuracy reflects a significant deficit. Long-term memory can usually be determined as the patient describes past events, but many patients have learned to accommodate to their memory loss and may become convincing but inaccurate historians. For a more objective test, the patient can be asked dates of birth, of marriage, or of certain remote events, such as beginning work or retirement. The capacity for abstract thinking can be tested by asking the person to classify objects into a common category. For example, the patient is asked, "In what way are an apple and a pear similar?" Difficulty in performing tests of abstract thinking is a frequent early sign of organic mental disorder.

A physical and neurologic examination including an assessment of blood pressure, is essential in the workup for dementia. The laboratory workup of an obviously demented individual in whom no apparent secondary clinical cause can be identified should include a complete blood cell count, serologic tests for syphilis, a thyroid panel, urinalysis, chest roentgenography, computed tomography of the brain, and possibly a dexamethasone suppression test if there is serious question regarding a differential diagnosis between depression and dementia. Psychological testing in early forms of dementia can identify selective memory problems in the context of normal intelligence as against the general cognitive decline of dementia. All of these laboratory tests are specific for disorders that must be eliminated in the differential diagnosis of the Alzheimer type of dementia. Therefore, they are necessarily specific but usually insensitive. For example, the computed tomographic scan may demonstrate an infarct or a cerebral tumor (*e.g.*, a meningioma), but the yield is low. Computed tomographic scans are not specific for Alzheimer's disease because cortical atrophy and widening of the lateral ventricles can be seen in the normal aging brain. Nevertheless, the tests are valuable in establishing the high probability of Alzheimer's disease (given the absence of other findings) as

well as ruling out some infrequent but potentially treatable forms of dementia.

The first step in making a differential diagnosis of an organic mental disorder is to distinguish delirium (an acute or subacute disorder manifested by widespread dysfunction of nerve tissue and characterized primarily by confusion and attentional problems) from dementia, which is characterized by chronicity, with impairment of all cognitive functions, especially memory. Once it has been determined that the individual is suffering from a dementia, the disorders to be considered are, in decreasing frequency, primary degenerative dementia, senile onset; SDAT multi-infarct dementia (cerebrovascular disease); primary degenerative dementia, presenile onset (presenile dementia or Alzheimer's disease); alcohol amnestic disorder (Wernicke-Korsakoff syndrome); dementia secondary to Parkinson's disease; and Huntington's chorea. Pick's disease and other conditions mentioned previously are very rare in late life; indeed they are rare at all stages of the life cycle. The clinical picture of each of these conditions overlaps significantly, so, before autopsy, the clinician never can be certain that he is managing true Alzheimer's disease, a combination of Alzheimer's disease and multi-infarct dementia, Pick's disease, and so on. Nevertheless, certain clinical characteristics assist somewhat in making the differential diagnosis. Multi-infarct dementia may be associated with cardiovascular disease and an uneven course over the duration of the disease. The erythrocyte sedimentation rate may also be elevated. Creutzfeldt-Jakob disease can generally be distinguished by its relatively rapid course. Dementia associated with Parkinson's disease occurs late in the course of the disease, and the extrapyramidal symptoms are obvious. Huntington's disease can be diagnosed by the peculiar writhing movements and the usual family history. Normal pressure hydrocephalus, rare but potentially reversible, presents with dementia, ataxia and urinary incontinence. The CT scan easily identifies the dilated ventricles, which appear ballooned. "Pseudodementias," psychiatric disorders that present with a primary problem of memory, include depressive disorders, anxiety disorders, and chronic schizophrenia. Many older persons are convinced they have contracted this dread disorder because of slippage in their memory capacity. The symptoms of Alzheimer's disease are usually distinct from the more benign forgetfulness that may be troublesome but not incapacitating. For example, the normal older adult may forget, but usually notices that he or she has forgotten and eventually remembers the forgotten information. Those who suffer from SDAT forget, do not realize they forget, and frequently could not care less that they have forgotten. In fact, the Alzheimer patient is remarkable for a capacity to deny the severity of the memory loss.

Treatment

No definitive treatment is available at this time for the primary degenerative dementias. Nevertheless, the clinician should not assume that no treatment is available. By establishing a cooperative and helpful relationship with the patient and the family coupled with a thorough diagnostic workup, the physician frequently can relieve many of their concerns. Frequently, other physical and psychiatric problems accompany the dementia. Therefore a "tune-up" of organ systems, improving cardiac and pulmonary function along with the elimination of nonessential medications, may improve the demented older adult. The physician should also make every effort to minimize sensory impairments, especially impairments in vision and hearing.

There is no known primary treatment of the underlying dementia process. Hydergine, a product containing ergoloid mesylates, is the only drug available in the United States. In one review it was found that most control studies using this agent do demonstrate some improvement in overall functioning.[28] One of the difficulties in evaluation has been the inability of most investigators to control for emotional and behavioral factors when attempting to measure acute changes in cognitive functioning.

If one accepts the cholinergic hypothesis of organic mental disorders, therapeutic agents containing choline (such as lecithin) or anticholinergic blocking agents such as physostigmine could be beneficial. Preliminary trials are being conducted with these agents. Most trials have not found lecithin to be effective. In a few trials, physostigmine has been of some benefit, but it has many potential adverse side-effects.

Pharmacologic agents are certainly indicated in the control of many secondary symptoms of the primary degenerative dementias, such as agitation and paranoia. These symptoms are often effectively controlled by low doses of phenothiazines or butyrophenones, such as thioridazine (Mellaril), haloperidol (Haldol). Usual doses would be haloperidol, 0.5 mg, or thioridazine, 10 mg, orally three times a day. The clinician must be aware of the frequent extrapyramidal side-effects, such as parkinsonian tremors and dyskinesias. Some re-

port the occurrence of these symptoms to increase with age. The most dreaded side-effect is tardive dyskinesia, which also increases in frequency with age. Unlike the extrapyramidal effects, the tardive dyskinesias do not always reverse with age; usually about 50% experience a significant remission in symptoms 1 year following cessation of the medication. The most frequent tardive symptom is dyskinetic and uncontrollable movement of the tongue, which not only is embarrassing but also may interfere with dietary intake. Insomnia and anxiety should not be treated with the benzodiazepines (such as flurazepam or diazepam) but rather with the antipsychotic agents, such as thioridazine, despite the adverse reactions of the latter agent. The benzodiazepines increase confusion and therefore lead to a paradoxic agitation.

The family can be a great asset in managing patients suffering from dementia. Not only can the physician demonstrate empathy for the family and attempt to educate the family concerning the illness, but suggestions can be made regarding the management of many of the typical behavioral problems that accompany dementia. An excellent detailed guide for family members in managing such problems is found in the book by Mace and Rabins.[18] Families can also be referred to a nationwide network of support groups.* For example, the management of wandering may include obtaining a necklace or bracelet with the name and phone number of the patient along with the statement "memory impairment." Reassurance offered to the disoriented patient may decrease attempts to "find where he belongs" or "find my wife." Exercise may also reduce restlessness. Keeping the doors locked at night coupled with the removal of dangerous equipment (such as unplugging the stove at night) may alleviate the concerns of the family managing the nocturnal wanderer.

DEPRESSION: TREATABILITY OF PSYCHOPATHOLOGY IN LATE LIFE

Since depression is one of the most common emotional problems, and the leading cause of suicide among the elderly, it should be regarded as a clinical entity of major concern. The recalcitrant dysphoric affect of some older adults, however, has biased the health care provider and thus denied many severely depressed older adults access to treatment modalities that are most effective.

* The Alzheimer's Disease and Related Disorders Association, Inc., 360 North Michigan Avenue, Suite 601, Chicago, IL 60601.

Epidemiology and Etiology

The prevalence of depressive symptoms in the community is quite high—15% of the elderly population in most studies.[4] The symptoms are about equally distributed between males and females and may be the result of a number of causes. Grief reactions, which are more frequent in late life than at other stages of the life cycle, cannot be distinguished from major depressive episodes. Only the identification of a significant loss enables the clinician to diagnose bereavement. Depressive symptoms may also accompany major life adjustments, including a change in residence, retirement, decline in physical health, or decline in economic resources. Yet the prevalence of major depressive episodes in late life is surprisingly low, actually lower than at any other stage of the adult life cycle. Most studies demonstrate a current prevalence of major depressive episodes in community populations of between 1% and 3%.[4,27] As suggested previously, depressive symptoms may be ubiquitous with increasing age, since the very term *depression* is ambiguous. In its broadest, most popular meaning, depression refers to everyday normal experiences of feeling "low," "blue," or simply "down in the dumps." Given the inevitability of loss and forced adjustments in late life, these symptoms are not infrequently encountered by those who care for older adults. Yet at the same time these older adults may not complain of being "depressed" (a relatively new psychological construct that has made a prominent entrance into the general vocabulary of the population only in recent times). Nevertheless, most of the dysphoric episodes encountered in late life are transient and the older person recovers spontaneously. These transient depressive episodes require little intervention by the clinician, other than support and possibly the short-term use of the benzodiazepines for the symptomatic control of agitation and sleep disturbances. The use of short-acting agents, such as oxazepam 15 mg, or alprazolam, 0.5 mg orally twice daily for agitation and temazepam, 15 mg, or triazolam, 0.25 mg, for sleep disturbance is usually sufficient. If these agents must be used for longer than 2 weeks, the clinician must reevaluate the symptoms and avoid the potential for tolerance if they are prescribed regularly over a longer period of time.

Of much greater importance are the major depressive disorders that occur for the first time in late life (or that recur in late life after having first occurred at earlier stages of the life cycle). These "clinical depressions" are characterized by the severity of their symptoms and duration of the pro-found depressed mood and would typically be diagnosed in the *DSM–III* as a major depressive episode with melancholia and/or psychotic features. The diagnostic criteria are presented below:

DSM–III DIAGNOSTIC CRITERIA FOR A MAJOR DEPRESSIVE EPISODE* (ANNOTATED FOR THE ELDERLY)

A sad or depressed mood (Frequently, older persons will only complain of being tired or "down in the dumps.")

Duration for at least 2 weeks, with four of the following symptoms present to a significant degree:

Poor appetite or significant weight loss (very common in the elderly) or weight gain (rare)

Insomnia (almost universal in the depressed elderly)

Loss of energy (very common in the depressed elderly)

Psychomotor agitation (the usual feature) or retardation (characteristic of the more severe late-onset depressives)

Loss of interest or pleasure in usual activities (common) or decrease in sexual drive (an infrequent complaint in late life)

Feelings of self-reproach or inappropriate guilt (infrequent in the elderly)

Diminished ability to think or concentrate, such as slowed thinking (a common complaint)

Suicidal thoughts (Older persons are less likely to report such thoughts, but the risk of suicide is greatest in late life depressives.)

*Adapted from Diagnostic and Statistical Manual of Mental Disorders, 3rd ed, pp 213–214. Washington, DC, American Psychiatric Association, 1980

These symptoms must be distinguished from a normal grief reaction or other conditions, such as an organic mental disorder, which may include appreciable depressive symptomatology. A genetic predisposition is probable, although the contribution of heredity to the disorder is undoubtedly less than at earlier stages of the life cycle.[16] Certain neurophysiologic changes that accompany normal aging may predispose the older person to the development of major depression. For example, older persons have a relative increase in levels of monoamine oxidase in the brain, which may contribute to a decrease in the catecholamine level. Such decreases have been implicated in depressive disorders in all stages of the life cycle.[24] The endocrine system may also undergo changes with aging, and increased emphasis has been placed on the connection between neuroendocrine alterations and a propensity to develop an endogenous depressive disorder. This is best evidenced by the findings of Carroll and colleagues[5] of nonsuppression of cortisol secretion following administration of dexamethasone in individuals suffering from major depressive episodes. No evidence suggests that older healthy persons are less likely to exhibit suppression by dexamethasone than persons at earlier stages of the life cycle. This suggests that the dexamethasone suppression test may be just as applicable in late life as at other stages of the life cycle.[25] Finally, sleep disturbances traditionally associated with depression, such as shortened rapid eye movement (REM) latency, decreased sleep efficiency, and shortened overall sleep time, are also found more frequently in late life. Therefore, distinguishing the sleep patterns of a normal older adult from a depressed person at earlier stages of the life cycle can be most difficult. A disruption of circadian rhythms that occurs normally in late life may predispose the older person to the development of a major depressive disorder.

Finally, most persons who comment on the depressions of late life emphasize the stress that older persons inevitably face. In fact, older persons are less likely to encounter stressful life events when measured by typical scales, such as the *Schedule of Recent Events*.[15] Nevertheless, common experience suggests that older persons do experience frequent exit events, such as the loss of spouse, siblings, and friends. Even in adapting to these losses, however, older persons may have unique advantages. Neugarten[19] suggests that older persons have "rehearsed" expected exit events, such as the death of a spouse, and therefore are better prepared to accept and adapt to this change. It is important for events to be anticipated, expected, or "on time" during the life cycle; unanticipated events are more likely to be traumatic.

Diagnosis

The diagnosis of depressive disorders in late life is not easy. Many clinicians have suggested that older persons mask their depressive symptoms. Symptoms of depression are thought to be highest among persons over the age of 65, but many of these are "somatic" symptoms, including sleep disturbance, decreased appetite, lethargy, and discouragement about the future, in contrast to a decrease in self-esteem, guilt, or delusions of per-

secution. An especially complicating symptom is the complaint of "difficulty concentrating." Depressed individuals with difficulty concentrating and memory loss are often thought of as suffering from "pseudodementia." Means by which pseudodementia can be distinguished from a true dementing illness are presented in Table 34-2. The most common instances of depressive symptoms in late life are the simple and transient dysphorias described previously (which may not have an obvious etiology) and are best diagnosed in the category of atypical depressive disorder in the *DSM-III*. Bereavement is probably the second most common cause of depressive symptomatology and generally can be recognized by the clinician who has gathered a suitable history. Depressive neuroses (dysthymic disorder) occur less commonly, rarely have their onset for the first time in late life, and usually are recognized by their intractability and resistance to usual modes of therapy.

Depressive symptoms often accompany medical illnesses and in fact are the direct result of these illnesses. Most commonly encountered in the elderly are depressive symptoms secondary to hypothyroidism, Cushing's disease, occult malignancy, and malnutrition (especially vitamin B_{12} deficiency). These depressive syndromes are generally more severe than those seen with a transient dysphoric mood and usually are diagnosed during a thorough medical workup. Medications frequently prescribed to older adults can also lead to significant depressive symptomatology, especially sedative hypnotic agents, antianxiety agents, antihypertensive agents (*e.g.*, guanethidine, reserpine, and propranolol), and corticosteroids. Depressive symptoms may also accompany the early stages of a true primary degenerative dementia but generally disappear as the dementia progresses.

The "clinical depressions" or major depressive disorders are characterized by the severity of their symptoms and the duration of the profound depressed mood as described above. Clinicians must acquire the capacity to recognize severe depressions, which can potentially eventuate in a suicide attempt or even a successful suicide.

Unfortunately, severe depressions frequently remained undetected and therefore older adults suffer unnecessarily from the burden of depressive symptoms. Occasionally, the clinician will encounter an older adult suffering from a bipolar affective disorder (with both manic and depressive episodes), but usually manic episodes in late life are less frequent and are not typical of mania at earlier stages of the life cycle. Manic episodes are not characterized by a jovial mood but rather by increased irritability and agitation.

TABLE 34-2 Clinical Characteristics of Depression (Pseudodementia) and Dementia

Dementia	Depression
Onset is slow and indeterminate.	Rapid onset that can usually be dated is noted.
Mental impairment is relatively stable.	Cognitive function fluctuates markedly.
Mood is typically shallow and fluctuates.	Mood is consistently depressed.
The patient tends to cover disabilities.	The patient tends to exaggerate disabilities.
"Near miss" answers and evasion are typical responses on the mental status examination.	"Don't know" answers are typical on the mental status examination.

(Modified from Wells CE: Dementia, pseudodementia, and dementia praecox. In Fann WE et al (eds): Phenomenology and Treatment of Schizophrenia. New York, Spectrum Publishing, 1978)

Treatment

Major depressive disorders in late life are eminently treatable. Appropriate medications, such as the tricyclic antidepressants, can reverse the symptomatology in over 70% of persons so affected. Physicians who prescribe medications to the older adult must always be aware of the potential for adverse side-effects, and antidepressant drugs are among those that produce frequent side-effects. Of special concern are the anticholinergic side-effects that may interfere with the memory of an already compromised older adult. By adjusting dosage downward, and monitoring the drug use carefully, most depressed older adults can tolerate these medications without difficulty. The depressed older adult should not be denied these powerful therapeutic agents because their severe depressions are not recognized or physicians are not skilled in prescribing them appropriately. An example would be the prescription of nortriptyline, usually beginning at a dosage of 50 mg, orally H.S. A therapeutic effect can often be attained at a dosage of between 75 mg and 100 mg orally H.S. in the elderly (in contrast to the 150-mg threshold usually recommended for younger persons). Desipramine in a dosage of 25 mg orally twice daily is excellent for the less common retarded major depressions in late life. Trazodone, because of the virtual absence of anticholinergic side-effects, has been recommended for late life depressions but is not without side-effects and is often not well tolerated. The clinician must take care to identify persons who suffer from postural hypotension on these medications. Syncope and falls are not uncommon in these older adults.

When medications fail, electroconvulsive therapy (ECT) may be an effective treatment. The negative public image of ECT alone renders this therapy one that is selected only in the most resistant and severe cases. It must be prescribed with care for older adults, since health problems and difficulties with memory may complicate the course. Nevertheless, ECT, when administered properly, is safe and may be extremely effective. In tricyclic antidepressant–resistive severe depressions, unilateral, nondominant ECT is effective in over 70% of the cases.[26]

Finally, older persons should not be denied access to psychotherapy for depressive illnesses that are less severe, especially those who do not present to the clinician with the more "biological symptoms and signs." Freud[12] believed that psychotherapy was ineffective in later years (later life for him being over the age of 40). Interestingly, he continued to "self-analyze" himself until well into his advanced years. Although the more traditional insight-oriented psychotherapies probably are less effective in the elderly, psychotherapeutic intervention should not be dismissed summarily. Studies suggest that short-term, cognitive and behaviorally oriented therapies can be effective in treating depressed older adults and that these improvements are not transient.[13] These psychotherapies combine supportive and educational components, are well tolerated by older persons, and are beneficial in changing adaptive styles to stressful life situations.

HYPOCHONDRIASIS: THE DISTINCTION BETWEEN PHYSICAL AND PSYCHIATRIC SYMPTOMS

The essence of hypochondriasis is a clinical picture in which the predominant disturbance is an unrealistic interpretation of physical signs or sensations as abnormal; this in turn leads to a preoccupation with the fear or belief of having a serious disease.[10] Even a thorough physical examination and laboratory workup that do not support the diagnosis and reassurance by the physician do little to alleviate the patient's anxiety. Therefore, hypochondriasis emerges as one of the most perplexing, frustrating, and difficult conditions to clinicians in a busy medical practice. Frequently an older patient (who may have exhausted the patience of many caretakers in the past) arrives in the clinician's office with a full inventory of new and used complaints, and protestation of a miraculous belief that there is at last someone who will bring relief.

Epidemiology

Most studies suggest that the prevalence of exaggerated physical complaints is between 10% and 20% of elderly people. In a community survey in Durham, North Carolina, approximately 10% of the elderly perceived their physical health to be poorer than it was when rated objectively.[2] It was of interest that an equal proportion of the older adults believed their health to be better than it measured objectively while most perceived their health to be near what was objectively evaluated. A separate study found that 53.6% of older persons thought themselves to be in better health than other older persons. Thirty-one percent believed their own health to be about the same as others, and only 9.8% considered their health to be worse than that of older persons their own age.[20] Therefore the assumption that older persons are uniquely predisposed to hypochondriacal symptoms and a poor evaluation of their health status is not verified in community studies. Probably excessive demands on physicians by these patients leads to the misconception that they typify older adults; they may indeed represent a significant proportion of the practice of the clinician.

Etiology

Hypochondriasis is of psychogenic etiology and has countless psychiatric interpretations. It has been thought to be a symbol of the older person's sense of decreased effectiveness and deterioration; a means of communicating and interacting with others; a device for transferring anxiety from other areas of concern to the body; a way of identifying with a deceased loved one who had similar physical symptoms; a means by which guilt can be assuaged through self-punishment; and an attention-getting device. Because these individuals require so much time and energy and demand so much from the clinicians, they undoubtedly obtain considerable secondary gain. Nevertheless, true physical illness can occur and must be monitored carefully.

Diagnosis

Although most older people are relatively healthy, many have contracted at least one chronic, if not disabling, physical illness. In addition, older persons frequently have not been "educated" in the language of either medicine or psychiatry. Sifting through the ever-present but poorly described array of complaints can be an arduous task. First, the older person cannot automatically be assumed to be a "chronic complainer" because physicians in the past have been unable to uncover a specific physical disorder to account for the complaints. For example, silent myocardial infarction, vitamin deficiencies, or thyroid dysfunction may produce diffuse, nondescript symptoms that can be labeled as "hypochondriacal," only later to progress to a more readily diagnosable level. Therefore, the busy clinician must, first of all, listen patiently to the description of symptoms, look for changing patterns in their presentation, assess the degree of suffering experienced, and perform a thorough physical examination.

Further phenomena complicate the ability of clinicians to understand the meaning of physical symptoms. The "cohort phenomenon" well known to students of the psychology of late life, is frequently overlooked by the health care provider. Older persons are not only subject to inevitable physical problems but also are products of the culture in which they were raised and through which they passed into adulthood. For example, one cannot automatically assume that the larger number of physical complaints by older adults compared with younger individuals is a constant manifestation of an aging process. In fact, evidence suggests the contrary. The cohorts of older adults who do complain most frequently of physical symptoms (especially the more aged cohorts in the 1980s) have, to the best of our knowledge, always complained of more physical symptoms. Longitudinal studies suggest that the level of symptom complaint increases very little with time itself. One explanation is that older persons were products of a childhood devoid of "psychological insights" available to persons aged 40 and under, that is, the elderly did not have the "advantage" of child rearing during the psychological society—"the age of Dr. Spock." Emotional distress is therefore frequently verbalized as physical symptomatology.

Concern with bowel habits and certain other changes in bodily function are also typical of birth cohorts who are aged today.

Following a thorough workup, the physician is in a position to determine if the patient is indeed suffering from hypochondriasis. The diagnosis is suggested when the predominant disturbance is an unrealistic interpretation of physical signs or sensations as abnormal and a preoccupation with the fear or belief of having an undiagnosed disease, although mild chronic physical problems may co-exist. Persistence of the unrealistic fears or beliefs in spite of medical reassurance not only leads to increased visits to the physician but also causes impairment in social, occupational, and recreational functioning.

The hypochondriacal preoccupation must be distinguished from schizophrenia as well as affective, somatization, and anxiety disorders.[10] In the psychotic disorders such as schizophrenia or major depression with psychotic features, there may be somatic delusions (*i.e.,* delusions of having a disease such as a cancer) whereas in hypoochondriasis the concern does not have the fixed characteristic of a delusion. In major depression or generalized anxiety disorder, the hypochondriacal preoccupation may appear but usually is not the predominant disturbance. For example, these individuals readily discuss their depressed or anxious affect and present a picture of some desperation. Clues in differentiating hypochondriasis from the depressive disorders are presented in Table 34-3. Somatization disorder, a less frequent syndrome, by definition does not have its onset in late life. It can be diagnosed only when the multiple somatic symptoms appear before the age of 40. In addition, patients suffering from a somatization disorder are more preoccupied with their symptoms than with a fear of having a specific disease, as is seen in the hypochondriacal patient.

Treatment

Treating the individual suffering from hypchondriasis is not easy, but certain guidelines can be helpful in management.[3] First, the physician must recognize that the patient is "ill" and express a professional interest in the patient. Regardless of the particular reason that drives a patient to the physician's office, a commitment should be made to help that patient through the suffering experienced. Listening attentively to the description of symptoms is essential in establishing rapport. During the initial visit, it is important to perform a thorough physical examination. Only routine screening laboratory tests should be performed. Medications such as analgesics or mild tranquilizers can be helpful in supporting the therapeutic relationship, but the potential for addiction in the hypochondriacal individual is high. Therefore, such drugs must be used with caution.

The key to management is the structure of the long-term relationship. These patients initially require rather frequent visits (often bimonthly) but, with time, visits should decrease in frequency. During the return visit, a specific amount of time, usually about 20 minutes, should be alloted. A brief interval history can be obtained from the patient and a very brief (5 minutes) physical examination performed. The remainder of the ses-

TABLE 34-3   Clinical Clues for Differentiating Hypochondriasis From the Depressive Disorders in the Elderly

Hypochondriasis	Depressive Disorders
Patients do not appear to be suffering, despite the frequent report of physical symptoms.	Patients suffer from both their physical and psychiatric symptoms.
Anger is directed toward others.	Anger is more likely to be directed toward self.
Patients are very sensitive to the side-effects of medications.	Patients tolerate the side-effects of medications as well as other elderly patients.
A history of physical problems in mid life is common.	Mid-life physical complaints are less common.
Social participation is hampered but not dysfunctional.	Decreased social participation is prominent and frequently dysfunctional.

(Modified from Blazer DG, Siegler IC: A Family Approach to Health Care of the Elderly, p 145. Menlo Park, CA, Addison-Wesley, 1984)

sion should be used to encourage the patient to discuss personal or social issues and deemphasize concern with somatic problems. The hypochondriacal patient is most manipulative with time, and therefore the clinician must terminate each visit promptly, regardless of how "important" the patient believes certain information is that is revealed toward the end of the visit. Eventually, patients can be "trained" to report essential information within the limits of the return visit. Physicians should not venture a diagnosis or prognosis of the patient's condition but at the same time should avoid interpretations such as, "it's all in your head." Frequently hypochondriacal patients will attack previous health care providers. The physician should neither defend nor criticize these providers but enable the patient to concentrate on the present relationship. With these demanding patients it is easy for physicians to wish to retaliate or argue with them regarding their symptoms or history of health care. Nevertheless, the physician should avoid confrontations with such patients whenever possible. In like manner, the physician should avoid unrealistic promises to "cure" the patient's illness. In general, these patients are best managed in the office of the primary care physician and referral to a specialist is to be avoided whenever possible.

As can be seen, the goals of "managing" the hypochondriacal patient are much different from the goals of treating other physical and psychiatric conditions. Although hypochondriacal symptoms may occasionally remit, hypochondriasis is more chronic than most psychiatric (and even physical) disorders encountered in older adults, but it has not proved to be as disabling over time as such disorders. Structuring the relationship between the patient and the primary care physician is the key for achieving successful therapeutic intervention. The time of visits, nature of the interaction, and physician expectations must be structured and maintained. This consistency is of great comfort to the patient because he recognizes that a degree of dependency can be transferred to the physician but only within certain limits.

PARANOID DISORDERS IN LATE LIFE: FAMILY INTERVENTION

Although overt paranoid psychoses are much less common in late life than dementia and the depressive disorders, paranoid symptoms are frequently encountered. Older persons often have the reputation of being morose, rigid, and suspicious

of anything new or unusual. Health care providers are likely to encounter certain older persons who are narrow minded, quarrelsome, unsociable, insensitive, withdrawn, and cold. They leave those with whom they come into contact tense and angry. Nevertheless, the paranoid older adult frequently requires medical treatment and the proper management of paranoid and suspicious behavior is critical to implementing other medical therapies.

Epidemiology

Lowenthal and Berkman, in a community sample of older persons in San Francisco, found of those rated psychiatrically impaired 17% had symptoms of suspiciousness and 13% of delusions.[17] In the entire sample, only 2.5% showed suspiciousness and 2% had delusions. Christenson and Blazer[6] found the prevalence of generalized persecutory ideation to be 4% in a community population. Sensory deficits, social isolation, medical illness, cognitive impairment, and the aging process itself are thought to place older persons at higher risk for persecutory thoughts. Cooper[7] and colleagues found a high frequency of deafness in patients with paranoid psychosis when compared with controls with affective psychosis. In the study by Christenson and Blazer,[6] sensory deficits and cognitive impairments were significant risk factors for the development of persecutory ideation. This ideation was also associated with impairments in physical health, social and economic resources, and activities of daily living.

Roth and his co-workers[23] found that approximately 10% of the elderly admitted for the first time to psychiatric institutions were basically "schizophrenic" and invariably had paranoid symptoms. The symptoms were typical of the schizophrenic disorders and included thought disorders, constriction and blunting of mood, and decreased volition. However, these individuals did not conform to the usual schizophrenic clinical picture because their personalities did not deteriorate rapidly, they maintained excellent cognitive functioning, and the percentage of first-degree relatives also suffering from schizophrenia was lower than for other types of schizophrenia.

Etiology

Paranoid symptoms in older persons may derive from several sources. First, paranoid behavior may be a way in which some older persons cope with their social environment. All persons continually scan the environment through their senses. Subconsciously, this scanning process enables individuals to integrate information and gives clues as to how to react to the environment. With advancing age, many perceptual abilities decrease (such as hearing) and the scanning process becomes less functional. Gaps appear in the individual's perception of the environment. Cognitive impairment may further complicate this problem.

Older persons may react to these gaps in at least two ways. First, they may decrease the range of their social environment. For examples, persons who suffer from cognitive impairment or perceptual difficulties may constrict their sphere of social activity to their neighborhood, their house, or even to one room in the house. The older person feels capable of mastering the sensory input from the more limited environment. Second, older persons may fill the gaps in perception with fantasy or other unconscious material. Fantasies enable them to explain situations and events that are not easily understood. As this fantasy material is integrated, it may lead to a frankly delusional orientation to the social environment. For example, an older woman who lives alone may interpret the numerous sights and sounds from the street as war maneuvers or other clandestine activities. Accompanying reactions to gaps in perceiving the social environment may include narrow-minded and rigid opinions of the environment. Therefore, the older person will not accept another explanation of misperceived events, even after the most logical explanation by the health care provider or family member. To the contrary, anyone who challenges the view is automatically not to be trusted. As mistrust of individuals increases, unsociable behavior develops, which leads in turn to increased withdrawal.

A less common disturbance of late life paranoid symptoms has been termed *late life paraphrenia.* Persons suffering from this schizophreniclike disorder are generally cognitively intact but are frankly delusional. Their personalities do not tend to deteriorate as rapidly as is seen in earlier life, and they may maintain excellent cognitive and perceptual functioning. Their thinking is frankly delusional and easily detected by the primary care physician. A mixed variety of these paranoid syndromes can certainly be seen in the elderly.

Diagnosis

Many factors can lead to paranoid symptomatology in late life. The list includes all the causes that may lead to organic mental disorders, including primary degenerative dementia of senile onset;

multi-infarct dementia; alcohol-related organic mental disorders, transitory or permanent (the alcohol amnestic syndrome); medications; and the delirium or organic hallucinosis of impaired physical functioning (*e.g.,* chronic obstructive pulmonary disease). Paranoid symptoms may emerge in the context of the schizophreniclike picture described previously but also may be seen in major depressive episodes with psychotic features. Finally, a chronic paranoid personality disorder that begins in childhood or early adolescence may persist into late life and may be exaggerated by changes in the environment of the older adult.

Therefore, the diagnostic workup of patients with paranoid symptoms must include a thorough history, mental status and physical examinations, a neurologic examination, laboratory procedures when appropriate (especially those that relate to identifying an acute delirium), and drug screens (for excessive levels of antianxiety or sedative hypnotic agents or even amphetaminelike drugs). Caution must be used when performing a mental status examination and physical examination. The formal mental status examination should be limited to areas not accessible through history, including items on memory and knowledge. Questions should always be prefaced by statements such as, "I'm now going to ask you a group of questions that I ask all persons whom I talk with. Some of the answers may be very easy and others may be quite hard. Just do the best you can. Please do not be insulted if the answers appear too easy." Most older persons with paranoid symptoms will cooperate with this portion of the examination if even a minimal relationship has been developed with the clinician. The physical examination should usually be performed in the presence of a third party, especially when paranoid symptoms are significant. Examination of the rectum and genitals generally can be avoided unless absolutely necessary, even with members of the same sex.

Even with the more uncooperative patient, the presence or absence of a significant organic mental disorder is usually apparent to the evaluating clinician. If present, this disorder must be evaluated further for possible reversible causes (such as drug intoxication).

Treatment

The most important step in treating the paranoid older person is developing a therapeutic relationship. Unlike paranoid individuals at earlier stages of the life cycle, older paranoid patients frequently accept the physician as a friend and confidant and will openly express fears, concerns, and beliefs about the social environment. The physician is often amazed at his ability to escape inclusion into the patient's delusional system. Yet if the clinician is perceived to be a mental health worker or psychiatrist, this positive relationship can easily deteriorate. A positive relationship can be facilitated therefore by maintaining an initial medical orientation and by directing honest attention and concern toward the physical and emotional distress experienced by the patient as a result of the perception that the environment is threatening. Taking blood pressure, checking the pulse, and inquiring about physical health in some detail facilitates the primary care physician's working relationship.

Dishonest approaches to the patient, such as superficially agreeing with the delusional thought, will most likely lead to conflict if the delusions become the topic of conversation. The physician should also avoid directly attacking or attempting to reason with the patient regarding an obviously unreasonable orientation to the social environment. A pharmacologic agent can generally be beneficial in improving symptomatology. The introduction of the phenothiazines or butyrophenones (thioridazine or haloperidol) in low but gradually increasing doses may produce dramatic results. Unfortunately, medication compliance is often a problem. These individuals do not enjoy taking medications in general, and the potential anticholinergic or parkinsonian side-effects can be quite disturbing. Careful education of the patients regarding the side-effects and an explanation of their causes can often prevent noncompliance, especially in the cognitively intact older adult.

As might be expected, working with the family of the paranoid patient is essential. Of all the behaviors encountered by families, frank paranoid ideation can be the most disturbing, even more disturbing than memory loss. Paranoid symptoms not only point to problems in the older person but are a direct attack on the integrity and motives of family members themselves. The potential for conflicts and distress is therefore great.

Health care providers who work with older adults recognize the importance of the family in ensuring that older persons are properly cared for. How can families be supported in their interaction with paranoid elders? First, the clinician must identify family members or friends whom the patient trusts, who are usually, although not always, those who accompany the patient to the clinician's office. When the paranoid patient comes with family members, it is important that the patient be

seen first so that any immediate suspicion regarding the intent of the clinician can be thwarted. During this interview, the clinician should request that members of the family be interviewed separately. Rarely does the older person refuse to grant this permission.

In the interview with the family, members should be encouraged to express their frustrations, fears, and guilt. The physician can help to alleviate family frustrations by emphasizing the difficulty in managing the paranoid individual and can explain the origin and expected outcome of the patient's condition. Fortunately, in the more schizophreniclike syndromes leading to paranoid symptoms in late life, the prognosis is relatively good. Other factors that suggest a positive outcome are presented below:

FACTORS THAT SUGGEST A MORE POSITIVE OUTCOME IN PARANOID PATIENTS

Married
Younger age
Good premorbid relationship
Absence of cognitive impairment
Good response to antipsychotic medication
Insight into symptoms after therapy
Absence of disturbing side-effects to medication
Adequate social network

This encouraging message can be of great relief to family members. In other situations, such as paranoid delusions that frequently accompany dementia, the prognosis is not as positive. In such situations, the clinicians must attempt to alleviate family guilt by explaining the nature of the paranoid process and help them to gain some distance from the accusations and withdrawal of the older paranoid patient. Practical means can frequently be suggested regarding ways in which family members might appropriately interact with the paranoid older adult. Regardless, the family is essential in the treatment of the paranoid older adult.[3]

REFERENCES

1. Blazer DG: The epidemiology of psychiatric disorder in the elderly population. In Grinspoon L (ed): Introduction to Psychiatry Update, vol II, pp 87–97. Washington, DC, American Psychiatric Press, 1983
2. Blazer DG, Houpt JL: Perception of poor health in the healthy older adult. J Am Geriatr Soc 27:330–334, 1979

3. Blazer DG, Siegler IC: A Family Approach to Health Care of the Elderly, pp 140–156, 219–220. Menlo Park, CA, Addison-Wesley, 1984

4. Blazer DG, Williams CD: The epidemiology of dysphoria and depression in an elderly population. Am J Psychiatry 137:439, 1980

5. Carroll BJ, Feinberg M, Greden JF et al: A specific laboratory test for the diagnosis of melancholia: Standardized validation and clinical utility. Arch Gen Psychiatry 38:15–22, 1981

6. Christenson RM, Blazer DG: Epidemiology of persecutory ideation in an elderly community population. Am J Psychiatry 141:1088–1091, 1984

7. Cooper AF, Curry AR, Kay DWK et al: Hearing loss in paranoid and affective disorders of the elderly. Lancet 2:851–854, 1974

8. Coyle JT, Price DL, DeLong MR: Alzheimer's disease: A disorder of cortical cholinergic innervation. Science 219:1184–1190, 1983

9. Davies P: Neurotransmitter-related enzymes in senile dementia of the Alzheimer's type. Brain Res 171:319–327, 1979

10. Diagnostic and Statistical Manual of Mental Disorders, 3rd ed. Washington, DC, American Psychiatric Association, 1980

11. Folstein MF, Folstein SE, McHugh PR: "Mini-mental state": A practical method for grading the mental state of patients for the clinician. J Psychiatric Res 12:189–198, 1975

12. Freud S: On psychotherapy (1904). In Collected Papers, vol 1, pp 249–263. London, Hogarth Press, 1950

13. Gallagher DE, Thompson LW: Effectiveness of psychotherapy for both endogenous and nonendogenous depression in older adult outpatients. J Gerontol 38:707–712, 1983

14. Heston LL, White JA: Dementia: A Practical Guide to Alzheimer's Disease and Related Illnesses. New York, WH Freeman, 1983

15. Holmes TH, Masuda M: Life change and illness susceptibility. In Dohrenwend BS, Dohrenwend BP (eds): Stressful Life Events: Their Nature and Effects. New York, John Wiley & Sons, 1974

16. Hopkinson G: A genetic study of affective illness in patients over 50. Br J Psychiatry 110:244, 1964

17. Lowenthal MF, Berkman PL: Aging and Mental Disorders in San Francisco. San Francisco, Jossey-Bass, 1967

18. Mace NT, Rabins PV: The 36 Hour Day: A Family Guide for Caring for Persons with Alzheimer's Disease. Baltimore, Johns Hopkins Press, 1981

19. Neugarten BL: Adaptation and the life cycle. J Geriatr Psychol 4:71, 1970

20. NIDA Services Research Report: A study of legal drug use by older Americans, (DAGW publication No. 77-495). Washington, DC, Department of Health, Education and Welfare, 1977

21. Palmore E (ed): Normal Aging. Durham, NC, Duke University Press, 1970

22. Palmore E (ed): Normal Aging II. Durham, NC, Duke University Press, 1974

23. Roth M: The natural history of mental disorders in old age. J Ment Sci 101:281–301, 1955

24. Samorajski T, Hartford JM: Brain physiology of aging. In Busse EW, Blazer DG (eds): Handbook of Geriatric Psychiatry, pp 46–82. New York, Van Nostrand Reinhold, 1980

25. Tourigny-Rivard MF, Raskind M, Rivard D: The dexamethasone suppression test in an elderly population. Biol Psychiatry 16:1177–1184, 1981

26. Weiner RD: The role of ECT in the treatment of depression in the elderly. J Am Geriatr Soc 30:710–712, 1982

27. Weissman MM, Myers JK: Affective disorders in a US urban community. Arch Gen Psychiatry 35:1304, 1978

28. Yesavage JA, Tinkleberg J, Hollister LE, Berger PA: Vasodilators in senile dementia: A review of the literature. Arch Gen Psychiatry 36:220–223, 1979

35 Psychological Aspects of Aging

Martha Storandt

In treating the geriatric patient it is important for the physician to be aware of what comprises normal aging in a psychological sense. In the first portion of this chapter changes in basic psychological functions with advancing age will be considered. For the interested reader, extensive reviews are available.[6,7]

The material presented here will refer to the generalized aged; this is not to imply that all older adults are alike. As in any other age-group, each older patient must be considered as an individual. This may prove difficult in the face of the tendency of many health care professionals to assign any person over age 65 to the classification "geriatric" and, often, to stereotype patients in terms of expected behaviors (*e.g.*, confusion, dementia, poor response to treatment). Each elderly patient comes to the physician with a unique psychological and social life history, with a set of values, needs, and resources unlike those of any other patient the physician will see. Consideration of this uniqueness will greatly influence the course of treatment in many instances.

The second portion of the chapter will deal with common forms of psychopathology in older adults and brief screening procedures to detect these problems. Although therapeutic procedures will not be covered here, it should be pointed out that the pessimism with which psychiatric treatment of geriatric patients is typically approached is unwarranted. The elderly can, and do, respond to treatment of many functional and organic disorders.[45]

Preparation of this chapter was supported in part by a research grant from the National Institute on Aging, AG 00535, and by the Edwin B. and Frances S. Behrend Memorial Fund.

NORMAL AGE CHANGES

Sensation and Perception

The ability to sense and perceive surroundings is basic to the interaction of a person with the environment. Age-related changes in sensation and perception can greatly influence the older adult's life. For example, changes in vision may isolate the person from the environment and lead to more complex psychological reactions such as depression, apathy, and social isolation. The common changes in vision, hearing, and the other senses that occur with increased age will be described here only briefly.

Vision

With increased age comes decreased pupil size, loss of lens transparency, increased thickness of the lens, and thickening of the capsule. These changes serve to reduce the amount of light that reaches the retina and thereby to raise the absolute visual threshold. Partial compensation may be achieved by increased illumination. As may be seen in Figure 35-1, a 60-year-old person requires approximately twice as much illumination as a 20-year-old person to compensate for decreased pupil size. The 75-year-old person requires three times as much.[14] Many older persons, however, develop cataracts. Until surgically removed, such lens opacity produces problems with glare, leading the person to avoid the bright light that would aid acuity. At the same time, older persons cannot adapt to dark as well as younger individuals, hence, the tendency to use night lights.

The elasticity of the lens also decreases with increased age, leading to increased farsightedness

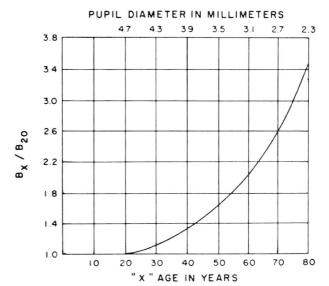

FIG. 35-1. Increases of brightness necessary to compensate for decrease in pupil size owing to advancing age. B_x = brightness required at x years; B_{20} = brightness required at 20 years. (Crouch CL: The relation between illumination and vision. Illuminating Engineering 40:747, 1945)

or presbyopia. The accommodative power of the lens is greatest (approximately 20 diopters) at about age 5 and decreases linearly until about age 60, reaching a value of approximately 0.5 diopter. Unless corrected by lenses, this leads to inability to focus on near objects, particularly reading materials. The ability to distinguish detail at far distances (visual acuity) also declines relatively rapidly in the later years—a change from a median Snellen decimal of 1.20 in the 40s to less than 0.50 at age 80.[52] This normal change also produces a need for corrective glasses.

Color discrimination, particularly for the hues at the blue end of the spectrum, decreases steadily after the 20s. This is related to the tendency of the lens to yellow with increasing age; the yellowed lens serves as a filter for the blues and violets.

Hearing

As shown in Figure 35-2, presbycusis (age-related hearing loss) is most severe for the high tones and more so in men than in women.[43] Not only does the absolute auditory threshold increase with age, but the difference limen (the ability to discriminate small changes in pitch) also increases greatly after approximately age 55.

Presbycusis influences speech intelligibility as well as pure tone thresholds. Consonants such as *s, z, t, f,* and *g,* which are largely composed of high frequency tones and carry little acoustic power, may prove to be indiscriminable. This may produce difficulties in the perception of normal conversation. The ability to perceive speech may

be hampered further if masking (a background sound or noise) is present or if the speech is distorted in some manner. Poor speech perception may also be due partly to reduced ability to process the information in the higher brain centers.

Taste and Smell

Early studies reported loss of taste buds and substantial decreased taste sensitivity in later life.[2,11] Studies suggest this decline may not be so great after all. It is now known that taste buds are replaced continually in adulthood. Studies of taste thresholds indicate that, although taste sensitivity may decline somewhat with age, the change is relatively small.[21,30]

The number of studies that have examined the olfactory sense as it changes with age is exceedingly small. The most recent studies suggest decreased sensitivity with age.[38–40] Deficits in smell may be more important with respect to eating habits of older adults than loss of the sense of taste. Of course, other factors such as lack of money or loneliness may also affect proper nutrition.

Touch, Vibration, and Pain

Sensitivity to touch and vibration appears to decrease with age.[47,50] There may be, however, great variability so that some older people may be more sensitive than some younger adults. Also, loss of sensitivity may not interfere in a major way with function.

The data with respect to pain are less clear; it

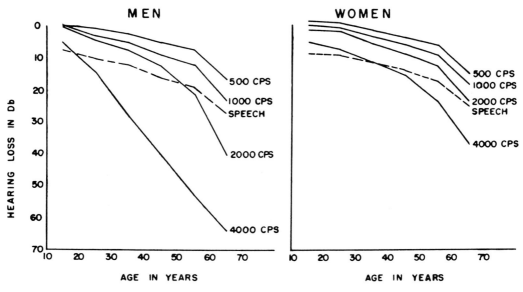

FIG. 35-2.   Average hearing loss by decades for men and women from ages 10 to 70. Median loss in right ear and median loss in left ear were averaged. Graphs are adapted from data collected by the Research Center, Subcommittee on Noise in Industry, American Academy of Ophthalmology and Otolaryngology, Wisconsin State Fair Survey, 1954. (Staloff J: Hearing Loss. Philadelphia, JB Lippincott, 1966)

may be that pain thresholds remain essentially unchanged throughout the life span. The clinical observation that older adults are less sensitive to pain may arise from the older person's hesitancy to report pain. Also, studies of the skin senses are made difficult by the methodologic problem that age-related threshold changes may vary as a function of body location.

Response Speed

Slower response time is undeniable in elderly adults. This appears to be largely a function of slowed central processing time, as opposed to increased peripheral nerve transmission times. Also, older persons may not feel the pressure to respond as rapidly as their busy, younger counterparts. The elderly are frequently described as cautious. Such cautiousness may reflect a tendency to withhold any type of response, even one likely to be correct, rather than to make a response that may be incorrect.

The importance of slower response speeds in older persons cannot be minimized. A rapid response is very important in many aspects of daily life: driving a car, crossing a street, and responding to various warning signals. It is also important to many of our measures of psychological function. For example, timed tests of intelligence have been

criticized as inappropriate for older adults for this very reason; the older adult is penalized in terms of test scores because the person takes longer to give an answer, whereas the young adult acts much more quickly. One study of the performance part of a standard test of intelligence, the Wechsler Adult Intelligence Scale (WAIS), found that a portion of the poorer scores of older adults was indeed due to slower initial responses.[44] Even when increased processing time is allowed, however, some deficit of intellectual performance remains, in comparison with younger adults.

It should be pointed out that there are many aspects of the person's life to which a rapid response to a stimulus may not be required: planting a garden, reading a book, and thinking through a problem in human relations. Most older adults recognize that they are not as fast as they were in their younger years and are quite adept in modifying activities and environments to allow for this slowing. The younger person who interacts with older adults should also be aware of this characteristic of old age.

Intelligence

The classic pattern of age-related intellectual performance may be described in terms of two separate curves, as shown in Figure 35-3. The first,

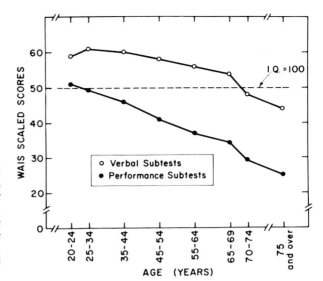

FIG. 35-3. Verbal and Performance WAIS scaled scores as a function of age. Data were obtained from Table 18 of the 1955 *Manual for the Wechsler Adult Intelligence Scale.* The broken line represents the conversion of the scaled scores to IQs of 100. Note the age credits that are necessary with the Performance subtests as compared with the Verbal subtests. (Botwinick J: Cognitive Processes in Maturity and Old Age. New York, Springer Publishing, 1967)

which declines relatively little throughout the adult life, represents verbal measures of intelligence and those functions that are based on stored information. Representative measures include the vocabulary and information subtests of the WAIS and the Mill Hill Vocabulary test. Horn and Cattell have described this type as crystallized intelligence and see it as representing the interaction of the person's biologically determined intellectual capabilities with that which is learned through acculturation and education.[23]

The second curve, which declines more precipitously, reflects perceptual-integrative intelligence. Representative tests of this function include the performance subtests of the WAIS, such as the digit symbol and block design subtests. Horn and Cattell call this type fluid intelligence, which is thought to be representative of the biologically determined capabilities of the person and is influenced by heredity and central nervous system injury.

There are many modifiers of intellectual performance (as opposed to capability). These include education, health status, occupation, test content, personality, practice, motivation, and the particular methods used to score the test. For example, those who have practiced a profession that emphasized scholastic skills (*e.g.,* teaching, the law) may perform better in old age on tests of intelligence because the majority of these measurement procedures also emphasize scholastic skills.

Learning and Memory

It is clear that even the most debilitated older adult retains the ability to learn. Although conditioned

responses may be acquired more slowly in the aged, they are acquired. In fact, many of the most promising psychological intervention techniques used with older adults are based on principles of operant conditioning, in which the individual learns to associate a particular behavior with a particular outcome. These relationships and the labels for the type of conditioning that are associated with them are shown in Figure 35-4.

Although conditioning represents the most basic step in learning, most of the research on learning and memory in later life has focused on more complex processes. The most current view of how learning and memory operate is called the depth of processing model.[12,13] Incoming information may be processed at different depths that are dependent on the degree of elaboration attached to the information. If the information is processed deeply, it will be remembered better than if it is processed at a shallow level. Deep or shallow processing may occur at the time of initial learning (encoding) or at the time of remembering (retrieval).

There is much evidence to indicate that older adults do not process information as deeply as do younger adults. For example, they do not organize the information into categories as well and do not form visual images as effectively. Both these techniques usually enhance information processing. In a practical sense, this would include the physician's instructions, items to be purchased at the store, and the names of new acquaintances.

A number of techniques have been suggested to assist the older adult with memory performance. These aids include note taking, categori-

Nature of outcome

		Positive	Negative
	Receives outcome	↑ Positive reinforcement	↓ Punishment
Result of response	Does not receive outcome	↓ Omission training	↑ Negative reinforcement (avoidance, escape)

FIG. 35-4. The four types of contingencies between outcomes and the results of a response. Arrows pointing up indicate increases in frequency of behavior; arrows pointing down indicate decreases in frequency of behavior. (Storandt M: Counseling and Therapy with Older Adults. Boston, Little, Brown, 1983)

zation and indexing, multimodal presentations, avoidance of interference from extraneous material, and mnemonic or mediational techniques. For example, one study used a self-help manual to train older persons who complained of memory difficulties (but were not brain damaged) in the use of mnemonic techniques, including imagery. Modest improvement was observed and was maintained at 1-month follow-up.[42]

Other research also suggests that the pace of learning and remembering may be important for older persons. For example, older adults may not spend enough time studying the material to begin with; if required to do so, their memory performances improve.[31] Similarly, numerous studies have indicated that the older person requires a longer response time to demonstrate memory.[1] If the material is paced at a relatively rapid rate, the older adult may omit a response just because there is not sufficient time to make it.

Motivation and Emotion

Much of the research that deals with basic motives such as hunger and thirst has, of ethical necessity, been conducted with animals. The ease with which we can generalize from these findings to humans is, of course, questionable. Also, many of the findings are contradictory, and the field is fraught with methodologic difficulties. It seems safe to say, however, that various levels of basic drive deprivation may be required for persons of differing ages in order to achieve comparable levels of motivation.[17]

With respect to more complex motivators and incentives, any generalization at all would be premature. The same is true with respect to the role of emotion in old age. Hypotheses concerning generalized anxiety levels in the old, the importance of task involvement and meaningfulness, fatigue, boredom, and aversive stimulation, as they relate to psychological functioning of the older adult, are being investigated. Results are as yet contradictory and no clear-cut statements can be made at this time.

Sexuality

In the past, sexual activity in the older adult was considered to be almost nonexistent, except perhaps in a pathologic sense. Older adults were counseled to accept reduced sexual drive as one of the unavoidable consequences of growing old. Based on the large-scale research activities of Kinsey and his colleagues,[25] of Masters and Johnson,[28] and of the investigators associated with the Duke Longitudinal Study,[36] however, it has been determined that many older adults are both interested in sex and sexually active.

Patterns of sexual activity throughout the life span appear to be different for men and women.[10,36,53] Men are most sexually active in early adulthood and they experience steadily declining levels of activity, and perhaps capability, thereafter. Women, on the other hand, appear to experience lower initial levels of coital activity in the postpubescent period but seem to maintain those levels throughout the life span, or at least until they experience the loss of an easily available partner, for example, through widowhood or impotence of the husband. It is difficult to know, however, if these differential patterns for men and women will be observed in future cohorts, given the introduction of the Pill and the accompanying sexual revolution of the 1960s.

Personality

At present there are three views about the relationship of personality to age: (1) personality does not change with age; (2) personality may appear to change with age but only because of generational differences in early experiences and environmental factors that lead to different preponderances of some traits or characteristics in one generation than in another; and (3) personality changes with age because there are various stages of development.

The first two positions are in essential agreement that once the personality is formed it remains relatively stable. If older persons today appear to be more conscientious, for example, it is not because they have become that way as they aged but because, as a group, they grew up in a time that emphasized this trait. Stage theorists, on the other hand, postulate a series of progressions determined by biological or maturational processes. Stage theories of personality in adulthood and later life have not been put to adequate empiric testing.

Erikson's theory of personality development provides an example of the third position as applied to older adults.[18] The first five stages in this theory apply to childhood and adolescence, the last three to adulthood. Each stage focuses on a central developmental task. In the final eighth stage, the task is the development of a sense of ego integrity, in which the individual experiences the life that was lived as the only one that could have been and develops a sense of oneness with those in other cultures and other historical periods. Failing this, the individual experiences despair that expresses itself as fear of death.

One of the unique realities of old age is that this period of life ends with death. This can be contrasted to earlier periods of the life cycle, in which one developmental stage is terminated by a transition to another one. In many instances, movement from one stage to another is looked forward to with great enthusiasm and positive expectations. Thus, unsuccessful resolution of Erikson's postulated final stage of personality development may be related to some of the depression observed in old age. On the other hand, many older adults seem reconciled to mortality and well prepared to face their own death. Most are concerned only that they have some measure of control over the circumstances under which this final part of living occurs.

Butler has described a therapeutic process of life review that builds on Erikson's theoretic view of the last stage of personality development.[9] Life review affords the person an opportunity to come to grips with past events and provides some measure of order to a life that is approaching its end.

Transitions

Stage theories should not be confused with the study of life transitions or adjustment to life events (*e.g.,* retirement, widowhood). Stage theories deal with universal maturational phenomena. Transitions may not happen to all (*e.g.,* widowhood), and adjustment to such life events as being old, as opposed to young or middle aged, vary from culture to culture.

Much effort has been directed toward defining and determining the correlates of successful aging. Prior to 1960, it was generally thought that to be happy in old age, a person should continue the activities and life-style followed in the middle years. Cumming and Henry,[15] however, in their theory of disengagement, suggested that successful aging involved the mutual withdrawal of the person from society and of society from the person, in preparation for the final disengagement of death. Reduced social activities were thought to reflect psychological involvement, which was postulated to change both in quantity and quality with increased age.

The theory of disengagement generated much controversy and research activity. Although some persons may age successfully by disengaging, it now appears that many either focus their activities on a smaller number, perhaps to husband their waning physical and psychic resources better, or maintain high levels of both psychological and social involvement and activity, demonstrating little, if any, disengagement in the later years.

It would seem that the health of the person mainly determines the level of morale in old age.[27] Other characteristics that also appear to be related to happiness include higher socioeconomic status; the presence of a confidante with whom the older adult may share intimate joys, worries, concerns, or cares; and previous life-style or personality characteristics.[26,32] It is probably true that the particular pattern of personality that the person carries into old age will influence adjustment to that life phase. The older person who has always been suspicious may appear to become quite paranoid in old age; reduced visual and auditory input no longer allows this person to check internal representations of the world with external reality. The person for whom occupation or career has formed a major component of the self-concept may experience depression on retirement.

Reichard and co-workers[37] described three

types of personality patterns in men that lead to
good adjustment in old age—the Mature, the
Rocking Chair, and the Armoured—as opposed to
two types that seem to produce poor adjustment—
the Angry and the Self-Haters. It is unknown how
well this typology would apply to women or how
complete it is. Furthermore, it has been observed
that the hostile, complaining geriatric patient, who
might correspond to the Angry type, is more likely
to survive in a nursing home environment.[49] Perhaps these outspoken ones receive more attention
and care! Thus, not only are life-style and personality important to adjustment in old age, but also
their influences may vary in impact as a function
of the setting and other external conditions.

PSYCHOPATHOLOGY

It has been estimated that approximately 15% of
older adults in the United States demonstrate at
least a moderate psychopathology.[35] Many do not
seek treatment for a variety of reasons: cultural
sanctions against admitting emotional problems,
lack of economic resources, unavailability of outpatient treatment facilities and trained personnel
to deal with the geriatric psychiatric patient, and
fear of institutionalization. Thus, it falls to the geriatrician to be cognizant of the common forms of
psychopathology of later life.

One study of 50 geriatric male patients admitted to medical and surgical wards reveals that 24%
had mental disorders that were not diagnosed by
their physicians.[41] The majority of the missed cases
were subsequently diagnosed as either alcoholism
or depression. Also, those who went undiagnosed
were largely older, unmarried (widowed, divorced,
single), or from a chronic care facility rather than
their own homes. Many had histories of circulatory problems, past mental hospitalization, or former imprisonments. The physician, by asking a
few simple questions at the time of the first interview, can elicit life history events that may suggest
the possibility of mental disorders in the older patient. Many of these psychological problems can
be treated.

The relatively common functional reactions of
depression, paranoia, and hypochondriasis will be
described here briefly. Other functional disorders
that the geriatrician may also observe in older patients include sleep disturbances, alcoholism, anxiety reactions, and transient situational adjustment
problems, for example, in the face of retirement,
widowhood, hospitalization, or changes in living
arrangements.

Functional Disorders

Depression

Depression in the elderly is frequently thought to
be reactive, as compared with the endogenous
depressions seen in younger patients. The elderly
experience many losses as they approach the end
of the life span (*e.g.*, widowhood, retirement, poor
health, and loss of social status). Depression is
probably related to the very high suicide rate of
older men (Fig. 35-5). Thus, this disturbance is to
be taken seriously when it occurs in an aged patient and treated actively, with a special emphasis
on dealing with the environmental precipitates of
the reaction. Too often suicide threats by older
individuals go unheeded by their families and physicians. One study reported that 77% of the white
male suicides studied saw a physician within 1
month prior to death.[29]

Furthermore, although Figure 35-5 clearly illustrates the need for active treatment of depressed
older men, depressed older women should not be
ignored. Their lower suicide rate may be a function
of fewer successful attempts, rather than less severe depression. Women tend to employ more passive modes of suicide (*e.g.*, drug overdoses) from
which they can be revived, as compared with men,
who tend to use active, irreversible methods (*e.g.*,
guns).

Symptoms of depression in old age are similar
to those in younger years. The physical signs may
be the first to appear. The more common ones
include loss of appetite, significant weight loss,
severe fatigue, and sleep difficulties, particularly
early awakening. These symptoms, however, must
be distinguished from the normal age-related
changes that appear in these indicators. The psychological indications of depression include sad-
ness, low activity and interest levels, severe pessimism, difficulty in making decisions, and
retarded speech and movement. Sometimes the
person cries a great deal or experiences severe guilt
and anxiety. The reasons for suicide in older adults
appear to be different than those of younger persons. The themes reflected in notes left by older
suicides in one study included health and isolation
or loneliness, as compared with themes of rejection in love relations and failures to cope with life
expressed by young and middle-aged adults.[16]

The physician may wish to include a brief test
of depression such as the 20-item Zung Self-Rating
Depression Scale or the Beck Depression Inventory
as a standard part of the initial workup of all older
patients.[4,54]

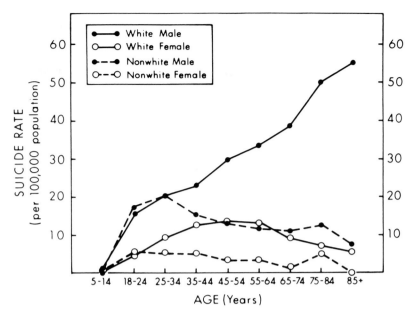

FIG. 35–5. Suicide rates by age, sex, and race in the United States, 1972. (Data from Vital Statistics of the United States, 1972, vol 2. Mortality Part A, US Department of Health, Education and Welfare, Public Health Service, National Center for Health Statistics, Rockville, Maryland, 1976)

The Zung Self-Rating Depression Scale can be administered by an office assistant and usually takes less than 5 minutes to complete. The form, illustrated in Figure 35-6, should be given to the patient with instructions to read each statement and put a check in the column that is most applicable at the present time. A patient on a diet will sometimes ask how to respond to question 5. The patient should be told to answer as if not on a diet.

When the patient has completed the questionnaire, the tester should look it over quickly to determine that the patient has not placed more than one check on each line. This sometimes happens with older persons who have difficulty with their vision, which can result in inaccurate responses to the remainder of the following items.

Items 1, 3, 4, 7, 8, 9, 13, 15, and 19 are scored as follows: a response of *none* or *a little of the time* receives a score of 1; *some of the time,* a score of 2; *good part of the time,* a score of 3; and *most* or *all of the time,* a score of 4.

Items 2, 5, 6, 11, 12, 14, 16, 17, 18, and 20 are scored as follows: a response of *none* or *a little of the time* receives a scores of 4; *some of the time,* a score of 3; *good part of the time,* a score of 2; and *most* or *all of the time,* a score of 1.

The raw score is obtained by summing the scores for each item. The total raw score is then converted to an SDS Index as in Table 35-1. Elderly patients with indices of 50 or more are exhibiting a significant degree of depressive symptomatology and should be referred for psychiatric evaluation and treatment. Cognitive-behavioral treatments have been shown to be effective in the treatment of depression in older adults.[19]

Paranoia

Another functional disorder seen in older adults is paranoia. As in depression, paranoia has a somewhat different character in the older adult than in the young, in whom it typically reflects a rather severe degree of personality disorganization. In the old person, however, paranoid reactions may result from social isolation or reduced cognitive and sensory capabilities and may reflect an attempt to make sense of a world no longer clearly represented through the eyes and ears.[5] For example, the person with hearing impairment may not be able to determine what is actually being said. Thus, the individual may make up these conversations and impart hostile motivations to those in the environment. Although paranoid reactions in the old

Name _____ Age _____ Sex _____ Date _____	None OR a Little of the Time	Some of the Time	Good Part of the Time	Most OR All of the Time
1. I feel down-hearted, blue and sad				
2. Morning is when I feel the best				
3. I have crying spells or feel like it				
4. I have trouble sleeping through the night				
5. I eat as much as I used to				
6. I enjoy looking at, talking to and being with attractive women/men				
7. I notice that I am losing weight				
8. I have trouble with constipation				
9. My heart beats faster than usual				
10. I get tired for no reason				
11. My mind is as clear as it used to be				
12. I find it easy to do the things I used to				
13. I am restless and can't keep still				
14. I feel hopeful about the future				
15. I am more irritable than usual				
16. I find it easy to make decisions				
17. I feel that I am useful and needed				
18. My life is pretty full				
19. I feel that others would be better off if I were dead				
20. I still enjoy the things I used to do				

Copyright © 1962, 1965, 1974 by **W.W.K. Zung.**

FIG. 35-6.   The Self-Rating Depression Scale. (Reproduced by permission of W.W.K. Zung)

may be more understandable, they still alienate the older person from family members, friends, and other human contacts. As in depression, paranoia should be treated actively, for example, by providing prosthetic devices to enhance sensory and cognitive capabilities and by providing an understanding environment.

Hypochondriasis

Another syndrome seen relatively frequently is excessive preoccupation with bodily functions and with the presence of physical disease in the absence of discernible physical cause. Patients tend to resist the explanation that the problems are psychological. Thus, the physician who makes this interpretation may cause the patient to make the rounds of physicians' offices in the search for someone who will indeed admit that the patient is ill.

Busse and Pfeiffer[8] have offered an interesting description of the dynamics of hypochondriasis as applied to older adults. The person experiences some failing in capabilities, common to old age. In our culture, however, the person who does not carry a share of the workload, who is not independent, productive, and capable, is seen in a negative light. On the other hand, the Judeo-Christian ethic requires us to care for the physically ill and disabled. Thus, the hypochondriacal patient attempts to explain inabilities on the basis of physical causes in order to gain approval and support from the environment. This attempt is doomed to failure because we have all played this game from time to time and are thus aware of the maneuver. The patient's family, friends, and acquaintances resent its overuse and react with hostility and anger.

Many of the psychological problems experienced by hypochondriacal patients are exacerbated by poor interpersonal relationships and ineffective communication with one or more family members. Thus, family therapy may be the treatment of choice. Frequently the first step of such a program involves separation of the family members in conflict, often by means of assignment of the identified aged patient to a day hospital program.

Organic Disorders

The bulk of studies comparing aging and brain damage would indicate that the two are not identical.[20,22,33] Application of the diagnosis of chronic brain syndrome to all impaired geriatric patients is quite inappropriate and is based on longstanding

TABLE 35-1 Conversion of Raw Scores to the SDS Index for the Zung Self-Rating Depression Scale

Raw Score	SDS Index	Raw Score	SDS Index	Raw Score	SDS Index
20	25	40	50	60	75
21	26	41	51	61	76
22	28	42	53	62	78
23	29	43	54	63	79
24	30	44	55	64	80
25	31	45	56	65	81
26	33	46	58	66	83
27	34	47	59	67	84
28	35	48	60	68	85
29	36	49	61	69	86
30	38	50	63	70	88
31	39	51	64	71	89
32	40	52	65	72	90
33	41	53	66	73	91
34	43	54	68	74	92
35	44	55	69	75	94
36	45	56	70	76	95
37	46	57	71	77	96
38	48	58	73	78	98
39	49	59	74	79	99
				80	100

misconceptions concerning the aging process. Furthermore, it is estimated that from 10% to 20% of older persons with organic disorders have acute, rather than chronic, syndromes.[35] Many reversible organic disorders in older adults are due to metabolic problems, drug intoxication, or treatable systemic disease.

The clinical symptoms of organic brain disease center around deficits in intellectual and cognitive performance, including disorientation, memory loss, poor visuomotor coordination, and an inability to assimilate new information, carry out sequential tasks, abstract information, or change set. The degree of impairment with respect to these functions is often associated with the severity of the disease. Also, the organic brain disorder may be accompanied by any of a wide range of emotional symptoms, especially in its early stages. These include anxiety, depression, hallucinations, delusions, emotional outbursts, withdrawal, or listlessness.

Organic brain disorders in older adults may be associated with specific histories. Examples of these include stroke, multi-infarct dementia, and alcoholism. Other organic disorders have specific symptoms (*e.g.*, Parkinson's disease) or clear diagnostic signs on computed tomography (*e.g.*, normal pressure hydrocephalus). The most common organic disorder in older adults, however, is Alzheimer's disease. The etiology of this primary neuronal degeneration is unknown and no successful treatment has yet been devised. The disease onset is gradual and the course is progressively downward.

Because of the pervasiveness of Alzheimer's disease and the difficulty in differentiating it from normal aging in the very early stages, a screening battery for mild senile dementia of the Alzheimer's type will be described. This brief (10-minute), easy-to-administer battery of four simple psychological tests correctly classified 98% of normal and mildly demented individuals.[46] It should be pointed out, however, that older persons suffering from other psychological and organic disorders were not included in the sample. Thus, persons suspected of other types of disorders should be administered additional diagnostic procedures (*e.g.*, neurologic studies, computed or positron emission tomography, tests for depression).

The screening battery comprises two subtests of the Wechsler Memory Scale (Mental Control and Logical Memory), a test of word fluency, and Form A of the Trailmaking Test, administered in that order.[51] The Wechsler Memory Scale can be purchased from the Psychological Corporation.* The Trailmaking Test may be obtained from the Neuropsychology Laboratory.†

The Mental Control subtest involves recall of well-practiced information such as the alphabet and counting by 3s. The Logical Memory subtest requires the individual to recall a brief prose passage that is read by the examiner. There are two such passages, and the score is the average number of memories recalled.

The word fluency procedure is from the Primary Mental Abilities Test.[48] The individual must name as many words as can be recalled that begin with the letter *s* within 60 seconds. Then the person is asked to do the same thing for words beginning with the letter *p*. The score on this test is the total number of words recalled.

The Trailmaking test is a simple paper and pencil task in which the person must draw lines connecting circles numbered 1 through 26, in order.[3] The score is the reciprocal of the time taken to complete the task (a maximum of 3 minutes is allowed) multiplied by 1000.

How the scores of the four tests of the battery are combined to produce a composite score is

* 304 East 45th Street, New York, NY 10017
† 1338 E. Edison Street, Tucson, AZ 85719

TABLE 35-2 Examples of Computation of Canonical Scores*

Test	Weight†	Subject 1 (Demented)		Subject 2 (Healthy)	
		Raw Score	*Wt. × Score*	*Raw Score*	*Wt. × Score*
Logical memory	−.445	2	−.890	9	−4.005
Trailmaking	−.066	12	−.792	60	−3.960
Word fluency	−.036	13	−.468	22	−.792
Mental control	.130	4	.520	7	.910
Constant	3.588		+3.588		+3.588
		Sum	1.958	Sum	−4.259

* If computed score is positive, classify as demented; if score is negative, classify as healthy.
† Unstandardized regression coefficients

demonstrated in Table 35-2. If the composite score is greater than 0, dementia is indicated. If the composite score is less than 0, normalcy is indicated. Only one normal and one demented person in the initial sample to which this battery was applied were misclassified using these simple procedures.

The physician may also want to use a brief mental status screening test. Two that are used commonly are the Mental Status Questionnaire and the Short Portable Mental Status Questionnaire.[24,34] Both of these procedures are sensitive to educational differences; the Short Portable Mental Status Questionnaire provides corrections for both education and race.

For more extensive neuropsychological evaluation, the physician may request the Halstead-Reitan or Luria-Nebraska neuropsychological batteries. In the hands of a trained neuropsychologist the Halstead-Reitan battery allows for relatively accurate localization of dysfunction, when such knowledge is required, and also can provide an indication of the progress of the disease or trauma. The pattern of deficits on this neuropsychological battery is generally different in the normal aged than the pattern seen in those with organic pathology. The Luria-Nebraska battery is somewhat shorter than the Halstead-Reitan and, therefore, may be tolerated better by the patient. It has not been in use as long as the Halstead-Reitan, and appropriate norms for older adults are just now beginning to appear. Also, fewer neuropsychologists may be trained in its use.

These are just a few of the assessment procedures used by psychologists. The list is too lengthy to describe in this chapter. The physician, however, should be aware that psychological testing is appropriate for older adults and seek consultation without hesitancy. Too often physicians do not refer their older patients for either assessment or

treatment of mental health problems. Presumably, the physician considers the patient merely to be old and, therefore, beyond help. The burgeoning literature on geriatric mental health clearly demonstrates that such is not the case.

REFERENCES

1. Arenberg D: Cognition and aging: Verbal learning, memory, and problem solving. In Eisdorfer C, Lawton MP (eds): The Psychology of Adult Development and Aging. Washington, DC, American Psychological Association, 1973
2. Arey LB, Tremaine MJ, Monzingo FL: The numerical and topographical relations of taste buds to human circumvallate papillae throughout the life span. Anat Rec 64:9, 1936
3. Armitage SG: An analysis of certain psychological tests used for the evaluation of brain injury. Psychol Monogr 60: No. 1 (Whole No. 277), 1946
4. Beck AT: Depression: Causes and Treatment. Philadelphia, University of Pennsylvania Press, 1977
5. Berger KS, Zarit SH: Late-life paranoid states: Assessment and treatment. Am J Orthopsychiatry 48:523, 1978
6. Birren JE, Schaie KW (eds): Handbook of the Psychology of Aging. New York, Van Nostrand Reinhold, 1977
7. Botwinick J: Aging and Behavior, 3rd ed. New York, Springer Publishing, 1984
8. Busse EW, Pfeiffer E: Functional psychiatric disorders in old age. In Busse EW, Pfeiffer E (eds): Behavior and Adaptation in Late Life. Boston, Little, Brown & Co, 1969
9. Butler RN: The life review: An interpretation of reminiscence in the aged. Psychiatry 26:65, 1973
10. Christenson CV, Gagnon JH: Sexual behavior in a group of older women. J Gerontol 20:351, 1965
11. Cooper RM, Bilash I, Zubek JP: The effects of age on taste sensitivity. J Gerontol 14:56, 1959
12. Craik FIM, Lockhart RS: Levels of processing: A

framework for memory research. J Verbal Learning Verbal Behav 11:671, 1972

13. Craik FIM, Simon E: Age differences in memory: The roles of attention and depth of processing. In Poon LW, Fozard JF, Cermak LS, Arenberg D, Thompson LW (eds): New Directions in Memory and Aging. Hillsdale, NJ, Lawrence Erlbaum Associates, 1980

14. Crouch CL: The relation between illumination and vision. Illuminating Engineering 40:747, 1945

15. Cumming E, Henry W: Growing Old: The Process of Disengagement. New York, Basic Books, 1961

16. Darbonne AR: Suicide and age: A suicide note analysis. J Consult Clin Psychol 33:46, 1969

17. Elias MF, Elias PK, Elias J: Basic Processes in Adult Developmental Psychology. St. Louis, CV Mosby, 1977

18. Erikson EH: Childhood and Society, 2nd ed. New York, WW Norton, 1963

19. Gallagher DE, Thompson LW: Treatment of major depressive disorder in older adult outpatients with brief psychotherapies. Psychotherapy 19:482, 1982

20. Goldstein G, Shelly CH: Similarities and differences between psychological deficit in aging and brain damage. J Gerontol 30:448, 1975

21. Grzegorczyk PB, Jones SW, Mistretta CM: Age-related differences in salt taste acuity. J Gerontol 34:834, 1979

22. Hallenbeck CE: Evidence for a multiple process view of mental deterioration. J Gerontol 19:357, 1964

23. Horn JL, Cattell RB: Age differences in primary mental ability factors. J Gerontol 21:210, 1966

24. Kahn RL, Pollack M, Goldfarb AI: Factors related to individual differences in mental status of institutionalized aged. In Hoch P, Zubin J (eds): Psychopathology of Aging. New York, Grune & Stratton, 1961

25. Kinsey AC, Pomeroy WB, Martin CE: Sexual Behavior in the Human Female. Philadelphia, WB Saunders, 1948

26. Lowenthal MF, Raven C: Interaction and adaptation: Intimacy as a critical variable. Am Sociol Rev 33:20, 1968

27. Maddox G, Eisdorfer C: Some correlates of activity and morale among the elderly. Social Forces 40:254, 1962

28. Masters WH, Johnson VE: Human Sexual Response. Boston, Little, Brown & Co, 1966

29. Miller M: Geriatric suicide: The Arizona study. Gerontologist 18:488, 1978

30. Moore LM, Niesen CR, Mistretta CM: Sucrose taste thresholds: Age-related differences. J Gerontol 37:64, 1982

31. Murphy MD, Sanders RE, Gabrieshski AS, Schmitt F: Metamemory in the aged. J Gerontol 36:185, 1981

32. Neugarten BL, Havighurst RJ, Tobin SS: Personality and patterns of aging. In Neugarten BL (ed): Middle Age and Aging. Chicago, University of Chicago Press, 1968

33. Overall JE, Gorham DR: Organicity versus old age

in objective and projective test performance. J Consult Clin Psychol 39:98, 1972

34. Pfeiffer E: A short portable mental status questionnaire for the assessment of organic brain deficit in elderly persons. J Am Geriatr Soc 23:433, 1975

35. Pfeiffer E: Psychopathology and social pathology. In Birren JE, Schaie KW (eds): Handbook of the Psychology of Aging. New York, Van Nostrand Reinhold, 1977

36. Pfeiffer E, Davis GC: Determinants of sexual behavior in middle and old age. Arch Gen Psychiatry 19:753, 1968

37. Reichard S, Livson F, Peterson PG: Aging and Personality. New York, John Wiley & Sons, 1962

38. Schemper T, Voss S, Cain WS: Odor identification in young and elderly persons: Sensory and cognitive limitations. J Gerontol 36:446, 1981

39. Schiffman S: Food recognition by the elderly. J Gerontol 32:586, 1977

40. Schiffman S, Pasternak M: Decreased discrimination of food odors in the elderly. J Gerontol 34:73, 1979

41. Schukit MA, Miller PL, Hahlbohm D: Unrecognized illness in elderly medical-surgical patients. J Gerontol 30:655, 1975

42. Scogin F: Memory Skills Training for the Elderly: The Efficacy of Self-Instructional Treatment on Memory Performance, Memory Complaints, and Depression. Unpublished doctoral dissertation, Washington University, 1983

43. Staloff J: Hearing Loss. Philadelphia, JB Lippincott, 1966

44. Storandt M: Age, ability level, and method of administering and scoring the WAIS. J Gerontol 32:175, 1977

45. Storandt M: Counseling and Therapy with Older Adults. Boston, Little, Brown & Co, 1983

46. Storandt M, Botwinick J, Danziger WL, Berg L, Hughes CP: Psychometric differentiation of mild senile dementia of the Alzheimer type. Arch Neurol 41:497, 1984

47. Thornbury J, Mistretta CM: Tactile sensitivity as a function of age. J Gerontol 36:34, 1981

48. Thurstone LL, Thurstone TG: Examiner Manual for the SRA Primary Mental Abilities Test. Chicago, Science Research Associates, 1949

49. Turner BF, Tobin SS, Lieberman MA: Personality traits as predictors of institutional adaptation among the aged. J Gerontol 27:61, 1972

50. Verrillo RT: Age-related changes in sensitivity to vibration. J Gerontol 35:185, 1980

51. Wechsler D, Stone CP: Manual: Wechsler Memory Scale. New York, Psychological Corporation, 1983

52. Weumouth FW: Effects of age on visual acuity. In Hirsch MJ, Wick RF (eds): Vision of the Aging Patient. Philadelphia, Chilton, 1960

53. Young WC: The hormones and mating behavior. In Young WC (ed): Sex and Internal Secretions. Baltimore, Williams & Wilkins, 1961

54. Zung WWK: Depression in the normal aged. Psychomatics 8:287, 1967

36

The Changing Role of the Physician with the Terminally Ill Elderly Person

Robert Kastenbaum and Beatrice Kastenbaum

Both the practice of medicine and the nature of American society continue to change in ways that affect the relationship between the physician and the terminally ill elderly person. It would be more difficult to identify factors that have remained invariant than to list dimensions of change. Diagnostic and treatment resources proliferate, but so do regulations, paperwork, and iatrogenic disorders. Medical advances must pass through the ever-tightening gauntlet of cost containment. What might have been counted as a great success—the survival of some 20 million Americans into their 60s and beyond—is shadowed by the unsolved challenge of serving those who have become highly dependent and debilitated as well as those who are rapidly approaching death.

EMERGING CONDITIONS AFFECTING THE OLDER PERSON

Geographic Dispersion of Families and the Decline of Neighborhoods

The terminally ill older person is less likely to have an intimate support network available. Although the average older American still has more contact with family members than might have been supposed,[27] the incessant mobility of our society has also taken its toll. It is not just younger family members who move about in search of educational and occupational opportunities. An increasing number of older people relocate after retire-

ment, most often attracted to the sunbelt states. When critical illness strikes, the relocated older person may lack family and close friends. This has led to a reverse migration trend as an older person in failing health comes home to die or a bereaved spouse moves back to a former community to seek comfort. However, the "neighborhoodliness" of communities remains under continuing pressure as economic and social change undermine traditional mutual support. The new planned communities do not invariably provide real neighborhood support, while the home town (whether urban or rural) is also likely to be changing in character. The physician, then, is more likely to be called on to help older people who have been deprived of intimate relationships even though a certain amount of superficial social involvement exists.

Fear of Dependency, Financial Ruin, and Burdening

Most older individuals have learned to give close attention to financial matters. They are also aware that medical expenses can quickly deplete the resources that have built up over the years. Furthermore, they realize that advances in medical care now make it possible for life to be extended (or dying prolonged) when there is little hope of restoring health. Motivation to prolong one's own life is often countered by the financial risk and by fear of becoming a burden on others. The most common theme I have heard from older patients

618

with life-threatening illnesses is the fear that they will be kept alive but useless over a prolonged period of time. This prospect can be especially distasteful to those who have worked long and hard to establish their independence and who pride themselves on not burdening others with their problems and obligations. Additionally, there is often the misgiving about spending funds on their last days that their spouse might need or that they would prefer to pass on to their heirs. Many of the elderly can tell us of the widow who was left penniless or even in debt after her husband's final illness. The physician, then, may become part of the older patient's own ambivalence about prolongation of life versus dependency, expense, and burdening others.

"Consumerism" and Unfinished Business

Older Americans have participated in many recent social trends, including the "consumerism" that now encompasses services as well as products. Today's older person is more likely to express strong preferences with respect to both medical care and funeral arrangements. There is increasing resistance to going along with routines and preconceptions that may be encountered in the medical care system. Furthermore, the elderly today often have activities and interests that belie the stereotype of "retirement living." This means that they also have more unfinished business to complete near the end of life. It would be a mistake to assume that the terminally ill older person has abandoned all interest in people and projects. The physician, then, will be expected to listen carefully to the preferences, needs, and expectations of the terminally ill older person and to help provide some "quality time" for completion of unfinished business.

The Survivor-in-Waiting

Because more persons now live to an advanced age, it is becoming increasingly common after a patient's death for there to be a surviving spouse. This is most often the wife, since the distance between female and male survival continues to broaden.[9] Frequently, the spouse is also highly involved in providing care and support for the terminally ill elder. She herself becomes vulnerable— to illness, accident, depression, and what is now fashionably called "burnout." Additionally, the transition from wife to widow can lead to new stress and confusion.[19] Although many elderly widows (and widowers) eventually achieve a

strong adjustment, there is often a crisis period in which impulsive actions, social isolation, and the prospect of a hastened mortality exist. The physician, then, may be called on to work sensitively with the spouse or other significant person, both to help share the burden of illness and to reduce the possibility of life-threatening danger when the spouse becomes a survivor.

THE HOSPICE ALTERNATIVE

The emergence of the hospice philosophy is leading to a series of changes in traditional care settings as well as in those that bear the hospice emblem as such. There is some uncertainty, ambiguity, even outright confusion about the hospice approach to terminal care. It is clear, however, that older patients are starting to make substantial use of this option. Among the nearly 4000 patients participating in year 1 of the Medicare Demonstration Cost Sample, 90% were 65 years of age or over.[20] Furthermore, the primary care person most often was an elderly spouse. The physician, then, may be called on to offer advice about the choice between traditional and hospice care and may be asked by the terminally ill older person to serve as medical leader of the hospice team. Because such situations are likely to become even more common as time goes on, we will now consider the hospice alternative in more detail.

Although hospice programs are relatively new to the United States, there is already a lining up of forces pro and con. Physicians can be found on both sides. The physician who has accepted the responsibility of serving as medical director of a hospice organization and the physician who refuses to refer any of his terminally ill patients to hospice have each other to contend with. Here we will simply review the basics of the hospice approach, note some of the more important research findings, and introduce a few considerations that might help physicians reach their own conclusions.

Hospice Basics

Hospice should be understood both as a philosophy of care and as an operational program. Although there is a close relationship between philosophy and program, the two are not interchangeable. It is possible for those who accept the hospice philosophy to achieve some of their objectives within more traditional programs of care while, at the same time, an operational hospice program may depart somewhat in practice from the stated goals.

The hospice philosophy takes as its primary goal the provision of care and support for persons in the last phases of incurable illness—and for their families. The intention is neither to hasten nor to postpone death. Rather, the intention is to enable patients to live as fully and comfortably as possible and in a manner consistent with their own lifestyles. The unit of care is the patient within the family. Family members are assisted to remain as active and involved as possible under the circumstances. Expert help from the outside is provided immediately as needed but is not intended to replace whatever natural support system might exist. This approach is responsive to complaints by many family members that they were excluded from the scene by medical personnel whose procedures took precedence over the needs and feelings of the family constellation.

Several key features of the hospice philosophy are emphasized by leaders in the field, as in a foundation document that led to current legislation:[10]

Remission of symptoms is a major treatment goal. Terminal status cannot be taken as a reason for neglect of symptom-control efforts. While pain control may be the most obvious specific goal here, the intention is to reduce all types of distress that can intensify the anguish of the dying person and reduce the opportunity for communication with loved ones.

The patient's intentions are to be respected as a primary determinant of the total pattern of management—from the first day of hospice care to the last.

Opportunities should be provided for leave-takings with the people most important to the patient and for experiencing the final moments in a way that is meaningful to the patient.

Family should have the opportunity to discuss treatment options, as well as dying, death, and related emotional needs with professional staff, and should have the opportunity for privacy with the dying person.

All caregivers should have adequate time to form and maintain personal relationships with the patient, and a mutual support network should exist among the staff, encompassing both the technical and the socioemotional dimensions of the situation.

These key components of the hospice philosophy do not specify the environment in which care should be provided. In practice, many patients and their families do prefer the home environment. From an economic and political standpoint, the reduction of in-hospital days is a goal of enabling legislation for the ongoing national hospice program. Nevertheless, the hospice philosophy does not of itself insist on the home environment. The more important point is that the patient be in the most appropriate environment at the moment, all factors taken into consideration. Principles of hospice care (theoretically, at least) can be carried out at home, in a hospital, or in a transitional respite care facility. Although the locus of care is important, hospice itself is a philosophy and system of care, not a place, nor is it demanded that the patient remain at home under all circumstances.

Hospice as a practical operation requires careful consideration in its own right. We will not deal here with historical aspects of hospice[26] but concentrate instead on the current (and ever-changing) picture.

Two general styles of hospice operation can be distinguished, as well as two most common types of organizational configuration. One style of hospice operation has been described (with some disparagement) as "hand-holding." The image here is of kindly volunteers stopping by to provide company and comfort for the patient and to assist the family in small ways. It is unfortunate that a number of professionals have chosen to look down on this type of arrangement. Social isolation of the dying person and unrelieved burden on the primary family caregiver cannot be considered as trivial matters. Nevertheless, this is a limited kind of service. Questions can be raised about the scope, availability, and accountability of hospice services within this model. Furthermore, hospice services of this type have difficulty in extending beyond the home environment. It is very difficult to maintain continuity of approach between the home and the hospital. The hospice philosophy may have no impact on treatment procedures when the patient is admitted to the hospital. It is not unusual for the patient and the family to face a critical choice: enter the hospital for a full range of services at the sacrifice of personal values and preferences or remain at home with inadequate services.

It is the other hospice model that is becoming increasingly dominant, however. The full-service hospice is the type that has been specified by the Hospice Care component of the Medicare program. A hospice that intends to obtain reimbursements under this act must demonstrate a broad range of capabilities. It should be noted that this model was not created by the law but, rather, won acceptance in competition with the more limited model. It should also be noted that a hospice organization can meet these requirements and yet not enroll in the Medicare reimbursement program. Some hospice directors judge that this reimbursement program is seriously underfunded and therefore have not elected to enroll. The critical point, then, is not whether a particular hospice organization happens to be enrolled in the Medicare reimbursement program but whether it has the strengths and attributes of a full-service operation.

What, then, are the characteristics a physician should look for? A functional and dependable hospice will have the following features.

Staffing

There will be an interdisciplinary team whose medical director has special knowledge of pain and other symptom control. The team will also include registered nurses knowledgeable in the care of the incurably ill who have the skills to teach and support family members in the area of end-of-life issues; qualified social workers to help patients and families cope with financial and emotional issues; members of the clergy with special skill in helping patients and families find peace and comfort and the opportunity to discuss their death-related hopes and fears; and a pool of carefully selected and thoroughly trained volunteers. The core staff should actually function as a team, sitting down regularly together to discuss cases in detail rather than each going their own way.

Availability

Hospice services are available 24 hours a day, every day of the year. In place is a dependable, fail-safe method for ensuring that immediate needs receive immediate response. Typically, a registered nurse is on call at all times and has quick access to the medical director when his or her services are required.

Continuity of Care

The hospice has established a firm and complete network of care that extends from in-hospital to in-home situations. The patient, then, can be moved from home to medical facility and back again without significant disruption in the philosophy of care. The attending physician plays a key role by writing orders that ensure continuity (*e.g.*, maintaining the pain-control regimen if it has been working).

Accountability

The hospice has a well-documented set of admission criteria and procedures that make clear the respective roles of patient, family, and physician. The hospice complies with applicable local, state, and federal laws and regulations that govern the organization and delivery of health care to patients and families. Accurate and current records are maintained on all patients and families, and a quality assurance program encompasses evaluation of services, regular chart audits, and organizational review.

These, in brief, are the characteristics of a full-service hospice. The attending physician continues to participate actively in case management and has the resources of the entire organization to supplement his efforts.

A full-service hospice can function well in either of two types of organizational configuration: hospital based or free standing. The challenges are somewhat different: the hospital-based hospice must develop the community and in-home components, while the free standing hospice must establish satisfactory relationships with hospitals. Evidence from the National Hospice Demonstration Project indicates that the goals of hospice management can be achieved by either type of organization.[8] There is a tendency for older patients and for patients with greater functional impairments to receive treatment in hospital-based hospices, although, as already noted, older patients predominate in all hospices. Studies suggest that hospice organizations seem to be achieving both the administrative goal of cost control and the human value goal of enabling patients to remain longer in the environments of their choice with significant reduction of symptomatic distress.[16,21] Subsequent studies will tell us more about the value of hospice in reducing the distress of the surviving caregivers.

Hospice Decisions

Increasingly, physicians will be called on to make decisions about hospice care for their patients. There are believed to be approximately 1200 hospice organizations in the United States,[8] although no definitive list has emerged. Many areas not yet served by a hospice are considering the development of such a service. Physicians will be expected to be well informed about their local hospice organizations and to offer sound advice when decision points arise. There is no substitute for in-depth knowledge of one's local hospice organization and those who operate it. A few general recommendations can be offered, however.

Consider the capabilities and limitations of the family as well as the patient. Could an enriched support network make the difference in enabling the patient to remain at home longer? Would skilled education by a hospice nurse help family members to provide much of the care without overtaxing their energies?

Consider the timing of possible enrollment in the hospice program. An unfortunate complication in hospice care has been the tendency of some physicians to wait until the patient is within a few days (or even hours) of death before recommending hospice care. These delayed actions give neither hospice nor the patient much of a chance. It must be said that physicians have at times shown a reluctance to acknowledge impending death and have also been known to wait until financial entitlements and resources have been depleted to recommend hospice care. An informed and active ''consumership'' is likely to place increasing pressure on decision making that is not really in the interests of patient and family.

Consider asking a well-informed social worker to explain the details of hospice enrollment to patient and family. Decisions should be based on the most recent and accurate information. It may be reassuring to patients and family members, for example, to learn that a decision is not binding; one can move in either direction, from hospice to traditional care or the reverse within certain limits.

Consider making it clear to patient and family that you, as physician, will remain actively involved in the care process and do all that can and should be done whether or not they favor enrollment in a hospice program. The physician–patient–family relationship remains an important one. The hospice philosophy was never intended to vitiate this relationship. Consider how you can be most helpful under either traditional or hospice arrangements and, therefore, save the patient from having to choose between you and hospice.

CHARACTERISTICS OF THE LAST PHASE OF LIFE IN OLDER ADULTS

There have always been situations in which it was difficult to specify either the beginning or the end of the dying process. The prospect of being buried alive, for example, once aroused considerable anxiety and had its occasional basis in fact.[13] Today new pressures have emerged that challenge the physician, the family, and the medicolegal system. Although more attention has been given to prob-

lems associated with the definition of death,[22,28] there are also difficulties and ambiguities with respect to the beginning of the terminal phase. Recent Medicare legislation requires that a patient be certified as having 6 months or less to live in order to receive hospice care. This legal requirement, however, is but a small part of the total picture. Classifying a person as terminally ill serves as a signal for complex change in the interpersonal forces at work. In one of our own experiments, those led to believe they were interacting with a man suffering from a fatal illness altered both verbal and nonverbal behavior as compared with their previous interactions with the same person.[30] The differences were in the direction of increasing both the physical and the psychological distance between the interviewer and the fatally ill person. Other studies have also supported the conclusion that we treat people differently when we believe their death to be imminent.[4,11]

Physician–Patient Communication

We will consider first the physician–patient communication process and then review selected social and behavioral clues to the onset of the terminal phase of life.

The physician is not the only person in the situation who has an opinion, but no one's words and actions carry more weight. The physician does not have to speak directly about prognosis for patients and families to draw their conclusions. Silence about prognosis, in fact, is often taken as an important clue, whether or not the clue is accurately interpreted.[12] ''Saying nothing'' is an option that is not really available to the physician: in a critical situation others will scan and evaluate the physician's words, silences, actions, and nonactions. With a life time of experience behind them, older people are often very good at ''reading'' the physician's attitude and conclusions. It is not unusual for an elderly man or woman to listen politely to the physician and seem to accept what has been said at face value only to remark a few minutes later that ''The doctor thinks I'm done for.'' We have witnessed many instances in which a terminally ill older person has attempted to spare the feelings of physicians and other staff members but has known his status full well.

It is understandable that physicians as well as others in the situation might wish to postpone announcement of ''the death sentence.'' Most commonly, the disinclination to speak openly of a fatal prognosis is rationalized as a way of keeping hope alive. However, this strategy can also be seen as an anxiety-reducing ploy on the part of those who withhold information and as a violation of the implicit trust between physician and patient.[25] Furthermore, clinical studies indicate that many patients comprehend their terminal status even when exposed to evasion and denial on the part of others.[29] The intended kindness can have the unfortunate effects of interfering with the dying person's opportunity to take care of unfinished business on both the practical and symbolic planes. In addition, hope is not necessarily destroyed by knowledge. Instead of hoping for prolongation of life under conditions of distress and serious dysfunction, one can emphasize other spheres of value.

Consider these recent examples that have come to the attention of one of us (R. K.) while working with medical residents in a large medical center. The physician in each instance had completed a follow-up examination of an elderly outpatient and shared the basic facts clearly, and directly, yet with sensitivity to the individual's feelings. In some instances the physician simply picked up on a comment by the patient to confirm what had already been surmised. One women turned immediately to her husband. "See, Charles, just what I told you! Now we can wrap things up!" The woman, suffering from painful radiation burns, expressed relief that treatment would now be limited to symptom relief and that she and her husband still had time to put some personal plans into operation instead of holding off until it might have been too late. A few weeks later they had completed a trip, and Charles reported progress in learning how to cook for himself. Although this woman was soon to die, she had the satisfaction of seeing several of her final projects completed. Another woman had become furious with herself for the inability to carry out obligations and promises. Realizing now that the problem was not in her willpower but in physical deterioration (primarily emphysema), she began to relieve herself of unrealistic burdens. Within a few minutes she was saying (with humor as well as purpose), "It's high time I did a few things for myself. They'll all have to find somebody else to do for them!" A tall, muscular man quietly thanked the physician for "levelling." He knew it must have been difficult for the doctor to give him the bad news, but she shouldn't worry too much. "Never did I think I'd have had such a good life. I've done most everything a man can do, and people have been just great to me." Like many other older people with progressive diseases and disabilities, he had gradually reconciled himself to death. He felt at peace with himself and secure in his religious beliefs. "Heaven would be just fine, if that's what God wants for me. Anything else God wants is OK with me, too."

The response to an unfavorable prognosis does not begin and end with the physician–patient interaction. Often the patient will have already considered the possibility before receiving the confirmation, and the cognitive and emotional processing continues afterward. The physician ordinarily is not in a position to observe the patient's (and family's) total response. It is safe to assume, however, that each individual will continue to work in his own style to integrate the fact of impending death into the overall world view. The attitude expressed on one occasion may be replaced by another as different aspects of the foreshortened life situation become dominant in the patient's mind. Most typically, the physician is valued as a listener but is not expected to work miracles. Patients are quite appreciative of the physician who not only "levels" with them but who also remains accessible and attentive throughout the entire terminal phase. In our own experience, older patients in general are especially appreciative of the opportunity to continue a supportive relationship with the physician while at the same time limit their expectations to what is reasonable under the circumstances.

Social and Behavioral Indices of the Last Phase of Life

The physician who is prepared to communicate openly and sensitively with terminally ill patients must still reach a judgment about when the last phase of life has begun. The medical picture alone can make this judgment complex and difficult. An aged person may be impaired, depleted, and vulnerable yet not at immediate risk—a situation that could change quickly. What appeared to be the final illness can be arrested in its course and the condition stabilized for an indefinite period. The situation is made even more complex by the fact that social and behavioral dimensions are closely related to physical ones. It may be useful for the physician to consider factors such as the following.

Cognitive and behavioral cues may be evident before biomedical indices make it clear that the person has entered on the final phase of life. The changes summarized below are not evidenced by every elderly man and woman for whom death is near. Furthermore, there are individual differences in expression as well as numerous false-positives. Nevertheless, experienced clinicians and researchers have learned to pay attention to certain changes and clues.

On the most general level, any abrupt change in thought and behavior can signal the advent of the terminal process in an elderly person who otherwise might appear to be in stable condition. Numerous observations of this kind were made in the course of a clinical research project in a large extended-care facility.[11,14,15] Some long-term residents suddenly approached friends or staff and pressed them to accept cherished possessions as gifts. One man, for example, handed over his pipe and tobacco (his "trademarks") to a friend and died before the day was over. He had not seemed to be in any immediate danger, although afflicted with several chronic conditions. Along with the gift-givers there were others who made a point of seeking out individuals for what proved to be final leave-takings. This included writing or telephoning relatives with whom they had not been in contact for years. As far as we could determine, these contacts usually did not involve direct discussion of impending death. Staff would be puzzled as to why this person was suddenly making the special effort to reach somebody who had never visited him; only in retrospect (stimulated by a psychological autopsy procedure[30]) did the out-of-character action make sense.

Other old men and women will put their premonitions of death into words. These communications can be either explicit or symbolic. Even the most direct expressions of a sense of impending death may not be "heard" or believed by the listener. "My time is up," a patient may say simply, and squeeze a nurse's hand. More directly yet, the message may be, "I won't be seeing you again. I'm going to die." The most typical reply to such utterances is reassurance, denial, or changing the subject:[11] "Oh, you're as healthy as a horse.... Don't talk that way.... You'll feel better in the morning.... Have you done everything the doctor told you?" Often the response does not acknowledge the nature of the communication at all; it is as though nothing had been said.

More subtle and indirect communications may also fall on deaf ears. "Good night, Charlie, see you Monday!" may be answered with "Goodbye," and a turning away. The communication may be oblique and idiosyncratic—a coded message that challenges the recipient. One example involved a 75-year-old former stonemason who had lived in the institution about 6 months and had participated actively in programs such as occupational and recreational therapy. He now appeared to have less vigor than previously but did not seem in peril for his life. However, one day he

said something peculiar, something out of character: could he please have directions to a certain cemetery near his former home? He was expecting the undertaker, you see. This communication was taken to make no sense and was therefore ignored. A few weeks later he reported that his former employer had called and wanted him to go back to work. There were graves to dig, eight of them. Staff were fond of this patient and humored him, without taking the communication seriously. Obviously, he was becoming a little "mental," yet his health remained stable and he did not present management difficulties.

This delusion persisted, however, and began to affect his behavior. He now refused to leave the ward: he did not want to be away when the people came to take him to the cemetery. The only physical problem evident at this time involved his teeth, which were receiving regular attention by the hospital dentist. It was judged that he needed and could easily withstand two extractions. These were performed in a routine manner without complications. But the old stonemason now insisted that he had to call his sisters—relatives he had never mentioned before. There still were no unusual physical complaints or major changes in his institutional behavior. Yet 2 days after the extractions and 1 month after the first cemetery inquiry, he died suddenly. His death was attributed to cerebral thrombosis.

This instance has been sketched in some detail to convey the circumstances in which preterminal changes in thought and behavior can be expressed repeatedly and yet not be registered as such. It was evident that this pleasant old man had become a bit "mental," so his unusual statements and the reluctance to leave the ward were simply minor problems to be worked around. However, the psychological autopsy procedure disclosed that he was in fact one of eight siblings.[30] The other seven had already died. With this significant bit of information now (belatedly) brought out, it was no longer such a mystery why he had specified that there were eight graves for the old stonemason to dig.

Lack of curiosity about the contents of a delusion or fixed idea often prevails when the stereotype of a confused or senile old person gains influence over us. It is entirely possible for a person to show cognitive impairment and yet still have a major theme to communicate. Learning from incidents such as this, the staff became more sensitive to "coded" communications and were thus in a better position to provide appropriate care, including psychosocial as well as biomedical.

Anxiety and depression are among the general

reactions that may signal the terminal phase of life. These states have other possible origins, of course, and there is no easy way to make the determination. We have a better chance of discerning preterminal implications when we do not fall victim to endemic assumptions about the nature of old age. The person who believes it is natural for the aged to be depressed or aimlessly agitated will not see anything that requires explanation.

Individual differences in response to preterminal changes make it unwise to focus on any single pattern of change. Each of us has our own way of reading these changes and integrating them into our lives. In a 5-year clinical study,[15] we had to abandon the assumption that there was a single pattern of thought and behavior change during the terminal process. The two most frequently observed patterns were actually mirror images of each other. Some old men and women became increasingly outgoing. They were talkative, sought interaction, and showed a heightened interest in the life that flowed around them. Meanwhile, other patients of similar age and medical status withdrew into themselves as they became aware of the increasing imminence of death. Affiliations were reduced, activities curtailed, and the remaining aspects of life were brought to resolution. Level of intellectual functioning and awareness of probable death were approximately the same for both sets of elders; it was their way of living with this prospect that differed.

Special attention should be given to cognitive changes that may signal the onset of the terminal phase. Decrements in performance on a battery of psychological tests have been found for institutionalized elderly who subsequently died sooner than their peers who did not show such decrements.[17,18] Their drawings, for example, became more constricted and disorganized several months before death. Major longitudinal studies have also found a greater mental decline for those who will die sooner than their peers. A pioneering research project by the National Institute of Mental Health drew a sample of old men who were highly selected for their good physical and mental health.[2] A decade later, a follow-up study found that the nonsurvivors had been inferior in cognitive performance to the survivors, even though all had been in relatively good intellectual status at the time of initial testing.[7] This suggests that even though a person may be thinking well enough, there may already be signs of accelerated decline that foretell earlier demise.

One of the best-controlled longitudinal studies has found that elders who decline to take tests of mental functioning as well as those who perform less adequately are more likely to die within the next 5 years.[23] A study of twins has also found that the member of a pair who shows a decline in mental functioning at one point in time is less likely to survive.[3] The tendency for reduced viability to show up in performances on psychological and behavioral tests has become well recognized in longitudinal research projects.[24] Taking large populations as the unit of analysis, it is possible to predict that elderly people with relatively greater cognitive impairment are closer to their deaths. This does not necessarily mean that the particular individual who stands in front of the physician will fit this pattern. There can be temporary and reversible drops in mental functioning in later life in association with insomnia, illness, nutritional problems, or depression.[5] Nevertheless, changes in the adequacy of mental functioning are properly regarded as possible clues to increased risk of death in old age. It is worth keeping in mind that the individual may remain aware of his situation and have significant personal values at stake even in the presence of cognitive loss.

There is more than one possible answer to the question: "When does dying begin?" Perhaps the most useful approach is to consider the onset of dying as a psychosocial event.[11] Four psychosocial contexts for the onset of dying are noted: (1) when the facts are recognized, (2) when they are communicated, (3) when the patient realizes or accepts the facts, and (4) when the judgment is made that nothing more can be done to prolong useful life. The assumption that there is an objective moment at which dying begins is highly questionable. Dying and living both occur within psychosocial contexts. The likelihood that each person in the situation may have a different version of reality does not detract from the importance of learning whether or not the dying process is perceived as impending or already in effect. As Glaser and Strauss and other have shown,[6] the behavior of caregivers is influenced by their perceptions, whether these be accurate or not. The same holds true for those of any age who find themselves in a life-threatening situation. There are important individual differences in the way that life and death are viewed: generalizing from yesterday's patient to today's can create problems all around. Awareness that one is now facing the terminal phase of life also has differential impact, depending on self-concept and personality, interpersonal support system, and many other factors. In a nontrivial sense, patient, physician, and family together construct a view of the last phase of life and proceed to function within it. Equipped both with technical expertise and the trust invested by patient and family, the physician is in an unique position to help shape coercive realities a little closer to the heart's desire.

REFERENCES

1. Birnbaum H, Kidder D, Coelen C, Goodrich N, Mor V: Hospice costs under the National Hospice Study Demonstration. Brown University Center for Health Care Research, 1984
2. Birren JE (ed): Human Aging: A Biological and Behavioral Study. Washington, DC, US Government Printing Office, 1963
3. Blum JE, Fosshage JL, Jarvik LF: Intellectual changes and sex differences in octogenarians: A twenty-year longitudinal study of aging. Dev Psychol 7:178, 1972
4. Bowers MK, Jackson E, Knight J, LeShan L: Counseling the Dying. New York, Thomas Nelson & Sons, 1964
5. Crook T, Cohen GD (eds): Physicians' Guide to the Diagnosis and Treatment of Depression in the Elderly. New Canaan, CT, Mark Powley Associates, 1983
6. Glaser BG, Strauss A: Awareness of Dying. Chicago, Aldine Publishing, 1965
7. Granick S, Patterson RD (eds): Human Aging, Part II, An Eleven-Year Followup Biomedical and Behavioral Study. Rockville, MD, US Department of Health, Education and Welfare, 1971
8. Health Care Financing Administration. Medicare program; Hospice Care: Proposed Rule. Federal Register, August 22, 1983, V. No. 163, 38146-38174.
9. Hendricks J, Hendricks CD: Aging in Mass Society, 2nd ed. Cambridge, MA, Winthrop Press, 1981
10. Kastenbaum R: Death, Society and Human Experience, 2nd ed. St. Louis, CV Mosby, 1981
11. Kastenbaum R: Multiple perspectives on a geriatric 'death valley.' Commun Mental Health J 67:100, 1967
12. Kastenbaum R: The New Psychology of Death. New York, Springer Publishing, in preparation
13. Kastenbaum R, Aisenberg RB: The Psychology of Death. New York, Springer Publishing, 1972
14. Kastenbaum R, Kastenbaum BK: Hope, survival, and the caring environment. In Palmore E, Jeffers FC (eds): Prediction of Life Span, pp 249–272. Lexington, MA, DC Heath & Co, 1971
15. Kastenbaum R, Weisman AD: The psychological autopsy as a research procedure in gerontology. In Kent DP, Kastenbaum R, Sherwood S (eds): Research, Planning, and Action for the Elderly, pp 210–217. New York, Behavioral Publications, 1972
16. Kidder D, Birnbaum H, Coelen C: Impact of hospice on the health care costs of terminal care patients. Brown University Center for Health Care Research, 1984
17. Lieberman M: Psychological correlates of impending death: Some preliminary observations. J Gerontol 20:181, 1965
18. Lieberman M, Caplan AS: Distance from death as a variable in the study of aging. Dev Psychol 2:71, 1970
19. Lopata HZ: Women as Widows: Support Systems. New York, Elsevier, 1979
20. Mor, V, Greer DS: Policy Implications of National Hospice Study Demonstration Findings. Brown University Hospice Study Center, 1984
21. Munley A: The Hospice Alternative. New York, Basic Books, 1983
22. President's Commission for the Study of Ethical Problems in Medicine and Biomedical and Behavioral Research: Defining Death. Washington, DC, US Government Printing Office, 1981
23. Riegel KF, Riegel RM, Myer M: A study of the dropout rate in longitudinal research on aging and the prediction of death. J Pers Soc Res 5:342, 1967
24. Schaie KW (ed): Longitudinal Studies of Adult Psychological Development. New York, Guilford Press, 1983
25. Schulz R, Aderman D: How the medical staff copes with dying patients: A critical review. Omega, Journal of Death and Dying 7:11, 1976
26. Stoddard S: The Hospice Movement. New York, Stein & Day, 1978
27. Troll L: Continuations: Adult Development and Aging. Monterey, CA, Brooks/Cole, 1982
28. Watson DN: Brain Death: Ethical Considerations. West Lafayette, IN, Purdue University Press, 1980
29. Weisman AD: On Dying and Denying. New York, Behavioral Publications, 1971
30. Weisman AD, Kastenbaum R: The Psychological Autopsy: A Study of the Terminal Phase of Life. New York, Behavioral Publications, 1968

VI

Special Topics in Geriatrics

37   Diabetes in the Elderly

Joan Albin, Herbert Ross, and Harold Rifkin

Diabetes detection, using oral glucose tolerance tests, reveals a distinct increase in the incidence of the metabolic disorder per decade of life beginning with the age of 50.[12] The fasting blood sugar value may remain normal, but the postglucose levels rise in a progressive and sustained manner. The result is a 2-hour sugar value that is usually as high or even higher than that attained at 1 hour.

A diagnosis of diabetes mellitus should not be made on the basis of a single glucose tolerance test because many factors apart from diabetes affect glucose tolerance. McDonald and co-workers,[27] in a study of the reproducibility of the oral glucose tolerance test, showed that many patients initially diagnosed as diabetics have, on subsequent testing, been reclassified as nondiabetics.

Careful attention should be paid to the dietary habits of the patient before the performance of the test. Perusal of various studies of glucose tolerance in the elderly reveal that the subjects were often inhabitants of nursing, convalescent, or old-age homes and were usually sedentary, chronically ill, or malnourished. These factors become increasingly significant in that severe carbohydrate restriction produces decreased glucose tolerance even in the normal person. The present recommendation is for patients to be given a minimum carbohydrate intake of 150 g/day for each of 3 days preceding the glucose tolerance test, provided that the subject has consumed a normal diet prior to this period. In elderly patients with poor nutritional status, a food intake of 250 g to 300 g of carbohydrate daily for 3 days is more appropriate.

Inactivity is an important contributory factor in decreasing glucose tolerance. Decreased glucose tolerance is frequently noted after acute stressful illnesses such as recent myocardial infarction, cerebrovascular accident, extensive burns, trauma, and surgical procedures. These events may occur in a previously undiagnosed diabetic, or the attendant stress may precipitate diabetes in a prediabetic person. It is conceivable that the abnormal glucose tolerance may be a temporary finding. Thus either acute illness, poor nutrition, or physical inactivity may be predisposing factors to glucose intolerance.

An abnormal glucose tolerance curve may result from endocrinopathies associated with increased secretion of various hormones (*e.g.,* thyrotoxicosis, hyperadrenocorticism, pheochromocytoma, and acromegaly). In addition, certain drugs frequently used by elderly patients decrease glucose tolerance. These include nicotinic acid and diuretic agents such as benzothiadiazines, furosemide, ethacrynic acid, L-dopa, β-blockers, tricyclic antidepressants, and phenothiazines. Other factors that affect the glucose tolerance include the time of testing, the size of the oral glucose load, and the activity of the subject during the test.[2]

Elderly age and old age are perhaps not to be construed as synonymous. Jackson and co-workers[20] have observed that diminution of glucose tolerance with age does not extend past 75 or 80 years. Patients between 75 and 84 years of age had no higher mean curves than those between ages 65 and 74. Actually, patients past age 85 have lower peaks and lower 2-hour blood sugar levels. Jackson succinctly states: "This suggests that old age is either less diabetogenic than elderly age or that most of the potential diabetics have already been diagnosed or died off."

A fundamental question is whether the deterioration of glucose tolerance with advancing age is a normal physiologic alteration or whether it relates to an increasing incidence of diabetes. Many solutions have been suggested to resolve this.

Andres and his associates[3] have performed 3-

hour glucose tolerance tests following administration of 1.75 g of oral glucose per kilogram of body weight to normal adult males. They confirmed the precious observations that blood glucose levels rise with age, particularly at the second hour. A nomogram was constructed using age-adjusted criteria for physiologic blood glucose levels at a crucial diagnostic time. This enables the physician to ascertain the significance of the patient's 2-hour value compared with that of others in a similar age-group. The nomogram appears to be useful for screening purposes.

Similarly, within the past decade, O'Sullivan and Mahan[30] designed a study to determine whether standards for interpreting blood sugar levels should be modified for each age-group. This would be valid if the rise in blood glucose levels with advancing age is accepted as a normal physiologic change. Two criteria were used to evaluate 1946 blood sugar data from the population of Oxford, Massachusetts. A single criterion based on the population's 92nd percentile for each of 7 decades were chosen. Confirmation of diabetes during the subsequent 20 years was used to evaluate the relative merits of the two approaches. The 92nd percentile for initial venous 1- to 2-hour postprandial blood sugar in the Oxford population was 140 mg/dl, whereas the corresponding percentiles for each decade group varied from 130 mg to 160 mg/dl.

Twenty-three percent of persons initially rated abnormal developed diabetes during the next 20 years, whereas the corresponding proportion for those initially abnormal by the age-adjusted criteria was 16%. In general, their criterion was of special value for patients under 40, but the age-adjusted criteria had the disadvantage of including more false positives. The single criterion appeared more favorable for those over 40, because 23% of the group judged abnormal by this criterion and normal by the age-adjusted criteria were found to have diabetes on subsequent observations.

A 4-year study of Pima Indians in Central Arizona revealed an age-related sharply rising mean blood glucose curve, which was primarily the result of an increasing proportion of diabetes rather than a physiologic deterioration of glucose tolerance with increasing age. Bennett and co-workers[4] observed the emergence of a significant bimodal pattern in the distribution of post–glucose-load tolerance levels among Indians ranging from 5 to 74 years of age. This pattern indicated that the population could be divided into subpopulations. The first group represented the majority of normal Indians and showed only a slight rise of mean

plasma glucose levels with age. The second group consisted of a subpopulation of diabetic Indians with higher blood glucose levels whose size increased with advancing age.

Review of these studies on the effect of aging on blood glucose and of other epidemiologic studies has increased our appreciation of the heterogeneity of diabetes and the lack of consistency in the definition of diabetes. In 1978, the National Diabetes Data Group was formed to propose a new scheme for the classification and diagnosis of diabetes, so as to provide a uniform framework for clinical and epidemiologic research.[29]

CLASSIFICATION OF DIABETES MELLITUS AND OTHER CATEGORIES OF GLUCOSE INTOLERANCE

Diabetes Mellitus
   Type I or Insulin Dependent Type (IDDM)
   Type II or Non-insulin Dependent Type (NIDDM)
     Obese
     Nonobese
   Other Types (hyperglycemia associated with certain conditions or syndromes)
Impaired Glucose Tolerance (IGT)
Gestational Diabetes (GDM)
Statistical Risk Classes
   Previous abnormality of glucose tolerance (Prev AGTT)
   Potential abnormality of glucose tolerance (Pot AGTT)

The subclassification of idiopathic diabetes mellitus separates the insulin-dependent patients (type I) from those who are non–insulin dependent (type II) regardless of age. The third subclassification of idiopathic diabetes mellitus is termed "other types" and refers to the association of hyperglycemia with a variety of genetic syndromes, pancreatic diseases, hormonal abnormalities, drug or chemical exposures, and insulin receptor abnormalities. Type I, or insulin-dependent diabetes (IDDM), is characterized clinically by an abrupt onset of symptoms, insulinopenia, proneness to ketosis, and dependence on injected insulin to sustain life.

In type II, or non–insulin-dependent diabetes (NIDDM), the onset of disease is usually insidious and there may be low, normal, or high levels of insulin associated with insulin resistance. Patients with NIDDM are not prone to ketosis and not dependent on insulin treatment to sustain life.

They may require insulin, however, for correction of hyperglycemia if this cannot be achieved with diet or oral agents.

The term *impaired glucose tolerance* (IGT) was introduced to describe those individuals with plasma glucose levels intermediate between those considered normal and those considered diabetic. Previous terms applied to this group include *chemical, borderline, latent,* or *subclinical diabetes.* The elevated postprandial glucose levels in elderly subjects with normal fasting plasma glucose levels would qualify for the category of impaired glucose tolerance. In most patients IGT does not progress to overt diabetes but either reverts to normal or remains impaired. Patients with IGT have an insignificant risk for the development of specific microvascular complications, but studies have shown an increased risk for macrovascular complications, especially when IGT is associated with other risk factors such as hypertension, hyperlipidemia, obesity, and cigarette smoking. It is unknown if this observation applies to the seventh, eighth, or ninth decades.

The last two categories refer to persons with normal glucose tolerance who have had previous or potential abnormalities of glucose tolerance. The long-term prognosis of patients in these statistical risk classes is unknown. The diagnostic criteria for categories of glucose intolerance are listed in Table 37-1. If a patient has symptoms of polyuria, polydipsia, and polyphagia or has a fasting plasma glucose level of greater than 140 mg/dl on more than one occasion, there is no need to do an oral glucose tolerance test.

The oral glucose tolerance test is done either for purposes of clinical research or when the diagnosis is in doubt. The current criteria are standardized with an oral glucose challenge of 75 g in nonpregnant adults.

The possible mechanisms of the impaired glucose tolerance of aging are impaired insulin release and/or impaired insulin action at target tissues. The data on insulin release in aging are conflicting, and numerous studies report increased, decreased, or normal insulin responses to oral or intravenous glucose. In contrast, most recent studies indicate that insulin resistance accounts for the impaired glucose tolerance of aging. DeFronzo studied 84 healthy volunteers between the ages of 21 and 84 years.[13] He found a highly significant inverse correlation between glucose metabolism in response to endogenous or infused insulin and advancing age. In this same group, the insulin response to infused glucose was similar in all age-groups. Other investigators, using different experimental techniques to study glucose metabolism, have also shown that reduced glucose tolerance of the elderly is due to insulin resistance. They concluded that the probable site of impaired insulin action was in skeletal muscle.[38] Insulin binding to cellular receptors in aging has been shown to be normal.[18] Diminished binding of insulin to its receptor in aged muscle has not been demonstrated. Therefore it is likely that insulin resistance is associated with a defect in glucose transport into cells or in some aspect of insulin-mediated intracellular glucose metabolism (post-receptor defect). Alternatively, the defect in glucose disposal may be related to the well-documented and significant reduction in muscle mass with aging.[10]

CLINICAL FEATURES

The elderly diabetic may present with few or no clinical symptoms and signs. Frequently, the complications are the heralding manifestations of the illness. In general, the elderly diabetic is obese and does not require insulin except perhaps during acute medical or surgical situations. He can frequently be managed by diet alone or with oral hypoglycemic agents. A smaller number of elderly diabetics are insulin dependent and ketosis prone, frequently exhibiting alternating swings between hypoglycemia and hyperglycemia. Occasionally,

TABLE 37-1 Diagnostic Criteria for Classification of Glucose Tolerance in Adults*

Criteria	Diabetes Mellitus	Impaired Glucose Tolerance
Fasting venous plasma glucose (mg/dl)	$\geq$ 140	< 140
1-hour venous plasma glucose (or ½ hr or 1½ hr)	> 200	$\geq$ 200
2-hour venous plasma glucose	$\geq$ 200	$\geq$ 140
		< 200

* 75 g glucose load

during acute stress, acidosis or rapidly developing coma may be the first indication of diabetes.

The complications of diabetes may be the significant clinical findings in the elderly patient. Cataracts are probably more frequent in the diabetic, although this has been challenged by some clinical investigators. The nature of the cataract is similar in both diabetics and nondiabetics. It may develop at an earlier age and may tend to mature more rapidly in the elderly diabetic. The development of cataract in diabetics is related to osmotic swelling of the lens fibers secondary to the accumulation of sorbitol during hyperglycemia.[9]

Similarly the pathogenesis of retinopathy is thought to involve osmotic damage to the intramural pericytes of the retinal capillaries by accumulation of sorbitol. In general, retinopathy is noted in 35% to 45% of diabetic patients over 60 years of age. Background retinopathy including microaneurysms, hemorrhages, macular edema, venous dilation and beading, and soft cotton wool and hard exudates are the usual findings.

Retinitis proliferans is a serious complication. The probability of visual impairment sufficient to cause difficulty in employment increases from 3% in patients under 30 years at the time of diagnosis of diabetes, to 32% in patients diagnosed over age 60.[8] Duration of diabetes is a major contributing factor, since the chance of blindness in younger patients is only 3% after 5 years of illness, in contrast to 20% in patients over 60 at the time of diagnosis. In patients with established retinopathy, control of diabetes does not appear to improve the prognosis.[25] Hypertension may accelerate progression of retinopathy. Therefore, control of high blood pressure is an important part of the management of these patients. Laser photocoagulation therapy for proliferative retinopathy is an effective method of preserving vision.[15]

Skin Disorders

Several skin conditions should alert the clinician to suspect diabetes in the older patient. Generalized itching has been noted and described by various physicians. Pruritus vulvae is a common complaint in elderly diabetic patients, but atrophic, dry, scaly, and lichenified vulvae with resultant pruritus is common in older women without diabetes.

Dupuytren's contracture is more common in the elderly diabetic than in the nondiabetic. Facial rubeosis and vascular changes in the skin of the feet may be found in patients who have had diabetes for 20 years or longer. The changes in the feet include a thin and delicate skin, atrophy of

the subcutaneous tissue, and associated plantar rubeosis. Xanthelasma palpebrarum, planar xanthomatous plaques of the skin (upper trunk), eruptive xanthomas, and necrobiosis lipoidica diabeticorum are seen both in the older and younger diabetic patients. It has been stated that bacterial infections producing furuncles, folliculitis, carbuncles, ecthyma, and streptodermatitis should alert the clinician to suspect diabetes.

Fungal skin infection, although not more common in the older age-group, may lead to more serious sequelae. These include candidiasis and mucormycosis. Candidiasis may lead to local intertriginous infection, paronychia, balanitis, and vulvovaginitis. Systemic dissemination may be catastrophic. Orbital cellulitis, cavernous sinus thrombosis, and fulminating meningitis may be the ultimate outcome of mucormycosis.

A cutaneous lesion, possibly specific for diabetes mellitus, is called diabetic dermopathy. It has also been described as atrophic pretibial macules. The plaques are usually small, oval or round, measuring 0.5 cm to 1.0 cm in diameter and occasionally crusted. The edges are usually well defined. The skin between the plaques is normal. The most frequent location of these lesions is on the anterior and lateral aspects of the lower extremities. They can also be observed below the external malleolus and on the forearms. When the lesions heal, they result in round or oval pigmented scars. These healed lesions are observed in elderly patients with longstanding diabetes.

Reactive perforating collagenosis characterized by the appearance of umbilicated hyperpigmented papules through which strands of collagen are extruded has been described in diabetics with retinal and renal complications.[34] This disorder had been previously described only in nondiabetic children with no evidence of renal disease.

Diabetic Neuropathy

The elderly diabetic patient may manifest combinations of peripheral neuropathies, visceral neuropathies, and cranial nerve palsies. Peripheral neuropathy may be chronic or subacute. The findings are most frequently symmetrical, confined to the lower extremities, and sensory. However, the upper extremities may also be involved. Loss of tactile sense and two-point discrimination in the fingers may be serious problems for a blind diabetic who relies on Braille. Absent ankle jerks and, somewhat less frequently, absent knee jerks may be the only indications of peripheral neuropathy. Diminution or complete loss of vibratory sense is relatively common. Pain and burning sensations in the feet with severe hyperesthesia may also occur. Remissions are common, but relapses frequently occur.

Although symptoms may decrease and actually disappear, loss of deep tendon reflexes and diminished vibratory sense persist. Absent perception of heat, cold, and touch may be noted in more severe cases. Deep pain, with hyperalgesia and tender muscles, is noted in advanced cases. Plantar ulcers can be a major cause of disability in the elderly diabetic. Neuropathy characterized by sensory loss and motor dysfunction of the intrinsic muscles of the foot is the predisposing factor. Neuropathic arthropathy, known as "Charcot's joints," usually involves the ankle and may be noted in patients with diabetes of long duration.

Diabetic amyotrophy or plexopathy is characterized by progressive weakness, muscle wasting, and pain involving the pelvic girdle and thigh muscles. The quadriceps femoris is most commonly affected. The amyotrophy is characteristically asymmetric with little or no sensory involvement. Older males with mild diabetes are commonly affected. Fortunately, the syndrome usually resolves completely in a few months to a year.

Ischemic mononeuropathy frequently involves cranial, median, ulnar, radial, femoral, and peroneal nerves. There is a sudden onset of weakness and pain followed by atrophy of the affected muscles. Resolution usually occurs in weeks to months. Diabetic truncal mononeuropathy presents as a sudden onset of severe pain that may mimic pleural, cardiac, or intra-abdominal disease. Cranial mononeuropathy presents as extraocular muscle palsies of the third, sixth, and fourth cranial nerves, in order of frequency. Pupillary function is characteristically spared. In the elderly diabetic, the most common condition to be excluded is aneurysm of the internal carotid artery.

Manifestations of visceral neuropathy develop in the elderly diabetic in the same fashion as in the younger patient. Involvement of the gastrointestinal tract is manifested by development of either esophageal dysfunction, gastroparesis diabeticorum, or diabetic enteropathy with a typical malabsorption syndrome or diarrhea. Constipation is a frequent symptom of the elderly and may also result from diabetic enteropathy. These conditions frequently lead to nutritional inadequacies, electrolyte and fluid imbalances, vitamin deficiencies, anemia, difficulty in diabetes control, and ultimately generalized weakness and debility. The vomiting and abdominal discomfort of diabetic gastropathy is often relieved by metoclopramide, a dopaminergic antagonist.

Neurogenic vesical dysfunction may be a presenting sign of diabetes. Buch and co-workers[7] found a high prevalence of bladder dysfunction by urodynamic measurements in asymptomatic newly diagnosed diabetics with hypotonic dilated bladders. Sonography of the bladder before and after voiding is a useful, noninvasive method for evaluating bladder dysfunction in these patients. This complication is especially serious because it may lead to infection of the bladder urine, ascending pyelonephritis, bilateral ureterocaliectasis, and pyonephrosis. In the elderly diabetic with preexisting arterial and arteriolar nephrosclerosis and diabetic intercapillary glomerulosclerosis, complications following neurogenic vesical dysfunction may lead to rapidly developing uremia and death. Retrograde ejaculation and impotence probably are of lesser consequence in the elderly diabetic, although the newer studies affirm the continuity and desirability of sexual functioning into old age.

Other manifestations of autonomic neuropathy are anhidrosis and gustatory sweating. The clinical cardiovascular effects of diabetic autonomic neuropathy include postural hypotension and resting tachycardia. Postural hypotension may have dire consequences in elderly patients with underlying arterosclerotic heart or cerebrovascular disease.

Simple noninvasive tests, such as heart rate response to Valsalva maneuver, respiratory beat to beat heart rate variation, heart rate response to standing, and blood pressure response to sustained handgrip and cold may provide valuable information in this group of patients at high risk for autonomic neuropathy. The presence of abnormal responses to the above tests in symptomatic diabetic patients has been found to correlate with a poor prognosis for long-term survival.[17] This group may also be at increased risk for sudden death for cardiac or respiratory causes.

A peculiar manifestation of neuropathy is characterized by profound loss of weight, anorexia, depression, and impotence.[16] The patients are older males whose diabetes is relatively mild inasmuch as they rarely require insulin. The picture has been observed to remit within 1 year in all six patients described. Clearly the major diagnostic problem presented by these patients is differentiation from malignancy, amyloidosis, lymphoma, and chronic infection.

The pathogenesis of diabetic neuropathy is not clearly understood. Microangiopathy of the vasa nervorum and infarction of peripheral nerves occurs in mononeuropathy. Metabolic alterations due to intracellular accumulation of sorbitol and fructose in the hyperglycemic subject lead to osmotically induced swelling of the myelin sheaths and decreased neural concentrations of myoinositol.[41] Normalization of blood glucose decreases this polyol pathway by decreasing aldose reductase activity.

Since most forms of diabetic peripheral neuropathy are characterized by remission and exacerbation, the efficacy of treatment is difficult to evaluate. Phenytoin and carbamazepine have been advocated.

In our experience, the results of the use of these drugs have been disappointing. Control of hyperglycemia is sometimes beneficial. Drugs such as tricyclic antidepressants, fluphenazine, and clonazepam are often effective in relieving pain and paresthesia. They have no effect on associated motor dysfunction. A new approach to therapy is the use of aldose reductase inhibitors, which decrease intraneuronal sorbitol accumulation and increase nerve myoinositol content. Sorbinil, an aldose reductase inhibitor, has been shown to improve motor nerve conduction velocity and is in active clinical trials for the treatment of painful neuropathy.[23]

Renovascular Disease

Diabetic renal disease increases with the duration of diabetes. The clinical manifestations may include hypertension, edema (nephrotic or cardiac in origin), azotemia, hypoproteinemia, hypercholesterolemia, proteinuria, and double-refractile lipiduria. The pathologic factors in diabetic nephropathy include diffuse and nodular intercapillary glomerulosclerosis, arterial and arteriolar nephrosclerosis, and chronic (interstitial) pyelonephritis. The clinical findings may relate more to the diffuse membranous changes than to the nodular lesion. The prognosis is guarded. The usual duration of life following the onset of proteinuria is considered to be between 5 and 8 years. Extrarenal factors may determine the ultimate outcome. These include recurrent attacks of congestive heart failure, systemic infection with sepsis, rigid salt restriction, or excessive use of diuretic agents. Dehydration and electrolyte loss secondary to prolonged vomiting, diarrhea, or a salt-losing renal process may throw the patient into intractable uremia. Acute pyelonephritis, gouty nephropathy, or necrotizing papillitis may precipitate renal failure. Patients with end-stage nephropathy may also develop superimposed uremic neuropathy. This must be borne in mind particularly because dialysis may

result in amelioration of this neuropathic component.

Diabetes in the aged is characterized by a relatively high incidence and severity of complications involving the medium-sized and large blood vessels. Between 50% and 70% of nontraumatic amputations in the United States occur in diabetics.[5] Clear understanding of the pathophysiology, vigorous patient education, and preventive measures would undoubtedly reduce the number of amputations. The most common manifestation of diabetic neuropathy is loss of sensation in the feet. The anhidrosis associated with diabetes results in cracking of the skin and allows entry of bacteria. The motor neuropathy causes typical foot deformity with exposure of metatarsal heads and ends of toes to the constant pressure of weight bearing. The insensitive, deformed, dry diabetic foot is subject to repeated asymptomatic and undetected lesions that may become infected. Occlusive peripheral vascular disease and microangiopathy delays wound healing and increases the risk for gangrene. Infection spreads rapidly along fascial planes of the foot and frequently involves the bone. Therefore, it is imperative that the feet be examined daily by the patient and at each visit by the physician. Preventive therapy with proper shoes and orthotic devices will reduce the daily trauma of walking. Daily inspection of the foot will reduce the risk of suspected lesions in a foot with abnormal sensation. Small, innocuous-looking plantar lesions may conceal widespread infection because of the impaired inflammatory response in the ischemic foot. These lesions should be debrided aggressively. Bed rest and antibiotics are essential. After the acute signs and symptoms have subsided, chronic ulcers may be effectively treated by total contact casting.

Ketoacidosis

A small group of insulin-dependent elderly diabetics may develop ketoacidosis as a result of infection, trauma, intercurrent illness, or other stresses.

Hyperglycemia and ketonemia result in an osmotic diuresis, with loss of water and electrolytes in the urine. If unchecked, hypovolemia and hypotension may develop. In general, water losses of 3 to 5 liters or more can be incurred. Patients usually exhibit some degree of hyperosmolality, indicating that water has been lost in excess of salts.

Salt deficits of 7 mEq to 10 mEq/kg occur in severe ketosis. Hyponatremia is common. Urinary losses account for the bulk of the deficit, but a variable loss may result from shifting of Na^+ into cells.

Serum potassium may be normal or elevated on admission, although most patients have sustained potassium deficits of up to 5 mEq/kg. The correlation of serum potassium with total body potassium is poor owing to a shift of K^+ out of the intracellular water in acidosis. Indeed, patients presenting with normal or low serum potassium levels in severe ketoacidosis have sustained substantial K^+ losses.

The degree of acidosis is variable. Deficits of HCO_3^- may equal 4 mEq to 5 mEq/kg. Arterial pH may be as low as 6.9, with an associated depression in arterial Pco_2. Deficits of Ca^{2+}, PO_4, and Mg^{2+} have also been recorded. Patients are usually in negative nitrogen balance, a condition that may persist for several days after the start of treatment.

In the elderly, the preceding events have a much greater impact on homeostasis than in the young patient. Kidneys whose nephron population may be reduced by longstanding renal disease do not readily handle the increased load of H^+ presented. Furthermore, renal function may become seriously impaired by reduced renal blood flow in acidotic patients presenting with hypovolemia or hypotension.

The primary aim of therapy is to stop production of endogenous acid and restore and maintain extracellular and intracellular fluid volume and electrolyte content. An individual approach to therapy is mandatory in the elderly. The duration and severity of ketosis, the existing cardiopulmonary and renal state, and the presence and type of infection are all factors that should be considered.

Recently, several studies have demonstrated the efficacy of continuous low-dose infusion of insulin in the treatment of diabetic ketoacidosis.[32] By infusing insulin at a rate as low as 5 units per hour, all abnormal parameters of disturbed metabolism were corrected. The frequency of hypoglycemia was considerably reduced. A similar response can be obtained by administering insulin intramuscularly in doses as small as 10 units/hr.

Hypernatremia and hyperosmolality occur more commonly after isotonic or hypertonic replacement fluids are used. In the elderly, especially when cardiac disease is present, hypotonic solutions may be administered with less danger of precipitating congestive heart failure. Isotonic solutions should be used, however, in the presence of hypotension attributable to depletion of intravascular volume. When heart failure is present, the monitoring of central venous pressure is helpful in guiding the physician. Over the first 8 to 12 hours, 3 to 4 liters of 0.45% NaCl is usually administered. Serum electrolytes, blood urea nitrogen, glucose, and arterial pH are determined initially along with a semiquantitative determination of serum and urinary ketones (Acetest) and urine glucose. These measurements are repeated at least every 4 hours.

Potassium is usually given as the serum level reaches normal unless electrocardiographic evidence of hypokalemia occurs before serum analyses are reported. This usually occurs by the fourth or sixth hour of treatment. Not more than 20 mEq/hr is given, especially in the elderly in whom cardiorenal problems may supervene.

During the early treatment phase of diabetic ketoacidosis, insulin therapy induces an intracellular shift of both potassium and phosphates. The decreased serum phosphate level affects total red blood cell phosphate concentration and indirectly lowers red blood cell 2,3-diphosphoglycerate content.[24] The latter nucleotide plays an essential role in regulating hemoglobin–oxygen affinity, facilitating oxygen release. Consideration should be given to replacing phosphates as well as potassium during the initial 24 hours of intensive therapy.

The use of bicarbonate has become a target of criticism, particularly since the danger of paradoxic cerebrospinal fluid acidosis has been reported.[35] We have not found this to be an absolute contraindication to the use of bicarbonate in severe ketoacidosis (HCO_3^- below 10 mEq/liter; pH below 7.1), but an awareness of this phenomenon is essential to its recognition. Moreover, bicarbonate should be considered in the elderly because severe acidosis with hyperkalemia may be followed by sudden cardiac arrest.

Administration of 5% glucose is usually begun when the blood sugar level reaches 250 mg/dl or less and is continued as 5% dextrose in 0.9% saline with potassium acetate or phosphate as indicated through the remainder of the acute phase of treatment. It is prudent to avoid lowering the blood sugar level below 250 mg/dl in the acute phase.

Within 12 to 24 hours, patients are usually able to eat and are given fluids and solid food. Regular insulin administration may be replaced by longer-acting preparations after 24 to 48 hours.

LACTIC ACIDOSIS

Elevations of resting blood lactate may occur in patients with diabetes mellitus. The presence of an excess of lactate is thought to represent cellular anoxia. This has been described with shock, hemorrhage, and exacerbations of chronic obstructive pulmonary disease and in patients for whom no apparent predisposing cause could be found.[1]

Clinically, the patient usually presents with a severe metabolic acidosis of sudden onset. Rapid development of stupor with Kussmaul-type respiration is usually present. Plasma lactate levels are high, usually above 7 mmol/liter. The level may not correlate well with the observed *p*H, however, because the degree of renal and respiratory compensation may vary in different patients. Nevertheless, plasma bicarbonate levels are frequently low. The serum potassium value is often elevated. Serum sodium concentration varies, but the serum chloride level is often reduced, creating the anion gap (serum sodium plus potassium minus chloride and bicarbonate: normal, 15 mmol to 17 mmol/liter) characteristic of this state. The serum phosphate value may be elevated, but the calcium level is normal.

The treatment of lactic acidosis is difficult. Because the etiology is frequently not clear, specific therapy designed to inhibit the endogenous production of hydrogen ions is not available. The situation has been likened to that of treatment of ketoacidosis in the preinsulin era. Treatment of shock, infection, dehydration, and correction of hypoxemia is mandatory and may indeed be the significant factors leading to a favorable outcome.

HYPEROSMOLAR NONKETOTIC COMA

The clinical picture of hyperosmolar nonketotic coma is characterized by thirst, polyuria, dehydration, progressive mental obtundation, and coma. Focal and generalized seizures, unresponsive to phenytoin or phenobarbital, have been reported. Delay in recognition and institution of proper management may be responsible for the continuing high mortality rate in many centers.

The alteration in mental status may range from lethargy to frank coma. The depth of coma seems to parallel the degree of hyperosmolarity.[19] It has also been suggested that the depth of coma also relates to the rapidity of dehydration.

The syndrome may occur spontaneously in a middle-aged or elderly patient who is usually mildly diabetic, requiring only dietary management or oral hypoglycemics or not even previously known to be diabetic. The syndrome has been described after burns, hypothermia, and the use of

steroids, alone or together with immunosuppressive agents or anticonvulsants such as phenytoin, and after peritonal dialysis or hemodialysis. We have observed this syndrome during an attempt at preoperative parenteral hyperalimentation in an elderly patient with pyloric obstruction.

The blood sugar level may rise as high as 2700 mg/dl, and the accompanying glycosuria leads to polyuria and dehydration, with more water being lost than solutes. Increased water intake usually follows, but it is usually insufficient to prevent the increase in osmolality that accompanies fluid losses and increasing blood sugar. As osmolality increases, intracellular dehydration, including that of the brain, occurs. Water intake diminishes as lethargy increases. Impairment of thirst may also play a role.

Renal function is frequently impaired as blood volume diminishes, impeding the elimination of excessive glucose still further. Because these patients are older, preexistent renovascular involvement is an additive factor.

The serum sodium level may be normal or diminished or elevated. Serum potassium levels are often somewhat elevated, the potassium stores are frequently depleted. Patients may exhibit mild acidosis with elevated blood lactate and ketone levels.

Therapy should be designed to restore normal plasma volume and to reduce the blood sugar level. The reported requirement for insulin has varied widely, from zero to hundreds of units. Dosage must be determined individually, and changes in plasma glucose, electrolytes, and osmolality should be monitored every 2 hours initially.

The choice of fluids for replacement is a matter of varying opinion. Isotonic saline and hypotonic saline have been advocated. Hypotonic solutions such as 0.45% saline are used at Montefiore Hospital and Medical Center. Infusion of 300 ml to 1000 ml/hr may be used initially. When severe preexistent caridac or renal disease is present, invasive monitoring of intracardiac pressures may be helpful. The need for potassium replacement is determined by the monitoring of serum levels and the frequent recording of the electrocardiogram.

Alcohol-induced ketoacidosis is generally a disorder of younger patients. Clinically, the patient is a mildly to moderately ill women presenting with nausea, vomiting, and abdominal pain after a heavy drinking binge. The blood sugar level may be low, normal, or mildly elevated in association with minimal glycosuria and marked ketoacidosis. Characteristically, the syndrome is self-limiting and easily correctable with fluid replacement.[11]

MANAGEMENT OF ELDERLY DIABETIC PATIENTS

The general principles of management differ somewhat in the elderly from those in younger patients. Problems in the elderly are more often related to the existing complications of the illness rather than to any symptoms attributable to the metabolic derangement.

The elderly patient has emotional and physical problems apart from diabetes. Rigid control may cause unwarranted anxieties relating to an enforced change in life-style. The elderly patient may be depressed, anorectic, tense, or agitated or suffering from malnutrition or insufficient physical and recreational activity. He frequently lives alone. Motivation to prepare meals according to dietary prescription is frequently minimal. Visual difficulties, memory deficits relating to cerebrovascular or Alzheimer's disease, and problems of ambulation due to neuropathy, stroke, or peripheral vascular disease compound the problems.

Nevertheless a nihilistic attitude toward dietary prescription is equally unwarranted. It is necessary only to bear in mind that one's goals in therapy must be limited by a realistic assessment of what can be achieved. One cannot change the eating patterns of a life time. Ethnic and individual considerations must not be disregarded in constructing a dietary program. Care should be taken by trained persons to learn these preferences and to incorporate them into the prescription. Attention must be paid to the patient's ability to afford what is prescribed. It is essential that the patient understand the instructions in detail if he is to be expected to carry them out.

If, as is frequently the case, the patient is overweight, caloric restriction should be encouraged. Dietary protein should be adequate in quantity and quality with minimum of 0.7 g/kg/day of high quality protein. Sucrose should be restricted. Cereals, breads, vegetables, rice, or noodles should be used as sources of carbohydrate. The glycemic response to different complex carbohydrates has been shown to be highly variable. The physical form as well as fiber content of the food may be important in determining the blood glucose response.[21]

Earlier enthusiasm for limiting carbohydrate content in favor of fats has long since been dissipated by the demonstration of the importance of hyperlipidemias as risk factors in the development of vascular disease. Recent emphasis has been on increasing carbohydrate in the form of starches to 50% to 55% of total calorie intake because of the demonstration by several workers that in mild maturity-onset diabetes, glucose tolerance is improved while hyperinsulinemia is either unchanged or ameliorated on this regimen.[6] However if the fasting blood glucose is above 200 mg/dl, a high carbohydrate diet may worsen the blood glucose response to meals.

Aggravation of hypertriglyceridemia usually does not occur in patients ingesting this diet.[40] High fiber diets have become fashionable in the dietary management of diabetes. Addition of fiber to standard meals has been shown to lower postprandial glucose and insulin levels in nondiabetic subjects as well as non-insulin-dependent diabetics.[22] In insulin-treated patients, increase in fiber content of the diet may result in lowering of postprandial glucose levels.[28] At higher levels of fiber intake, the patient may need less insulin.

Regular exercise to the limit of comfortable tolerance may contribute to a heightened sense of well-being in the elderly. However, in our opinion there is no evidence that structured programs of vigorous exercise are either practical or beneficial in improving blood glucose control. In fact, if patients have blood glucose values greater than 250 mg/dl, vigorous exercise may further aggravate the hyperglycemia.[37]

Diet alone may not be sufficient for adequate control. Oral hypoglycemic agents or insulin may be necessary. Increasing visual impairment, diabetic neuropathy, and dementia make insulin injections difficult or even hazardous. Insulin, however, is necessary in emergencies such as acidosis, infection, stroke, and other stresses or during and following surgery. Its use beyond the acute stress should not be automatic. Hypoglycemia may be a more serious threat than ketosis, which is less common in the elderly diabetic. In those elderly diabetic persons who require insulin, the goals of treatment should be defined. The reduced life expectancy of the elderly, the presence of other medical problems, and the risk of hypoglycemia must all be considered in establishing reasonable goals of therapy. The rationale for meticulous glycemic control is the prevention or delay of microvascular retinal and renal complications, which tend to occur after 15 to 20 years of diabetes. Since the elderly or chronically ill patients have a reduced life expectancy, they may not be at a serious risk for the development of microvascular disease. Evidence suggests that tight control in the presence of established microvascular disease is not beneficial and may actually accelerate progression.[25]

Therefore, in our opinion we would aim for a range of blood sugar levels to decrease the risk of hypoglycemia and avoid hyperglycemic symptoms. Generally a blood glucose range between 150 mg and 250 mg/dl fulfills these aims.

The criteria for the selection of insulin preparations in the elderly are similar to those in other age-groups. Human insulin or purified pork insulin should be used for patients with local or systemic allergy to conventional insulin, lipodystrophy, and immunoresistance (defined as insulin requirements greater than 100 units/day) and in patients with intermittent need for insulin therapy.

Therapy With Oral Agents

Sulfonylureas are used in type II diabetic patients who are not ketosis prone and who, therefore, have preserved pancreatic insulin reserves. The combined use of sulfonylurea derivatives and insulin in such patients has been considered to be of little value. This form of therapy is being re-evaluated.

Mechanism of Action

In short-term studies, sulfonylureas have been shown to stimulate insulin secretion and to potentiate the insulin response to nonglucose stimuli.[33] Long-term studies show improved glucose levels without increased insulin levels. Thus, chronic effects of sulfonylureas appear to be mediated by extrapancreatic mechanisms.[14] A peripheral action on adipose tissue and skeletal muscle has been postulated. Sulfonylureas increase the number of insulin receptors and improve sensitivity to insulin at target tissues by postreceptor mechanisms.[31] An inhibition of hepatic gluconeogenesis by sulfonylureas has also been demonstrated.

The sulfonylureas are generally well tolerated with minimal side-effects. Gastrointestinal, dermatologic, and hematologic side-effects occur rarely. Hyponatremia, due to inappropriate antidiuretic hormone effect, occurs most commonly with chlorpropamide. Prolonged and severe hypoglycemia is a serious potential risk of all the preparations and requires hospitalization for intravenous administration of glucose for several days.

Since many elderly diabetics are taking other medications, it is important to be aware of drug interactions.[26] Several drugs potentiate or prolong the action of the sulfonylureas. Phenylbutazone delays the renal excretion of hydroxyhexamide, an active metabolite of acetohexamide. Salicylates

have a mild hypoglycemic action and may enhance that of tolbutamide. Sulfonamides, antithyroid drugs, probenecid, monoamine oxidase inhibitors, and dicumarol also produce hypoglycemia in combination with sulfonylureas. Alcohol, when taken with sulfonylureas, may produce a reaction similar to that seen with disulfiram, resulting in sudden collapse. Antagonism to the action of the oral agents has been noted with use of diuretics, corticosteroids, and high doses of nicotinic acid.

The oral sulfonylureas in current use include tolbutamide, acetohexamide, chlorpropamide, and tolazamide. Tolbutamide is rapidly absorbed and reaches a peak concentration in 3 to 5 hours. It is excreted mainly as the carboxymethyl and hydroxymethyl metabolites. Its peak hypoglycemic activity occurs 4 to 6 hours after ingestion.

Acetohexamide is also rapidly absorbed from the gastrointestinal tract. Its half-life in plasma is short—1.3 hours. However, it is converted to a very active metabolite, hydroxyhexamide, which has a biologic half-life of 5.3 hours. The hypoglycemic action of acetohexamide becomes maximal in 3 hours and lasts 12 to 24 hours.

Although absorption of chlorpropamide is rapid, the biologic half-life is 33 hours because it circulates bound to plasma albumin. It is eliminated in the urine. The hypoglycemic effect of a single dose lasts 24 hours or longer.

Tolazamide is slowly absorbed from the gastrointestinal tract, with peak plasma levels 8 to 12 hours after ingestion. The half-life in plasma is 7 hours. Its onset of hypoglycemic action occurs at 4 to 6 hours and is maximal for about 10 hours. Eighty-five percent of the administered dose appears as urinary metabolites.

Maximal accepted daily doses for the sulfonylureas are as follows: tolbutamide, 3 g; acetohexamide, 1 g; chlorpropamide, 750 mg; and tolazamide, 1 g.

A new class of sulfonylurea agents has been approved for use. The advantages of glyburide and glipizide are increased potency, once-a-day dosage, absence of hyponatremia, and fewer drug interactions. Since the second-generation agents are bound to albumin by nonionic forces, those drug interactions due to displacement of sulfonylureas from albumin are not observed. The dose range for glyburide is 2.5 mg to 20 mg/day and for glipizide, 2.5 mg to 40 mg/day.

The findings of the University Group Diabetes Program (UGDP) should be discussed briefly here.[36] The purpose of UGDP was to determine whether or not control of blood glucose levels would help prevent or delay vascular disease in non-insulin-requiring diabetes. After 8½ years of follow-up at 12 university-affiliated treatment centers, "the findings indicate that a combination of diet and tolbutamide therapy is no more effective than diet alone in prolonging life. Moreover, the findings suggest that tolbutamide and diet may be less effective than diet alone or diet and insulin, at least insofar as cardiovascular mortality is concerned." The debate on the validity of this study is continuing. A number of criticisms have been leveled against the study by diabetologists, epidemiologists, and statisticians. These include inappropriate patient selection and randomization; higher risk factors at the outset of the study among those taking tolbutamide; manipulation of electrocardiographic data; risk factors such as smoking and hypertension not measured or monitored; use of fixed drug dose; preponderance of mortality in a small number of participating clinics; use of "patient data" against "computerized data"; neglect of "co-morbidity"; contradiction of these findings by those of other studies here and abroad; and the danger of extrapolation of the UGDP findings to other sulfonylurea compounds. In our opinion, the use of sulfonylureas has not been shown to be associated with an increased risk of cardiovascular mortality.

HYPOGLYCEMIA

Hypoglycemia is an avoidable risk in the elderly diabetic. It may occur in patients taking either oral agents or insulin. Because chlorpropamide possesses a long half-life in plasma and a long duration of action, cumulative effects may result in severe and prolonged hypoglycemia. However, this complication has also been reported with tolbutamide and indeed may occur with all oral agents now in use.

The onset of severe or even fatal lowering of blood sugar levels in the elderly may not be heralded by the usual symptoms and signs of increased epinephrine output seen in the young. Many patients do not experience tachycardia, nervousness, anxiety, or sweating. They may become unconscious without warning. Episodes of bizarre psychotic behavior, slurring of speech, convulsive seizures, disorientation, confusion, and somnolence are sometimes mistaken as signs of advanced cerebral arteriosclerosis. Nocturnal headache, nightmares, crying out during sleep, unusual sleep posture, and inability to be easily aroused should be viewed with the utmost suspicion. Chronic organic mental syndrome of severe degree may result from repeated unrecognized episodes and may yet be reversible with correction of the cause.

In long-term insulin-treated diabetes, there may be abnormal secretion of epinephrine and glucagon in response to hypoglycemia. This will increase the duration and severity of hypoglycemic episodes and may in part explain the lack of warning symptoms. This risk of insulin therapy must be weighed against the questionable benefits of tight control in the elderly.[39]

REFERENCES

1. Alberti KGMM, Nattress M: Lactic acidosis. Lancet 2:25, 1977
2. American Diabetes Association, Committee on Statistics: Standardization of oral glucose tolerance test. Diabetes 18:299, 1969
3. Andres R: Relation of physiologic changes in ageing to medical changes of disease in the aged. Mayo Clin Proc 42:674, 1967
4. Bennett PH et al: Diabetes in the Pima Indians: Evidence of bimodality in glucose tolerance distributions. Diabetes 187 (suppl 1):333, 1969
5. Brand, PW: The diabetic foot. In Ellenberg M, Rifkin H (eds): Diabetes Mellitus Theory and Practice, 3rd ed, pp 829–849. New Hyde Park, NY, Medical Examination Publishing Company, 1983
6. Brunzell JD et al: Improved glucose tolerance with high carbohydrate feeding in mild diabetes. N Engl J Med 284:521, 1974
7. Buch AC et al: Bladder dysfunction and uropathy in diabetes. Diabetologia 12:251, 1976
8. Caird FI: Diabetic Retinopathy as a Cause of Visual Impairment. In Symposium on Treatment of Diabetic Retinopathy, p 41. US Public Health Service publication No. 1890, Washington, DC. US Government Printing Office, 1968
9. Cogan DG, Kinoshita JH, Kador PF, Robison G, Datilis M, Cobo M, Kupfer C: Aldose reductase and complications of diabetes. Ann Intern Med 101:82–91, 1984
10. Cohen SH, Vartsky D, Yasumura S, Sawitsky A, Zanzi I, Vaswani A, Ellis KJ: Compartmental body composition based on total body nitrogen, potassium and calcium. Am J Physiol 239:524–530, 1980
11. Cooperman MT et al: Clinical studies of alcoholic ketoacidoses. Diabetes 23:433, 1974
12. Davidson MD: The effect of aging on carbohydrate metabolism: A review of the English literature and a practical approach to the diagnosis of diabetes in the elderly. Metabolism 28:688–705, 1979
13. DeFronzo RA: Glucose intolerance and aging: Evi-

dence for tissue insensitivity to insulin. Diabetes 29:1095, 1979

14. DeFronzo RA, Ferrannini E, Koivisto V: New concepts in the pathogenesis and treatment of non-insulin-dependent diabetes mellitus. Am J Med (Suppl 1A) 74:52–81, 1983

15. Diabetic Retinopathy Study Research Group: Photocoagulation treatment of proliferative retinopathy: The second report of the Diabetic Research study findings. Am J Ophthalmol 85:82–98, 1978

16. Ellenberg M: Diabetic neuropathic cachexia. Diabetes 23:418, 1974

17. Ewing DJ, Campbell IM, Clarke BF: Assessment of cardiovascular effects of diabetic autonomic neuropathy and prognostic implications. Ann Intern Med 92:308–311, 1980

18. Fink RI, Kolterman OG, Griffin J, Olefsky JM: Mechanisms of insulin resistance of aging. J Clin Invest 71:1523, 1983

19. Fulop M, Rosenblatt A, Kreitzer SN, Gerstenhaber E: Hyperosmolar nature of diabetic coma. Diabetes 24:594, 1975

20. Jackson WPU, Vinick AI: Hyperglycemia and diabetes in the elderly. In Ellenberg M, Rifkin H (eds): Diabetes Mellitus, Theory and Practice. New York, McGraw-Hill, 1970

21. Jenkins DJ, Wolever T, Jenkins A, Lee R, Wong G, Josse R: Glycemic response to wheat products: Reduced response to pasta but no effect on fiber. Diabetes Care 6:155–159, 1983

22. Jenkins DJA, Leeds AR, Gassull MA: Decrease in postprandial insulin and glucose concentrations by guar and pectin. Ann Intern Med 86:20–23, 1977

23. Judzewitsch RG, Jaspan JB, Polonsky KS et al: Aldose reductase inhibition improves nerve conduct velocity in diabetic patients. N Engl J Med 308:119–124, 1983

24. Kantor Y, Gerson JR, Bessman AN: 2,3-Diphosphoglycerates, nucleotide phosphate and organic and inorganic phosphate levels during early phases of diabetic ketoacidosis. Diabetes 26:429, 1977

25. Lauritzen T, Frost-Larsen K, Larsen HW, Deckert T and Steno Study Group: Continuous subcutaneous insulin. Lancet 1:1445–1446, 1983

26. Lebovitz HE, Feinglos MN: The oral hypoglycemic agents in diabetes mellitus. In Ellenberg M, Rifkin H (eds): Diabetes Mellitus, Theory and Practice, 3rd ed, pp 591–610. New Hyde Park, NY, Medical Examination Company, 1983

27. McDonald GW, Fisher GW, Burnham C: Repro-

ducibility of the oral glucose tolerance test. Diabetes 14:473, 1965

28. Miranda PM, Horowitz DL: High fiber diets in the treatment of diabetes mellitus. Ann Intern Med 88:482–486, 1978

29. National Diabetes Data Group Classification and Diagnosis of Diabetes Mellitus and Other Categories of Glucose Intolerance. Diabetes 28:1039, 1979

30. O'Sullivan JB, Mahan C: Relationship of age to diagnostic blood glucose levels. Diabetes 18 (suppl 1):332, 1969

31. Olefsky JM, Reaven GM: Effects of sulfonylurea therapy on insulin binding to mononuclear leukocytes of diabetic patients. Am J Med 60:89, 1976

32. Page MM et al: Treatment of diabetic coma with continuous low-dose infusion of insulin. Br Med J 2:687, 1974

33. Pfeifer MA, Halter JB, Graf R, Porte JD: Potentiation of insulin secretion to nonglucose stimuli in normal man by tolbutamide. Diabetes 29:335–340, 1980

34. Poliak SG, Lebwohl MG, Parris A, Prioleau PG: Reactive perforating collagenosis associated with Diabetes mellitus. N Engl J Med 306:81–83, 1982

35. Posner JB, Plum F: Spinal fluid pH and neurologic symptoms in systemic acidosis. N Engl J Med 277:603, 1967

36. Prout TE, Goldner MG: A study of the effects of hypoglycemic agents on vascular complications in patients with adult-onset diabetes: II. Mortality results, University Group Diabetes Program. Diabetes (suppl 2) 19:787, 1970

37. Richter E, Ruderman NB, Schneider SN: Diabetes and exercise. Am J Med 70:201–209, 1981

38. Robert JJ, Cummins JC, Wolfe RR, Durkot M, Matthens DE, Zhao XH, Bier M, Young VR: Quantitative aspects of glucose production and metabolism in healthy elderly subjects. Diabetes 31:203, 1982

39. Unger RH: Special Comment: Meticulous control of diabetes, benefits, risks and precautions. Diabetes 31:479–484, 1982

40. Weinsur RL et al: High and low carbohydrate diets in Diabetes mellitus. Ann Intern Med 80:332, 1974

41. Winegrad AK, Greene DA: Diabetic polyneuropathy: The importance of insulin deficiency, hyperglycemia and alterations in myoinositol metabolism in its pathogenesis. N Engl J Med 295:1416, 1976

38 Hypertension in the Elderly

Marvin Moser and Henry Black

One of the medical success stories of the 20th century is the reduction in mortality and morbidity that has accompanied the successful efforts to control elevated blood pressure. The concept that hypertension is a major independent risk factor for cardiovascular disease and death in persons over 65 years of age can no longer be seriously questioned, and we can no longer accept the dictum that "normal" systolic blood pressure (SBP) is 100 mm Hg plus a person's age. With so many Americans in this age-group with a blood pressure outside a normal range, it is important to review the methods of study and management for the elderly patient with high blood pressure. Newer data have appeared that require an update of earlier reviews.

Epidemiologic data, especially from the Framingham Study and repeatedly confirmed by others, have clearly shown that an elevated blood pressure is an important and perhaps the most ubiquitous risk factor for cardiovascular disease at any age (Table 38-1).[6] Furthermore, elderly persons with normal blood pressures (<140/90 mm Hg) have an increased longevity when compared with those with higher readings. Data are also clear that an elevated SBP is just as important as an elevated diastolic blood pressure (DBP) in determining prognosis in both sexes at all ages (Fig. 38-1). Contrary to previous beliefs, postmenopausal women do not "tolerate" hypertension better than men; elderly women with a normal DBP but borderline or elevated SBP have a 50% greater risk of developing cardiovascular disease than those with normal SBP. We must, therefore, define hypertension in the elderly; review and analyze the data regarding its potential as a risk factor; summarize the methods of evaluating and treating elderly patients with hypertension and contrast these to our approach in younger patients; and review and evaluate the results of therapy in patients in this age-group to determine whether treatment reduces mortality and the risk of cardiovascular complications.

Hypertension in the elderly has been classified in two different ways: (1) isolated systolic hypertension (ISH), in which SBP is greater than 160 mm Hg while DBP is less than 90 mm Hg, and (2) diastolic and systolic hypertension, in which DBP is greater than 90 mm Hg and SBP is usually greater than 160 mm Hg. The need to divide hypertension in the elderly into ISH and typical hypertension (diastolic-systolic hypertension) relates to the concept that ISH was believed to result from loss of elasticity in large vessels from arteriosclerosis in the aging population and does not have the same implications for morbidity or mortality or require the same therapy as combined systolic and diastolic hypertension. Certain factors, as elaborated by epidemiologic data, tend to dispute this theory. As in a younger population, the diagnosis of hypertension should not be made on the basis of one set of readings but rather after averaging several sets of determinations performed on different occasions.[5]

HYPERTENSION AS A RISK FACTOR IN THE ELDERLY

Diastolic Blood Pressure Elevations

Diastolic hypertension is common in persons over 60 years of age. The Community Hypertension Evaluation Clinic (CHEC) Program screened more than 1 million Americans using a single sitting blood pressure measurement and showed that

TABLE 38-1. **Average Annual Cardiovascular Incidents Per 1000 Population**

		Diastolic		
	Age	*<90 mm Hg*	*90–109 mm Hg*	*≥110 mm Hg*
Men	45–54	9.5	17.7	33.6
	55–64	18.0	37.7	62.2
	65–74	24.2	42.9	55.6
Women	45–54	3.0	5.9	13.6
	55–64	10.2	15.6	39.4
	65–74	17.2	32.4	54.5

(Data from Framingham Heart Study. [Castelli WP: CHD risk factors in the elderly. Hosp Pract 11:113, 1976])

18.2% of white men and 14.9% of white women, aged 60 to 64, had a DBP greater than 95 mm Hg while 4.2% and 3.2% had a DBP greater than 110 mm Hg (Fig. 38-2).[42] In blacks, the prevalence was even greater. Thirty-two percent of black men, aged 60 to 64, had DBP greater than 95 mm Hg, and 31% of black women of this age had these readings. The prevalence of more severe hypertension (greater than 110 mm Hg) was impressive, with 11.8% of black men and 11.2% of black women being affected. The prevalence was actually less than among subjects aged 50 to 59, which suggests that many hypertensives may die before they reach their seventh decade. More recent surveys in Milwaukee[18] and the Hypertension Detection and Follow-Up Program (HDFP)[8] found similar results. Do these elevations of blood pressure cause any problems?

Studies have established that hypertension is an important independent risk factor for cardio-vascular disease, particularly cerebrovascular accidents (CVA), congestive heart failure (CHF), and coronary artery disease (CAD) in young and middle-aged persons. A risk factor is a characteristic that is positively associated with the future development of a disease or condition. Its presence will help predict whether an individual will get a certain condition, but it is not necessarily an etiologic factor, catalyst, or preclinical stage of that condition or disease. Data from Framingham and elsewhere[36] show that the prevalence of hypertensive heart disease and hypertension-related conditions also increases sharply in hypertensive, compared with normotensive, individuals over 65 years of age. Increasing levels of blood pressure for both men and women increase the risk of cardiovascular disease for each decade of age; thus, hypertension is just as important a cardiovascular risk factor in the elderly as it is in younger persons, particularly if the DBP is greater than 110 mm Hg.

Systolic Blood Pressure Elevations

Isolated systolic hypertension is a common finding in the elderly population; it is unusual in persons under 45 to 50 years of age. In Framingham, the prevalence of ISH, here defined as greater than or equal to 160/less than 95 mm Hg, rose from about 5% for the 60- to 64-year-age-group to 30% for those over 80.[21] In Milwaukee, the majority of subjects screened over the age of 65 had systolic hypertension. Systolic pressure continued to rise with age while mean DBP for this population peaked in the sixth and seventh decades and fell thereafter. This had also been found in the Community Hypertension Evaluation Clinic (CHEC) Program.[42] Should life expectancy continue to increase, we can expect an increasingly large number of otherwise healthy elderly citizens to have ISH.

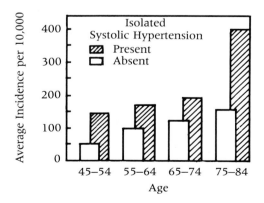

FIG. 38-1. Risk of myocardial infarction with isolated systolic hypertension (≥160/<95). (Data from Framingham Heart Study. [Castelli WP: CHD risk factors in the elderly. Hosp Pract 11:113, 1976])

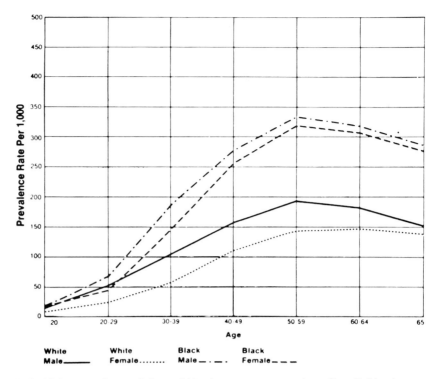

FIG. 38-2. Prevalence of elevated blood pressure at screening—diastolic blood pressure 95 mm Hg. (Stamler J, Stamler R, Riedlinger WF, Algera G, Roberts RH: Hypertension screening of 1 million Americans: Community Hypertension Evaluation Clinic [CHEC] Program, 1973 through 1975. JAMA 234:2299, 1976)

Until recently, many[38] but not all[12,26] investigators believed that an elevation in SBP without associated diastolic hypertension was merely a consequence of decreased aortic compliance and conferred little risk to the patient. In the early 1960s, however, that view began to change. The 1959 Build and Blood Pressure Study done by the Society of Actuaries showed that mortality increased rapidly as SBP rose above 137 mm Hg.[28] In the early 1970s, the Framingham study showed that while many factors increased the likelihood that an individual would get cardiovascular disease, hypertension was unquestionably the most important one for strokes.[19,25] Furthermore, the level of SBP was actually a better predictor than the diastolic or mean blood pressure (MBP) of a CVA, CHF, or CAD regardless of the patient's age.[20,23,24] Thus, elevations in SBP in the elderly do not appear to be a benign consequence of aging. Colandrea and the Chicago People's Gas Company Study also reported an increase in cardiovascular morbidity and mortality in a group of patients with isolated systolic hypertension.[7,9] The Chicago Stroke Study also showed that not only was the rate of all strokes and nonembolic brain infarctions increased about twofold in hypertensives (> 160/ 95 mm Hg on one casual sitting blood pressure measurement) but also that, as in the Framingham study and other studies, the increased risk was more accurately predicted by systolic than diastolic blood pressure.[23,33–35,39] The rate of all strokes increased dramatically as blood pressure rose (Table 38-2). In this study, subjects with ISH (SBP ≥ 160 mm Hg with DBP ≤ 79 mm Hg) had an overall stroke rate of 110 per 1000, compared with a rate of 42 per 1000 in those with an SBP less than or equal to 139 mm Hg and DBP less than or equal to 79 mm Hg.

These studies also showed that the greater the rise in SBP during the 5 years before a stroke occurred, the greater the mortality from the stroke.[11,33,35] The 1979 Build and Blood Pressure Study confirmed the results of the 1959 study and again showed that mortality rises as SBP rises for both men and women.[4]

In the group with blood pressures of 138 to

TABLE 38-2 Risk of Stroke (Per 1000 Persons) With Increasing Levels of Blood Pressure (mm Hg)

Systolic	Rate	Diastolic	Rate
<129	47	<69	52
144–179	65	>95	92
>180	135		

(Data from Framingham Heart Study. [Kannel WB: Current status of the epidemiology of brain infarction associated with occlusive arterial disease. Stroke 2:295, 1971])

147/83 to 92 mm Hg, mortality was increased 40% over expected in men and 25% in women; in individuals with blood pressures of 148 to 157/88 to 97 mm Hg, mortality was increased by 76% in men and 46% in women; and in persons with higher systolic pressures, 148 to 167/78 to 87 mm Hg, mortality was increased by 59% in men and 51% in women.

The Framingham data were reanalyzed and confirmed that stroke rates increased as SBP rose, especially to levels of 160 mm Hg or higher, in a group with a DBP less than 95 mm Hg.[24] In this paper, the degree of aortic compliance was measured by pulse wave recordings and subjects were classified into four groups based on the prominence of the dicrotic notch. Although more subjects with ISH had reduced aortic compliance as measured by this indirect technique (absence of the dicrotic notch), an elevated SBP was strongly correlated with an increased likelihood of stroke, regardless of the degree of reduction in aortic compliance.

It is now clear that ISH is not merely a result of large vessel arterial disease. We now know that subjects with this finding face an increased risk of degenerative cardiovascular disease, but as yet we have little definitive data on whether lowering the pressure will reduce mortality and morbidity. Most of the clinical investgations that proved that antihypertensive treatment was beneficial and safe did not include elderly patients with ISH.

It is tempting, based on available data, to conclude that lowering of blood pressure would be helpful in reducing risk. In favor of this concept is the argument that the pressure elevation itself results in further acceleration of the process of arteriosclerosis, increased myocardial muscle work, increased oxygen consumption, left ventricular hypertrophy, and possible cardiac failure.

Lowering blood pressure, therefore, which in some cases may etiologically be secondary to arteriosclerosis, may actually prevent hypertensive heart disease and acceleration of the process of atherogenesis.

TREATMENT OF HYPERTENSION IN THE ELDERLY

There is considerable uncertainty about whether, when, and how to treat elderly hypertensives. The clinician has a particular problem in deciding what to do in this population. First, the elderly hypertensive may have special physiologic problems different from those in younger hypertensives. In elderly patients autoregulation in various blood vessel beds is less effective than in younger persons, and vital organ function is often considerably decreased. For example, renal function decreases with age and by age 70 the glomerular filtration rate (GFR) may be reduced by as much as 40% to 50%. In deciding specific antihypertensive therapy, this fact must be considered. Myocardial contractility and cardiac output is reduced in the elderly as a result of myocardial cell changes, and cardiac reserve may be decreased by the presence of CAD. Oxygen demand may be increased by an increased cardiac mass and systolic wall tension associated with aging, with ISH, or with systolic and diastolic hypertension. Oxygen supply may be compromised further in an elderly hypertensive patient who experiences a sudden or dramatic reduction in blood pressure as a result of excessively vigorous therapy. Cerebrovascular disease, with a decreasing ability of blood vessels to adjust to sudden changes in volume or pressure, may also lead to difficulties in management.

Secondly, until recently there have been relatively little data on the effect of therapy on hypertension in the elderly. We do have some data, however, relating to this problem.[14–16,44–46] Twenty-three hundred seventy-six of the subjects in the HDFP study were over 60 years of age. In this study, mortality for subjects 60 to 69 years of age at entry was reduced by 16.4% for those in the stepped or special (SC) group compared with the referred care (RC) group, with no reported increase in side-effects or adverse reactions. Blood pressure was lowered to a greater degree in a higher percentage of patients in the SC compared with the RC group. There was a 45.5% reduction in fatal and nonfatal strokes in the SC group.[16]

The reduction in overall mortality in the stepped-care group was significantly greater than in the RC group even in those patients with pretreatment diastolic blood pressures of 90 mm Hg to 95 mm Hg and without evidence of target organ damage (the truly mild hypertensive).[17] The age-adjusted stroke incidence was reduced overall by 50% in the SC group of mild hypertensives (DBP, 90 mm Hg to 104 mm Hg) with no end organ damage. These impressive findings, however, do not answer the question regarding treatment of ISH.

The European Working Party on High Blood Pressure in the Elderly recently reported their findings in a group of subjects 60 years of age or older (average age 71) with both systolic and diastolic hypertension. Eight hundred forty people with average pretreatment blood pressures of 182-183/101 mm Hg were randomized to a treatment or placebo group. The use of one capsule/day containing 25 mg of hydrochlorothiazide and 50 mg of triamterene was sufficient to lower blood pressure to goal levels in 51% of the patients: 45% required two or more capsules; only 35% required the addition of methyldopa. Serum potassium decreased by only 0.1 mEq/L to 0.2 mEq/L and side effects were generally not significant.

Blood pressures were reduced by $-10/-6$ mm Hg in the placebo group and $-32/-13$ mm Hg in the treated group at the end of the first year, with only a slight additional decrease in blood pressure in the treated group over the next 4 to 5 years. A decrease of 27% in total cardiovascular mortality, 38% in cardiac mortality, and 32% in deaths from cerebrovascular disease was noted in the treated compared to placebo patients (differences in deaths from cerebrovascular disease did not achieve statistical significance presumably because of the small number of cases involved).

Both the European and the HDFP studies showed that elderly subjects can participate in and are adherent to a study regimen and can be treated successfully and safely. This is in contrast to the many anecdotal reports of poor adherence in the elderly because of memory or hearing problems and the reports of serious adverse reactions to therapy. Many of these have resulted from a poor choice of or too much medication. A pilot study on ISH in the elderly has been completed.[37] This demonstrated that goal blood pressure can be achieved in over 75% of elderly subjects by the use of low doses of a diuretic (chlorthalidone, 12.5 mg to 25 mg/day) with few serious adverse reactions or side-effects.

In view of the epidemiologic data that show increased risk and the results of the studies demonstrating benefit of treatment with relatively limited risk, the following approach to managing hypertension in the elderly is suggested.

Diagnostic studies should be limited in the elderly as in younger patients; most secondary causes of hypertension are generally less common or less often correctable. Endocrine disorders that produce hypertension, such as pheochromocytoma, Cushing's syndrome, or primary aldosteronism and other mineralocorticoid excess states are extremely rare, although not unheard of in this population. Renal parenchymal disease as a cause of hypertension may be present but can be diagnosed with a minimum of testing and is rarely curable at this stage. Iatrogenic hypertension can occur in the elderly, occasionally as a result of the use of nonsteroidal anti-inflammatory agents. Coarctation of the aorta will almost certainly have been diagnosed earlier in life.

Renovascular hypertension, on the other hand, may be more common in this population than in younger patients, with the diagnosis often suggested by the history. Generally, the patient will either be newly diagnosed as hypertensive late in life or will have had mild and easily controllable high blood pressure that becomes difficult to manage. In our experience, elderly patients with renovascular hypertension are almost exclusively white, often have significant vascular disease elsewhere (cerebrovascular disease, peripheral vascular disease and/or CAD), are or have been heavy smokers, and usually have treatment-resistant hypertension.

The specific diagnosis of this condition must be tempered by several factors. First, normotensive elderly persons often have identical renal artery lesions with those seen in patients with renovascular hypertension.[13] Second, a nephrectomy or a successful vascular procedure that reestablishes blood flow to the ischemic kidney does not always cure the hypertension,[40,41] and many patients still will require medical therapy.[47] Because the duration of the hypertension is inversely related to the degree of success of the surgery, the longer the history of hypertension the poorer the surgical results. Lastly and most importantly, the risk of surgery is increased in this population, especially if significant co-morbid disease is present. If blood pressure can be controlled with medication, without significant side-effects, it is often prudent to continue treatment and not investigate for renovascular disease. If control becomes difficult, further studies are indicated.

Newer diagnostic techniques have simplified the case finding and treatment of renovascular hypertension. Digital angiography may enable us to visualize the renal arteries with a venous injection: it can be done on an outpatient basis, and cost and morbidity are less than with standard arteriography. Unfortunately, this technique may not be accurate enough to distinguish lesions in the secondary or tertiary renal vessels, but these are of less importance in the elderly. Significant amounts of contrast material, with its attendant risks, must also be used. We have begun doing digital intra-arterial studies by puncturing the artery with a small catheter and injecting a small bolus of dye into the arterial circulation. This technique gives clearer pictures, and subjects can still be studied as outpatients. These procedures give more definitive information than the hypertensive intravenous urogram or any type of renal radionuclide study. Once a lesion has been demonstrated, its physiologic significance should be determined by doing bilateral renal vein renin studies, although not all investigators believe that these determinations are necessary.

Percutaneous transluminal angioplasty has changed the treatment of renovascular hypertension.[10] This technique has made it possible to increase renal artery lumen size and renal blood flow without surgery. Complications are usually minimal and acceptable, especially in high-risk patients. *The results, however, have been disappointing in our experience.* Some lesions are not dilatable, especially in patients with bilateral disease and ostial stenoses, and lesions recur in many, often within 6 months or less following the procedure. Of late, larger balloons are being used to dilate the lesions, but it is too early to tell whether this modification will increase the success rate. Fortunately, only a relatively small number of hypertensives, even in the elderly group, will have to be studied or treated for this entity.

We would recommend that evaluation of elderly patients, like all hypertensives, be directed at assessing end organ damage, discovering co-morbidity, and excluding secondary causes of hypertension. Many of these recommendations are contained in the recently released Third Joint National Committee Report on Detection, Evaluation, and Treatment of High Blood Pressure.[31] Much of this can be done with a careful history and physical examination. Pretreatment workup should include measurement of serum potassium, glucose, cholesterol, uric acid, and creatinine levels (an automated blood chemistry determination), a complete blood cell count. both macroscopic and micro-

scopic urinalysis, and an electrocardiogram. In some patients, a chest roentgenogram will be useful, and in rare instances an echocardiogram will add information about cardiac function and hypertrophy. *We do not believe* that ambulatory blood pressure monitoring, routine echocardiography, or stress testing are very helpful, either in evaluating or in planning therapy for these patients. Although some additional information may be obtained, treatment is rarely changed by the results of these tests. Hospitalization is rarely, if ever, required unless the patient has accelerated or malignant hypertension, an extremely uncommon occurrence in this age-group.

DIAGNOSTIC EVALUATION OF THE ELDERLY HYPERTENSIVE PATIENT

Indicated in Every Patient

Complete history and physical examination directed at determining the etiology of the patient's hypertension, degree of end-organ damage, and amount of co-morbidity
Serum potassium
Serum creatinine
Serum glucose
Urinalysis (both macroscopic and microscopic)
Complete blood cell count
12-lead electrocardiogram

Indicated in Most Patients

Serum cholesterol
Serum uric acid

Rarely Indicated

Cardiac echocardiogram
Digital subtraction angiography
24-hour urinary catecholamines and/or metabolites
Plasma renin activity
Plasma catecholamines

Specific Therapy

Treatment is indicated in elderly hypertensives with elevations of both SBP and DBP (140/90 mm Hg or higher). We agree with the recommendations of the Third Joint National Committee that this is a reasonable approach if nonpharmacologic therapy does not work. The report also recommends specific therapy in patients with isolated SBPs greater than or equal to 180 mm Hg, and we believe that patients with SBPs between 160 and 179 mm Hg, without DBP elevations, probably should also be treated, although, as noted, benefit of treatment has not been proven. The goal of therapy should be to reduce blood pressure to less than 140/90 mm Hg if possible for those with elevations of both SBP and DBP. In patients with ISH, a reduction of at least 20 mm Hg or to as low a blood pressure as can be achieved without significant side effects should be attempted. Although some elderly patients tolerate systolic pressures of 130 mm Hg to 140 mm Hg, many may not feel well at these levels.

The key to successful treatment of hypertension in the elderly is to be patient. The regimen should begin with lower doses than in younger patients and proceed more slowly at each step in the titration process. Aggressive treatment with resultant hypotension and inadequate organ perfusion may be a greater short-term risk than the elevated blood pressure.

Nondrug Methods

Nondrug treatment of hypertension has been recommended since the beginning of the 20th century. Many different approaches, including modification of the amount of some nutrients in the diet, weight loss, exercise, and behavioral changes have been proposed.[3] It is important to put these methods in perspective, especially in the elderly patient in whom the risk-benefit ratio of therapy with antihypertensive drugs is more difficult to prove. Although there has been some question about the value of sodium restriction in treating high blood pressure, most researchers agree that modest sodium restriction (60 mEq to 100 mEq day) is probably safe and will reduce blood pressure in some patients. Many elderly persons, however, have a lifelong habit of eating salt and have trouble reducing their intake even to this level. In fact, many younger individuals are unable to achieve and maintain this level of sodium intake. Furthermore, some older persons may not be able to afford to buy or find low-sodium foods despite the new Food and Drug Administration recommendations that foods be labeled with their sodium content. Patients should be told not to add salt while cooking or after it is prepared and to avoid heavily salted foods. Recent suggestions that potassium depletion may increase blood pressure or that augmenting dietary potassium may reduce blood pressure are interesting but not proven. The patient with renal insufficiency must be especially careful if this approach is taken. It is probably a

good idea to suggest a 60 μg to 100 μg/day intake of potassium with an increased intake of fresh fruits and vegetables, although cost of some of these foods may make them unaffordable to some persons. Examples of some high sodium, foods are listed below:

SOME FOODS WITH A HIGH SALT OR SODIUM CONTENT THAT SHOULD BE AVOIDED OR LIMITED

Potato chips	Bouillon
Pretzels	Ham
Salted crackers	Sausages
Biscuits	Frankfurters
Pancakes	Smoked meats or fish
Pastries or cakes made from self-rising flour mixes	Sardines
	Tomato juice (canned)
	Frozen lima beans
Pickles	Frozen peas
Sauerkraut	Canned spinach
Soy sauce	Canned carrots
Catsup	Many kinds of cheese
Olives	"Fast foods"
Commercially prepared soups or stews	

Calcium deficiency has also been implicated as a possible etiologic factor in hypertension,[27] although the data are far from convincing. Calcium supplements may be useful in elderly women with osteoporosis but have not as yet been definitely shown to reduce blood pressure. There are even less good data on the value of magnesium supplements or the use of diets high in polyunsaturated fats as treatment for hypertension, although these treatments have been suggested. A reasonably tolerated low-fat diet is probably a good idea in all patients, but we should remember that cholesterol elevations are not as strong a cardiovascular risk factor in elderly patients. It should also be remembered that some high cholesterol foods, such as eggs and milk, are nutritious, easy to prepare, and relatively inexpensive.

Weight loss may help to lower blood pressure in the obese hypertensive, but obesity is less of a problem in the elderly and weight reduction is difficult to accomplish. Exercise may assist in losing weight and, if modified to the patient, can and should be recommended in patients over 60. Although exercise may improve fitness and make patients feel better, there are few good data to demonstrate that exercise alone will reduce blood pressure over time in these patients. Behavioral methods, such as relaxation and biofeedback, are interesting approaches to antihypertensive therapy but probably unlikely to be very useful in the elderly population.

Nonpharmacologic methods of reducing blood pressure have the advantage of not exposing the patient to any of the possible risks of drug therapy, but they are generally not effective enough to substitute for drug treatment in most elderly patients. We do, however, recommend that some of these approaches be used, especially in elderly mild hypertensives, before initiating drug treatment. Often, specific medications can be started simultaneously with a weight and sodium reduction program. If this latter approach is successful, medication can be stopped after 6 months to judge whether or not lowering of blood pressure can be sustained without it.

Pharmacologic Therapy

If nondrug therapy fails, as it often does, medication should be started (Tables 38-3 and 38-4). There are abundant data to confirm that diuretics are probably the first-step drug of choice in most elderly patients. The Third Joint National Committee on Detection, Evaluation, and Treatment of High Blood Pressure has again suggested this approach.[31] Low doses of hydrochlorothiazide (HCTZ, 12.5 mg/day), or chlorthalidone (12.5 mg/day) may be effective, although, in our experience, a starting dose of 25 mg/day is usually more effective. Potassium supplements are usually not needed at this dosage but may be required should the dose be raised. If the blood pressure goal for the patient has not been reached after 4 to 8 weeks, then the dosage should be doubled (Table 38-5). Patients on digitalis, with evidence of ectopy, or those with diabetes may require potassium supplements at the outset or, in many cases, it may be more appropriate to begin therapy with combination diuretics such as HCTZ/triamterene (Dyazide), which contains 25 mg of hydrochlorothiazide, or if necessary with HCTZ/amiloride (Moduretic), which contains 50 mg of hydrochlorothiazide. The use of specific potassium supplements adds to the cost and complexity of the regimen, and supplementation with foods high in potassium (*e.g.,* orange juice, bananas, raisins, vegetables) may also add cost and unwanted calories. Hypokalemia should be suspected in patients who complain of weakness, muscle cramps, palpitations, or dizziness and should be looked for and corrected if present. A decrease of more than

TABLE 38-3 Antihypertensive Therapy in Elderly Patients

Step	Therapy
I	Small doses of diuretics
II	Full doses of diuretics plus potassium supplements or combination diuretic-potassium sparing therapy
III	Addition of a β-blocker or substitution or addition of hydralazine, α-methyldopa, clonidine, guanabenz, prazosin, captopril, or calcium entry blocker
IV	Substitution or addition of guanethidine or guanadrel

0.5 mEq to 0.6 mEq/liter from baseline or an absolute value of below 3.5 mEq/liter should be corrected.

Although thiazides increase uric acid, gout is not a common complication of therapy, except in those with a preexisting gouty diathesis. Cholesterol levels are elevated by 5 mg to 10 mg/dl initially but eventually return to near baseline levels and remain there despite continuation of therapy. If patients are placed on a reasonably low fat diet and a diuretic is prescribed, little change in lipid levels will be noted. Triglyceride levels will also be elevated by diuretics (and β-blocker therapy), but there is no evidence that induced elevations have an adverse prognostic significance. Thiazides may also elevate the serum glucose value and decrease insulin secretion, probably secondary to potassium depletion, but these changes may also not be of clinical significance. Although other agents can be successfully used as monotherapy in some patients (β-blockers, calcium channel blockers, converting enzyme inhibitors, and α-blockers), the thiazides appear to be first-step drugs of choice because of efficacy, ease of administration, lack of subjective side-effects, and cost.

Should blood pressure not be successfully controlled in a reasonable time (3 to 4 months) with appropriate doses of diuretics, a second agent should be added. β-Blockers are probably the best choice, although these medications are less effective in the elderly than in young patients. There are seven β-blockers available in the United States. Four of the available agents (propranolol, pindolol, timolol, and nadolol) block both the β1- and β2-adrenergic receptors and so are deemed noncardioselective, and three drugs (atenolol, metoprolol and acebutolol) primarily block β1-receptors and are thus cardioselective. Neither of these, however, completely spares the β2 receptors, especially in high doses. Labetalol is a β-blocker and also has some α-blocking activity. Pindolol and acebutolol have intrinsic sympathomimetic activity (ISA). Five of the agents (atenolol, metoprolol, nadolol, propranolol-LA and acebutolol) can be given once a day.

β-Blockers have distinct advantages and disadvantages in the elderly. All but pindolol lower cardiac output. This is a problem in the elderly since cardiac output is often low before treatment. Drugs with ISA are partial β-agonists in addition to being β-adrenergic inhibiting drugs when the patient is at rest and so tend to maintain cardiac output. Many older persons also have cardiac conduction disease and resting bradycardias that may be worsened by β-blockers. Drugs with ISA may be useful in these patients since these drugs do not reduce heart rate further. Since many elderly hypertensives also have peripheral vascular disease, which is often exacerbated by β-blockers (especially the noncardioselective ones), these drugs should be used with caution. Noncardioselective agents will also block β2-receptors in the pancreas and may reduce insulin secretion and worsen diabetes in type II or insulin-dependent diabetics; on the other hand, they may reduce the potassium-lowering effects of catecholamine excess, a potentially beneficial effect in the elderly patient with ischemic heart disease and/or ectopy.

In spite of some problems, β-blockers are useful in the elderly. Myocardial oxygen consumption, heart rate, and cardiac work are reduced when β-blockers are given. Angina pectoris, which is common in elderly patients, is often decreased. Several large trials throughout the world have demonstrated that the use of β-blockers will reduce the infarction rate and death in patients who have survived an initial acute myocardial infarction.[2,32] Thus, β-blockers have a definite place in the treatment of hypertension in the elderly. They should be used with great care, if at all, in patients with a history of CHF, asthma, chronic obstructive pulmonary disease, significant degrees of atrioventricular block, insulin-dependent diabetes, and symptomatic peripheral vascular disease. In general, cardioselective agents may be preferred, and drugs that can be given on a once-a-day basis facilitate compliance. Several thiazide–β-blocker combination tablets are now available and also make adherence to a program easier.

Rauwolfia drugs, in combination with diuretics, are effective in mild to moderate hypertensives regardless of age.[30] Many physicians no longer use these drugs, especially in the elderly, because of their central nervous system side-effects. There is no question that many are "slowed down" by reserpine, and some patients become depressed. This can be an especially troublesome problem in those with cerebrovascular disease or mild but compensated Alzheimer's disease. However, reserpine is inexpensive, is effective in a once-a-day dosage, comes in a number of single daily dose combinations with thiazides to improve compliance, and can be safe if used in selected patients. Its use should be avoided in the elderly who live alone, have been depressed, or have any evidence of dementia.

Should these medications be ineffective, many other drugs are now available for lowering blood pressure. Central α-agonists, such as α-methyldopa, clonidine, and guanabenz, can be used. α-Methyldopa was the step-two agent used in the European Study with good results.[1] This agent may cause postural hypotension, fatigue, and depression and may reduce mental acuity. α-Methyldopa may also rarely cause hepatitis or Coombs'-positive hemolytic anemia. Clonidine is likely to cause drowsiness and dry mouth and is often poorly tolerated by the elderly. It may, however, be more effective as a blood pressure–lowering drug than α-methyldopa in some patients especially if given at bedtime. Guanabenz is a newer agent with many of the same problems as clonidine.

α-Adrenergic blocking agents, such as prazosin, may be useful in elderly patients. These drugs will improve cardiac function by reducing afterload initially, but this beneficial effect may not be sustained with long-term treatment. Although generally well tolerated, prazosin and other as yet unapproved members of this class of agents such as terazosin may cause significant dizziness and even syncope when the drug is begun or when the dose is increased. The patient must be warned to be careful when he or she stands, especially in a hot room, after eating a large meal, or after drinking an alcoholic beverage. If low doses (1.0 mg) are used to start, this "first dose phenomenon" can usually be prevented. A combination of a small dose of a diuretic and prazosin may be effective in some elderly patients who have not responded to other medications, or the addition of prazosin to a thiazide and reserpine or thiazide–β-blocker regimen may produce goal blood pressures, that is, less than 140/90 mm Hg or the lowest pressure that can be achieved without significant side-effects.

Converting enzyme inhibitors are relatively new drugs. Captopril was the first released, and enalapril will be available soon. These medications

TABLE 38-4 Drugs Available as Antihypertensive Therapy for Elderly Patients

	Minimum Dose (mg)	Maximum Dose (mg)	Dose Frequency (times per day)	Cost
Diuretics				
Hydrochlorothiazide and similar compounds	25	50	qd–bid	Low
Chlorthalidone	25	50	qd	Moderate
Metolazone	2.5	5.0	qd	Moderate
Indapamide	2.5	5.0	qd	High
Furosemide	20	?	bid–qid	Moderate
Ethacrynic acid	25	100	bid–qid	Moderate
Bumetanide	0.5	2.0	qd	Moderate
Spironolactone	25	200	qd–qid	High
Amiloride	5	20	qd	Moderate
Triamterene	25	200	bid	Moderate
Combinations*				
Dyazide (HCTZ/triamterene)	1 tablet	2 tablets	bid	Moderate
Moduretic (HCTZ/amiloride)	1 tablet	2 tablets	qd	Moderate
Aldactazide (HCTZ/spironolactone)	1 tablet	4 tablets	qd–qid	High
Beta Blockers				
Noncardioselective				
Propranolol	40	240	bid	Moderate
Propranolol-LA	40	240	qd	High
Nadolol	40	240	qd	High
Timolol	10	40	bid	High
Pindolol (with ISA)	10	40	bid	High
Labetalol (with α-blocking activity)	100	400	bid	High
Cardioselective				
Acebutolol (with ISA)	400	800	qd	High
Metoprolol	50	150	qd–bid	High
Atenolol	25	100	qd	High
Combinations with diuretics				
Central α-Agonists				
α-Methyldopa	500	1500	bid	Moderate
Clonidine	0.2	1.2	bid	Moderate
Guanabenz	8	16	bid	High
Combinations with diuretics				
Vasodilators				
Hydralazine	25–50	200	bid	Low
Minoxidil	2.5	20	qd–bid	Moderate
Converting Enzyme Inhibitors				
Captopril	12.5–25	150	bid	High
Enalapril	Not yet available in the United States			
Rauwolfia Alkaloids				
Reserpine	0.1	0.25	qd	Low
Combinations*				
Peripheral Sympathetic Blockers				
Guanethidine	10	100–150	qd	Moderate
Guanadrel	10	100–150	bid	Moderate

TABLE 38-4 Continued

	Minimum Daily Dose (mg)	Maximum Dose (mg)	Dose Frequency (times per day)	Cost
Calcium Channel Blockers				
Nifedipine	30	120	tid	High
Diltiazem	90	180	tid	High
Verapamil	240	480	tid	High
α-Blockers				
Prazosin	2	15	bid–tid	Moderate
Trimazosin		Not yet available in the United States		
Terazosin		Not yet available in the United States		
Combinations with diuretics				

* For combinations, see?

are useful as second-step agents to treat moderately severe hypertension. Captopril will also improve cardiac function and is effective in treating patients with heart failure resistant to diuretics and digitalis. Few studies have been done in treating hypertension in the elderly with converting enzyme inhibitors. However, if the dose is kept low (*e.g.*, starting with 12.5 mg of captopril twice daily and going to a maximum of 50 mg/bid) and if these drugs are used with great care in patients with renal failure, they are effective, either alone or usually with a diuretic. They may be especially useful in the elderly with heart failure, but they are expensive.

Calcium channel blockers (*i.e.*, nifedipine, diltiazem, verapamil) have not yet been approved as antihypertensive agents; however, they are being used for this indication. Of the group, nifedipine reduces blood pressure most effectively and may also improve cardiac output. Side-effects may be troublesome, with headaches, flushing, and edema occurring in 10% to 15% of patients. Diltiazem is almost as effective and often better tolerated. Verapamil may have an adverse effect on atrioventricular conduction. The beneficial cardiac effect of some of these drugs may make them useful in the elderly, but at present experience is limited. Our initial experience with these agents as well as with nitrendipine, a new entry blocker, has, however, been favorable. These medications are also expensive.

Direct-acting vasodilators may also be useful as

TABLE 38-5 Dosages of Antihypertensive Drugs in the Elderly

Drugs	↓ Kidney Function	Liver Disease or ↓ Function
Thiazides	↓	NC
Furosemide	NC or ↑	NC
Potassium-sparing diuretics	↓	↓
Propranolol	NC	↓
Atenolol	↓	NC
α-Methyldopa	NC	↓
Prazosin	NC	↓
Hydralazine	NC	↓
Clonidine	NC	NC
Guanabenz	NC	NC

(↑, increase dosage; ↓, decrease dosage; NC, no change)
(Moser M: Management of cardiovascular disease in the elderly. J Am Geriatr Soc [Suppl 30]11:20–28, 1982)

adjuncts to diuretics. In younger patients, hydralazine often causes tachycardia and occasionally angina when given without an adrenergic-inhibiting agent. This problem is often not seen in the elderly because of reduced baroreceptor sensitivity. Hydralazine will reduce afterload and thus may improve cardiac output. Data have suggested that vasodilators, when used alone, may not be effective in reducing left ventricular hypertrophy even if blood pressure is reduced.[43] When they are given in combination with a diutetic and an adrenergic inhibitor, however, LVH can be prevented or reversed. Minoxidil is an excellent drug for resistant hypertensives but has too many side-effects (*e.g.*, edema, hirsutism, tachycardia) to be of great use in the management of hypertension in the elderly.

Peripheral sympathetic blockers, such as guanethidine and guanadrel, are effective antihypertensive agents but can cause significant postural hypotension and diarrhea. These problems may be more pronounced with the longer-acting preparation, guanethidine, than with guanadrel. These agents have the advantage of reducing blood pressure without any central nervous system side-effects, an important advantage in this population, but they must be used with great care. In general, a majority of elderly patients will respond with a satisfactory reduction in blood pressure following the use of a diuretic and one of the adrenergic-inhibiting agents. Some, however, will be unable to tolerate therapy or blood pressure lowering.

Special Therapeutic Problems

The elderly hypertensive, more so than younger patients, presents special management problems. None of these is insurmountable, but they do require attention and often adjustments in the choices of drugs or the doses used (Table 38-6).

Social and Logistical Problems

Many elderly live on fixed incomes and are not as mobile as younger patients. Many live alone or have few friends or family members on whom to depend. In these patients, the regimen chosen should be as simple and inexpensive as possible, and agents that may cause depression or worsen dementia should be avoided. Appointment schedules should be adjusted so that these patients can come during the middle of the day when transportation services are available. In our experience, once blood pressure has been controlled excellent results have been achieved with only three to four visits a year. Checking blood pressures in the elderly on a once-a-month basis is generally unnecessary. It is important that these patients understand the reasons for various medications, how to take them, and what to do if they experience side-effects. Patient-education booklets, such as "How You Can Help Your Doctor Treat Your High Blood Pressure"* and "High Blood Pressure and What You Can Do about It,"† help in this necessary educational effort.

Elderly Patients With Coronary Artery Disease

Many older persons have angina, a history of a myocardial infarction, or ischemic cardiomyopathy. In these patients care must be exercised to avoid excessive or rapid lowering of blood pressure. Diuretics are almost always needed and β-blocking and calcium channel blockers may be especially useful. If patients are on digoxin or have arrhythmias, special attention should be paid to serum potassium levels. For those with heart failure, whether it is due to ischemic or hypertensive heart disease and congestive cardiomyopathy, drugs that reduce afterload (vasodilators) preload (nitrates and diuretics), or both afterload and preload (converting enzyme inhibitors, α-blockers) may be especially useful. β-Blockers should usually be avoided in these patients, but they can be used in patients whose heart failure is compensated. The fact that β-blockers may prevent reinfarction or death in patients with previous myocardial infarctions may outweigh the risks in some of these patients.[2,32]

Elderly Patients With Cerebrovascular Disease and/or Prior Strokes

As indicated earlier, data from the VA, the HDFP, and the EWPWE studies have shown that the rate of cerebrovascular accidents is reduced in the elderly by the lowering of blood pressure. As in the case of CAD, special care must be taken to avoid overaggressive treatment and excessively rapid lowering of blood pressure. Although not all studies have demonstrated a reduction in stroke recurrence in patients who have had a previous CVA, none has demonstrated that treatment increased the risk of strokes by lowering blood pressure.[36] Most studies have demonstrated benefit of

*Available through local heart associations.
†Available from the National High Blood Pressure Information Center, 120/80, National Institutes of Health, Bethesda, Maryland, 22205

TABLE 38-6 Agents to Favor and Avoid in Special Situations in the Elderly

Situation	Favor	Avoid or Use With Caution
With coronary artery disease	β-Blockers Calcium channel blockers	Vasodilators as monotherapy

With congestive failure	Diuretics
	Converting enzyme inhibitors
	Some calcium channel
	    blockers
	Vasodilators
	α-Blockers
	Central α-agonists
		β-blockers
		Some calcium channel
		    blockers

With renal insufficiency	Loop diuretics Central α-agonists Vasodilators	Converting enzyme inhibi- tors?

With cerebrovascular disease	Diuretics
	Converting enzyme inhibitors
	Some calcium channel
	    blockers
		Some β-blockers
		Peripheral sympathetic
		    blockers
		Central α-agonists
		Rauwolfia alkaloids
		α-blockers

With peripheral vascular disease		Some β-blockers

With diabetes	Potassium-sparing diuretics
	    and combinations
	? Calcium channel blockers
		Some β-blockers (especially in
		    insulin-dependent patients)

With depression		*Rauwolfia* alkaloids Central α-agonists Some β-blockers

lowering the blood pressure. The fear that treatment of hypertension will increase the occurrence of strokes is unwarranted in our opinion. Agents that will decrease blood pressure slowly should be favored and those that cause postural hypotension (central α-agonists, peripheral sympathetic blockers, and α-blockers) should be used with caution.

Elderly Patients With Renal Insufficiency

It is common for renal function to decrease with age. As in younger patients, thiazide diuretics may not be effective in patients with reduced glomerular filtration, and loop active agents like furosemide, ethacrynic acid, or bumetanide may be required. In the elderly, the serum creatinine value may appear to be in the normal range but because muscle mass is reduced, a serum creatinine value that is "normal" for a younger patient may actually indicate some renal insufficiency. A timed creatinine clearance may have to be done in some cases to establish the patient's actual renal function; this is usually not necessary. Although there was once considerable controversy about the dan-

ger of lowering blood pressure in patients with renal insufficiency, there is no longer any question that the decrease in function noted initially as blood pressure is lowered is transient and the overall long-term effect of reducing blood pressure is beneficial. The doses of some drugs, particularly captopril, nadolol, and atenolol, which are excreted by the kidney, often need to be reduced, however, in patients with renal insufficiency. Possible changes that may have to be made in dosages of antihypertensive drugs in the elderly, in whom both renal function and microsomal activity in the liver may be decreased with a decreased ability to metabolize certain medications, are shown in Table 38-5.[29]

Elderly Hypertensives With Diabetes

The combination of hypertension and diabetes increases cardiovascular risk significantly, and many elderly patients have both diseases. Treatment to maintain blood pressure at normal levels is important to prevent strokes, CHF, and progressive renal insufficiency. In the diabetic, particular attention should be paid to maintaining total body potassium levels at as near normal as possible, but overaggressive correction of potassium loss should be avoided in those diabetics with renal insufficiency and in those with renal tubular acidosis. These patients have a potassium-secreting defect and are at risk for hyperkalemia. Drugs that may exacerbate the diabetic's tendency to postural hypotension and impotence should also be avoided if possible.

Other Concomitant Conditions

Elderly patients with gout may need thiazide diuretic therapy to control their blood pressure and so may be at risk of having additional gouty attacks. Although some other agents may be effective as monotherapy, none is as useful in as many patients as a diuretic. We routinely treat hypertensives with gout who need thiazides with either probenecid or allopurinol as well to prevent new attacks. Asymptomatic hyperuricemia *per se*, even with levels of 10 mg to 11 mg/dl, is usually not a cause for concern.

CONCLUSIONS

Hypertension in the elderly is common. Progressive elevation of blood pressure is noted in each decade in both sexes and all races. Combined systolic and diastolic blood pressure elevations in patients 65 years of age or over represent a significant risk factor, and lowering of blood pressure has been shown to be beneficial in those patients.

Isolated systolic pressure elevation is also a risk factor, but a more cautious approach should be taken. Data are not yet clear that lowering the pressure will increase longevity and reduce or eliminate complications. In this group, the risk, expense, and inconvenience of therapy must be weighed against the still unproven benefit of lowering blood pressure to normotensive or near normotensive levels. At present, it seems reasonable to attempt to lower pressure if this can be achieved without significant inconvenience or side-effects.

Evaluation of elderly hypertensive patients need not be complex and should be limited to studies defining target-organ involvement and searching for causes of secondary hypertension by means of a history, physical examination, and a few simple laboratory tests.

There are now numerous drugs available to choose from to treat hypertension. Although diuretics have proved effective in many elderly pa-

tients, the use of other agents, either alone or in combination with diuretics, will probably increase the percentage of responders. The precept of "go slow and not too low" must be kept in mind at all times in this group of patients. Even a partial reduction of blood pressure may significantly reduce risk.

REFERENCES

1. Amery A, Berthaux P, Birkenhager W et al. Antihypertensive therapy in patients above age 60 years (Fourth Interim Report of the European Working Party on High Blood Pressure in Elderly [EWPHE]). Clin Sci Mol Med 55:263s, 1978
2. Beta-Blocker Heart Attack Trial Research Group: A randomized trial or propranolol in patients with acute myocardial infarction: I. Mortality results. JAMA 247:1707–1714, 1982
3. Black HR: Non-drug treatment of hypertension. In Amery A, Fagard R, Staessen J (eds): Hypertensive Cardiovascular Disease: Pathophysiology and Treatment, pp 692–707. The Hague, Martinus Hijhoff Publishers, 1982
4. Blood pressure study 1979. Published by Society of Actuaries and Association of Life Insurance Medical Directors of America, 1980
5. Carey RM, Reid RA, Ayers CR, Lynch SS, McLain WL, Vaughan D: The Charlottesville blood-pressure survey. JAMA 236:847–851, 1976
6. Castelli WP: CHD risk factors in the elderly. Hosp Pract 11:113, 1976
7. Colandrea MA, Friedman GD, Nichaman MZ, Lynd CN: Systolic hypertension in the elderly. Circulation 41:239, 1970
8. Daugherty SA: Description of the enumerated and screened population. Hypertension 5:IV-1–IV-43, 1983
9. Dyer AR, Stamler J, Shekelle RB et al. Hypertension in the elderly. Med Clin North Am 61:513, 1977
10. Franklin SS, Young JD Jr, Maxwell MH et al: Operative morbidity and mortality in renovascular disease. JAMA 231:1148–1153, 1975
11. Fujishima M, Omae T, Takeya Y et al: Prognosis of occlusive cerebrovascular diseases in normotensive and hypertensive subjects. Stroke 7:472, 1976
12. Gubner RS: Systolic hypertension: A pathogenetic entity. Am J Cardiol 9:773, 1962
13. Holley KE, Hunt JC, Brown AL Jr et al: Renal artery stenosis: A clinical-pathologic study in normotensive and hypertensive patients. Am J Med 37:14–22, 1964
14. Hypertension Detection and Follow-up Program: I. Reduction in mortality of persons with high blood pressure, including mild hypertension. JAMA 242:2562, 1979
15. Hypertension Detection and Follow-up Program:

II. Mortality by race, sex and age. JAMA 242:2572, 1979

16. Hypertension Detection and Follow-up Program: III. Reduction in stroke incidence among persons with high blood pressure. JAMA 247:633, 1982

17. Hypertension Detection and Follow-up Program: The effect of treatment on mortality in "mild" hypertension. N Engl J Med 307:976, 1982

18. Itskovitz HD, Kochar MS, Anderson AJ, Rimm AA: Patterns of blood pressure in Milwaukee. JAMA 238:864, 1977

19. Kannel WB: Current status of the epidemiology of brain infarction associated with occlusive arterial disease. Stroke 2:295, 1971

20. Kannel WB, Castelli WP, McNamara PM et al: Role of blood pressure in the development of congestive heart failure. N Engl J Med 287:781, 1972

21. Kannel WB, Dawber TR, McGee DL: Perspectives on systolic hypertension: The Framingham Study. Circulation 61:1179, 1980

22. Kannel WB, Dawber TR, Sorlie P, Wolf PA: Components of blood pressure and risk of atherothrombotic brain infarction: The Framingham Study. Stroke 7:327, 1976

23. Kannel WB, Gordon T, Schwartz MJ: Systolic versus diastolic blood pressure and risk of coronary heart disease: The Framingham Study. Am J Cardiol 27:335, 1971

24. Kannel WB, Wolf PA, McGee DL et al: Systolic blood pressure, arterial rigidity, and risk of stroke: The Framingham Study. JAMA 245:1225, 1981

25. Kannel WB, Wolf PA, Verter J, McNamara PM: Epidemiologic assessment of the role of blood pressure in stroke: The Framingham Study. JAMA 214:301, 1970

26. Koch-Weser J: Correlation of pathophysiology and pharmacotherapy in primary hypertension. Am J Cardiol 32:499, 1973

27. McCarron DA, Morris CD, Cole C: Dietary calcium in human hypertension. Science 217:267–269, 1982

28. Morton PA: Ordinary insurance: The build and blood pressure study. Trans Soc Actuaries 11:987, 1959

29. Moser M: Management of Cardiovascular disease in the elderly. J Am Geriatr Soc (suppl 30)11:20–28, 1982

30. Moser M: Prognosis of effectively treated hypertension. In Onesti G, Lowenthal DT (eds): The Spectrum of Antihypertensive Drug Therapy, p 1. New York, Biomedical Information Corp, 1977

31. The 1984 Report of the Joint National Committee on Detection, Evaluation and Treatment of High Blood Pressure. Arch Intern Med 144:1045–1057, 1984

32. Norwegian Multicenter Study Group. Timolol-induced reduction in mortality and reinfarction in patients surviving acute myocardial infarction. N Engl J Med 304:801–807, 1981

33. Rabkin SW, Mathewson FAL, Tate RB: Long-term changes in blood pressure and risk of cerebrovascular disease. Stroke 9:319, 1978

34. Rabkin SW, Mathewson FAL, Tate RB: Predicting risk of ischemic heart disease and cerebrovascular disease from systolic and diastolic blood pressures. Ann Intern Med 88:342, 1978

35. Rabkin SW, Mathewson FAL, Tate RB: The relation of blood pressure to stroke prognosis. Ann Intern Med 89:1520, 1978

36. Radin AM, Black HR: Hypertension in the elderly: The time has come to treat. J Am Geriatr Soc 29:193–200, 1981

37. Schnaper HW, Furberg CD, Kuller LH et al: The response of isolated systolic hypertension to diuretic therapy. CVD Epidemiol Newsl 33:30, 1983

38. Sellers MD: Significance and management of systolic hypertension. Am J Cardiol 17:648, 1966

39. Shekelle RB, Ostfeld AM, Klawans HL: Hypertension and risk of stroke in an elderly population. Stroke 5:71, 1974

40. Smith HW: Unilateral nephrectomy in hypertensive disease. J Urol 76:685–701, 1956

41. Sos TA, Pickering TG, Sniderman K et al: Percutaneous transluminal renal angioplasty in renovascular hypertension due to atheroma or fibromuscular dysplasia. N Engl J Med 309:274–279, 1983

42. Stamler J, Stamler R, Riedlinger W et al: Hypertension screening of 1 million Americans: Community Hypertension Evaluation Clinic (CHEC) Program, 1973 through 1975. JAMA 235:2299–2306, 1976

43. Tarazi RC: Regression of left ventricular hypertrophy by medical treatment: Present status and possible implications. Am J Med 75(3A):80–86, 1983

44. Veterans Administration: Effects of treatment on morbidity in hypertension: I. Results in patients with diastolic blood pressures averaging 115 through 129 mm Hg. JAMA 202:116, 1967

45. Veterans Administration: Effects of treatment on morbidity in hypertension: II. Results in patients with diastolic blood pressure averaging 90 through 114 mm Hg. JAMA 213:1143, 1970

46. Veterans Administration: Effects of treatment on morbidity in hypertension: III. Influence of age, diastolic pressure and prior cardiovascular disease; further analysis of side effects. Circulation 45:991, 1972

47. Whelton PK, Harris AP, Russell RP et al: Renovascular hypertension: Results of medical and surgical therapy. Johns Hopkins Med J 149:213–219, 1981

39

The Oral Cavity

Leo Zach* and Norman Trieger

Age-associated changes in the oral cavity and surrounding face are sufficiently marked to make them prime factors in any evaluation of aging.[48] This is best indicated by that classic symbolization of aging, "long in the tooth." In addition, the many complaints and problems, whether of pain, difficulty in chewing, or xerostomia or of the varied benign and neoplastic lesions, make this region one of basic importance to the geriatrician.

In round numbers, 11 million of a pool of 23 million persons over age 65 have no teeth at all.[57] Above 90% of the edentulous group will have had dentures fitted, 25% of whom will not wear them. Thirty-three percent of the denture wearers demonstrate lesions attributable to the denture and changes in the underlying tissues. The lesions may range from ulceration of the mucosa to fibrous hyperplasia producing redundant tissue flaps around the denture peripheries. Elderly persons who manage to retain teeth are not spared discomfort or danger. At least 70% will show dental root caries, decay that follows breakdown of the root-supporting tissues, the periodontal structures.[27] Periodontal disease is a more potent factor than caries in causing tooth mortality in aged dentitions.[41,58]

Apart from the purely dental problems, the aged are increasingly prone to disorders arising in other oral tissues: gingiva, mucosa, salivary glands, lips and musculature, and jaw bones. An interesting change is the diminished sensory level to pain of tooth origin.[25] This is due to a continuing deposition of secondary dentin with metamorphic changes in sensory dentinal fibrils.[4] The clinical sequela is that older patients are impelled to seek treatment because of dental pain when disease is more advanced than in the younger group. A beneficial consequence is that they experience less pain during manipulations such as grinding and drilling.

Providing dental treatment for the aged patient is made more difficult by other attendant systemic diseases. Often, medical consultation is needed for patients with cardiovascular, neurologic, and metabolic disorders who are receiving multiple medications.

Problems in the oral cavity and perioral regions have engaged the attention of the geriatrician to a growing extent. Dentists, as well, are increasingly receiving special training in the oral diseases of the aged. These are developments that bode well for diagnosis and service to this growing population.

THE TEETH

Teeth in old age are markedly different from young teeth. Most of the macroscopic changes are illustrated in Figure 39-1. Reference is made to the numbers on the drawing. At (*27*) on the "old tooth" segment, attritional wear at the height of the cusp has diminished the height of the anatomical crown, the portion covered by enamel. Indeed, the enamel is shown to have been completely penetrated, exposing the underlying dentinal core. This dentin (*26*), which composes most of the bulk of the tooth substance, is shown darker than its counterpart (*4*) in the young tooth. Exposed, aged dentin is less permeable than covered dentin and is sclerotic, literally harder, and less pain conductive than young dentin.[42] These changes are secondary to mild stimuli such as continued wear or slow caries and in no way jeopardize retention in

---

* Deceased.

the jawbones. Considerably softer than enamel, this exposed dentin is usually depressed in relation to the surrounding ridge of enamel. Its color varies from yellow through tones of brown and even black, by incorporation of exogenous pigments that extend 1 mm or more deep. Derived mainly from food pigments, salivary constituents (mucins, salts), and the "tar" components of tobacco smoke or juice, such discolorations cannot be removed by surface cleansing.

Dental Attrition

Although variations in the hardness (Brinnell number) of enamel from person to person are of small order, attrition can range from minimal faceting of the cusps to extreme loss of tooth substance, sometimes extending to the gingival crest.[75] Some of the contributory factors are as follows:

Men exhibit greater wear than women, probably because of the greater power of masticatory muscles.

Attrition is greatly enhanced by night grinding or bruxism, considered a tension-related mechanism. Continued nocturnal grinding may ultimately loosen teeth. Treatment may range from the construction of a soft nightguard worn over the teeth at night as a stress-absorbing cushion, to linking loosened teeth together by means of

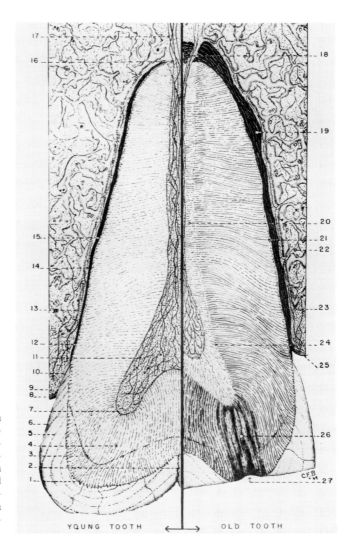

FIG. 39-1. Diagrammatic cross section through a maxillary premolar tooth and supporting structures, showing normal (physiologic) age changes. Numbered areas are referred to in the text. Note particularly abrasion (27), diminution of pulp (11), and increased cemental thickness (19). (Bodecker CF: University of The State of New York: Examination for Dentists in Histology. New York, State Education Department, 1944)

conjoined dental crowns. Diazepam (Valium), 5 mg, 1 hour before bedtime, or psychiatric consultation may be useful.

Abrasive foods produce accelerated wear and loss of tooth height. In rural Mexico, for example, elderly persons often display teeth worn down to the root, because of a lifetime of chewing cornmeal products ground on rapidly abrading stone mortars. Elderly Eskimo women exhibit a similar wearing away from the practice of softening leather hides by chewing on them. Such tooth wear shortens the inferior third of the face with the diminished jaw height universally judged to be old-looking. Mobility and attrition on the mesial and distal sides of the teeth increases the spacing between the teeth and diminishes dental arch diameter.[52]

Xerostomia in varying degrees also contributes to dental attrition in the aged. Diminished salivary secretion, whether in the healthy aged or secondary to disease such as Sjögren's syndrome or irradiation for neoplasm, diminishes lubrication of the food bolus and increases wear. Sognnaes[63] cites the case of an 18-year-old girl with total xerostomia whose teeth were wore down to the gum line so that "she had the appearance of an old Eskimo."

Functional wearing of the teeth, usually pronounced in old age may be greatly enhanced by environmental conditions, many associated with occupation. Schour and Sarnat[54] list the following occupations as contributing to excessive attrition: masons and stoneworkers as a result of the dust and grit-laden atmosphere, confectionery workers as a result of powdered sugar, polishers, blasters, carpenters, and many others.

A lengthy list of mechanical habits abrade and distort both the shape and position of the teeth.[10] These include faulty or overzealous toothbrushing,[28] particularly marked when coarsely abrasive dentifrices are used on a hard-bristled brush,[40] the long continued clenching of pipe-stems between the teeth, and the biting of thread in sewing.

Chemical erosion also plays a role in dissolution of tooth substance, especially when the destructive substrate has had many years to act. These substrates include acids from citrus fruits and soft drinks.[21,29] Lemon juice in warm or hot water often used by the elderly as an aid to digestion or a source of ascorbic acid is particularly pernicious. Lemon juice has a much lower pH than other common juices (orange, grapefruit), and its enamel-decalcifying effect is enhanced by warming.

Various medications can significantly decrease salivary flow: drugs that are given to decrease gastric and intestinal motility; antihypertensive agents; diuretics; tricyclic antidepressants; antihistamines; tranquilizers and muscle relaxants; levodopa; and others.

Dentin Changes

In Figure 39-1, secondary dentin (20) is indicated as having replaced most of the volume of the dental pulp or "nerve" (11) of the young tooth. Deposition of calcified, tubular dentin occurs throughout life with the pulp becoming a thin filament represented as a fine line in roentgenograms. This diminution in pulpal diameter is shown in Figure 39-2. Note also that post-formation dentin has occluded the incisal portion of the pulp chamber, leaving the residual pulp tissue almost wholly confined to the root. This progressive walling-in of the pulp canals and chambers is a surer sign of aging than the more variable attrition of the surficial hard dental tissues.[7]

The secondary dentinal deposition and resulting smaller pulps in the elderly provide a greater barrier to the penetration of a carious lesion. Also, preparation of the tooth to receive a crown or a deep filling may be performed with less danger of encroaching on or exposing this delicate, inner tissue. The thermal effects of drilling are lessened in older drilled teeth and lead less frequently to pulpitis than equivalent tooth-cutting procedures in young teeth.[77,78] Thus, some procedures may be undertaken without recourse to local anesthetics.[53]

The laying-down of secondary dentin is an exceedingly slow process throughout life. The process bursts into a flurry of matrix deposition, frequently structurally disorganized, when the vital pulp tissue is assaulted by events more aggressive than aging. The stimulus may be thermomechanical, such as tooth grinding; bacterial, as in dental decay; chemical, as in the placing of medicaments or fillings within a tooth; or traumatic, as from a blow to the teeth or jaws. In Figure 39-3, a thermally produced bulbous mass of so-called tertiary, irritational, or scar dentin (RD) is seen protruding into the well-vascularized, stellate, fibrous connective tissue of the pulp.[34,81] Quantitative aspects of the formation of reparative dentin are reported by Stanley and co-workers.[66] Labeling the cells of the fibroblastic pulp with tritiated thymidine demonstrated their migration and histodifferentiation into tubule-producing odontoblasts.[82] But if the injury is too great, the pulp undergoes necrosis, which, in turn, may lead to dentoalveolar abscess;

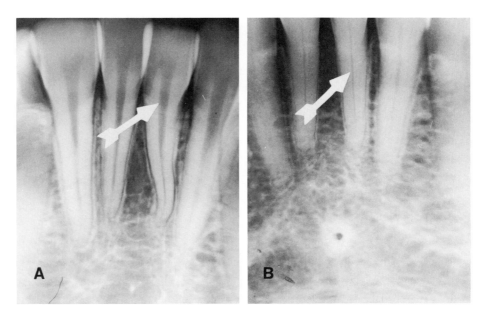

FIG. 39-2. Periapical roentgenograms showing the progressive diminution of pulpal diameter (*arrows*) in two women aged 13 (*A*) and 72 (*B*). Note also the lack of pulpal tissue in the crown portions of the incisors in the aged teeth.

cellulitis, which may wedge through the fascial planes; and even osteomyelitis and septicemia. The progress of these infections of odontogenic origin is particularly noted in the debilitated and terminally ill elderly patient.[3,12] The diminished immunologic response to opportunistic infection also plays a role in preventing localization of these infections.[49]

Cementum Thickening

In Figure 39-1, a comparison of the black areas surrounding the tooth root (*15*) and (*19*) demonstrates the markedly thickened layer of cementum that invests the root of the old tooth as compared with the young tooth in which dentin is close to alveolar bone. Like its counterpart of secondary dentin formation on the pulpal walls, cementum is also a tissue that manifests continuous matricial deposition and calcification throughout life, sometimes achieving extraordinary proliferation in the elderly. An almost linear relationship holds between average cementum thickness and age. Zander and associates[84] found a threefold increase in the thickness of the cemental lining of single-rooted teeth from early adolescence to advanced old age.

Excessive deposition of cementum, or true hypercementosis, is much more common in the aged

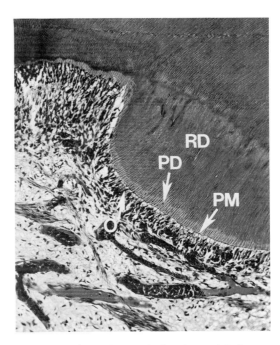

FIG. 39-3. Photomicrograph showing a globular protrusion of scar dentin (*RD*) protruding into the dental pulp. The formative odontoblasts (*O*) have a distinct basement membrane (*PM*) and begin again to form tubular predentin (*PD*) after an injury to the tooth has subsided. (× 200)

because the laying-down of cemental lamellae is essentially a slow process. Multipotential fibroblasts of the peridental ligament (Fig. 39-1, *14*) histodifferentiate to form cementoblasts, which produce a bonelike cementum matrix.[62] The cementoblasts become enclaved in the matrix of their own production and remain within lucunae in a manner that exactly parallels the osteocytes. Apart from periapical cemental dysplasias and truly neoplastic cementomas, hypercementosis results in a milk-bottle–like bulbous root. Early hypercementosis (Fig. 39-4) on its way to producing the clubbed root is evident in the roentgenogram of a 74-year-old patient shown in Figure 39-5. Teeth of the elderly with an orderly hypercementosis are generally firmer in their alveolar sockets and should not be considered pathologic. When advanced disease requires extraction, the expanded anatomy of the roots may cause the oral surgeon considerable difficulty.[43] A casual approach usually leads to fractured teeth with retained roots and need for secondary surgical revision. The situation is further compounded by

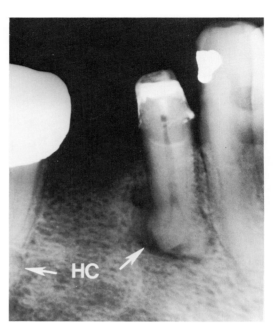

FIG. 39-5. Roentgenogram showing considerable hypercementosis (*HC*) surrounding the apical root portions, producing cemental clubbing in a 74-year-old man.

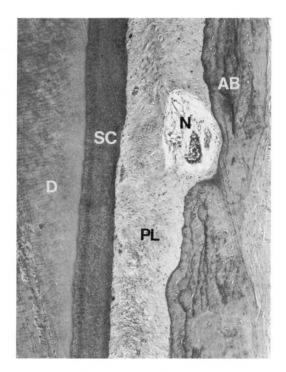

FIG. 39-4. Photomicrograph through the supporting structures of the tooth demonstrating secondary cementum formation (*SC*) between the dentin (*D*) and peridental ligament (*PL*). A neurovascular bundle (*N*) is seen adjacent to the socket wall of alveolar bone (*AB*). (×250)

senile osteoporosis, so that excessive torquing of the tooth with forceps may produce mandibular fracture or the separation of a considerable portion of the maxilla when the root is finally avulsed. The elevation of mucoperiosteal flaps and the division of multirooted teeth, particularly when the roots are widely divergent, assist in making the oral surgery minimally traumatic to the older patient.[26]

Although much hypercementosis is idiopathic, certain conditions such as Paget's disease are known to favor if not actually to induce cemental overproduction. These include periapical infection, hyperelongation of the tooth in the alveolar socket secondary to loss of an antagonist, lack of function, peridontitis, and root fracture.[74] Excessive function (traumatic occlusion), on the other hand, has not been implicated as a causative factor.

THE SUPPORTING STRUCTURES (PERIODONTIUM)

The incidence of advanced periodontal disease in the aged is truly appalling, with a linear progression through the advancing years. In Johnson's study[31] of American males, in the 18- to 24-year age-group the incidence of advanced periodontal disease marked by alveolar bone loss was 10.3%, rose linearly to the 45- to 54-year-age-group (36.9%), and peaked at 58.4% in the 64- to 74-year age-group. Gupta's Indian survey[23] of over 1600 persons reported an insignificant incidence in children from age 5 to 14 (0.6%), with an alarming increase to 27.2% in adolescents and young adults ages 15 to 29. The incidence was 75.2% in the 30- to 39-year age-group, and the group 41 years and older demonstrated an almost universal incidence of 96.9%. The enormously greater incidence reported in the Indian study represents lack of access of the population to dental care and to the whole complex of nutritional, sanitary, genetic, and socioeconomic conditions that describe human existence on the subcontinent.

With over 50% of American males over age 65 (the incidence is slightly less in females) showing advanced periodontal disease, breakdown of the tooth-supporting structures is responsible for more oral disease and loss of teeth than any other pathosis, dental decay included, in the elderly. In Figure 39-1, it is evident that the attachment of the gingiva to the root (*25*) in the old tooth extends considerably higher than on the young tooth (*8*), where the gum tissue is in contact with enamel at its crest. With the passage of years, a migration of gingival epithelial attachment in the direction of the apex occurs, even in the absence of clinically evident periodontitis. There is still conjecture as to whether this visible elongation of the exposed tooth is physiologic or represents a pathologic process.[68] This passive migration of the dentogingival junction involves detachment of the epithelium from root cementum, lysis of gingival submucosal collagen, and atrophy, with progressive lowering of the apical crest of supporting alveolar bone[18] (*23* in Fig. 39-1).

This slow exposure of the roots does not result *per se* in loss of teeth, but when the additive effect of periodontitis is superposed the dentition may be ravaged. Many local factors in the aged combine to produce destructive periodontitis, factors that are considered extrinsic in contrast to a host of intrinsic factors that describe the tissue and metabolic state of the aged patient.[65]

ETIOLOGIC OR CONTRIBUTORY FACTORS IN PERIODONTAL BREAKDOWN IN THE AGED

Extrinsic (Local) Factors

Bacterial
Accumulation of dental plaque

Peridental invasion by specific gram-negative anaerobes
Adherent calculus
Enzymes and decomposition products, exudates
Materia alba (mucinous food debris)
Food impaction
Mechanical
Calculus
Food impaction and retention
Open and loose interdental contacts
Mobility and spreading (spacing) of teeth
Wedging antagonistic cusps (plunger cusps)
Overhanging edges (margins) of fillings and crowns
Poorly designed or fitting prostheses (bridges and dentures)
Excessively soft or sticky consistency of diet
Mouth breathing; incomplete closure of lips
Improper or inadequate oral hygiene (home care)
Injurious habits (tongue-thrust, pencil chewing)
Improper dental treatment methods (iatrogenic)
Accidental trauma
Anatomical Predispositions
Tooth malalignment, malposition, or altered anatomy (malocclusion)
Abnormally high frena and muscle insertions
Shallow mucobuccal vestibules
Functionally insufficient area of attached gingiva
Thin gingival mucosa
Thick, bulbous gingival margins
Bony exostoses or ledges
Very thin labial or buccal alveolar bone plates
Unfavorable crown-root ratio (extended crown, diminished root)

Intrinsic (Systemic) Factors

Endocrine Dysfunctions
Postmenopausal (osteoporosis)
Acromegaly
Hyperparathyroidism (primary and secondary)
Metabolic and Other Diseases
Protein-deficient diet
Avitaminoses (ascorbic acid)
Diabetes mellitus
Hyperkeratosis palmoplantaris
Marfan's syndrome
Xerostomia secondary to many causes
Cyclic neutropenia
Leukemias and lymphomas (Hodgkin's disease)
Autoimmune diseases
Hypophosphatasia
Paget's disease
Systemic debilitating disease in general
Emotional or Psychosomatic Disorders
Leading to neuromuscular insufficiency to maintain oral hygiene
Bruxism (tooth clenching or grinding)
Organic brain syndrome
Cerebrovascular accident

Incapacitating psychoses
Drugs and Metallic Poisons
Phenytoin
Heavy metals (bismuth, arsenic, lead, mercury)
Cytotoxic agents (methotrexate, vincristine sulfate)
Allergic responses
Marrow suppressants
Nondemonstrable
Poor resistance and repair
Age
Fatigue
Stress
Bone "factor"

(Grant DS, Stern IB, Everett FG: Orban's Periodontics, A Concept—Theory and Practise. St. Louis, CV Mosby, 1972)

A more detailed survey of the correlates that operate between systemic disease and periodontal disease is offered by Kerr.[33]

Diabetes mellitus, both juvenile and late onset, offers the most striking example of periodontal response to metabolic disease. Since the pioneering work of Sheppard[60] some 50 years ago, there is ample documentation of progressive deepening of the gingival crevice, lysis of periodontal ligament, and destruction of alveolar bony support of the teeth in the uncontrolled diabetic. This progresses to a fulminating suppurative periodontitis with periodontal abscesses and, not infrequently, to serious facial cellulitis.[79] Microangiopathic changes, similar to those found in diabetic retinopathy, have been observed in periodontal ligament and gingiva of diabetics: luminal diminution with disruption of endothelial cells and a periodic acid–Schiff (PAS)-positive subendothelial infiltrate.[38] Motility and phagocytosis of polymorphonuclear leukocytes have been found to be abnormal in type I and some type II diabetes. The sudden onset of pyogenic infections about the teeth of the aged, especially if multiple and recurrent despite incision and drainage, is a well-recognized symptom and should alert the physician or dentist to the possibility of diabetic etiology. The diabetic patient who wears dentures, particularly if under poor control, is overly susceptible to denture stomatitis, especially if the dental prosthesis is not scrupulously clean. Edema, redness, and even ulceration are evident on the tissue-bearing surfaces under the dentures, often in sharp contrast to normal mucosa peripheral to the denture. Overgrowth of *Candida albicans* (candidiasis) is a frequent association in the elderly. In geriatric institutions, or with any aged population with neuromuscular or mental impairment, staff must make efforts to cleanse the dentures at regular intervals.

The roentgenogram in Figure 39-6 illustrates the advanced horizontal alveolar bone loss in a 71-year-old man with periodontitis. The maxillary incisors were moderately mobile to the extent that any cutting or tearing form of incision, as in eating an apple, produced pain. The cumulative effect of local factors acting on an impaired tissue substrate to produce overwhelming periodontal breakdown is shown in Figure 39-7. This roentgenogram of a 62-year-old woman with uncontrolled diabetes demonstrates extreme loss of supporting bone so that only root apices are imnbedded in bone. Small triangular radiopaque spurs *(C)* are evident protruding from many of the roots about midway down their length: these represent circumferential collars of the subgingival and supragingival calculus (tartar). This deposit is essentially calcified dental plaque that has undergone mineralization in the supersaturated oral fluids.[39] It adheres to dentures and other dental restorations from which

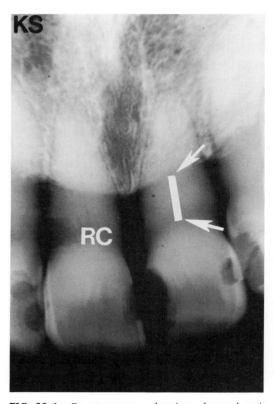

FIG. 39-6. Roentgenogram showing advanced periodontosis with horizontal loss of bone level (white line between arrows) in a 71-year-old man. Root decay is evident *(RC)*.

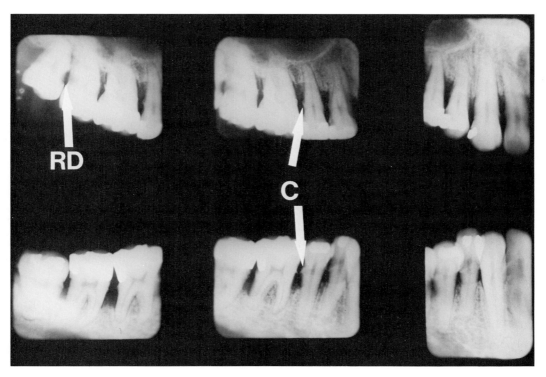

FIG. 39-7. Roentgenogram of the right side of both dental arches in a 62-year-old woman with uncontrolled diabetes. Extreme bone loss is generalized, aided by adherent calculus (*C*) and exposing root surfaces that become susceptible to decay (*RD*).

plaque is not regularly removed. Rate of formation, a considerable variable, increases on average with age. Root decay within periodontal pockets is shown (*RD*).

Calculus and precursor plaque are the prime extrinsic factors in destructive dental disease in the aged population. It leads to atrophy of the supporting structures of the tooth as a result of inflammatory enzymes, vertical lysis of bone, and ultimate loss of the tooth.[8] Experimental studies[50] accompanied by an intensely plasmacytic inflammatory exudate, strongly hint at the role of immune-defense mechanisms. The osteolysis that produces extreme periodontal pocket formation is illustrated in Figure 39-8, a roentgenogram of a 67-year-old woman with vertical, wedge-shaped bony defects particularly well marked (at the end of the arrow) where loss of supporting bone extends almost to the root apex of the maxillary molar tooth. Failure to eliminate infection and calculus, evident (just below the arrow) as a fuzzy, opaque mass adhering to root, has destroyed tooth support.

The prevention and treatment of periodontal disease is the key to the preservation of teeth in the elderly. Plaque control and calculus removal by scaling, using either hand or ultrasonic instruments,[67] are the initial steps. Instruction in home care is given, including proper tooth brushing, use of dental floss, and oral irrigation devices. Treatment directed at decreasing periodontal pockets is instituted: curettage of the pocket wall; the adjunctive use of systemic antibiotics (*e.g.*, clindamycin) effective against gram-negative anaerobic pathogens has been found to be highly efficaceous.[70] Gingival flap operations to expose root–alveolar bone relationships are frequently resorted to[36] and allow direct observation and evaluation of the degree of supportive structure loss. Removal of necrotic debris and granulation tissue is followed by gingival recontouring.[47]

A number of other useful procedures, including autogenous bone transplants, may be applicable.[24] Prognosis of teeth that can be luxated within their reduced sockets depends, among other factors, on the degree of mobility measured angularly and on whether the mobility may be arrested or stabilized by appropriate treatment. Teeth may loosen as a result of trauma, whether produced by pathologic drifting and a faulty occlusion (bite relationship)

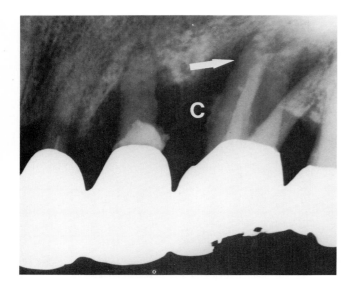

FIG. 39-8. Roentgenogram of maxillary posterior teeth of a 67-year-old woman with deep, vertical periodontal pocket formation almost reaching the apices of the roots (*arrow*). Calculus (*C*) is one of the causative extrinsic agents. The teeth on either side of the arrow have a hopeless prognosis.

or by an acute blow, and is particularly evident in uncontrolled diabetes, avitaminosis C, protein malnutrition, postconvulsive seizure, and as a result of acute oral (dentoalveolar) infection.[45] Teeth that may be depressed in their sockets are considered to have a hopeless prognosis and are not acceptable for attempted immobilization by means of splinting.

Dental Caries

The geriatric population is subject to decay of the crown portions of the teeth and is afflicted with a high rate of root caries as well, a type of decay almost unique to older age-groups.[2] When root surfaces are exposed, whether by physiologic or peridontal atrophy, the caries attack rate is high on the uncovered cementum or dentin (see Fig. 39-7). Root caries may band the root circumferentially and penetrate to such depth that fracture of the tooth leads to loss of its coronal portion. The root stump on roentgenography will usually demonstrate a periapical radiolucency indicative of a granuloma or a cyst. Retained roots may remain in the jawbones for years painlessly but may represent a chronic infected focus, which may flare up at any time. In Figure 39-9, a roentgenogram from a 66-year-old man, the apical lucency represents bone replacement with chronic granulation tissue seeded with small foci of pus. The second molar tooth also shows considerable periapical infection. The third molar is impacted.

Contrary to popular belief, then, dental caries is far from being restricted to the young. Older persons may have many susceptible tooth surfaces

already filled because of previous decay and still remain highly exposed to both coronal and root decay.[46] Treatment of cavities in useful teeth with a reasonable prognosis periodontally may require great dexterity but represents an important service to elderly patients who usually have lost several or many teeth already. Each remaining tooth assumes greater significance because it may serve as an abutment or stress barrier for a bridge or a partial denture.

Dental caries is an infectious disease primarily attributed in humans to *Streptococcus mutans*. Increased caries activity in the elderly is abetted by several factors: foremost is diminished oral hygiene stemming from the difficulty of removing plaque from denuded roots and psychological or physical impairments. Abraded dentin surfaces, clasps on partial dentures, bridgework, periodontal disease, and tipped teeth all contribute to the caries rate.[30] Changes in the diet, such as the sucking of lozenges or candies to stimulate salivary flow in xerostomia, greatly increase the ambient, intraoral bacterial count and caries attack rate. Xerostomia itself, through loss of ptyalin and caries-inhibiting buffers in lessened salivary volume, also results in increasing caries susceptibility,[6] occasionally to the rampant stage of generalized severe decay. The prescribing of a daily or weekly fluoride rinse for home use exerts a distinct anticariogenic effect.[59] Several different techniques for establishing a fluoride-induced caries-arresting regimen are available:

Mouthrinses: sodium fluoride, 0.025% to 0.2% (much greater concentration of fluoride than in toothpastes)

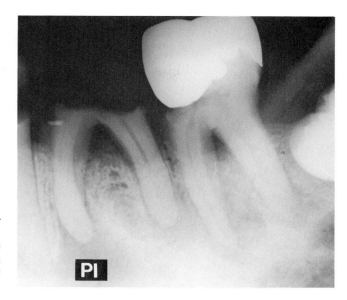

FIG. 39-9. Roentgenogram of posterior mandibular teeth with retained roots and periapical infection (PI). Infection of bone is also evident in the tooth to the right, as well as an impacted wisdom tooth. All three molars were extracted.

Toothbrushing: acidulated phosphate fluoride gel, 0.5%; stannous fluoride gel, 0.4%; sodium fluoride gel, 1.1%

Chewable tablets and lozenges: sodium fluoride, 0.25 mg to 1.0 mg

Use of custom fitted trays (plastic molds to hold the fluoride solution)[17]

Maxilla and Mandible

Vertical dimension of the lower third of the face diminishes markedly in the edentulous older patient. Loss of alveolar bone height produces the collapsed facies and a sunken-lipped, "pursestring" mouth with radiating skin fissures typical of the elderly who do not wear dental prostheses. Resorption of the alveolar processes occurs in two dimensions, vertically and labiobuccally, resulting in loss of height and an osseous retreat from the covering lips and cheeks. Resorption is greater in the mandible than the maxilla, and, when severe, it constitutes a major problem in the fitting of conventional dentures.[64] The residual bony ridge may become thin and knifelike, unable to withstand the downward compressive forces of a functional denture. Mandibular resorption may progress to the level of the mental foramen of the inferior alveolar neurovascular bundle, externalizing these structures as they exit from the jawbone and requiring modification of a lower denture to prevent pain or lip-chin paresthesia. In Figure 39-10*A*, a roentgenogram of the full superior-inferior dimension of the mandible in a 71-year-old woman edentulous for 16 years, the men-

tal foramen (arrow) appears as an ovoid lucency at the crest of the alveolar ridge. The mandibular height may be compared with that in Figure 39-10*B*, which shows a roentgenogram of a 51-year-old woman of approximately the same height and weight. In the maxilla, alveolar resorption may proceed to such an extent that only an eggshell-thin rim of cortical bone separates the oral cavity from the floor of the maxillary antrum. The presence of functioning tooth roots, then, is the major factor in preserving the osseous architecture of the lower face. Correction of atrophy by well-designed dentures frequently produces dramatic change in appearance, a more varied nutrition, and better phonation. That loss of vertical dimension of occlusion adversely affects speech intelligibility has been demonstrated in patients whose speech patterns were evaluated for clarity while wearing dentures that varied only in degree of closure.[61]

Other gross changes are recorded in the jawbones of the elderly. It has long been assumed that the mandibular angle from body to ramus is flattened with advancing age, most markedly in edentulous patients.[37] It is now held that angle measurements are of such variability that they reflect functional bone remodeling rather than progressive, age-related alterations. Mandibular blood supply changes from an essentially centrifugal feed through the inferior alveolar to a centripetal source by way of facial, lingual, and buccal arteries. Atherosclerotic changes in the alveolar artery are compensated for by the mandibular peripheral vessels entering through periosteum.[11] Postextraction remodeling of jawbones in the elderly reveals that

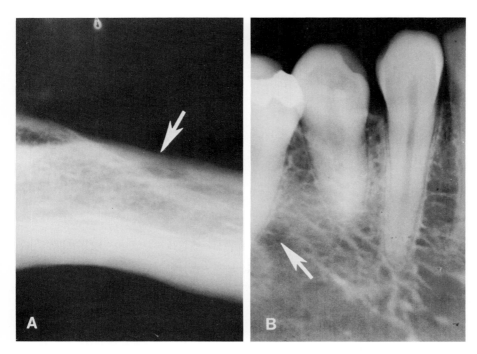

FIG. 39-10. Roentgenograms of full mandibular height of a 71-year-old woman (*A*) contrasted to a 51-year-old woman who retained her dentition (*B*). The mental foramen in *A* lies on the crest of the alveolar ridge (*arrow*), with normal position evident at the arrow in *B*. The anatomical basis for the sunken-faced, aged look is evident.

loss of osseous tissue is greatest in the labiobuccal aspects of the maxilla, while in the mandible, conversely, it occurs at the expense of the lingual side of the alveolar ridge. The net result is that many elderly edentulous persons develop an acquired prognathism especially evident when the lower jaw is thrust forward by the pterygoid muscles so that the anterior ridges can appose while chewing.

The jawbones share senile osteoporotic changes with the rest of the skeleton. Loss of coarse trabeculation, cortical thinning, and general diminution occur in the jawbones through disuse atrophy in the edentulous patient. Superimposition of hormonal osteoporosis on jawbones that no longer have functional stress-stimulation may lead to the supposition that the mandible, particularly, shows an earlier and more exaggerated porosity than other bones, especially in females.[1] The mandible, as one of the non-weight-supporting bones, rarely shows spontaneous fracture except when secondary to rarefying lesions such as cysts, tumors, and hyperparathyroidism. Oral surgeons are mindful of the increased osseous fragility in the elderly and will frequently dissect a hypercementosed, infected tooth rather than avulse it with forceps. Healing

of fractures and extraction wounds in the aged patient is slowed by a reduction in cellular osteogenic potential, with nonunion of fractures increasing in incidence with age. The incidence of dry socket after extractions, essentially a localized alveolar osteitis related to breakdown and necrosis rather than endothelialization and fibrosis of the fibrin clot, also increases. Small alveolar sequestra may be passed.

The Temporomandibular Joint

The temporomandibular joint is a complex, diarthrodial joint capable of both swinging (hingelike) and sliding motions in many axes. It undergoes functional remodeling throughout life, usually in response to changes in articulation of the teeth with which it constitutes a tripodal functional limit. Most of these changes, such as deepening of the glenoid fossa of the temporal bone or flattening of the eminentia articularis, are not considered degenerative but adaptive.[44] Thinning, sometimes progressing to perforation of the articular disk (meniscus), occurs with advancing age but infrequently leads to joint malfunction or pain. Flattening of the articular surfaces and nodular articular calcifications, with some evidence of lipping, are not important clinically, although they are common in the aged. Bearing stress to only a limited degree, the temporomandibular joint is fortunately spared most of the disabling consequences of osteoarthritis. Some pain and tenderness together with crepitation on movement are not uncommon, but seldom is there reduction in mobility. Joint clicking and snapping are frequent complaints in the aged, thought to be caused by disturbed synchronization of intra-articular disk and condylar movements of jaw opening, and, again, this is usually painless. Subluxation and dislocation following a blow to the jaw, as well as fracture of the thinned condylar head, are more frequent in the aged, usually ascribed to increase laxity of the circumferential articular ligament. Ankylosis occurs but rarely, usually following serious pyogenic infection secondary to crushing trauma.

Costen's syndrome[14] is a controversial symptom-complex attributed to overclosure of the temporomandibular joint in elderly edentulous patients. According to its propounder, posterior-superior displacement of the condylar head results in a wide variety of symptoms: tinnitus, otalgia, vertex headache, dizziness, and glossodynia. Many aged patients complain of one or more of these symptoms. The anatomical basis for relating them to mechanical pressures in the fossa seem vague and ill-conceived. The postulated chronic joint trauma has been replaced by the myofacial pain-dysfunction syndrome,[55] which stresses the role of muscle fatigue in producing the myriad symptoms. Prosthetic appliances, muscular overextension and overcontraction, grinding and clenching, severely altered occlusal patterns, and a strong psychological overlay are now considered factors in the symptom complex. It is noteworthy that 80% to 90% of these patients are female and that palpation of the joint through the auditory meatus fails to elicit pain. Injection of sclerosing solutions, meniscectomy, and reconstructive procedures have all been attempted and rejected. Minimal intervention with avoidance of irreversible or complicated procedures should be the therapeutic guide. Muscle relaxants and tranquilizers, anti-inflammatory agents, local heat, correction of gross bite dysharmonies, and reassurance are variably effective. Attention to psychological stress factors will frequently serve to alleviate symptoms.

Polyarticular rheumatoid arthritis bypasses the temporomandibular articulation in 80% of cases.[16] The joint may become involved simultaneously with or subsequent to other joint inflammations. Few patients suffer severe limitation of motion, and ankylosis is rare.

Lips and Oral Mucosa

The oral mucosa undergoes aging changes comparable to other mucocutaneous areas. These make the tissue more abradable, slower to heal, and less able to resist stress through denture loading or rub. The epithelium is grossly thinner with fewer layers of prickle cells, although eukeratinization and parakeratinization levels remain about the same.[83] Focal hyperkeratoses, distinct from the dyskeratosis owing to altered maturational progression and cellular instability, are common in denture wearers. These white patches, frequently rough in texture, occur in elderly edentulous patients who masticate food with the mucosa overlying the residual alveolar ridges. Crusty white patches in unstressed mucosal areas are best biopsied to rule out dyskeratoses and carcinoma *in situ*. The term *leukoplakia* signifies "white patch" and is best discarded in favor of specifying a histologic entity. Of greater prognostic importance is the finding of erythroplasia either isolated or part of the leukoplakic patch. These areas have been shown to represent dysplastic changes and carcinoma *in situ*. Clinical diagnosis without biopsy is treacherous.

The oral membranes of the elderly are usually pale and dry. Arteriolar sclerosis and diminution of the capillary bed accounts for the pallor. The xerostomia is secondary to diminished salivary flow of both the major and minor glands. Submucosal changes include a gross thinning based on collagen diminution with concomitant hyalinization and increase in fibroblast density.[51] The mucopolysaccharide concentration in the ground substance and the number of mast cells are increased. Cellular kinetic studies indicate a diminished proliferation. Elastic tissue generally diminishes but may increase in the lips, referred to as senile elastosis. In this degenerative change, there is frequently a blurring of the vermilion border, which may seem to merge imperceptibly with perilabial skin. The lips may appear hyperplastic and nodular.[5] Treatment is neither effective nor necessary.

Solar cheilitis is common especially in the sunbelt; the lips are parched and wrinkled, hyperkeratotic, and not easily stretched. Irreversible changes leading to squamous cell carcinoma are not uncommon in the lower lip, while most nonhealing sores of the upper lip are basal cell carcinomas. Avoidance of solar radiation to the lips is basic. Sunscreen ointments should be strongly recommended for the lips, as well as the forehead, infraorbital ridges, zygoma, and ears. Prompt biopsy of labial ulcers with early detection of carcinoma improves prognosis and reduces mutilative surgery.

In the oral mucosa, neoplasia especially shows an advancing incidence with increased age. Discussion will of necessity be brief. Epidermoid (squamous cell) carcinoma is by far the most common intraoral malignant neoplasm. The US Public Health Service reports an incidence of 19.4 per 100,000 males and 5.2 per 100,000 females,[76] with a rising incidence. There are age, sex, and geographic variations: in parts of India intraoral cancer in men is more common than bronchogenic, gastric, or prostatic cancer. The bulk of patients are between 55 and 75 years of age with peak incidence around 65. Predisposing factors are as follows:

Smoking, especially of pipes and cigars, cigarettes and tobacco chewing to a lesser degree

Alcohol, particularly with daily ingestion over 7 ounces of hard liquor (Keller[32] confirmed Trieger's[71] findings of a greatly increased incidence in cirrhosis of the liver)

Syphilis, especially in cancer of the lips and anterior tongue

Nutritional deficiency (Plummer-Vinson syndrome)

Sunlight and weather exposure

Despite common belief, trauma and irritation from broken teeth and ill-fitting dentures have seldom been definitely related to oral carcinoma; oral dilapidation does seem to carry a positive correlation. Genetic predisposition is mediated through viruses, with Epstein-Barr virus implication. Multiple lesions are not uncommon as examples of "field cancerization."

Epidermoid carcinoma of the lip is overwhelmingly a disease of males (98%) and occurs on the lower lip in over 90% of cases.[15] Of all oral malignancies, it carries the most favorable prognosis, with block dissection and cobalt-60 radiation offering up to 80% 5-year survival rates. Incidence in other sites is as follows: tongue, 52%; floor of mouth, 16%; alveolar mucosa (gingiva), 12%; palate, 1%; and buccal mucosa (cheeks), 9%.

Prognosis for these sites is poor with 5-year survivals of 30% for tongue to less than 20% for floor of mouth. Preexisting and co-existing liver disease further prejudices the prognosis.[71] The extensive lymphatic drainage to sublingual and submandibular nodes promotes early metastasis. Antral carcinoma, frequently undetected until far advanced, has the poorest prognosis of all with less than 10% 5-year survival.

Indolent oral mucosal lesions and nonhealing ulcerations, particularly with raised borders or cracking keratinization, should be regarded as carcinoma unless biopsy proves otherwise. Oral carcinoma in fairly early stages is illustrated in Figures 39-11 through 39-13.

The full gamut of malignant neoplasia occurs in the aged, but aside from epidermoid carcinoma and some salivary gland lesions such as malignant pleomorphic adenoma and benign oncocytoma, they usually occur with no greater frequency than in other age-groups. Another exception is oral melanoma, which, unlike its counterpart on the skin, occurs twice as frequently in males as in females. The average age at detection is 50, with site predilection for the palate and maxillary alveolar mucosa.[73] Pigmented lesions with the pos-

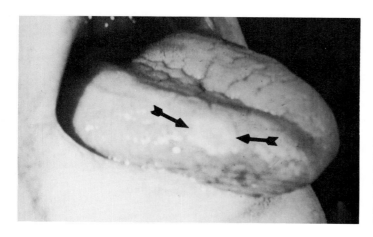

FIG. 39-11. Early squamous cell carcinoma on lateral border of the tongue in a 67-year-old man. The lesion has a keratotic surface and is just beginning to ulcerate in its center. Prognosis is fairly good at this stage, especially without nodal involvement.

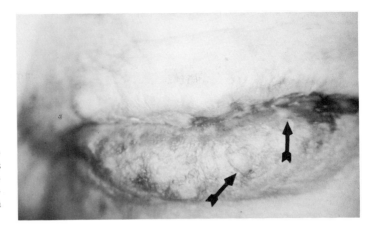

FIG. 39-12. Multiple lesions (field concerization) at an early stage of squamous cell carcinoma in the lower lip of a 79-year-old man. Despite the wide area involved, radiation therapy and dissection offer an excellent 5-year cure rate.

sible exception of lip ephelides and the obvious gingival pigmentation of blacks should be biopsied because malignant transformation of nevi, especially of the junctional variety, is not uncommon.

The sarcomas are fortunately rare, although osteosarcoma in longstanding Paget's disease has been frequently reported in the maxilla. Multiple myeloma is often evident in the jawbones, usually in the mandible, and many cases have been detected in routine dental roentgenograms. Discrete, punched-out lucencies that cannot be ascribed definitely to odontogenic infections or cysts should call for biopsy or bone survey.

Benign neoplasms and neoplasmlike reactive hyperplasia include redundant flaps of fibrotic oral membrane surrounding the borders of old dentures to fibrous polyps induced by chronic trauma such as sucking on the cheeks. Papillomas, small, whitish, cauliflowerlike lesions, are observed in all portions of the mucosa but especially the palate. Lipomas, usually of the cheeks, and hemangiomas

are also seen. Grapelike, tortuous, varicosed vessels on the floor of the mouth and below the tongue should not be confused with vascular neoplasm. They are a common adaptation to increased venous pressure. Unlike esophageal varices, they do not spontaneously rupture, nor do they become aneurysmal. No treatment is indicated. Hereditary hemorrhagic telangiectasia (Osler-Weber-Rendu) is marked by spiderlike, red lesions almost anywhere on oral and lip mucosa. They hemorrhage easily and make oral surgical procedures more difficult.

Walnutlike bony excrescences of the palate, the buccal aspect of the maxillary alveolar ridges, and the lingual aspects of the lower jaw are collectively referred to as tori. These cortical osseous hyperplasias, usually developmental, should not be termed *osteomas*, although histologically indistinguishable from benign bone tumors. Their protrusion into the oral cavity may lead to mucosal ulceration, especially in the edentulous older patient.

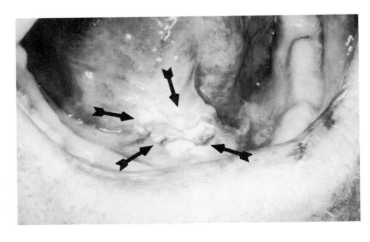

FIG. 39-13. Deeply invasive squamous cell carcinoma in the floor of the mouth of a 66-year-old, alcoholic (cirrhotic) man. The lesion is indurated and has raised borders and an ulcerated center. The patient died 9 months after massive excision and irradiation. Epidermoid carcinoma at this site carries the gravest prognosis.

Surgical removal is difficult and seldom indicated unless dentures must be made.

Metastatic tumors to the oral regions may be intraosseous or to soft tissues. The most common primary sites are breast, lung, kidney, thyroid, prostate, and colon.[13] Metastases are four times more frequent in the mandible than in the maxilla, and paresthesia of the lip is a frequent presenting symptom.

The increasing incidence of oral mucous membrane lesions with age makes them a particular concern to the geriatrician. Thus amyloidosis commonly becomes manifest in the gingiva and tongue, whether primary, secondary, tumor, or myleoma-associated. Gingival biopsy using Congo red as the amyloid-specific stain is diagnostic. Nodular macroglossia, occasionally with ulceration, is a frequent symptom in advanced amyloidosis in the aged.[9]

Recurrent aphthous stomatitis, often confused with herpetic stomatitis, afflicts many elderly patients. Scopp and Valauri[56] estimate that one in seven persons suffers from these ulcerations. They appear singly or multiply, most frequently in the mucobuccal fold but also on the palate, tongue, and buccal mucosa. They are more common in females. The lesion starts as an erythematous macule, which undergoes necrosis and quickly becomes a painful, shallow, sharply defined ulcer. Pain may interfere with eating, swallowing, and tongue movements. When secondarily infected, there may be submandibular and cervical lymphadenopathy. The ulcers heal in a period of 10 days to 2 weeks, invariably without scarring. After a variable period of remission, new lesions may develop at other sites. Recurrence may be irregular or periodic, with new ulcers developing in "crops."

The etiology of recurrent aphthous ulceration (RAU) is still unclear. Most investigators favor an autoimmune phenomenon as the result of a mucosal cell-mediated mechanism.[35] Both stable and transitional L-form streptococci have been isolated from the ulcers. These are thought to become pathogenic when stress lowers host resistance.[20] Nutrition, emotional stress, and a plethora of psychosomatic factors have been suggested, but the evidence is scanty at best. Of interest is the negative correlation of RAU with smoking.

Treatment is palliative because neither cure nor prevention exists. Topical corticosteroids such as 0.1% triamcinolone acetonide in an adherent vehicle are helpful in hastening involution and reducing pain. Surface protection with tincture of myrrh and benzoin or Orabase is useful. Severe attacks may require a topical anesthetic such as viscous lidocaine to make chewing and swallowing possible. Chlortetracycline mouthrinses (0.5% four times daily) have been reported helpful. Whichever of these is chosen, the use of escharotics to burn out RAU and other lesions should be avoided. Silver nitrate, phenol, and chromic acid have no place in the armamentarium of oral mucosal disease because their most common effect is to mask or exacerbate lesions. Cauterization is often an overtreatment that traumatizes the submucosa.

The geriatrician is frequently consulted for a variety of tongue complaints. Vague and usually transitory glossodynia is a frequent complaint of aged women. In the absence of papillary atrophy or specific mucosal lesions, glossodynia is most often of psychological origin and may be regarded as a "depressive equivalent." Reassurance and management of the underlying depression is indicated. A smooth, atrophic, and superficially hypersensitive tongue is often seen. Papillary atrophy and erythema are frequent findings in protein malnutrition, iron deficiency anemia, multiple vitamin B deficiency, malabsorption syndromes, and in the classic syndromes of pellagra and beri-beri. Elderly food faddists, even from favored socioeconomic groups, on marginal diets notable for their nutritional exclusions rather than inclusions are prone to atrophic glossitis. The geriatrician confronted with these complaints or findings should consider gross nutritional deficiency in his evaluation.

Anatomical variants such as plicate, scrotal, and lobed tongues may become noticeable to the elderly patient because of tongue enlargement, which accompanies loss of teeth. Geographic tongue ("wandering rash" and glossitis atrophica areata) requires no treatment, but patients frequently need reassurance for it and the variants mentioned above. Bluish tongue lesions are usually mucus-retention cysts if superficial and hemangiomas if deep seated. With hemangiomas, lingual arterial ligation may be required before excision.

Salivary Glands

Most forms of salivary gland disease, infectious, obstructive, metabolic, autoimmune, and neoplastic (with the exception of epidemic viral parotitis), are more common in the aged. Acute pyogenic sialadenitis, usually of the parotid gland, may be unilateral or bilateral. The usual route of infection is through Stensen's duct with acute swelling and pain on the sides of the face. Retrograde sialography shows pooling of injected dye within necrotic locules of destroyed acinar structure. Compression of the gland and "milking" may evacuate pus from the duct, with some relief. Recurrent infection may require partial or total parotidectomy. Great expertise is required to avoid transecting branches of the facial nerve, which course over and through the substance of the parotid. Conditions favoring xerostomia, such as dehydration or irradiation, contribute to sialadenitis. Keeping the patient well hydrated is a simple therapeutic measure.[19]

Chronic sialadenitis, more common than the acute form, is usually due to sialolithiasis. The parotid and submaxillary are most commonly affected with multiple small stones rather than a single large one as cause of obstruction. Presenting symptoms are a waxing and waning enlargement; pain, especially while eating or even thinking of food; and a thickened discharge from either Stensen's or Wharton's duct. Dilatation and necrosis distal to the obstruction may necessitate varying degrees of sialectomy. Dissection of the stone, particularly if single and large, is frequently successful.

REFERENCES

1. Atkinson PJ, Woodhead C: Changes in human mandibular structure with age. Arch Oral Biol 13:1453, 1968
2. Banting DW, Courtright PN: Distribution and natural history of carious lesions on roots of teeth. J Can Dent Assoc 41:45, 1975
3. Bender IB, Pressman RS: Factors in dental bacteremia. J Am Dent Assoc 32:836, 1945
4. Bernick S: Differences in nerve distribution between erupted and non-erupted human teeth. J Dent Res 43:406, 1964
5. Bernier JL, Reynolds MC: The relationship of senile elastosis to actinic radiation and to squamous cell carcinoma of the lip. Milit Med 117:209, 1955
6. Bertram U: Xerostomia. Acta Odontol Scand [Suppl] 25:4, 1967
7. Bevelander G, Benzer S: Morphology and incidence of secondary dentin in human teeth. J Am Dent Assoc 30:1075, 1943
8. Bjorby A, Löe H: The relative significance of different local factors in the initiation and development of periodontal inflammation. J Periodont Res 2:76, 1967
9. Bhaskar SN: Synopsis of Oral Pathology, 3rd ed, p 523. St. Louis, CV Mosby, 1969
10. Bodecker CF: Editorial: Again, erosion—abrasion. NY State Dent J 19:154, 1953
11. Bradley JC: Age changes in the vascular supply of the mandible. Br Dent J 132:142, 1972
12. Burnet GW: The microbiology of dental infections. Dent Clin North Am 14:681, 1970
13. Clausen F, Poulsen H: Metastatic carcinoma to the jaws. Acta Pathol Microbiol Scand 57:361, 1963
14. Costen JB: A syndrome of ear and sinus symptoms dependent upon disturbed function of the temporomandibular joint. Ann Otol Rhinol Laryngol 43:1, 1934
15. Cross JE, Guralnick E, Doland EM: Carcinoma of the lip. Surg Gynecol Obstet 87:153, 1948
16. Crum RJ, Loiselle RI: Incidence of temporomandibular joint symptoms in male patients with rheumatoid arthritis. J Am Dent Assoc 81:129, 1970
17. Englander HR, Keyes PH, Gestwicki M: Clinical anticaries effect of repeated topical sodium fluoride application by mouth rinses. J Am Dent Assoc 75:638, 1967
18. Gargiulo A, Wentz FM, Orban B: Dimensions and relation of the dentinogingival junction in humans. J Periodontal 32:261, 1961
19. Goldberg MH, Harrigan WF: Acute suppurative parotitis. Oral Surg 20:281, 1965
20. Gorlin RJ: Summary of workshop on ulcerative and bullous lesions of the orofacial region. J Dent Res 50:797, 1971
21. Gortner RA Jr, Kenigsberg RK: Factors concerned with different erosive effects of grapefruit juice on rats' molar teeth. J Nutr 46:133, 1952
22. Grant DS, Stern IB, Everett FG: Orban's Periodontics, A Concept—Theory and Practise, pp 149-150. St. Louis, CV Mosby, 1972
23. Gupta OP: An epidemiological study of periodontal disease in Trivandrum. J Dent Res 43:876, 1964
24. Hagerty PC, Maida I: Autogenous bone grafts, a revolution in the treatment of vertical bone defects. J Periodontal 42:626, 1971
25. Harkins SW, Chapman CR: The perception of induced dental pain in young and elderly women. J Gerontol 32:4, 1977
26. Hayward JR: Oral Surgery, p 58. Springfield, IL, Charles C Thomas, 1976
27. Hazen SP, Chilton NW, Mumma RD Jr: The problem of root caries: I. Literature review and clinical description. J Am Dent Assoc 86:137, 1973
28. Hirschfeld I: Abnormalities of the tooth surface induced by toothbrushing. Dent Items Interest 58:28, 1936
29. Holloway PJ, Mellanby M, Stewart RJC: Fruit drinks and tooth erosion. Br Dent J 104:305, 1958
30. Jackson D, Burch PRJ: Dental caries as a degenerative disease. Gerontology 15:203, 1969
31. Johnson ES, Kelly JE, VanKirk LE: Selected dental findings in adults by age, race and sex: United States—1960–1962. Vital Health Stat 11:1, 1965
32. Keller AZ: Cirrhosis of the liver, alcoholism and heavy smoking associated with cancer of the mouth and pharynx. Cancer 20:1015, 1967
33. Kerr DA: Relationships between periodontal disease and systemic disease. J Dent Res 41:302, 1962
34. Kutler Y: Classification of dentin into primary, secondary and tertiary. Oral Surg 12:996, 1959
35. Lehner T: Autoimmunity and management of recurrent oral ulceration. Br Dent J 122:15, 1967

36. Levine HL, Stahl SS: Periodontal flap surgery with gingival fiber retention. J Periodontol 43:91, 1972

37. Lonberg P: Changes in the Size of the Lower Jaw on Account of Age and Loss of Teeth. Stockholm, Private Press, 1951

38. McMullen JA, Legg M, Gottsegen R, Camerini-Davalos R: Microangiopathy in the gingival tissues of prediabetics with special reference to the prediabetic state. Periodont 5:61, 1967

39. Mandel ID: Histochemical and biochemical aspects of plaque formation. Periodont 1:43, 1963

40. Manly RS: The abrasion of cementum and dentin by modern dentifrices. J Dent Res 20:583, 1941

41. Marshall-Day CD, Stephens RG, Quigley LF Jr: Periodontal disease: Prevalence and incidence. J Periodontol 26:185, 1955

42. Miles AEW: Ageing in the teeth and oral tissues. In Bourne GH (ed): Structural Aspects of Ageing, pp 352–397. New York, Hofner Publishers, 1961

43. Mitchell DF, Standish SM, Fast TB: Oral Diagnosis/Oral Medicine, p 125. Philadelphia, Lea & Febiger, 1969

44. Mongini F: Remodelling of the mandibular condyle in the adult and its relationship to the condition of the dental arches. Acta Anat (Base 1) 82:437, 1972

45. Mühleman HR: Tooth mobility, a review of clinical aspects and research findings. J Periodontol 38:686, 1967

46. Osborn J, Briel N, Hedegard B: The nature of prosthetic dentistry. Int Dent J 16:509, 1966

47. Persson P: The regeneration of the marginal periodontium after flap operation. Acta Odontol Scand 20:43, 1962

48. Pickett HG, Appleby RG, Osborn MO: Changes in the denture supporting tissues associated with the aging process. J Prosthet Dent 27:257, 1972

49. Ram JS: Aging and immunologic phenomena: A review. J Gerontol 22;92, 1967

50. Rifkin B: Observations on alveolar bone resorption in periodontitis of beagle dogs. Preprinted abstracts presented at the Annual Meeting of the International Association of Dental Research, #408, 1977

51. Ring JR: Histological and histochemical age changes in oral subepithelial connective tissues. In Shock NW (ed): Ageing—Social and Biological Aspects. Washington, DC, American Association for the Advancement of Science, 1960

52. Robinson HBG: Abrasion, attrition and erosion of the teeth. Health Center Journal (Ohio State University) 3:21, 1949

53. Rosenthal SL: Dental problems of age. J Dent Med 15:4, 1960

54. Schour I, Sarnat BG: Oral manifestations of occupational origin. JAMA 120:1197, 1942

55. Schwartz L: Disorders of the Temporomandibular Joint. Philadelphia, WB Saunders, 1959

56. Scopp IW, Valauri AJ: Diseases of the oral mucosa. J Dermatol Surg 2:246, 1976

57. Scott DE: Opportunities for research in aging. Opening remarks presented at Symposium: The geriatric patient—dentistry's growing challenge, Boston, 1977

58. Shafer WG, Hine MK, Levy BM: A Textbook of Oral Pathology, 2nd ed. Philadelphia, WB Saunders, 1966

59. Shannon IL: A new approach to oral hygiene for the cerebral palsy patient. Bull Dent Guid Counc Cerebral Palsy 12:12, 1972

60. Sheppard IM: Alveolar resorption in diabetes mellitus. Dent Cosmos 78:1075, 1936

61. Sherman H: Phonetic capability as a function of vertical dimension in complete denture wearers—a preliminary report. J Prosthet Dent 23:621, 1970

62. Sicher H, Bhaskar SN (eds): Orban's Oral Histology and Embryology, p 161. St. Louis, CV Mosby, 1972

63. Soggnaes RF: Dental hard tissue destruction. In Soggnaes RF (ed): Mechanisms of Hard Tissue Destruction, p 94. Washington, DC, American Association for the Advancement of Science, 1963

64. Stafne EC: Oral Roentgenographic Diagnosis, 2nd ed, p 134. Philadelphia, WB Saunders, 1963

65. Stahl SS: The etiology of periodontal disease. In Ramfjord SP, Kerr DA, Ash M (eds): World Workshop in Periodontics. Ann Arbor, University of Michigan Press, 1966

66. Stanley HR, White CL, McCray L: The rate of tertiary (reparative) dentine formation in the human tooth. Oral Surg 21:180, 1966

67. Stewart JL, Drisko RR, Herlach AD: Comparison of ultrasonic and hand instruments for the removal of calculus. J Am Dent Assoc 75:153, 1967

68. Ten Cate AR: Development of the periodontium. In Melcher AH, Bowen R (eds): Biology of the Periodontium. New York, Academic Press, 1969

69. Tiecke RW, Bernier JL: Statistical and morphologic analysis of four hundred and one cases of intraoral squamous cell carcinoma. J Am Dent Assoc 49:684, 1954

70. Trieger N, Chomenko A: New concepts in the treatment of periodontitis. J Oral Maxillofac Surg 40:701–708, 1982

71. Trieger N, Ship II, Taylor GW, Weisberger D: Cirrhosis and other predisposing factors in cancer of the tongue. Cancer 11:357, 1958

72. Trieger N, Taylor GW, Weisberger D: Significance of liver dysfunction in mouth cancer. Surg Gynecol Obstet 108:230–234, 1959

73. Trodahl JN, Sprague WG: Benign and malignant melanocytic lesions of the oral mucosa: An analysis of one hundred and thirty-five cases. Cancer 25:812, 1970

74. Weinberger A: The clinical significance of hypercementosis. Oral Surg 7:79, 1954

75. Weinberger A: Attritioning of teeth. Oral Surg 8:1048, 1955

76. Wynder EL, Bross IJ, Feldman RM: A study of the etiological factors in cancer of the mouth. Cancer 10:1300, 1957

77. Zach L: Thermogenesis in operative technics. J Prosthet Dent 12:977, 1962

78. Zach L: Pulpal lability and repair: Effect of restorative procedures. Oral Surg 33:111, 1972

79. Zach L: Diabetes and dentistry: A review of some correlates. NY J Dent 46:229, 1976

80. Zach L, Cohen G: Ultrasonic cavity preparation: The effect on the immature dentition. J Prosthet Dent 8:139, 1958

81. Zach, L, Cohen G: Pulp response to externally applied heat. Oral Surg 19:515, 1965

82. Zach L, Topal R, Cohen G: The radioautographic demonstration of pulpal repair using H^3 thymidine. Program and Abstracts presented at the 43rd Meeting of the International Association of Dental Research, 1965

83. Zachinsky L: Range of histologic variation in clinically normal gingiva. J Dent Res 33:580, 1954

84. Zander HA, Hürzeler B: Continuous cementum apposition. J Dent Res 37:1035, 1958

40 Ultrasound in Geriatrics

Fred Winsberg

Ultrasound is an attractive means of examining the geriatric patient because of its noninvasive nature. The applications of ultrasonic imaging have greatly expanded in the past few years because of technologic developments that have resulted in improved image quality and less dependence on operator technique. However, ultrasound remains a technique that requires a skilled operator and can be time consuming because the body is imaged in slices.

There are currently two main types of ultrasonic B-scanners: (1) those in which the transducer is moved by the operator, called contact B-scanners, and (2) those in which the beam scanning is electronically or mechanically accomplished by the machine. The technique has undergone a rapid period of technologic growth, and the second type has largely replaced the first. Both methods are referred to as B-scanning, and both methods have intensity modulation that has been called gray scale.

The automatic scanning devices are generally referred to as real-time scanners because the operator can interact with the image and the image rate is fast enough to identify motion. In cardiac imaging a single beam may be used for recording motion and making certain measurements. This is referred to as M mode. However, the automated real-time B-scanner has assumed an increasingly important role in cardiac imaging because spatial relationships are much less ambiguous than with the classic M-mode echocardiogram. Modern instruments combine two-dimensional real-time imaging with M-mode imaging, and many also incorporate Doppler flow information. The latter makes possible the diagnosis of valve incompetence and shunts with precision. A new technologic development, not yet commercially available, is the combination of spatial and flow information. The flow information is displayed in color and shows the flow of blood across valves and shunts in real time.

CENTRAL NERVOUS SYSTEM

The use of echoencephalography has diminished in the past few years because of the general availability of computed tomography. At the present time most users believe that classic single beam echoencephalography is too subjective to be reliable except in very experienced hands.

Ultrasound imaging of the central nervous system has, however, attained considerable importance in the operating room, where the neurosurgeon can use it to guide him in directing biopsies or aspirations. It has also been extensively used intraoperatively in examining the spine for tumors and disk herniations.

EXTRACEREBRAL VASCULAR SYSTEM

Extracerebral vascular disease is a major problem since it contributes heavily to strokes. Several noninvasive methods of detection of carotid disease are available. Indirect techniques include oculoplethysmography and periorbital Doppler ultrasound, but these examinations are only sensitive for very high-grade stenoses or occlusions.

The simplest systems for direct examination of the carotid bifurcation employ continuous-wave Doppler ultrasound. The relative velocity of a column of blood with respect to an ultrasonic beam results in a difference in the frequency of the reflected sound from the emitted sound. This difference frequency is proportional to the velocity of blood flow and can be continuously monitored so that one has a curve of blood velocity versus time. This curve is modified by obstructive disease or by changes in the resistance of the intracerebral circulation owing to generalized arteriosclerosis. A skilled operator can detect a hemodynamically significant lesion (greater than 60%) involving the common carotid, internal carotid, subclavian, and vertebral arteries. Improvement in sensitivity has resulted from the coupling of Doppler ultrasound to the spectrum analyzer, which analyzes the frequency content of the sound, much as the ear detects the sound of familiar voices or instruments by recognizing their frequency content. Normal arterial flow is characterized by laminar movement of red blood cells in which there is a narrow band of frequencies. With relatively minor disease, flow disturbance resulting in broadening of this spectrum occurs before there is significant increase in peak velocity. Spectrum analysis can also be applied to pulsed Doppler ultrasound. The latter limits velocity information to a specific depth and thus location within the vessel. The marriage of pulsed Doppler ultrasound to real-time imaging results in what is called the duplex imager, in which one images the carotid with a high-resolution ultrasound imager (Fig. 40-1) and records flow information from selected sample volumes within the vessel. The location of the sample volume is indicated on the image and thus the visible lesion may be related to the velocity disturbance it produces. A considerable body of experience has now been built up with duplex imaging, and it has a high degree of sensitivity and specificity for lesions around the carotid bifurcation. In general, imaging is most reliable for the detection of early disease and in the discrimination of ulcerated or hemorrhagic plaque from smooth plaque, whereas Doppler ultrasound is often better than imaging for measurement of the degree of stenosis when stenosis is severe or there is heavy calcification. During the period of enthusiasm for intravenous digital subtraction angiography (IVDSA) some believed that it would replace ultrasound, but that has not proved to be the case. Ultrasound remains simpler, safer, and comparable in accuracy with IVDSA.

HEART

In the past decade, echocardiography has become an important and mature field. It has greatly contributed to the understanding of a variety of car-

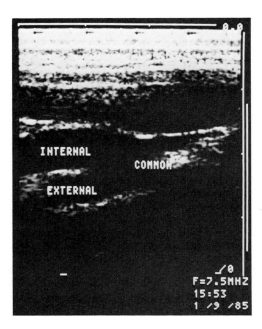

FIG. 40-1. High-frequency ultrasound image of a normal carotid bifurcation.

diac problems, including valvular disease, cardiomyopathy, and, to a lesser extent, coronary artery disease.

It is, of course, difficult to segregate geriatric from other age groups in evaluating cardiac disease. I have even seen a few atrial septal defects that went undiagnosed until the seventh or eighth decade. There are, however, a few problems that occur with sufficient frequency to merit specific comment:

The heart is enlarged and/or the patient is in heart failure. Most often the explanation is simply a dilated, poorly functioning left ventricle, and this is readily ascertained by echocardiography, obviating the need for further investigation. Pericardial fluid is relatively rare in the elderly except as a consequence of myocardial infarction (Dressler's syndrome) or secondary to congestive failure or uremia.

Another common indication for study is atrial fibrillation. Usually a specific cause is not identified. Occasionally, one finds unsuspected mitral stenosis.

Patients with murmurs are often referred for ultrasound study. A surprisingly large amount of aortic valve disease will be disclosed in echocardiograms of the elderly. The valve and aortic root are often calcified, and there may be varying degrees of restriction of opening of the valve. A crit-

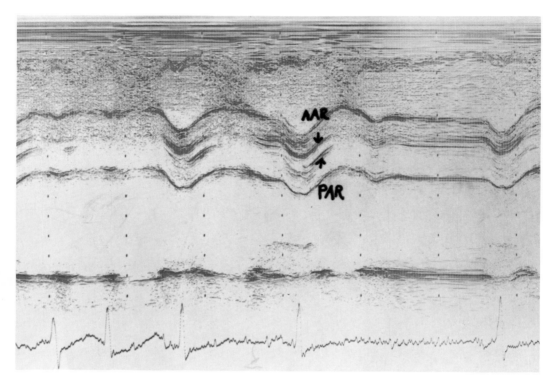

FIG. 40-2. Calcific aortic stenosis in a 78-year-old woman. Arrows show narrow opening of aortic valve. (*AAR,* anterior aortic root; *PAR,* posterior aortic root)

ical degree of aortic stenosis may be signaled by angina or cerebral ischemia, and it is of significance to detect this lesion because aortic valve replacement is now feasible even in a 70-year-old person. Doppler ultrasound has become the preferred means to evaluate aortic stensosis. The velocity across the valve is easily related to the gradient by a simple formula:

$$\text{gradient in mm Hg} = 4 \times V^2$$

Skillful use of Doppler ultrasound obviates the need for cardiac catheterization in patients with aortic stenosis.

A common complex is aortic stenosis and/or regurgitation and mitral annulus calcification. For reasons unknown, this diagnosis is not considered often enough by the clinician. It may produce multiple murmurs, both systolic (ejection and holosystolic) and diastolic. The degrees of left atrial enlargement, mitral regurgitation, and aortic valve disease are extremely variable, but this combination of lesions is extremely common in elderly patients (Figs. 40-2 and 40-3). Usually the hemodynamic consequences are not important, but the combination of significant aortic stenosis and mitral regurgitation places an intolerable burden on the left ventricle.

Other systolic murmurs commonly encountered in elderly patients are due to a variety of mitral valve dysfunctions. The most frequent is secondary to left ventricular dysfunction and is characterized echographically (in two-dimensional studies) by a reduced surface of systolic contact of the anterior and posterior leaflets. Normally the two leaflets touch as a pair of clapped hands, whereas in left ventricular dysfunction only the fingertips touch. A less common but still important syndrome is the floppy or flail mitral valve. In the elderly, this may be due to longstanding prolapse, infective endocarditis, chordal rupture, and even rupture of papillary muscles. When a flail leaflet is discovered, the patient should be considered for valve replacement if left ventricular function is conserved. Some cardiac surgeons are skilled at repairing flail leaflets, and this avoids some of the complications of valve replacement.

The aging heart tends to hypertrophy symmetrically, but one also encounters asymmetric hypertrophy with or without obstructive cardiomyopathy in a relatively asymptomatic elderly patient.

Since hypertrophic cardiomyopathy is a disease with considerable variability in its clinical manifestations, some elderly patients may present in

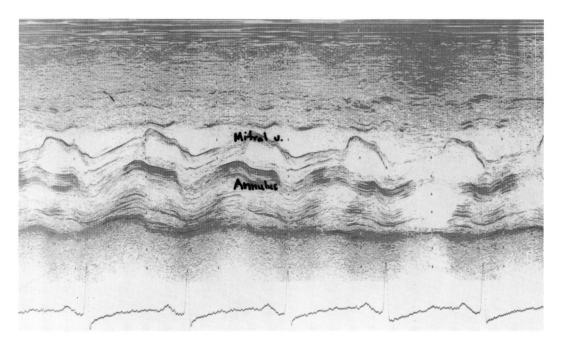

FIG. 40-3. Same patient as Figure 40-2. The mitral annulus is heavily calcified. The mitral valve can be seen in front of it. There is symmetric left ventricular hypertrophy.

mild failure or with angina. If their echocardiograms suggest asymmetric hypertrophy it is useful to examine other members of the family to establish the fact that one is indeed dealing with the hereditary form of asymmetric hypertrophy.

Cardiac tumors are rare and even more rarely diagnosed clinically. The most common is the left atrial myxoma, which is easily displayed by ultrasound and usually confused clinically with mitral stenosis. Right atrial myxomas and a variety of primary and metastatic tumors are also seen.

Left atrial thrombus is difficult to demonstrate by ultrasound and is not usually detected. Some vegetations are visible and occasionally infective endocarditis is detected by echocardiography before a clinical diagnosis has been made.

Patients with embolic episodes are frequently referred for echocardiography to find a possible source. In my experience, this is rarely rewarding.

ABDOMINAL B-SCANS

There has been a great increase in the use of ultrasonic abdominal imaging since 1974 when the television scan converter was introduced, permitting reasonably reliable intensity modulation in two dimensional images (gray scale). Of particular interest in the geriatric patient are the following problems:

Liver and Biliary Tree

In the past, radionuclide scintigraphy was considered the best screening method for hepatic lesions. However, the development of high-quality real-time scanners has made ultrasound a better and more cost-effective approach. In addition, ultrasound provides a more precise diagnosis and can distinguish cysts and inflammatory diseases from neoplasms (Figs. 40-4 and 40-5). Liver cysts are quite common in the elderly and may attain considerable size. Drainage of very large cysts that contain as much as 2 liters of fluid may be carried out under ultrasound control if they produce significant symptoms, such as nausea and vomiting due to compression of the stomach or jaundice due to compression of the biliary tree. Liver abscess, either single or multiple, is not rare in elderly patients. Predisposing factors include previous surgery, neoplasm, cholelithiasis, and immune deficiency. Puncture and drainage of liver abscesses under ultrasound control permits a precise bacteriologic diagnosis and can be lifesaving. The importance of the diagnostic and therapeutic role of ultrasound for liver abscess cannot be overemphasized.

In the jaundiced patient, ultrasound is the first study that should be performed to distinguish medical from surgical jaundice. The bile ducts contain protein-free liquid and are readily visible. The

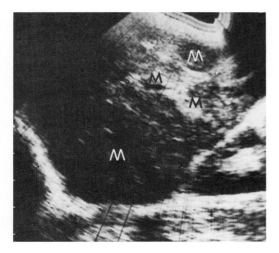

FIG. 40-4. Sagittal section of the liver showing multiple metastatic lesions (*M*).

differentiation of bile ducts from portal veins requires some experience but is not difficult to learn. Computed tomography is also useful in identifying dilated bile ducts but is a much more expensive examination.

Dilatation of the intrahepatic biliary tree and/or extrahepatic bile ducts indicates the level of obstruction and the need for surgical relief. Depending on the clinical situation and the facilities of the hospital, demonstration of obstructive jaundice by ultrasound may be followed by percutaneous transhepatic cholangiography, surgery, or retrograde study (endoscopic retrograde cholangiopancreatography [ERCP], Fig. 40-6).

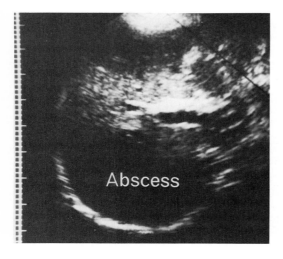

FIG. 40-5. Subphrenic abcess. The dense echo below the abcess is the hemidiaphragm.

Gallbladder

Real-time sonography is now the accepted method of diagnosing cholelithiasis and has largely replaced the oral cholecystogram. Ultrasound is also useful in diagnosis of acute cholelithiasis associated with calculous disease. Its role in acalculous cholecystitis is less clear, but the latter diagnosis seems resistant to diagnosis by imaging of any kind and is often a puzzling clinical problem. Unfortunately, edema of the gallbladder, which is the ultrasonic indicator of cholecystitis, also occurs with hypoalbuminemia, congestive failure, and hepatitis. Thus it is not a specific finding. Pericholecystic abscess, particularly if associated with calculi, is a specific finding. The sonographer should try to evaluate the presence of tenderness localized to the gallbladder. However, this finding is difficult to elicit in the debilitated, sedated, or narcotized patient (Fig. 40-7). The ultrasonic diagnosis of hydrops of the gallbladder may prevent the unhappy complication of perforation of the gallbladder, which is all too common in the geriatric age-group.

Right Upper Quadrant

Ultrasonic examination of the right upper quadrant may show subphrenic and subhhepatic collections (see Fig. 40-5). A commonly palpated "mass" in elderly women is the right kidney, which may lie in an anterior position just beneath the liver (Fig. 40-8). It is surprising how often a patient is referred for ascites and a large liver with a presumptive diagnosis of metastatic carcinoma who is in fact suffering from congestive heart failure. The characteristic swollen liver and dilated vena cava are readily evident with ultrasonic examination. Perhaps even more surprising is the fact that owing to tricuspid regurgitation in a patient with congestive failure the dilated pulsatile vena cava may be mistaken for an aortic aneurysm!

Pancreas

Until the advent of ultrasound and computed tomography, the pancreas could only be examined indirectly. Even though direct visualization of pancreatic neoplasms is now possible, it is doubtful that increased survival from this dreadful disease has occurred. However, early diagnosis may at least permit more expeditious management of the patient. One strategy that is being employed with increasing frequency is fine needle aspiration biopsy followed by chemotherapy and radiation therapy without surgery.

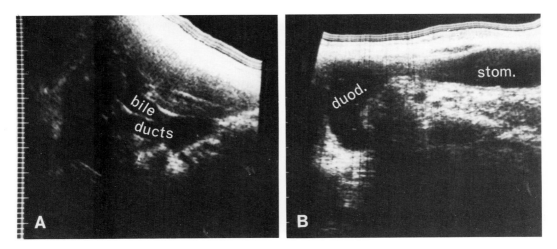

FIG. 40-6. (*A*) Dilated bile ducts are shown within the liver. (*B*) Transverse cut showing distended stomach and duodenum. This patient, aged 84, was admitted with sudden vomiting and jaundice that was due to a carcinoma of the duodenum in the region of the ampulla.

Obstructive juandice is frequently the presenting symptom in tumors of the pancreatic head and as indicated in the previous section is readily diagnosed. Gallstones are coincidentally present so that the discovery of stones does not exclude carcinoma.

Kidney

Renal masses in the elderly are very likely cystic. This diagnosis is made with great accuracy by ultrasound, and angiography may be avoided. When there is reason to do so, cyst puncture is readily carried out with ultrasonic guidance. This can be accomplished with a 22-gauge needle without anesthesia as an outpatient procedure. The fluid may be sent for cytologic examination but there is an increasing tendency to abstain from renal puncture in patients over age 60 who have characteristic ultrasound findings of renal cyst because renal cysts are ubiquitous. If a renal mass cannot be clearly identified with ultrasound or is not definitely cystic, computed tomography or angiography is indicated. The rare situation of a cyst adjacent to a carcinoma must be kept in mind, but cysts containing clear fluid are, for practical pur-

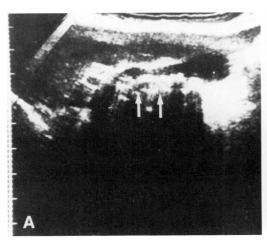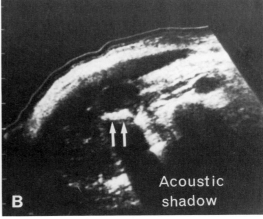

FIG. 40-7. (*A*) Sagittal and (*B*) transverse cuts of right upper quadrant in an elderly woman with multiple gallstones (*arrows*). Characteristic acoustic shadowing is shown.

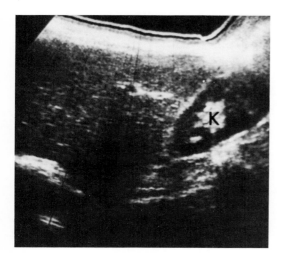

FIG. 40-8. Sagittal cut of right upper quadrant in a thin old woman in whom the clinician felt a "mass." The kidney (*K*) lies just under the skin.

poses, never malignant. If, on the other hand, puncture shows old blood, the cyst must be considered malignant, and cytological study is superfluous.

Renal Failure

Ultrasound is extremely useful in the evaluation of patients with renal failure. One may find obstructive uropathy, abnormal-appearing kidneys that may be normal in size or atrophic, or normal-appearing kidneys. If hydronephrosis is encountered, percutaneous nephrostomy may be carried out with ultrasound guidance to relieve obstruction and appropriate palliative or therapeutic action can be taken after this temporizing procedure. If the kidneys are atrophic, it is useless to carry out further diagnostic procedures. If they are normal in size, renal biopsy may be indicated.

Lower Urinary Tract

A simple but useful role for ultrasound is the evaluation of retained urine in the bladder after voiding. Although the prostate can be imaged from the abdomen through a full bladder there has been increasing interest in transrectal imaging of the prostate in order to detect occult carcinoma or to guide biopsy of palpable lesions. Another technique that may gain wider acceptance is the use of transrectal ultrasound to guide placement of radioactive nuclides for treatment of prostate cancer.

Aortic Aneurysm

Aortic aneurysm is a common lesion in the elderly. Criteria for surgical therapy vary in different institutions, but it is generally agreed that a painless aneurysm less than 5 cm in diameter may be safely followed. Aneurysms 5 cm or greater may be watched if the patient's cardiovascular or cerebral status is generally compromised, but in an institution in which the surgical mortality of elective resection approaches zero, elective resection is preferable to emergency resection, at which time the mortality is about 50%.

Aortic aneurysms are easy to identify with ultrasound. Their dimensions may be accurately measured, and the entire lumen is displayed including intraluminal thrombus, whereas only the blood-filled portion is displayed on angiograms. Only half of aortic aneurysms are detected on plain roentgenograms by their characteristic calcification.

With older equipment, it was not possible to determine the relation of the aneurysm to the renal arteries, but this problem will probably disappear because the vascular anatomy of the branches of the aorta is well displayed with the newest high-resolution gray-scale machines (Fig. 40-9). Involvement of the iliac arteries is relatively easy to display. Occasionally, an isolated iliac aneurysm may be demonstrated.

Elderly patients, particularly women, frequently have an exaggerated lumbar lordosis,

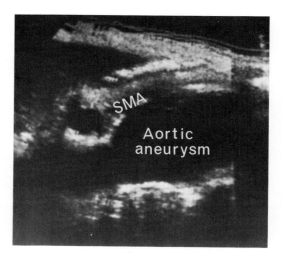

FIG. 40-9. Sagittal cut of the aorta showing an aortic aneurysm and its relation to the superior mesenteric artery (*SMA*).

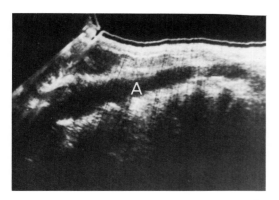

FIG. 40-10. Thin elderly patient with very superficial aorta: (*A*) sagittal cut.

which displaces the aorta anteriorly. The aorta thus becomes a subcutaneous organ, easily palpable and easily confused with an aneurysm (Fig. 40-10).

Female Pelvis

The female pelvis is relatively easily examined by ultrasound. The full bladder serves as an acoustic window and permits visualization of the uterus and adnexae.

Sonography can demonstrate a variety of neoplastic and inflammatory conditions. It can also reassure the clinician when physical examination is difficult or equivocal.

Ovarian tumors are notoriously occult clinically and are too often discovered when treatment is only palliative. Systematic screening for early detection of ovarian tumors is currently under consideration.

Lower Extremities

The arteries of the lower extremities are easily examined with continuous wave Doppler techniques, and hemodynamically significant lesions can be detected (Fig. 40-11). However, before surgical intervention is undertaken contrast visualization must be done. Popliteal aneurysms may be demonstrated by B-scanning.

One may also use the Doppler technique to measure the blood pressure in the lower extremities, and the pressure may be monitored after exercise to evaluate the functional significance of an occlusive lesion or set of lesions. It is also a useful technique for follow-up after surgery.

Doppler ultrasound has proved disappointing in diagnosing venous disease.

Breast

Breast ultrasound is of limited value for diagnosing breast disease. Cystic lesions are clearly seen and easily distinguished from solid masses. There is interest in developing a practical machine for ultrasonic mammography, but it is not yet a suitable means of screening.

Thyroid

Cystic lesions of the thyroid are common in some geographical regions and may be readily displayed by ultrasound. It is reasonable to aspirate a cyst of the thyroid even though malignancy is not entirely excluded.

Eyes

Ultrasound has proved very useful in ophthalmology. Of particular interest in the geriatric patient

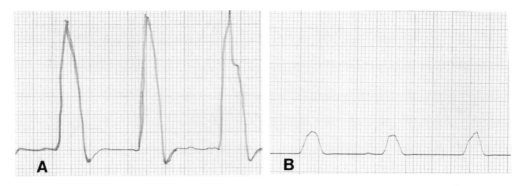

FIG. 40-11. Doppler study in patient with obstruction at the origin of the superficial femoral artery. (*A*) Normal tracing from the common femoral. (*B*) Damped velocity curve in the superficial femoral.

is the demonstration of a normal retina and vitreous in the eye containing a cataract. Ultrasonic examination of the eyes should be carried out before cataract removal to exclude a detached retina or extensive vitreous opacification. Ultrasound is also used to measure the length of the eye so that a lens implant of correct focal length may be selected.

BIBLIOGRAPHY

Alani SE, Hutchinson JE III, Schwartz MJ: Replacing the aortic valve in the 9th decade of life. Geriatrics 32:100, 1977

Coleman DJ, Lizzi FL, Jack RL: Ultrasonography of the Eye and Orbit. Philadelphia, Lea & Febiger, 1977

Curati WL, Petitclerc R, Winsberg F: Ultrasonic features of mitral annulus calcification: Report of 21 cases. Radiology 122:215, 1977

Goldberg SJ, Allen HD, Marx GR, Flinn CJ: Doppler Echocardiography. Philadelphia, Lea & Febiger, 1985

Kempezinski RF, Yao JST: Practical Noninvasive Vascular Diagnosis. Chicago, Year Book Medical Publishers, 1982

Stephenson LW, MacVaugh H III, Edmunds LH: Surgery using cardiopulmonary bypass in the elderly. Circulation 58:250, 1978

Winsberg F, Cooperberg PL: Real Time Ultrasonography. New York, Churchill Livingstone, 1982

41   Falls

Ronald D.T. Cape

Joseph Sheldon,[20] in 1948, was the first physician to highlight the importance of a fall to an elderly person. He wrote the following:

> The fact that old people are liable to tumble and hurt themselves is a matter of common knowledge, and indeed accidental injuries formed the second largest item amongst the previous illnesses considered by the subject to be affecting their present health, almost equalling rheumatic disease in incidence. Not only may the injuries resulting from these falls be of great severity, but in really old people a fall may have the effect of precipitating a senile decay. Apart altogether, however, from its social importance, the liability of old people to fall presents problems of the greatest clinical interest. It is odd that this has attracted so little curiosity, and it is greatly to be hoped that a more intensive study of the question may be made in the future.

Sheldon later undertook a study of 500 falls in 202 individuals[21] and initiated research into the subject that has continued with increasing momentum during the past 35 years.

It is easy to understand that a fall that causes a fracture or other serious injury can be of great significance to the old person. It is also true that the effect of the many falls, more than ten times as many as cause fractures, create a serious loss of confidence in the person's ability to walk. As Sudarsky and Lonthal[23] have noted, fear of falling may occur not only after an incident but also in old people who are finding it difficult to walk for neurologic reasons. There is little doubt that if physicians were able to abolish this problem, they would make an enormous contribution toward reducing morbidity and encouraging the maintenance of independence in the elderly.

EPIDEMIOLOGY

In Sheldon's survey, 279 answers from 90 men and 189 women indicated that 21% of men and 43% of women were liable to fall, with this liability increasing with age (Table 41-1). Sheldon suggested three main reasons for this high incidence in the elderly: (1) an increased liability to trip over trivial objects; (2) difficulty in maintaining the erect posture once balance has been disturbed; and (3) susceptibility to a sudden collapse of the postural controlling mechanism leading to a "drop attack." In the nine pages devoted to this subject in his classic text there are innumerable vignettes of falls sustained by many of his subjects. Almost 40 years since Sheldon produced his work, its clarity and definition of the problem remain excellent.

In 1968, Clark[6] published a study of fractured hips and described in detail the falls that resulted in the injuries. All the patients in his study were women. Exton-Smith[7] reported in 1977 on an investigation of the incidence of falls in 963 individuals over the age of 65. This study confirmed the fact that women fall twice as often as men, the incidence increasing linearly with age, from 30% in the 65- to 69-year age-group to over 50% in those between 85 and 90. For men, the proportion increases from 13% in the younger age-group to about 30% in the 80- to 84-year age-group. Beyond that age, there was a reduction in incidence (Fig. 41-1). Two groups of factors of separate origins were shown to play a role. The first arose in the environment, where irregularities of floor surface, objects left lying about, or awkward sidewalk steps may result in an accidental fall; the second group stems from the functioning of the individual who falls. Feelings of faintness, loss of balance, inability to right oneself, blackouts, or a sudden

TABLE 41-1   Liability to Fall (%)

Age Category (Years)	Women	Men
60–64	34	
65–69	27	10
70–74	47	19
75–79	60	25
80–84	77	38
≥85	69	33
Total	43	21

(Sheldon JH: The Social Medicine of Old Age, pp 96–105. London, Oxford University Press, 1948)

giving way of the legs all may arise due to an inherent happening, transient or permanent, in the individual.

Gryfe and his colleagues[10] carried out a prospective study of all falls in the Jewish Home for the Aged in Toronto over a 5-year period. Of 441 residents, 69% were women and 73% were betweens the ages 75 and 90 years, with almost a third aged 80 to 84 years. The female rate of falling was more than twice as great as men in all age-groups. In 83% of the 651 falls the resulting morbidity was negligible, but in 6% there were fractures, and 11% had soft tissue injuries that required suturing.

Perhaps the most complete epidemiologic study comes from the town of Gisborne, New Zealand. There, Campbell and co-workers[3] analyzed falls experienced by a population sample of 553 subjects who were 65 years of age and over. This sample included 1:20 of the population aged 65 to 74 years, 1:6 of the population aged 75 to 79 years, and everyone who was aged 80 years and over. Of a total of 589 identified in this way, only 30 (5.1%) refused to participate. The sample included people living in their own homes (469), those in residential group homes (75), and a small number in hospitals (15). The prevalence of falling is seen in Figure 41-2 with a steady increase from 25% at the ages of 65 to 75 to 56% beyond the age of 90. This study also demonstrated that trips or accidental falls diminish with increasing age, a finding that agreed with those of Overstall and colleagues,[17] and attributed this reduction to diminishing activity. On the other hand, the number of falls caused by patient factors increased steadily in both series.

Epidemiologic data thus demonstrate that falling is common in the elderly, occurring in approximately one third of everyone over the age of 65 years in any 1 year. It is twice as common in women as in men; only 5% to 15% of patients will sustain significant injuries as a result of the fall. Purely accidental falls due to walking on uneven surfaces, slipping on greasy or wet floors, or tripping over rugs, pets, or other obstructions become less common in the very old, while falls due to patient factors become increasingly frequent.

ETIOLOGY

Control of Posture

One of the unique features of humans is their adoption of an erect posture. This allows the use

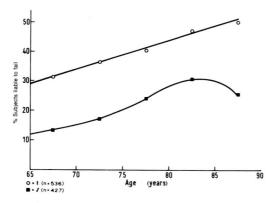

FIG. 41-1. Age incidence of falls in elderly men and women.

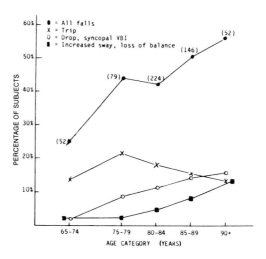

FIG. 41-2. Type of fall by age-group. (Campbell AJ, Reinken J: Falls in old age: A study of frequency and related clinical factors. Age Ageing 10:164, 1981)

of hands and arms for more skillful activities than is possible by four-legged creatures. The upright posture, however, demands a well-organized and elaborate central nervous arrangement to give it stability and reliability. It is based on sensory receptors throughout the body feeding information into the central nervous system, which then processes it and organizes appropriate motor neuron responses (Fig. 41-3).

Sheldon was the first to study posture by measuring the involuntary movements, which occur all the time when an individual attempts to stand still. He devised a light aluminum frame that was secured on a person's shoulders and had a triangular projecting element with a spring-loaded pencil.[22] The subject was then invited to stand as still as possible for 1 minute with the pencil resting on a piece of graph paper. The object of the test was to measure how far and how much the pencil deviated from its original spot. Sheldon carried out this simple maneuver with the subject's eyes either open or closed and the feet apart or together. He was able to make an approximate quantitative assessment of the degree of sway, which he then plotted in a graph. Figure 41-4 is taken from this study and illustrates sample tracings from childhood to old age. Sheldon claimed that postural control was a skill acquired early in life, which achieved stability by the mid teens and began to be less effective beyond the age of 60.

Others[11,17] have confirmed the general validity of Sheldon's observations. Overstall and co-workers noted that the degree of sway of individuals who experienced accidental falls was no greater than that of control subjects who had not fallen. On the other hand, individuals who had fallen because of loss of balance, vertigo, drop attacks, or other reasons associated with the patient did have a statistically greater degree of sway. Attempts are being made to develop more sophisticated methods of assessing sway; Kirshen and associates[14] have used multivariate analysis to generate a profile of falls and to develop a predictive equation that would identify subjects liable to fall. Results were inconclusive, but such criteria may be an important element in attempts to prevent falls in the future.

Key centers for postural control are in two regions: the neck and the inner ear. The relative importance of cervical mechanoreceptors and the endolymph of the semicircular canals is a matter of continuing debate. Wyke[24] has suggested that during evolution the change from quadruped to upright posture was accompanied by an increased importance in the reflexogenic significance of cervical mechanoreceptors as compared with those located in the vestibule. He suggests that changes in the cervical spine that commonly accompany aging, such as osteoarthritis, decrease in cervical intervertebral disk height, or cervical vertebral col-

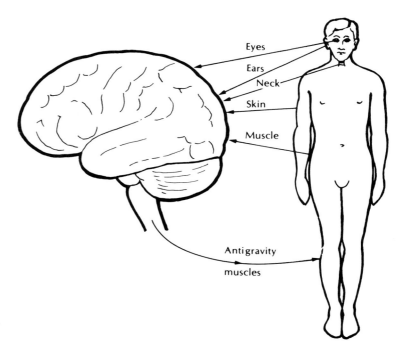

FIG. 41-3. Sensory and motor pathways that control posture.

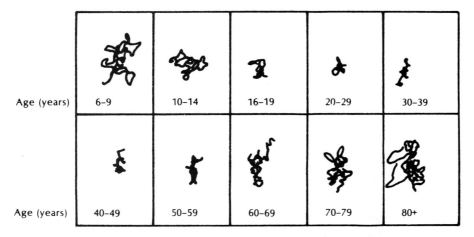

| Age (years) | 6–9 | 10–14 | 16–19 | 20–29 | 30–39 |
| Age (years) | 40–49 | 50–59 | 60–69 | 70–79 | 80+ |

FIG. 41-4. Effect of age on sway as revealed by tracings in Sheldon's study. (Sheldon JH: The effect of age on the control of sway. Gerontol Clin 5:129–138, 1963)

CAUSES OF FALLING

PRECIPITATING CAUSES OF FALLS

Accidental*

Trips
Slips
Misjudging steps
Poor visibility on stairs
Overreaching
Loose slip rugs
Obstructions on floor

Medical

Drop-attacks
Due to cardiovascular disorder
    Postural hypotension
    Arrhythmias (tachy + brady)
    Carotid sinus syndrome
    Aortic stenosis
Due to neurologic disorders
    Epilepsy
    Vertigo
    Parkinsonism
    Hemiplegia
    Motor neuron disease
General weakness
Occult hemorrhage
Iatrogenesis

*Some falls result from both accidental and medical factors.

lapse, result in feelings of postural instability, unsteadiness of gait, or vertigo. Hazell,[12] on the other hand, emphasizes the need for careful evaluation of vestibular function in such cases. The caloric test can give useful information on whether a central or peripheral lesion is involved. It excludes vestibular disease when the result is normal, in which case, one might reasonably attribute symptoms to cervical mechanoreceptor disturbance.

Falls usually occur with walking or running rather than standing. Some attempts to study gait have focused on the reasons why falls occur. Imms and Edholm[13] describe a technique to assess gait and showed some interesting differences between groups of elderly subjects who were either housebound or able to take limited or unlimited activity outdoors. Sudarsky and Ronthal[23] assessed 50 patients (mean age 79.5) who presented with gait disorders. In 56% they were able to reach a single neurologic causal diagnosis. Although efforts to investigate postural sway and gait are new and will improve, data are slowly being accumulated that should lead to developing techniques to reduce sway, improve gait, and prevent falls.

Accidental Falls

By definition accidental falls occur because the individual encounters an environmental hazard. This results in a trip or slip. Such episodes account for almost half of all falls in individuals over the age of 65 years. Clark[6] noted that one fourth of the fractured hips in his subjects occurred purely as a result of accidents that might have been prevented had the environment been satisfactory. Half of his subjects sustained falls that he suspected might have been prevented by careful consideration of both the environment and the nature of the medical factors. Only in the final fourth of his 450 cases did he believe the fall was inevitable.

To avoid accidental falls, the environment in which an old person lives should be clear and uncluttered by small items of furniture situated in awkward positions. Slip rugs and low stools are to be discouraged, but many elderly persons like to have their own belongings around them, and it may take careful counseling from the physician to achieve the desired objective. Even a pet is a risk factor. A second important aspect is light; vision is an integral part of the postural control mechanism, and a dim, dull light with gray, brown, or fawn coloring to walls, carpeting, and furniture makes for a dim environment in which it is hazardous to maneuver.

Stairs are a major hazard, as has been demonstrated by both Sheldon and Clark. Stairs should be clear of all obstructions, be well lit, and, if at all possible, have a bannister on each side. Similar care with furniture and potential obstructions is necessary in both bedroom and bathroom. The provision of a suitable night light to avoid total darkness on attempts to reach the bathroom is also a sensible precaution. Finally, handrails, grab bars, and other similar aids to safe mobility should be placed in strategic positions. When there is concern about the potential danger to a patient of a particular environment, it is helpful to have an occupational therapist study the milieu and advise on appropriate changes.

Medical Falls

It is difficult to know how to describe the second major group of causes of falls. Because medical falls are attributable to a disability or disordered function in the patient, it is appropriate to associate them with the individual. Since they are caused in many cases by potentially treatable conditions, the nonspecific title of medical falls seems appropriate. It is convenient to divide them into four groups: (1) drop attacks, (2) falls due to cardiovascular causes, (3) falls due to neurologic causes, and (4) general causes.

Drop Attacks

There is some debate as to whether a drop attack does indeed constitute a specific type of fall. Such falls have been extensively and carefully described by Kremer,[15] Sheldon,[21] Clark,[6] and others. The drop attack is characterized by its unexpectedness and sudden nature. Sheldon[21] pointed out that

many individuals who have sustained such an episode affirm that they were "at their avocations and feeling in good health at the time." Because of the suddenness of the episode there is no time for the individual to attempt to prevent or break the fall. There is no loss of consciousness, although inevitably there may be a dazed or stunned feeling immediately following the drop to the ground. An 86-year-old woman described by Sheldon was peeling a potato when she suddenly fell and found herself on the floor with a potato in one hand and the knife in the other. A woman, aged 61, was walking to church with a friend on each side when, as she says, she suddenly found herself on the pavement. She records her friends' reaction of surprise as they said, "whatever are you doing down there?"

The second major feature of the drop attack is that many subjects may be totally unable to rise from the ground. Individuals who go to their aid may have great difficulty in helping these persons back to their feet. There appears to be an inert seemingly paralyzed state of the antigravity muscles of limbs and trunk. An intelligent daughter reported that the main difficulty in helping her father, aged 84, back to his feet after such an event was that of lifting his trunk for "he has no strength in the body." Two things appear to be helpful. The first is that there is power retained in the arms and, if the person is able to lay hands on a chair, he may be able to hoist himself back to his feet. The second feature is that pressure exerted on the soles of the feet either by the individual being close to a wall or by a third person appears to restore neurologic integrity and to make it possible to get up again. For a fuller description of drop attacks with several case examples, one or two of which have been quoted previously, the reader is referred to Sheldon's article.[21]

Falls Due to Cardiovascular Causes

Postural hypotension, arrhythmias, carotid sinus syndrome, and aortic stenosis are the four principal causes of syncopal attacks and falls from cardiovascular disturbance.

Although responsible for only 4% of falls in both Sheldon's[21] and Clark's[6] series, *postural hypotension* is an important cause that may be eradicated by successful treatment. The diagnosis is straightforward and a widely recognized complication of the use of antihypertensive medications. It may also be initiated by other drugs such as tricyclic antidepressants, phenothiazines, diuretics, and benzodiazepines, all of which are quite commonly given to elderly patients. What may be less well known is that significant numbers of older people suffer from postural hypotension unrelated to drugs. Twenty-four percent of a group of almost 500 elderly people examined by Caird and co-workers[2] demonstrated a fall in systolic blood pressure of 20 mm Hg or more when moving from the recumbent to erect posture. By age, 16% between 65 and 74 years and 30% over the age of 70 years had such evidence of orthostatic hypotension. These changes in blood pressure were noted when readings were taken 1 minute after adopting the erect posture. More severe degrees of postural hypotension are associated with neurologic conditions such as parkinsonism or peripheral neuropathy. Although the condition is relatively common, it is equally true that many elderly people adjust to it and learn to pause in moving from one posture to another. Those with potential difficulties will complain of dizziness or swimming of their heads when they make such moves.

Arrhythmias include both fast and slow changes in heart rate. On occasion the individual may experience wide variations of heart rate with short periods of tachyarrhythmia and periods of marked bradycardia that may make diagnosis difficult. One such case occurred in an 80-year-old woman who was receiving digoxin because of a known tendency to rapid irregular fibrillation. It was not until she had been studied by 24-hour cardiac monitoring that it was realized that she was also having periods of extreme bradycardia resulting in lethargy, excessive fatigue, and falls. When she had a pacemaker implanted and continued with digoxin therapy, she became asymptomatic.[5]

It has become fashionable to submit any individual with recurrent falls to 24-hour cardiac monitoring.[9] Kirshen and associates,[14] however, found that the value of routine monitoring was limited. Lipsitz[16] has commented that the evaluation of syncopal attacks requires a careful history and physical examination to identify common conditions and physiologic stresses. Laboratory studies have, on the whole, had a low sensitivity and specificity in elderly patients with this complaint and should be ordered selectively.

The carotid sinus syndrome results from apparent oversensitivity of the carotid sinus to stimulation, resulting in an undue slowing of the heart and a syncopal attack. It occurs more commonly in elderly men than women. This fact has been attributed to the effect of wearing firm collars so that movements of the neck may stimulate the carotid sinus to slow the heart and produce the attack. This is not a common type of syncope. In the course of physical examination one can massage the carotid sinus and estimate the sensitivity of the response by measuring the heart rate. On occasions this may result in a fainting attack; this once occurred when I, much to my embarrassment, was examining a colleague's father. To avoid firm neck collars and be careful with neck movements is probably as sound advice as can be given to most sufferers.

Aortic stenosis has been known for many years to precipitate syncope. Ross[19] suggests that this may be the first symptom of the condition and that it is likely caused by a transient arrhythmia or fall in blood pressure during or immediately following exercise.

Neurologic Causes of Falls

Epilepsy is a condition usually associated with younger persons who sustain petit mal or grand mal convulsions. In the elderly, it most commonly occurs following cerebrovascular accidents and hemiplegia. Not infrequently, 1 or 2 years following hemiplegia, Jacksonian seizures may occur stimulated by the scar or cyst left by a preceding thrombosis. Some years ago Fine[8] recorded 40 cases of epileptic syndromes in the elderly that he had personally encountered. Of those, 18, or almost half, followed hemiplegias, 11 were attributed to "generalized cerebral arteriosclerosis" in all of which there were electroencephalographic changes. Five patients had convulsions, and six experienced blackouts only, followed by a period of confusion. This study suggested that for every three post-stroke hemiplegic cases there may well be a fourth in whom seizure activity is not obvious, and the invididual may develop what appear to be syncopal attacks that result in falls. Unfortunately, the electroencephalogram has not proved of much diagnostic value, but recognition of the disorder raises the possibility of using anticonvulsive drugs to prevent further episodes. Clues to the occurrence of this type of latent epilepsy may be the accompaniment of incontinence with the syncopal attack and a period of either mild confusion or lethargy during the postictal phase.

Vertigo is a common complaint of elderly patients who often describe it as dizziness. This is a difficult symptom for clear description: there may be a sensation of spinning round, veering to one side, falling forward or backward, or being fuzzy or "swimmy" in the head. Clues may develop from a carefully taken history, such as onset associated with first getting up from bed or after sudden movements of the neck. Sheldon[20] found that half his subjects in the 1948 survey suffered from vertigo in one form or another, although there was a greater incidence in women than men (60% vs. 40%). He attributed this chiefly to disease of the ear and vestibule, but it is likely that both postural hypotension and deterioration of cervical mechanoreceptor function play a significant role.

Other central nervous conditions that predispose to falls include parkinsonism, because of bradykinesia and a festinating gait; typically, these result in a fall that pitches the victim forward. Hemiplegia and motor neuron disease by creating weakness in one or both lower limbs may also be responsible for a number of falls.

General Causes

Of Sheldon's 1948 sample 12.1% suffered from weakness, which had a higher incidence in women. This situation may arise as a result of continuing reduced activity, rendering the individual progressively weaker. Bortz[1] has written eloquently of the effects of disuse and, unfortunately, many elderly people cease to use their legs as frequently or regularly as they should, resulting in muscles wasting and becoming weaker. One fall, by inducing fear of further similar episodes, may initiate this sequence of events, as may chronic painful musculoskeletal conditions such as osteoarthritis.

A second situation that occurs from time to time is a hidden or latent systemic problem that manifests itself as a fall. A typical example would be an individual who sustains a gastrointestinal hemorrhage, which is not at first obvious, or in whom an anemia has developed over a period of time. Both of these situations can cause weakness or faintness and result in a fall. Such episodes emphasize the need for careful investigation of everyone who falls.

Finally, as in almost any topic related to the elderly, the possibility of an iatrogenic condition should always be considered. Some iatrogenic falls will be mediated by mechanisms already discussed, such as postural hypotension. The high prevalence of iatrogenic disease in the elderly patient makes it wise to emphasize that drugs and associated substances may play a major role in producing unsteadiness of gait and falls. Alcohol is the most widely consumed drug, and overindulgence can quickly cause total loss of postural control. The older individual is less able to metabolize and excrete alcohol. The elderly patient should be warned of this potential danger, and a careful history of alcohol consumption should always be carried out. The 60- to 70-year-old chronic alcoholic is a problem, but the octogenarian who has found some solace in the sherry bottle is perhaps an even greater one because, partly from benign senescent forgetfulness and partly from the instinctive cunning of the addict, the history of consumption may be difficult to elicit.

In North America there is a wide belief in the efficacy of pills. This unfortunate trait leads to many awkward situations, and the only satisfactory method of obtaining full information on what drugs an individual is taking is to have all of the bottles brought to the office or undertake a personal search on a home visit. Psychoneurotic anxiety, depression, or other affective symptoms lead physicians to prescribe psychotropic preparations of one kind and another. Serious difficulties may arise when one individual takes two or three of these drugs. Blunting of judgment and reduced efficacy of postural mechanisms can lead to either accidental or medical falls. No list of general causes, therefore, would be complete without reference to iatrogenesis.

DIAGNOSIS

History

Any elderly person who voluntarily or on questioning admits to falling should have this fact noted and added to the problem list. It is wise to include specific questions because many elderly persons accept falling as one of the penalties brought about by increasing age. In one major study of a large number of elderly referrals to a geriatric department,[4] no specific question was asked about falls and the incidence recorded was just under half that noted by Sheldon, Exton-Smith, and others. It is strongly recommended, therefore, in the assessment of elderly persons that they should be asked when they last fell or if they have fallen during the past few months.

Having established such an occurrence, the second point is to make careful notes of the sequence of events leading up to, during, and following the episode. This will be a time-consuming process but is nonetheless critical if one is to reach a satisfactory explanation for the falls and create a plan to prevent further similar episodes. The ideal is to obtain an eyewitness account from someone who saw the incident. Unfortunately, such witnesses are seldom available. The time of day when the

690   *Falls*

fall occurred will indicate whether rising from bed was a factor that might suggest orthostatic hypotension. Falls in the bathroom may suggest the possibility of micturition or defecation syncope.

Having documented the circumstances of the fall, one can then decide whether it was due to environmental factors and, therefore, an accident or whether it had a medical cause. The next step will be to concentrate questions on obtaining information about cardiovascular and neurologic function. By this means one would hope to obtain evidence pointing to an arrhythmia or gait disturbance, which would require further investigation. Finally, a general review of the health of the individual and of all drugs currently taken should complete this part of the examination.

Physical Examination

A complete careful routine examination is required. Attention will be focused on cardiovascular and neurologic parameters. Blood pressure should be measured both recumbent and either sitting up with the legs dangling for 1 minute or standing to determine whether a postural drop of significance occurs. Some degrees of drop will frequently be encountered, and one should also note any symptoms produced by moving from the recumbent to the erect position. For this to be of value, the individual should obviously have been in the recumbent position for at least 5 to 10 minutes.

Having completed the standard examination, it is important to observe the gait of the individual. Sudarsky and Ronthal[23] examined a series of 50 patients whose age was about 80 years for undiagnosed gait disorders and were able to establish a diagnosis in just over half, as shown in Table 41-2. The features of an essential gait disorder, which these authors described, were short steps, a wide base, and a tendency to be easily displaced backward. The latter can be tested by pressure on the sternum. With this gait, there was no spasticity or cerebellar ataxia and Romberg's test was normal. Many patients also experience difficulty in attempting to walk on a straight line. A useful description of the impaired gait of the elderly has been given by Rodstein.[18]

Investigations

Routine investigations should include a complete blood cell count to establish the presence of anemia or leukocytosis, either of which would suggest

TABLE 41-2   Diagnosis of Gait Disorders in 50 Elderly Patients

Principal Diagnosis	No. (%) of Patients
Myelopathy	8 (16)
Parkinson's disease	5 (10)
Hydrocephalus	2 (4)
Multiple cerebral infarcts	8 (16)
Cerebellar atrophy	4 (8)
Sensory disorders	9 (18)
Essential gait disorder	7 (14)
Other disorders	7 (14)

(Sudarsky L, Ronthal M: Gait disorders among elderly patients. Arch Neurol 40:740–743, 1983)

systemic disease. Latent bleeding or anemia or acute or subacute infection by causing systemic upset may initiate falls. Serum electrolyte studies will be useful: hypokalemia may cause weakness, and either hyponatremia or hypernatremia with dehydration may cause postural hypotension. An electrocardiogram should establish the cardiac rhythm and whether there is evidence of ischemic heart disease that might cause episodes of arrhythmia. If there are grounds for believing that the individual has significant heart disease and the history suggests the possibility of arrhythmias, 24-hour cardiac monitoring should be carried out.

A roentgenogram of the cervical spine in all cases suggestive of drop attacks is useful. Reduction in space between the vertebrae or cervical vertebral collapse causes abnormal stress to cervical apophyseal joints. Most elderly patients will exhibit degenerative change in the cervical spine, but attention to detail in this area is important because of the presence of vital mechanoreceptors. Occasional normal findings can also point elsewhere for the cause of the fall. Hypoglycemia is a potential cause of loss of consciousness and falls and should be borne in mind; Doppler studies of the vessels in the neck are developing in sophistication and value and may indicate whether there is any suggestion of narrowing in the carotid systems that might in turn point to transient ischemic attacks as a possible explanation for a fall. Although epilepsy remains one of the causes to be considered, electroencephalography has proved somewhat unrewarding but could be included as a potential provider of information. Finally, the development of techniques to evaluate the sway pattern of individuals who fall may offer help in the future.

TREATMENT

Falling represents a catastrophic episode to the patient and a clear statement from the physician of his concern and determination to discover the cause if possible is very important. Having completed the examination and investigation of the patient, it is important to describe the result of these to the patient and attempt to allay anxieties and explain, as well as is possible, the cause of the falls.

For accidental falls the important element will be to ensure that the environment in which the individual is living is made as "fall-free" as possible. Suggestions about how to achieve this have already been given.

To manage drop attacks the only positive steps that can be taken at the present time are the use of cervical collars and possibly, in some cases, gentle neck traction. The work of Wyke[24] emphasizes the critical importance of the neck in postural control, and experience suggests that immobilizing the neck may help to prevent drop attacks. The scientific basis for this line of treatment remains somewhat suspect, but I would claim success in more than half the cases in which it has been tried. I should add, however, that if the faithful wearing of an appropriate cervical collar for 1 or 2 months does not prevent episodes, there is no point in continuing to use the collar.

The treatment of falls due to cardiovascular causes will depend on the nature of the cause. Individuals who are liable to tachyarrythmias will require appropriate treatment with digoxin or other antiarrhythmic medication. Those who fall and prove to have a brady- or tachyarrhythmia syndrome will require treatment with antiarrhythmics and with a pacemaker. Sufferers from carotid sinus syndrome must be advised to take care with sudden neck movements but, at the present time, there are no more positive steps that can be taken to control such attacks. Aortic valve disease will require cardiologic advice on whether it is appropriate to take surgical measures. Whether this in turn will prevent falls is a moot point.

When postural hypotension can clearly be attributed to antihypertensive treatment, adjustment of that treatment may be all that is required. If, on the other hand, it is due to autonomic peripheral neuropathy or is associated with failure of baroreceptor mechanisms, it may be necessary to use fludrocortisone and add salt to the diet in an attempt to maintain blood pressure levels when the subject is in the upright position. Usually, fludrocortisone in a dose of 0.1 mg/day given by mouth will have a significant effect on postural hypotension and may be sufficient to prevent symptoms, although it may not completely abolish the condition.

When there is reasonable evidence to suggest the possibility that seizure activity may be responsible for blackouts with falls, the trial of phenytoin or other anticonvulsant medication should be tried. Because a foolproof method of determining the validity of the diagnosis is not available, a therapeutic trial seems the only other alternative. Preventing further falls justifies this rather nonscientific approach; if the use of such medication is effective, the patient will be greatly assisted in maintaining independence and the diagnosis of falls due to epileptiform activity is confirmed.

Vision is of vital importance in maintaining our postural mechanisms as Sheldon and others have demonstrated. There will be occasions when falls may occur because of the uncertainty of an individual's vision. With this or with persistent complaints of vertigo or dizziness, the views of ophthalmologists and otorhinolaryngologists should be sought.

Finally, for all patients and particularly for those in whom general weakness is the cause of the fall, suitable physiotherapeutic programs aimed at strengthening the muscles, particularly of the lower limb and trunk, and improving postural control should be attempted. One must persuade the elderly patient that the only way to increase strength is by using muscles. For too long, the present elderly generation have assumed that, if something is painful, it is best to rest. The message in the future should be that, whatever else happens and however poorly one feels, regular exercise and use of limbs is absolutely imperative.

CONCLUSION

Falling is an important and frequent complication of many illnesses in the elderly and represents one of geriatric medicine's most common and most recalcitrant problems. There are a number of causes for falling. Postural control, which is a function of the central nervous system, becomes less effective in old age; there are obvious risks of accidental falls that can be prevented by appropriate actions; and there are a number of medical factors, many of which can be treated and prevented. The only way of attempting to help patients with a falling problem is to give that problem as much intensity of consideration and investigation as any other. By providing interest, understanding, and an attempted solution to the problem, in many cases its worst features can be alleviated and elderly patients can be helped to remain independent.

REFERENCES

1. Bortz W: Disuse and aging. JAMA 248:1203–1207, 1982
2. Caird FI, Andrews GR, Kennedy RD: Effect of posture on blood pressure in the elderly. Br Heart J 35:527–530, 1973
3. Campbell AJ, Reinken J, Allan BC, Martinez GS: Falls in old age: A study of frequency and related clinical factors. Age Ageing 10:264–270, 1981
4. Cape RDT: A geriatric service. Report to Birmingham, England, Regional Hospital Board, August 1968
5. Cape RDT: Aging: Its Complex Management, pp 119–129. Hagerstown, MD, Harper & Row, 1978
6. Clark ANG: Factors in fracture of the female: Clinical study of the environmental, physical, medical and preventive aspects of injury. Gerontol Clin 10:257–270, 1968
7. Exton-Smith AN: Clinical manifestations. In Exton-Smith AN, Evans JG (eds): Care of the Elderly, pp 41–52. London, Academic Press, 1977
8. Fine W: Epileptic syndromes in the elderly. Gerontol Clin 8:121–133, 1966
9. Gordon M: Occult cardiac arrhythmias associated with falls and dizziness in the elderly: Detention by Holter monitoring. J Am Geriatr Soc 26:418–423, 1978
10. Gryfe CI, Amies A, Ashley MJ: A longitudinal study of falls in an elderly population I incidence and morbidity. Age Ageing 6:201–210, 1977
11. Hasselkus BR, Shambes GM: Aging and postural sway in women. J Gerontol 30:661–667, 1975
12. Hazell JWP: Vestibular problems of balance. Age Ageing 8:258–260, 1979
13. Imms FJ, Edholm OG: The assessment of gait and mobility in the elderly. Age Aging 8:261–267, 1979
14. Kirshen AJ, Cape RDT, Hayes KC, Spencer JD: Postural sway and cardiovascular parameters associated with falls in the elderly. J Clin Exper Gerontol 6:291–307, 1984
15. Kremer M: Sitting, standing and walking. Br Med J 2:121–124, 1958
16. Lipsitz LA: Syncope in the elderly. Ann Intern Med 99:92–105, 1983
17. Overstall PW, Exton-Smith AN, Imms FJ, Johnson AL: Falls in the elderly related to postural imbalance. Br Med J 1:261–264, 1977
18. Rodstein M: Falls by the aged. In Cape RDT, Coe RM, Rossman I (eds): Fundamentals of Geriatric Medicine, pp 109–116. New York, Raven Press, 1983
19. Ross J Jr: Acquired Valvular Heart Disease. In Beeson PB, McDermitt W, Wyngaarden JB (eds): Cecil Textbook of Medicine, 15th ed, pp 1190–1194. Philadelphia, WB Saunders, 1979
20. Sheldon JH: The Social Medicine of Old Age, pp 96–105. London, Oxford University Press, 1948
21. Sheldon JH: On the natural history of falls in old age. Br Med J II:1685–1690, 1960
22. Sheldon JH: The effect of age on the control of sway. Gerontol Clin 5:129–138, 1963
23. Sudarsky L, Ronthal M: Gait disorders among elderly patients. Arch Neurol 40:740–743, 1983
24. Wyke BD: Cervical articular contributions to posture and gait: Their relation to senile disequilibrium. Age Ageing 8:251–258, 1979

42

Sleep Disorders and Sleep Dysfunctions in the Elderly

Charles P. Pollak

The prevalence of sleep problems among the elderly is shown by the disproportionate use of hypnotic/sedative drugs by this population. One study found that of the 62% of the elderly residing in the community who receive prescription drugs daily, 13.6% were receiving sedative-tranquilizers.[19] As many as one half of those over 65 may use sleeping pills "frequently."[31] Of 1,075,800 nursing home residents surveyed in 1973–1974, 34% had received a hypnotic-sedative during the previous week and 48% had received a tranquilizer, with tranquilizers often being prescribed at bedtime.[20]

Complaints about sleep also become more common with increasing age and have been found by survey in 25% to 40% of persons over the age of 60.[5,23] Focused surveys of sleep and its related disorders in the community elderly are underway at several centers. The significance of such disorders goes beyond the elderly subject to the family caretakers, caretaking institutions, and society at large. Sleep disturbances such as night wandering, frequent micturition, and shouting have been cited by the caretakers of elderly patients as the most frequent and least well tolerated of all problems, outranking even (daytime) incontinence and dangerous behavior.[42] The night-time disturbances produce fatigue in the family members[37] and have been cited as the most frequent problems relieved by hospitalization of the elderly family member.[18] Since many disabled elderly who would qualify for institutional care have traditionally been cared for at home, the burden of nocturnal disturbances that disrupt the sleep of family members probably accounts for a sizable (but as yet undetermined) share of family decisions to resort to institutional care, expected to cost 75 billion dollars by 1990.[7]

The Association of Sleep Disorders Centers has published an official nosology of sleep disorders based on major symptom categories:

Disorders of initiating and maintaining sleep (the insomnias)
Disorders of excessive somnolence
Disorders of the sleep-wake schedule
Dysfunctions associated with sleep, sleep stages, or partial arousals (parasomnias)

The nosology includes descriptions of almost every known sleep disorder and can serve as a short textbook.[4] Additional general references will be found at the end of this chapter.

Some of the disorders encompassed by this field are disorders of sleep itself, while others are induced by or confined to the state of sleep. This distinction is heuristically useful and will be used to organize this chapter.

DISORDERS OF SLEEP

In this section, the ways in which sleep—more accurately, the sleep-wake process—can become disordered will be reviewed. In contrast to disorders induced by the state of sleep, which may not be apparent to the patient, disorders of the sleep and waking states are usually upsetting or disabling and may bring the elderly person to the physician's office or, more often, to the pharmacy.

Acute Disorders of Sleep

As a biologic process common to birds and mammals, sleep differs from stupor and coma by being easy to interrupt. Otherwise, the sleeping organism would make easy prey. A wide variety of environmental and internal stimuli cause arousal by stimulating a common mechanism, the reticular activating system, and it is likely that most acute sleep-wake disturbances are caused by the activation of this mechanism. (Acute disturbances of the timing of sleep and wakefulness, represented by jet lag, are an exception.)

Situational Insomnia

Situational insomnia occurs in anticipation of, or in consequence of, an emotionally significant event. It is by definition transient, lasting no longer than about 3 weeks after the event. It is experienced by everyone from time to time and should not be considered a disorder requiring medical attention unless it recurs frequently, occurs in the absence of events with obvious strong meanings, or is severe (total sleeplessness). A form of situational insomnia is frequently recorded in sleep laboratories because of the novelty of the setting to most patients ("first night effect"[1]). It is this type of sleep disturbance that probably motivates most purchases of over-the-counter hypnotics, yet little is known about its prevalence, precipitating factors, duration, and contribution to the development of chronic insomnias.

It is a matter of clinical judgment whether to use hypnotic drugs to manage situational insomnia in elderly patients. Hypnotics provide symptomatic relief at night but can also lead to impairments of alertness, memory, judgment, and coordination the next day or during the night if the patient happens to awaken. It is possible that prompt control of situational sleeplessness can prevent the development of chronic insomnia by preventing the development of anticipatory anxiety and other mechanisms that sustain insomnia; these mechanisms will be discussed in the next section.

The preferred hypnotics are the new, short-acting benzodiazepines such as temazepam and possibly triazolam. They should be given in small trial doses and then raised to an effective and well-tolerated level. Drugs with long half-lives, such as flurazepam, produce round-the-clock effects on the central nervous system and can accumulate when used nightly. Drugs that have abuse potential or produce rapid tolerance and dependency, such as alcohol in any form, barbiturates, methaqualone, glutethimide, and methyprylon should also be avoided. Doses should never be escalated once a satisfactory response has been achieved, even if the response disappears. The total period of administration should not exceed a few weeks;

if sleeping problems persist, an explanation beyond the immediate cause should be searched for.

Virtually all effective hypnotics affect sleep in some way. Barbiturates and alcohol, for example, suppress rapid eye movement sleep and alter the sleep electroencephalogram, while benzodiazepines suppress slow-wave sleep and may increase sleep spindles. It is not known whether such changes in sleep "quality" are of clinical importance, but they do illustrate that sleep is a complex, coordinated set of processes dependent for its initiation and maintenance on an endogenous timing system or biological clock. Sleep cannot be forced. Safe and effective use of hypnotics in the elderly requires that they be administered with a delicate touch.

Bereavement

A special form of insomnia precipitated by a life event is caused by object loss. The elderly are particularly exposed to the death of loved ones, and the resulting bereavement has all the features of major depression, including severe insomnia. Indeed, sleep disturbance ranks second to crying as the most common symptom in bereavement and can remain prominent for 1 year or more.[8]

Medical, Toxic, and Environmental Causes

Any disorder that produces strong afferent stimulation of the reticular activating system may be associated with a symptomatic sleep disturbance. Patients may report pain, paresthesias, pruritus, dyspnea, cough, or strangury. Examination may show fever, alveolar hypoventilation, or other metabolic derangements. To the degree that the causative disease is chronic, the sleep disorder may also be chronic. Medical causes of insomnia, including the effects of many drugs used by the elderly, are presumably more common in the elderly, but not much systematic data are available.[9] Several general reviews are available.[4,15,17,41,47]

Jet Lag

An acute, limited bout of poor sleep is a prominent symptom of "jet lag." It is attributed to the slowness with which the biologic timing system responsible for the sleep-wake rhythm is reset after rapid travel to a new time zone. The role of resetting may be even slower in the elderly, since tolerance of shiftwork (which requires repeated resetting of biological clocks) decreases with age.[14,39]

Chronic Sleep-Wake Disturbances

The diagnosis of persistent insomnia should start with a careful definition of the complaint. The following are the most common and useful categories of presenting complaint:

Difficulty initiating sleep
Difficulty maintaining sleep
Altered quality of sleep
Combinations of the above

Defining the complaint in chronic sleep disorders of patients may be surprisingly difficult and is fraught with pitfalls. One type of patient often regarded as "insomniac" complains of feeling "tired" or "fatigued" in the daytime and infers that sleep must have been disturbed the preceding night. The physician hearing such complaints should not simply accept the patient's explanation but should ask about sleep difficulties directly: "How often do you find it difficult to fall asleep?" "How long does it take to fall asleep?" "How often do you awaken or have difficulty returning to sleep?" If answered vaguely, such questions should lead to other questions that will often relate the dysphoric symptoms to something other than sleep disturbance, such as depression or a medical/surgical illness with systemic manifestations. Significant dysphoric symptoms affect nearly 15% of the elderly.[6]

Incidentally, although patients with dysphoria usually deny prominent sleepiness, sleep apnea should be kept in mind as a diagnostic possibility. A similar pitfall is presented by the patient who complains, "I cannot sleep unless I take. . . ." Unless the clinician inquires into sleep difficulties unrelated to drug withdrawal, as well as the effects of attempts to stop the medication, he may believe with the patient that a medication to which the patient has become tolerant is continuing to exert a beneficial effect.

Even the explicit complaint of difficulty initiating and maintaining sleep should be interpreted with caution, since polygraphic laboratory sleep recordings (polysomnography) often show sleep disturbances that are less severe than reported. Even normal, asymptomatic volunteers awakened directly from polygraphically monitored sleep frequently report that they were awake at the time they were called.[43] This in no way invalidates the patient's complaint, since the patient may be perceiving an internal state that the sleep clinician cannot detect. The pathogenesis of insomnia complaints remains a subject for research.

To see how chronic insomnia arises, one may first consider the same emotional factors important in situational insomnias—anxiety and depression. Recognizable depression is present in over 5% of the elderly,[6] and depressive illnesses are often associated with insomnia, often including a specific constellation of polygraphic sleep abnormalities.[26] It is therefore not surprising that depression can frequently be detected in association with chronic insomnia in the elderly.[40] It is important to consider the diagnostic possibility of depression, since the elderly commonly "mask" the symptoms of depression with somatic concerns, including sleep disturbances.[27] The patient may say, "It is depressing not to be able to sleep." Inappropriate hypnotic drug treatment of insomnia related to depression may produce cognitive defects that are attributed to senile dementia.[48] Whenever underlying depressive illness is suspected in the elderly insomniac, treatment should be aimed against the depression; if the sleep disturbance is related, it should clear as the depression responds to treatment.

Although depression is of special importance in the elderly, new factors also come into the picture that sometimes represent misguided efforts to lessen symptoms and instead are responsible for sustaining the insomnia over long periods of time:

Sleep schedule changes (especially, excessive time in bed)
Hypnotic drug use/dependency
Adverse conditioning

Sleeplessness itself may cause worry, especially if the experiences of a long life have shown a susceptibility to insomnia. In some personalities, the worry about sleep may begin hours before bedtime and mount as the time approaches. Even after falling asleep, a nocturnal awakening may reactivate worries about returning to sleep, turning what would ordinarily have been a brief arousal into a new bout of sleeplessness. Adverse conditioning to the circumstances of sleep may close the circle of sleeplessness, anxiety about sleeplessness, arousal, and further sleeplessness. Such self-reinforcing patterns of sleeplessness can be broken with a hypnotic drug and are an indication for the use of sleeping pills.

Use of a hypnotic should be limited to a few weeks since many if not all hypnotics produce pharmacologic tolerance of their sleep-inducing and sleep-maintaining effects. Once partial or complete drug tolerance has developed, the user may continue to complain of insomnia. Continued symptoms of sleeplessness are, of course, grounds for discontinuing the ineffective hypnotic. It may not be so obvious that the absence of symptoms is also grounds for discontinuation, especially if the drug user complains that efforts to reduce the dose lead to sleeplessness (rebound insomnia). Drug withdrawal by tapering is usually the correct course of action.

Fortunately, the total volume of hypnotics prescribed for the US population decreased during the 1970s,[21] and clinical experience shows that many patients minimize the use of such drugs: they use smaller and less frequent doses than prescribed and rotate drugs on different nights. Drug withdrawal can therefore be carried out safely with few withdrawal symptoms in the unhospitalized patient. After withdrawal, sleep is no worse than when the patient was using the hypnotic (or alcohol), demonstrating to physician and patient that the hypnotic had indeed been ineffective and that the sleep disturbance for which the hypnotic was begun is gone. Such cases show that bouts of sleeplessness triggered by sudden reductions in dosage should be attributed to the withdrawal of the drug (rebound insomnia), not to a recurrent sleep disturbance. In this sense, hypnotic drug dependence can be considered a cause of recurrent insomnia.

As already mentioned, patients who present themselves as "insomniac" because of hypnotic drug dependence should be asked whether they experience difficulty initiating or maintaining sleep or only fear the return of insomnia should the hypnotic be stopped. Tapering of the drug should be considered as an early step in management; it may be the only measure required.

Although not well documented by community-based surveys of sleep practices and patterns, the use of sleep logs has revealed that many elderly patients spend at least as much time in bed as they ever did in their adult lives. The reasons for excessive time in bed include an expectation of "8 hours" of sleep, lack of working hours after retirement, and dysphoria or depression ("I have nothing to get up for"). Nightly total sleep time decreases with age, however, resulting in many unnecessary wakeful hours in bed.[31] The consequences for sleep patterns have not yet been systematically investigated, but it seems likely that the hours of wakefulness become distributed throughout the night-time hours. It is known that the frequency of nocturnal awakenings is greater in the elderly,[31] even under controlled laboratory conditions and isolation from environmental time cues.[46]

By restricting the patient's time in bed, and therefore the opportunity for sleep, the physician can quickly eliminate much of the experience of sleeplessness. The method is as follows. From a home sleep log* kept by the patient for 10 to 14 days, the physician should calculate the average total sleep time and assign a total period in bed that slightly exceeds this average. Exact clock hours for retiring and arising should then be selected to position the sleep period to enable the patient to follow desired evening and morning activities, consistent with the habits of other household members. Some patients do better with an afternoon nap (1 to 2 hours around 3 PM), but the night-time period in bed should then be reduced accordingly. Regular hours of sleep should also be encouraged to avoid resettings of the biological clock, especially on weekends, that might increase sleeplessness.

Another age-related change in sleep-wake pattern is a tendency to fall asleep earlier and wake up earlier (phase advance). This may be related to shortening of the length of sleep-wake and other cycles observed when elderly subjects are isolated from external time cues. Indeed, insomnia patterns analogous to those observed in the elderly have been produced in our laboratory by placing young normal subjects on scheduled sleep-wake cycles that are longer than 24 hours.[13]

Along with fragmented nocturnal sleep, an increase in daytime napping has been described in the elderly.[29] It has been proposed that the shift from a circadian (about 24 hour) rhythm of sleep and wakefulness to a pattern of multiple daily naps and waking episodes may be caused by neuronal aging of the circadian timing systems of the brain.[45] In support of this idea, patients with Alzheimer's disease show a greater degree of sleep fragmentation and napping than normals of similar age.[36] The institutionalized demented elderly often display confusion, hallucinations, agitation, and wandering during the night. This has been referred to as "sundowning."[35,38] Some nursing home residents are probably confused and agitated at night because the physical and social stimuli that normally maintain alertness and orientation are reduced. The waning effects of hypnotic/sedative drugs taken at the institution's "bedtime" may sometimes contribute to such problems.[45] It is likely that some "abnormal" nocturnal behaviors are virtually the same behaviors as those considered normal in the daytime. Disturbances of the

*Available from Metrodesign Associates, 81 S. Main St, Homer, NY 13077.

circadian sleep-wake pattern have simply translated these behaviors into the night, when staff is less likely to tolerate them.

Disturbed circadian sleep-wake patterns may be found in other neurologic diseases. Patients with Parkinson's disease may have episodes of nocturnal rigidity with difficulty changing position in bed. This can sometimes be controlled by levodopa taken at bedtime or during the night,[45] but other patients appear to have lost a circadian sleep-wake pattern: sleep and waking episodes are scattered throughout the 24-hour day without any visible pattern. A similar loss of circadian pattern was reported in a patient with progressive supranuclear palsy.[44] Total sleep time over 24-hour periods was normal.

It often seems to the caretakers of such patients that day and night have become "reversed": the patient sleeps by day and wakes by night, but true inversion of the sleep-wake cycle is probably less common than a breakdown of the circadian pattern by fragmentation of nocturnal sleep plus daytime napping. It is likely that institutional living is often deficient in the time cues normally supplied by light of outdoor intensity, occupational demands, and social stimulation, while sensory and cognitive defects reduce the effectiveness of those timing cues that are available. As a result, the institutionalized elderly may develop non-24-hour sleep-wake periodicities similar to the free running rhythms produced in laboratories from which environmental time cues have been eliminated[3] or as found in occasional persons living in society.[25,32]

The management of such problems should include the use of consistent, firm but not harsh synchronizing events (*e.g.,* getting undressed for bed, lying down and turning the lights down at a regular clock hour). Bedtime and waketime should have a 24-hour pattern. For patients with a strongly fragmented sleep-wake pattern, however, the time in bed at night should be short and should be supplemented by one or more daytime naps. Although such multiphasic routines place additional demands on the staff, they reduce the prolonged periods of nocturnal wakefulness that can disorient the patient and can cause angry reactions from the caretakers.

Dysfunctions Associated With Sleep (Parasomnias)

In this section several common physiologic disturbances induced by the state of sleep will be discussed. That such disturbances exist at all is remarkable and has only been known since the discovery of sleep apnea in 1965.[16,22] It has been observed that scarcely any functions remain unchanged during sleep and that virtually a new branch of internal medicine is needed for sleep in parallel to the medicine of wakefulness, for it is during wakefulness that nearly all medical diagnostic procedures are currently performed.

Of the many dysfunctions induced or worsened by sleep, several increase with age: sleep apnea, restless legs syndrome, periodic movements in sleep, sleep-related cardiovascular symptoms caused by congestive heart failure such as paroxysmal nocturnal dyspnea and orthopnea, nocturnal agnina, and perhaps certain cardiac arrhythmias. A few of these will be discussed.

Sleep Apnea

The term *sleep apnea* refers to an abnormal event—marked reduction or cessation of air flow during sleep. The event generally lasts from 20 to 40 seconds. It is caused by varying combinations of reduced central respiratory drive and functional obstruction of air flow at the pharynx. Each event is terminated by arousal. In obstructive cases, loud snoring may be heard as air flow resumes.

Sleep apnea increases with age but may be clinically inapparent in the elderly. Recent home recordings of breathing during sleep have revealed sleep apnea in 28% of a representative sample of community elderly. Half of the cases were obstructive. A higher frequency of apneas was associated with more reports of global depression and nocturnal confusion or wandering at night.[2] Additional health implications of asymptomatic sleep apnea are suggested by two independent studies demonstrating more frequent hypertension in individuals with multiple symptoms of obstructive sleep apnea, especially loud snoring.[30,33]

Most cases of sleep apnea appear to be mild. In the most severe cases, the apnea events are sequential and there may be no sleep that is free of apnea. When obstructive sleep apnea produces symptoms, they often include daytime sleepiness. This is not surprising, considering that partial arousal is necessary to terminate each of hundreds of nightly episodes of apnea. The sleepiness may be of disabling severity. Some apneics complain of insomnia as well. The spouses of apneics should be questioned, since they are likely to be aware of loud snoring, episodes of shallow breathing or struggling (asphyxia), or such nocturnal signs of sleep apnea as profuse sleeptalking, sleepwalking, or sleeping in odd positions.

Symptomatic obstructive sleep apnea (the hypersomnia–sleep apnea syndrome) is mainly a disease of middle-aged males. Its prevalence parallels that of snoring, which increases from childhood to the 50s and 60s and may decrease afterward. If the decrease is caused by selective mortality, elderly males can be regarded as survivors of the disease process associated with snoring and apneas during sleep. Postmenopausal females, however, may also develop the disorder.

Chronic daytime sleepiness is most often caused by sleep apnea,[9] but drug toxicity should always be considered. Other less common causes of chronic sleepiness in the elderly are sleep schedule disturbances, lifelong narcolepsy, and medical disorders.

Obstructive sleep apnea may be position dependent (it is usually worse in the supine position) and may therefore come and go throughout the night. This, plus a tendency for sleep apnea to increase later in the night,[28] makes it necessary to record the sleep and breathing pattern for at least one full night to assess the presence and the severity of sleep apnea. Numerous treatment options for sleep apnea are now available. They include permanent tracheostomy, uvulopalatopharyngoplasty, mandibular lengthening operations, nasal positive airway pressure, nocturnal oxygen, medroxyprogesterone, weight loss, and nonintervention.

A prudent choice of management depends on an accurate assessment of the severity of the condition, its potential for causing behavioral or cardiovascular consequences, and the psychosocial background of the patient. Measures of severity include the type, number, and duration of apneas; the degree of oxyhemoglobin desaturation; and the frequency and type of associated cardiac arrhythmias. The crucial consequences of sleep apnea are daytime sleepiness and other behavioral changes such as irritability and depression, as well as progressive pulmonary hypertension and its cardiovascular effects. Important psychosocial considerations in selecting treatment include the effects of sleepiness and irritability on the patient's occupation, family, and ability to drive safely; likelihood of losing weight if obese; and capacity to cooperate with treatment.

When mild, sleep apnea may be of little further concern. Otherwise, polysomnograms should be repeated several times a year, along with reassessments of daytime sleepiness and general health. Patients should be informed that respiratory depressants and central nervous system depressants in general may increase the severity of sleep apnea. Alcohol should therefore be avoided close to bed-

time, as should most hypnotics. Benzodiazepines, however, in small doses and in absence of other drugs with which they may interact, can be safe.[34] If general anesthesia is required, the responsible surgeon and anesthesiologist should be aware that hypoventilation or apnea may develop during the postoperative period, especially during the night when vigilance in the recovery room may be at its low point. Treatment consists of arousing and ventilating the patient with air (not oxygen, which can depress respiratory drive further).

Restless Legs Syndrome and Periodic Movements in Sleep

The restless legs syndrome (RLS) is a chronic neurologic disorder that is more frequent and severe in older age-groups. The symptoms develop when the patient is sitting or lying down and may be especially severe while trying to fall asleep at night. Sufferers describe odd creeping, crawling sensations in the legs or arms, together with an irresistible urge to move.[12] Sufferers pace the floor rapidly, stomp their feet, or massage their legs until relief is obtained. The relief is only temporary, however, and the sensations return when a new attempt is made to fall asleep. Fortunately, the condition is often episodic, with asymptomatic intervals of weeks to months or longer.

Once sleep is initiated, periodic movements usually develop in the legs and occasionally in the arms. The movements may easily be recorded polygraphically with surface electromyogram electrodes over the anterior tibialis or other muscles. They are highly periodic and take the form of partial or full triple flexion withdrawals. Although each movement is often associated with a brief electroencephalographic arousal, there is no specific association with insomnia or other sleep disorder.[10] Indeed, periodic movements in sleep may be totally asymptomatic. Occasionally, the spouse complains of being kicked in bed.

Like RLS, periodic movements in sleep are more common in older patients. No reliable treatment is available. There may be benefit from mild opioids such as propoxyphene (Darvon).[24]

REFERENCES

1. Agnew HW, Webb WB, Williams RL: The first night effect: An EEG study of sleep. Psychophysiology 2:263–266, 1966
2. Ancoli-Israel S, Kripke DF, Mason WJ: Obstructive sleep apnea in a senior population. Sleep Res 13:130, 1984

3. Aschoff J: Circadian systems in man and their implications. Hosp Pract 11:51, 1976
4. Association of Sleep Disorders Centers and the Association for the Psychophysiological Study of Sleep: Diagnostic classification of sleep and arousal disorders. Sleep 2:1–137,, 1979
5. Bixler E, Kales A, Soldatos C et al: Prevalence of sleep disorders in the Los Angeles metropolitan area. Am J Psychiatry 136:1257, 1979
6. Blazer D, Williams CD: Epidemiology of dysphoria and depression in an elderly population. Am J Psychiatry 137:439–444, 1980
7. Butler RN: The Medicine of the Future—Geriatrics. Presented at the 33rd Annual Meeting of the Gerontological Society, Joseph T. Freeman Lecture, 1980; Quoted by Besdine RW: Health and illness behavior in the elderly. In Health, Behavior and Aging, Institute of Medicine, National Academy Press, 1981
8. Clayton PJ: Bereavement. In Paykel ES (ed): Handbook of Affective Disorders, pp 403–415. New York, Guilford Press, 1982
9. Coleman RM, Miles LE, Guilleminault CC, Zarcone VP, van den Hoed J, Dement WC: Sleep-wake disorders in the elderly: A polysomnographic analysis. J Am Geriatr Soc 29:289–296, 1981
10. Coleman R, Pollak C, Weitzman E: Periodic movements in sleep (nocturnal myoclonus): A case series analysis. Ann Neurol 8:416–421, 1979
11. Deleted.
12. Ekbom RA: Restless legs syndrome. Neurology 10:868–873, 1960
13. Fookson JE, Kronauer RE, Weitzman ED, Monk TH, Moline ML, Hoey E: Induction of insomnia on non-24 Hour sleep-wake schedules. Sleep Research 13:220, 1984
14. Foret J, Bensimon G, Benoit O, Vieux N: Quality of sleep as a function of age and shift work. In Reinberg A, Vieux N, Andlauer P (eds): Night and Shift Work: Biological and Social Aspects, pp 149–160. Oxford, Pergamon Press, 1981
15. Freemon FR: Sleep in patients with organic disease of the nervous system. In Williams RL, Karacan I (eds): Sleep Disorders: Diagnosis and Treatment, pp 261–283. New York, John Wiley & Sons, 1978
16. Gastaut H, Tassinari C, Duron B: Etude polygraphique des manifestations épisodiques (hypniques et respiratoires) du syndrome de pickwick. Rev Neurol 112:568–579, 1965
17. Gerard P, Collins K, Dore C, Exton-Smith A: Subject characteristics of sleep in the elderly. Age Ageing 7(suppl):55–63, 1978
18. Grad J, Sainsbury P: Mental illness and the family. Lancet 1:544–547, 1963
19. Guttman D: A survey of drug-taking behavior of the elderly. In Services Research Report, National Institute on Drug Abuse, 1977; Cited in Institute of Medicine: Sleeping Pills, Insomnia, and Medical Practice. Washington, DC, National Academy of Sciences, 1979
20. Hing, E: Characteristics of Nursing Home Residents, Health Status, and Care Received: National Nursing Home Survey. Vital and Health Statistics: Series 13, Data from the National Health Survey, No. 51. Department of Health and Human Services, publication No. (PHS) 81-1712
21. Institute of Medicine. Report of a Study: Sleeping Pills, Insomnia, and Medical Practice. Washington, DC, National Academy of Sciences, 1979
22. Jung R, Kuhlo W: Neurophysiological studies of abnormal night sleep and the pickwickian syndrome. Prog Brain Res 18:140–159, 1965
23. Karacan I, Thornby J, Anch M et al: Prevalence of sleep disturbance in primarily urban Florida County. Soc Sci Med 10:239, 1976
24. Kavey: Personal communication
25. Kokkoris C, Weitzman E, Pollak C et al: Long-term ambulatory temperature monitoring in a subject with a hypernychthemeral sleep-wake disturbance. Sleep 1:177, 1978
26. Kupfer DJ, Foster FG, Coble P, McPartland RJ, Ulrich RF: The application of EEG sleep for the differential diagnosis of affective disorders. Am J Psychiatry 135:69, 1978
27. Lassler LB, Gauiria M: Depression in old age. J Am Geriatr Soc 26:471–475, 1978
28. Deleted.
29. Lewis S: Sleep patterns during afternoon naps in the young and elderly. Br J Psychiatry 115:107, 1969
30. Lugaresi E, Coccagna G, Cirignotta F: Snoring and its clinical implications. In Guilleminault C, Dement W (eds): Sleep Apnea Syndromes, p 13. New York, Alan R Liss, 1978
31. Miles LE, Dement WC: Sleep and aging. Sleep 3:119–220, 1980
32. Miles LM, Raynal DM, Wilson MA: Blind man living in normal society has circadian rhythms of 24.9 hours. Science 198:421–423, 1977
33. Pollak CP, Bradlow HC, Spielman AJ, Weitzman ED: A pilot survey of the symptoms of hypersomnia-sleep apnea syndrome as possible risk factors for hypertension. Sleep Res 8:210, 1980
34. Pollak CP, Pressman MR, Appel D, Spielman AJ, Chervin RD, Weitzman ED: Sleep apnea in elderly insomniacs and effects of flurazepam. Sleep Res 10:222, 1981
35. Prinz P, Raskind M: Aging and sleep disorders. In Williams R, Karacan I (eds): Sleep Disorders: Diagnosis and Treatment, pp 303–321. New York, John Wiley & Sons, 1978
36. Prinz PN et al: Changes in the sleep and waking EEGs of nondemented and demented elderly subjects. J Am Geriatr Soc 30:86–93, 1982
37. Rabins RV, Mace NL, Lucas MJ: The impact of dementia on the family. JAMA 248:333–335, 1982
38. Raskind M, Eisdorfer C: When elderly patients can't sleep. Drug Ther 7:44, 1977
39. Reinberg A, Andlauer P, Guillet P et al: Oral temperature, circadian rhythm amplitude, aging, and tolerance to shiftwork. Ergonomics 23:55–64, 1980

40. Reynolds CF, Coble PA, Black RS, Holzer B, Carroll R, Kupfer DJ: Sleep disturbances in a series of elderly patients: Polysomnographic findings. J Am Geriatr Soc 28:164–170, 1980
41. Roehrs T, Zorick F, Roth T: Sleep Disorders in the Elderly. Geriatr Med Today 3:6:76–86, 1984
42. Sanford JRA: Tolerance of debility in elderly dependents by supports at home: Its significance for hospital practice. Br Med J 3:471–473, 1975
43. Sewitch DE, Pollak CP, Weitzman ED, Antrobus JS, Clark WC: Sleep-wake perception in normal sleep. Sleep Res 11:95, 1982
44. Wagner DR, Pollak CP, Moline ML, Fookson JE, Monk TH: Sleep in progressive supranuclear palsy. Sleep Res 13:184, 1984
45. Weitzman ED: Sleep and aging. In Katzman R (ed): Neurology of Aging, pp 167–188. Philadelphia, FA Davis, 1983
46. Weitzman ED, Moline ML, Czeisler CA, Zimmerman JC: Chronobiology of aging: Temperature, sleep-wake rhythms and entrainment. Neurobiol Aging 3:299–309, 1982
47. Williams RL: Sleep disturbances in various medical and surgical conditions. In Williams RL, Karacan I (eds): Sleep Disorders: Diagnosis and Treatment, pp 285–301. New York, John Wiley & Sons, 1978
48. Williamson J: Depression in the elderly. Age Aging 7(suppl):35–40, 1978

BIBLIOGRAPHY

Association of Sleep Disorders Centers and the Association for the Psychophysiological Study of Sleep: Diagnostic classification of sleep and arousal disorders. Sleep 2:1–137, 1979

Guilleminault C (ed): Sleep and Waking Disorders: Indications and Techniques. Menlo Park, CA, Addison-Wesley, 1982

Miles LE, Dement WC: Sleep and aging. Sleep 3:119–220, 1980

Mendelson W: The Use and Misuse of Sleeping Pills. New York, Plenum Press, 1978

Wagner DR, Weitzman ED: Sleep and arousal disorders. In Rosenberg R (ed): The Clinical Neurosciences. New York, Churchill-Livingstone, 1983

Weitzman ED: Sleep and aging. In Katzman R (ed): Neurology of Aging, pp 167–188. Philadelphia, FA Davis, 1983

Williams RL, Karacan I (eds): Sleep Disorders Diagnosis and Treatment. New York, John Wiley & Sons, 1978

43 Urinary Incontinence

Mark E. Williams

Urinary incontinence is the involuntary loss of sufficient quantities of urine to produce a social or hygienic problem. Clinically significant urinary incontinence is probably present in 5% to 10% of older persons living in the community.[21,31] In the institutional setting the prevalence may approach 50%.[15,21] The prevalence of urinary incontinence increases with physical disability, neurologic disease, gynecologic and urologic surgery, hospital admission, and use of medication. No convincing associations have been demonstrated between incontinence and sex, increasing age, or urinary tract infection.

NEUROLOGIC CONTROL OF MICTURITION

The central nervous system interactions with the bladder, urethral sphincters, and pelvic floor muscles have been organized into four loops.[2] Loop I allows modulation of the primary reflex arc (loop II) through cortical, thalamic, and cerebellar inputs. The primary reflex arc, loop II, is composed of sensory nerves that travel from the bladder to the brain stem and corresponding motor neurons that originate in the brain stem and descend through the spinal cord to the sacral spinal pudendal motor nucleus and then to the bladder. Loop III allows passive relaxation of the pelvic floor muscles during bladder filling, while loop IV provides volitional control over the pelvic floor musculature and the external urethral sphincters. These loops communicate the bladder volume to the brain, modulate the reflex arc, and coordinate relaxation of the pelvic muscles to permit room for the bladder to fill. When the bladder becomes distended, detrusor contractions develop (loop II), which must be inhibited (loop I) to avoid abrupt

bladder emptying. As the bladder fills, the pelvic muscles relax (loop III) and a person becomes aware of the urge to void (probably loop IV).

The identification and localization of adrenergic and cholinergic neuroreceptors within the bladder and urethra have increased our understanding of lower urinary tract function and form the basis of pharmacologic therapy.[3,17,25] α-Adrenergic receptors, abundant in the bladder outlet and along the urethra, increase urethral resistance when they are stimulated. β-Adrenergic receptors, predominant in the body and dome of the bladder, produce detrusor relaxation. Stimulation of cholinergic neuroreceptors, located throughout the bladder and urethra, cause detrusor contractions. Because of this arrangement of adrenergic and cholinergic receptors, bladder filling can be viewed as a sympathetic nervous system activity, producing increased urethral resistance and allowing relaxation of the bladder, while voiding is essentially a parasympathetic activity by mediating bladder contractions and inhibiting sympathetic activity.

NORMAL PHYSIOLOGY

To maintain urinary continence, the pressure within the bladder must remain below intraurethral pressure. Intravesicular pressure is influenced by intra-abdominal pressure, the amount of urine contained in the bladder, and the contractile state of the detrusor muscle.[18,26] Detrusor tone is augmented by cholinergic stimulation, β-adrenergic inhibition, increased afferent stimulation, and decreased central nervous system activity. Factors diminishing detrusor tone include cholinergic inhibition, muscle relaxants, and decreased afferent stimulation.

Bladder outlet and urethral resistance are related to the smooth muscle tone of the urethra and bladder neck, the urethral mucosal thickness, and the maintenance of the posterior urethrovesical angle.[1,12,28] The external urethral sphincter (which allows voluntary cessation of urine flow) is not necessary for continence. Factors that increase smooth muscle tone and bladder outlet resistance include prostatic hypertrophy and α-sympathetic stimulation. Smooth muscle contractions are diminished by α-sympathetic blockade, muscle relaxants (such as diazepam), and postsurgical manipulation of the pelvis, bladder, or urethra. Thickness of the urethral mucosa in women is maintained by estrogens and appreciably thins in estrogen deficiency. Finally, distortion of the posterior urethrovesical angle (normally 90° to 100°) produced by bladder prolapse, masses surgery, or other conditions can reduce bladder outlet resistance by decreasing the sphincter's mechanical advantage.

PATHOPHYSIOLOGY

Regardless of the precipitating cause, bladder pressure sufficient to overcome sphincter resistance is the sine qua non of urinary incontinence. The disproportion between bladder pressure and sphincter competence can be classified as follows:[30] detrusor instability refers to bladder contractions of sufficient magnitude to overcome urethral resistance. Overflow incontinence, when urine flow occurs only at very high bladder volumes, results from either a diminution of bladder tone or an elevation of sphincter resistance. Sphincter weakness or stress incontinence occurs when bladder outlet resistance is reduced. Functional incontinence refers to urologically normal individuals (frequently with compromised mobility) who cannot or will not reach the toilet in time to avoid an accident. Finally, iatrogenic incontinence describes incontinence resulting from medications, physical restraints, or other factors controlled by physicians. The clinical characteristics of these pathophysiologic categories are outlined in Table 43-1.

DIAGNOSTIC APPROACH

The rationale for the clinical evaluation of incontinent persons is to document the problem, identify individuals who require immediate urodynamic investigation, and classify the disproportion between bladder pressure and sphincter resistance.

Those individuals who cannot be classified may be empirically treated for detrusor instability, reserving urodynamic studies for persons who do not respond to initial treatment.

No data are available to address the sensitivity, specificity, or predictive value of the various components of the clinical evaluation.[29] The problem of false-positive tests is particularly poignant in urodynamic studies in which continent individuals (especially elderly women) may show significant abnormalities, usually associated with incontinence.[4]

Documentation of urinary incontinence is most easily accomplished by having the patient or caregiver keep an incontinence chart. The chart records observations made every 2 hours as to whether the person is wet or dry and any associated symptoms or circumstances. By obtaining this record over 48 to 72 hours, the number and timing of urinary accidents can be observed. The voiding pattern can be diagnostically important. For example, incontinence following the ingestion of potent diuretics suggests iatrogenic incontinence. Although uncommon, some individuals will be completely continent when the chart is maintained.[8,14] Knowledge of the voiding pattern can assist bladder retraining programs. Because successful bladder training often depends on estimating when the bladder is full, the incontinence chart provides a useful way to determine bladder status and thus to devise an effective training schedule and to modify staffing schedules.[11]

The medical history is usually insufficient to discriminate various pathophysiologic conditions because urinary complaints are common in older persons and symptoms are generally nonspecific. [5,14] Small volume urine loss uniquely associated with increases in intra-abdominal pressure strongly suggests stress incontinence.[7,10] Individuals with a history of recent pelvic or urologic surgery should undergo urodynamic evaluation because multiple pathophysiologic mechanisms may exist. Finally, a comprehensive review of all a patient's medications is especially important. Behavioral problems uncovered during the history may be causal or may have resulted from the stresses produced by incontinence.

The goal of the physical examination is to identify causes precipitating incontinence and to help establish the urinary pathophysiology. Estrogen deficiency, fecal impaction, neoplasia, prostatic hypertrophy, and cystitis represent potential causative factors to be explored on examination. A few clinical signs are related to specific pathophysiologic abnormalities. For example, palpable fun-

TABLE 43-1 Clinical Features of Specific Urinary Pathophysiology

Category	Mechanism	Cause	Clinical Findings
Detrusor instability	Uninhibited detrusor contractions sufficient to overcome urethral resistance	Defects in CNS inhibition (loop I) Hyperexcitability of afferent pathways (loop II) Deconditioned micturition reflexes	Most common type (up to 70%) No characteristic features on history or physical examination More common in the setting of neurologic disease Characteristic urodynamic findings, but the specificity of these findings is unknown
Overflow incontinence	Intravesicular pressure cannot exceed intra-urethral pressure	Bladder outlet obstruction Destrusor inadequacy Impaired afferent sensation	Palpable or percussable bladder after voiding (highly specific) Postvoid bladder residual greater than 50 ml Urine flow rate less than 15 ml/sec Characteristic urodynamic profile
Sphincter insufficiency	Intraurethral pressure falls below intravesicular pressure	Inadequate estrogen to maintain urethral mucosa in women Weakness of pelvic and urethral muscles Urinary infections	History of urine loss only after situations that abruptly increase abdominal pressure Previous pelvic or urologic surgery Atrophic vaginitis on pelvic examination Demonstrable urine loss on provocative testing Urodynamic findings are usually normal
Functional incontinence	Inability to reach toilet in time	Impaired mobility, inconvenient facilities, inflexible staff schedules Psychological factors	Unfamiliar surroundings or lack of convenient toileting facilities History of accidents on the way to the bathroom Musculoskeletal limitations often present Urodynamic studies usually normal
Iatrogenic incontinence	Multiple mechanisms including loss of awareness to bladder cues; decreased bladder or sphincter tone; inability to reach toilet in time	Various drugs, especially diuretics, sedatives, and autonomic nervous system agents Physical restraints	History of polypharmacy Presence of physical restraints

neling of the bladder neck suggests stress inconti-nence,[27] while a palpable bladder identifies overflow incontinence.[14] The presence of severe musculoskeletal disability or physical restraints should alert the clinician to functional or iatro-genic incontinence. Finally, signs of central ner-vous system disease should prompt a comprehen-sive neurologic evaluation.

Signs of uterine prolapse, cystoceles, and atrophic vaginitis should be pursued on pelvic ex-amination. Atrophic vaginitis is suggested by vul-val and vaginal atrophy, reddened mucosa, and a scant watery discharge. A mucosal smear showing intermediate and parabasal epithelial cells con-firms the diagnosis. As previously mentioned, stress incontinence is suggested by palpable fun-neling of the bladder outlet demonstrated on pel-vic examination. If two fingers placed along the urethra to restore the posterior urethrovesical an-gle can stop the incontinence, then a favorable response to surgery can be anticipated.[12]

A careful functional evaluation complements other health observations and frequently uncovers conditions predisposing to incontinence. Gener-ally, the evaluation includes mobility testing, quantifying the time and effort an individual must expend to toilet successfully, and observing the patient's ability to overcome any physical con-straints such as doors or stairs that interfere with toilet use. Complete evaluation of these environ-mental factors may require a home visit by a pro-fessional.

Routine laboratory studies should include uri-nalysis, serum electrolytes, and tests for urea ni-trogen, glucose, and calcium levels to exclude polyuric syndromes. An abnormal urinalysis sug-gests local disease and further evaluation is war-ranted. Bladder catheterization immediately fol-lowing urination is a recommended procedure to determine residual urine volume. Residual vol-umes greater than 50 ml are abnormal and may indicate obstruction or an adynamic detrusor. Urine flow studies, especially useful in evaluating elderly men, are easy to perform and require min-imal equipment. Peak flow rates less than 15 ml/sec imply bladder outlet obstruction or detrusor inadequacy.[14,19] False-negative tests can occur be-cause some patients can artificially increase blad-der pressure by contracting their abdominal mus-cles.

The specific contribution of urodynamic studies and their place in the evaluation of urinary incon-tinence remains undefined. Although widely rec-ommended, little evidence exists regarding the in-dications, sensitivity, specificity, and predictive value of urodynamic studies, especially in elderly persons. Many continent older persons exhibit di-agnostic abnormalities on urodynamic testing; conversely some incontinent persons have normal studies. Furthermore, many urodynamic proce-dures introduce artifacts such as lack of privacy, unnatural voiding positions, or uncomfortable re-cording equipment. The magnitude of these arti-facts and their clinical implications (if any) remain to be established.

Professional experience in geriatric inconti-nence clinics and urodynamic studies in the elderly have been published only recently. Unfortunately, most reports have limited value for physicians be-cause they describe highly selected patient sub-groups referred because of treatment failure. No reports have documented an increased effective-ness of urodynamic studies over traditional clinical evaluation. One investigator retrospectively devel-oped an algorithm to identify elderly women un-likely to benefit from urodynamic studies.[14] Deci-sion rules could correctly classify most of the 100 patients according to urodynamic diagnosis by us-ing historical and physical examination informa-tion. Findings pathognomonic of urinary patho-physiology were seen in 15% of the sample, and 46% of the population could have been treated empirically for detrusor instability. Only 39% would have required cystometric studies to con-firm a specific diagnosis.

The role of urodynamic studies in elderly men is more controversial. Incontinent men usually have detrusor instability from detectable condi-tions: incontinence following surgery, or overflow incontinence detectable on physical examination or with urine flow studies.[13,22,24] Stress inconti-nence in men is uncommon; even after urologic surgery, most of these individuals have detrusor instability.[20] Men with abnormal urinalysis, large prostates, palpable bladders, or postoperative con-ditions generally require urodynamic and/or cys-toscopic evaluation. Patients not exhibiting these findings usually have detrusor instability and may be candidates for empiric treatment, reserving uro-dynamic studies for treatment failures.

The performance of urodynamic studies in the elderly presents a number of unique difficulties. Coexistent physical and mental limitations may compromise an elderly person's ability to tolerate the rigors of a full urodynamic evaluation. Com-plete cooperation with urodynamic studies may be impossible for some individuals without increasing the attendant risk of the procedure. Given the number of affected older people, the costs of com-plete urologic evaluation, and the small but unavoidable risk of invasive studies, the definition of elderly patient subgroups most likely to benefit from urodynamic evaluation remains an important clinical challenge.

TREATMENT

Most ambulatory patients can expect complete resolution of incontinence with optimal management. Consequently, an optimistic and supportive outlook is appropriate. An accurate determination of the urinary pathophysiology greatly increases the likelihood of successful treatment. The specific treatment goals and therapeutic options for each pathophysiologic classification are outlined in Table 43-2. There are no age-specific strategies; but in older persons, it is particularly important to look for iatrogenic causes and occult urinary tract infection. Approximately 30% of incontinent older

persons experience spontaneous recovery within a few weeks.[15]

Behavioral treatments are useful adjuncts to any pharmacologic regimen. Most strategies are predicted on a knowledge of the incontinence pattern. Regular checks every 2 hours recorded on incontinence charts can help define the patient's pattern of urinary accidents. Once the incontinence pattern is identified, the daily schedule can be altered to allow toilet use at a time when the bladder is most likely to be full. Bladder retraining requires establishing a micturition schedule and then increasing the voiding interval by having the patient consciously delay urinating. Several studies using either prospective cohorts or randomized controls have reported improvement or cure in 50% to 70% or women using this technique.[9,11,16,23]

Palliative measures such as absorbent pads or indwelling catheters are appropriate only for tem-

TABLE 43-2   Initial Treatment Approaches for Specific Types of Urinary Incontinence

Category	Therapeutic Goal	Therapeutic Options	Comments*
Detrusor instability	Block detrusor contractions; increase bladder capacity; reduce symptoms of urgency; increase confidence and self-esteem	Behavior therapy *plus* anticholinergic agents *or* calcium channel blockers *or* antispasmodic agents	Behavioral therapy *plus* imipramine, 25 mg qhs *or* oxybutynin, 5 mg tid
Overflow incontinence	Provide complete bladder drainage	Surgical intervention; pharmacologic agents; intermittent catheterization	Depends on the cause of the overflow incontinence
Sphincter weakness	Increase urethral resistance	Pelvic exercises; estrogen replacement; α-sympathetic agonists; surgical intervention	Estrogens in post-menopausal women *plus* phenylpropanolamine, 25 mg bid, *or* imipramine, 25 mg qhs
Functional incontinence	Minimize obstacles to expeditious voiding	Environmental modification; improving mobility; resolving psychological difficulties; modifying staffing schedules; minimizing unpleasant conditions	Requires an individualized approach
Iatrogenic incontinence	Reduce physician-controlled factors	Modify medications; minimize use of physical restraints; effectively treat underlying illnesses	Requires an individualized approach

Note: bid = twice a day; qhs = at bedtime; tid = three times a day.
* Initial oral doses of medications are given. Higher doses are frequently required and must be titrated to the clinical response and side-effects. Treatment recommendations are rapidly changing, and these options are provided only for basic guidelines and not definitive therapy.

porary control or as last resort options. These measures must be socially acceptable (*i.e.*, must control the urinous smell while not being excessively bulky under the clothing) and must keep the patient dry. Strategies meeting these requirements are the use of rubber or plastic pants with absorbent pads or superabsorbent chemicals (such as carboxymethyl cellulose), intermittent self-catheterization discussed above, or collection devices. Again, it must be emphasized that indwelling catheters and collection systems are last resort options.

CONCLUSIONS

In evaluating incontinent elderly patients, the real challenge is to classify the form of urologic dysfunction. Reversible disease processes such as local pelvic abnormalities (*e.g.*, fecal impaction, urinary tract infection, or atrophic vaginitis), polyuric syndromes, and drug effects are readily apparent from the history, physical examination, and simple laboratory procedures and account for less than 10% of cases of urinary incontinence.[6,14] Most patients can be successfully treated on the basis of the functional urologic abnormality; the cause usually does not provide useful information. For example, the treatment of detrusor instability focuses on reducing bladder contractions, increasing bladder capacity, and improving confidence and self-esteem. Treatment does not depend on knowing whether the bladder instability is due to brain trauma, multiple sclerosis, Alzheimer's dementia, or other irreversible disease. Thus, knowledge of the urologic mechanisms producing urinary incontinence allows the physician to manage the incontinence and help the patient expeditiously and successfully, while avoiding the disappointment and frustration (for both the physician and the patient) of not being able to define or cure the primary disease underlying the urinary incontinence.

Although it is recognized that age-associated conditions are becoming more prevalent and more expensive to treat, the fundamental motivation to improve our skills is our perception of the personal impact produced by urinary incontinence. The degree to which we, as physicians, can assist incontinent older patients may largely reflect our understanding of human discomfort and our sensitivity to personal distress. From this perspective, it is unacceptable that over one half of incontinent older persons believe they have to hide their difficulties and are not receiving treatment. It is unacceptable that some incontinent persons choose incontinence over the side-effects of our

present treatments. Finally, it is unacceptable that many physicians prefer using palliative measures such as plastic pants and indwelling catheters to performing a comprehensive evaluation, which will usually result in a cure for a majority of affected individuals.

Until these basic issues are examined and resolved, urinary incontinence will continue to compromise the freedom and quality of life of older persons and will continue to drain precious health resources.

REFERENCES

1. Bors E, Comarr AE: Neurological Urology, pp 45–60. Baltimore, University Park Press, 1971
2. Bradley WE: Innervation of the male urinary bladder. Urol Clin North Am 5:279–293, 1978
3. Bradley WE, Rockswold GL, Timm GW, Scott FB: Neurology of micturition. J Urol 115:481–486, 1976
4. Brocklehurst JC, Dillane JB: Studies of the female bladder in old age: I. Cystometrograms in non-incontinent women. Gerontol Clin 8:285–305, 1966
5. Brocklehurst JC, Dillane JB, Griffiths L, Fry J: The prevalence and symptomatology of urinary infection in an aged population. Gerontol Clin 10:242–253, 1968
6. Castleden CM, Duffin HM, Ashner MJ: Clinical and urodynamic studies in 100 elderly patients. Br Med J 282:1103–1105, 1981
7. Drutz HP, Mandel F: Urodynamic analysis of urinary incontinence symptoms in women. Am J Obstet Gynecol 134:789–792, 1979
8. Eastwood HDH: Urodynamic studies in the management of urinary incontinence in the elderly. Age Ageing 8:41–48, 1979
9. Elder DD, Stephenson TP: An assessment of the Frewen regime in the treatment of detrusor dysfunction in females. Br J Urol 52:467–471, 1980
10. Farrar DJ, Whiteside CG, Osborne JL, Turner-Warwick RT: A urodynamic analysis of micturition symptoms in the female. Surg Gynecol Obstet 141:875–881, 1975
11. Frewen W: Role of bladder training in the treatment of the unstable bladder in the female. Urol Clin North Am 6:273–277, 1979
12. Green TH Jr: Urinary stress incontinence: Differential diagnosis, pathophysiology and management. Am J Obstet Gynecol 122:368–400, 1975
13. Harui D: Post-prostatectomy incontinence. Urol Res 6:113–118, 1978
14. Hilton P, Stanton SL: Algorithmic method for assessing urinary incontinence in elderly women. Br Med J 282:940–942, 1981
15. Isaacs B, Walkey FA: A survey of incontinence in elderly hospital patients. Gerontol Clin 6:367–376, 1964

16. Jarvis G, Millar DR: Controlled trial of bladder drill for detrusor instability. Br J Urol 281:1322–1323, 1980
17. Khanna OP: Disorders of micturition: Neuropharmacologic basis and results of drug therapy. Urology 8:316–328, 1976
18. Kuru M: Nervous control of micturition. Physiol Rev 45:425–494, 1965
19. Layton TN, Drach GW: Selectivity of peak versus average male urinary flow rates. J Urol 125:839–841, 1981
20. Mayo ME, Ansell JS: Urodynamic assessment of incontinence after prostatectomy. J Urol 122:60–61, 1979
21. Milne JS: Prevalence of incontinence in elderly age groups. In Willington WL (ed): Incontinence in the Elderly, pp 9–21. London, Academic Press, 1976
22. Overstall PW, Rounce K, Palmer JH: Experience with an incontinence clinic. J Am Geriatr Soc 28:535–538, 1980
23. Pengelly AW, Booth CM: A prospective trial of bladder training as treatment for detrusor instability. Br J Urol 52:463–466, 1980
24. Raz S: Diagnosis of urinary incontinence in the male. Urol Clin North Am 5:305–322, 1978
25. Raz S: Pharmacological treatment of lower urinary tract dysfunction. Urol Clin North Am 5:323–334, 1978
26. Tang PC, Ruch TC. Non-neurogenic basis of bladder tonus. Am J Physiol 181:249–257, 1955
27. VanRooyen AJL, Liebenberg HC. A clinical approach to urinary incontinence in the female. Obstet Gynecol 53:1–7, 1979
28. Wein AJ, Raezer DM: Physiology of micturition. In Krane RJ, Siroky MD (eds): Clinical Neuro-Urology, pp 1–34. Boston, Little, Brown, 1979
29. Williams ME: A critical evaluation of the assessment technology for urinary continence in older persons. J Am Geriatr Soc 31:657–664, 1983
30. Williams ME, Pannill FCP: Urinary incontinence in the elderly. Ann Intern Med 97:895–907, 1982
31. Yarnell JWG, St. Leger AS: The prevalence, severity and factors associated with urinary incontinence in a random sample of the elderly. Age Ageing 8:81–85, 1979

44

Environments of Geriatric Care

Isadore Rossman

Increasing survivorship and decreasing fertility rates are skewing the US population towards middle- and old age, with major social and medical consequences. The over-65 age-group has grown from 9 million in 1940 to 25.7 million in 1980 and is projected at around 35.7 million for the year 2000. Hospital stays, medical expenditures, chronic illnesses, and the need for custodial care are disproportionately higher for this group. It has come to be generally realized that many aspects of geriatric care have been poorly thought through, resulting in unpleasant repercussions throughout the medical care establishment. About a third of all hospital days are ascribable to the over-65 age-group, and the number of nursing-home beds doubled after passage of Medicare-Medicaid legislation, to more than 1.3 million. Geriatric care founded on the twin pillars of hospital and nursing home was overall expensive, unsatisfactory, and often inappropriate.

The planning and selection of appropriate geriatric environments must recognize that the aged present composites of frailty, impairment, and illness that form a complex of needs.[2,14,22] Heretofore environments of care have been limited in availability and often chosen in an almost random or fortuitous manner.[9,23] As an illustration, consider a prototype male, aged 75, with general atherosclerosis, controllable cardiac failure, with moderate stiffness owing to parkinsonism, presenting with an organic mental syndrome and episodic nocturnal confusion. Depending on his doctor, family, and community settings, this patient could be treated for long or indefinite periods at home, in a hospital, in a nursing home, or even in a psychiatric institution.

What is true in one decade may not be so in a subsequent one, and patterns of geriatric care remain in flux. At one point in the 1960s, elderly patients with organic mental syndromes constituted the single largest group being admitted to state psychiatric hospitals. For complex reasons these hospitals fell into disfavor and many of their inmates were transferred out into the community or into nursing homes.[20] Widely varying policies in the different states and communities have also contributed to a shifting scene. The day care or home care available in one locale may be inadequate or nonexistent in another. It is predictable, however, that more attention and financing will be expended on geriatric environments, and the wise use of them will call for knowledge of their special features, and most important, their limitations and drawbacks.

GERIATRIC TRIAGE

In most younger patients, decisions regarding hospitalization, convalescence, and return to home or to work are relatively uncomplicated. In the geriatric group, the many variations on the theme of ability and disability make triage problems far more complex. A single fateful flaw such as incontinence or assaultive tendencies may close many doors that would otherwise be open and may be the overriding factor in what would otherwise be an uncomplicated decision. Because many of the factors to be weighed are only quasi-medical or purely social, some physicians are automatically disinterested or even repelled by disposition problems. Unfortunately, the physician who turns such problems over to a social worker, a nurse, or a family member may be projecting a problem with many technical aspects onto others with only an inaccurate grasp of the medical totality. Environ-

708

mental decisions are often made with a stroke of the pen and are based on assumptions that do not accord with reality. Thus, the surgical house officer who unwittingly sends an old man with a good repair of a strangulated hernia out to a poor nursing home is sometimes astonished to see him return several weeks later with a large decubitus ulcer and bacteremia. However tedious the selection of an appropriate medical environment may be, it can reverse, hamper, or be in harmony with preceding medical efforts. Hence, it can be as important as any other basic medical or surgical decision.

So great are the variations in community resources that an environmental decision appropriate to one locality may not be possible in another. The florid and unplanned proliferation of intermediate and long-term facilities is emphasized by the diverse character of the agencies responsible for their construction. They have included city, county, state, and federal governments, religious and philanthropic organizations, and private profitmaking corporations. Criteria for admission have often been fundamentally nonmedical and may even have an arbitrary or capricious character. They include age (the extended-care facility [ECF]), armed forces service (Veterans Administration hospitals), poverty ("county poor house"), presence of a specific disease (tuberculosis, arthritis, cancer), and even poor prognosis (home for incurable invalids). Even where the choices include good out-of-hospital facilities, far too great a range persists. Some communities have excellent hospital-based coordinated home care programs that have made possible earlier discharge and prolonged, if not indefinite, stays at home. Yet despite the admitted success of these programs, which have been in operation for some 35 years, they are scattered about chiefly in cities, with a relatively low daily census. Even for such a basic structure in the medical care pattern as a hospital, local and geographic factors may play a determinant role, as when patients reside in distant, rural, or mountain settings. Generally, the geriatrician has at least a choice of the hospital, a nursing home facility, and the home itself. The differences in these three environments are such that their pros and cons should be carefully pondered.

THE HOSPITAL

Virtually all the profession's training, from medical school through residency, takes place in the hospital. Hence, this is the major medical environment

with which, perhaps too exclusively, the practitioner is familiar. The modern hospital has dominated medical thinking and practice to such an extent that it has all but eclipsed other medical environments. This eclipse has thrown its shadow on the medical school curriculum until very recently. In contrast to other medical environments, the modern hospital has had the lion's share of resources and financing. Because modern medical practice has reached its acme in the hospital setting, reasons for hospitalization, whether for ferreting out the diagnosis or initiation of complex surgical and medical treatments, seldom need defense. Most practitioners think too readily of hospitalization, think too highly of its benefits, and tend to overestimate its returns.

Although much geriatric hospitalization is born of necessity, some is less than mandatory, and some is certainly at the discretion and convenience of the practitioner. Thus, some important factors influencing hospitalization may result from the practitioner's concern as much or more than they do from the patient's disease. There may be a transformation of uncertainty into certainty by use of the hospital's diagnostic resources. This may not alter or improve treatment or prognosis, but it unquestionably contributes to the relief of the practitioner's anxiety by defining the nature of the problem. A hospital work-up can yield an impressive collection of relevant—and occasionally irrelevant—data, although such data collection has an unreckoned cost in pain, morbidity, and even mortality. The studies of Reichel and Gillick and colleagues[5,10] are among the few that call attention to the iatrogenic morbid consequences in the elderly of going to the hospital. Another important reason for hospitalization may be to disperse some of the burdensome aspects of the patient's problems by the involvement of others at the hospital level. The heavy responsibility the physician may feel in facing a sick elderly person in an out-of-hospital setting can be thus resolved.

Emotional reactions to hospitalization are significant in all age-groups, but in some respects they may be more intense in the elderly. Unless the patient is cortically impaired, anxiety and depression may be prominent. For many, disorientation and increased agitation can be the consequence (Fig. 44-1).

Anxiety

There are few patients who do not experience significant anxiety with hospitalization. Occasionally a patient with asthma or a similar disorder obtains

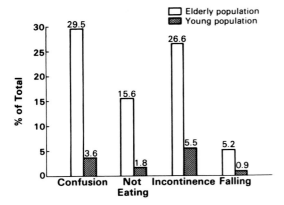

FIG. 44-1. Incidence of four functional alterations associated with hospitalization in an elderly (> 70) population compared to a younger (< 70) group. (Gillick MR, Serrell NA, Gillick LS: Adverse consequences of hospitalization in the elderly. Soc Sci Med 16:1033, 1982 [Reprinted with permission from Pergamon Press Ltd.])

prompt and gratifying relief in a hospital and looks on it with unalloyed positive feelings. Far more regard the hospital as a way station on the road to eternity. The need to go to the hospital may be interpreted, correctly or otherwise, as evidence of a serious or worsening disorder. With most hospitalized geriatric patients, one can correctly assume fears of dying and death. The feelings of helplessness and of injury that the hospitalization induces may accentuate these fears. The everyday routines of the hospital with their many symbolic overtones—puncturing for blood, the drinking of barium, the fecal sampling—may all contribute to anxiety. It is not always recognized that the laity innocently assume that the more the diagnostic maneuvers, the weightier the disease process being pursued. Even the many patients in whom benign or minor disorders are under diagnostic consideration grimly go through procedures secretly convinced that malignant disorders and other serious conditions are being sought. Even when a brief clarification of the meaning or intent of procedures could have enormous reassurance value, hospital personnel are found to be derelict.

Duff and Hollingshead[4] describe in distressing detail the failures of a modern teaching hospital to grapple with the anxieties of patients. They state: "Anxiety [is] a characteristic response from the time a person learned he had to be hospitalized until he was discharged. Even when he returned home he might still be fearful." The neglect of even the most hectic anxiety is noted by the same authors: "For the most part, the anguish and fears of the patients were outside the interest of the physicians and nurses. No ward patient thought there was a physician to whom he could talk about his fears of hospitalization, illness, or treatment."

Hospital routine may appear to its personnel as a smooth and rational sequence of medical events. To the patient, the same routine appears baffling, irrational, and trying. It confers a jerked-about quality on the way of life in hospitals and repeatedly contributes to the startle reactions most patients experience. Wheelchairs and stretchers appear unexpectedly with silent attendants. There are early morning awakenings for no weightier procedure than temperature taking. Paging systems blare forth unexpectedly. Even the fundamental routines involved in the serving of meals are prone to unexpected omissions, changes, or delays. Occupants of adjacent beds may scream in pain, cry out in confusion, or die despite the efforts of the cardiac arrest team. An alternative, the private room, may lead to feelings of isolation and depersonalization. In the battle against the undesirable and even disastrous impact of hospitalization, the geriatrician has a major role: he can forewarn, explain, reassure, soothe, and sedate.

Depression

Hospitalization may produce a reactive depression or increase the depth of a preexisting one. It may be difficult to dispel such depressions, because grossly realistic factors may be present. Because most geriatric patients suffer from chronic or progressive diseases, each hospitalization may emphasize deterioration, increased disability, or worsening pain. Although hospital personnel may perceive clearly the possible gains of their treatment and its place in a useful pattern of medical care, the same perception may not be shared by the patient. Rather, a process of negative conditioning occurs and for patients who have had mastectomies, colostomies, amputations, and other grave assaults, a negativism emerges toward hospitalization that exacerbates the impact of the admission.

One depressing consequence of hospitalization, especially if long or repeated, is the role loss that occurs. Even a disabled woman functioning to only a minor degree as a homemaker or mother must surrender such roles in the hospital. A man reduced to semi-helplessness, either by his illness or the hospital environment, may react profoundly to the loss of usual role relationships. In contrast to maintenance at home, the hospital has a blighting effect on supportive interpersonal relationships and dilutes or abolishes even longstanding paternal or maternal roles. This, combined with weakness, helplessness, and feelings of isolation, is often summated in the production of depression.

Disorientation and Agitation

Some elderly patients, generally with organic mental syndromes, are confused by almost any change in environment, and they thus may decompensate because of hospitalization. In one study on a general medical ward 29.5% of patients over 70 demonstrated functional confusion (see Fig. 44-1). Confusion may occur promptly on transfer into the hospital or grow more gradually following admission. Operative procedures and anesthesia, which may perhaps be associated with an increment of cerebral ischemia, can be aggravating factors. The onset of a more serious disorientation may be heralded by reports of episodic confusion at night, which are sometimes forgotten or denied the next morning by the patient. The attentive geriatrician must, therefore, read the night nurse's notes.

It is not always advisable to place certain elderly impaired patients into private rooms where isolation phenomena are increased. Impaired vision and hearing may further contribute to the deprivation that occurs after transfer from a familiar environment with its loss of the usual orienting visual, auditory, tactile, and even olfactory cues. Because even healthy young adults deprived of sensory cues become disoriented and may even hallucinate, similar phenomena in the elderly should not be regarded as unique. Old patients unattended for long periods often complain of an ill-defined malaise. This can progress to an obvious confusion. The confusion produced by hospitalization is not specific to this environment. It occurs with equal readiness on transfer to other unfamiliar settings such as nursing homes. Whether it occurs to the same degree on transfer back to a familiar home setting has not been studied. Experiences on a home care program indicate that even after a considerable absence, the home environment exerts a favorable rather than unfavorable effect on orientation and confusion.

Other more specific aspects of the hospital, however much they may be taken for granted, are not likely to contribute to the geriatric patient's sense of well-being. Hospital rooms are generally cheerless, and some have the forbidding quality of cells. Meaningful relationships may be placed in abeyance or in jeopardy by regulations that limit visiting or, as with young children, forbid them altogether. This kind of deprivation emphasizes the essentially alienating process inherent in hospitalization. Even in a few instances, in which prolonged visiting or bedside nursing by relatives is encouraged, the hospital environment functions in a constrictive fashion. The customary semi-private status abolishes all privacy. The observer familiar with the continuing relationships within a family will generally observe a reticence when the same family members are seen interacting during visiting hours.

Other of the procrustean aspects of hospitalization are well known. To patients who have managed to achieve sleep with difficulty, early arousal for a trivial procedure justly seems irrational. Although the early morning bedpan may be desirable for nurses and early rounds suitable for surgeons, the patient finds little that is suited to him. The cardiac patient may unhappily resign himself to a salt-free diet, but there is no persuasive reason why the average patient should resign himself to food that is generally drab and has that institutional flavor. A nutritional problem can result if a patient chooses poorly when he outlines a day's menu; alternative selections may not be available. With a geriatric patient who is often anorexic, there may be little drive to battle for more calories, resulting in weight loss from the hospital stay. That anorexia is not a fixed aspect of an illness or of old age is often clearly demonstrated when the patient goes home and gains weight, sometimes to an unexpected degree. This observation, often reported by home care programs, has been made even with cancer patients. The geriatrician can employ several countermeasures for his hospitalized patient: ordering multiple dishes and desserts, which enhance range of choice; ordering between meal supplements such as juices, milk shakes, and eggnogs; and even encouraging family members to bring in items known to have special appeal. The feeding process blends therapeutic needs with primitive pleasures and has important affective overtones. A bedside consultation with a nutritionist and coaxing the patient with a catering diet may convey to the patient important feelings of warmth and concern.

Any patient of any age who has had several hospitalizations is likely to possess a catalogue of major and minor annoyances, derelictions, and other difficulties. Some of these are apparently trivial, such as the painful needling for blood samples followed by extravasation or the prolonged wait for bedpanning. But beyond the accumulation of minor grievances are the major events that might perhaps have been prevented. A fall from a hospital bed with fracture is always a major disaster. Development of incontinence in a slightly confused elderly patient put to bed in the hospital may be a major retrogressive event. Forbidding ambulation because of concern over falls may have severe effects also, as described by one observer[19]: "In the hospital . . . we often find the patient safely confined to bed. An organization of brisk, efficient nurses feed him, bathe him, and toilet him, all administered in bed. Any locomotor initiative the patient may possess tends to be smothered in this womb-like environment, and before long we find him curled up in a reminiscently fetal position with flexion contractures."

The geriatric group is frail, borderline in its residual capacities, the least adaptable to the difficulties consequent to hospitalization. The experienced geriatrician seldom hospitalizes his patients without hesitation, and uses measures to diminish the unfavorable impact of the hospital environment. Although perhaps not applicable to every case, some measures may be of help:

Visit the patient frequently, especially in the beginning of hospitalization. Encourage the nursing staff to be supportive; perhaps have the nutritionist drop in. A warm supportive private duty nurse sometimes can be of great help.

Orient the patient regarding hospital routines such as the drawing of blood, the holding up of breakfasts, the wherefores of bowel cleansing, and the expectations regarding diagnostic procedures (*e.g.*, the radiographic table is hard and may be a little uncomfortable, the barium mixture is thick and chalky but harmless).

Explain the rationale for the various steps, specifically in terms of the gains in diagnosis and treatment that will follow.

Use drugs appropriately and judiciously for the treatment of anxiety, agitation, and insomnia.

Anticipate common mishaps such as nocturnal falls by prophylactic measues: low beds, side rails, a urinal within easy reach, a night light, and mild restraints.

Start discharge planning on the day of admission.

OTHER HOSPITAL FACILITIES

There are several chronic and long-term hospitals scattered about the country with patient populations somewhat intermediate between those of the general hospital and of the nursing home. The classic tuberculosis hospitals that were all but disbanded by advances in chemotherapy are good examples of the role such facilities could play. They were equipped to do necessary laboratory and radiographic services in relation to tuberculosis and also to perform repeated pneumothorax, and even thoracoplasty. Long-term nursing care was, of course, a primary consideration. Similar long-term hospitals, not restricted to the therapy of a single disease, are still found, particularly in urban areas. Many Veterans Administration hospitals run the gamut from acute general hospitals to long-term specialized ones. In the latter are many patients one could equally well encounter in a nursing home. With a basic eligibility criterion—that of being a veteran of the US armed forces—most VA hospitals tend more to take care of the chronically ill or permanently incapacitated male. Most of these hospitals built after World War II were designed to have working relationships with a nearby medical school or teaching hospital, with considerable upgrading in their levels of care. They often offer useful solutions to some of the problems encountered by the geriatrician. Needless to say, his professional relationship with the patient terminates, at least for the time, when the patient is admitted to the VA hospital.

Still another example of a specialized hospital to which referral may be made is the state mental hospital. Here, too, the patient is detached from the usual paths of medical practice on admittance. For many elderly psychotics, such a hospital is often the end of the line. One perceives that a valuable function of the proprietary nursing home is the custodial care it gives to elderly psychotics, many indistinguishable from those who have been sent to state mental hospitals.[20]

The drawbacks of these hospitals are well known and have been frequently aired. Some are huge institutions, swamped under the weight of thousands of patients and located long distances from the cities and other centers of population from which their patients came. Shortages of personnel at all levels, a poverty of rehabilitation and work facilities, and frank deficiencies in psychiatric care are found in the hospital systems in all but a few states. Although treatment improved with the advent of shock therapy and the phenothiazines, most elderly patients in these hospitals generally do not respond well to these modalities. Most, at least at the present time, present generally irreversible states of derangement. Partly as a consequence of financial stringency, and in part because of legal decisions holding that patients in psychiatric institutions could not be kept there in the absence of psychiatric care, a steady outflow from these state hospitals began in the early 1970s. A large number of the patients wound up in nursing homes. In one study, one third of nursing-home patients had a psychiatric diagnosis, with one half of this group deemed psychotic.[20]

INSTITUTIONAL FACILITIES

In retrospect, one of the initial errors committed after the passage of Medicare legislation was the explosive development of proprietary nursing homes.[9,14] Patients with very diverse incapacities and illnesses were sent into these homes often with inadequate evaluation or consideration of the alternatives.[14,17,23] An irrational mix of frail ambulants, those with severe organic mental syndromes, and the preterminally ill could thus be grouped together. As daily costs rose and the patient census soared, enormous expenditures resulted. In some homes poor care became notorious and downright fraud became scandalous.[9] A wave of reform followed, which included the emergence of classification systems to place patients in settings appropriate to their needs. These vary somewhat in different locales, but generally three types of care facilities can be distinguished:

1. A skilled nursing facility (SNF) in which the sicker and most disabled patients are cared for. Many patients may be bedfast or wheelchair-bound and require a variety of medications and nursing procedures; even those who are ambulatory have disorders that require close supervision (Fig 44-2).
2. An intermediate care facility (ICF), also known as a health-related facility (HRF), for a less impaired group. Patients are usually able to ambulate to a dining room, may or may not require supervision in taking daily medications, and require few nursing procedures.
3. A domiciliary facility (DCF) for a custodial care group. These are essentially bed-and-board environments with no medical or nursing care called for. Foster home placement is essentially similar and has been advocated for certain geropsychiatric patients.[11]

Scoring systems have been devised to match patient to facility with factors such as being bedfast, disoriented, in need of feeding, and incontinent being the more highly weighted ones. This and other classification systems are of importance not only in ensuring proper placement of patients but in cost-effectiveness accounting because costs vary downward with decreasing levels of care.

Some of the better facilities can be compared with the good community hospital in the sense that transfer from one to the other is not a difficult

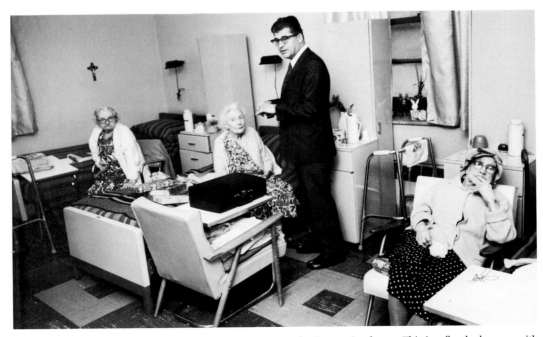

FIG. 44-2. Three "frail ambulants" in a New York City nursing home. This is a five-bed room, with space between beds and other dimensions defined by the city's nursing code. The packages on the middle bed are gifts for the patient's 94th birthday.

transition. Under the impact of Medicare financing, more luxurious nursing homes are being erected. Ninety-two percent of nursing home patients are aged 65 or over; thus, the financing of care for the elderly is the dominant factor in this area.

Medicare has awakened interest in the therapeutic possibilities of nursing homes and has led to new assessments of their roles in decreasing some of the pressure on the modern hospital, as well as complementing them in programs of progressive patient care. Traditionally, the nursing home stood apart from the usual pathways to the extent that the physician, neither in his training nor for years thereafter, was likely to enter a nursing home. The physician who for some reason did stray off the beaten path would, at least until recently, encounter a dismaying scene: end-of-the-line patients, in a drab setting, many incontinent or psychotic. There were other severe limitations in this environment: no laboratory facilities, even for such elementary procedures as a urinalysis or blood cell count, and inadequate supplies of basic items such as catheters, dressings, and injectables.

The sole service the geriatrician can count on in most homes is nursing, occasionally some elementary physical medicine, and little more. If time and nursing care can ameliorate or resolve the patient's presenting condition, the nursing home can fit into the pattern of medical care without significant difficulty. Perhaps more typically, the nursing home serves as a repository for incapacitated patients who for myriad medical and social reasons have no alternative for necessary custodial care. A nursing home may have a stable population of patients who remain not only for months but for years. The adaptations that some patients develop in these settings can be a tribute to their flexibility and defenses. Not only is privacy surrendered, but new ways of relating to a group not of one's choosing must also be developed. There is little that one can do if he finds his neighbors, not to mention nurses or attendants, not to his liking. Some attempts to sort patients out into compatible, or at least nondissonant, groups may occur. Thus, the more oriented and ambulatory patients are to be encountered on the ground floor of the institution, with the confused, the wandering and the incontinent patients somewhat more distantly located. There may or may not be a modest amount of space given to recreational and diversionary therapy. The television set is undoubtedly the chief contribution to the whiling away of time, with reading, playing bingo, or knitting as occasional alternatives.

It is obvious that the geriatrician is considerably hampered in this kind of setting. Insofar as diagnostic measures are concerned, either the patient must be brought to a laboratory or hospital or samples of blood, urine, stool, and others are taken at the site and brought to the appropriate laboratory or facility. A lack of medications, especially parenteral ones, can be quite hampering. The physician in a nursing home learns to carry supplementary articles in his bag. Paucity of diagnostic facilities makes trips by the patient necessary, some of which are poorly tolerated. The typical nursing home has no provision for giving intravenous fluids. Therefore, patients with relatively easily reversed states of dehydration or electrolyte abnormalities must return to the hospital for such procedures. Many nursing homes seem unable to cope with the demands for inhalation equipment in chronic pulmonary insufficiency. Some balk over patients requiring feedings through nasogastric tubes or through gastrostomies. Although most nursing homes have access to physical therapists, necessary instruments and facilities are generally limited. Further limiting treatment is the difficulty in obtaining specialist consultations. The geriatrician willing to follow his patient into the ECF may find his hospital colleagues drawing the line for one or another reason. Thus, the physician in a nursing home is rather like an outlying sentry: he has to be watchful and patient, he is bound to feel isolated from the center of activities, and often he has to fall back on a sense of duty to comfort his mild sensations of malaise.

HOME CARE

The home care program developed as a contribution to the therapeutic needs of a significant number of hospitalized patients. Collectively, they were patients with a chronic illness for whom in-hospital procedures were no longer mandatory but who still required a considerable amount of skilled medical, nursing, and other forms of treatment. At its maximum, the team that could be brought into the patient's home consisted of a doctor, nurse, social worker, physiotherapist, occupational therapist, home health aide, and homemaker. Consultant services representing the various specialties were available in the hospital and occasionally were extended to the home. Where personnel, administration, and funding arose in the hospital, the programs were referred to as hospital-based. Because of the high degree of liaison and communication made possible by the team concept, they have also been defined as coordinated home care programs.[3]

These programs have clearly demonstrated the usefulness of relating home care to hospital care, particularly with the chronically ill patient, and the desirability of ready transfer from one to the other of these environments as dictated by the fluctuating needs of the patient. The collective experience of these home care programs and their impact on the fabric of medical care might be summarized as follows:

Sharpened Definition of the Hospital Patient

Home care programs have clearly defined the elements of hospital care that can be transferred to the home and have thereby redefined or delimited the concept of the in-hospital patient. Almost any kind of home care program can demonstrably shorten hospital stays. In a sample of 200 patients in a large general hospital in New York City lacking a home care program, an evaluation team consisting of an experienced physician and social worker found 12% to 14% of the patients could have been transferred to such a program. Experience indicates that many patients, rather sooner than many hospital personnel are aware, reach a stage in which further care can be continued extramurally. One of the unforeseen ripple effects of this experience was to set the stage for the federal capping program known as the diagnosis-related group (DRG) prospective remuneration system.

Desirable Extension of Medical Care

Patients with continuing therapeutic needs, particularly those who are homebound or can get to the hospital or doctor's office only with difficulty or great pain, have been able to receive continuing care of good quality. For some patients, this has meant the maintenance of gains achieved in the hospital that otherwise were lost. Prior to the advent of home care, it was not uncommon to find that the homebound patient had lost such important capacities as the ability to ambulate or to transfer or other important aspects of activities of daily living. By bringing equipment to the home on long-term loan, by offering various forms of therapy, or even simply by instruction of those in the home setting and supervision of the patient's course, it was found that regression can be prevented. In a variety of chronic or severe illnesses, such as very advanced cancer, the skilled medical and nursing services brought into the home and support given to the family demonstrably helped to remedy previous situations of inadequate care. An important and somewhat unexpected finding was that many patients and families preferred home care to hospital care.

Value of the Family as a Medical Resource

Although patients who live alone may be cared for on home care programs, a usual requirement is that a responsible family member be at home much, if not all, of the time. A number of cross-national studies have shown that a majority of the ill elderly are in fact cared for at home.[21,22] The importance of the caring relative is underlined by the fact that many rejections for assignment to home care programs have been for social rather than medical reasons. What appears to the hospital staff to be a fumbling, inadequate, or even somewhat trying relative may in the home care setting turn out to be a prize medical resource. Elaborate programs of care based on the responsible relative's contribution have been set up at home. It is not at all difficult to teach some caring relatives to give general nursing care of a high order, including hypodermic injections, irrigations, tube feedings, and oxygen administration. That famous ingredient, tender loving care, that hospitals have such difficulty in generating, may be present in generous amounts in the home setting.

Prevention of Institutionalization

It is a common experience of home care programs that when a battery of services is delivered to the home, and the family is supported through the trials of a chronic care program, push for transfer into a nursing home or similar institution is diminished or prevented. Many of the patients who have been cared for on home care programs are at least as sick and disabled as many of those in nursing homes. A home care program that skillfully marshals and increases its services and support can successfully care for even a completely bedridden moribund patient. The wish and the need to care for one's family members and the dread or abhorrence with which patient and family may view institutionalization can thus be resolved by home care (Fig. 44-3).

High Level of Cost Effectiveness

In contrast to the rising costs of institutional care, whether hospital, nursing home, extended care

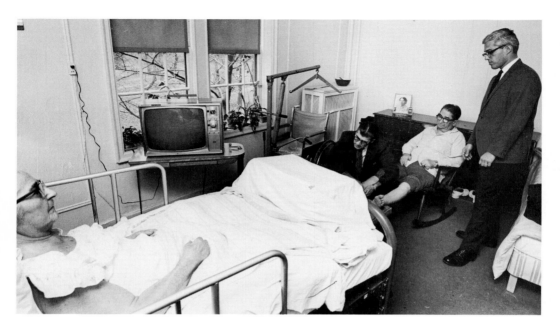

FIG. 44-3. A Medicare couple at home. The wife, aged 79, has diabetes and parkinsonism, and is a bilateral amputee. Her husband, aged 75, has arteriosclerotic heart disease, Class IIIC. The visiting physicians are examining his edematous legs, in which Kaposi's sarcoma has developed—this diagnosis was made at home. Note the hospital bed, Hoyer lift, and wheelchair—paraphernalia supplied by the Home Care Program.

facility, or even homes for the aged, home care, even when elaborate, is comparatively inexpensive. If one figures in the cost of food, laundry, proportional share of rent, and so on, total cost for a patient in a home care setting is approximately that of care for an ambulatory patient in an HRF. It is, on average, considerably less than the cost of care in the hospital. The cost advantages favoring home care have continued undiminished over 3 decades of inflation and soaring medical costs. These facts indicate the economic importance of the home care provisions written into the Medicare Act, especially in large urban hospitals where hospital costs of more than $500 a day have become commonplace. This was the economic force behind the DRGs, in an attempt to shorten hospital stays by earlier discharge home. When a chronically ill patient can remain at home with the bulk of care furnished gratis by family members, the cost advantage of home care continues. But as some homebound patients become increasingly dependent and require attendants, costs do rise. This led Ginzberg and associates in a recent extensive review to declare: "On balance, it appears that if avoidance of institutionalization is the goal, home care is the locus of choice; if savings is the criterion, it has not been determined whether home care is ultimately more economical."[5a]

CRITERIA FOR HOME CARE

Despite the many advantages just cited, errors can be made in embarking on the home care of patients. Sometimes the geriatrician must turn a deaf ear either to the patient's entreaties or to the family's wishes. To avoid occasional medical or social disasters, a correct assessment of patient and family should be made. Among the factors to be kept in mind are the following:

Medical

Can the patient's medical needs be met adequately or reasonably in the home setting? The patient who requires daily or almost daily medical visits, monitoring of blood chemistries, or intravenous fluid therapy may be too taxing to be successfully manageable at home. Most home care patients require a doctor's visit no more than once or twice a week and sometimes as little as once a month.

Occasionally, the need for the doctor is minimal, whereas the need for other kinds of services is predominant. A further consideration is the location of the home, which, if at a considerable distance, may prevent efficient delivery of home medical services.

Nursing Needs

If the patient requires a great deal of nursing care, the family may face an exhausting requirement that cannot be met. Some deteriorating patients require round-the-clock nursing care, and although some devoted family members have met such needs, most of these patients are generally regarded as ineligible for home care. With patients already at home, as the patient's condition deteriorates, the increase in nursing requirements may be managed by stepping up the quantity of services delivered. At some point, however, especially in progressing illnesses, it may become apparent that the treatment program should be transferred into another setting such as a nursing home.

Social Aspects

For the typical home care patient, the need for a responsible, cooperative, caring relative at home cannot be bypassed. If the family is unwilling or indifferent, even though medical and nursing needs are acceptable, home care may be impossible or tenuous. Experienced social workers evaluating the family sometimes find that what appears to be negativism is only hestitation or anxiety. When these are successfully resolved by the doctor, nurse, or social worker, a successful home care program may be launched. However, home care may be a test of the success of preceding interpersonal relations. A poor marriage relationship wherein one can elicit past patterns of neglect, hostility, or infidelity may make it impossible to carry out home care successfully. It is rather rare that the physical setup militates against home care. Occasionally, overcrowding and gross inadequacy, however customary in the family's style of life, may prevent such care. Except where the most impoverished conditions are found, dietary patterns in the home are suitable for the average patient; indeed, in many instances they are more suitable than those in the hospital.

Occasionally, the geriatrician finds himself in the somewhat troubled situation of agreeing to home care for an elderly patient who is alone. Some elderly patients are adamant in their refusal of hospitalization or institutionalization. Some

draw themselves up to their full height (however diminished by age) and proclaim their unalterable decision to stay at home. The physician is sometimes faced with the dilemma of either withdrawing his services and abandoning the patient at home or reluctantly going along with home care after tossing out some of his prized criteria for selection. Some of these patients admitted to home care programs are frail, weak, dizzy, ataxic, episodically confused, or otherwise "unsuitable." However, once the physician accepts the risk inherent in such a situation, a fair percentage of such patients can be maintained at home for long periods.

As an illustration, one 78-year-old woman with an organic mental syndrome was maintained in her usual habitat for almost 2 years. A few of her needs, such as shopping, were met by the intervention of a compassionate Home Care secretary. Many similar cases over the years indicate that even experienced home care personnel may overemphasize the dangers inherent in living alone. Certainly, the precautions that dominate thinking in the hospital setting need not be so strictly applied in the home. For example, home care patients virtually never take deliberate overdosages of drugs (two cases in 2000 patients), and the free use of oxygen at home has turned out to be quite safe.

An important feature of the team delivery of medical services into the home is the altered quality of the interpersonal relationships. It is perhaps relevant that royalty has often insisted on home care to the extent that surgical and obstetric procedures have been brought to the royal bedroom. Some of the same implications of unstinted giving and special privilege may be generated in the home. The suspicious attitudes that many hospitalized patients have regarding the intent of those about them, the meaning of procedures, and the ideas of "experimentation" disappear, even when the same physicians and procedures are brought to the home. Another double-edged aspect is that patients on home care programs almost inevitably become more dependent. This dependency can be shared with various members of the team, although some physicians are uncomfortable when cast in the mixed role of father figure, rich donor, and rescuing hero.

Despite the demonstrable usefulness and desirability of such hospital-based home care programs, barely a hundred or so were set up in the 2 decades following the demonstration at Montefiore Hospital. Some obstacles including finanical hurdles have been cleared away by the Medicare endorsement of home health agencies. These were defined by this legislation as agencies for delivering nursing and at least one other service into the home of the discharged hospital patient, and it has made possible the delivery of millions of services in a home setting. Most of them have been funneled through visiting nurse associations or similar agencies, and future expansion probably will be chiefly through such organizations. Liaison with physicians is maintained by written communication or telephone. Weakness of liaison is perhaps the major difficulty such home health agencies have encountered, compared to the hospital-based programs.

Some look askance at home care programs, maintaining that most patients sick enough to require house calls can be taken care of better in the hospital emergency department or in an institution. This viewpoint confuses emergency medical care with the after-care of discharged patients. The discharged hospital patient may have many medical and nursing needs that are more reasonably and efficiently delivered to the home. Institutionalizing such patients to obtain medical care has obvious drawbacks. The extent of the problem is underlined by one international study (1968): In the US, 6% of the total elderly population were homebound, and 2% more were bedfast. In Britain, 13% of the total elderly population were either homebound or bedfast. The authors of the study declared: "The proportion of people over 65 who are bedfast, homebound, or limited in mobility, who are living at home and who must be considered in planning a broad program of services, are roughly 24% in Denmark, 21% in Britain, and 14% in the United States."[22] Granting that most of the needs of the elderly homebound patient may be for nursing and similar services, there still seems to be no escape from the obligation on the part of physicians to make some home visits.

OTHER ALTERNATIVES TO INSTITUTIONALIZATION

After Care Program (ACP)

Still another alternative for the homebound ill patient was launched at New York's Montefiore Hospital in 1972. Referred to as the After Care Program (ACP), it was generated in part by difficulties in expanding home care programming: shortages of personnel, time and safety considerations, and cost-savings. Intended to parallel the original home care services, homebound patients are brought to the hospital in a van equipped for the

wheelchair-bound and are given a 3-hour package of services. These include physical, occupational, and recreational therapies; an opportunity to see nurse, physician, social worker, and laboratory services; and a group-socialization aspect that is highly regarded by patients. The values of this program as compared with traditional home care have been found to make it a viable alternative for many patients, one that is perhaps more applicable to present patterns of practice.[15,17] In contrast to day care centers no need for meal preparation or rest periods exists, and patients with active ongoing needs rather than custodial problems are the target group.

Day Care Centers

A considerable number of elderly disabled patients require care during the day, with variable components of active, supervisory, and custodial care.[1,2,7] The British experience described by Brocklehurst[1] indicates that hemiplegia, arthritis, amputation, and organic mental syndromes are the more common diagnostic categories. Such a center may enable the breadwinner at home to go out to work without breaking up the family unit and may also help avoid the need for institutionalization. In Oxford, England, Cosin has added the further feature of "floating beds" that provides for admission to hospital of a homebound or day-center patient so as to enable family members to go off for vacation.

The range of facilities existing here and abroad illustrates the spectrum of geriatric needs and the need for multiple solutions.[2,14,21] Home care, after care, and day care are representative of solutions that can be appropriately invoked as alternatives to institutionalization for selected patients. The varieties of institutions—SNF, HRF, DCF—again emphasize the view that an elderly population have disabilities and capabilities mixed in such a fashion that a diversity of institutional settings are required to match the needs.

Hospice

Hospice programs have spread over the past 15 years because of increasing recognition that the needs of many terminal patients were not best met in the modern hospital. Hospice has been defined as, "A coordinated program of home and inpatient care which treats the terminally ill patient and family as a unit, employing an interdisciplinary team under the direction of an autonomous hospice administration. The program provides palliative and supportive care to meet the special needs arising out of physical, psychological, spiritual, social and economic stresses that are experienced during the final stages of illness and during dying and bereavement."[8] Apart from the emphasis on bereavement care and the use in some programs of a special facility or a specific in-hospital area, hospice in concept and execution closely follows the Montefiore Home Care Program, half of whose original patient group had advanced cancer.[3],[12-14] In the early years of home care, cost considerations had not risen to paramount status and readmission to hospital was easy and prompt and was determined by balanced consideration of the patient's needs and the family burden. Even then it became clear that the bulk of care days for the terminally ill patients was in the home setting.

As had been predicted by one of the early physicians in the home care movement, "If we are not driven in the home care direction by compassion, then we will be by fiscal pressure."[16] This indeed was codified into federal law in 1982: legislation specified that Medicare patients could have a maximum of 210 days of hospice care, and of the total care days, no more than 20% could be as an inpatient. Reimbursement for hospice care was limited to no more than 40% of the costs of care for terminal illness in non-hospice settings. A feasibility study in New York State indicated that some hospice programs were able to meet such a cap, others did not; considerable variation in cost levels were reported in different parts of the state. The study concluded that patient and family satisfaction with hospice were noteworthy, costs were often less than other forms of terminal care, and the programs were pronounced a success.[8] Somewhat in contrast, the randomized controlled trial reported by Kane and colleagues[6] found no significant differences between patient groups in measures of pain, symptoms, activities of daily living, or affect. Also hospice care was not associated with a reduced use of hospital inpatient days or therapeutic procedures and was no less expensive than conventional care. Since hospice patients and caregivers expressed greater satisfaction with hospice, Kane and colleagues thought it should be made available as an option. Other aspects of hospice care are dealt with elsewhere in this text (see Chapter 36).

SELECTING THE ENVIRONMENT

It is apparent that there may be multiple and troublesome aspects to the selection of the appropriate environment for a patient. The older pattern based on the three-generation household, in which elders were cared for by their descendants, persists in many parts of the world but not in the "more advanced" countries. Some geriatric patients are so denuded of significant relationships that the physician may find himself invested to an uncomfortable extent with roles that might more logically have been attached to sons, daughters, or trusted friends. If the physician becomes the patient's advocate, he may find himself arrayed against reluctant hospitals, stony-hearted nursing homes, myopic house staffs, and perhaps detached sons and daughters. Since nowhere else in medicine is the selection of environments as important as in geriatrics, the geriatrician will continue to be concerned in the choices.

REFERENCES

1. Brocklehurst JC: The Geriatric Day Hospital, p 100. London, King Edward's Hospital Fund for London, 1970
2. Brocklehurst JC (ed): Geriatric Care in Advanced Societies, p 155. Baltimore, University Park Press, 1975
3. Cherkasky M: The Montefiore Hospital home care program. Am J Public Health 39:163, 1949
4. Duff RS, Hollingshead AB: Sickness and Society, pp 273, 277. New York, Harper & Row, 1968
5. Gillick MR, Serrell NA, Gillick LS: Adverse consequences of hospitalization in the elderly. Soc Sci Med 16:1033, 1982
5a. Ginzberg E, Balinsky W, Ostow M: Home Health Care. Its Role in the Changing Health Services Market. Totowa, NJ, Rowman & Allanheld, 1984
6. Kane RL, Wales J, Bernstein L, Leidowitz A, Kaplan S: A randomized controlled trial of hospice care. Lancet 1:890, 1984
7. Lurie E, Kalish RA, Wexler R, Ansak M: On Lok Senior Health Center, a case study. Gerontologist 16:39, 1976
8. New York State Department of Health: An analysis and evaluation of the New York State Hospice demonstration program. Albany NY, 1982
9. New York State Moreland Act Commission on Nursing Homes and Residential Facilities Report, Albany, NY 1976
10. Reichel W: Complications in the care of five hundred elderly hospitalized patients. J Am Geriatr Soc 13:973, 1965
11. Risdorfer EN, Primanis G, Dozoretz L: Family care as a useful alternative to the long-term hospital confinement of geropsychiatric patients. J Am Geriatr Soc 19:150, 1971
12. Rossman I: Treatment of cancer on a home care program. JAMA 156:827, 1954
13. Rossman I: Suitability of home care for the cancer patient. Geriatrics 11:407, 1956

14. Rossman I: Alternatives to institutional care. Bull NY Acad Med 49:1084, 1973

15. Rossman I: The after care project: A viable alternative to home care. Med Care 12:534, 1974

16. Rossman I: Long-term home care of chronic illness. Clin Med 84:9, 1977

17. Rossman I: Options for care of the aged sick. Hosp Pract 12:107, 1977

18. Rossman I: Home care of the cancer patient. In Home care: Living with Dying. New York, Columbia University Press, 1979

19. Rossman I, Clarke M, Rudnick B: Total rehabilitation in a home care setting. NY State J Med 62:1215, 1962

20. Schmidt LJ, Reinhardt AM, Kane RL, Olsen DM: The mentally ill in nursing homes: New back wards in the community. Arch Gen Psychiatry 34:687, 1977

21. Shanas E, Maddox GL: Aging, health, and the organization of health resources. In Binstock RH, Shanas E (eds): Handbook of Aging and the Social Sciences. New York, Van Nostrand Reinhold, 1976

22. Shanas E et al: Old People in Three Industrial Societies. New York, Atherton Press, 1968

23. Williams TF, Hill JG, Fairbank ME, Knox KG: Appropriate placement of the chronically ill and aged. JAMA 226:1332, 1973

Index